# CONTENTS

# PREFACE

It is almost ten years since the publication of the first edition of the Clinical Radiation Oncology. With rapid changes in the field, the need for an updated version is obvious.

Many chapters in this edition have been completely rewritten and/or updated. Because of limited space, some chapters from the first edition were eliminated. This is not a reference book; instead it is a text that contains practical ideas and information for the general radiation oncologists for their daily practice. It may also provide pertinent information for the medical oncologists, surgeons, and primary care physicians managing patients with malignant diseases.

I wish to express my profound gratitude to the contributors of the chapters of this book. The cooperation of the editor and staff at John Wiley & Sons, Inc. is deeply appreciated.

C. C. Wang

# CHAPTER 1

# BASIC CONCEPTS OF CLINICAL RADIATION ONCOLOGY

C.C. WANG

Oncology is generally referred to as the study of tumors of a malignant nature with the potentiality for causing death. Morbidity and mortality from cancer constitutes a major socioeconomic problem; indeed, in the United States, deaths from cancer are exceeded only by those resulting from heart disease. In 1998 approximately 1,228,600 new cases of cancer were newly diagnosed, with 564,800 deaths or 46% mortality as reported.[1]

Surgery, radiation therapy, and chemotherapy are the three principal modalities available for treatment of malignant disease. It is being demonstrated that the best therapeutic results ensue when treatment policy decisions are made by a multidisciplinary team rather than by an individual specialist. It is also to be noted that some cancers that were considered incurable by earlier standards have been found to be curable by a modern treatment technique or combination of therapeutic modalities, that is, radiation therapy, surgery, and/or chemotherapy. The specialists in these fields therefore must participate in decision-making for therapy from the very outset. Because there is seldom a second chance to effect a cure, the choice of initial treatment must be the correct one, made after careful consideration of all clinical features in the individual patient. This clearly requires that surgeons, medical oncologists, and radiation oncologists know the strengths and weaknesses of the opposing disciplines and be thoroughly informed of the limitations of their chosen specialties. The welfare of patients with malignant disease lies in the complementary and cooperative efforts of the team.

It is estimated that, during their illnesses, 50% to 60% of patients afflicted with cancer will require radiation therapy, either for cure or palliation. Radiation oncology therefore is a medical specialty of major oncologic importance. Such a specialty demands a working knowledge of the clinical and biologic course, both treated and untreated, of various cancers, a knowledge of the clinical staging of the disease and of the efficacy of various methods of treatment, an awareness of the significance of rehabilitation and follow-up, and an appreciation of the clinical application of the physical and biologic aspects of ionizing radiation. The administration of ionizing radiation to patients is only a part of the specialty of radiation oncology. Major efforts of the radiation oncologist include the preevaluation of patients regarding the indications for radiation therapy, medical attention to patients during and after irradiation, and assessment of therapeutic results through follow-up examinations. Cancers arising from various anatomical sites of the body possess different biologic characteristics.

*Clinical Radiation Oncology: Indications, Techniques, and Results, 2nd ed.* Edited by C.C. Wang.
ISBN: 0-471-23803-1   Copyright © 2000 Wiley-Liss, Inc.

Each has its own natural history, a distinct biologic behavior, a separate mode of tumor growth and spread, and a characteristic response to radiation therapy. The therapeutic management and results may differ greatly.

The prognosis of the patients with malignant diseases depends on many factors, such as the cell type, tumor grade, stage of the primary disease, and presence or absence of regional or distant metastases. When the tumor is confined to the site of origin, the local control rates by radiation therapy are higher than when the lesions have extended into the adjacent organs, for example, cancer of the cervix, skin, and head and neck. Of course, treatment techniques determine the ultimate outcome of patient survival if other factors remain unchanged.

## PLANNING AND PREPARATION FOR RADIATION THERAPY

After radiation therapy has been elected, treatment should be carefully planned and executed. In the modern practice of radiation therapy, treatment planning is based on the nature, size, and location of the tumor, the volume of tissue to be encompassed, the normal organ to be spared, and the intent of treatment (i.e., curative or palliative). The proposed course is carried out with the aid of a simulator and a dedicated computer prior to actual treatment. All workups should be complete, including evaluation of the extent of the primary lesion by physical examination, as well as various diagnostic means such as radiographic imaging studies, contrast studies, and CT or MRI scans. In certain cases, such as tumors in gynecological, genitourinary, and head and neck areas, the patient is under general anesthesia during evaluation of the tumor sites. The distant soft tissues and bony parts are evaluated for metastases, including chest x-rays and bone scans.

Except for a few situations in which biopsy is considered unwise, impractical, and perhaps harmful, confirmation of malignancy should be obtained from a pathologist before treatment. Needless to say, a complete physical examination, including blood and urine studies and liver profile, is highly desirable for appraisal of the patient's physical status. Anemia, weight loss, or electrolyte imbalance should be corrected before treatment is begun.

With a few exceptions, most radiation therapy is given with megavoltage linear accelerators machines ranging from 4 MV to 10 MV x-rays and higher for deeply situated tumors, such as pelvic lesions. For skin and superficial lesions, low energy x-rays (e.g., 50–100 kV) may be used, but such conditions can well be managed by low energy electrons from the linear accelerators. The basic physical properties of radiation are reviewed in Chapter 3.

Other treatment modalities include radiation from cyclotrons of particulates such as protons and neutrons. These novel treatment machines are scarce in the United States, hence are not readily available for daily radiation therapy for the vast majority of patients; this equipment is mostly reserved for a few special lesions.

The total dose to be given is determined by the total treatment time (protraction), the number and dose of daily fractions (fractionation), the cell type, the tolerance of the tumor bed, and, most important, the response of the tumor and the patient to treatment. In general, the radioresponsive tumors such as germ cell tumors, lymphomas and Hodgkin disease treated with intent to cure require a dose of between 30 and 45 Gy in 4 to 5 weeks. For squamous cell carcinoma and adenocarcinoma, a total dose for cure ranges between 65 and 70 Gy in a period of 7 to 8 weeks. For radioinsensitive or resistant tumors such as bone and soft tissue sarcoma, a dose greater than 70 to 75 Gy in 7 to 8 weeks is required.

For the past 15 years, radiation therapy programs have undergone significant changes with altered fractionation based on sound radiobiologic ground. Fractionation schedule, dose per fraction and number of fractions per day, total treatment time, and doses are among the factors that may affect the treatment results in some tumors. Readers are referred to the section of Chapter 15 entitled Altered Fractionation.

## INTENT OF RADIATION THERAPY

The intent of radiation therapy can be divided into three categories: (1) curative, (2) palliative, and (3) adjunctive to surgery. Curative radiation therapy is not without morbidity and should be performed with care and justification. In curative radiation therapy, the treatment course is usually prolonged and physically taxing. Radiation reactions, both local and systemic, may be severe, but should be accepted as an inevitable price for the possibility of cure. As a matter of fact, the discomfort suffered by the patients is not less and is perhaps sometimes more than that from radical surgery. A patient who is physically unfit for radical curative surgery because of severe anemia, cachexia, and rapid deterioration of physical condition is equally unfit for curative radiation therapy. The aims of palliative therapy are to alleviate symptoms and to provide comfort and, if justified, prolongation of meaningful survival.

## COMBINED RADIATION THERAPY AND SURGERY

Surgery and radiation therapy are effective in eradicating small, limited human cancers. Each has its merits, indications, and limitations. Radiation therapy has the advantage of being able to control the disease in situ, thus avoiding removal of a useful and necessary part as well as preserving bodily function. Therefore, radiation therapy must be considered to be the best tissue- and organ-sparing procedure presently available. On the other hand, for certain early lesions situated in less strategic locations, surgery is preferred because it can be carried out expediently and effectively without functional and cosmetic mutilation.

In the management of advanced carcinomas, surgical failures are often due to inability to remove unrecognized microscopic tumor projections at the periphery, thus resulting in marginal recurrence. Tumor seeding in the wound and metastases via lymphatic or hematogenous routes are additional means to account for therapeutic failures after surgery. Large tumor masses often contain hypoxic cells in the center, which are insensitive to radiation therapy. In contrast, tumor cells at the periphery of the tumor mass are actively proliferating, well oxygenated, well nourished, and therefore radioresponsive and controllable by irradiation. Local failures from radiation therapy are therefore central rather than marginal, as in surgery. Distant metastases through the lymphatic and hematogenous routes also constitute failures of local irradiation in a significant number of patients.

Radiobiologically, it is known that an approximately exponential relationship exists between the dose of ionizing radiation administered to a cell population and the surviving fraction of cells. Experimental studies have demonstrated that relatively low doses of radiation will inactivate a vast number of cells in a tumor. $D_{37}$, the dose that reduces the survival cell population to the original 37%, ranges from 1.0 to 2.5 Gy in most biologic systems.[2–5] Other factors influencing cell survival include the capacity for sublethal repair after radiation injury, the environment of oxygenation[6,7] or hypoxia, total dose and dose per treatment (fraction size), and the quality of radiation. Clinical observations indicate that in better than 90% of cases, small microscopic aggregates of tumor cells, so-called subclinical disease, which cannot be detected on physical examination and yet are known from experience to be microscopically and histopathologically detectable, can be controlled with a dose of 45 to 50 Gy in 5 weeks.[8,9] However, for grossly palpable tumors, much higher doses, such as 65 to 70 Gy in 7 weeks or more, are required for inactivation or eradication of the entire cell population to maximize the possibility of local control. For far advanced tumors, radiation therapy is handicapped not only by excessive cell population but also by the presence of a large number of radioresistant hypoxic cells.[10] The radiation dose level must be markedly increased (i.e., 75–80 Gy, and sometimes beyond the limits of tolerance of normal vasculoconnective tissues), thus resulting in radiation necrosis. Therefore eradication of a far advanced tumor by radiation therapy is highly improbable. Readers are referred to Chapter 2.

Based on knowledge of radiobiology and of the mechanisms of treatment failures, the major strength of radiation therapy is to eradicate the radiosensitive, actively growing, well-nourished, and well-oxygenated cells in the periphery of the tumor, or the subclinical disease that is implanted in the wound or lymph nodes. The strength of surgery, on the other hand, is to remove the centrally situated tumor core containing radioresistant hypoxic cells. Therefore, for the advanced, extensive tumors that are rarely curable by either method alone, the logical approach is a combination of radiation therapy and surgery.

Two conceptual approaches to combined radiation therapy and surgery are preoperative and postoperative radiation therapy.[11]

## Preoperative Radiation Therapy

The aims of preoperative radiation therapy are to destroy unrecognized peripheral projections of the tumor, to control subclinical disease in the primary site or in the lymph nodes, or to convert technically inoperable tumors into operable ones. This form of combined approach has been found to decrease iatrogenic scar implant, local or marginal recurrences, and the incidence of distant metastases.

The disadvantages of preoperative radiation therapy are as follows: (1) the exact tumor extent is obscured because of shrinkage and destruction of the radiosensitive components of the lesion prior to surgery; (2) the delay of surgery creates a great deal of anxiety on the part of some patients; and (3) the risk of postoperative complications is increased. The dosage employed in this form of conventional preoperative radiation therapy program is usually moderate (i.e., 45–50 Gy in one month). This is followed in 3 to 4 weeks by radical surgery according to the original extent of the disease, as though radiation therapy had not been given. The program is applicable to medium-sized or advanced tumors of the head and neck, colorectum, bladder, soft tissue sarcomas, and so on, and is commonly not associated with significant postoperative morbidity and mortality.

Low dose, short-course preoperative radiation therapy, that is, 10 Gy divided into four or five daily fractions or 25 Gy in five fractions followed immediately by surgery, has been used in some tumor sites such as pancreas, bladder, and colorectum. This regimen has been found to be effective in preventing scar implant and decreasing distant metastases as well as providing improved local control and survival.

## Postoperative Radiation Therapy

The aims of postoperative radiation therapy are to eradicate residual disease remaining at the resected peripheral margins and to control subclinical disease implanted in the wound or in the lymph nodes.[12,13] The procedure is usually carried out approximately 3 to 4 weeks after surgery when the wound is healed. Generally, a dose of 55 to 60 Gy in 6 weeks is planned[14] if the surgery is radical in extent. On the other hand, if the surgery is primarily a partial resection with gross residual disease remaining, high dose radiation therapy must be given, that is, 65 to 70 Gy in 7 weeks, administered by means of the shrinking field technique to the area of known disease.

The question of preoperative versus postoperative radiation therapy is unresolved, each method having its advantages and disadvantages, proponents and opponents. The decision should be made on an individual basis, including personal preference and experience. Theoretically, preoperative radiation therapy performed with the cancer cells undisturbed and in their maximum stage of oxygenation possesses a possible advantage over irradiation in the postoperative hypoxic condition. Additionally, there are times at which moderately advanced lesions, such as bladder, colorectal, and some head and neck tumors, respond unexpectedly well to radiation therapy and concurrent chemotherapy after 45 Gy, and therefore the planned combined surgery program is terminated. Many patients benefit from continuation of radiation therapy to a curative level and have their mutilative surgery aborted.

Randomized trials of some head and neck lesions indicated that the postoperative radiation therapy can improve local control with some increased distant metastases.[15–17]

For far advanced tumors, a combined program may be given by means of the "sandwich technique," which refers to planned therapies administered both prior to and after surgery.

## RADIORESPONSIVENESS AND RADIOCURABLE TUMORS

Clinically, radioresponsiveness refers to the rate of gross tumor shrinkage and restitution of anatomical parts and functional changes following a given treatment program of dose–time–volume relationship. Tumor shrinkage, a common denominator of radioresponsiveness, is determined by many factors such as innate cell sensitivity related to tissues of origin and cell kinetics of a tumor, including rate of cellular proliferation, cell death and absorption, and the amount of vasculoconnective tissues in or about the tumor. Human tumors are extremely complex. An aggregate of cancerous growth represents an enormous biologic disorder. Various cells that will grow differently are intermingled with various amounts of connective vascular tissues. A wide range of biologic factors affects the radiation response in different histopathologic types of malignancies. In spite of this complicated tumor biology and composition, clinically some tumors respond to radiation therapy better than others, and some respond to much lower amounts of radiation.

Within each category, the response of an individual tumor to radiation may vary greatly according to tumor size, stage, tumor bed (i.e., the adjacent environment), and immunologic status of the patient. Other factors, such as

method of delivery of radiation, total dose, and fractionation scheme, may influence the response of the tumor to radiation therapy.

Radiocurability means that the tumor–normal tissue relationship is such that a tumor control dose of radiation may be delivered to eradicate the growth without permanently damaging the adjacent normal tissue. These tumors, when diagnosed and treated in an early stage without distant metastases, are highly curable by radiation therapy and are often termed radiocurable tumors. Included in this category are the following:

1. Carcinoma of the skin and the lip
2. Carcinoma of the head and neck
3. Carcinoma of the breast
4. Carcinoma of the cervix and endometrium
5. Carcinoma of the prostate
6. Hodgkin disease, and localized extranodal lymphoma
7. Seminoma of testis and dysgerminoma of ovary
8. Medulloblastoma, pineal germinoma, and ependymoma
9. Retinoblastoma
10. Choroidal melanoma (treated by proton particle beam or [198]Au plaque)

Other tumors with limited radioresponsiveness may be included in this group as curable tumors through combined therapies, that is, radiation therapy, surgery, and/or chemotherapy. These include the following:

1. Wilms tumor
2. Rhabdomyosarcoma
3. Colorectal carcinoma
4. Soft tissue sarcoma
5. Embryonal carcinoma of testis

Most other malignant neoplasms carry an unfavorable prognosis and cannot be claimed as curable lesions because of inability to diagnose early or lack of a favorable therapeutic ratio. Examples include tumors arising from or involving adjacent organs highly vulnerable to radiation injury and tumors with a propensity to develop distant metastases. In some instances, however, a limited number of cures may be obtained unexpectedly following surgery, irradiation, or combination of both.

## RADIOSENSITIVITY AND TUMOR CONTROL PROBABILITY

Clinically, "radiosensitivity" is often used interchangeably with "radioresponsiveness." Radiobiologically, the former term is used to indicate the innate sensitivity of the cells to radiation. As shown in dose–survival curves, the radiosensitivity for various normal and malignant mammalian cell lines is related to the slope of the curve or the $D_0$ ranging between 1 to 2.5 Gy in the oxygenated environment. (See Chapter 2). The factors that may influence radiosensitivity include the ability to repair sublethal damage after radiation injury, the degree of oxygenation or hypoxia, the total dose and dose per treatment, the fractionation scheme, and the quality of radiation. These are discussed in the subsections that follow.

### Therapeutic Ratio

The probability of tumor control and normal tissue complications versus radiation dose are related by a sigmoid curve, but with different slopes (Figure 1-1) in various tissues. The relative positions of these curves or their differential comprise the *therapeutic ratio*. It is this ratio that determines whether any particular tumor related to the adjacent normal tissue or tumor bed can he treated easily, with difficulty, or not at all. This is the foundation of clinical radiation oncology. Since the tumor control probability curve is located to the left of that for normal tissue complications, there is an increased or favorable therapeutic ratio. To the contrary, any tumor with a control probability curve to the right of the normal tissue

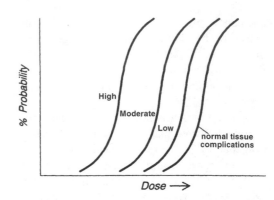

**FIGURE 1-1** Therapeutic ratio, a foundation of radiation oncology, showing tumor control and normal tissue complication probabilities versus radiation doses. The tumors are divided into radiosensitive, moderately sensitive, and resistant.

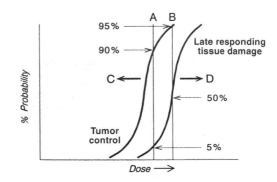

**FIGURE 1-2** Definition of optimal tumor control dose. **(A)** 90% tumor control probability and 5% complications. **(B)** A further increase of dose tumor control probability is increased to 95% (5% improvement) with 50% complications. Methods to shift tumor control curve to the left **(C)** or complicated curve to the right **(D)** may improve therapeutic results.

complications carries a negative therapeutic ratio, and radiation therapy benefits are nil; such tumors rarely are treated successfully by radiation therapy alone (Figure 1-2). All therapeutic techniques must exploit this differential between tumor control and normal tissue complications versus dose. No improved therapeutic gains can be expected by shifting all sigmoid curves in the same direction and to the same degree.

## Linear Energy Transfer (LET) and Relative Biologic Effectiveness (RBE)

Factors affecting the radiosensitivity include the quality of radiation, which is measured as linear energy transfer (LET). The LET is designated as the average energy deposited in each linear unit of track of secondary electron as ionization (or other charged particles) and is measured in electron volts per micrometer (eV/$\mu$m), or more practically, in kilovoltage (keV/$\mu$m). Fast neutrons and other forms of particulate radiation have dense ionization and high LET. X-rays and high energy electrons have sparse ionization and low LET. Biologic damage to cells is related to LET. In a general way, high LET radiation is more likely to produce substantial damage in a given volume of living matter and does not depend on the oxygen environment similarly in both tumor and normal tissues. Since there is no significant differential repair of sublethal damage between various tissues, the benefits of fractionated radiation therapy are voided; both radiation damage to the adjacent normal tissues and local tumor control are somewhat higher than with conventional x-ray therapy. With an admixture of x-ray and neutron beam therapy, some increase in therapeutic ratio may be obtained, with resultant improvement in local control and a decrease in complications.

RBE is used to compare the biologic effectiveness of different radiation relative to 200 kV x-rays as the standard. For the low LET radiation such as $^{60}$Co $\gamma$ rays or low megavoltage x-rays, the RBE is slightly less than unity. While the higher LET radiations have greater RBE, up to 3.5, the increased RBE does not continue indefinitely. With radiation of extremely high LET, more energy is deposited in the target than is needed to produce even the maximum biologic effect. Such radiation deposits excessive energies, resulting in overkill, and therefore is wasted. This phenomenon generally occurs in radiation with LET exceeding 100 keV/$\mu$m. The RBE of electrons probably ranges from unity to below unity, that is, from 0.85 to 0.90 compared to $^{60}$Co radiation. Because the contribution of the electron beam in daily radiation therapy is only one-third or one-fourth of the total dose, the value of RBE as 1.0 (unity) is used in dose calculation.

## Oxygen Enhancement Ratio (OER)

In most biologic systems under both normal and malignant conditions, the radiation effects of x-rays or $\gamma$-rays are greater when the cells are irradiated under oxygenated conditions than under hypoxic conditions. The difference in radiosensitivity under oxygenated conditions is in the neighborhood of two- to threefold and is called the oxygen enhancement ratio (OER). For the oxygen to be a radiation sensitizer, it must be present in the cells during irradiation. The mechanism of oxygen-enhancing radiosensitivity is believed to develop when oxygen combines with radiation-induced radicals, initiating a chain of events that finally result in biologic damage. The biologic damage by dense ionizing radiation, such as fast neutrons, is indeed so dense in the target site that lethal events occur directly and therefore are not mediated by oxygen. Neutrons or other dense ionizing radiation therefore have a lower OER.

All cells in the tumor are not benefited to the same extent by increased amounts of oxygenation. Markedly increasing radiosensitivity associated with increasing intracellular oxygen occurs when the cells are hypoxic, but such enhancement of radiosensitivity is much less or nonexistent if the cells are already fully oxygenated. In clinicopathologic conditions, a tumor core more than 150 to 180 $\mu$m distant from functional capillaries often contains hypoxic cells, which are insensitive to radiation therapy.[10] To overcome the cellular hypoxia, radiation therapy was carried out with hyperbaric oxygen[7] or in conjunction with hypoxic cell sensitizers, but the therapeutic gains have been disappointing, and such clinical research has not come to fruition.

In clinical situations, the availability of oxygen to the tumor can be altered by a variety of changes inside the body such as impaired circulation from radical surgery, fibrosis from earlier irradiation, and anemia secondary to hemorrhage. Studies indicate that local tumor control is decreased in patients with low hemoglobin levels, for example, in carcinoma of the cervix and in some head and neck carcinomas.

## Fractionation and Fraction Size (Dose per Treatment)

The radiation effects produced by a single dose of x-rays or γ-rays are more pronounced than those produced by the same amount delivered in divided daily fractionated doses over a longer period of time. The decreased response with daily fractionation, which is due to cell recovery or repair from sublethal damage occurring between dose fractions, accounts for most of the increased dose necessary with conventional clinical fractionation. With fractionated x-irradiation given in small daily increments, sublethal damage is repaired daily, often in less than 24 hours and perhaps within 4 to 6 hours.[3,18] The shoulder of the survival curve is therefore duplicated (at least in part) with each daily fraction. This type of recovery occurs predominantly in normal oxygenated tissues, both acute and late-responding tissues, and is possibly less marked or absent in some chronically hypoxic tumor cells.[19,20] After radiation injury, the regenerative process is followed by the resumption of mitotic activity of the normal cell and repopulation from the stem cells. The malignant cells may exhibit regenerative capability to a similar but lesser degree. Fractionation therefore is relatively sparing of normal tissue and results in more damage to tumor cell population from radiation. During fractionation and protraction of radiation therapy, the radiosensitive oxygenated cells are destroyed, with subsequent reduction in the tumor size. The radioresistant hypoxic cells, which were distant from the functional vasculature, became closer to the blood supply and therefore were reoxygenated. The result is a transfer of hypoxic cells to a more oxygenated compartment and enhancement of the overall radiosensitivity and radiocurability of the entire tumor, leading to eventual complete sterilization of the tumor without significant injury to the adjacent normal tissues. This concept is applied routinely in clinical radiation therapy.

Conventional radiation therapy generally is given with one fraction per day (QD) for a certain number of days in the total treatment days. Such programs were derived from experience with satisfactory control of some human cancers. Based on the modern radiobiologic knowledge, such QD schedules may not be the best for treatment of human cancers. For the past two decades, radiation therapy fractionation programs have been changed greatly.[14,21] The readers are referred to Chapter 15B.

## FACTORS IMPROVING QUALITY OF RADIATION THERAPY

### Shrinking Field Concept

It is generally recognized that the larger the tumor mass, the larger the radiation therapy field required, the lower the total dose that can be tolerated, and subsequently the lower the probability of achieving tumor control. Radiobiologically, the peripheral extension of tumor mass containing mostly microscopic disease can be controlled by a relatively lower dose of radiation, that is, 50 Gy in 5 weeks.[8,9] After this dose level has been achieved with tumor shrinkage, the residual mass with hypoxic cells can be irradiated with smaller fields to the desired level of higher dose without undue damage to the adjacent normal tissues. This concept is routinely applied in the treatment of most squamous cell carcinomas (e.g., head and neck, gynecological, lung, gastrointestinal malignancies) with improved local control and decreased complications (Figure 1-3).

### Time–Dose–Fraction (TDF) Relationship

The biologic effects of radiation injuries of the normal tissues are closely related to total treat-

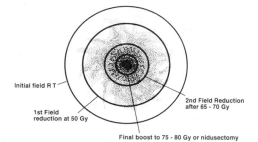

Initial field R T

1st Field
reduction at 50 Gy

2nd Field Reduction
after 65 - 70 Gy

Final boost to 75 - 80 Gy or nidusectomy

**FIGURE 1-3** Diagram showing shrinking field radiation therapy (RT) with various components of a solid tumor with microscopic disease at the periphery requiring 50 Gy in 5 weeks for eradication; gross disease, 65 to 70 Gy, and residual disease treated by nidusectomy or highest dose by interstitial implant or intraoral cone.

ment time, amount of total radiation dose, and number of daily fractions.[22,23] The result of such a relationship is designated as a value number, the nominal standard dose (NSD) or TDF, and is used as a general guide to treatment planning for normal tissue tolerance, that is, to the isobioeffect. The NSD or TDF value is an estimate of isobioeffect only within the radiotherapeutic range of fraction size, that is, 1.5 to 3.0 Gy per treatment. The acute and late effects may be different, even with identical NSD or TDF values. Any value after an extremely large or smaller fraction size must be interpreted with great caution and may not be clinically applicable. Likewise, the formula has different tolerance values for nervous tissues and for normal vasculoconnective tissues. Since the tumor control dose in any part of the body is limited by the tolerance of the normal tissue adjacent to the tumor, the NSD or TDF values may also be used to designate the tumor control dose, and the values can be used to compare various treatment schemes with different total dose and time, fraction size, and number of fractions. For a small squamous cell carcinoma, generally a TDF value of 110 is considered to be adequate for tumor control and is equated to approximately 65 Gy divided into 32 daily fractions, 5 fractions a week. However, for a much larger tumor, a higher TDF value (e.g., 120 or 130) is often needed.

In daily radiation practice, external beam radiation therapy and interstitial or intracavitary implant are commonly combined. In such instances, combined TDF values may be calculated,[24] but care must be taken in the use of unusual techniques, fractions, or protraction. Calculated TDF values are useful to the experienced clinician who has a clear understanding of the limitations of the isobioeffect formulations. To keep the daily and total doses within the limits of normal tissue tolerance, the TDF should be frequently consulted for any change of dose per fraction or alteration of fractionation of the treatment program.

## Daily Multifield Treatment

When the parallel opposing portal technique is used for the treatment of deep-seated tumors, it is important that all fields be treated each day.[25,26] This is particularly true when a lesion situated in separation greater than 20 cm in diameter is treated by low megavoltage radiation. The increased peripheral dose may produce radiation injuries to the overlying normal tissue, resulting in severe subcutaneous fibrosis, ulceration, or greater injury to the peripheral organs. This deleterious phenomenon, designated the "edge effect," is magnified by treating 3 or 4 days a week (with same weekly dose) instead of 5 days a week, owing to the necessity of increasing the fraction size to keep the weekly dose constant. On the other hand, for a smaller separation (< 6 cm: e.g., in carcinoma of the vocal cord), the isobioeffect does not differ significantly between the midline tumor and the peripheral normal tissues, and therefore it would not be absolutely necessary to treat all fields each day as in the wider separation.

## RADIATION COMPLICATIONS

The acute effects of radiation therapy often accompany curative radiotherapeutic procedures. These are not to be considered as radiation complications; rather, they are normal radiation reactions, deliberately produced for therapeutic reasons, and in most cases reversible, though normally not to the full extent. Acute effects are related to total dose and total treatment time. When the cell renewal mechanism of normal tissues is altered—that is, when cell death exceeds cell production—the acute effects will be severe. Reduction in dose per fraction with prolonging of the treatment course or a small treatment break can diminish this severity, however.

The late effects of radiation therapy depend primarily on the late-responding tissues of the vasculoconnective stroma and the slowly proliferating, reacting parenchymal tissues. Late effects are related to significantly fraction size, number of fractions, and total dose, as well as to tissues and treatment volume irradiated, and are not necessarily proportional to the extent of the acute effects despite similar nominal standard dose or time–dose–fraction values.

When the effects on the vasculoconnective tissues become unduly severe, late complications of radiation therapy occur, some of which may be symptomatic and require corrective treatment measures. As shown in Figure 1-2, dose A is associated with 90% of probability of local tumor control and 5% of complications. A further small increase of dose (from A to B) is accompanied by much higher complications, that is, 50%, and yet the percentage of local control is not proportionately increased. In the clinical practice of radiation therapy, a total of 70 to 75 Gy of external beam therapy with 2 Gy per day in 7 to 8 weeks, or 70 Gy continuous brachytherapy irradiation in 7 days, is considered to be the maximal dose normal late-responding tissues can tolerate.

The definition of an "optimal" tumor control dose is different for each individual radiation oncologist. Only the physician's clinical expertise and experience can yield a valid judgment regarding acceptable dose level and normal tissue complication in return for a probability of improved tumor control, that is, the reward–risk ratio. In certain instances, the increased risk of complications such as transverse myelitis or temporal bone necrosis is to-

tally unacceptable and should be avoided. On the other hand, soft tissue necrosis, osteoradionecrosis of the mandible, and radiation pneumonitis of limited extent can be corrected by surgery or are relatively asymptomatic, and thus such risks are worth taking if significant tumor control can be achieved with higher doses of radiation therapy.

For the patient with a curable tumor or an incurable tumor with a prospect of prolonged survival, radiation therapy with a fraction size larger than 2.5 or 3.0 Gy for 5 days a week is not considered to be optimal because the likelihood of late complications in long-term survivors is higher. This is particularly important in dealing with CNS, optic nerve, or chiasm and spinal cord lesions, which may significantly increase the incidence of neuropathy.[27] Likewise, the treatment of inoperable carcinoma of the breast, or head and neck tumors with a large fraction size (i.e., 4 Gy per fraction per day and/or a reduced number of fractions per week) results in marked increase in late complications such as severe fibrosis or rib fractures or osteoradionecrosis of the mandible. There is an exception to this statement, however: the treatment of small cancers of the skin (1–2 cm in diameter), for which a daily fraction of 4 to 5 Gy is a common practice in our institution.

When a rapid, high daily dose of radiation therapy is needed, the logical approach is multifraction-per-day (MFD) radiation therapy, that is, two or three fractions of 1.6 to 1.8 Gy per fraction daily, with 4 to 6 hours between fractions. At the present time this program is commonly practiced for patients with superior cava syndrome, spinal cord compression, and other conditions.

For the highest level of local control, radiation complications may occur in a small percentage of patients treated by curative radiation therapy. If complications are cause for concern, the radiation oncologist may have to reduce the dose level, and this in turn may result in decrease of local control and patient survival. However, the experience of frequent and repeated occurrences of severe complications (i.e., > 10%) is not regarded as good radiation therapy and should prompt review of dose calculations and treatment policy, as well as an investigation of radiation techniques and modalities. Not infrequently, severe complications are the result of an unrealistic and unjustifiable decision by a physician to treat a biologically radioinsensitive tumor too vigorously, or to re-treat recurrences in areas already heavily irradiated with high radiation doses.

## PRINCIPLES OF PALLIATIVE RADIATION THERAPY

In daily clinical practice the optimal decision between curative and palliative radiation therapy may not always be easy or possible. Many patients who appear to be beyond possible cure may respond so favorably to palliation therapy that long-term, apparently cancer-free survival may result. It is therefore important to note that if palliative radiation therapy is offered, one must be reasonably certain that the patient has an incurable lesion and is not denied the chance of cure by curative radiation therapy or other means. Failure to approach a still-curable lesion in a manner likely to produce a cure is unacceptable; it is even worse than pursuing curative efforts in a patient with apparently incurable cancer by means of high doses, to the general detriment of the patient, with resultant severe radiation symptomatic necrosis and complications. The general philosophies of palliative radiation therapy were admirably discussed in the literature by Paterson[28] and Schulz.[29] The following points are worthy of observation.

1. The selection of patients for palliative radiation therapy must be exercised with good judgment.
2. The expectation of relief should equal or exceed that possible from other palliative measures.
3. The duration of radiation therapy should not consume a major portion of the patient's remaining life, and the patient must be in a position to enjoy whatever

benefits the palliation is expected to produce.
4. Palliative radiation therapy should not cause great distress to the patient, nor should it make the existing condition worse.
5. If neither cure nor palliation appears to be possible, no irradiation should be given.

The techniques of palliative radiation therapy need not be highly demanding or elaborate but must be tailored to the patient's condition. For the patient in excellent physical shape with a limited lesion, who appears to have hope of prolonged survival, the goal of palliative radiation therapy is to achieve lasting local control, ridding the patient of the regional difficulties and providing prolongation of life and comfortable existence, with restoration of some degree of health and happiness. The radiation therapy technique must be sophisticated, somewhat similar to curative radiation therapy.

Although the treatment time should be as short as possible, the principles of using proper fraction size for daily radiation therapy as discussed in Chapter 15B, Altered Fractionation Radiation Therapy, should always be kept in mind. For patients with extensive cancer, and with rapidly progressive tumors for which only short-term survival is anticipated, the radiation therapy course can be markedly accelerated, with treatment to be completed in a short period of time. On the other hand, for the patient whose condition (e.g., metastatic breast carcinoma in bone, indolent tumors, solitary metastasis) offers a good prospect of prolonged survival, or in patients with high performance status or extensive local–regional disease without other demonstrable distant metastases, the treatment course should be more protracted, with conventional fraction size and doses that do not result in severe late radiation sequelae. Likewise, radiation damage to the spinal cord or brain, even in patients with incurable cancer, must be avoided at all costs. Between the two extremes, an intermediate course may be considered, which probably is used mostly in the daily practice of radiation therapy.

For the epitheliomatous lesions, the dose employed for palliative radiation therapy can be divided into three categories: (1) accelerated treatment with a daily fraction of 5 Gy for 5 days or 8 to 10 Gy for 2 days, (2) intermediate treatment with a daily fraction of 2.5 to 3.0 Gy for 10 to 15 fractions, and (3) conventional fractionated treatment with 2.0 to 2.25 Gy per fraction for a total dose of 45 to 50 Gy. Each has its merits and advocates. For the large daily fraction program, such late radiation therapy effects in normal tissues[30] as severe fibrosis and vascular damage, or serious brain or spinal cord damage, may not be apparent for months or years following completion of irradiation, should the patient survive. The radiation therapy schemes are further modified by the histologic type and location of the tumor, and normal tissue tolerance of the involved organ (brain, spinal cord, lung, kidney, gastrointestinal tract, skin, breast, etc.). In general, a lasting palliation for squamous cell carcinoma and adenocarcinoma calls for a tumor dose of approximately 50 Gy. For the highly responsive tumors, such as lymphomas and germ cell tumors, a dose of 25 to 30 Gy should suffice. For mesenchymal sarcomas, a much higher dose is required (i.e., 55–60 Gy), and the palliative value is still questionable.

Other chapters in this book cover conditions of clinical importance commonly seen in a general hospital, including spinal cord compression,[31] superior venae cavae syndrome,[32,33] metastases to the brain,[34] skeleton with severe pain, and/or inpending pathologic fracture,[35] or others,[36,37] which may call for the immediate use of palliative radiation therapy.

## SUMMARY

The modern practice of radiation therapy, either for cure or for palliation, demands extreme technical sophistication and justification. The use of various treatment modalities and techniques, or a combination of photons and electrons intermingled with isotopic brachytherapy, has greatly reduced the incidence of most of the major irreparable radiation injuries of the bone and soft tissues that were commonly seen in the past kilovoltage era, and salvage surgery often can be performed without significant postoperative complications. In spite of recent advances in radiation oncology, however, the cure rates of most cancers have reached a plateau. Further improvement of treatment results must depend on further progress in the use of combined therapies, including surgery, chemotherapy, or refinement of altered fractionation schemes, particulate radiation, and other approaches.

## REFERENCES

1. American Cancer Society: *CA: Cancer J Clin* 1998;48, no 1.
2. Hewitt HB, Wilson CW: Survival curve for mammalian leukemia cells irradiated in vivo. *Br J Cancer* 1959;13:69–75.
3. Elkind MM, Whitmore GF: *The Radiobiology of Cultured Mammalian Cells.* New York, Gordon & Breach, 1967, pp 7–143.
4. Fowler JF: Differences in survival curve shapes for formal multi-target and multi-hit models. *Phys Med Biol* 1964;9:177–188.
5. Puck TT, Marcus PI: Actions of x-rays on mammalian cells. *J Exp Med* 1956;103:653–666.
6. Gray LH: Radiobiologic basis of oxygen as modifying factor in radiation therapy. *Am J Roentgenol* 1961;85:803–815.
7. Glassburn JR, Brady LW, Plenk: Hyperbaric oxygen in radiation therapy. *Cancer* 1977;39:751–765.
8. Fletcher GH: Elective irradiation of subclinical disease in cancers of the head and neck. *Cancer* 1972;29:1450.
9. Fletcher GH: Lucy Wortham James Lecture: Subclinical disease. *Cancer* 1984;53:1274–1284.
10. Thomlinson RH, Gray LH: The histological structure of some human lung cancers and the possible implications for radiotherapy. *Br J Cancer* 1955;9:539–549.
11. Powers WE, Palmer LA: Biologic basis of preoperative radiation treatment. *Am J Roentgenol* 1968;102:176–192.
12. Looser KJ, Shah JP, Strong EW: The significance of "positive" margins in surgically re-

sected epidermoid carcinomas. *Head Neck Surg* 1978;1:107–111.

13. Johnson JT, Barnes EL, Myers EN, Schramm L, Borochovitz D, Sigler BA: The extracapsular spread of tumors in cervical node metastasis. *Arch Otolaryngol* 1981;107:725–729.

14. Peters LJ, Ang KK: The role of altered fractionation in head and neck cancers. *Semin Radiat Oncol* 1992;2(3):180–194.

15. Kramer S, Gelber RD, Snow JB, Marcial VA, Lowry LD, Davis LW, Chandler R: Combined radiation therapy and surgery in the management of advanced head and neck cancer: Final report of 73-03 of the radiation therapy oncology group. *Head Neck Surg* 1987;10:19–30.

16. Tupchong L, Scott CB, Blitzer PH, Marcial VA, Lowry LD, Jacobs JR, Stetz J, Davis LW, Snow JR, Chandler R, Kramer S, Pajak TF: Randomized study of preoperative versus postoperative radiation therapy in advanced head and neck carcinoma: Long-term follow-up of RTOG study 73-03. *Int J Radiat Oncol Biol Phys* 1991;20:21–28.

17. Vandenbrouch C, Sancho H, LeFur R: Results of randomized clinical trial of preoperative irradiation versus postoperative in treatment of tumors of the hypopharynx. *Cancer* 1977;39:1445–1449.

18. Elkind MM, Sutton G, Moses WB, et al: Sublethal and lethal radiation damage. *Nature* 1967;214:1088–1092.

19. Suit HD, Urano M: Radiation biology for radiation therapy, in CC Wang (ed): *Clinical Radiation Oncology Indications, Techniques and Results,* 1st ed. Littleton, MA, PSG Inc, 1988, pp 17–55.

20. Suit HD, Urano M: Repair of sublethal radiation injury in hypoxic cells of a C3H mouse mammary carcinoma. *Radiat Res* 1969;37:422–434.

21. Wang CC, Blitzer PH, Suit HD: Twice-a-day radiation therapy for cancer of the head and neck. *Cancer* 1985;55:2100–2104.

22. Ellis F: Nominal standard dose and the RET. *Br J Radiol* 1971;44:101–108.

23. Orton CG, Ellis F: A simplification of the use of NSD concept in practical radiotherapy. *Br J Radiol* 1973;46:529–537.

24. Ellis F, Sorenson A: A method of estimating biological effect of combined intracavitary low dose rate radiation with external radiation in carcinoma of the cervix uteri. *Radiology* 1974;110:681–686.

25. Wilson CS, Hall EJ: On the advisability of treating all fields at each radiotherapy session. *Radiology* 1971;98:419.

26. Gitterman M, Littman P, Doppke K, et al: Rethinking the necessity of treating all fields in each radiotherapy session. *Radiology* 1975;117:419–424.

27. Harris JR, Levene MB: Visual complications following irradiation for pituitary adenomas and craniopharyngiomas. *Radiology* 1976;120:167–171.

28. Paterson R: Use and abuse of palliative radiotherapy. *J Fac Radiol* 1957;8:235–238.

29. Schulz MD: Radiotherapy in advanced and incurable malignant disease. *Radiology* 1957;69:321–323.

30. Cox JD: Large-dose fractionation (hypofractionation). *Cancer* 1985;55:2105–2111.

31. Rubin P, Mayer E, Poulter C: Extradural spinal cord compression by tumor. Part 11: High daily dose experience without laminectomy. *Radiology* 1969;93:1248–1260.

32. Rubin R, et al: Superior venae caval syndrome: Slow low-dose versus rapid high-dose schedules. *Radiology* 1963;388–401.

33. Davenport D, Ferree C, Blake D, et al: Response of superior venae caval syndrome to radiation therapy. *Cancer* 1976;1577–1580.

34. Posner JB: Diagnosis of treatment of metastases to brain. *Clin Bull* 1974;4:47.

35. Blitzer P: Reanalysis of the RTOG study of the palliation of symptomatic osseous metastasis. *Cancer* 1985;55:1468–1472.

36. Prasad B, Lee M, Hendrickson FR: Irradiation of hepatic metastases. *Int J Radiat Oncol Biol Phys* 1977;2:129–132.

37. Turek-Marscherder M, Kazem I: Palliative irradiation for liver metastases. *JAMA* 1975;232:625–628.

# CHAPTER 2

# RADIATION BIOLOGY FOR RADIATION ONCOLOGISTS

SIMON N. POWELL and HERMAN D. SUIT

Successful radiation treatment requires not only that all tumor cells be inactivated or killed but that sufficient cells of the irradiated normal tissues survive and proliferate to reconstitute the damaged tissue and carry on normal or near-normal functions. This means that a differential response between tumor and normal tissue which favors the latter is a prerequisite for an effective radiation treatment strategy. Efforts directed at improving the efficacy of radiation therapy endeavor to (1) increase that differential, (2) increase radiation dose to the tumor tissue and/or reduce dose to normal tissues, and (3) predict the response of the tumor, to ensure selection of the optimal treatment protocol. The reaction of a tissue or organ to radiation represents the integrated response of the cellular constituents and their functional organization in the tissues.

Radiation damage to cells may be lethal or nonlethal. Lethality is determined by whether the damage is reparable or nonreparable, which in turn is dependent on the type, site, and timing of the damage inflicted. The lethal response is of greatest interest to the clinician because of the requirement that to cure a cancer patient, all tumor cells be killed. A lethal response or loss of cell viability means the loss of capacity for sustained proliferation or for the production of a continuously expanding progeny. A nonviable cell, in this sense,

may retain metabolic integrity for a long period after irradiation and indeed may pass through several after postirradiation divisions before its metabolic death. Such a cell should be of no consequence to the patient. Figures 2-1A and 2-1B demonstrate pedigrees of irradiated L59 fibroblasts determined by microcinematographic studies.[1] For the pedigree in Figure 2-1A, a dose of 2.16 Gy was administered to an L59 cell 13.5 hours after mitosis. As shown, the cell divided after a total of 29.5 hours. This represents a major delay in cell division for this cell line. One of the daughters was able to establish a pedigree sector that underwent several postirradiation divisions; by the sixth postradiation division, all progeny had become pyknotic or the interdivision times exceedingly prolonged. This colony would, almost certainly, be abortive. A colony that expands to a population of more than 50 cells is usually viable. The second sector was short-lived. The posttreatment pedigree shown in Figure 2-1B demonstrates establishment of a viable colony by a cell that did survive the irradiation through the successful proliferation of cells in one pedigree sector.

The pedigrees of Figure 2-1 demonstrate that following radiation there is a prolonged interdivisional interval and an increased probability of daughter cell death among progeny of surviving cells, and that a sector

*Clinical Radiation Oncology: Indications, Techniques, and Results, 2nd ed.* Edited by C.C. Wang.
ISBN: 0-471-23803-1   Copyright © 2000 Wiley-Liss, Inc.

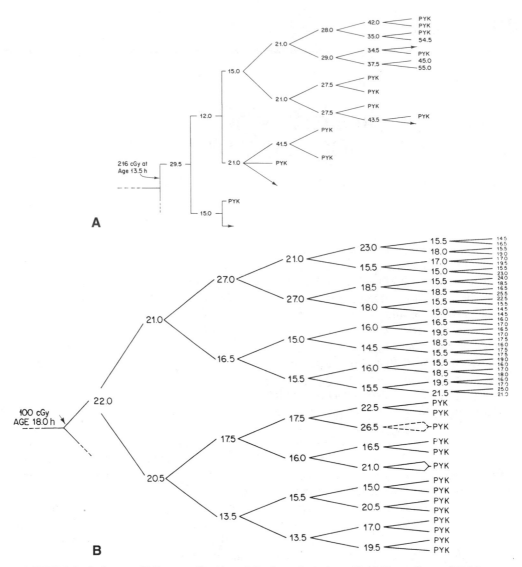

**FIGURE 2-1**   Pedigrees of L59 mouse fibroblasts following a single dose of 2.16 Gy at cell age of 13.5 hours **(A)** and 1 Gy at cell age of 18 hours **(B)**: PYK, pyknotic. (Reproduced from Thompson and Suit.[1])

or indeed an entire colony may die after several postirradiation divisions. This complex set of observations is still not fully understood at a molecular and genetic level, but many of the factors determining cell death or radiation sensitivity, as well as the mechanistic basis of cell division delay, have been established in the last 10 years. A still more complex observation is that cell lines developed from Chinese hamster cells that survive ~15 Gy exhibit heritable nonlethal damage.[2]

This was characterized by morphologic changes in chromosomes, small cell size, increased probability of death of daughter cells, and an increased radiation sensitivity. These heritable changes were maintained through repeated cell passages up to 80 cell generations. The clinical consequence of this type of surviving cell is not clear. Much of the remainder of this chapter addresses determinants of death or survival after exposure to ionizing radiation.

## BIOLOGY OF RESPONSE TO IONIZING RADIATION

The observed response of a tissue or organ to radiation will be determined by the proportion of cells that have lost viability, the time course for pyknosis and lysis of the radiation-killed cells, and the proliferative activity and functional integrity of the surviving cells. The time of appearance of gross or symptomatic change of the tissue or organ is principally a function of the cellularity of the tissues and the proliferation kinetics of the cellular constituents. For example, changes in bone marrow are prompt because marrow is composed of actively dividing cells and is highly cellular. In contrast, changes in mature muscle are seen only at times remote from the radiation treatments; this is because muscle is composed predominantly of stroma and the constituent cells have an extremely slow turnover. Thus, there may be vastly different time courses for the appearance of damage in two diverse tissues, even if the fraction of cells killed was the same for each tissue. An end point for tissue reaction—for example, a specific level of severity of skin reaction—is the consequence of radiation treatment that achieves a particular survival fraction among the constituent cells of the tissue of interest.

### Cell Viability

Therefore, fundamental knowledge for the radiation oncologist is the relationship between radiation dose and probability of cell kill. Cell survival curves, that is, the relationship between the fraction of surviving cells and radiation dose, were established for viruses and bacteria in the 1940s and 1950s. Such information could not be generated for mammalian cells until techniques were developed for culturing of individual mammalian cells in vitro, which permitted the use of colony formation as the measure of cell viability in the same manner as had been employed for viruses and bacteria. This was accomplished by Puck and Marcus in 1955,[3] using cells derived from human squa-

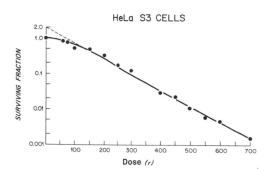

**FIGURE 2-2** Radiation cell survival curve for single-dose irradiation of HeLa cells in vitro under aerobic conditions. (Reproduced from Puck and Marcus.[4])

mous cell carcinoma of the uterine cervix (HeLa cells). This constituted an extraordinary valuable development for the biological sciences. These authors followed in 1956 with a paper inaugurating the era of quantitative mammalian cellular radiation biology in which they described the first radiation cell survival curve for mammalian cells.[4] This curve is reproduced as Figure 2-2: a plot of log survival fraction (SF) versus dose $D$. The resultant curve was characterized by a shoulder region followed by a straight line. Puck and co-workers subsequently published similar survival curves for cells derived from diverse normal and malignant tissues (human and nonhuman; cells maintained for short or long periods in vitro; and for aneuploid and euploid cells).[5]

### Target for Loss of Cell Viability

Cell death is thought to occur as a result of one or more biochemical lesions in a critical region of DNA which cannot be repaired, or cannot be repaired correctly. There may be repair of such damaged sites, but misrepair of critical genes would be inadequate for cell survival. Of course, damage to noncritical genes may go unrepaired or be misrepaired with no manifest impact on normal cell function or the whole organism; the resultant nonlethal damage would be heritable. The biochemical changes in the DNA are directly or indirectly due to the radiation. In the former, damage results from ionization produced directly by the photons or particles of the radiation beam. Indirect effect means damage secondary to biochemical intermediates, predominantly highly reactive species produced in water, especially OH radicals.

For a given radiation dose, a specific amount of energy is deposited in cells, tissues, or water and results in ionization damage to DNA. Differences in cell sensitivity to radiation are due to differences in the chemical and biological processing of that damage, collectively called "repair." Repair in this wide definition covers a broad range of subjects: the physics of energy deposition by ionizing radiation, the initial measurable damage inflicted in the DNA, the chemical and biological modification of this damage, and finally the biological consequences of residual radiation-induced damage.

Many lines of evidence point to DNA as the target for loss of cell viability due to ionizing radiations. Extremely narrow beams of particulate radiation cause cell death when aimed at the nucleus but not the cytoplasm.[6] Cells that have incorporated tritiated thymidine ([3]HTdR) into their DNA are killed by the effects of the extremely low energy electrons produced with decay of the tritium. These are absorbed predominantly in adjacent DNA.[7] In contrast, tritiated uridine, which is incorporated into RNA, is much less toxic to cells. Analogs of thymidine (e.g., BrdUrd and IdUrd), increase radiation sensitivity.[8,9] This has been further substantiated by studies of Warters et al.,[10] who showed that iodine-125 was vastly more damaging to Chinese hamster ovary cells if incorporated into DNA as [125]I deoxyuridine than if attached to the cell membrane as [[125]I]concanavalin A (con A).

### Physical Energy Deposition

Energy is deposited in a variety of ionization densities. For 1 Gy absorbed dose of [60]Co irradiation, approximately 1000 sparse ionizations, 20 to 100 moderate clusters, 4 to 40 large clusters, and 0 to 4 very large clusters occur.[11] Radiations of different qualities produce different relative amounts of ionization densities. The relative number of ionization clusters tends to match the relative biological effectiveness (RBE) and are thus thought to be biologically more relevant. RBE is the ratio of the dose from standard low linear energy transfer (LET) radiation to produce a defined biological effect, relative to the dose from a test radiation needed to produce the same effect.

### Immediate Biochemical Modification of Induced Damage

Certain rapid biochemical mechanisms can modify the conversion of ionizations into biologically relevant damage. For example, one immediate effect of ionization is loss of hydrogen atoms from DNA, and this could be reversed rapidly by hydrogen donor molecules such as those containing sulfydryl groups. These molecules would need access to damaged sites and necessarily would be either small or already present adjacent to DNA. Reduced glutathione (the most abundant sulfydryl hydrogen donor molecule) and cysteamine are potent modifiers of DNA damage. A correlation between sulfydryl levels and radiosensitivity would be expected. This has been found in some cases, but not universally. Artificial manipulation of thiol levels has a clear effect on measurable initial DNA damage, which is the damage that can be measured in cells after energy deposition and immediate modification. Another mechanism of "immediate" biochemical modification of DNA damage is rapid enzymatic metabolism of the products of water radiolysis. Hydrogen peroxide is generated from hydroxyl radicals, and is converted to water and oxygen by catalase, or to water and dehydrogenated cosubstrate by peroxidases. Superoxide radicals are catalyzed by superoxide dismutase. Thus, levels of these enzymes can affect the amount of DNA damage sustained. The conformation of DNA may influence how much damage it sustains, but the evidence for this is conflicting. Cells grown as multicellular spheroids can be more radioresistant than the same cells in monolayer culture. The ability of DNA to unwind is greater in monolayer cultured cells. This may be explained by a tighter packing of chromatin in the cells of spheroids, which results in less damage being inflicted.

## Initial DNA Damage After Irradiation

Initial DNA damage is defined as the measured DNA damage in the cell after immediate biochemical modification has occurred but before biological processing (i.e., enzymatic reactions of relatively long half-time) has taken place. In practical terms, this means the measured DNA damage when cells are irradiated on ice, preventing repair. A variety of types of DNA damage have been detected, and the main types are summarized in Table 2-1. Many techniques are available to measure lesions in DNA. The measurement of single- or double-strand breaks is based on DNA fragmentation in alkaline (denaturing) or neutral conditions, respectively. DNA fragments can be separated according to size by a variety of means: velocity sedimentation, filter elution, or pulsed-field gel electrophoresis. DNA protein cross-links are quantified by the reduction in strand breaks detected when no protein digestion is allowed in the preparation of the test DNA. By contrast, base damage can be measured and characterized by chemical methods, and these have, for example, detected more than 20 radiation products of thymine. Specific antibodies have been made to recognize certain types of base damage, and such information can indicate alternative means of measurement of these specific classes of DNA damage.

Of the radiation-induced lesions listed, the double-strand break (dsb) appears to be associated most closely with cell lethality. The word "association" should be stressed: correlation exists between the number of dsb and lethal events, but this neither shows which dsb are lethal nor excludes the possibility that some other lesion produced in proportion to dsb is the critical lesion. The ratio of dsb to ssb can be varied by altering the damaging agent. With hydrogen peroxide the dsb:ssb ratio is reduced and this causes less cell lethality per lesion, while with bleomycin the ratio is increased and more cell death per lesion is found. The absolute number of double-strand breaks correlates well with the cell survival probability, irrespective of the agent used to cause those breaks. Hence, it is concluded that the dsb is the more important lesion biologically. Could two independently produced ssb combine to form a dsb? For radiation doses in the clinical range, the answer is "Only with an extremely low probability."

Although the majority of DNA dsb (i.e., DNA fragments) are rejoined, the fidelity or accuracy of the repair process is less than perfect in many instances. The consequence is that although the dsb is rejoined, it may not have corrected the function of a critical gene, and the consequence of the damage and repair process is cell lethality. Residual lesions can remain because of either saturation of repair processes leading to a failure to rejoin in the available time, or misrepair of the broken ends. Specific subsets of dsb, either by nature or position, may have a higher probability of repair failure. One

**TABLE 2-1   Principal Types of DNA Damage**

| Type of Lesion | Damage | Number of Grays per Diploid Cell |
|---|---|---|
| Double-strand break | | 40 |
| Single-strand break | | 500–1000 |
| Base damage | | 1000–2000 |
| Sugar damage | | 800–1600 |
| DNA–DNA cross-links | | 30 |
| DNA–protein cross-links | | 150 |

proposal is that the ability to repair a DNA dsb may be influenced by the presence of other minor types of damage in the immediate vicinity (i.e., within 10 base pairs or one helical turn of the site of cleavage). Such effects produce what is called a locally multiply damaged site (LMDS),[13] at which a cluster of ionizations has caused a group of lesions to form close together, which can result in a greater probability of loss of genetic material and cell death.

## The Processing of Initial Radiation Damage

Cells have developed a wide variety of repair mechanisms for dealing with the many different types of DNA damage. Repair pathways appear to operate a repair hierarchy: (1) reversal of damage, (2) excision repair, for damage confined to a single strand, and (3) repair for double-strand damage by recombination or end joining. These three mechanisms repair the diverse types of lesion, from small simple lesions to large complex lesions that necessitate tissue restoration. If the function of one component is defective, repair defaults to the next stage in the hierarchy. For example, in xeroderma pigmentosum cells, which are defective in excision repair, single-strand damage due to ultraviolet light triggers a high frequency of recombinational repair events, since the lesions are not removed by excision repair.

The reversal of damage in DNA is the most direct mode of DNA repair. Examples of this mechanism of repair include enzymatic photoreactivation of pyrimidine dimers, repair of guanine alkylation by alkyltransferase, repair of single-strand breaks by direct rejoining, and repair of sites of base loss by direct insertion. For most of these examples, a single gene is required for a specific function. At first sight, this seems to be an economic use of genetic information compared with the multiple gene products required for the more complex repair processes. However, since there is a large variety of DNA lesions induced, this type of specific direct reversal of damage is likely to apply to lesions produced frequently and sponta-

neously. These repair mechanisms maintain the integrity of the DNA sequence: a so-called housekeeping function.

## Excision Repair

Excision repair involves cleavage of the sugar–phosphate backbone to remove the site of damage, which requires either single nucleotide excision (base excision repair) or patch excision (nucleotide excision repair). Single nucleotide excision occurs by the following sequence: a glycosylase removes the base damage and leaves an apurinic or apyrimidinic (a.p.) site; an a.p. endonuclease cuts 5′ to the a.p. site; the baseless deoxyribophosphate residue is removed by a specific 5′-phosphatase enzyme. This enzyme is distinct from the 5′-to-3′ exonuclease activity of DNA polymerase I. Patch excision involves a different set of enzymes: protein complexes are involved in damage binding and cleavage as well as DNA unwinding. The mechanisms of damage recognition have been largely unknown, but recent evidence for nucleotide excision repair suggests that two different mechanisms operate.[14] Damage in transcribed genes is recognized by a stalled RNA polymerase; damage in nontranscribed regions involves a specific protein, XP-C. Recognition of damage is followed by local unwinding of the DNA in the region of damage, which allows access of repair enzymes. The damaged patch is removed, and the space is resynthesized by the action of DNA polymerase and joined by ligase (see Fig. 2-3). The exonuclease activity of DNA polymerase makes the length of the resynthesized patch considerably larger than the size of the patch initially excised.

Excision repair is a multistep process and occurs less rapidly than the single-step actions involved in the direct reversal of damage. The precise kinetics of excision repair is difficult to define, because, for the removal of pyrimidine dimers resulting from ultraviolet light, the rate of removal depends on whether the sequence is actively transcribed or even whether it is the sense strand or the antisense strand. There is a

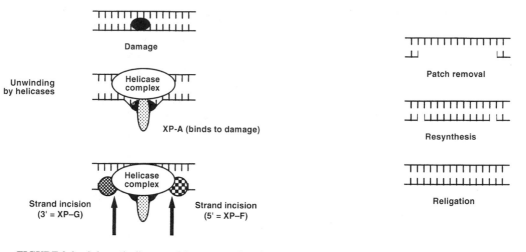

**FIGURE 2-3**  Schematic diagram of the process of nucleotide excision repair. Damage affecting a single strand recruits proteins to the site of damage. This results in incision of the affected strand upstream and downstream from the site of damage, and removal of an oligonucleotide patch. Resynthesis results in correction of the damage site.

well-established connection between transcription and excision repair demonstrated by the genetic syndromes of xeroderma pigmentosum groups B, D, and G.[14] These diseases demonstrate ultraviolet light sensitivity and general impairment of transcription: they are linked by impaired unwinding of the DNA (i.e., the genes encode helicases) required for both transcription and repair.

## Mismatch Repair

Mismatch repair has certain similarities to excision repair in that the repair requires single-strand cleavage around the site of the mismatch of base pairs. This is a type of housekeeping function, inasmuch as base-pairing errors can occur as part of every replication cycle. However, because the types of mispairing can be numerous, a single protein machinery is used to deal with the multiple types of lesion, which include not only base mismatches but also misalignment loops (replication slippage). The proteins involved in mismatch repair are separate from excision repair, and the recognition enzymes can distinguish mismatches from misalignments (resulting in small single-stranded loops). The human homologs of the bacterial mismatch repair genes, *mutS* and *mutL*, have shown remarkable evolutionary conservation of this repair pathway. There are numerous homologs of the mutS proteins (termed MSH), and it is the combination of MSH2 and MSH3, which recognize misalignments, and MSH2 and MSH6, which recognize mismatches.[15] Both the bacterial and human cells lacking functional *mutS* or *mutL* exhibit high rates of mutation. In humans, defects in these genes account for hereditary nonpolyposis colon cancer. There are differences in the mechanism of cleavage between bacteria and humans: cleavage is directed opposite a methylated base in bacteria, but is directed more by secondary structure of the DNA in eukaryotes (see Fig. 2-4).

## Repair of Double-Strand Damage: Rejoining or Recombination?

When double-stranded DNA damage is induced in cells, the first step in the removal of that damage is to "clean up" the damaged region. As a minimum, this will involve the excision of at least one nucleotide from each strand, by the action of specific endonucleases. Double-stranded DNA damage is in close proximity on

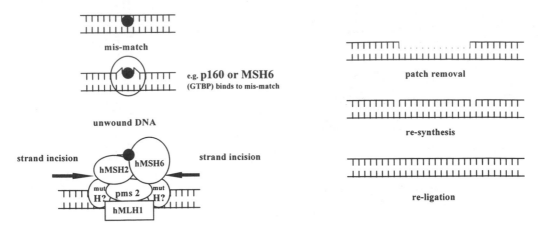

**FIGURE 2-4** Schema of mismatch repair in a representation analogous to that of Figure 2-3. The mismatch results in recruitment of different proteins from those used in nucleotide excision repair, but incision both sides of the mismatch results in patch excision and resynthesis.

each strand (suggested by the clustering of ionizations), and excision repair of both strands will lead to a loss of sequence. Simple blunt-ended religation of strand breaks can be demonstrated in vitro, but this will not restore the sequence. Although ligase can rejoin breaks, the lack of this enzyme in yeast leads to hypermutability rather than increased radiosensitivity. Bloom syndrome is a rare human disease characterized by ligase deficiency, early onset of cancer, and hypermutability, but cell killing from radiation occurs only at the sensitive end of the normal spectrum.[16] This suggests that simple rejoining may not be the dominant mechanism for closing double-strand breaks.

The association of radiation sensitivity with a lack of DNA recombination (defined as a strand exchange resulting in a junction between two sites of a DNA double helix) was initially made in the *rad52* mutant of the budding yeast, *Saccharomyces cerevisiae,* but this association has now extended to mammalian cells with the observation of radiation sensitivity in *scid* mice [severe combined immune deficiency as a result of impaired V(D)J recombination].[17] Fibroblasts from *scid* mice were also found to be deficient in double-strand break repair upon subjection to two damage assays, pulsed-field gel electrophoresis and neutral filter elution,

thus associating double-strand damage processing with recombination.[18,19]

Recombination in yeast is dominated by homologous recombination; that is, DNA strand exchange occurs at sites of sequence similarity, which is often the homologous chromosome in diploid cells. By contrast, nonhomologous recombination is frequent in mammalian cells. Nonhomologous recombination means that little or no apparent homology exists at the site of DNA strand exchange. Homologous recombination does occur in mammalian cells, as demonstrated by gene targeting or knockout experiments, but there are usually more opportunities for nonhomologous recombination when the entire mammalian genome is available. It is suspected that nonhomologous recombination involves short sequence homology, maybe as few as 2 to 6 base pairs. Any recombination event will result in at least short sequences of heteroduplex DNA at the site of strand exchange, and thus mismatch repair. Long tracts of heteroduplex are therefore likely to result in nonviable cells.

Rejoining involves the ligation of exposed DNA termini; recombination is strand exchange between two double-stranded sequences (see Fig. 2-5). If the recombination process involves short sequence homology at the broken

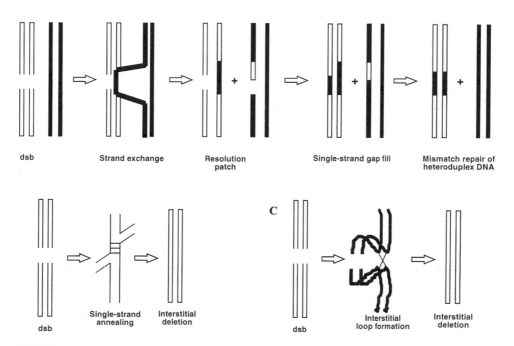

**FIGURE 2-5**  Recombinational repair involves strand exchange between two separate regions of double-stranded DNA. **(A)** A double-strand break can stimulate strand exchange with a homologous region of DNA (such as the homologous chromatid or chromosome, or another region of sequence similarity). Resolution of the strand exchange results in a donation sequence proceeding from the undamaged DNA to the site of damage. Both DNA sequences can be restored as a result of having a single-stranded template, and any heteroduplex DNA created can be corrected by means of mismatch repair. The repair process in **(A)** is sequence preserving, but a frequent consequence of ionizing radiation is to produce an interstitial deletion. The production of an interstitial deletion by single-stranded annealing **(B)**, and by recombination between an upstream and a downstream sequence **(C)** are two different mechanisms to produce this sequence alteration.

ends, distinguishing recombination from end rejoining is difficult. It may be that broken ends can be protected from exonuclease degradation if the broken end can be induced to fold over and form a hairpin end. There is evidence that V(D)J recombination uses this mechanism. Because of the genetic overlap between V(D)J recombination and double-strand break repair, it is thought that x-ray damage may be processed similarly.

## Residual DNA Damage

All changes in radiosensitivity cannot be attributed to the efficiency of double-strand break rejoining or the extent of residual DNA damage, although this is characteristic of certain well-described rodent cell mutants also defective in

V(D)J recombination.[20] Many mutant cell lines that differ in radiosensitivity from their parent line demonstrate no differences in double-strand break rejoining. Some of these may be explained by defects in homologous recombination, which has been suggested recently by discovering that another class of radiosensitive mutants are deficient in proteins related to Rad51. Rad51 is a homolog of the bacterial protein RecA, which plays a critical role in homologous recombination. One radiosensitive hamster cell mutant has shown a defect in repair fidelity (the accuracy with which a break is rejoined), a characteristic that may explain radiosensitivity in this as well as other cell lines. A similar defect is shown by cells from patients with the disease ataxia-telangiectasia (A-T),[21,22] which has long been of interest to radiation biologists because of x-ray sensitivity and a lack of cell cycle arrest in response to DNA damage. A-T cells also show no impairment of double-strand break rejoining.

Tumor cells do not as a rule differ in radiosensitivity because of obvious differences in double-strand break rejoining, as in the radiosensitive mutants just described. A correlation of rejoining kinetics with radiation response has been reported occasionally, but often tumors differing in sensitivity have no difference in double-strand break rejoining. The frequency with which strand breaks are misrepaired has also been reported to show a correlation with radiosensitivity.[23] The measurement of DNA damage remaining, after repair has reached its maximum effect, might be the most significant measure of damage. The removal of double-strand breaks may occur to different extents in different cell lines studied, but, like rejoining kinetics, it does not discriminate well between lines of differing radiosensitivity.

Chromosomal aberrations, by contrast, consistently correlate well with cell survival. One of the main problems with techniques to measure DNA damage is that they measure rejoining of fragments and not functional repair. That is, they measure the extent to which a break has been removed but they do not indicate whether the functional integrity of the DNA has been restored. Chromosome aberrations identify many lesions in which the fragmentation in DNA has been resolved but clear abnormalities remain. Many of the exchange events reduce fragmentation, including the intrachromosomal translocation (e.g., inversion) and the interchromosomal translocation. The mechanism by which chromosome aberrations arise remains hotly debated, and in essence reflects the debate between proponents of rejoining and recombination.

## Radiation Sensitivity, the Cell Cycle, and Signal Transduction

The relationship between x-ray sensitivity, DNA damage, cell cycle progression, and signal transduction has not been resolved. The main problem is knowing whether a lack of cell cycle arrest is a cause of radiation sensitivity, or another consequence of the defect predisposing to radiosensitivity. Many of the yeast genes controlling radiation sensitivity are not DNA repair genes and may prove to be links in a pathway that signals DNA damage. The control of cell cycle and damage signaling are rapidly enlarging subjects, recently given a large stimulus by the cloning of the gene mutated in ataxia-telangiectasia (*ATM*). Yeast genes that control both x-ray sensitivity and cell cycle arrest will most likely find homologs in mammalian cells. The concept of cell cycle checkpoints was derived from the discovery of the *rad9* mutant in *S. cerevisiae.* X-ray sensitivity could be overcome by chemical blockade of entry into mitosis, thus allowing time for otherwise normal repair.

DNA constitutes a uniquely important molecule in the cell, and there is virtually no redundancy for certain gene functions. Hence, damage to an essential segment of a DNA molecule (e.g., to an essential gene) that is not repaired could be fatal to the cell. This is not to say that unrepaired damage to other cellular constituents (e.g., nuclear or perhaps cellular membranes) is unimportant, but to emphasize that DNA is the important target for cell lethality. The proteins involved in the repair of double-stranded DNA damage caused by ionizing radiation are involved in the complex mediating of a certain type of DNA rejoining/recombination, and may not be specific to double-strand breaks in DNA. Identifying other proteins involved in this complex and the actions performed by the complex will be areas of intense interest over the next few years.

## MODELS FOR DESCRIBING CELL SURVIVAL

The two models in common usage to describe cell survival are the multitarget, single-hit model and the linear–quadratic model. The multitarget model was used almost exclusively from the 1950s to the mid-1980s. Then, use of the linear–quadratic model became favored because of the better fit to survival data in the low dose range. In the high dose range, with cell survival out to less than 0.001, the multitarget model still works effectively, and the survival curve becomes a straight line.

## Multitarget, Single-Hit Model

Survival curves of the general shape described by Puck and Marcus for HeLa cells (Fig. 2-2) have been found for nearly all mammalian cells studied in vitro. Cell survival curves of this shape are most commonly described in terms of the two parameters of the multitarget single-hit model, namely, $D_0$ and $n$, by the equation:

$$SF1 - \left[1 - \exp\left(\frac{-D}{D_0}\right)\right]^n$$

where SF is the surviving fraction. According to this model, each cell has $n$ targets, all of the same size, and for cell death to occur, all $n$ targets must be hit (inactivated). The width of the shoulder is reflected by $n$, the intercept with the ordinate of a back-extrapolation of the straight-line portion of the curve, as illustrated in Fig. 2-6. The curve becomes a straight line at surviving fractions less than 0.1, where on the average only one undamaged target remains per cell. Hence, in this distal portion of the curve, cell killing follows first-order kinetics. The slope of the straight-line portion of the curve is described in terms of the $D_0$ or the dose that reduces the surviving fraction to 0.37 (kills 0.63 of the cells); this is the reciprocal of the slope. With reference to the model, $D_0$ corresponds to the dose that on the average produces one hit in one target. In the exponential portion of the curve, a unit of dose achieves a constant fractional cell kill. For example, after a dose that yields an SF of 0.1, further radiation in the amount of $1.0D_0$ reduces SF to 0.037, $2.3D_0$ would reduce SF to 0.01. Thus, as radiation dose is increased, there is a constant fractional cell kill, although the absolute number of cells killed per unit of dose is constantly diminishing. Also shown in Figure 2-6 is the parameter

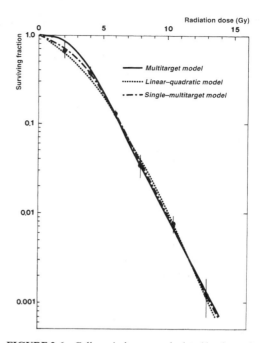

**FIGURE 2-6**  Cell survival curves calculated by the multitarget, single-hit model; the single-target modification of the multitarget, single-hit model (single and multitarget); and the linear–quadratic model. For survival fractions (SF) from $10^{-1}$ to $10^{-3}$, the three curves fit experimental data equally well. For SF $> 0.1$, the best fit of survival data is by the linear–quadratic model or the single-target and multitarget single-hit models. The fit by the simple multitarget model is less good. For cell surviving fractions down to $< 10^{-8}$, the multitarget model becomes the best estimate of experimental data.

$D_q$, the dose at which the back-extrapolation of the straight-line portion of the curve intersects SF = 1.0. The "quasi-threshold" dose $D_q$ is a measure of the "shoulder" width and serves as an indicator of the capacity of the cell to accumulate sublethal radiation damage.

This multitarget, single-hit model has been a good descriptor of results in many studies designed to derive surviving fractions for cells subjected to large single doses of radiation. A selected tabulation of $D_0$ and $n$ values from the literature for irradiation of mammalian cell lines in vivo are presented in Table 2-2.[24–45] Average values for several human tumor cell lines studied in vitro are given in Table 2-3.[46] The range of $D_0$ values for aerobic cells is 1.2 to 2.2 Gy for epithelial and mesenchymal cells

TABLE 2-2   $D_0$ and $n$ Values for Cells of Several Normal and Malignant Rodent Tissues Irradiated In Vivo

| Tissue | $D_0$ (Gy) | $n$ | Ref. |
|---|---|---|---|
| NORMAL | | | |
| Bone marrow | 1.05 | 2.0 | Till and McCulloch[23] |
| Cartilage | 1.65 | 6.0 | Kember[24] |
| Skin | 1.35 | | Withers[25] |
| Jejunal crypt | 1.43 | 20.4 | Withers et al.[26,27] |
| Lymph node | 0.74 | 2.7 | Smith and Vos[28] |
| Gastric mucosa | 1.37 | 5.2 | Chen and Withers[29] |
| Colon | 1.42 | | Withers and Mason[30] |
| Capillary endothelium | 1.68 | 6.0 | Reinhold and Buisman[31] |
| Thyroid | 1.95 | 4.0 | Mulcahy et al.[32] |
| Lung cells | 1.49 | 6.1 | Guichard et al.[33] |
| | 1.58 | 3.9 | Deschavonne et al.[34] |
| Kidney (tubular cells) | 1.53 | | Withers et al.[35] |
| Hair follicle cells | | | |
| (resting monoblasts) | 2.19 | 6.7 | Potten and Chase[36] |
| Testis | 1.79 | | Withers et al.[37] |
| MALIGNANT | | | |
| CBA leukemia | 1.62 | 2.0 | Hewitt and Wilson[38] |
| P-388 leukemia | 1.60 | 1.6 | Berry and Andrews[39] |
| Lymphoma | 1.14 | 0.7 | Bush and Bruce[40] |
| Gardner lymphoma | 1.10 | 1.2 | Powers and Tolmach[41] |
| Rhabdomyosarcoma | 1.20 | 10.2 | Reinhold[42] |
| Mammary carcinoma | 1.35 | 4.8 | Urano et al.[43] |
| Fibrosarcoma, FSaII | 2.12 | 2.9 | Urano et al.[44] |
| Squamous cell carcinoma | 1.20 | 10.0 | Urano et al.[45] |

TABLE 2-3   Values for Parameters of Radiation Response of Human Tumor Cell Lines Studied In Vitro

| Tumor Type | Number of Cell Lines (Gy) | $D_0$ | $n$ | $\alpha$ | $\beta$ | Surviving Fraction (2 Gy) |
|---|---|---|---|---|---|---|
| Glioblastoma | 5 | 1.44 | 12 | 0.241 | 0.029 | 0.58 |
| Melanoma | 19 | 1.04 | 73 | 0.255 | 0.053 | 0.51 |
| Squamous cell carcinoma | 6 | 1.28 | 5.0 | 0.273 | 0.045 | 0.49 |
| Adenocarcinoma | 6 | 1.04 | 37 | 0.311 | 0.055 | 0.48 |
| Lymphoma | 7 | 1.48 | 1.8 | 0.451 | 0.051 | 0.34 |
| Oat cell carcinoma | 6 | 1.51 | 1.8 | 0.650 | 0.081 | 0.22 |

*Source:* Adapted from Malaise et al.[46]

and 0.7 to 1.1 Gy for cells of bone marrow and lymphoid origin; the corresponding values for $n$ are 2 to 20 and 1 to 2 for cells of the two classes of tissues. Cells of tumors tend to have $D_0$ and $n$ values comparable to those of the cells of the tissue of origin. This simple model has been unsatisfactory at low doses ($< 0.5D_0$), where it predicts surviving fractions of greater than 0.99. Experimental data for mammalian cells consistently document some cell kill at such doses.[47] The multitarget, single-hit model may be modified to provide a good fit to the data at low doses by assuming that in a proportion of the cells there is a single target and in the other cells there are multiple targets; $D_0$ is assumed to be the same for all targets in all cells.

## Linear–Quadratic Model

For many cell lines, the data relating surviving fraction to low radiation doses are described more accurately by a continuously downbending curve than by a straight line.[48] In this setting a linear–quadratic (LQ) model has been used to describe the relationship SF = $\exp[-(\alpha D + \beta D^2)]$, where $\alpha$ and $\beta$ are constants. The $\alpha$ component is due to single-event killing and is proportional to dose. The $\beta$ component reflects events that interact, and thus the effect is proportional to dose squared. The SF data in Figure 2-6 are fitted equally well by the modified multitarget, single-hit and the linear–quadratic models over the SF range 0.1–0.001. The LQ model is now commonly employed in discussions of the effectiveness of fractionated irradiation, namely, multiple small doses (see below). Determination of $\alpha$ and $\beta$ have been made for a variety of human and rodent cell systems, studied in vitro or in vivo (Tables 2-3 and 2-4).[49–53]

## Cell Survival Curves for Cells Irradiated In Vivo

In 1959, 3 years after Puck and Marcus published the survival curves for HeLa cells irradiated in vitro, Hewitt and Wilson[38] reported the first radiation cell survival curve for mammalian cells irradiated in vivo and viability assessed in vivo. These authors determined the number of CBA leukemia cells, which on average would be expected to transplant the disease into half the isologous recipients, the $TD_{50}$, as a function of radiation dose. Log surviving fractions ($TD_{50}$ normal cells/$TD_{50}$ irradiated cells) were plotted versus dose; the $D_0$ and $n$ from the resultant curve were 1.6 Gy and 2.0 for cobalt-60 irradiation.

In 1961 the first survival curves for cells of normal tissue were published. Till and McCulloch[24] determined that the $D_0$ for murine bone marrow cells was 1 Gy. They had developed a technique analogous to that employed by Hewitt and Wilson except that the number of bone marrow colony-forming units was reflected by the number of nodules in the spleen of mice that had been lethally irradiated prior to intravenous (IV) injection of normal or irradiated bone marrow cell suspensions. Shortly thereafter, techniques that did not require the disruption of tissue integrity were used to obtain $D_0$ for

TABLE 2-4   Values for $\alpha$, $\beta$, $\alpha/\beta$, and Surviving Fraction After Single-Dose Irradiation ($SF^2$) for Several Rodent Cell Systems

| Cell System | Radiation | $\alpha$ | $\beta$ | $\alpha/\beta$ | $SF^2$ | Ref. |
|---|---|---|---|---|---|---|
| Tumor | | | | | | |
| FSaII fibrosarcoma | [60]Co | 0.201 | 0.0161 | 12.5 | 0.627 | Urano et al.[49] |
| Normal tissue | | | | | | |
| Jejunal crypt cells | X | 0.233 | 0.0177 | 13.2 | 0.645 | Thames et al.[27] |
| Colon | [137]Cs | 0.147 | 0.0173 | 8.50 | 0.695 | Tucker et al.[50] |
| Testes | [137]Cs | 0.215 | 0.0172 | 12.5 | 0.607 | Thames and Ang[51] |
| Cultured cells | | | | | | |
| V79 hamster | [60]Co | 0.180 | 0.0196 | 9.2 | 0.645 | Millar et al.[52] |
| CHO cells | [60]Co | 0.219 | 0.0255 | 8.6 | 0.583 | Urano et al.[49] |
| 10T1/2 cells (contact inhibited) | [137]Cs | 0.179 | 0.0170 | 10.5 | 0.653 | Zeman and Bedford[53] |

several normal tissues, including skin, jejunal crypt, hair follicle cells, gastric cells, colon cells, and cartilage. The estimated $D_0$ values are presented in Table 2-2 for these and other studies including $D_0$ values of malignant tissues.

## Sublethal Damage Repair (SLDR)

Early in radiation therapy, investigators observed that the radiation dose resulting in a given reaction is substantially higher when the radiation is administered as a series of treatments rather than as a large single dose. This means that radiation damage is being corrected: either repair of damage in the individual cell or repopulation of the irradiated tissue. Elkind and Sutton, in 1959,[54] first described quantitatively the repair of radiation damage by mammalian cells studied in vitro. This is illustrated by Figure 2-7, in which the surviving fraction of V79 Chinese hamster cells increased following a total dose of 14 Gy given as two doses instead of a single dose. The surviving fraction increased from 0.02 to 0.07 as the time between the two doses increased from zero to 2 hours. As intertreatment interval increased from 2 to 6 hours, surviving fraction decreased. This did not reflect a loss of repair but rather an increase in sensitivity of the surviving cells as the cells progressed from more resistant into more sensitive phases of the cell

cycle (reflecting the partial synchrony induced by the first dose). At longer intervals, cell proliferation occurring before the second dose would cause the surviving fraction to increase.

This phenomenon of a higher surviving fraction for two-dose treatment has been confirmed repeatedly for diverse cells studied in vitro and in vivo. Repair observed by the split-dose technique is designated repair of sublethal damage (SLDR). The result is a near-complete restoration of the shoulder with no change in slope of the survival curve. Repair is thus partial; that is, the surviving cells are not restored to a pretreatment status. The half-time for SLDR by mammalian cells irradiated in vivo or in vitro is 0.25 to 1.0 hour.[29,55] For example, Chen and Withers[29] determined SLDR for intervals between the first and second dose of 5, 10, 20, 60, and 120 minutes for cells of the mouse stomach; the repair half-time was 26 minutes.

## Potentially Lethal Damage Repair (PLDR)

Functional repair of radiation damage, observed by an increase in cell survival, may also be demonstrated by altering conditions of the cells following single radiation doses.[56] For example, the surviving fraction of cells in plateau phase culture is increased by delaying the time between irradiation and replating of the cells.[57] This is designated *repair of potentially lethal damage* (PLDR), namely, damage that would be lethal if not repaired. The consequence is an increase in cell survival. Cells placed in fresh media promptly enter into a phase of active cell proliferation, and procedures that bring cells into active proliferation are usually associated with a reduced repair, hence greater cell kill for a specified radiation dose. Little et al.[58] showed that the survival curve for cells irradiated while in plateau phase was significantly less steep (higher $D_0$) if the cells were subcultured at 6 or 12 hours rather than immediately. The same phenomenon has been observed for tumor cells irradiated in vivo. Radiation resistance of human tumors has been tentatively attributed to an increased capacity for PLDR,[59] although since tumor cells often have defects in cell cy-

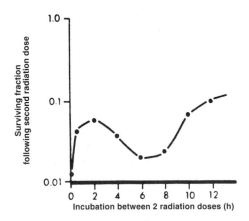

**FIGURE 2-7** Survival fractions for radiation administered as a single dose or as two doses (749 rads, followed by 650 rads) separated by variable times in hours. (Reproduced from Elkind and Sutton.[34])

cle checkpoints, it is surprising to see improved cell survival due to conditions that favor growth arrest.

The repair half-times for PLDR are approximately the same as for SLDR. In the study by Winans et al.,[55] the repair half-time by S-phase Chinese hamster ovary cells was 15 minutes for SLDR and PLDR. The dominant effect of PLDR is to increase $D_0$, in distinction from SLDR, which reconstitutes the shoulder of the survival curve. The biochemical processes responsible for SLDR and PLDR are not defined; the extent to which they constitute fundamentally different processes, as distinct from reflecting different experimental procedures, has not been determined. With reference to clinical radiation therapy, the observed response of tissues treated by multifraction irradiation allows for repair of both SLDR and PLDR; that is, the tissues are not disrupted and the cells remain in situ for the duration of treatment and, of course, afterward.

## BIOLOGICAL FACTORS THAT INFLUENCE CELL SURVIVAL AND RADIATION SENSITIVITY

### Oxygen Tension

The most powerful modifier of radiation sensitivity of mammalian cells is molecular oxygen. The oxygen enhancement ratio (OER), defined as the ratio of radiation doses in anoxic to oxic conditions required to produce equal effect, is in the range of 2.5 to 3.3.[60] This sensitizing effect of oxygen is of particular interest to the clinician because oxygen is maximally sensitizing at physiologic concentrations; the $P_{O_2}$ in normal tissues is in the range of 15 to 100 mmHg; the $P_{O_2}$ of venous blood is 40 mmHg.[61] In fact, radiation resistance does not begin to appear until $P_{O_2}$ falls below approximately 20 mmHg. These findings have powerfully stimulated research interest in tumor radiation biology and radiation therapy because of the report in 1955 by Thomlinson and Gray,[62] that the distance between capillaries and microscopically demonstrated necrosis in human lung cancer

corresponded to the predicted diffusion length of oxygen, namely, the distance from the capillary at which the $P_{O_2}$ would be zero. This was based on assumed values for capillary $P_{O_2}$, length, and blood flow rate; oxygen diffusion coefficient in tumor cells; and $O_2$ consumption for tumor and stromal cells. Their finding implies that there are hypoxic but viable cells adjacent to the necrotic areas. Hence the tumor would comprise viable cells that are aerobic and hypoxic, resulting in heterogeneity of radiosensitivity as a consequence of differences in cellular $P_{O_2}$. Powers and Tolmach[41] were the first to demonstrate the presence of aerobic and hypoxic cells in a rodent tumor by analysis of cell survival curve shapes. Of course, tumor cells are not simply aerobic or hypoxic; rather, there would be a gradient of $P_{O_2}$, hence radiosensitivity, from the capillary to the necrotic zone. For convenience, we talk of the hypoxic fraction as the fraction of cells that respond as would hypoxic cells. The proportion of cells of solid tumors that are hypoxic in a radiobiologic sense varies from 0% to 50%. The hypoxic tumor cells would be radiation resistant relative to the cells of normal tissue (aerobic). Provided hypoxic and viable cells were present in human tumors, they might be the cause of some of the local failures of conventional radiation treatment.

There is an extensive literature on the relationship between $P_{O_2}$ and radiation sensitivity. A series of cell survival curves for Chinese hamster ovary cells, equilibrated with variable oxygen tensions from 0.0001% to 100% oxygen, is presented in Figure 2-8.[63] For these CHO cells irradiated under acutely hypoxic and full media conditions, oxygen was dose modifying. When the multitarget model was used, the $D_0$ was dependent and $n$ was independent of $P_{O_2}$. In these experiments $n$ was constant at 7 for all conditions at irradiation. The importance of hypoxic cells to radiation therapy is, of course, dependent on the extent to which hypoxic tumor cells in vivo exhibit radiation resistance. To assess the sensitivity of hypoxic tumor cells in vivo requires an understanding of the role of severity of the hypoxia, the duration of the hypoxia, and the levels of

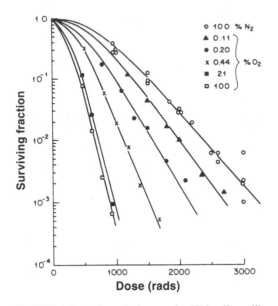

**FIGURE 2-8**   Cell survival curves for CHO cells equilibrated with oxygen at various oxygen pressures. (Reproduced from Ling et al.[63])

other metabolites on the radiation sensitivity of hypoxic cells.

There is evidence for some cell lines that $n$ approaches 1.0 under conditions of extreme hypoxia.[64] This is important because the smaller shoulder on the survival curve for hypoxic cells means that OER decreases progressively with a reduction in dose or dose per fraction. The lesser $n$ for hypoxic CHO cells, in the research by Paicic et al., was associated with a decrease in OER from 2.0 to 1.6 as dose decreased from 2.0 to 0.3 Gy; at 10 Gy, the OER was 2.7. Taylor and Brown[65] reported that for 20 doses of 1.7 Gy (12 h between treatments) to contact inhibited C3H-10T1/2 cells the OER was 1.34. For the same cell system, the OER for single-dose irradiation and at a dose of 5 Gy was 3.0. This low OER for multiple small fractions was attributed to a reduced repair of sublethal damage by the hypoxic cells. Others have also found low OER values for radiation administered in small doses.[66]

Knowledge of the shape of the survival curve at low doses is important in applying the findings of radiation biology to radiation therapy, where small doses per fraction are em-

ployed. Further, the laboratory model systems need to be pertinent to the application in mind. In the Thomlinson–Gray model, hypoxia develops gradually as the cells are displaced away from the capillaries. This results not only in the low $P_{O_2}$ values but in reduced levels of other metabolites (glucose, glutamine, ATP, etc.) and an increase in catabolites (e.g., lactate). Hence, such chronically hypoxic tissues may be characterized not only by hypoxia but also by low levels of nutrients, low pH, and so on. Recent evidence has suggested that hypoxia may result in clonal selection of cells deficient in the tumor suppressor p53.[67] Hypoxia can lead to the activation of p53[68] in intact cells and trigger programmed cell death. Tumor cells deficient in the function of p53 do not exhibit this response; rather, they survive to proliferate and dominate the surviving population. It is now recognized that hypoxia is a potent stress signal, which can lead to a marked change in the pattern of gene expression.[69]

There is accumulating evidence that prolonged exposure to low oxygen tension under conditions of general metabolic deprivation induces less radiation resistance than acute hypoxia with normal metabolite availability, namely, a smaller $D_0$ and a lesser repair of radiation damage. Spiro et al.[70] reported that hypoxic V79 cells were unable to repair sublethal damage if maintained at $10^{-5}$ ppm oxygen in a simple balanced salt solution (e.g., no glucose). If glucose were present, repair was about half that for normal culture conditions (aerobic, full media). Gupta et al.[71] found that Ehrlich ascites and P388 tumor cells had OERs of 1.22 and 1.17, respectively, if maintained at 0.1% oxygen during and following irradiation. The respective values were 2.51 and 2.87, however, for cells incubated in oxygen after irradiation. In studies on a C3H mouse mammary carcinoma, repair of SLD was reduced in the chronically hypoxic cells.[73]

Some observations indicate that blood flow through tumor capillaries is intermittent; that is, for variable time periods flow through a particular capillary may be markedly reduced or stopped.[73–75] Thus, $P_{O_2}$ of tumor cells adjacent to such a capillary would be reduced to virtually zero, hence would be acutely hypoxic. Such cells should exhibit full hypoxic resistance, namely, maximum $D_0$ and $n$. If acutely hypoxic cells occur in human tumors, they might constitute a more serious problem for the success of radiation therapy than the chronically hypoxic cells of the Thomlinson–Gray model. An important fact to remember is: hypoxic cells, acutely and chronically, are more resistant than aerobic cells.

During the course of fractionated irradiation there is often an improvement in the tissue $P_{O_2}$, a process called reoxygenation.[76,77] This could occur as a consequence of tumor regression with reduction of intercapillary distances, decrease in number of metabolically active (oxygen-consuming) cells, and decreased intratumoral pressure, with an associated improved blood flow. Accordingly, the radiotherapeutic importance of the hypoxic cells as visualized in the model proposed by Thomlinson and Gray remains undefined.

## Cell Proliferation Kinetics and the Cell Cycle

The replication cycle for somatic cells was described as four stages by Howard and Pelc (radiation biologists at the Hammersmith Hospital in London) in 1952.[78] From their study of the incorporation of $^{32}P$ into the nuclei of growing root tips of the broad bean *Vicia faba,* the four stages are: M, or mitosis; S, or the phase during which DNA is replicated; $G_1$, the period or gap between M and S; and $G_2$, the period between S and M. The cell cycle is illustrated diagrammatically in Fig. 2-9A. The cell cycle time (the interval between the end of one mitosis to the end of the next) exhibits wide variation. For mammalian cells, there is a relatively narrow distribution of times of S, $G_2$, and M phases, but $G_1$ may exhibit wide variation, especially for cells in vivo. There is a $G_0$ phase for cells of several normal tissues; they are not in active cell cycle but are brought back into active proliferation by homeostatic control mechanisms. $G_0$ cells are in most instances subpopulations of $G_1$ cells; they reenter the cell cycle after an appropriate signal at a point within $G_1$, and

shortly after they enter S phase. Tissues with prominent $G_0$ populations include liver, periosteum, and skin, as shown by the rapid increase in proportion of S-phase cells following partial hepatectomy, fracture, or incision through skin. Recent advances in tumor biology have shown that transformed cells are often characterized by loss of the normal regulation of cell cycle, particularly affecting the $G_1$ phase of the cell cycle.[79] Figure 2-9B shows cell survival curves for Chinese hamster cells irradiated at various points of the cell replication cycle.

The sequence of discoveries that led to our current understanding of cell cycle control is a remarkable story of the convergence of two different disciplines, biochemistry and genetics. Masui[80] and Smith and Pardee[81] in 1970 independently identified a substance in frog eggs called maturation promoting factor (MPF), which controls when mitosis (and meiosis) begin. The same factor was active in a wide range of cells from yeast to mammalian cells. Injection of a crude extract of MPF could trigger mitosis even after protein synthesis inhibition. The genetics of cell cycle research existed independently of cellular biochemistry initially. Leland Hartwell[82] identified mutant forms of yeast that were "stuck" at specific points in the cell cycle, and the genes were termed cell division cycle (*cdc*) genes. Paul Nurse, working with fission yeast (*Schizosaccharomyces pombe*), highlighted the *cdc2* gene as being required for entry into mitosis.[83] The question at the time was whether the *cdc2* gene was the biochemical factor MPF.

In 1988 MPF was purified and found to consist of two protein molecules.[84] One of these proteins, CDC2, was found to be present and constant through the cell cycle. What was the second component of MPF, and how did this make MPF active only in mitosis? A protein, which had been discovered in 1971, abruptly disappeared after mitosis only to accumulate during interphase; it was termed cyclin.[85] A series of experiments demonstrating the failure to synthesize cyclin led to a block of entry into mitosis. The failure to degrade cyclin also results in a cell cycle block: the exit from mitosis.[86] A combination of *cdc2* and cyclin was

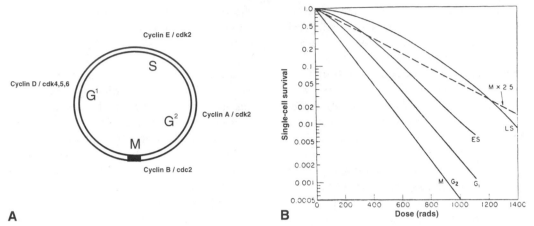

**A**

**B**

**FIGURE 2-9** **(A)** The four stages in the replication cycle for somatic cells. For mammalian cells, there is only a slight variation in the duration of S, $G_2$, and M phases of the cycle, whereas the $G_1$ phase may be extremely variable. The cyclin and cyclin-dependent kinase associated with each phase of the cell cycle are shown. **(B)** Cell survival curves for Chinese hamster cells irradiated (single dose) at M, $G_1$, early S, and late S of the cell replication cycle. (Reproduced from Sinclair.[91])

confirmed to be MPF, but not necessarily active MPF. Other proteins are important in its activation or suppression. However, the fundamental biochemical and genetic components of the cell cycle had now been identified: the cyclin and the cyclin-dependent kinase (CDK). More recent work has identified a whole series of cyclin–CDK complexes that occur throughout the cell cycle. The complex series of proteins that regulate the activity of the cyclin–CDK complex are more diverse between species, and are the means by which tumor cells develop disorders of cell cycle control.

The concept of cell cycle checkpoints was derived from experiments seeking to identify genes responsible for controlling entry into mitosis. Ionizing radiation leads to an accumulation of cells predominantly in $G_1$ and $G_2$. There is also a direct inhibition of replicon initiation and elongation, resulting in a transient arrest in S phase. The *rad9* mutant of *S. cerevisiae* shows a lack of $G_2$ arrest (and is radiation sensitive), but if time for repair is given artificially (by chemical blockade) the *rad9* cells are no longer radiosensitive. Hence the term checkpoint.[87] Mammalian cells that lack the function of the tumor suppressor p53 show a lack of $G_1$ arrest in response to DNA damage[88]: they too have a defective cell cycle checkpoint. As evidence

that the observed radiation sensitivity is determined by a complex of gene functions, loss of p53 function does not necessarily translate into radiation sensitivity,[89] and some p53 mutant cells have increased radiation resistance.

Just when cell cycle control seemed to be understandable, it has blossomed into increasing complexity. *Cdc2* is not one gene, but a family of genes now termed cyclin-dependent kinases (*cdk*). Monoclonal antibodies have allowed distinction of a family of *cdc2*-like proteins. Many of these have a proven cyclin association: *cdc2* (now *cdk1*) associates with cyclin B; *cdk2* is a 33 kDa protein that appears to be more closely associated with $G_1$/S cyclins (E and A). *Cdk3* rescues *cdc2* mutants, but is otherwise not abundant in cells. *Cdk4* and *cdk6* associate with D-type cyclins, and their function is to phosphorylate the retinoblastoma protein, pRb. The complex is active earlier in $G_1$ and *cdk4* does not complement the *cdc2* mutants of yeast. The cyclin–*cdk* complexes associated with $G_1$/S transition are under intensive investigation for association with tumor suppressor genes.

Terasima and Tolmach[90] were the first to demonstrate that radiation sensitivity varies with the cell's position in the cell cycle. Sinclair[91] and many others have fully documented this phenomenon. Figure 2-9B shows cell survival curves for synchronized Chinese hamster cells irradiated at M, $G_1$, early S, or late S phase of the cell cycle. The cells in M showed the greatest sensitivity. The survival curve for M-stage cells was a simple exponential with little or no shoulder, whereas cells in late S had a very broad shoulder and a less steep straight-line portion. Cells in $G_1$ and early S were intermediate. More recent studies have shown that these, but not all, cells at the transition between $G_1$ and S are also quite radiosensitive, but less so than M-phase cells.

Accordingly, the effect of a single dose of radiation on a population of asynchronously dividing cells will depend on the distribution of cells according to age in the cell replication cycle (age-density distribution) and the variation in sensitivity with cell age (age–response function). For fractionated irradiation, the survivors of a first dose of radiation will predominantly be the cells that were in a relatively resistant phase of the cell cycle at irradiation. Following irradiation, the surviving and relatively resistant cells progress into more sensitive phases. There is a delay in progression of the cells through the cell replication cycle, which can occur in all phases of the cell cycle. The delay is dependent on cell line, dose, and cell age at irradiation; the delay is maximum for cells in $G_2$. The result is a rapid decline in the mitotic index, essentially to zero as cells accumulate in $G_2$ but cannot enter M. After a period, which depends on cell line and radiation dose, the surviving cells begin to progress through the cell cycle and the mitotic index returns to control levels. Thus, a radiation dose kills the more sensitive cells and results in partial synchrony, such that most of surviving cells are in a relatively resistant phase. Because of the broad distribution of cell cycle times, the partial synchrony is rapidly dampened and then lost. However, even the partial synchrony may be of consequence to response to highly fractionated irradiation. Proliferation of surviving clonogens during each intertreatment interval increases the number of clonogens that must be inactivated to achieve a specific response—for example, tumor control or defined reaction by

a normal tissue. Clonogen proliferation for a particular cell population between treatments will be a function of time between fractions and dose per fraction. Accordingly, the optimal fractionation pattern will be dependent on the differential proliferation kinetics of the cells of tumor and the critical normal tissues.

For tumor tissues, three parameters of cell proliferation kinetics are important to an understanding of the biology of tumor growth: mean cell cycle time ($T_c$), growth fraction (GF), and cell loss factor ($\phi$). Kinetics of proliferation are assayed by labeling cells in S phase by a pulse or continuous exposure to [$^3$H]-TdR or BrdUrd, and then determining the proportion of cells in S during the exposure to the label.[92–94] From such data the GF, $\phi$, and $T_c$, may be derived. In tumor tissue, only a proportion of the cells are in active cell cycle (i.e., GF $< 1.0$). The importance of GF on growth rate may be considered by this example: a cell population has $1 \times 10^6$ cells and GF $= 0.6$. After one cell cycle, there would be $(0.6 \times 10^6) \times 2 + 0.4 \times 10^6 = 1.6 \times 10^6$ cells; this assumes no cell loss. The potential doubling time ($T_{pot}$) is the doubling time for a cell population with GF less than 1.0 and no cell loss. If there were a constant proportion of the progeny of each cell cycle remaining in the growth fraction, $T_{pot}$ could be estimated as follows:

$$T_{pot} = \frac{\ln 2}{\ln(1 + GF)} T_c$$

In the example with GF $= 0.6$, $T_{pot} = 1.47 \times T_c$. The $\phi$ is the fractional loss in the expected increment in cell number after one cell cycle time. For example, if there were $10^6$ cells and all were in cell cycle (GF $= 1.0$), after one cell cycle $2 \times 10^6$ cells would be expected, namely, the increment should be $1 \times 10^6$. If the observed total number of cells after one cell cycle were $1.1 \times 10^6$, the increment would have been 0.1 instead of $1.0 \times 10^6$. Hence $0.9 \times 10^6$ or 90% of expected increment were lost (i.e., $\phi = 0.9$). The tumor doubling time, $T_D$, is related to $T_c$ by:

$$T_D = \frac{T_{pot}}{1 - \phi}$$

thus, for $\phi = 0.9$ and GF $= 0.6$, $T_D = 14.7 \times T_c$.

The observed volume or cell population doubling time of tumors is usually much longer than the measured mean cell cycle time. In fact, the difference may be quite large. Among human tumors, $T_D$ may be many months but $T_c$, is usually 1 to 3 days. This discrepancy is due primarily to large φ and to a lesser extent small GFs. For example, φ may exceed 0.9 and indeed be close to 1.0. During tumor growth, there is a progressive broadening of distribution of $T_c$, an increase in φ, and a decrease in GF. This results in progressively slower growth of tumor, with increasing tumor age.

## PHYSICAL PARAMETERS AFFECTING RADIATION RESPONSE

### Dose Rate

The rate of irradiation is an important determinant of the response to photons. This has long been recognized because clinical observations revealed that tissues tolerated 50 to 70 Gy given in 5 to 10 days by low dose rate continuous irradiation (e.g., via a radium mold), whereas with high dose rate external beam irradiation the time required to administer comparable doses and have tolerable reactions was 6 to 7 weeks. Hall[95] showed for HeLa cells that $D_0$ increased by a factor of 2 as dose rate decreased from 1.0 Gy/min to 0.01 Gy/min; $n$ decreased to 1.0 with a decrease in dose rate to 0.1 Gy/min. Survival curves for V79 cells in plateau phase that were irradiated at 1.43 Gy/min and at 1.54 and 0.55 Gy/h are shown in Figure 2-10. The survival curves at high dose rate had $D_0$ and $n$ values of 2.7 Gy and 5.0, while at low dose rates the $D_0$ and $n$ values were 5.6 and 2.0. The slope of the low dose rate curve approximates that of the slope of the initial part of the high dose rate curve and reflects cell inactivation by single-hit events (e.g., the α component of the LQ model). Indeed, many observers suggest that low dose rate effects are clear evidence of the superiority of the LQ model over the multitarget, single-hit model. The extrapolation number approaches but does not reach 1 at the low dose rates in fed or unfed plateau V79 cells.[96]

The generally held view for the reduced effect of radiation at lesser dose rates is that repair of radiation damage occurs during the period of irradiation. The magnitude of the dose rate effect correlates with the extent of sublethal damage repair observed with split-dose radiation studies. Response to radiation is modified only slightly as dose rates extend outside the range of 0.01–1 Gy/min. Several studies have shown only small dose rate effects (or even an inverse dose rate effect) because the dose rate was adequate to block cell proliferation, with the consequent accumulation of cells in $G_2$, a radiation-sensitive phase.[97] The OER is reduced at low dose rates[98] and constitutes a potential advantage of low dose rate radiation in treating hypoxic tumors. However, the true molecular genetic basis for low dose rate effects is not really understood and will be a complex mixture of the effect of repair, cell cycle arrest, and possibly reoxygenation.

## Linear Energy Transfer and Relative Biological Effectiveness

Linear energy transfer (LET) is a parameter of beam quality and refers to the transfer of energy

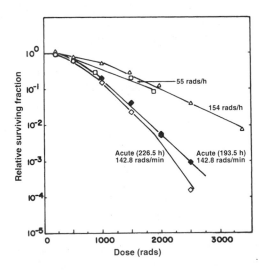

**FIGURE 2-10**   Cell survival curves for plateau phase and fed V79 cells irradiated at 1.43 rad/min and at 1.54 and 0.55 rad/h$^{-1}$. For acute exposures the irradiations were performed at 193.5 and at 226.5 hours into the experiment. (Reproduced from Mitchell et al.[96])

to the irradiated material per unit path length of the photon or particle. For example, for $^{60}$Co radiation the average LET is about 0.6 keV per micrometer of path. This means that along the photon path there is, on the average, a transfer of 0.6 keV to the irradiated material in each micrometer of photon path length. For fast neutrons, LET is much higher, for example, 5 to 10 keV/$\mu$m; they are referred to as high LET radiations. At the upper end of the range of LET, heavy particle radiations have an LET up to 100 to 1000 keV/$\mu$m. As LET increases there is a de-

creasing distance between ionization events. For $^{60}$Co and fast neutron radiation there are 17 and 150 to 200 ion pairs per micrometer, respectively. The average energy for production of an ion pair is 34 eV. The variation in density of ionization events along the photon or particle path with LET is illustrated by Figure 2-11A, for electrons and neutrons in a Wilson cloud chamber.[99]

Ionizations produced by radiation are not randomly distributed throughout the irradiated material: they occur along photon or particle paths. Along such a path they are not distrib-

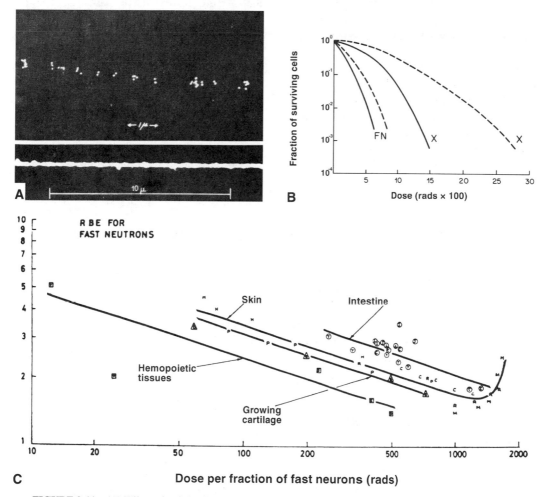

**FIGURE 2-11** (**A**) Wilson cloud chamber tract of a fast electron (upper panel) illustrates that ionization occurs in clusters, with the clusters clearly separated; in contrast, fast neutrons (lower panel) show the ionizations to be a continuous track. (Reproduced with permission from Bacq and Alexander.[99]) (**B**) Cell survival curve for rat rhabdomyosarcoma R1 cells subjected to 300 kV(p) x-ray (X) or 15 MeV fast neutron (FN) irradiation[103] under aerobic (solid line) or hypoxic (dashed line) conditions. (**C**) Relative biologic effectiveness (RBE) as a function of neutron dose for various tissues. (Reproduced from Field and Hornsey.[104])

uted randomly but occur in clusters. Further, the ionizations along a path are produced at virtually the same instant. Accordingly, for high LET radiation, there are likely to be ionizations at nearly the same site and at exactly the same time, with resultant massive local damage. Such concentrated damage is likely to be more difficult to repair, although whether there are types of damage that are irreparable is not clear. SLDR and PLDR are sharply reduced or absent following fast neutron irradiation or radiation with higher LET particles.[45,100,101] OER and cell cycle effects are also decreased with high LET radiations. OER for low LET photons is 3 and approaches 1 at LET greater than 200 keV/$\mu$m. For fast neutron radiations OER is 1.5 to 2.0. Furthermore, cell-cycle-dependent radiation sensitivity (age–response function) decreases following high LET radiation.[102] Also, the effectiveness of radiation response modifiers (e.g., sensitizers and radiation protectors) is diminished or absent for high LET radiation.

The relative biological effectiveness (RBE) of various beams is described in terms of the ratio of doses to produce a defined level of damage or cell surviving fraction for the new beam to that for a conventional beam, usually 250 kV$_p$ (kilovolt-peak) X-rays or $^{60}$Co photons. Cell survival curves are presented in Figure 2-11B for cells irradiated in vitro by 300 kV$_p$ x-ray and 15 MeV neutrons.[103] Because of the very small $n$ for neutron irradiation, the RBE is highly dependent on dose, and increases inversely with dose. This dependence of RBE on dose or dose per fraction is shown by Figure 2-11C.[104]

## TISSUE RESPONSES TO IONIZING RADIATION

The response of a tissue, organ, or tumor to radiation is determined by the proportion and absolute number of cells that survive in each constituent tissue, the ability of the surviving cells to proliferate and reconstitute the damaged tissue, the number and time course of the

postradiation divisions of the killed cells, and the time course for the metabolically dead cells to undergo lysis and their cellular debris to be removed from the site.

### Tumor Tissue Response

In the design of a treatment strategy, consideration is given to the expected shapes of the dose–response curves for tumor and normal tissue and their relative position along the dose axes. Under favorable circumstances, the dose–response for tumor control is to the left of that for the normal tissue damage. From an analysis of the two curves, the proportion of subjects expected to achieve tumor control and be free of normal tissue damage can be derived. This is illustrated by Figure 2-12, which presents dose–response curves for control of carcinoma of the skin and for skin damage.[105] There is some overlap of the two curves; hence the proportion of tumor-free and complication-free patients begins to decrease as doses increase beyond a certain point. A general relationship of this type obtains for virtually all treatment strategies.

### Tumor Cell Radiation Sensitivity

Radiation response characteristics of many tumor cell lines derived from human tumors have been studied in vitro. Results from several of these are presented in Figure 2-13 in terms of surviving fractions following 2 Gy or SF$_2$.[106–109] The striking feature of these data is the broad distribution of SF$_2$. Furthermore,

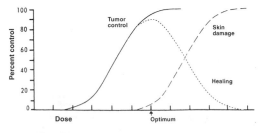

**FIGURE 2-12**  Dose–response curves for tumor and for serious skin damage. (Reproduced from Fletcher[105] as drawn from Holthusen, with permission.)

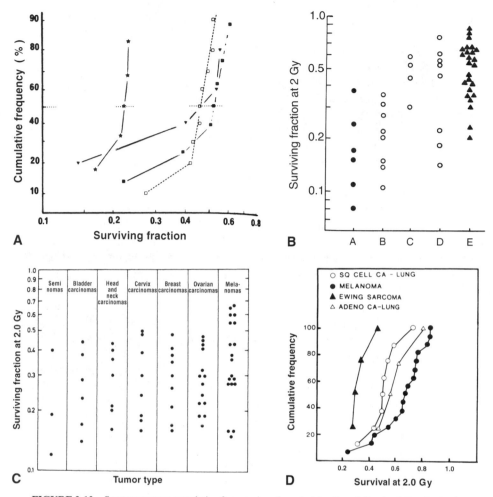

**FIGURE 2-13**   Scattergrams or cumulative frequencies of survival fractions following 2 Gy given to human tumor cell lines growing in vitro. **(A)** Cumulative frequency of survival fraction (SF) at 2 Gy: stars, fibroblasts; triangles, colorectal carcinomas; solid squares, melanomas; open squares, HeLa assayed by different authors. (Reproduced from Fertil and Malaise.[106]) **(B)** SF at 2 Gy for various cell lines from the laboratory of Deacon et al.[107] and from literature. Tumor cell lines are grouped according to "clinical radiation sensitivity": A, Burkitt lymphoma, neuroblastoma, myeloma; B, small cell, medulloblastoma; C, breast, bladder, cervix; D, pancreas, colon, rectum, lung; E, glioblastoma, melanoma, osteosarcoma, renal carcinoma. **(C)** $SF_2$ at 2 Gy data for various human tumor cell lines from the laboratory of Rofstad et al.[108] **(D)** $SF_2$ at 2 Gy data for various human tumor cell lines from the laboratory of Brock et al.[109]; these are not derived from assays of colony formation (as in **A–C**): open circles, squamous cell carcinoma (lung); solid circles, melanoma; solid triangles, Ewing sarcoma; open triangles, adenocarcinoma (lung).

there is substantial overlap in $SF_2$ between the various tumor groups. Note that $SF_2$ for melanoma extended from less than 0.2 to 0.9. The relatively sensitive small cell carcinoma of lung overlapped the values for melanoma. The extensive data from Rofstad et al.[108] in Figure 2-13C exhibit broad and overlapping distribu-

tions in $SF_2$ for each of the seven categories of tumors studied; these data are of special interest in that they are derived from cell lines studied in a single laboratory. Broad distribution of $SF_2$ is also shown by the work of Brock et al. (Fig. 2-13D), again produced in a single laboratory.[109] These investigators did not use colony formation as the end point, but rather a measure of cell proliferation postradiation.

The importance of relatively small differences in surviving fraction after repeated doses of 2 Gy is emphasized by the results of calculations shown in Table 2-5 (these assume that SF is constant for all 30 treatments). For example, if the surviving fraction after a single dose of 2 Gy were 0.8, after 30 equal doses the surviving fraction would be $1.2 \times 10^{-3}$. In contrast, for a cell line having $SF_2 = 0.2$, the surviving fraction after 30 equal doses of 2 Gy would be $1.1 \times 10^{-21}$. At present, the degree of heterogeneity of intrinsic cellular sensitivity throughout an individual tumor is unknown. The degree of heterogeneity of radiation sensitivity of tumor cells of different tumors is almost certainly not as broad as indicated by Figure 2-13; the $SF_2$ (in vitro) probably serves as a crude indicator of sensitivity. Knowledge of $SF_2$ for the tumor in the individual patient might prove to be of value in more effective planning of treatment. However, the last decade of research on this topic has been overshadowed by problems of measuring the $SF_2$ with reliability. Some series have shown a good correlation of in vitro $SF_2$ with tumor control rate,[110] but others have not.[111] Indeed, there have been problems in ascertaining that the cells growing from the tumor biopsy samples and being assayed for radiation sensitivity are indeed tumor cells and not fibroblasts.[112,113] There is possibly greater clinical value in determining whether a patient is relatively radiosensitive, which has led to interest in determining the normal tissue sensitivity before treatment rather than the tumor cell sensitivity. There is evidence that the radiation sensitivity of tumor clonogens tracks that of the normal tissues. In A-T patients, there are reports of local control and standard normal tissue reactions after doses that were ~0.3 of the conventional doses administered to apparently normal patients. In laboratory studies, fibrosarcomas were induced by methylcholanthrene in C3H/Sed and *scid* mice. The cell lines derived from the C3H/Sed mice had radiation sensitivity ~2.5 times greater than the *scid* tumor cell lines.[114] This is approximately the differential

**TABLE 2-5  Surviving Fractions (SF) After Treatment of a Model Cell Population with One or with 30 Equal Doses**

| | SF | |
|---|---|---|
| After One Dose | | After 30 Equal Doses |
| 0.8 | | $1.2 \times 10^{-3}$ |
| 0.6 | | $2.2 \times 10^{-7}$ |
| 0.4 | | $1.2 \times 10^{-12}$ |
| 0.2 | | $1.1 \times 10^{-21}$ |

radiation sensitivity that obtains for normal tissues for these two mouse strains.

Radiation sensitivity of rodent tumor cells irradiated in vivo has been assayed using in vivo and in vitro techniques[38,42,115] (see Tables 2-2 and 2-4). These techniques require the excision of the irradiated tumor, preparation of a cell suspension, and the injection of graded numbers of cells into isologous recipients, or the plating of the cells in vitro. Studies based on such methods have resulted in valuable data and improved understanding of tumor radiation biology. These are not discussed in detail here, as we direct our attention to in situ assays based on in vivo responses of intact tumors.

The response of a solid tumor in vivo to local irradiation is not simply the response of a pure colony of tumor cells. Rather, the response reflects the direct action of radiation to kill tumor cells, and to an undefined extent there is an indirect effect of the radiation to kill stromal and capillary endothelial cells with secondary production of microinfarctions. Based on the results of an experiment in which human tumor xenotransplants were studied in nude and *scid* mice, the latter effect appears to be quite small in tumor inactivation by radiation.[116] The dose to produce a defined level of normal tissue damage in the normally radiation-sensitive nude mice was 2.5 that for the comparable reaction in *scid* mice. Similar studies were performed on spontaneous tumors of the C3H/Sed mice, on isotransplants into C3H mice, and on allotransplants in *scid* mice. The finding was that the values of the median tissue culture dose ($TCD_{50}$) were no lower for tumors in the *scid,* whose capillary endothelial cells are radiation sensitive, than for tumors with normally sensitive endothelial cells. The clear implication is that radiation killing of endothelial cells makes at most a minor impact on tumor control probability by radiation. Some cells will be inactivated because of metabolic inadequacies (e.g., severe hypoxia, hypoglycemia), host-specific or nonspecific immune rejection reaction against tumor cells, and cell loss due to factors that promote cell differentiation (i.e., remove the cell from the proliferating population). The control of tumor angiogenesis has recently become an area of intense study. Antiangiogenesis agents have moved into phase I clinical trials. Two recently discovered regulators of angiogenesis, angiostatin and endostatin, have demonstrated striking effects in the control of mouse tumors.[117,118] The importance of vascular targets as mechanisms for controlling spontaneous tumors of man remains to be determined.

## Dose–Response Curves for Tumors Irrradiated In Situ

Following irradiation, tumors are retarded in growth rate. The tumor growth curve may show a flattening or may exhibit temporary regression followed by regrowth. There may be complete regression followed by regrowth. The most desired response is, of course, complete and permanent regression. The two end points that have been used extensively in experimental radiation therapy have been tumor growth delay (TGD) and tumor control probability (TCP). "Tumor control" means complete and permanent regression or absence of growth for the period of observation. Thus, even though regression is incomplete, tumor control would be scored provided there was no growth during the study period.

***Tumor Growth Delay*** One example of the progressively longer delay in tumor growth with increasing radiation dose is shown in Figure 2-14A for the RIB5, a benzpyrene-induced fibrosarcoma of the rat.[119] There is an increase

in the delay of tumor growth with radiation dose, and the slope of the regrowth curve is progressively less steep. Figure 2-14B plots tumor growth delay as a function of radiation dose for the RIB5 tumor irradiated under conditions of clamp hypoxia (a clamp placed around the root of the flap of tissue bearing the tumor), air (0.2 atm $O_2$), or hyperbaric oxygen.[120] The TGD for air closely follows that for hyperbaric oxygen in the low dose range, indicating that the response to low doses is determined by the aerobic cells of the tumor. At higher doses, the TGD curve follows that for irradiation under clamp hypoxia, implying that at high dose levels the response is determined by the hypoxic cells. An enhancement ratio (ER) for hyperbaric oxygen can be derived from the ratio of doses—for example, (hyperbaric oxygen)/air—to achieve a specified TGD. Obviously, the ER would be dose dependent.

***Tumor Bed Effect*** Analysis of tumor growth delay curves is complicated by the effects of radiation on the stroma as well as tumor cells. That is, TGD is not a simple function of the fraction of tumor cells surviving at each dose level. With increasing radiation dose there are (1) progressively longer mean cell cycle times, (2) increasing probabilities of unsuccessful division, and (3) changes in the normal tissues (especially a growing capillary network) of the tumor bed, namely, they become less able to expand enough to support tumor growth. The effect on the irradiated stroma, called the tumor bed effect (TBE), is most easily demonstrated by observing the time for tumor to grow to a specified size following transplantation into normal or irradiated tissue. At 50 days posttransplantation, the $TD_{50}$ (the number of tumor cells required to produce a tumor in 50% of the inoculations) for the spontaneous mammary carcinoma MCaIV transplanted into unirradiated tissues was $2 \times 10^4$.[121] In contrast, there were virtually no tumors when the tumor cells were inoculated into the legs irradiated to 35 Gy. However, 200 to 250 days after irradiating the tumor bed site, the $TD_{50}$ values were comparable for transplantation into normal or irra-

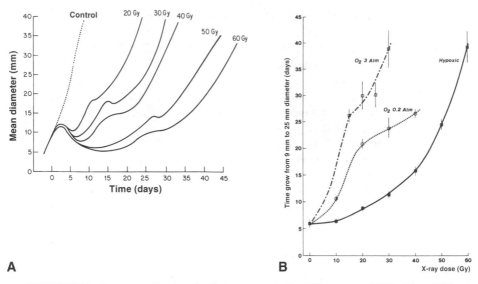

**FIGURE 2-14** Tumor growth curves for the benzpyrene-induced fibrosarcoma RIB5 of the rat following single radiation doses given to air-breathing animals with no restriction in blood flow to the tumor. (Reproduced from Thomlinson.[119]) **(B)** Tumor growth delay versus radiation dose after irradiation of RIB5 under air, hyperbaric oxygen, and clamp hypoxic conditions. (Reproduced from Thomlinson.[120])

diated legs. A tumor bed effect is not observed for all tumor systems: similar studies using a fibrosarcoma showed no TBE. Milas et al.[122] reported that sarcomas, in contrast to adenocarcinomas, exhibit little or no such effect. The point for emphasis is that irradiation of normal tissue retards the growth of some transplanted tumors, but does not affect transplantability in normal and irradiated tissue. Thus, TBE cannot be considered to be a component of the response to radiation that contributes to tumor control. However, TBE may complicate the use of TGD as an end point. In such studies the role of TBE has to be considered explicitly.

***Tumor Control Assays***   Tumor control or local control is the end point of greatest relevance to clinical radiation therapy. This end point is also attractive in that scoring yes or no for local control is unambiguous in nearly every instance. From dose–response assays for tumor control, the $TCD_{50}$ and slope can be defined. The $TCD_{50}$ is the dose that would be expected to achieve tumor control in half the irradiated tumors, for the time specified.

The dose–response curve for a model tumor is characterized as (1) $M$ clonogens; (2) clonogens that die only of direct radiation effect (i.e., no clonogen death due to the host reaction against tumor or secondary to damage to the tumor vascular system, etc.); or (3) inevitable tumor recurrence if one or more clonogens survive treatment. Accordingly, TCP or tumor control probability will be a reflection of the probability that all clonogens are inactivated. For example, $TCD_{50}$ means that in half the irradiated tumors no clonogens survive and in the other half one or more cells survive. The relationship between TCP, surviving fraction, and clonogen number is:

$$TCP = \exp\{-(SF \times M)\}$$
$$\therefore \quad \ln TCP = SF \times M$$

The natural logarithm of TCP represents the average number of surviving cells per tumor; thus, TCPs of 0.1, 0.37, and 0.5 mean that the average number of surviving cells would be 2.3, 1.0, and 0.693. Hence, at the $TCP_{50}$, the average number of cells surviving per tumor is not 1 but 0.693. This is because in some tumors there are two, three, four, or more surviving cells. These results are fascinating because they indicate that there is an extremely small number of cells that survive radiation treatment in tumors that recur. For example, even after treatments yielding a TCP of only 0.1, more than 90% of all recurrences develop from one to four surviving cells. This suggests that the difference between success and failure of treatment is only one or a very few surviving cells. At $TCD_{50}$ and $TCD_{37}$ dose levels, the average numbers of cells surviving among tumors that recur are 1.39 and 1.58, respectively.

Following a particular treatment there is a probability of inactivation of all tumor cells, that is, killing all tumor cells in a proportion ($P$) of the tumors. This proportion can be very high: for example, greater than .99 but never 1.00. Accordingly, the term "tumoricidal dose" has no meaning. Rather, the radiation oncologist should think in terms of probability of tumor control by a given treatment. The relationship between radiation dose and tumor control probability for single-dose irradiation can be approximated by[123]:

$$TCD_P = D_0[\ln M + \ln n - \ln(-\ln P)]$$

According to this relationship, the $TCD_{50}$ for tumors comprising a particular cell population (uniform $D_0$, $n$) will increase with $D_0[\ln M]$. For tumors of a particular clonogen number ($M$), $D_0$, and $n$, $TCD_P$ increases with $(D_0)[-\ln(-\ln P)]$. Thus, the dose increment required to raise TCP from 0.1 to 0.9 would be $3.08 \times D_0$. The relationship for fractionated irradiation is more complex and is not discussed here.

Performance of a dose–response assay for tumor control usually accords with the following general protocol:

1. The tumor system is selected (for a desired histopathologic type, growth rate, metastatic aggressiveness, immunogenicity, etc.). For experimental radiation oncology, the optimal tumor system is a spontaneous tumor studied either as the autochthonous in situ tumor or as early generation isotransplants.

2. The size of tumor at which radiation is to be administered is selected.

3. The animals are allocated by a random number scheme to the doses to be employed.

4. A tumor is accessed into an experiment on the day that the tumor achieves the size specified by the experimental protocol.

5. Tumor diameters are measured at appropriate frequency following treatment so as to permit the construction of tumor growth curves, if desired.

6. The period of observation permits at least 90% of the regrowths to be scored (usually 100–200 days for rodent tumors).

7. At completion, tumor control results are plotted and a regression line is fitted to allow computation of the $TCD_{50}$ and the slope of the curve at the $TCD_{50}$.[123]

8. Animals are scored for deaths (due to intercurrent disease, induced tumors, findings at autopsy, etc.).

Figure 2-15 shows the dose–response curve for control at 120 days, of 8 mm MCaIV isotransplants, subjected to single-dose irradiation under clamp hypoxia.[124] The tumors in this assay were highly uniform: 8 mm diameter or 250 mm³ in volume; all cells in all tumors were hypoxic; tumors were nonimmunogenic[125]; and radiation dose was highly uniform. There was virtually no likelihood of equivocal scoring of local control. These data are derived essentially from one tumor. The tumor had been cloned into several hundred virtually identical subjects and treated in an extremely uniform manner. In Figure 2-15A the data are plotted on a linear–linear grid; the dose–response curve is S-shaped, being quite steep in the TCP range of 5 and 40% and less steep in the range above 60%. The same data are plotted on a probability (logit) ordinate versus log dose in Figure 2-15B, yielding a nearly straight line that approaches closely that expected from the

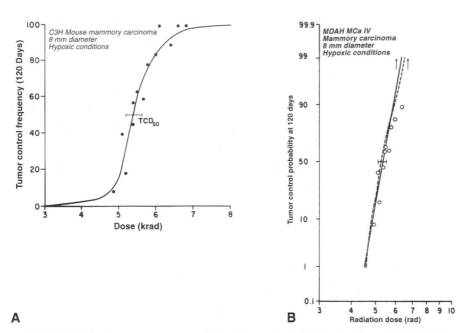

A

B

**FIGURE 2-15**   Dose–response curves for local control at 120 days, of an 8 mm MCaIV third-generation iso-transplant treated by single-dose 250 kV(p) x-radiation under clamp hypoxia. (Reproduced from Suit.[124]) **(A)** Data plotted on a standard linear grid. **(B)** Same data plotted on a logit of tumor control versus log dose: solid line, logit regression line through the data points; dashed line, that predicted by the multitarget model.

equation above, and assigning realistic values for the parameters $D_0$, $n$, and $M$.

### Slope of Dose–Response Curve and Heterogeneity Among Treated Tumors

To illustrate the dependence of slope of dose–response curve on the heterogeneity of the tumors included in the dose–response assays, Figure 2-16 was prepared. Here, independently determined dose–response curves for MCaIV are shown for tumors of 4 to 5, 8, and 12 mm diameter. The solid line is the resultant and relatively flat curve if all data from the 4 to 5, 8, and 12 mm tumors were pooled. Heterogeneity of whatever origin will result in a flattening of the curve.

**Tumor Volume and $TCD_{50}$**   The experience in virtually all clinical radiation therapy demonstrates that tumor volume at irradiation is an important determinant of the likelihood of success following a particular total dose and fractionation schedule. This has been observed

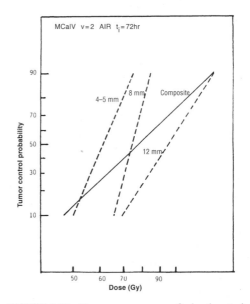

**FIGURE 2-16**   Dose–response curves for local control of MCaIV treated under air by two equal doses of [137]Cs radiation separated by 72 hours; the tumors were 4 to 5, 8, or 12 mm in diameter. The solid line is the calculated dose–response curve if all data from the three assays were pooled.

unarguably for tumors in experimental animal systems. The $TCD_{50}$ values for a series of transplanted and spontaneous autochthonous mammary carcinomas subjected to single-dose irradiation under clamp hypoxia exhibit an orderly increase with tumor volume.[123] The observed data points fit within a band that would be expected with a $D_0$ of 3.0 to 3.25 Gy and an extrapolation number of 1 to 6. In a subsequent study on MCaIV, radiation was administered under oxic conditions to microcolonies (site of injection of $10^5$ cells) and to tumors of 0.6 and 250 mm$^3$. The $TCD_{50}$ values were 15.2, 22.0, and 54.3 Gy, respectively.[126] The extremely steep increase in $TCD_{50}$ between 0.6 and 250 mm$^3$ tumor volumes strongly suggests that the tumor growth was accompanied by a deterioration of metabolic conditions in the tumor: a significant fraction of tumor clonogens became hypoxic. These data conform to an expectation of increasing $TCD_{50}$ with tumor volume due to increasing number of clonogens and the appearance of relatively radiation-resistant foci of cells as tumors achieve large size.

**Recurrent Tumors** As described earlier, cells that survive large radiation doses have heritable changes, including *increased* radiation sensitivity. Experiments have been performed to assess the radiation response of tumors derived from failures after high doses. For example, a C3H mouse mammary carcinoma that had recurred following a single radiation dose (the $TCD_{95}$) was transplanted into fresh isologous recipients. This tumor grew slowly: the volume doubling time was 17 days, compared with 3 to 4 days for the untreated tumor growing in untreated tissue. The $TCD_{50}$ at 240 days was 59.9 Gy for the control tumor but 51.3 Gy for the recurrent tumor growing in unirradiated tissue. The difference between these two $TCD_{50}$ values, which were measured concurrently, was significant at $p < .01$.[127] The treatments were performed under conditions of clamp hypoxia to obviate concern regarding the status of oxygenation in the primary and the recurrent tumors. Ando et al.[128] reported similar findings in their study of a recurrent fi-

brosarcoma. A recurrent tumor may be comprised of cells of greater sensitivity than the original tumor, but this does not mean that the gross response would be greater for the recurrent tumor than for the primary. The recurrent tumor would be growing in an irradiated tumor bed with attendant vascular system inadequacies and probably a higher proportion of hypoxic cells.

In the clinic, recurrent lesions are usually not subjected to full dose levels because of the limited tolerance of the normal tissues. The infrequency of good clinical results in the treatment of local failures cannot be taken as proof of an increased inherent radiation resistance of the tumor cells. Interestingly, induction of radiation resistance by repeated treatment is extraordinarily uncommon. This contrasts with the rapid appearance of drug-resistant mutants in tumor cell populations exposed to drug treatment. An additional observation is that drug-resistant mutants do not appear in cells of normal tissues, reflecting the stable genome of normal cells and the heterogeneity in tumors generated by an unstable genome.

**Immune Rejection Reaction and Tumor Response** The potential of an immune rejection reaction to cause partial or complete rejection of a tumor has been studied comprehensively in experimental animal tumor systems. These have been based primarily on tumors induced by chemicals (methylcholanthrene, benzypyrene) or viruses (e.g., SV40). The immunogenicity of these tumors is well shown by the effect of specific immunization against a particular tumor on the $TD_{50}$ and $TCD_{50}$. The first demonstration of an immune reaction by an inbred mouse against an isologous tumor was reported by Foley[129] for the methylcholanthrene-induced fibrosarcoma. Foley found that if a mouse had been exposed to the tumor antigen by transplantation of the tumor followed by excision of the transplanted tumor at an appropriate size, the animal was able to reject subsequent tumor challenge. In our laboratory, when the $TD_{50}$ assay was used with isotransplantation of a methylcholanthrene-induced fibrosarcoma, FSal, the $TD_{50}$ was significantly increased by previous immunization and significantly decreased by whole-body irradiation (WBI) before transplantation.[130] Similarly, the $TCD_{50}$ values were 34.8, 25.9, and 43.1 Gy for control mice, and for mice that had been immunized or given 4 Gy WBI prior to transplantation, respectively.

## Normal Tissue Response

There is an extensive literature on the effects of ionizing radiation on diverse normal tissues, organs, and organisms. The work was vigorously supported by the U.S. Atomic Energy Commission and the Department of Defense during the early years of the era of nuclear weapons. That work generated a vast array of dose–response assays for death following shortly after irradiation, employing a wide variety of species. Those studies were based primarily on conventional photons at various dose rates, which were complemented by comprehensive determinations of life shortening and causes of death versus dose for different species.

Over the past 30 years there has been intensive study in experimental animals of the response of normal tissues to localized irradiation. The effort has been directed at evaluating the response of tissues to radiation under conditions similar to those employed in clinical radiation therapy. These studies have been performed principally on mouse, rat, and miniature pig. For many tissues, ingenious experimental strategies have permitted the derivation of values for the parameters of survival curves including $D_0$, $n$, and $\alpha/\beta$ ratio (see Tables 2-2 and 2-6). An observation by Withers[131] that has had great importance to clinical radiation therapy was that the total dose to produce a specified level of damage was much more dependent on dose per fraction in late-responding than in acute-responding tissues. This is illustrated in Figure 2-17, a plot of dose to produce the defined effects versus dose per fraction. Slopes of the curves are steeper for the late-responding tissues (e.g., spinal cord, kidney, lung) than for the acutely responding

**TABLE 2-6  Values of $\alpha/\beta$ Ratios for Various Normal Tissues Determined from Multifraction Experiments on Animals**

| Effects | $\alpha/\beta$ (Gy) |
|---|---|
| ACUTE | |
| Skin desquamation | |
| Mouse | 8–14 |
| Rat | 9–10 |
| Pig | 8–11 |
| Human | 9–11 |
| Jejunal clones | 6–11 |
| Colon clones | 8–9 |
| Colon weight loss | 12–13 |
| Testis clones | 9–13 |
| Mouse tail necrosis | 7–26 |
| Mouse $LD_{50}$ (30 days) | |
| LATE | |
| Rat spinal cord | |
| Cervical | 1.0–2.7 |
| Lumbar | 2.3–4.9 |
| Kidney | |
| Rabbit | 1.7–2 |
| Pig | 1.7–2 |
| Mouse | 1.0–3.5 |
| Lung, mouse | 2.0–6.3 |
| Bladder, mouse | 3.5–7 |
| Pig skin, late contraction | 2.0–5 |

*Source:* Adapted from Fowler.[134]

tissues (skin, testes, jejunal crypt cells). A review by Williams et al.[132] indicates that the $\alpha/\beta$ ratios for tumors are comparable to those for acutely responding normal tissues. Thus, the $\alpha/\beta$ ratio is high ($> 5$) for acutely responding tissues and tumors and low ($< 5$) for most late-responding normal tissues. The major implication for radiation therapy is to use small doses per fraction ($\leq 2$ Gy) where late-responding normal tissues are to receive the full dose in a radical course of treatment. In other words, when the dose-limiting toxicity is the late-responding normal tissue (e.g., spinal cord) the optimum therapeutic ratio is obtained by the use of small doses per fraction.

The radiation biology of each of the various important normal tissues cannot be reviewed

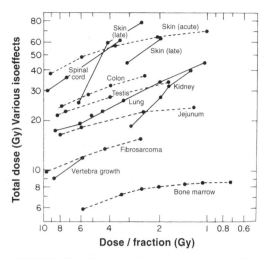

**FIGURE 2-17**  Plots of total dose to produce a specified effect versus dose per fraction for various late- and acute-responding (solid and dsahed lines, respectively) tissues. (Reproduced from Withers.[131])

comprehensively in this introductory chapter. Details relevant to each site and tumor type are included in the chapters covering specific concerns. The response of normal tissues to a course of radiation depends on number of stem cells, total dose, number of fractions, time between fractions, dose per fraction, inherent cellular radiation sensitivity, the micrometabolic milieu of the cells of the constituent tissues, cell proliferative activity, cell divisions during treatment, cellular age redistribution during treatment, and capacity and kinetics of repair of radiation damage.

## ATTEMPTS TO REDUCE THE IMPACT OF HYPOXIC CELLS ON TUMOR RESISTANCE

In virtually all solid tumor systems of experimental animals, reoxygenation results in a decrease, during the course of fractionated irradiation, in the proportion of cells that are hypoxic. Even so, the available evidence indicates that hypoxic cells can persist and are the major determinants of the dose required for tumor inactivation. That is, reoxygenation does

not appear to be complete in tumors of experimental animals. A large part of preclinical laboratory and clinical research in radiation therapy has been directed toward reduction of the number and/or importance of hypoxic cells in tumors and hence improve the efficacy of radiation therapy.[133,134] These approaches include (1) dose fractionation, (2) blood transfusion, (3) respiration of oxygen at higher concentrations than air, or even a high pressure (hyperbaric oxygen), (4) use of chemical sensitizers of hypoxic cells, (5) suppression of $Q_{O_2}$, (6) increase of tumor blood flow, (7) decrease of blood viscosity, (8) erythrocyte rigidity, (9) irradiation under the condition of tourniquet hypoxia, that is, rendering all the cells of the normal tissue as well as the tumor hypoxic, (10) high LET radiation, and (11) hyperthermia. The magnitude of the gain achieved by a new treatment may be described in terms of the therapeutic gain factor (TGF), which is the enhancement ratio (ER) of the tumor, divided by the ER of normal tissue.

The presence of hypoxic regions in previously untreated rodent and human tumors has been demonstrated. Studies on human tumors have employed UV cryophotometric methods to determine the oxy–deoxyhemoglobin ratio of individual erythrocytes in capillaries of histologic sections prepared and studied under cryogenic conditions.[135,136] Thus, there is unambiguous evidence of the presence of hypoxic cells in at least some untreated solid tumors of experimental animals and man. Furthermore, hyperbaric oxygen improves tumor tissue $P_{O_2}$, in rodents.[137] Figure 2-18 demonstrates the effect of clamp hypoxia or hyperbaric oxygen [respiration of 100% oxygen at 3 atm pressure absolute $(O_2\text{-}3\text{ATA})$] on the dose–response curve for local control of 8 mm MCaIV tumor, treated in five equal fractions.[138] The three dose–response curves are steep, parallel, and widely and significantly separated. The enhancement ratio for $TCD_{50}$ clamped versus $O_2\text{-}3\text{ATA}$ was 2.3. This indicates that $P_{O_2}$ of all tumor cells, even under hyperbaric conditions and fractionated irradiation, was not at normal tissue levels; if so, the ratio should have been in

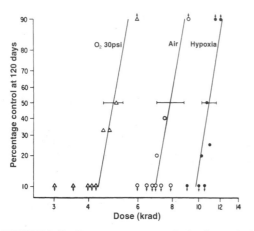

**FIGURE 2-18** Dose–response curves for local control of 8 mm MCaIV isotransplants treated by five equal doses (one day between treatments) given under air, clamp hypoxia, or hyperbaric ($O_2$ 3 ATA) conditions. (Reproduced from Howes and Suit.[138])

the range 2.5–3.0. Hyperbaric oxygen also achieved a large reduction in $TCD_{50}$ over that for air conditions, with an ER of 1.75. Hyperbaric oxygen has increased the response to fractionated radiation of virtually every solid tumor of rodents tested.

Clinical trials have been conducted using several of these approaches. Henk[139] reported the absolute 5-year results from the Medical Research Council trial of hyperbaric oxygen (respiration of oxygen at 3 ATA) in the radiation treatment of squamous cell carcinoma of the oral cavity and oropharynx. There was significant gain both in local control and survival. Bush et al.[140] demonstrated a gain in survival of anemic (10–12 g/dL) patients with stage III carcinoma of the uterine cervix by transfusing and maintaining Hgb at 12 g/dL or more. Overgaard et al.[141] reported a gain in local control with the use of nimorazole, the radiation sensitizer of hypoxic cells, in the Danish head and neck trial; this gain was found for all subcategories analyzed (sex, site, stage, Hgb). Many other trials of radiation sensitizers such as misonidazole have yielded equivocal results. Currently, neither radiation sensitizers (oxygen mimetics) nor hyperbaric oxygen is in routine clinical use, despite the findings of clinically significant benefits in randomized trials. The reasons for this are not entirely clear: there is circumstantial evidence to support the view that the effects of oxygen are less, the more radiation therapy is fractionated, just as dose rate lessens the OER.

## DOSE FRACTIONATION AND TISSUE RESPONSE

A major area of clinical research in radiation therapy is the study of dose fractionation pattern and tissue response. The standard dose fractionation of radical treatments employed in 1999 in the United States in definitive treatment of patients with solid tumors remains 1.8 to 2.0 Gy per fraction, with five fractions per week, the total dose being 60 to 75 Gy. For combinations of radiation with surgery or drugs or both, the total dose is usually reduced, and in many instances the dose per fraction may also be cut back. However, in the last 10 years, there has been an increasing trend to altered fractionation schemes (see Chapter 15B). Planning new fractionation protocols is based on the biologic and radiobiologic characteristics of the cells of the tumor and the critical normal tissues, such as repair capacity, cellular sensitivity, and proliferative kinetics.

The improving metabolic status of tumor cells, which may occur as fractionated treatment progresses, may cause cells to enter into active cell cycle, hence to increase cell number between fractions. This has been designated proliferative response or recruitment. The effect of such a process would be to increase the tumor control dose. An important proportion of the tumor cells are in a prolonged $G_1$ phase as a result of metabolic insufficiency, and as this is alleviated, the cells resume proliferation. The result is a reduction in mean cell cycle time and cell loss factor combined with a higher growth fraction. Consequently, there is an acceleration of clonogen population growth. These findings support the notion that in the treatment of some tumors shortened overall times of treatment might be of greater effectiveness.

As a general rule, for fast-growing tumors such as squamous carcinoma of the head and neck, accelerated fractionation (reduction in the overall treatment time) helps to offset the problems of proliferation during treatment.[142] However, acceleration cannot be achieved simply by giving a larger fraction size per day: this would result in a greater risk of complications in late-responding tissues, as explained earlier. Therefore, the acceleration is achieved by delivering two smaller fractions of treatment per day, making the total dose per day higher. This approach usually adopts 1.5 to 1.6 Gy twice a day, reaching doses of 55 to 60 Gy in 3.5 to 4 weeks, before acute toxicity demands a gap in therapy.[143,144] Even with a short break in therapy, the overall treatment time for the delivery of doses in the range of 70 Gy can be 5.5 to 6 weeks. A randomized trial of accelerated fractionation was undertaken in the study done by the European Organization for Research on the Treatment of Cancer (EORTC) of head and neck cancer.[145] Actuarial survival at 5 years was 13% better in the accelerated arm compared with the standard arm, a significant improvement in survival. Subgroup analysis suggested that the greatest benefit was seen in the tumors with fast proliferation kinetics (short $T_{pot}$).[146] One way to try to improve the acute tolerance of accelerated fractionation is to use a concomitant boost. This means treat the large field (tumor and regional nodes) once a day and the small field (tumor volume only) once a day, resulting in the tumor being treated twice daily and the regional nodes daily. This may be suitable if the regional nodes are being treated electively, but less appropriate if there is detectable disease in the nodes.

The alternative manipulation of the fractionation schedule is to increase the total radiation dose, and achieve this by giving small doses per fraction, known as hyperfractionation. The rate of delivery of treatment is usually around 2 Gy/day, 1 Gy twice a day or 1.2 Gy twice a day being the most commonly used schemes. A randomized trial in the treatment of bladder cancer[147] showed an improvement in outcome with 84 Gy, 1.2 Gy twice a day over 7 weeks, compared with 64 Gy, 2 Gy daily. The treatment of CNS tumors, such as pediatric brain stem gliomas, is thought to benefit from hyperfractionation, and doses of 1 Gy twice a day to 72 Gy have been used.[148]

For both types of twice-a-day therapy, the intertreatment interval is usually set at 4 to 6 hours between fractions. The optimum intertreatment interval remains uncertain. The recovery of tumor cells in cell culture in split-dose experiments appears to be complete in ~6 hours. For late-responding tissues (e.g., spinal cord), 6 to 12 hours may be essential to realize the full benefit of hyperfractionation. Since clinical therapy is designed to produce side effects to the spinal cord at an extremely low frequency, it will be difficult to distinguish between an intertreatment interval of, for example, 6 and 12 hours. Animal data may help bring some insight, but characteristics for the tolerance of rodent spinal cord may not answer such a specific question. The tolerance of the monkey spinal cord has been evaluated to provide important additional information.[149]

The strategies of acceleration and hyperfractionation may be combined. A rigorous test of this general strategy was conducted by Dische and Saunders[150] in the United Kingdom on patients with cancer of the lung and cancer of the head and neck region. The investigators employed 1.4 Gy initially, and then 1.5 Gy, three times a day with 6 hours between fractions, in 36 fractions over a 12-day period; this has meant treatment through the weekend. The total dose was 50.4 Gy, escalating to 54 Gy in 12 days. Because the preliminary data gave encouraging results, the United Kingdom Medical Research Council sponsored two randomized trials, which were reported recently.[151] Both trials showed improvement in overall survival when CHART (**c**ontinuous **h**yperfractionated **a**ccelerated **r**adiation **t**herapy) was used.

The ultimate test of hyperfractionation is low dose rate continuous radiation therapy. Pierquin et al.[152] have investigated this approach using 8 to 10 Gy/day at 1 Gy/h for total treatment times of several weeks. Preliminary results from a clinical trial of low dose rate continuous therapy versus conventional fractionated treatment for oral cavity–oropharyngeal squamous cell carcinomas indicated a gain for the low dose rate therapy technique.

## Models for Fractionation Dependence

Radiobiologic characterizations of tissues for assessing the fractionation dependence is increasingly done in terms of the $\alpha/\beta$ ratio. Use of this ratio must be made with explicit recognition that there is no allowance for the time factor. This is an important consideration for treatment protracted over more than 3 to 4 weeks, because there may be a proliferative response in the acutely responding tissues (malignant and normal). The reason for the increasing use of the $\alpha/\beta$ ratio is its simplicity in equating different doses per fraction ($d$) and total dose ($D$):

$$D_1 = \frac{D_2(d_2 + \alpha/\beta)}{d_1 + \alpha/\beta}$$

If $d_2 = 2$ Gy per fraction, and $D_2 = 60$ Gy total dose, and the fraction size is increased to 3 Gy per fraction, what is the equivalent total dose?

For $\alpha/\beta$ ratio = 2 Gy, such as for spinal cord, $D_1 = 60 \times 4/5 = 48$ Gy.

For $\alpha/\beta$ ratio = 10 Gy, such as for a tumor, $D_1 = 60 \times 12/13 = \sim55$ Gy.

There is general use of nomograms to estimate doses that yield comparable levels of response for treatment given in different total times or different number of fractions, for example, nominal standard dose (NSD)[153] and time dose fractionation (TDF).[154] These measures are being refined and modified to employ exponents of dose per fraction and time more appropriate to the normal tissue of concern. The formulas must be accepted only as guidelines, not rules, for small deviations from established practice. This point needs emphasis because there have been untoward reactions when major extrapolations or extensions from conventional treatments have been based on these formulas. The exact values of the parameters are not necessarily constant. Certainly for acutely responding tissues the exponent for the time factor depends on the total overall time of treatment, small to zero for highly accelerated treatments (without a break), but larger for highly protracted treatments. Our policy is to apply these guidelines only for quite small shifts from standard practice.

## COMBINATION OF RADIATION AND CHEMOTHERAPEUTIC AGENTS: CYTOTOXICS, SENSITIZERS, AND PROTECTORS

The current practice of clinical oncology places high proportions of patients with stage $M_0$ disease on chemotherapy. Accordingly, knowledge of the mechanism of action of chemotherapeutic agents and the manner in which cellular response to radiation is modified by chemotherapeutic drugs is important. The effect of such combinations depends on five factors:

1. The pharmacokinetics of the drug: the time course of drug concentration in the various tissues.
2. The cell cycle dependence of the drug: some drugs affect cells at specific phases in the cell cycle (e.g., vincristine and vinblastine arrest cells in $G_2/M$), whereas other agents affect cells at all stages in the cell cycle (e.g., an alkylating agent such as cyclophosphamide).
3. The mechanism of action in terms of direct cytotoxicity or sensitization of radiation effect.
4. The timing and magnitude of a drug-induced proliferative response.
5. The dose–response relationships.

Table 2-7 lists the more commonly employed chemotherapeutic agents according to mechanism of action.

**TABLE 2-7    Chemotherapeutic Drugs in Common Usage: Mechanism of Action**

| Drug | Mechanism of Action |
|---|---|
| Cyclophosphamide | Alkylating agent |
| Melphalan | Alkylating agent |
| Chlorambucil | Alkylating agent |
| Cisplatin | Bifunctional alkylating agent |
| Carboplatinum | Bifunctional alkylating agent |
| Bleomycin | Free radicals and strand breaks |
| Doxorubicin (Adriamycin) | Topoisomerase II inhibitor + ?other |
| Etoposide | Topoisomerase II inhibitor (proliferating cells) |
| 5-Fluorouracil | Antimetabolite: thymidylate synthase inhibitor (S-phase) |
| Methotrexate | Antimetabolite: tetrahydrofolate inhibitor (S-phase) |
| Cytarabine | Antimetabolite: cytosine analog (S-phase specific) |
| Actinomycin D | RNA polymerase inhibitor |
| Vincristine | Depolymerizes microtubules (M-phase specific) |
| Vinblastine | Depolymerizes microtubules (M-phase specific) |
| Paclitaxel (taxol) | Stabilizes microtubules (M-phase) |
| Docetaxel (taxotere) | Stabilizes microtubules (M-phase) |

The chemotherapeutic agent may act as a cytotoxic agent and/or modify the response to radiation. Sensitization is used by Steel[155] to refer to an enhanced response where the chemical agent is not cytotoxic at the dose level employed. This is explained by Figure 2-19. The first survival curve (Fig. 2-19A) is for cells treated by an agent that does not reduce survival on its own but does reduce $D_0$. Drugs may reduce either $n$ or $D_0$ or both. An example of such an agent is 1UdR.[156] In Figure 2-19B, the drug reduced the surviving fraction but did not affect the cell's response to radiation; the two curves are identical in shape. The effect here is defined as additive. The radiation cell survival curve for previously untreated cells is the upper curve; the lower curve represents cells treated by a cytotoxic chemotherapeutic agent. "Chemoenhancement" refers to the situation of a cytotoxic chemical agent that reduces $D_0$ and/or $n$ (Fig. 2-19C). Of course, modification of response can be protective. The ER for a particular drug–radiation treatment is the ratio of radiation doses to produce a specified effect for radiation alone to that for radiation plus drug.

The observed ER depends on the timing of the radiation in relation to administration of the

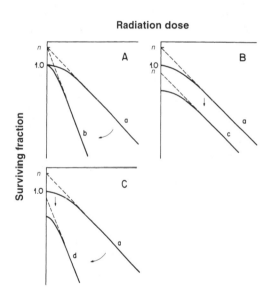

**FIGURE 2-19**    Cell survival curves for cells treated by radiation alone or combined with a radiation response modifier. **(A)** Curve a, treatment by radiation alone; curve b, treatment by radiation and a chemical sensitizer that reduces $D_0$ but does not affect $n$. This agent is not cytotoxic at the concentrations used. **(B)** Curve a, radiation alone; curve c, radiation combined with a chemical that is cytotoxic and at the concentration employed reduces survival fraction but does not modify the shape of the cell survival curve for cells that survive the chemical treatment. **(C)** Curve d; cells treated by a chemical that is cytotoxic as in B but also reduces $D_0$.

drug, the drug and radiation dose, the pharmacokinetics, the nature of the drug-damaged site, and the kinetics of repair of the drug and radiation damage. There can be a major effect, even though the drug is given at a remote time after the radiation, if the drug produces cytoxicity in the recovering tissues. This has been shown to be particularly true for actinomycin D and doxorubicin (Adriamycin), as seen clinically affecting normal tissues (e.g., the skin) in the "recall" phenomenon. Steel[155] uses the term "spatial" cooperation or interaction to refer to effective treatment at a different site (e.g., radiation for the primary lesion and a chemotherapeutic agent for metastatic foci).

Maase and Overgaard[157] have evaluated the ER for a spectrum of chemotherapeutic agents combined with single-dose irradiation of a C3H mouse mammary carcinoma. They reported that doxorubicin, cyclophosphamide, and mitomycin C yield large ER values. Several other agents (bleomycin, 5-fluorouracil, methotrexate, and cisplatin) effected large tumor growth delays but did not alter the $TCD_{50}$. This result is interesting in providing evidence that a good "response" to a drug does not necessarily mean that combining the drug with radiation will produce an increase in local control probability.

Important clinical gains have been realized by combining chemotherapy and radiation therapy in the treatment of patients with embryonal rhabdomyosarcoma, Ewing sarcoma, Wilms tumor, lymphomas (including lymphoma of bone), and nonseminomatous testicular tumors. Indeed, the effectiveness of chemotherapy in these conditions has obviated the need for radiation therapy at all, for certain stages of disease. Until recently, trials of the combined approach for solid tumors in adult patients have yielded limited evidence of clinical gains. Combined modality therapy has become standard for stage III breast cancer, with evidence in favor of a survival benefit for adjuvant chemoradiation.[158] The recent publications assessing postmastectomy radiation therapy for node-positive breast cancer[159,160] have supported the principle that the best results are obtained by the combination

of the best chemotherapy with radiation therapy. However, the optimum sequencing of treatment has still to be determined. Knowledge of the mechanism of action of drugs and radiation will help predict favorable and unfavorable combinations.

However, this observation is not universal in oncology. To date, most trials in head and neck or cervix cancer have shown no survival advantage from the use of chemotherapy in addition to radiation therapy.[161] This failure may have resulted partly because the drugs are used to induce regression before the start of radiation therapy. If a major proliferative response has been initiated prior to the start of radiation (despite an impressive clinical regression), a gain is less likely. This raises the whole question of the optimum timing of the two modalities of chemotherapy and radiation therapy: it may be that in certain situations, synchronous therapy will have an advantage over initial chemotherapy to eliminate the effect of proliferation. These forms of trials are still ongoing for many disease sites.

## Radiation Protectors

Considerable research has been devoted to the design or identification of drugs that can protect normal tissues against the effects of ionizing radiation. The goal is to concentrate an effective protector in normal tissue but not in tumor tissue. The principal approaches have been directed toward drugs that inactivate radiation-produced radicals. Sulfhydryl-containing compounds have been shown to be effective in this capacity. Several decades ago, cysteine and cysteamine were found to be powerful protectors of bone marrow in rodents. These compounds were highly toxic to man at doses that were protective against radiation. One sulfhydryl compound has been identified as a potent protector and is much less toxic: WR-2721 [$S$-2-(3 aminopropyl amino)ethylphosphorothiofic acid—now known as amifostine]. Laboratory studies have demonstrated a significant protective effect by WR-2721 at nontoxic doses for a variety of normal tissues, including bone marrow, jejunal crypt cells, intestine, lung, testis, spinal cord, and hair follicles.[162–166] The critical question is whether the drug protects tumors from cytotoxicity. Protection has not been observed for large rodent tumors. However, Milas et al.[164] reported that WR-2721 did protect micrometastases in the lungs from a C3H mouse fibrosarcoma. Clinical studies of WR-2721 have observed protection of human bone marrow by tolerable doses of WR-2721 in patients receiving half-body irradiation. There might be an important clinical role for the topical or regional application (e.g., intra-arterial administration) of radiation protectors to tissues in the treatment volume but outside the target volume.

## The Rationale for the Combination of Surgery and Radiation Therapy

The goals in combining irradiation and surgery are (1) to reduce the extent of surgery and dose of radiation; (2) to achieve a tumor control probability at least as good as with radical surgery or radical irradiation alone; and (3) to achieve a superior cosmetic and functional result. The surgical strategy for the treatment of malignant disease has evolved from local excision to radical resection because of the demonstration that there are microscopic extensions beyond the clinically or radiographically evident lesion. Hence, successful surgery requires that the surgical specimen be enlarged substantially enough to include all the microscopic extensions.

Conservative surgery would remove the grossly evident lesion. Radical surgery includes all the tissues suspected of involvement by subclinical disease. The radiographically evident mass could be resected easily, becoming associated with less functional or cosmetic loss than would obtain for resection of all tissue likely to be involved by subclinical disease. The reverse obtains for the success of radiation therapy. Radiation at moderate dose levels would be expected to inactivate the microscopic extensions of disease, but radical or very high dose levels would be required to kill all cells of the principal tumor mass. Hence, combining moderate dose radiation and conservative surgery should produce a result equivalent to that achieved by extending the surgical procedure from simple excision to radical resection. Combining radiation and surgery on a planned basis has been successful for several anatomical sites—for example, early-stage carcinoma of the breast, sarcoma of soft tissue, and cervical lymph node disease. For patients with carcinoma of the urinary bladder or carcinoma of the rectum, resection still requires removal of the bladder or rectum, but the microscopic extensions are inactivated and the local failure rate is reduced.

The exact strategy for combining irradiation and surgery depends on the local circumstances for the individual anatomical site. The irradiation may be given before, after, or during the surgical procedure. Preoperative irradiation has several advantages:

1. The radiation oncologist and the surgeons plan the overall treatment jointly.
2. Radiation given preoperatively is designed to include only tissues known or suspected of involvement with a clinically significant probability, whereas radiation given postoperatively must include not only the tissues of the tumor bed but all tissues handled during the surgical procedure, including the drain wound. The consequence is that irradiation given postoperatively will in most instances require larger treatment fields. This is particularly the case for complex treatment plans undertaken to minimize the coverage of uninvolved normal tissues.
3. At surgery, there will usually be evident some regression of tumor; the smaller tumor mass facilitates a planned conservative resection.
4. Preoperative irradiation in the amount of about 50 Gy can be confidently expected to inactivate virtually all tumor cells in the microscopic extensions of tumor.

Hence the probability of autotransplantation of tumor in the tumor bed or establishment of metastasis as a consequence of exfoliation of viable tumor cells into the blood vascular spaces is virtually eliminated.

5. There is no delay in the start of irradiation. When radiation is given postoperatively, there may well be a significant delay because of problems in wound healing. The fresh surgical bed should provide excellent growth conditions for residual tumor cells. If there is a substantial delay, there will be an increase in the tumor cell number and thus a decrease in the likelihood of a successful treatment.

The principal disadvantage of giving radiation preoperatively is that there may be increased difficulty in achieving satisfactory primary wound healing. An advantage of radiation given postoperatively is that the entire surgical specimen is available for histopathologic study for determining the histologic grade and pattern of microscopic extensions.

Experiments have been performed to evaluate the effectiveness of preoperative irradiation combined with conservative or radical resectional surgery or amputation in the treatment of C3H mice bearing early-generation isotransplants of the spontaneous fibrosarcoma, FSaII. Figure 2-20A presents dose–response curves (probability of tumor control versus log dose) for single-dose irradiation of 8 mm FSaII isotransplants treated by irradiation alone or irradiation followed by local excision or en bloc excision.[167] There is a sharp shift of the dose–response curve to the left when irradiation is combined with surgery. The displacement in the dose–response curve by going from conservative to radical resection is slight. Figure 2-20B plots the extent of leg shortening against tumor control probability for irradiation given alone or in combination with local or en bloc resection. In this experimental system there was a small but definite gain for irradiation combined with local rather than en bloc resection. Such experimental results, of course, do not represent a perfect model for clinical studies but do indicate that combined-modality treatment results in a

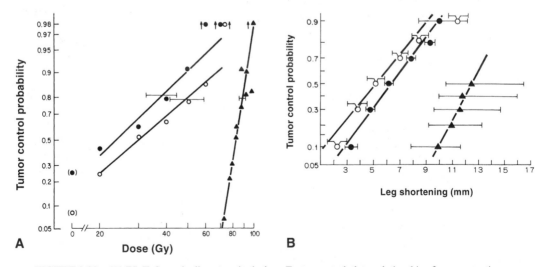

**FIGURE 2-20**  **(A)** FSaII, 8 mm in diameter, single dose. Tumor control–dose relationship after preoperative radiation or radiation alone as treatment of 8 mm tumor. Solid circles, en bloc resection 4 days after radiation; open circles, local resection 4 days after radiation; open circle with parenthesis, local resection alone; solid triangles, radiation alone. The 95% confidence limit is shown at 80% tumor control level. **(B)** Tumor control versus leg shortening for 8 mm tumors, with three different treatment options as shown in **(A)**.

major reduction in dose required to achieve a given tumor control probability.

## NEW APPROACHES TO OPTIMIZE RADIATION THERAPY

### Modulation of Apoptosis to Increase Tumor Cell Kill or Protect Normal Tissues

The tumor suppressor gene *p53* is critically involved in both $G_1$ arrest and apoptosis induction in response to DNA damage.[168] The ultimate importance of apoptosis to radiation-induced loss of clonogenicity remains to be clarified. Based on the initial observations that cells without wild-type *p53* function did not undergo $G_1$ arrest,[88] it was expected that cells with mutant or no *p53* would be radiation sensitive because they would replicate prior to repairing their DNA.[169] Although a few reports have shown increased radiation sensitivity in association with loss of wild-type *p53* function, most reports have shown no difference or increased radiation resistance with the loss of wild-type *p53* function.[89] The increased resistance is predominantly due to the lack of radiation-induced apoptosis. This conclusion stems from studying cells of hematopoietic origin[170,171] or transformed fibroblasts.[172] Human uroepithelial cells, immortalized by the E6 protein of human papillomavirus, have low or no detectable *p53* and do not exhibit radiation-induced apoptosis, while their E7-immortalized counterparts, with wild-type *p53,* do undergo apoptosis when exposed to ionizing radiation.[173] This last study is particularly interesting because the authors report that the normal, E6- and E7-immortalized cells had similar survival, based on 96-hour trypan blue exclusion, despite the differences in apoptosis levels. This suggests that the presence of functional p53 protein may change the mode of cell death, but not the ultimate amount of cell death after irradiation. This possibility raises problems about the validity of the end point when only apoptosis after exposure to a genotoxic agent is scored.

What is the clinical relevance of apoptosis in radiation oncology? Because of the observations in murine tumors that increased pretreatment apoptosis levels correlate with increased radiation-induced apoptosis, longer tumor growth delays, and lower $TCD_{50}$ values, studies were undertaken to determine whether the pretreatment apoptotic index correlates with response of patients' tumors to radiotherapy. Thus far, results are contradictory. Two papers, one on cervical adenocarcinoma and one on transitional cell carcinoma of the bladder, have concluded that the higher the pretreatment apoptosis level in biopsy samples from patients' tumors, the better the response to radiotherapy.[174,175] In contrast, another report on cervical carcinoma concluded that patients whose biopsy samples showed pretherapy apoptosis levels above the median had worse survival rates than patients with apoptosis indices below the median.[176]

When considering the relevance of apoptosis to radiation therapy for cancer, many questions remain: Do some tumor types that were thought not to undergo apoptosis after irradiation in fact die by that mode but after longer times? Do proliferating cells that undergo late apoptosis divide one or more times between the radiation exposure and expression of apoptosis? Are these cells responding to a persistent lesion that remains in the cells through one or more cell cycles or to a lesion created by replication of damaged DNA? Are proliferating cells more susceptible to radiation-induced apoptosis than quiescent cells, or vice versa? Does apoptosis contribute significantly to the loss of clonogenic cell survival or to tumor cure at long times after radiation exposure?

An example of the potential significance of these questions is apparent in recent clinical studies undertaken by the Radiation Therapy Oncology Group (RTOG). In a randomized prospective trial, this group has shown increased local control of advanced prostate tumors and improved survival in patients treated with combined androgen deprivation and ionizing radiation.[177] It is well documented that androgen deprivation causes apoptosis in normal prostatic tissue,[178,179] and prostate tumor cells have been shown to undergo apoptosis after radiation exposure.[180] In the clinical setting, important questions regarding the timing and duration of hormone treatment relative to radiation treatment are unanswered, but are the subject of ongoing protocols.

Manipulation of apoptosis in concert with radiation therapy might have therapeutic benefit, but obtaining additional biological information about radiation-induced apoptosis will be important in the design of new treatment regimens. This paradigm has been explored by Fuks and others, who have demonstrated that basic fibroblast growth factor can protect the lung against radiation-induced injury mediated via apoptosis.[181] The other goal will be to devise methods to increase radiation-induced apoptosis in tumors. Hormonal manipulations will be useful in only a proportion of tumors, or perhaps in only a subset of cells within any individual tumor. Understanding the mechanism of radiation-induced apoptosis will become increasingly important: membrane manipulations via ceramide and sphingomyelinase have been reported to play a major role.[182,183] An additional variable is in vivo versus in vitro irradiation: studies published to date suggest that cells irradiated in vivo undergo apoptosis much more rapidly than cells irradiated in vitro. The factors, presumably including environmental factors (cytokines, hormones, oxygenation, etc.) that may be involved in this difference have yet to be determined.

## Tumor Angiogenesis as a Target for Therapy

Tumor hypervascularity was initially thought to reflect inflammatory vasodilation of preexisting host vessels, a response to tumor metabolites and necrotic tumor products that was of no benefit to the tumor. Another point of view was that tumor growth and metastasis depend on angiogenesis and that a chemical signal from tumor cells can shift resting endothelial cells into a phase of rapid growth. These ideas were not widely accepted at first, but a clear concept of the role of angiogenesis in cancer and other diseases has now emerged.[184]

Most tumors in humans persist in situ for months to years without neovascularization but become vascularized when a subgroup of cells in the tumor "switches" to an angiogenic phenotype. In the prevascular phase, the tumor is rarely larger than 2 to 3 mm and may contain a million or more cells. Such asymptomatic lesions are sometimes directly visible on the skin or cervix or in the bladder, but usually they are clinically undetectable. Cells in prevascular tumors or dormant micrometastases may replicate as rapidly as those in expanding, vascularized tumors; but without the growth of new vessels, the rate of proliferation of such cells reaches equilibrium with their rate of death.

The switch to the angiogenic phenotype involves a change in the local equilibrium between positive and negative regulators of the growth of microvessels. Tumor cells may overexpress one or more of the positive regulators of angiogenesis, may mobilize an angiogenic protein from the extracellular matrix, may recruit host cells such as macrophages (which produce their own angiogenic proteins), or may engage in a combination of these processes. Of the known angiogenic proteins, those most commonly found in tumors appear to be basic fibroblast growth factor (bFGF) and vascular endothelial growth factor (also known as vascular permeability factor). The angiogenic activities of these two factors can be synergistic. Upregulation of an angiogenic factor is not sufficient in itself for a tumor cell to become angiogenic. Certain negative regulators or inhibitors of vessel growth may need to be downregulated. These endogenous inhibitors defend the vascular endothelium from mitogenic stimuli. More than a trillion endothelial cells line the inside of blood vessels and cover an area of approximately $1000 \text{ m}^2$ in a 70 kg adult. The turnover time of these normally quiescent cells can exceed 1000 days; during angiogenesis, however, capillary endothelial cells can proliferate as rapidly as bone marrow cells, which have a mean turnover time of 5 days.

From a clinical perspective, neovascularization permits tumors to grow and metastasize; it also heralds the onset of symptoms. Most tumors become symptomatic and clinically detectable only after neovascularization. It should be emphasized, however, that the switch to the angiogenic phenotype does not always result in a rapidly proliferating tumor. Moreover, in distant metastases, angiogenesis may be suppressed by circulating inhibitors from a primary tumor and may become apparent only after its removal.

Paradoxically, neovascularization gradually reduces a tumor's accessibility to chemotherapeutic drugs. Tumors do not outgrow their blood supply but instead compress it. By the time they are clinically detectable, increased interstitial pressure from leaky vessels in the tumor, and the relative absence of intratumor lymphatics, cause vascular compression and eventually central necrosis. Thus, it is not surprising that in rodents antiangiogenic therapy increases the delivery of chemotherapy to a tumor, probably by lowering interstitial pressure and unpacking the mass of tumor cells. Recent evidence has shown that antiangiogenesis strategies can achieve complete and long-term regression for murine tumors and result in prolonged tumor regression in the absence of cytotoxic chemotherapy.[185] The application of this approach to the treatment of human cancer is eagerly awaited.

# REFERENCES

1. Thompson LH, Suit HD: Proliferation kinetics of x-irradiated mouse L cells studied with time lapse photography methods and data analysis. *Int J Radiat Biol* 1967;13:391–397.

2. Morgan WF, Day JP, Kaplan MI, McGhee EM, Limoli CL: Genomic instability induced by ionizing radiation. *Radiat Res* 1996;146(3):247–258.

3. Puck TT, Marcus PI: A rapid method for viable cell titration and clone production with HeLa cells in tissue culture: The use of x-irradiated cells to supply conditioning factors. *Proc Natl Acad Sci USA* 1955; 41: 432–437.

4. Puck TT, Marcus PI: Action of x-rays on mammalian cells. *J Exp Med* 1956;105:653–666.

5. Puck TT, Morkovin D, Marcus PI, et al: Action of x-rays on mammalian cells: Survival curves of cells from normal human tissues. *J Exp Med* 1957;485–500.

6. Rogers RW, von Borstel RC: Alpha-particle bombardment of the *Habrobracon* egg. 1. Sensitivity of the nucleus. *Radiat Res* 1957;7: 484–490.

7. Person S: Comparative killing efficiencies for decays of tritiated compounds incorporated into *E. coli. Biophys J* 1963;3:183–187.

8. Djordjevic B, Szybalski W: Genetics of human cell lines. III: Incorporation of 5-bromo- and 5-iodo-deoxyuridine into the deoxyribonucleic acid of human cells and its effect on radiation sensitivity. *J Exp Med* 1960; 112:509–531.

9. Kaplan HS, Smith KC, Tomlin PA: Radiosensitization of *E. coli* by purine and pyrimidine analogues incorporated in deoxyribonucleic acid. *Nature* 1961;190:794–796.

10. Warters RL, Hofer KG, Harris CR: Radionuclide toxicity in cultured mammalian cells: Elucidation of the primary site of radiation damage. *Curr Top Radiat Res Q* 1977;12:389–407.

11. Nikjoo H, Uehara S, Wilson WE, Hoshi M, Goodhead DT: Track structure in radiation biology: Theory and applications. *Int J Radiat Biol* 1998;73(4):355–364.

12. Sham E, Durand RE: Cell kinetics and repopulation mechanisms during multifraction irradiation of spheroids. *Radiother Oncol* 1998;46(2):201–207.

13. Ward JF: Biochemistry of DNA lesions. *Radiat Res Suppl* 1985;8:S103–S111.

14. Bootsma D, Hoeijmakers JH: DNA repair. Engagement with transcription. *Nature* 1993;363 (6425):114–115.

15. Kolodner R: Biochemistry and genetics of eukaryotic mismatch repair. *Genes Dev* 1996;10(12):1433–1442.

16. Aurias A, Antoine JL, Assathiany R, Odievre M, Dutrillaux B: Radiation sensitivity of Bloom's syndrome lymphocytes during S and G2 phases. *Cancer Genet Cytogenet* 1985;16(2):131–136.

17. Fulop GM, Phillips RA: The *scid* mutation in mice causes a general defect in DNA repair. *Nature* 1990;347:479–482.

18. Biedermann KA, Sun JR, Giaccia AJ, Tosto LM, Brown JM: *scid* mutation in mice confers hypersensitivity to ionizing radiation and a deficiency in DNA double-strand break repair. *Proc Natl Acad Sci USA* 1991;88(4):1394–1397.

19. Hendrickson EA, Qin XQ, Bump EA, Schatz DG, Oettinger M, Weaver DT: A link between double-strand break-related repair and V(D)J recombination: The *scid* mutation. *Proc Natl Acad Sci USA* 1991;88(10):4061–4065.

20. Jeggo PA: DNA–PK: At the cross-roads of biochemistry and genetics. *Mutat Res* 1997; 384(1):1–14.

21. Cox R, Debenham PG, Masson WK, et al: Ataxia-telangiectasia: A human mutation giving high-frequency mis-repair of DNA double-stranded scissions. *Mol Biol Med* 1986;3:229–244.

22. Powell S, Whitaker S, Peacock J, McMillan T: Ataxia telangiectasia: An investigation of the repair defect in the cell line AT5BIVA by plasmid reconstitution. *Mutat Res* 1993;294(1): 9–20.

23. Powell SN, McMillan TJ: The repair fidelity of restriction enzyme-induced double strand breaks in plasmid DNA correlates with radioresistance in human tumor cell lines. *Int J Radiat Oncol Biol Phys* 1994;29(5):1035–1040.

24. Till JE, McCulloch EA: A direct measurement of the radiation sensitivity of normal mouse bone marrow cells. *Radiat Res* 1961;14:213–222.

25. Withers HR: Recovery and repopulation in vivo by mouse skin epithelial cells during fractionated irradiation. *Radiat Res* 1967;32:227–239.

26. Withers HR, Elkind MM: Radiosensitivity and fractionation response of crypt cells of mouse jejunum. *Radiat Res* 1969;38:598–613.

27. Thames HD, Withers R, Mason KA, et al: Dose–survival characteristics of mouse jejunal crypt cells. *Int J Radiat Oncol Biol Phys* 1981;7:1591–1597.

28. Smith LH, Vos O: Radiation sensitivity of mouse lymph node cells relative to their proliferative capacity in vivo. *Radiat Res* 1963;19:485–491.

29. Chen KY, Withers HR: Survival characteristics of stem cells of gastric mucosa in C3H mice subjected to localized gamma irradiation. *Int J Radiat Biol* 1972;21:521–534.

30. Withers HR, Mason KA:The kinetics of recovery in irradiated colonic mucosa of the mouse. *Cancer* 1974;34:896–903.

31. Reinhold HS, Buisman GH: Repair of radiation damage to capillary endothelium. *Br J Radiol* 1975;48:727–731.

32. Mulcahy RT, Gould MN, Clifton KH: The survival of thyroid cells: In vivo irradiation and in situ repair. *Radiat Res* 1980;84:523–528.

33. Guichard M, Deschavanne PJ, Malaise EP: Radiosensitivity of mouse lung cells measured using an in vitro colony method. *Int J Radiat Oncol Biol Phys* 1980;6:441–447.

34. Deschavanne PH, Guichard M, Malaise EP: Repair of sublethal and potentially lethal damage in lung cells using an in vitro colony method. *Br J Radiol* 1981;54:973–977.

35. Withers HR, Mason KA, Thames HD: Late radiation response of kidney assayed by tubule cell survival. *Br J Radiol* 1986;59:587–595.

36. Porten CS, Chase HB: Radiation depigmentation of mouse hair: Split-dose experiments and metanocyte precursors (amelanotic melanoblasts) in the resting hair follicle. *Radiat Res* 1970;42:305–319.

37. Withers HR, Hunter N, Barkley HT, et al: Radiation survival and regeneration characteristics of spermatogenic stem cells of mouse testis. *Radiat Res* 1974;57:88–103.

38. Hewitt HB, Wilson CW: A survival curve for mammalian leukemia cells irradiated in vivo. *Br J Cancer* 1959;13:69–75.

39. Berry RJ, Andrews JR: Quantitative relationships between radiation dose and the reproductive capacity of tumor cells in a mammalian system in vivo. *Radiology* 1961;77:824–830.

40. Bush RS, Bruce WR: The radiation sensitivity of transplanted lymphoma cells as determined by the spleen colony method. *Radiat Res* 1964;21:612–621.

41. Powers WE, Tolmach LJ: Demonstration of an anoxic component in a mouse tumor-cell population by in vivo assay of survival following irradition. *Radiology* 1964;83:328–336.

42. Reinhold HS: Quantitative evaluation of the radiosensitivity of cells of a transplantable rhabdomyosarcoma in the rat. *Eur J Cancer* 1966;2:33–42.

43. Urano M, Fukada N, Ando K, et al: Tumor control and regrowth probability after a single

radiation of experimental animal tumors. *J Natl Cancer Inst* 1974;53:517–524.

44. Urano M, Goitein M, Verhey L, et al: Relative biological effectiveness of a high energy modulated proton beam using a spontaneous murine tumor in vivo. *Int J Radiat Oncol Biol Phys* 1984;10:509–514.

45. Urano M, Nesumi N, Ando K, et al: Repair of potentially lethal radiation damage in acute and chronically hypoxic tumor cells in vivo. *Radiology* 1976;118:447–451.

46. Malaise E, Fertil B, Chavaudra N, et al: Distribution of radiation sensitivities for human tumor cells of specific histological types: Comparison of in vitro to in vivo data. *Int J Radiat Oncol Biol Phys* 1986;12:617–634.

47. Palcic B, Brosing JW, Skarsgard LD: Survival measurements at low doses: Oxygen enhancement ratio. *Br J Cancer* 1982;46:980–984.

48. Chapman JD, Gillespie CJ, Reuvers AP, et al: The inactivation of Chinese hamster cells by x-rays: The effects of chemical modifiers on single and double-events. *Radiat Res* 1975;64:365–375.

49. Urano M, Kahn J, Kenton LA: Unpublished data, 1987.

50. Tucker SL, Withers HR, Mason KA, et al: A dose–surviving fraction curve for mouse colonic mucosa. *Eur J Cancer* 1983;19:433–437.

51. Thames HD, Ang KK: Altered fractionation: Radiobiological principles, clinical results, and potential for dose escalation. *Cancer Treat Res* 1998;93:101–128.

52. Millar BC, Fielden EM, Miller JL: Interpretation of survival-curve data for Chinese hamster cells, V-79, using the multi-target with initial slope and $\alpha,\beta$ equation. *Int J Radiat Oneol Biol Phys* 1978;33:599–603.

53. Zeman EM, Bedford JS: Dose rate effects in mammalian cells: V. Dose fractionation effects in non-cycling C3H 10T 1/2 Cells. *Int J Radiat Oncol Biol Phys* 1984;10:2089–2098.

54. Elkind MM, Sutton H: X-ray damage and recovery in mammalian cells in culture. *Nature* 1959;184:1293–1295.

55. Winans LF, Dewey WC, Dettor CM: Repair of sublethal and potentially lethal x-ray damage in synchronous Chinese hamster cells. *Radiat Res* 1972;52:333–351.

56. Phillips RA, Tolmach LJ: Repair of potentially lethal damage in X-irradiated HeLa cells. *Radiat Res* 1966;29:413–432.

57. Little JB: Repair of sub-lethal and potentially lethal radiation damage in plateau phase cultures of human cells. *Nature* 1969;224:804–806.

58. Little JB, Hahn GM, Frindel E, et al: Repair of potentially lethal radiation damage in vitro and in vivo. *Radiology* 1973;106:689–694.

59. Weichselbaum RR: Radioresistant and repair-proficient cells may determine radiocurability in human tumors. *Int J Radiat Oncol Biol Phys* 1986;12:637–639.

60. Gray LH: The concentration of oxygen dissolved in tissue at the time of radiation as a factor in radiotherapy. *Br J Radiol* 1953;26:638–648.

61. Guyton AC: *Textbook of Medical Physiology.* Philadephia, Saunders, 1976, p 545.

62. Thomlinson RH, Gray LH: Histological structure of some human lung cancers and possible implications for radiotherapy. *Br J Cancer* 1955;9:539–549.

63. Ling CC, Michaels HB, Gerweck L, et al: Oxygen sensitization of mammalian cells under different irradiation conditions. *Radiat Res* 1981;86:325–340.

64. Revesz L, Paicic B: Radiation dose dependence on the sensitization by oxygen and oxygen mimic sensitizers. *Acta Radiol* 1985;24:209–217.

65. Taylor YC, Brown JM: Radiosensitization in multifraction schedules. I. Evidence for an extremely low oxygen enhancement ratio. *Radiat Res* 1987;112:124–133.

66. Dasu A, Denekamp J: New insights into factors influencing the clinically relevant oxygen enhancement ratio. *Radiother Oncol* 1998;46(3):269–277.

67. Graeber TG, Peterson JF, Tsai M, Monica K, Fornace AJ Jr, Giaccia AJ: Hypoxia induces accumulation of p53 protein, but activation of a G1-phase checkpoint by low-oxygen conditions is independent of p53 status. *Mol Cell Biol* 1994;14(9):6264–6277.

68. Graeber TG, Osmanian C, Jacks T, Housman DE, Koch CJ, Lowe SW, Giaccia AJ: Hypoxia-mediated selection of cells with diminished

apoptotic potential in solid tumors. *Nature* 1996;379:88–91.

69. Ratcliffe PJ, O'Rourke JF, Maxwell PH, Pugh CW: Oxygen sensing, hypoxia-inducible factor-1 and the regulation of mammalian gene expression. *J Exp Biol* 1998;201:1153–1162.

70. Spiro IJ, Kennedy KA, Stickler R, et al: Cellular and molecular repair of x-ray induced damage: Dependence on oxygen tension and nutritional status. *Radiat Res* 1985;101:144–155.

71. Gupta V, Rangata NS, Belli JA: Enhancement of radiation sensitivity by postradiation hypoxia. *Radiat Res* 1986;106:132–136.

72. Suit HD, Urano M: Repair of sublethal radiation injury in hypoxic cells of a C3H mouse mammary carcinoma. *Radiat Res* 1969;37:423–443.

73. Brown JM: Evidence for acutely hypoxic cells in mouse turnouts, and a possible mechanism of reoxygenation. *Br J Radiol* 1979;52:650–656.

74. Jain RK: Integrative pathophysiology of solid tumors: role in detection and treatment. *Sci Am* 1998;4 suppl 1: S48–S57.

75. Jain RK: 1995 Whitaker Lecture: Delivery of molecules, particles, and cells to solid tumors. *Ann Biomed Eng* 1996;24(4):457–473.

76. Thomlinson RH: The effect of fractionated irradiation on the proportion of anoxic cells in an intact experimental turnout. *Br J Radiol* 1966;39:158.

77. Kaltman RF: The phenomenon of reoxygenation and its implication for fractionated radiotherapy. *Radiology* 1972;105:135–142.

78. Howard A, Pelc SR: Synthesis of deoxyribonucleic acid in normal and irradiated cells in its relationship to chromosome breakage. *Heredity* 1952;6(suppl):216.

79. Hartwell LH, Kastan MB: Cell cycle control and cancer. *Science* 1994;266:1821–1828.

80. Masui Y: A quest for cytoplasmic factors that control the cell cycle. *Prog Cell Cycle Res* 1996;2:1–13.

81. Smith HS, Pardee AB: Accumulation of a protein required for division during the cell cycle of *Escherichia coli*. *J Bacteriol* 1970;101(3):901–909.

82. Hartwell LH: *Saccharomyces cerevisiae* cell cycle. *Bacteriol Rev* 1974;38(2):164–198.

83. Nurse P: Genetic control of cell size at cell division in yeast. *Nature* 1975;256(5518):457–461.

84. Maller JL: MPF and cell cycle control. *Adv Second Mess Phosphoprotein Res* 1990;24:323–328.

85. Evans T, Rosenthal ET, Youngblom J, Distel D, Hunt T: Cyclin: A protein specified by maternal mRNA in sea urchin eggs that is destroyed at each cleavage division. *Cell* 1983;33(2):389–396.

86. Murray AW, Solomon MJ, Kirschner MW: The role of cyclin synthesis and degradation in the control of maturation promoting factor activity. *Nature* 1989;339: 280–286.

87. Weinert TA, Hartwell LH: The *RAD9* gene controls the cell cycle response to DNA damage in *Saccharomyces cerevisiae*. *Science* 1988;241:317–322.

88. Kastan MB, Onyekwere O, Sidransky D, Vogelstein B, Craig RW: Participation of p53 protein in the cellular response to DNA damage. *Cancer Res* 1991;51:6304–6411.

89. Bristow RG, Benchimol S, Hill RP: The *p53* gene as a modifier of intrinsic radiosensitivity: Implications for radiotherapy. *Radiother Oncol* 1996;40(3):197–223.

90. Terasima T, Tolmach LJ: Variations in several responses of HeLa cells to x-irradiation during the division cycle. *Biophys J* 1963;3:11–33.

91. Sinclair WK: Cyclic x-ray responses in mammalian cells in vitro. *Radiat Res* 1968;33: 620–643.

92. Steel GG: *Growth Kinetics of Tumours*. Oxford, Clarendon Press, 1977.

93. Gray JW, Dolbeare F, Pallavicini MG, et al: Cell cycle analysis using flow cytometry. *Int J Radiat Biol* 1986;49:237–255.

94. Porten CS: Cell cycles in cell hierarchies. *Int J Radiat Biol* 1986;49:257–278.

95. Hall EJ: Radiation dose-rate: A factor of importance in radiobiology and radiotherapy (review). *Br J Radiol* 1972;45:81–97.

96. Mitchell JB, Bedford JS, Bailey SM: Dose-rate effects in plateau-phase cultures of S3 HeLa and V79 Cells. *Radiat Res* 1979;79: 552–567.

97. Mitchell JB, Bedford JS, Bailey SM: Dose rate effects in mammalian cells in culture. III. Comparison of cell killing and cell proliferation during continuous irradiation for six different cell lines. *Radiat Res* 1979;79: 537–551.

98. Steel GG: The ESTRO Breur Lecture. Cellular sensitivity to low dose-rate irradiation focuses the problem of tumour radioresistance. *Radiother Oncol* 1991;20(2):71–83.

99. Bacq Z, Alexander P: *Fundamentals of Radiobiology,* 2nd ed. New York, Pergamon Press, 1961, p 22.

100. Shipley WU, Stanley JA, Courtenay VD, et al: Repair of radiation damage in Lewis lung carcinoma cells following in situ treatment with fast neutrons and x-rays. *Cancer Res* 1975;35:932–938.

101. Hall EJ, Roizin-Towle L, Theus RB, et al: Radiobiological properties of high-energy cyclotron-produced neutrons used for radiotherapy. *Radiology* 1975;117:173–178.

102. Raju MR, Bain E, Carpenter SG, et al: Effects of argon ions on synchronized Chinese hamster cells. *Radiat Res* 1980;84:152–157.

103. Barendsen GW: Res tumours and normal different linear energy, in A Howard (ed): *Current Research,* vol 4. Amsterdam, 1968, pp 283.

104. Field SB, Hornsey S: Tissue, in GW Barendsen et al (eds): *High LET Radiotherapy.* Oxford, pp 181–186.

105. Fletcher GH: *Textbook of Radiotherapy,* 2nd ed, Philadelphia, Lea & Febiger, 1975, p 145.

106. Fertil B, Malaise EP: Inherent cellular radiosensitivity as a basic concept for human tumor radiotherapy. *Int J Radiat Oncol Biol Phys* 1981;7:621–629.

107. Deacon J, Peckham MH, Steel GG: The radioresponsiveness of human turnouts and the initial slope of the cell survival curve. *Radiother Oncol* 1984;2:317–323.

108. Rofstad EK, Wahl A, Brustad T: Radiation sensitivity in vitro of cells isolated from human tumor surgical specimens. *Cancer Res* 1987;47:106–110.

109. Brock WA, Baker F, Peters LJ: Radiosensitivity of human head and neck squamous cell carcinomas in primary culture and its potential as a predictive assay of tumor radiocurability. *Int J Radiat Biol* 1989;56:751–760.

110. West CM, Davidson SE, Elyan SA, Swindell R, Roberts SA, Orton CJ, Coyle CA, Valentine H, Wilks DP, Hunter RD, Hendry JH: The intrinsic radiosensitivity of normal and tumour cells. *Int J Radiat Biol* 1998;73(4):409–413.

111. Taghian A, Ramsay J, Allalunis-Turner J, Budach W, Gioioso D, Pardo F, Okunieff P, Bleehen N, Urtasun R, Suit H: Intrinsic radiation sensitivity may not be the major determinant of the poor clinical outcome of glioblastoma multiforme. *Int J Radiat Oncol Biol Phys* 1993;25(2):243–249.

112. Geara FB, Peters LJ, Ang KK, Wike JL, Sivon SS, Guttenberger R, Callender DL, Malaise EP, Brock WA: Intrinsic radiosensitivity of normal human fibroblasts and lymphocytes after high- and low-dose-rate irradiation. *Cancer Res* 1992;52(22):6348–6352.

113. Price P, McMillan TJ: Use of the tetrazolium assay in measuring the response of human tumor cells to ionizing radiation. *Cancer Res* 1990;50(5):1392–1396.

114. Budach W, Hartford A, Gioioso D, Freeman J, Taghian A, Suit HD: Tumors arising in SCID mice share enhanced radiation sensitivity of SCID normal tissues. *Cancer Res* 1992;52(22):6292–6296.

115. Hill RP, Bush RS: A lung-colony assay to determine the radiosensitivity of the cells of a solid tumor. *Int J Radiat Biol* 1969;15:435–444.

116. Budach W, Taghian A, Freeman J, Gioioso D, Suit HD: Impact of stromal sensitivity on radiation response of tumors. *J Natl Cancer Inst* 1993;85(12):988–993.

117. O'Reilly MS, Boehm T, Shing Y, Fukai N, Vasios G, Lane WS, Flynn E, Birkhead JR, Olsen BR, Folkman J: Endostatin: An endogenous inhibitor of angiogenesis and tumor growth. *Cell* 1997;88(2):277–285.

118. O'Reilly MS, Holmgren L, Shing Y, Chen C, Rosenthal RA, Moses M, Lane WS, Cao Y, Sage EH, Folkman J: Angiostatin: A novel angiogenesis inhibitor that mediates the suppression of metastases by a Lewis lung carcinoma. *Cell* 1994;79(2):315–328.

119. Thomlinson RH: The oxygen effect in mammals, in *Brookhaven Symposia in Biology,* no 14; *Fundamental Aspects of Radiosensitivity.* Upton, NY, Brookhaven National Laboratory, 1961, p 675(C-31) (Biology and Medicine TlD 4500, ed 16).

120. Thomlinson RH: Oxygen therapy—Biological considerations, in TJ Deeley, and CAP Wood (eds): *Modern Trends in Radiotherapy.* London, Camelot Press, 1967, pp 52–72.

121. Urano M, Suit HD: Experimental evaluation of tumor bed effect of C3H mouse mammary carcinoma and for C3H mouse fibrosarcoma. *Radiat Res* 1971;45:41–49.

122. Milas L, Ito H, Hunter N, et al: Retardation of tumor growth in mice caused by radiation-induced injury of tumor bed stroma: Dependency on tumor type. *Cancer Res* 1996;46:723–727.

123. Suit HD, Shalek RJ, Wette R: Radiation response of C3H mouse mammary carcinoma evaluated in terms of cellular radiation sensitivity, in RJ Shalek, et al (eds): *Cellular Radiation Biology.* Baltimore, Williams & Wilkins, 1965, pp 514–530.

124. Suit HD: Radiation biology: A basis for radiotherapy, in GH Fletcher (ed): *Textbook of Radiotherapy.* Philadelphia, Lea & Febiger, 1973, pp 75–121.

125. Suit HD, Silobrcic V: Tumor-specific antigen(s) in a spontaneous mammary carcinoma of C3H mice. 11. Active immunization of mammary tumor agent free mice. *J Natl Cancer Inst* 1967;39:1121–1128.

126. Suit HD, Maeda M: Hyperbaric oxygen and radiobiology of a C3H mouse mammary carcinoma. *J Natl Cancer Inst* 1967;39:639–652.

127. Suit HD: Response to x-irradiation of a tumor recurring after a TCD95 radiation dose. *Nature* 1966;211:996–997.

128. Ando K, Koike S, Ikehira H, et al: Increased radiosensitivity of a recurrent murine fibresarcoma following radiotherapy. *Jpn J Cancer Res* 1985;76:99–103.

129. Foley EJ: Antigenic properties of methylcholanthrene-induced tumors in mice of the strain of origin. *Cancer Res* 1953;13:835–837.

130. Suit HD, Kastelan A: Immunologic status of host and response of a methylcholanthrene-induced sarcoma to local x-irradiation. *Cancer* 1970;26:232–238.

131. Withers HR: Biologic basis for altered fractionation schemes. *Cancer* 1985;55:2086–2095.

132. Williams MV, Denekamp J, Fowler JF: A review of alpha/beta ratios for experimental tumors: Implications for clinical studies of altered fractionation. *Int J Radiat Oncol Biol Phys* 1985;11:87–96.

133. Suit HD: Modification of radiation response. *Int J Radiat Oncol Biol Phys* 1984;10:101–108.

134. Fowler JF: La ronde—Radiation sciences and medical Radiology. *Radiother Oncol* 1983;1:1–22.

135. Mueller-Klieser W, Vaupel P, Manz R, et al: Intracapillary oxyhemoglobin saturation of malignant tumors in humans. *Int J Radiat Oncol Biol Phys* 1981;7:1397–1404.

136. Wendling P, Manz R, Thews G, et al: Heterogeneous oxygenation of rectal carcinomas in humans: A critical parameter for preoperative irradiation? in D Bruley, HI Bieber, and D Roneau (eds): *Oxygen Transport to Tissue,* vol 6. New York, Plenum Publishing, 1985, pp 293–300.

137. Mueller-Klieser W, Vaupel P: Tumour oxygenation under normobaric and hyperbaric conditions. *Br J Radiol* 1983;56:559–564.

138. Howes AE, Suit HD: The effect of time between fractions on the response of tumors to irradiation. *Radiat Res* 1974;57:342–348.

139. Henk JM: Late results of a trial of hyperbaric oxygen and radiotherapy in head and neck cancer. A rationale for hypoxic cell sensitizers? *Int J Radiat Oncol Biol Phys* 1986;12:1339–1341.

140. Bush RS, Jenkin RDT, Allt WEC, et al: Definitive evidence for hypoxic cells influencing cure in cancer therapy. *Br J Cancer* 1978; 37(suppl 111):302–306.

141. Overgaard J, Hansen HS, Jorgensen K, et al: Primary radiotherapy of larynx and pharynx carcinoma—An analysis of some factors influencing local control and survival. *Int J Radiat Oncol Biol Phys* 1986;12:515–521.

142. Fowler JF: Fractionated radiation therapy after Strandqvist. *Acta Radiol Oncol* 1984;23(4):209–216.

143. Wang CC: Local control of oropharyngeal carcinoma after two accelerated hyperfractionation radiation therapy schemes. *Int J Radiat Oncol Biol Phys* 1988;14(6):1143–1146.

144. Garden AS, Morrison WH, Ang KK, Peters LJ: Hyperfractionated radiation in the treatment of squamous cell carcinomas of the head and neck: A comparison of two fractionation schedules. *Int J Radiat Oncol Biol Phys* 1995;31(3):493–502.

145. Horiot JC, Bontemps P, van den Bogaert W, Le Fur R, van den Weijngaert D, Bolla M,

Bernier J, Lusinchi A, Stuschke M, Lopez-Torrecilla J, Begg AC, Pierart M, Collette L: Accelerated fractionation (AF) compared to conventional fractionation (CF) improves loco regional control in the radiotherapy of advanced head and neck cancers: results of the EORTC 22851 randomized trial. *Radiother Oncol* 1997;44(2):111–121.

146. Begg AC, Hofland I, Moonen L, Bartelink H, Schraub S, Bontemps P, Le Fur R, Van Den Bogaert W, Caspers R, Van Glabbeke M, et al: The predictive value of cell kinetic measurements in a European trial of accelerated fractionation in advanced head and neck tumors: An interim report. *Int J Radiat Oncol Biol Phys* 1990;19(6):1449–1453.

147. Littbrand B, Edsmyr F, Revesz L: A low dose-fractionation scheme for the radiotherapy of carcinoma of the bladder. Experimental background and preliminary results. *Bull Cancer* 1975;62(3):241–248.

148. Fallai C, Olmi P: Hyperfractionated and accelerated radiation therapy in central nervous system tumors (malignant gliomas, pediatric tumors, and brain metastases). *Radiother Oncol* 1997;43(3):235–246.

149. Ang KK, Price RE, Stephens LC, Jiang GL, Feng Y, Schultheiss TE, Peters LJ: The tolerance of primate spinal cord to re-irradiation. *Int J Radiat Oncol Biol Phys* 1993;25(3):459–464.

150. Dische SN, Saunders MI: Continuous, hyperfractionated, accelerated radiotherapy (CHART): An interim report upon late morbidity. *Radiother Oncol* 1989;16(1):65–72.

151. Saunders M, Dische S, Barrett A, Harvey A, Gibson D, Parmar M: Continuous hyperfractionated accelerated radiotherapy (CHART) versus conventional radiotherapy in non-small-cell lung cancer: A randomised multicentre trial. CHART Steering Committee. *Lancet* 1997;350(9072):161–165; Dische S, Saunders M, Barrett A, Harvey A, Gibson D, Parmar M: A randomised multicentre trial of CHART versus conventional radiotherapy in head and neck cancer. *Radiother Oncol* 1997;44(2):123–136.

152. Pierquin B, Calitchi E, Mazeron JJ, Le Bourgeois JP, Leung S: Update on low dose rate irradiation for cancers of the oropharynx—May 1986. *Int J Radiat Oncol Biol Phys* 1987; 13(2):259–261.

153. Ellis F: Nominal standard dose and the ret. *Br J Radiol* 1971;44(518):101–108.

154. Ulmer W: On the problem of time, dose and fractionation (TDF) in the linear–quadratic model. *Strahlentherapie* 1985;161(3):177–185.

155. Steel GG: Terminology in the description of drug-radiation interactions. *Int J Radiat Oncol Biol Phys* 1979;5:1145–1150.

156. Mitchell JB, Russo A, Kinsella TJ, et al: The use of non-hypoxic cell sensitizers in radiobiology and radiotherapy. *Int J Radiat Biol Oncol Phys* 1986;12:1513–1518.

157. Maase H, Overgaard J: Interactions of radiation and cancer chemotherapeutic drugs in a C3H mouse mammary carcinoma. *Acta Radiol Oncol* 1985;24:181–187.

158. Hortobagyi GN: Comprehensive management of locally advanced breast cancer. *Cancer* 1990;66(6 suppl):1387–1391.

159. Overgaard M, Hansen PS, Overgaard J, Rose C, Andersson M, Bach F, Kjaer M, Gadeberg CC, Mouridsen HT, Jensen MB, Zedeler K: Postoperative radiotherapy in high-risk premenopausal women with breast cancer who receive adjuvant chemotherapy. Danish Breast Cancer Cooperative Group 82b Trial. *N Eng J Med* 1997;337(14):949–955.

160. Ragaz J, Jackson SM, Le N, Plenderleith IH, Spinelli JJ, Basco VE, Wilson KS, Knowling MA, Coppin CM, Paradis M, Coldman AJ, Olivotto IA: Adjuvant radiotherapy and chemotherapy in node-positive premenopausal women with breast cancer. *N Eng J Med* 1997;337(14):956–962.

161. Tannock IF, Browman G: Lack of evidence for a role of chemotherapy in the routine management of locally advanced head and neck cancer. *J Clin Oncol* 1986;4:1121–1126.

162. Yuhas JM: Biological factors affecting the radioprotective efficiency of doses. *Radiat Res* 1970;44:621–628.

163. Yuhas JM: Radiotherapy of experimental lung tumors in the presence and absence of a radioprotective drug, S-2-(2 aminopropylamino)ethylphosphorothioic acid (WR-2721). *J Natl Cancer Inst* 1973;50:69–78.

164. Milas L, Hunter N, Reid BO, et al: Protective effects of S-2-(3-aminopropylamino) ethylphosphorothioic acid against radiation damage

of normal tissues and a fibrosarcoma in mice. *Cancer Res* 1982;42:1888–1897.

165. Spence AM, Krohn KA, Edmonson SW, et al: Radioprotection in rat spinal cord with WR-2721 following cerebral lateral intraventricular injection. *Int J Radiat Oncol Biol Phys* 1986;12:1479–1482.

166. Marchese MJ, Minarik L, Hall EJ, et al: Potentially lethal damage repair in cell lines of radioresistant human tumors and normal skin fibroblasts. *Int J Radiat Biol* 1985;48:431–439.

167. Todoroki T, Suit HD: Therapeutic advantage in preoperative single-dose radiation combined with conservative and radical surgery in different size murine fibrosarcoma. *J Surg Oncol* 1985;29:207–215.

168. Vogetstein B, Kinzler KW: p53 function and dysfunction. *Cell* 1992;70:523–526.

169. Lane DP: Cancer. p53, guardian of the genome. *Nature* 1992;358(6381):15–16.

170. Lowe SW, Schmitt EM, Smith SW, Osborne BA, Jacks T: p53 is required for radiation-induced apoptosis in mouse thymocytes. *Nature* 1993;362:847–849.

171. Clarke AR, Purdie CA, Harrison DJ, et al: Thymocyte apoptosis induced by p53-dependent and independent pathways. *Nature* 1993;362:849–852.

172. Lowe SW, Bodis S, McClatchey A, et al: p53 status and the efficacy of cancer therapy in vivo. *Science* 1994;266:807–810.

173. Puthenveettil JA, Frederickson SA, Reznikoff CA: Apoptosis in human papillomavirus 16 E7-, but not E6-immortalized human uroepithelial cells. *Oncogene* 1996;13:1123–1131.

174. Wheeler JA, Stephens LC, Tornos C, et al: ASTRO research fellowship: Apoptosis as a predictor of tumor response to radiation in stage IB cervical carcinoma. *Int J Radiat Oncol Biol Phys* 1995;32:1487–1493.

175. Chyle V, Pollack A, Czerniak B, et al: Apoptosis and downstaging after preoperative radiotherapy for muscle-invasive bladder cancer. *Int J Radiat Oncol Biol Phys* 1996;35:281–287.

176. Levine EL, Renehan A, Gossiel R, et al: Apoptosis, intrinsic radiosensitivity and prediction of radiotherapy response in cervical carcinoma. *Radiother Oncol* 1995;37:1–9.

177. Pilepich MV, Krall J, Al-Sarraf M, et al: A phase III trial of androgen suppression before and during radiation therapy (RT) for locally advanced prostate carcinoma: A preliminary report of RTOG protocol 86 1 0. *Proc ASCO* 1993;12:229 (abstract).

178. Colombel M, Olsson CA, Ng P-Y, Buttyan R: Hormone-regulated apoptosis results from reentry of differentiated prostate cells into a defective cell cycle. *Cancer Res* 1992;52:4313–4319.

179. Berges RR, Furuya Y, Remington L, English HF, Jacks T, Isaacs JT: Cell proliferation, DNA repair, and p53 function are not required for programmed death of prostatic glandular cells induced by androgen ablation. *Proc Natl Acad Sci USA* 1993;90:8910–8914.

180. Algan O, Stobbe CC, Helt AM, Hanks GE, Chapman JD: Radiation inactivation of human prostate cancer cells: The role of apoptosis. *Radiat Res* 1996;146:267–275.

181. Fuks Z, Alfieri A, Haimovitz-Friedman A, Seddon A, Cordon-Cardo C: Intravenous basic fibroblast growth factor protects the lung but not the mediastinal organs against radiation-induced apoptosis in vivo. *Cancer J* 1995;1:62–72.

182. Haimovitz-Friedman A, Kan C, Ehleiter D, et al: Ionizing radiation acts on cellular membranes to generate ceramide and initiate apoptosis. *J Exp Med* 1994;180:525–535.

183. Santana P, Pena LA, Haimovitz-Friedman A, et al: Acid sphingomyelinase–deficient human lymphoblasts and mice are defective in radiation-induced apoptosis. *Cell* 1996;86:189–199.

184. Folkman J: Angiogenesis and angiogenesis inhibition: An overview. *EXS* 1997;79:1–8.

185. Boehm T, Folkman J, Browder T, O'Reilly MS: Antiangiogenic therapy of experimental cancer does not induce acquired drug resistance. *Nature* 1997;390(6658):404–407.

# CHAPTER 3

# PHYSICAL ASPECTS OF RADIATION THERAPY

KAREN P. DOPPKE

## DOSIMETRY

Radiation therapy treatment units are calibrated to deliver a specific dose to water or muscle at a defined point in the reference field, either per monitor unit or per minute. It is from the measured dose in water under calibration conditions that the dose in the patient is determined. The transfer of dose from the water phantom to the patient requires the development of a dosimetry system or systems for calculating the dose in the patient. The actual dose delivered to the patient's actual tumor volume or normal tissues during treatment is usually not measured.

## Dosimetry Systems

Several dosimetry systems have evolved and are now used routinely in most radiation oncology centers. These systems are based on the determination of dose in a scattering medium simulating tissue, such as water. For all megavoltage beams the recommended method of calibration is the measurement of ionization with an ionization chamber in a water phantom. The evolution and description of the various dosimetry systems can be found in a number of radiation physics textbooks.[1–3] We begin with a review of the standard systems, as a reference for material presented later in the chapter.

*Percentage Depth Dose*  The dosimetry system that is probably most often used is the ratio of the dose at depth to the dose measured at the depth of the dose maximum, expressed as a percent. The percentage depth dose (%DD) is defined as follows:

$$\%\text{DD} \ (F,Q,A,d) = \frac{\text{dose}(F,Q,A,d)}{\text{dose} \ (F,Q,A,d_{\text{max}})} \times 100$$

where $F$ = standard treatment distance
 $Q$ = energy of the beam
 $A$ = radiation field area at $F$
 $d$ = depth of the point of interest
This dosimetry system is used for all energy photon and electron treatment beams and often is the standard by which the energies of the various treatment beams are compared.

*Tissue–Air Ratio*  A dosimetry system was developed in the 1953 by Johns et al. for use in rotational or moving beam therapy for cobalt-60 and other low energy photon beams.[4] This system is based on the tissue–air ratio (TAR), which is the ratio of a dose at a point in a scattering medium such as water to the dose measured at the same point in space with the scattering medium removed. The TAR is dependent on the depth of the point of measurement in the medium, the quality of the x-ray beam, and the field area at the point of mea-

*Clinical Radiation Oncology: Indications, Techniques, and Results, 2nd ed.*  Edited by C.C. Wang.
ISBN: 0-471-23803-1   Copyright © 2000 Wiley-Liss, Inc.

surement, but it is not dependent on the surface source distance (SSD).

$$\text{TAR } (Q,A,d) = \frac{\text{dose } (Q,A,d)}{\text{dose in air } (Q,A)}$$

This dosimetry function is the ratio of doses at a point located the same distance from the radiation source, and can be used with different source–skin distances with only small differences in dose, usually less than 2%.[5]

Most radiation therapy machines are designed and built with gantry mounting for rotational and isocentric techniques. Therefore, the TAR system is probably one of the systems most often used for cobalt-60 and other low energy x-ray beams.

An extension of the TAR system was developed for rotational and isocentric treatment techniques using high energy photon beams. The measurement of "dose in air" for the TAR relationship requires that electronic equilibrium be present. For $^{60}$Co and other low energy photon beams, the equilibrium thickness is equal to or less than 1 cm. Thus even for relatively small treatment fields this measurement in air is really a measurement of dose to a small phantom in air. But for photon beams where the dose maximum is greater than 2 cm, the phantom required to provide equilibrium thickness is often as large as the treatment field. Under these conditions the relationship developed for the TAR dosimetry system cannot be assumed. This limitation of the TAR system is overcome if the point of measurement of the dose in air is replaced by the measurement of dose in a scattering medium at a defined reference depth at the same distance from the source.

**Tissue–Phantom Ratio**  A dosimetry system for high energy photon beams, which is independent of SSD, is the tissue–phantom ratio (TPR), suggested and developed by Karzmark et al.[6] The TPR is the ratio of the dose at the depth of interest to that of the dose at the reference depth. It is dependent on the quality of the radiation beam $Q$, the area of the field at the

point of measurement $A$, and the depth $d$ of the point of interests in the phantom.

$$\text{TPR } (Q,A,d) = \frac{\text{dose } (Q,A,d)}{\text{dose } (Q,A,d_{\text{ref}})}$$

The recommended depth in water for the reference depth is 5 cm for most low and medium energy beams up to 10 MV; for treatment beams with the depth of maximum dose greater than 3 cm, the reference depth is usually the same depth recommended for the calibration of the high energy photon beam 7 cm or greater.[7,8]

**Tissue–Maximum Ratio**  A similar dosimetry system based on measurements in a phantom has been developed using the reference depth as the depth of dose maximum. This system, suggested and developed by Holt et al.,[9] is called the tissue–maximum ratio (TMR). The depth of dose maximum is the reference depth for all field sizes. Often the depth of dose maximum changes with field size for high energy photon beams; therefore the maximum depth is usually specifically chosen—normally it is the depth maximum for the smallest clinical field size. TMR is the ratio of the dose at depth to that of the dose at dose maximum, and under clinical geometry it is independent of source–skin distance.

$$\text{TMR } (Q,A,d) = \frac{\text{dose } (Q,A,d)}{\text{dose } (Q,A,d_{\text{max}})}$$

The TMR is dependent on quality of the beam $Q$, the area of the field $A$, and the depth $d$. This system is used as frequently as tissue phantom ratios for high energy photon beams.

## Dosimetry Measurements

The measurement of %DD, TAR, or TPR for a therapy machine requires the measurement of dose on the central axis for a large number of field sizes and depths. These relative dose measurements are usually determined from ionization measurements in a water phantom. The measured data then are used to determine the dose on the central axis for field sizes and depths not measured by means of interpolation. Using the dosimetry systems above and the measured data, the dose can be calculated on the central axis in a uniform medium to within ±3% for most square and rectangular treatment fields.[10] Published data should not be used for patient treatment unless measurements have verified the data. The *British Journal of Radiology* has published central axis data for a number of photon and electron treatment beams for many different energies.[11]

The foregoing dosimetry systems cannot be used to predict the dose in the treatment field at points not on the central axis unless additional information about the radiation field is available. The calculational method most often used to determine the dose not on the central axis separates the dose at the point of interest into primary and scattered radiation and is referred to as the Clarkson method.[12,13] The primary beam contribution to the dose-off axis is modified to account for effects due to effective source size, collimator/head scatter, and transmission, which depend on the treatment unit. The scatter component is determined separately by finding the effective area of field at depth. These calculations are normally done by treatment planning computer programs and can generate complete dose distributions. Newer commercial treatment planning systems are now providing dose calculation algorithms that take into account the transport of scattered photons and electrons in the patient. These methods should provide a better method of dose calculation, especially in regions exhibiting changes in patient density. The dose distributions calculated using all calculational methods should be carefully evaluated to assure that they match measured data.

***Patient Measurements*** The measurement of the actual dose delivered to the patient and the tumor volume is not always simple, but every effort should be made to ensure that calculated doses are verified. If patient measurements are not to be done routinely, a set of check measurements should be performed in phantoms for a number of clinically relevant treatment techniques. The measurements are taken to ensure that the measured and calculated doses are within acceptable limits of ±3% for phantoms of uniform density. Patient measurements should be utilized to verify the dose delivered to the patient when the treatment fields are significantly modified by unusual treatment situations or devices. Several types of radiation detector can be used to monitor the dose delivered to the patient during treatment.

Direct-reading devices such as ionization chambers can be used to measure the dose during treatment on the patient's skin surface, or within the patient if the chamber is small. The ionization readings need to be corrected, using the appropriate factors to determine the dose. The measurements can be evaluated before further treatment is given. If significant differences exist between the expected readings and the actual readings, the treatment plan and the dosimetry can be reviewed before further treatment is given. Ionization chambers are relatively expensive and need careful handling, but they do not have significant energy dependence for photon beams in the megavoltage regions.[1]

Another type of ionization chamber that has been used to evaluate patient dose is the transmission chamber. A number of isocentric therapy units have area ionization chambers built into the beam interceptor; this has been especially true of $^{60}$Co units. This type of ionization chamber measures the radiation exiting the patient over a defined area centered on the central axis of the beam.[14] This transmission measurement can be used to check calculations that would predict the amount of radiation exiting the patient. Transmission measurements vary with field size and thickness of the patient.

A radiation detector that is frequently used for patient dosimetry is the solid state silicon diode. Such devices are relatively small and less delicate than ionization chambers, making them somewhat more acceptable for routine quality control and patient measurements. The diode is usually placed on the patient's surface (or intracavitarily for new treatment fields) and the output is compared to expected readings. The diode must be calibrated because its sensitivity changes with energy and can have a significant directional dependence. The response is often dependent on previous radiation exposure and temperature.[1] Calibration procedures need to be reviewed routinely to ensure that the correction factors applied to the readings are appropriate. Commercial systems designed to monitor patient dose are available, and often these devices can be used in quality control procedures.

The major advantage of the detectors just described is that there is no delay in obtaining the measured patient results. Therefore errors in the patient treatment information (e.g., patient thickness measurements, patient positioning, machine setup, dose calculations) can be discovered before additional treatments are given.

Another type of dosimeter used for patient dosimetry is the solid state thermoluminescent crystal. These detectors can be very small and can be inserted into holders or catheters for dose measurements. The solid state crystals, which are commercially available in thicknesses of a millimeter or less, can be used in the powdered form to determine the size and thickness of the detector. The most frequently used thermoluminescent dosimeters are lithium fluoride and lithium borate; occasionally calcium fluoride is selected. Lithium fluoride and lithium borate have effective atomic numbers that are similar to soft tissue, and for most high energy photon beams their energy dependence and relative sensitivity are similar. Calcium fluoride is not used as often because of its higher effective atomic number, but its increased sensitivity makes it an excellent dosimeter for low dose measurements.

Thermoluminescent materials need to be calibrated in the therapy beams with which they will be used. Careful annealing and reading procedures need be followed to obtain an accuracy of approximately $\pm 3\%$.[15] Because of their small physical size they can be used to measure dose at the air–surface interface and in regions of rapid dose changes. These dosimeters are also frequently used in phantoms for electron beam therapy or in brachytherapy because of their small size. Several dosimeters can be positioned at different sites on the patient during treatment, and therefore a number of dose measurements can be obtained during one treatment session. The results of the measurements are not immediately available, and thus there will be some delay in the evaluation of the patient dose.

Another integrating dosimeter that can be used for patient dosimetry is radiographic film. The film can be placed to measure the radiation field leaving the patient, much as is done in a transmission ionization chamber. Using a calibration curve for the film (i.e., optical density vs. dose) permits the estimation of the dose variation in the treatment field. The results will vary with field size and changes in the scattering conditions. Obtaining accurate patient measurements with this technique is difficult because of the variation of film darkening due to processing conditions, emulsion nonuniformity, and artifacts caused by the film holder and cassette.[1]

Film, in general is not recommended for routine patient measurement. With care and under controlled conditions, however, it is useful in evaluating the relative dose in a radiation field. Film is often used for photon and electron field dosimetry in phantoms because of its high spatial resolution. Film response is determined in the therapy beam of interest by means of standard geometry and phantoms; then relative dose distribution in the patient or modified radiation field can be determined.

The use of film for portal variation in some radiology departments is being replaced by the electronic portal imagers. These devices are primarily used to image the treatment fields electronically and to compare these images with simulation images or digitial reconstructed radiographs (DRR) of the planned fields. The images can then be compared by means of subtraction techniques, or modified to enhance contrast or edges. The use of the imaging systems for routine quality assurance of special treatment beams and the actual measurement of the exiting radiation field for patient dosimetry.

Radiation detectors should be available for patient measurements and quality assurance procedures in a radiation oncology department. The measurement of dose delivered to a patient under actual treatment conditions is recommended, especially when patient contour and/or treatment devices significantly modify the treatment field.

## TREATMENT BEAM CHARACTERISTICS

Radiation oncology departments can now choose from a large selection of treatment machines with many different photon energies, and most high energy accelerators have electron beams at multiple energies. With treatment beams available in increased numbers and types, the treatment field characteristics have become an important consideration in the choice of the treatment unit. A treatment beam is usually characterized by first defining the central axis depth dose and the relative dose profiles at depth. The area of the field that is encompassed by the 95% or 90% isodose level relative to the dose on the central axis at the depth of interest is the part of the beam that is used for treatment. The area of the beam that is changing rapidly over a small distance and is normally defined as the penumbra is usually of secondary interest when modern linear accelerators are used. These characteristics vary with the modality, the energy and geometric configuration of the source, the collimator, and the treatment distances.

Variation in the foregoing characteristics must be considered when treatment planning techniques are transferred to different treatment machines. Often one treatment planning technique can be moved to another energy and treatment machine without modification. More often, however, new techniques must be developed to match the new modality available.

## Photon Beams

***Depth Dose***   Variation of dose versus depth for photon beams is primarily dependent on the energy of the beam and the area of the field. Usually only small differences occur in the depth–dose profile for the same nominal beam energies, and these differences would be due to accelerator design, target, and flattening filter. Percent depth doses for 4, 10, and 25 MV x-ray beams for three field sizes at 100 cm SSD are shown in Table 3-1. The table shows the variation in percent depth dose relative to the energy of the photon beams and also the modification of the dose at depth relative to the area of the treatment field. The area of the treatment field for low energy photon beams significantly changes the depth–dose variation that is due to the increased scatter component at lower energies. The dose due to scattered radiation for high energy photon beams is relatively small, and therefore the effect of field size on the percent depth dose is small.

The change in relative dose in relation to energy and depth is shown in Figure 3-1. The dose is normalized at 12 cm depth for three different energy treatment beams for the same field area. The increased dose in tissues near the entrance surface for the $^{60}$Co beam, compared to the high energy beam, is significant and demonstrates the need for multifield treatment techniques for low and medium energy beams. To reduce the effect of increased dose on normal tissue near the surface for low energy photon beams, multifield and rotational techniques are required to deliver relative doses to lesions at depths greater than 5 cm. Most new treatment units are designed to be isocentric and are capable of delivering multiple fields at each treatment session without additional patient positioning; therefore the dose per treatment field to the normal tissue surrounding the target volume is reduced. The treatment of lesions with single fields should always be considered carefully; for example, the ratio of dose at a depth of 5 cm to the dose at depth maximum is greater than 1.25 for a 100 cm$^2$ $^{60}$Co field at 80 cm SSD.

TABLE 3-1  Comparison of Percent Dose for 4, 10, and 25 MV X-Rays at 100 cm Surface Source Distance Versus Field Size

| Depth (cm) | 4 MV X-Rays | | | 10 MV X-Rays | | | 25 MV X-Rays[a] | | |
|---|---|---|---|---|---|---|---|---|---|
| | 6 × 6 cm² | 10 × 10 cm² | 20 × 20 cm² | 6 × 6 cm² | 10 × 10 cm² | 20 × 20 cm² | 6 × 6 cm² | 10 × 10 cm² | 20 × 20 cm² |
| 5.0 | 82.9 | 84.9 | 86.8 | 90.3 | 90.8 | 91.3 | 100 | 100 | 100 |
| 7.0 | 73.5 | 76.0 | 79.0 | 82.2 | 83.2 | 84.3 | 95.8 | 95.5 | 94.3 |
| 10.0 | 61.0 | 64.3 | 68.0 | 71.2 | 73.0 | 74.8 | 86.3 | 86.0 | 85.3 |
| 20.0 | 31.8 | 35.0 | 39.8 | 43.1 | 45.3 | 48.3 | 58.3 | 59.0 | 59.2 |
| 30.0 | 16.6 | 18.8 | 22.7 | 26.0 | 27.8 | 31.0 | 39.6 | 40.2 | 41.3 |

[a] Percent depth dose normalized at a depth of 5 cm.

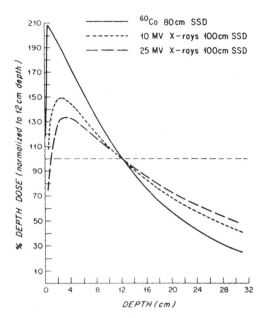

**FIGURE 3-1** Comparison of the relative increase in the superficial dose versus energy for $^{60}$Co, 10 MV x-rays, and 25 MV x-rays, all normalized at 12.0 cm depth in water.

The depth–dose characteristics of a radiation field are modified by the presence of lung, bone, fat, and air cavities in the patient. These tissues can change the penetration and also modify the scattering characteristics of the beam. For megavoltage beams the change in penetration of the beam is primarily due to the change in the relative electron density of these tissues to water. Lung tissue, with densities relative to water of 0.2 to 0.5 g/cm$^3$ and large volume, can significantly modify the standard depth–dose characteristics.

A number of standard calculational methods are used to estimate the modification of the dose deposited in the lung tissue and beyond. These techniques do not account for changes in scatter and cannot provide the appropriate corrections at locations where electronic equilibrium does not exist (e.g., at the interface between tissues of different densities) or in the presence of air cavities. The techniques used primarily modify the dose at depth by a ratio. The dose at depth in water is compared to the dose at that same point but with the depth modified by the product of the thickness of the inhomogeneity times the relative electron density of that tissue. The most frequently used methods are the effective depth method or the ratio of tissue–air ratios, the Batho power law method, and the isodose shift method.[16-18]

More sophisticated and accurate methods are available to account for some of the effects due to changes in scatter. These methods are available on some treatment planning computers.[19,20] A new generation of treatment planning computers have in addition to the standard dose calculation methods, the newer convolution algorithms, which model the spectrum of the treatment beam and provide methods of estimating the secondary electrons produced in the beam. With faster computers, "Monte Carlo" methods can be used directly to determine the dose distribution in individual patients. The calculation time is still long (determining the dose in complex beam arrangements requires several hours), but in special situations this type of calculation may be important for the development of special techniques.

**TABLE 3-2   Comparison of Change in Penumbra Region for 4, 10, and 25 MV X-Rays Due to Various Thicknesses of Cork (Electron Density = 0.22) Simulating Lung Tissue**[a]

| Cork Thickness (cm) | 4 MV X-Rays (cm) | 10 MV X-Rays (cm) | 25 MV X-Rays (cm) |
|---|---|---|---|
| At interface | 0.9 | 1.1 | 2.1 |
| 1.9 | 1.8 | 2.4 | 3.4 |
| 5.7 | 1.8 | 2.9 | 4.2 |
| 10.2 | 1.9 | 2.9 | 4.6 |

[a] Penumbra 90% to 10%; 10 × 10 cm$^2$ field at 100 cm source axis distance.

Estimated error ± 2.0 mm.

In general, the dose beyond lung increase with lung thickness and decrease with increasing energy and increasing field size. A dose correction factor for the tissue beyond 13.5 cm lung for a $10 \times 10$ cm$^2$ field, for example, would be 1.18 and 1.60 for 25 MV x-rays and $^{60}$Co, respectively.[21] Dose corrections for large inhomogenates should be considered, especially when computed tomography (CT) data provide information about the location and relative density of the anatomical structures.[20] Significant changes in the treatment beam profile in lung may be necessitated by the increased range of the secondary electrons. Table 3-2 indicates these changes in the penumbra for photon beams of three different energies. These data were measured in various thicknesses of cork with a polystyrene phantom above the cork to simulate the chest wall. At high energy, the distance between the central axis and the 90% and 95% isodose lines is substantially reduced. The effects of high energy photon beams should be considered in plan-

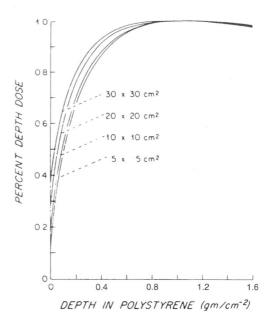

**FIGURE 3-3**  Buildup curves and surface dose for 4 MV x-rays versus field size at 100 cm SSD.

ning treatment. Normal beam profiles are reestablished at depth in the tissues beyond the lung. The modification of dose beyond bone and fat is relatively small for megavoltage photon beams. The differences expected due to the increased electron density of bone relative to water are approximately 3% to 5%. The absorbed dose in bone will increase as the energy of the beam increases above 10 MV because of the dependence on atomic number ($Z$) of pair production.[1]

The dose modification due to air cavities at the tissue–air interface is important if the treatment volume or the tumor is at the interface. This decrease in dose to the tissue is similar to the buildup effects at the surface. The dose at the interface decreases with increasing energy, decreasing field size, and increasing cavity size.[22] Figure 3-2 demonstrates this effect for a small field irradiating a long narrow cavity with 10 MV x-rays; the modification of the dose at the interface is 12.5%.

**Buildup Region**  The advantage of $^{60}$Co and higher energy photon beams is that there is

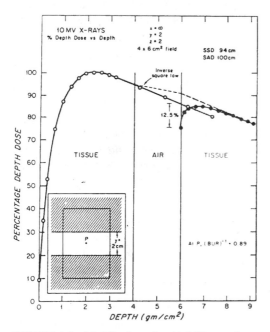

**FIGURE 3-2**  Modification of a 10 MV x-ray beam depth–dose profile due to presence of a long narrow air cavity: SSD, source surface distance; SAD, source axis distance. (From Epp et al.[22])

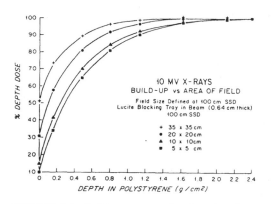

**FIGURE 3-4** Buildup curves and surface dose for 10 MV x-rays versus field size at 100 cm SSD; Lucite blocking tray in beam. (From Doppke et al.[25])

a region of superficial tissue that receives not the maximum dose but a significantly lower dose, owing to the range of the secondary electrons. The energy of the photon beam is the major factor determining the depth of dose maximum and the relative dose at the air interface, that is, the surface dose. The surface dose changes with the field size, the material and the thickness of the secondary devices in the beam, and the location of these devices relative to the patient surface. Figure 3-3 indicates the variation in dose in the buildup region for 4 MV x-rays versus field size at 100 cm SSD. Note that the depth of dose maximum is shifted toward the surface and that the surface dose increases as the field area increases.[23]

Measurements of the buildup region should be done at the normal treatment distance of the patient surface to source. For isocentric techniques the patient's skin surface can be as much as 20 cm closer to the source in the treatment of lesions in the chest or pelvis relative to isocenter. Therefore, if accurate surface dose is required, measurements should be done at that distance.

Loss of skin-sparing or modification of the dose in the buildup region can occur for low energy photon beams such as $^{60}$Co when the field sizes are large ($\geq 400$ cm$^2$) and when the collimators or blocking trays are located close to the surface. Modification of the depth of

dose maximum and the buildup region for high energy x-ray beams is probably not as clinically significant as it is with cobalt and other low energy photon beams. The buildup region versus the area of the field for 10 MV x-rays is shown in Figure 3-4. The variation of dose in the superficial regions for high energy photon beams of the same nominal energy can be different due to the design of the accelerator, for the newer treatment units the surface dose will be similar.

Blocking trays or other low $Z$ material in the radiation fields will produce electron contamination and increase the dose superficially, without changing the basic depth–dose characteristics of the beam beyond the depth of dose maximum. The modification of dose in this region due to the presence of a Lucite tray to support beam-shaping devices is shown in Figure 3-5 for the 4 MV x-ray beam. Table 3-3 indicates the change in percent depth dose that occurs in relation to distance with and without the presence of a blocking tray for 10 MV x-rays. Blocking trays and other low $Z$ materials positioned in the treatment beam also increase the dose outside the field edge in the buildup region.[24]

Often high energy beams are preferred for the treatment of certain lesions because of the penetrating characteristics of the beam, but if the treatment volume extends to or is near to

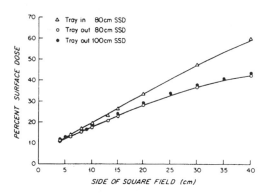

**FIGURE 3-5** Comparison of the percent surface dose for two different treatment distances for 4 MV x-rays with and without a blocking tray in the beam. (From Biggs et al.[23])

**TABLE 3-3**  Comparison of Percent Depth Dose for a $28 \times 28$ cm$^2$ Field in the Buildup Region for 10 MV X-Rays with and Without Blocking Trays in the Beam

| Depth of Polystyrene (g/cm$^2$) | 80 cm SCD | | | 150 cm SCD |
| | Wire Mesh No Tray (%) | Lucite Tray, Tray, 64 cm STD (%) | 64 cm STD (%) | Lucite Tray, 64 cm STD (%) |
| --- | --- | --- | --- | --- |
| Surface | 33.8 | 38.2 | 69.6 | 22.8 |
| 0.5 | 79.5 | 82.6 | 94.8 | 73.5 |
| 1.0 | 93.0 | 94.3 | 98.0 | 90.5 |
| 1.5 | 98.1 | 98.6 | 99.6 | 97.0 |

SCD = source chamber distance.

STD = standard treatment distance.

the surface of the patient, as in superficial nodal disease, a bolus may be required to modify the dose in the buildup region.

To increase the dose superficially without using bolus in high energy photon beams, Lucite or other low $Z$ materials can be positioned close to the patient under controlled conditions. Figure 3-6 shows the effect of Lucite sheet, 1.2 cm thick and 80.5 cm from the source in relation to the area for a 10 MV x-ray beam. The data are compared to the same relative dose and area without the Lucite sheet in place. Such devices are used to increase the dose to the superficial sites in the treatment of head and neck cancer with 10 MV x-rays. This device has been referred to as a "beam spoiler."[25]

A similar device has been used in the treatment of Hodgkin disease with 10 MV x-rays. Figure 3-7 shows the modification of the buildup region with a Lucite sheet 0.64 cm thick, at 125 cm from the source; the patient's surface is at 150 cm SSD. The beam spoiler is designed to increase the dose at 0.5 cm depth in tissue to 90% of the maximum dose and still maintain skin-sparing.

Wedges and other devices do not significantly modify the buildup region if they are fabricated from medium or high $Z$ materials. Often, medium $Z$ materials are used as filters in low energy beams such as $^{60}$Co to improve the buildup region by removing secondary electrons from the beam, especially for large fields.[26]

For extended treatment distances, as in whole-body radiation therapy with extremely large fields, the buildup region can be modified substantially from that measured at conventional treatment distances. For unusual and extended distance treatments, additional measurements are often necessary to evaluate the dose in the buildup region.

***Treatment Beam Profile***  The treatment field size is normally defined by the 50% isodose level relative to the dose on the central axis at the depth of dose maximum. The variation of dose in the treatment area normally encompassed by the 90% or 95% isodose level is determined by the size of the field, the energy

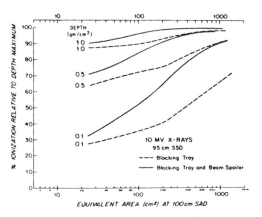

**FIGURE 3-6**  The relative dose at depth for 10 MV x-rays with and without beam spoiler in place. (From Doppke et al.[25])

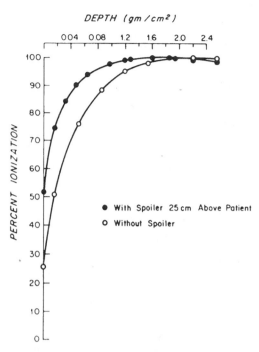

DEPTH (gm/cm²)

PERCENT IONIZATION

● With Spoiler 25 cm Above Patient

○ Without Spoiler

**FIGURE 3-7** Dose in the buildup region at 150 cm source surface distance for a 30 × 30 cm² field with and without beam spoiler for 10 MV x-rays.

of the beam, the depth, the design of the flattening filter for accelerators, and, to some extent, by the distances from source to collimator and source to skin or surface. Ideally, the dose across the treatment volume should not vary by more than ±5% (Table 3-4).

At depth, the flatness of a radiation field is modified owing to the variation in the attenuation of the beam relative to the central axis and in the change in the scattered radiation versus depth. Often, to obtain radiation fields that are flattened at depth (i.e., ≥ 10 cm) the flattening filters for accelerators are designed to have, at the depth of dose maximum, a substantially high dose near the edges of the field. This increase in dose can be greater than 10%. This is a characteristic of some accelerator-produced x-ray fields. The flatness of the largest treatment fields should be evaluated at depth and at the depth of dose maximum.

The beam profiles should be evaluated carefully before treatment techniques are transferred from, for example, a [60]Co unit to any x-ray accelerator. Figure 3-8 shows the beam profiles for large fields at the depths of dose maximum for [60]Co, 4 MV, and 10 MV x-rays. Often there is an increase in dose in the corner of the field along the diagonal relative to the dose along the primary axis, that is, parallel to the collimators. The beam profile for a 10 MV x-ray beam at dose maximum for the primary and diagonal axis is shown in Figure 3-9.

The improvement in field flatness by secondary blocking or the use of secondary trimmers is not significant for high energy photon beams. The source size and position of the secondary field-defining devices can modify the dose near the edges of the field for [60]Co. For most high energy accelerators flatness is not significantly modified by secondary blocking for routine clinical techniques.

***Penumbra Region*** The penumbra region is defined by the distance between isodose levels, usually 80% to 20% at the depth of dose maximum, but it is more important at depth. The variation in the penumbra is due to the geometry of source and collimator distances,

**TABLE 3-4  Distance (cm) from the Field Edge to the 95% or 98% Dose Level Relative to the Central Axis Dose for 5 and 10 cm Depth and Several Beam Energies**

| Energy | 5 cm Depth | | 10 cm Depth | |
|---|---|---|---|---|
| | 50%–98% | 50%–95% | 50%–98% | 50%–95% |
| [60]Co | 1.9 | 1.1 | 2.9 | 1.7 |
| 4 MV x-rays | 1.0 | 0.6 | 1.7 | 0.9 |
| 10 MV x-rays | 1.2 | 0.8 | 1.7 | 1.1 |
| 25 MV x-rays | 1.6 | 1.1 | 2.2 | 1.4 |

the energy of the beam, and the source size. The evaluation of the penumbra region for all available treatment beams is important in treatment planning and should be considered when the relative merits of various treatment units are compared. For example, if a sensitive structure is close to the treatment volume, the treatment beam with the smallest penumbra may be the one of choice if all other beam characteristics are similar. Table 3-5 compares the penumbrae for three different energy beams at 5 cm depth in water. For the standard treatment distances the treatment unit with the smallest effective source size would have the smallest penumbra. Secondary blocking or the use of secondary trimmers on cobalt units can reduce the width of the 90% to 10% isodose level by approximately 1 cm. The reduction of the penumbra by secondary blocking for high energy x-ray beams is not significant if the blocks are designed to match the divergence of the beam and are at the standard blocking distance of approximately half the SSD. A reduction in dose is seen outside the 20% level for secondary blocking when the collimators also define the treatment field edge.

For x-ray beams of high energy (i.e., > 10 MV), the penumbra region increases because the range of the secondary electrons produced in the field increases.[1] The loss of secondary

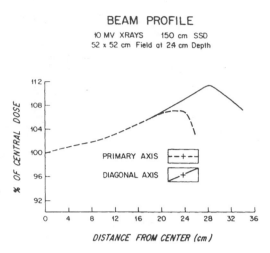

**FIGURE 3-9**   Comparison of the beam profiles along the primary and diagonal axes at the depth of dose maximum for 10 MV x-rays.

electrons from the field often causes a decrease in beam flatness for small fields at depth. The decrease in beam flatness often requires the use of fields of increased size, to reduce the dose variation across the treatment volume.[8] The use of additional field-flattening devices can be considered if the dose to adjacent sites needs to be kept at a minimum, and if the high energy beam is required because of the depth of the treatment volume. Such a device has been designed and described by Biggs et al. for small fields for high energy x-ray beam.[27]

The availability of computer-controlled multileaf collimators on newer linear accelerators has increased the flexibility of the treatment unit. Depending on their design and manufacture, these collimators either replace one of the major beam-defining jaws or are in addition to the standard jaw arrangement. Several major research centers and commercial vendors have developed computer programs to move the multileaf collimators during treatment to modify the intensity profile across the field and produce optimized dose distributions.

**Combination of Treatment Fields**   In most treatment situations the patient is irradi-

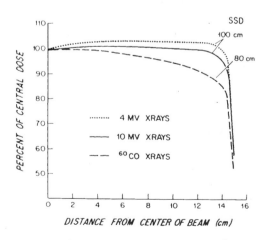

**FIGURE 3-8**   Beam profiles for a 30 × 30 cm² field at depth of dose maximum for ⁶⁰Co, 4 MV, and 10 MV x-rays.

**TABLE 3-5  Dosimetric Penumbra for a $^{60}$Co Beam and 10 and 25 MV X-Rays Measured at 5 cm Depth in Water (10 × 10 cm$^2$ Fields)**

| Treatment Unit | Distance Between 90% and 20% Isodose Level (cm) |
|---|---|
| $^{60}$Co unit, 80 cm SSD | |
|    No trimmers | 1.5 |
|    With trimmers | 0.9 |
| 10 MV x-rays 100 cm SSD | 0.7 |
| 25 MV x-rays 100 cm SSD | 1.2 |

SSD = source surface distance.

ated with a number of treatment fields. The actual combination of fields depends on the treatment site, the extent and location of the target volume, and often the clinician's treatment philosophy. In general, the aim is to maximize the dose to the tumor volume while minimizing the dose delivered to all other tissues.

The application of a single treatment field is usually associated with the treatment of superficial lesions by means of either lower energy x-rays or electrons. In these cases the dose across the target volume should not differ by more than ±5%, and the dose to the normal tissue should not exceed this dose by more than 10%.

Parallel opposed fields are not usually considered to be the optimum treatment arrangement for high dose radiation therapy except for small patient separations (Figure 3-10). Usually the superficial tissues receive a higher dose than the target volume. Normally, for treatment sites at depth, three or more fields provide a more uniform dose distribution in the target volume, and the dose to the normal tissues is reduced. The application of an increasing number of treatment fields usually decreases the dose to specific normal tissues in each of the treatment beams. The optimal number of treatment fields is probably dependent on the treatment site. But with the development of intensity-modulated beams, the final dose distribution may require fewer actual fields than are needed for similar distributions gener-

ated with unmodulated beams, thus reducing the dose to normal tissue.

Moving beam therapy is often used to minimize the dose to superficial tissues and to provide a uniform dose in the target volume. However, the dose distributions cannot be easily shaped for rotational techniques. With high energy photon beams, stationary field techniques can be used with equal planning success, the fields can be shaped to the target volume, and often sensitive normal tissues can be excluded entirely.

The beam intensity can be modulated during treatment by means of a specially designed planning system used in conjunction with special collimators. This system modifies the dose as the treatment unit rotates around the patient. The present commercial implementation of this technique requires a special collimator device that is designed to treat small tumor volumes in the brain or to implement boost techniques. Other moving beam techniques us-

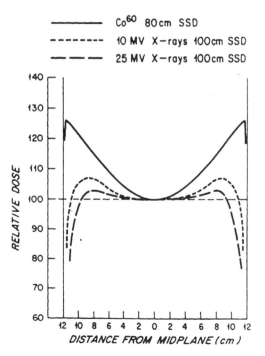

**FIGURE 3-10**  Comparison of the relative dose at depth to the superficial dose for parallel opposed fields for 25 MV, 20 MV, and $^{60}$Co photon beams.

ing dynamic beam therapy allow optimization of the dose distribution in the target volume, with the sparing of normal structures, by continually changing the collimator and the isocenter in the patient. This technique has been shown to be useful in treatment sites where the target volume varies substantially in size and location in the patient.[28]

Full-dose distributions are obtained by means of commercial treatment planning systems or computer software developed for the treatment center. Most treatment planning computers available allow for the use of CT data as an input of patient information. These CT data provide localization of structures within the patient in the entire treatment volume. The CT data are modified to electron densities, and dose calculations can be performed to correct for heterogeneity. For a discussion of treatment planning procedures and newer approaches, see Chapter 15. Specific treatment techniques are discussed in relation to the disease sites in the appropriate chapters.

**Matching Fields** Multiple fields are often necessary if the target volume is larger than the maximum field size available on the treatment unit of choice or if additional therapy is required directly outside a previously treated volume. Several standard techniques provide a uniform dose distribution in the region of the field junctions.

The most frequently used technique is to calculate the geometric divergence of the treatment beams at depth relative to the surface of the patient at the junction region. This junction or matching technique assumes that the geo-

FIELD JUNCTIONS
$^{60}$Co THERATRON-780     80 cm SAD

**A**     MATCHED FIELDS

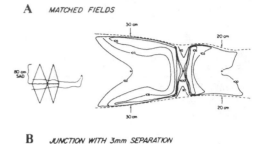

**B**     JUNCTION WITH 3mm SEPARATION

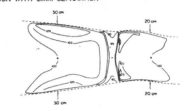

**FIGURE 3-12**   Dose distribution for two sets of parallel opposed to $^{60}$Co fields. **(A)** 50% isodose curves matched at depth **(B)** Dose distribution with 3 mm separation between the 50% isodose curves.

metric projection of the field edge defines the 50% isodose level at the depth of interest. Figure 3-11 shows the standard method of calculating the separation required for the fields on the patient's surface.

Beam divergence increases with field size, and if opposed matching fields are not of the same size there will be an area beyond the level of the junction in which the dose will be greater than the dose on the central axis at each depth in the patient. An increase in the treatment distance will decrease the beam divergence at depth so that again, if different treatment distances are used, areas of either over- or underdosing might occur. A solution to this difficulty is to ensure, if at all possible, that the required treatment beams have the same divergence. If the field sizes are different, the treatment distance can be modified to increase or decrease the divergence of the treatment beams.

Figure 3-12 shows the dose distribution for two sets of opposed $^{60}$Co fields matched at depth. The treatment distance is the same, but

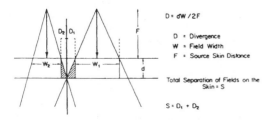

**FIGURE 3-11**   Method for calculating the geometric divergence of radiation fields in depth.

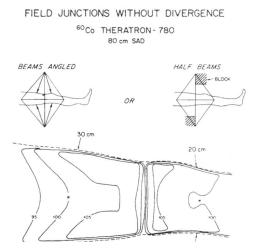

FIELD JUNCTIONS WITHOUT DIVERGENCE
$^{60}$Co THERATRON-780
80 cm SAD

BEAMS ANGLED          HALF BEAMS

OR

**FIGURE 3-13** Dose distribution for matched nondivergent $^{60}$Co beams.

the field lengths are 30 and 20 cm respectively. The dose distribution with an additional 3 mm separation between the fields is also shown. The reduced dose in the region above and below the matched level may not be acceptable clinically if the target volume is located in this region. Treatment beams that have no divergence are required if a uniform dose distribution is necessary to irradiate the entire volume.

Two techniques are routinely used to create nondivergent photon beams. The first method is to use a half-beam block or to position one of the primary collimators at the central axis. The centers of the two treatment fields are then used at the junction. These blocked fields are relatively easy to set up, but it must be remembered that there is radiation transmitted through the block; therefore, areas of the patient outside the treatment volume receive some additional radiation. For treatment machines with independent jaws, the transmission of radiation through jaw is the same as for standard fields, and the dose is reduced. Additional scattered radiation will be present in the treatment area.

Another method is to modify the angle of the beam entering the patient by the rotation of either gantry or couch so that the edge of the

beam is nondivergent at the junction region. Figure 3-13 shows the dose distribution if the beam edges are not divergent. In the region of the junction there can still be sharp variation in dose and if the nondivergent fields are not aligned properly, substantial over- or underdoses can occur.

One method of compensating for a possible patient or beam misalignment is to move the position of the junction by a fixed displacement (e.g., in 1 cm steps). The number of junction levels used in a particular situation depends on the beam penumbra and on the site. For example, for $^{60}$Co beams with large penumbrae, three levels may be sufficient, while for accelerator-produced x-ray beams with relatively small penumbrae, a larger number of levels would be recommended. The number of levels chosen should be related to the treatment site and the treatment beam characteristics. Figure 3-14 shows the dose distribution for

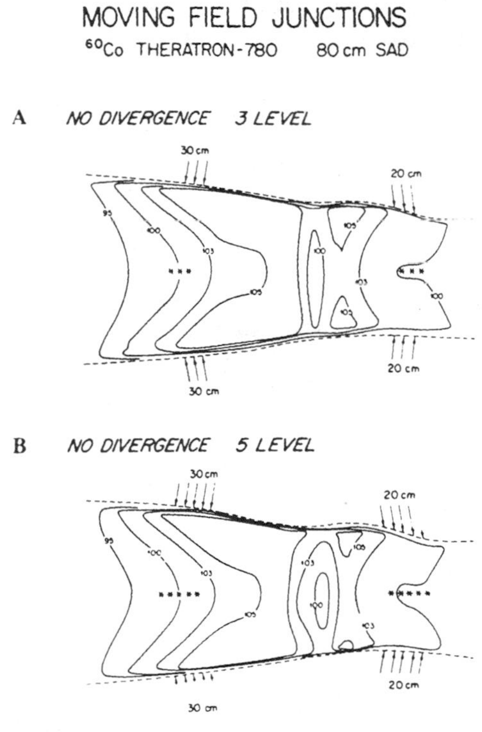

MOVING FIELD JUNCTIONS
$^{60}$Co THERATRON-780    80 cm SAD

A    NO DIVERGENCE    3 LEVEL

B    NO DIVERGENCE    5 LEVEL

**FIGURE 3-14** Comparison of three- and five-level moving junctions with nondivergent $^{60}$Co beams.

nondivergent beams with three- and five-level moving junctions.

Another method of modifying the junction region is to add a specially designed junction wedge to the treatment beam edge. At the Massachusetts General Hospital, we have used such a device for a number of years in the treatment of patients with Hodgkin disease. The device was designed to replace the standard five-level moving junction. A diagram of the technique is shown in Figure 3-15. The penumbra region was modified to be linear from the 90% to the 10% level over 5 cm. Figure 3-16 shows the beam profiles at depth through the junction region for divergent beams with and without the wedge in place. Also shown are the profiles with slight misplacements, which might occur in determining or locating the field edge at depth. For nondivergent beams, similar over- or underdosing will occur in all depths in the patient. The wedge technique or the moving junctions provide some additional safety in matching treatment fields. A number of other authors have designed similar field edge wedges, and Fraass et al. have published

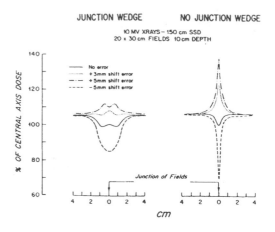

**FIGURE 3-16** The dose profile at 10 cm depth for matched fields in the junction region with and without the junction wedge. The dose profiles for small errors in field placement are also shown.

dose distributions for several sites and energies with a wedge in place.[29] The method used for field matching should be carefully reviewed, and it should be specific to the treatment beam and treatment site.

## ELECTRON BEAM DOSIMETRY

High energy electron beams are now available for routine therapy from high energy accelerators. Because the accelerators are of different designs, however, the electron beam characteristics are often substantially different even though the nominal accelerated energies are the same. The differences in characteristics are due primarily to the methods used to produce flattened electron fields and to the collimator designs. The major clinical advantage of electron beams is their limited range in tissues, which is determined by the energy of the beam.

The most frequently used electron beam energies are from 5 to 20 MV. Electrons provide the capability of treating superficial lesions to higher dose and limiting the dose to the normal tissues beyond the electron range. Electrons are often used to increase the local dose to the primary site when small-field techniques are em-

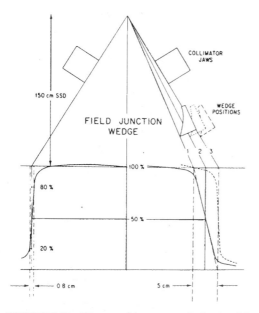

**FIGURE 3-15** Diagram of the geometry in the use of the junction wedge and the modification of the penumbra from 0.8 cm to 5.0 cm for a 10 MV x-ray beam.

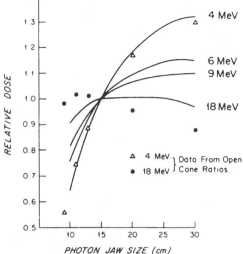

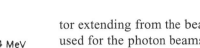

**FIGURE 3-17** Change in the relative dose at depth maximum versus photon jaw settings normalized to the recommended setting for a $10 \times 10$ cm$^2$ cone and for four electron energies. (From Biggs et al.[32])

ployed in combination with larger photon beams.

The treatment of superficial tumors with electron beams has almost completely replaced the need for medium energy x-ray units in a radiation therapy department. The treatment beam characteristics and the techniques described in this section are related to the experience in the Department of Radiation Oncology at Massachusetts General Hospital.

Electron beam dosimetry for stationary field treatment is normally based on central axis percent depth–dose data. Calibration of electron fields is done at the depth of dose maximum, and for most accelerators the treatment distances are at or near 100 cm SSD. The International Commission on Radiation Units and Measurements (ICRU) has published a report of a complete discussion of electron dosimetry and calibration techniques.[30]

## Electron Beams

Fields are defined by a series of treatment cones, or applicators, or by a variable collima-

tor extending from the beam-defining system used for the photon beams. These applicators or cones are designed to be positioned at or near the patient's surface. The location of the end of the applicator or cone relative to the patient's surface should not be modified substantially for routine therapy. The beam flatness and the dose at depth maximum is modified with changes in the separation between the end of the treatment cone and the patient surface, that is, the treatment distance.[31]

The cone or applicators used in defining the treatment field modify the dose at the depth of dose maximum and often the position. The opening of the photon-beam-defining jaws or collimators may also affect the dose in the electron field[32] (Figure 3-17). The photon jaws are interlocked with the electron applicators to a preset opening; this prevents large modifications of the expected dose during routine treatment. A standard set of electron applicators or a variable collimator is provided by the manufacturer of the accelerator. An output factor or cone ratio must be determined for each cone or for a series of field size settings for all beam

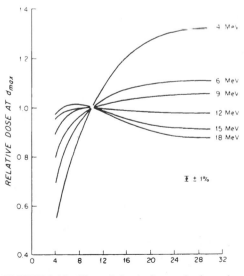

**FIGURE 3-18** The variation in dose at depth maximum for the treatment cones on the Varian Clinac 18 versus energy. (From Biggs et al.[32])

energies. The variation in dose versus field area for the electron beams from one accelerator is shown in Figure 3-18. Large changes in the dose at depth maximum can occur with the change in the size of the treatment field. The depth of maximum dose and the depth of the 90% dose level can decrease significantly for small fields. Representative depth–dose curves for various energies are shown in Figure 3-19.

Unlike most x-ray beams from high energy accelerators, the dose at the depth of dose maximum does not follow the standard inverse square relationship.[33] The dose at depth maximum should be measured for each cone size and for all electron energies relative to a standard treatment distance: that is, separation between the patient surface and the cone. Table 3-6 shows correction factors required relative to the standard treatment distance for a 12 MeV beam for three different cone sizes compared with an inverse square calculation assuming 100 cm SSD. If an effective source or virtual source position is determined for each energy and cone, a calculation of the inverse square type can be performed, but such a calculation should be used only over a limited range of treatment distances. If the extended treatment distances are used, certain significant changes in the beam penumbra and the beam flatness must be evaluated.

The central axis depth dose for electron beams does not change with the area of the field as it does for photon beams. For treatment fields that are smaller in diameter than the maximum range of the electrons, there may be a decrease in the dose along the central axis of

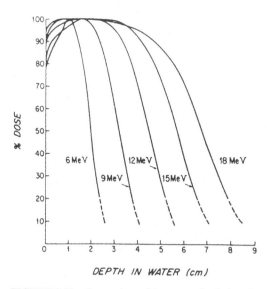

**FIGURE 3-19**  Comparison of the percent depth dose for five electron beams.

the beam and a change in the shape of the depth–dose curve. But for treatment fields with a diameter larger than the maximum range of the electrons, the relative dose at depth on the central axis will not change. Figure 3-20 shows the variation in depth of the 80% depth dose for six electron energies. At higher energies, such as 18 MeV, the change in depth of the 80% dose for 10 × 10 cm² field to a 4 × 4 cm² field is approximately 1 cm. More than one set of central axis depth–dose data is necessary for the routine use of electron beams.

***Buildup Region***   Electron beams exhibit a buildup region, but the relative dose at or near

**TABLE 3-6**   **Surface Source Distance (SSD) Correction Factors for 12 MV Electrons Versus Cone Size Compared with an Inverse Square Calculation Assuming 100 cm SSD**

| SSD (cm) | Treatment Field (100 cm SSD) | | | Inverse Square Calculation |
|---|---|---|---|---|
| | 4 × 4 cm² | 10 × 10 cm² | 25 × 25 cm² | |
| 95 | 1.165 | 1.086 | 1.110 | 1.106 |
| 100 | 1.00 | 1.00 | 1.00 | 1.00 |
| 105 | 0.856 | 0.892 | 0.907 | 0.909 |
| 115 | 0.672 | 0.723 | 0.750 | 0.760 |

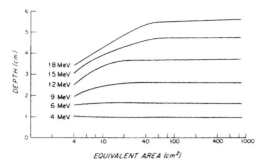

**FIGURE 3-20**  Variation in depth of the central axis 80% depth dose for square fields for six electron energies. (From Biggs et al.[32])

the surface usually increases slightly with electron beam energy. The percent depth dose at or near the surface of the patient is usually not less than 70% of dose at depth maximum for the lower energy beams; but for electron beams of 15 MeV or higher, the dose at the surface is usually near 90% of the dose at depth maximum. The variation in dose at the surface and in the buildup region is due primarily to the scattering characteristics of the electron beam upon entering the patient. Lower energy electrons have larger scattering angles, and therefore there is a sharper increase in the relative dose over a shorter range in tissue compared to an electron beam of higher energy. The buildup region is dependent on the type of accelerator, the electron-scattering foils, and the collimator design. Changes in field area can modify the dose at the surface. The surface dose usually increases for very small fields, and the depth of dose maximum is closer to the surface.

Often, bolus is required in the treatment of superficial skin lesions. The bolus material should always be placed on the patient's surface and should cover the area of interest. If bolus is used in only a section of the field, the edges of the bolus should be tapered or layered. Typical substances used as bolus materials are paraffin wax, polystyrene, and acrylic, but all materials used should be of low Z, similar to water. Super Flab and Super Stuff are commercially available products that have been used with electron beams as bolus material.[34]

**Photon Component**  All electron fields have a photon component that is dependent on the energy of the beam and on the design of the accelerator. Electrons interacting with scattering foils, monitoring ionization chambers, and the field defining cones produce x-rays that contribute dose to the patient. Some x-rays are produced in the patient, but most of the x-rays are produced from interactions with the higher Z materials. The x-ray contamination can be greater than 5% for some high energy electron beams. Newer accelerators have scattering foils that have reduced the photon component of electron beams. The x-ray component of the beam deposits dose beyond the maximum range of the electrons, and if multiple electron fields are used, such as in arc therapy or in designs featuring a number of intersecting or opposed beams, the total dose beyond the range of the electrons should be evaluated.

**Electron Beam Profile**  Flatness across the electron beam is dependent primarily on the field-flattening system, that is, the scattering foil system or the scanning beam design. Electron beams have lateral divergence, which is due to the scattering of electrons outside the field area; this expansion of the beam is especially true at the lower energy beams (Figure 3-21). The flatness of the electron beam is de-

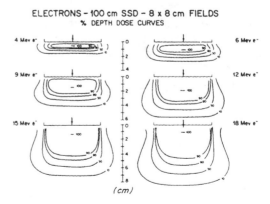

**FIGURE 3-21**  Comparison of isodose distributions for six electron energies; note the increased divergence of the 10% isodose curve relative to the central dose region of the 90% dose level.

pendent on depth in the patient and changes with energy. The area of the field at depth for small fields and for high energy beams can be much less than the field area indicated by the light field. Care needs to be taken to ensure that at the depth of the dose prescription, the area of the field encompasses the treatment volume. Often the field size needs to be increased by 1 cm or more to ensure that the treatment area is sufficient at depth. Figure 3-22 shows the variation in the width of 90% and 80% isodose levels for electron beams at six energies versus the nominal width of the field at the depth of dose maximum. For high energy beams at depth, especially for small fields, often the width of the 90% and 80% isodose curve becomes constricted. Table 3-7 shows the 90% width at the depth of the 90% isodose for several small fields at 9 and 18 MeV. The data presented are from the Varian Clinac 18. Other accelerators may have different characteristics, but the isodose distribution should be reviewed whenever the dose prescription is at depth.

### Electron Penumbra

The penumbra region for most electron fields changes with the depth because the mean energy of the beam is continually decreasing. The penumbra region for most electron beams is often larger than it is for most accelerator-produced photon beams. The width of the penumbra should be measured at the depth of dose maximum and at the depth of dose prescription, normally not less than the 90% depth. For example, the width of the 80% to 20% isodose level at the depth of dose maxim for 12 MeV electrons is 1 cm, and the difference between the 90% to 10% isodose is 1.7 cm. At the depth of the 85% isodose

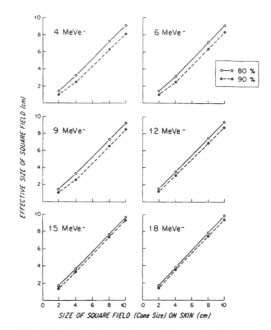

**FIGURE 3-22** Comparison of the nominal field size (cone size) with the actual distance in centimeters between the 90% or 80% isodose curve at depth maximum.

level, the 90% to 10% isodose level relative to the central axis dose becomes 2.7 cm wide. The penumbra region will vary somewhat with the design of the accelerator and the distance between the end of the cone or applicator and the patient's surface.

### Electron Field Shaping

The electron cones and applicators supplied by the accelerator manufacturer are usually standardized in shape and are rarely sufficient for routine electron beam therapy. The cones or applicators are usually designed to allow modification of the

**TABLE 3-7** Comparison of the Width of 90% Isodose Curve at the 90% Depth Versus Cone Size and for Two Energies

| Nominal Energy (MV) | | Cone Size (cm) | | |
|---|---|---|---|---|
| | | $6 \times 6$ cm$^2$ | $8 \times 8$ cm$^2$ | $10 \times 10$ cm$^2$ |
| 9 | 1.5 | 3.5 | 5.5 | 8.0 |
| 18 | 1.3 | 2.5 | 3.5 | 5.7 |

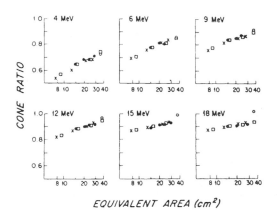

EQUIVALENT AREA (cm²)

**FIGURE 3-23** Changes in dose at depth maximum versus field size for several field shapes modifying a 6 × 6 cm² cone for six electron beam energies.

field shape by special inserts, or else the field shaping is done directly on the patient's surface, usually with lead. Field shaping can modify the output factor or the cone ratio normally associated with the unshaped field. If one or both field edges are reduced to less than the range of the electrons, modification of the central axis depth dose is also possible. Therefore measurements are often required for a number of electron fields beyond the standard set of cones or applicators. The cone ratios for the 6 × 6 cm² cone modified by inserts placed in the standard cone for a number of different field shapes are shown in Figure 3-23. Field shaping with lead or other material such as the low melting point alloys should be thick enough to allow only 5% or less transmission of the electron beams. The thickness required should be determined under clinical treatment geometry and for large fields at each energy. The thickness in millimeters of lead should be at least approximately equal to the energy in million electron volts divided by 2.[3]

**Internal Shielding**  With electron beams, field shaping often can be done not only to modify the area of the field but also to modify the range or penetration of the beam. The surface of the patient can be modified with a bolus to decrease the penetration of the beam in

the patient, and to increase the patient's surface dose. Internal shielding with high or low Z materials can reduce the penetration of the beam and protect tissues beyond the treatment volume. Lower Z materials are recommended for internal shielding if there is sufficient space for their placement in the patient. If high Z materials are to be used because of lack of space internally, backscattered electrons can significantly increase the dose to the adjacent tissue. Figure 3-24 indicates the increasing dose due to backscattered electrons relative to polystyrene for six electron energies measured with lithium fluoride crystals. Similar data were obtained with ionization chambers and are reported by Klevenhagen et. al.,[35] where $E_z$ is the mean energy of the electron beam at the lead interface and EBS is the electron backscatter factor:

$$EBS = I + 0.735 \exp(-0.052\, E_z)$$

The actual value of the backscatter factor depends on the characteristics of the electron beam at the interface. The equation can be used to estimate this effect due to lead.

The range of the backscattered electrons varies with energy, but a significant reduction in dose to the adjacent tissues can occur if low Z material is positioned between the tissue and the shielding material. Figure 3-25 indicates

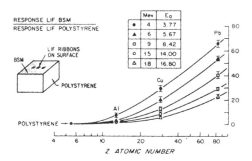

**FIGURE 3-24** Variation in the relative increase in backscattered electrons measured with lithium fluoride (LiF) crystals at the surface of various materials relative to electron beam energy: BSM, backscattering material.

the range of the backscattered electrons from lead in polystyrene for various energies measured with lithium fluoride crystals. If the thickness of the absorbing tissue equivalent material is too large to be positioned in the patient, other low $Z$ materials such as aluminum, copper, or tin should be considered. Eye shields used in electron beams should always be coated with low $Z$ material to avoid as much as possible the significant increases in dose to the adjacent tissues.

***Electron Beam Planning*** Full-isodose distribution should be available for all energies before treatment of patients. Most treatment centers can provide dose distributions for electron fields in water or tissue substitutes. Treatment of highly irregular surfaces can cause significant modifications in the dose distribution near the surface and at depth. The presence of bone, air cavities, and lung tissue modifies the range of the electron beam and often changes the dose in the surrounding tissues.[13] Computer treatment planning programs that use pencil beam algorithms and account for electron scattering can provide dose distributions with sufficient accuracy for most routine treatment situations. Dose distributions of electron beams in regions of tissue inhomogeneities, and irregular contours or in regions near bone and air cavities, should always be reviewed carefully and evaluated. Measurements should be done in a phantom to confirm as much as possible the dose distribution.

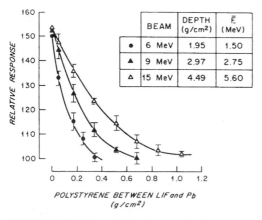

**FIGURE 3-25** The relative decrease in dose versus thickness of polystyrene away from a lead shield for three electron beams at depth.

## REFERENCES

1. Johns HE, Cunningham JR: *The Physics of Radiology,* 4th ed. Springfield, IL: Charles C Thomas, 1983.

2. Hendee WR: *Radiation Therapy Physics.* Chicago, Year Book Medical Publishers, 1981.

3. Khan FM: *The Physics of Radiation Therapy,* 2nd ed. Baltimore, Williams & Wilkins, 1992.

4. Johns HE, Whitmore GF, Watson TA, et al: A system of dosimetry for radiation therapy with typical rotation distributions. *J Can Assoc Radiol* 1953;4:1.

5. Johns HE, Bruce WR, Reid WB: The dependence of depth dose on focal skin distances. *Br J Radiol* 1958;31:254–260.

6. Karzmark CJ, Deurbert A, Loevinger R: Tissue phantom ratios—An aid to treatment planning. *Br J Radiol* 1965;38:158.

7. Determination of absorbed dose in a patient irradiated by beams of x or gamma rays, in *Radiotherapy Procedures.* US National Bureau of Standards ICRU Report 24, 1976.

8. American Association of Physicists in Medicine: A protocol for the determination of absorbed dose from high-energy photon and electron beams. *Med Phys* 1983;10:741–771.

9. Holt JG, Loughlin JS, Moroney JP: Extension of concept of tissue–air ratios (TAR) to high energy x-ray beams. *Radiology* 1970;96:437–446.

10. Measurement of absorbed dose in a phantom irradiated by a single beam of x or gamma rays in *Radiotherapy Procedures.* US National Bureau of Standards ICRU Report 23, 1973.

11. Hospital Physicists Association: Central axis depth dose data for use in radiotherapy. *Br J Radiol* 1996;983(suppl 25).

12. Clarkson JR: A note on depth doses in fields of irregular shape. *Br J Radiol* 1941;14:265–268.

13. Cunningham JR: Scattered-air ratios. *Phys Med Biol* 1972;17:42–51.

14. Federiek SO, Johns HE: Transmission dose measurement for cobalt-60 radiation with spe-

cial reference to rotation therapy. *Br J Radiol* 1957;30:190–195.

15. McKinlay AF: Thermoluminescence dosimetry, in *Medical Physics Handbooks,* vol 5. Bristol, England, Adam Hilger, 1981.

16. Batho HF: Lung corrections in cobalt-60 beam therapy. *J Can Assoc Radiol* 1974;15:79–83.

17. Young MEJ, Kornelsen RD: Dose corrections for low-density tissue inhomogeneities and air channels for 10-MV x-rays. *Med Phys* 1983;10:450–455.

18. Young MEJ, Gaylord JP: Experimental test of corrections for tissue inhomogeneities in radiotherapy. *Br J Radiol* 1970;43:349–355.

19. Cassell KJ, Hobby PA, Parker RP: The implementation of a generalized Batho inhomogeneity correction for radiotherapy planning with direct use of CT numbers. *Phys Med Biol* 1981;26:825–833.

20. Sontag MG, Cunningham JR: The equivalent tissue–air ratio method for making absorbed dose calculations in a heterogeneous medium. *Radiology* 1978;129:787–794.

21. Shimm DS, Doppke KP, Leong JCK, et al: Variation in the lung inhomogeneity correction factor with beam energy. *Acta Radiol Oncol* 1985;24:407–410.

22. Epp ER, Boyer AL, Doppke KP: Underdosing of lesions resulting from lack of electronic equilibrium in upper respiratory air cavities irradiated by 10 MV x-ray beams. *Int J Radiat Oncol Biol Phys* 1977;2:613.

23. Biggs PJ, Doppke KP, Leong JC, et al: Tissue phantom ratios for a Clinac 4/100. *Med Phys* 1982;9:753–757.

24. Horton JL: Dose in the buildup region outside of the primary beam. *Med Phys* 1984;11:331–334.

25. Doppke KP, Novack D, Wang CC: Physical considerations in the treatment of advanced carcinomas of the larynx and pyriform sinuses using 10 MV x-rays. *Int J Radiat Oncol Biol Phys* 1980;6:1251–1255.

26. Leung PMK, Johns HE: Use of electron filters to improve the buildup characteristics of large fields from cobalt-60 beams. *Med Phys* 1977;4:441.

27. Biggs PJ. Shipley WU: A beam width improving device for 25 MV x-ray beams. *Int J Radiat Oncol Biol Phys* 1986;12:131–135.

28. Chin LM, Kiyewski PK, Svensson GK, et al: A computer-controlled radiation therapy machine for pelvic and para-aortic nodal areas. *Int J Radiat Oncol Biol Phys* 1981;7:61–70.

29. Fraass BA, Tepper JE, Glatstein E, et al: Clinical use of a match-line wedge for adjacent megavoltage radiation field matching. *Int J Radiat Oncol Biol Phys* 1983;9:209–216.

30. *Radiation Dosimetry Electron Beams with Energies Between 1 and 50 MeV.* Bethesda, MD: International Commission on Radiation Units and Measurements, ICRU Report 35, 1984.

31. Mills MD, Hogstrom KR, Almond PR: Prediction of electron beam output factors. *Med Phys* 1982;9:60–68.

32. Biggs PJ, Boyer AL, Doppke KP: Electron dosimetry of electron fields on Clinac-18. *Int J Radiat Oncol Biol Phys* 1979;5:433–440.

33. Khan FM, Sewehand W, Levitt SH: Effect of air space on depth dose in electron beam therapy. *Radiology* 1978;126:249–251.

34. Shama SC, Derbel FC, Khan RM: Tissue equivalence of bolus materials for electron beam. *Radiology* 1983;146:854.

35. Klevenhagan SC, Lambert GD, Arbari A: Backscattering in electron beam therapy for energies between 3 and 35 MeV. *Phys Med Biol* 1982;27:363–373.

# CHAPTER 4

# CANCER OF THE SKIN

C.C. WANG

The skin has two layers: an outer epidermis and the inner dermis. The former consists of stratified squamous epithelium, the external layer of which is keratinized. The dermis contains connective tissue and elastic fibers and the subcutaneous tissue further down. The sebaceous glands and other glands of the skin are in the dermis and the adjacent subcutaneous tissue. All skin components can give rise to malignant tumors.

Malignant tumors arising from the skin of the head and neck region include basal cell carcinoma (BCC), squamous cell carcinoma (SCC), lymphoma, malignant melanoma, malignant fibrohistiocytoma, angiosarcoma, and skin appendage carcinoma. The adnexal tumors consist of sebaceous gland carcinoma and meibomian, eccrine, and apocrine gland carcinomas. The common basal cell carcinomas, so-called rodent ulcers, appear typically as pearly firm elevations with occasional central ulceration surrounded by minute capillaries, and are commonly found on the skin of the eyelids, nose, and nasolabial sulcus. BCC may manifest various forms, including superficial multicentric, nodular or noduloulcerative, pigmented, morphea or sclerosing, and adenoid cystic varieties. It is unreliable to differentiate between BCC and SCC on clinical grounds. It is, therefore, important that a tissue biopsy sample be obtained before any form of treatment is given.

Other uncommon tumors of the skin of the head and neck include mycosis fungoides, lymphomas, and leukemic infiltrates. These tumors involve multiple sites as a generalized process, and their local problems may require local radiation therapy.

The tumor, node, metastasis (TNM) staging system recommended by the American Joint Committee on Cancer[1] is as follows:

Tis Carcinoma in situ

T1 Tumor 2 cm or less in greatest dimension

T2 Tumor more than 2 cm but not more than 5 cm in greatest dimension

T3 Tumor more than 5 cm in greatest dimension

T4 Tumor invades deep extradermal structures (i.e., cartilage, skeletal muscle, or bone)

Nx Regional lymph nodes cannot be assessed

N0 No regional node metastases

N1 Regional node metastases

Cancers of the skin of radiotherapeutic interest and importance are mostly limited to the head and neck regions. Most of the skin cancers arising from the extremities and trunk are commonly managed by surgical means, and radiotherapy plays a role only as an adjuvant or palliative procedure.

Squamous cell carcinoma arising from the skin of the head and neck may metastasize to the

*Clinical Radiation Oncology: Indications, Techniques, and Results, 2nd ed.* Edited by C.C. Wang.
ISBN: 0-471-23803-1 Copyright © 2000 Wiley-Liss, Inc.

regional lymph nodes in about 5% of cases and more frequently in the advanced lesions. The squamous cell carcinomas in the extremities have a higher incidence of nodal metastases: approximately 20%.[2,3] Therefore, for the treatment of early, small, and well-differentiated carcinoma of the skin, elective nodal treatment either by radiation therapy or by surgery is not warranted if the regional nodal area is clinically negative. For the clinically positive nodes, however, radical node dissection with or without adjuvant radiation therapy is indicated if the primary carcinoma is controlled. Basosquamous cell carcinoma represents a microscopic pattern combining characteristics of both basal and squamous cell carcinoma. These lesions have biologic features similar to those of basal cell carcinoma and the management is essentially the same, except that the admixture of squamous cell carcinoma may occasionally metastasize to regional nodes. The metastasis of basal cell carcinoma to the regional nodes is extremely rare but may occur.

## SELECTION OF THERAPIES AND INDICATIONS

There are many ways to treat skin cancers. These include surgical excision, curettage, radiation therapy,[3–5] cryosurgery,[6] Mohs micrographic surgery,[7] and topical 5-FU cream.[8] Although Mohs procedure can be used for treatment of basal cell carcinoma of the skin, it is better reserved for the management of advanced lesions and/or recurrent tumors after curative surgery or radiation therapy. For early and moderately advanced lesions, surgery and irradiation remain the mainstays of curative procedures.

The selection of treatment modalities depends on the 4C's, which are:

Cure

Cosmesis

Cost

Convenience

Surgery is the treatment of choice under the following conditions:

1. Small lesions treated by excision expediently, without sequential dysfunction or aesthetic impairment
2. Small lesions of the neck and the scalp
3. Lesions of the dorsum of the hand or arising from scar, thermal burns, and chronic radiation dermatitis
4. Lesions arising in atrophic and aged skin, lupus vulgaris, and infected tumors in the pinna of the ear with chondritis
5. Large, destructive lesions, where extensive loss of soft tissue is evident and plastic repair will be necessary if radiation therapy is used for the cure
6. Extensive tumor infiltrating the underlying bone
7. Skin appendage carcinomas and invasive melanomas

Radiation therapy is treatment of choice under the following circumstances:

1. Carcinomas arising in the midline of the face, eyelids, nose, and lip, so-called facial triangle (Figure 4-1)

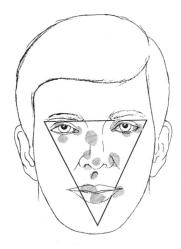

**FIGURE 4-1** The so-called facial triangle, illustrating various sites of cancer of the skin most suitable for radiation therapy.

2. Large, deeply infiltrative lesions of the skin of the face without bone involvement

3. BCC and SCC arising in the skin of the auricle

4. Lesions involving the commissure of the mouth

5. Lesions arising in the pre- and postauricular areas and in the nasolabial sulcus

## EVALUATION OF SKIN CANCERS

Before a radiotherapeutic procedure is considered, the size, thickness, and margins of any lesions must be carefully assessed. The margins are best evaluated under bright light with the aid of magnifying glasses. The lesion should be palpated gently. The surrounding hair follicles, skin texture, and color should be carefully compared with the normal skin and the lesion. The use of Woods lamp (ultraviolet) light may aid in differentiating between the tumor(s) and the adjacent normal skin. Unfortunately, carcinoma and keratosis cannot be differentiated by Woods lamp alone.

When the lesions are situated on the skin of the cheek and lip, bidigital palpation by gloved finger may be very informative with respect to the depth of infiltration of the lesion. When the lesions are fixed to the adjacent bone, appropriate radiographs, including CT scans, should be obtained to evaluate the possibility of bone involvement.

### Specific Considerations

1. The underlying structures such as cornea and lens of the eye, mandible, teeth, gum, and nasal septum must be protected with lead shields. For sites that cannot be protected by intervening lead shields, such as scalp, the area over the mastoid sinus, the temporomandibular joint, the brain, and the spinal cord, appropriate energies of x-rays, electrons, or implants or a combination of these should be selected.

2. In our practice, most radiation failures are due to geographic misses from insufficient margins; rarely is insufficient dose the cause of failure.

3. Radiotherapeutically, there is no allowance in difference of radiosensitivity between squamous cell carcinoma and basal cell carcinoma; but the former may involve the management of the primary lesion and occasionally metastatic nodes.

4. The radiation technique and total dose level are the same.

## RADIOTHERAPEUTIC MODALITIES AND ACCESSORIES

Most superficial cancers of the skin currently are treated by low energy electrons, commonly 6 to 9 MV electrons. Low megavoltage photons (4–6 MV) or sources of cobalt-60 radiation are used for treatment of large and thick invasive

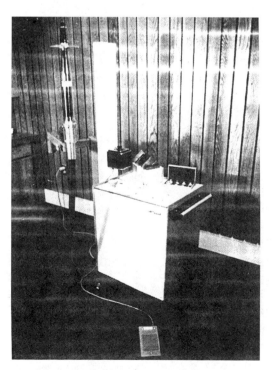

**FIGURE 4-2** A Phillips 50 kV contact machine for treatment of small carcinoma of the eyelid.

tumors and/or regional lymph node metastases. BCC of the eyelid is best treated by the low energy x-rays, such as the Phillips 50 kV(p) contact unit (Figure 4-2).

In addition to external beam therapy, brachytherapy can be employed. The preferred procedure, afterloading interstitial implant, uses angiocatheter applicators and $^{192}$Ir sources. For the past 4 years a high dose rate (HDR) $^{192}$Ir source has been available at the Massachusetts General Hospital (MGH); large fraction (i.e., 3–4 Gy/fraction, BID) is given as a boost, fractionated for 2 to 3 days.

As a general rule, lesions in a curved surface are preferably treated by electrons and lesions in a flat surface by brachytherapy alone or combined with electrons.

In radiation therapy of skin cancers, lead shields are used for proper exposure of the lesion and protection of the adjacent normal tissues. Individually made lead cutouts, specially for the eye, nose, and gum shields, are used for treatment of appropriate tumor (Figures 4-3 and 4-4). For electron beam therapy, 6 to 9 MV beams are frequently used. The low energy electrons have skin-sparing characteristics, and a thin layer of bolus must be added on the surface of the tumor to achieve $D_{max}$ on the skin, as shown in Figure 4-5. Individual Cerrobend cutouts with appropriate apertures are made to shape the lesion and placed under the window of the linear accelerator. These simple gadgets

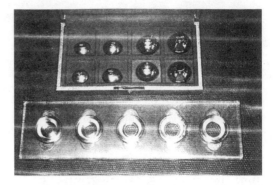

**FIGURE 4-4** **Top**: Lead eye shields for radiation therapy of eyelid. **Bottom**: Lead "nipple" cutouts suitable for treatment of cancer of the inner canthus of the eye.

are extremely important in the treatment of skin cancers.

## Radiation Therapy Dosages and Fraction Size

No lesion thicker than 1.0 cm can be treated satisfactorily by 50 or 100 kV x-radiations. Such lesions are treated either by low energy electrons or in combination with an interstitial implant. For external beam x-ray therapy, various time–dose–fraction schemes[9] are available and have proven to be effective. The cosmetic results are related to the fraction size and total dose. The fractionated radiation therapy data in Tables 4-1[3,10] and 4-2 are presented for lesions 1.5 to 2.0 and 5 to 6 cm in diameter.

One notes that the treatment schemes are extremely variable, depending on the availability of treatment machine time and the characteristics of the patient population (i.e., young or old, male or female, likelihood of patient's long-term survival). Our program of radiation therapy for skin cancer at the MGH, which has been used for the past 35 years, has proven to be highly effective, with acceptable cosmetic results. It is as follows:

1. For small lesions 0.5 to 1 cm in size, a single treatment of 24 Gy is curative. This regimen is rarely used, but may be

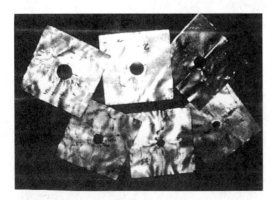

**FIGURE 4-3** Special lead sheets and cutouts to tailor the shape and size of the lesions for the 50 kV contact machine.

given to debilitated, aged patients who have difficulty attending daily radiation therapy sessions on an outpatient basis.

2. For lesions 1.5 to 2.5 cm in size, 45 Gy in five fractions or 45 Gy in nine fractions is commonly used, depending on the patient's skin and physical condition of the patient, age, and availability for daily sessions.

3. For a somewhat larger lesion, or highly desirable cosmeses, a prolonged course of treatment is prescribed (i.e., 52 Gy divided into 13 daily fractions).

4. Large tumors are treated with 60 Gy in 25 fractions.

5. For large lesions suitable for combined external beam and interstitial implants, generally a total dose between 65 and 70 Gy is planned (i.e., 30 Gy in 10 daily fractions by x-rays or electrons plus 30–35 Gy by implant).

6. Experience has shown that the isobioeffect of TDF value of 125 to 135 as shown in Figure 4-6 is required for permanent local control of most small- to medium-sized carcinomas of the skin. For a larger and thicker lesion, a higher dose is required.

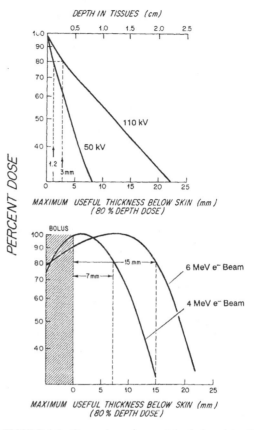

**FIGURE 4-5** Comparison of percent depth dose data of radiations versus maximal therapeutic thickness of the lesions suitable for radiation therapy.

**TABLE 4-1  Fractionationated radiation therapy schemes for skin carcinomas (1.5 to 2.0 cm in diameter)\***

| Total dose (Gy) | Dose/fraction | Time (days) (TDF) | Institution |
|---|---|---|---|
| 35 | 7 | 5 (113) | Princess Margaret Hosp |
| 45 | 3 | 15 (92) | U Oregon |
| 45 | 3 | 15 (92) | U Florida |
| 40 | 4 | 10 (96) | U Florida |
| 35 | 7 | 5 (113) | U Ariz |
| 40 | 5 | 8 (108) | U Ariz |
| 45 | 9 | 5 (167) | U Ala |
| 30 | 10 | 3 (123) | Christie Hospital |
| 20 | 20 | 1 | Christie Hospital |
| 45 | 9 | 5 (167) | Mass General Hosp |
| 45 | 5 | 9 (123) | MGH |
| 52 | 4 | 13 (125) | MGH |
| 20–23 | 20–23 | 1 (Rarely used) | MGH |

\*Data surveyed by Kyle Colvett, M.D., 1994.

**TABLE 4-2  Fractionationated radiation therapy schemes for skin carcinomas (5.0–6.0 cm in diameter)\***

| Total dose (Gy) | Dose/fraction | Time (days) (TDF) | Institution |
| --- | --- | --- | --- |
| 60 | 3 | 20 | Princess Margaret Hosp (PMH) |
| 40 | 4 | 10 | PMH |
| 45 | 3 | 15 plus implant | PMH |
| 60 | 3 | 20 | U Oregon |
| 45 | 1.8 | 35 | U Florida |
| 60 | 3 | 20 | U Ariz |
| 30 | 3 | 10 plus implant | U Ala |
| 35 | 7 | 5 plus implant | Christie Hospital |
| 60 | | Implant alone | Christie Hospital |
| 60 | 3 | 20 | Mass General Hosp |
| 52 | 4 | 13 | MGH |
| 30 | 3 | 10 plus implant | MGH |

\*Data surveyed by Kyle Colvett, M.D., 1994.

## Technical Pointers

1. Patient should be lying comfortably on the treatment couch but immobilized.

2. Underlying radiosensitive structures (e.g., cornea and lens of the eye, mandible, teeth, gums, nasal septum) must be protected with waxed lead shields. For sites that cannot be protected by intervening lead shields, select appropriate energies of x-rays, electrons, or implants or combination of various therapeutic modalities.

3. To compensate for surface-sparing effects of low energy electrons, "bolus" should be added over the tumor when a 6

**TABLE 4-3  6 MeV Electron Beam with 0.5 cm Bolus**[a]

| | Depth in patient (cm) | % DD |
| --- | --- | --- |
| Surface dose | 0.0 | 84 |
| Dose maximum | 0.5 | 100 |
| 0.5 cm bolus plus | 1.0 | 80 |
| 0.5 cm bolus plus | 2.0 | 40 |

[a] Varian 2100 C data.

to 9 MV electron beam is employed (see Figure 4-5).

4. For extensive lesions involving bone and muscle, consider surgery first, with adjuvant postoperative radiation therapy.

5. Use the same dose and treatment scheme for squamous cell carcinoma and basal cell carcinoma.

6. Always evaluate the lesion 2 weeks after treatment related to the skin reactions and radiation coverage. If the irradiated lesion and the adjacent tissue do not show brisk erythema to the point of moist desquamation, give an additional 9 to 10 Gy on top of the previously prescribed dose through a smaller field.

7. The lesion should heal in 4 to 6 weeks, leaving a smooth pliable scar. Any nodu-

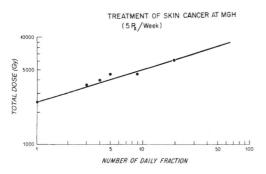

**FIGURE 4-6**  Isobioeffect line for treatment of small- to medium-sized cancers of the skin at the Massachusetts General Hospital, TDF values ranging between 125 and 135.

larity or ulceration in 6 months should be investigated by biopsy for recurrence.

Tables 4-3 and 4-4 give data related to 6 to 9 MeV electron dose distribution at depth (DD) for daily clinical management of skin carcinoma.

## RADIOTHERAPEUTIC RESULTS

Carcinoma of the skin is highly curable by radiation therapy, with local control rates of 90% or higher. When basal cell carcinoma involves bone, the local control rate is poor but the patient may live with the disease for many years, and therefore a relentless surgical approach could be rewarding. Metastatic squamous cell carcinoma of the skin to the regional nodes has a poor prognosis, with a 3-year NED (no evidence of disease) rate of approximately 30%.

Table 4-5 shows the results of treatment of skin as reported in the literature.[11–13]

## SPECIFIC SITES OF RADIOTHERAPEUTIC INTEREST

### Carcinoma of the Eyelid[10,14,15]

For all practical purposes, basal cell carcinomas of the eyelid are considered to be cancers of the skin and are treated as such. When a lesion involves the inner canthus, surgical removal would mean either plastic repair or damage to the lacrimal duct. Radiation therapy is preferred

**TABLE 4-5   Local Control After Treatment of Skin Cancer**

| | |
|---|---|
| Regato[11] | 594/654 pts–93% by RT |
| Lauritzen[12] | 2802/2900 pts–96.5% by S or RT |
| Freeman[13] | 2235/2288–98% by S or RT |

because it can often achieve a result that is good both functionally and cosmetically, as well as control of the disease comparable to that produced by a surgical procedure. Tumors of the canthi tend to involve the bony orbit rather early, especially at the inner canthus. When this occurs, control by radiation therapy is uncommon—about 25%—and therefore orbital exenteration may be required to save the patient's life. Postoperative radiation therapy may be considered as an adjuvant procedure.

Because of the superficial nature of most early cancer of the eyelid and the necessity for avoiding irradiation of the underlying radiosensitive structures of the eye, radiation therapy must be highly individualized. Radiations of low penetration are highly desirable, such as 4 to 6 MV electrons or 50 kV x-rays using the Phillips contact machine (the only kilovoltage machine used for clinical radiation therapy at the MGH at the present time).

The doses used for treatment of carcinoma of the eyelids are similar to radiation therapy for carcinoma of the skin: that is, for the small lesions, 45 Gy in 5 daily fractions; for moderately advanced lesions, 45 Gy in 2 weeks; and for large lesions, 4 Gy per fraction for 13 days.

### Technical Pointers

1. Because a smaller portal is used and because of the radiosensitive structures of the eye, the daily setup of treatment should be handled by the attending radiation oncologist.
2. An inner waxed lead eye shield or beam-blocking devices should be used to protect the cornea and lens.

**TABLE 4-4   9 MeV Electron Beam with 1.0 cm Bolus[a]**

| | Depth in patient (cm) | % DD |
|---|---|---|
| Surface dose | 0.0 | 90 |
| Dose maximum | 0.6 | 100 |
| 1.0 cm bolus plus | 1.0 | 82 |
| 1.0 cm bolus plus | 2.0 | 55 |

[a] Varian 2100 C data.

3. Topical anesthetic (0.5% paracaine hydrochloride) is applied to the eye. The eyeshield is cleaned with alcohol and then rinsed with saline solution or tap water. (The residue of the alcohol would be irritating to the conjunctiva.)

4. Individual cutouts with at least 0.5 cm visible normal margins are used.

5. The anesthetized eye is bandaged for about 30 minutes after each irradiation to prevent foreign bodies from gaining access to the eye.

Squamous cell carcinoma of the eyelid is an uncommon disease, and its management is identical to that for basal cell carcinoma in terms of extent of coverage and radiation dose and fractionation. Metastases from carcinoma of the eyelids occur in about 10% of cases and carry a grave prognosis. The parotid lymph nodes are the most common site of involvement. The management of such metastases is a combination of surgical resection and radiation therapy.

Sebaceous gland carcinoma of the eyelid is rare, with high incidence of regional lymph node and distant metastases (i.e., approximately 25%).[16] For the small lesion, radiation therapy is the treatment of choice with good local control and satisfactory cosmesis.[16] The large infiltrative tumors associated with orbital invasion are better managed by surgical resection with adjuvant postoperative radiation therapy. Owing to the high propensity of such carcinomas for lymph node metastases, elective ipsilateral parotid and neck irradiation with 45 to 50 Gy in 4 weeks appears worthwhile.

The results of radiation therapy carcinoma of the eyelid are shown in Table 4-6.

## Carcinoma of the Skin Overlying the Nasal Cartilage and the Nasolabial Sulcus[4,5]

Carcinomas arising from the bridge and tip of the nose and nasal alae present a difficult prob-

**TABLE 4-6  Local Control of Carcinoma of the Eyelid**

| | |
|---|---|
| Regato[14] | 108/117-92% |
| Wildermuth and Evan[15] | 67/71-93% |
| Fitzpatrick[10] | 1106/1166-95% |
| Wang (unpublished) | 290/300-97% |

lem for radiation dosimetry. The so-called saddle lesion, covering both nasal alae, would be better treated by a combination of low energy electrons and/or interstitial implant. The nasal cartilage has a high radiation tolerance: radiochondritis following a therapeutic dose of radiotherapy has not been encountered in our practice and is a mythical misconception in the literature.

Carcinoma arising from the nasolabial sulcus tends to burrow beneath the skin and into the premaxillary fossa and adipose tissue, with the result that the true tumor extension often escapes accurate detection. The treatment of choice for these lesions is a combination of external beam therapy and interstitial implant.

### Technical Pointers

1. Use 6 to 9 MV electrons and a 0.5 cm bolus over the lesion, treating 1 to 1.5 cm below the skin surface.

2. A lead shield is inserted into the nostrils to protect the nasal floor and the septum.

3. The underlying gum posterior to the upper lip is protected with a lead shield.

4. To accommodate the slope of both nasal alae with increase of distance from the electron target, the peripheral dose is constricted toward the center, with decrease of depth dose in the periphery. A portal considerably wider than those typical of photon therapy is used.

5. Dose and treatment schemes are the same as for skin in general.

6. For combined electrons and brachytherapy, give 30 Gy in 2 weeks and 35 Gy in 3 days, respectively.

## Carcinoma of the Skin of the Auricle of the Ear

When the lesion is infected and deeply ulcerative, exposing the cartilage, surgical excision is preferred. For early, superficial lesions arising from the pinna or concha of the ear, radiation therapy alone may be used with good local control and cosmetic results. Because of the irregular curvature of the surface of the auricle of the ear, x-ray therapy for this disease often results in "hot spots" and "cold spots" in the irradiated field, which may produce radiochondritis or local recurrence. Treatment of choice for these lesions is low energy electrons; the incidence of radiochondritis is much lessened.

### Technical Pointers

1. The middle ear can be protected by inserting a lead cylinder (in the shape of the auditory canal, so-called earplug).
2. The mastoid sinus can be protected by placing a waxed lead shield behind the auricle.
3. If the conchae of the ear are not involved, they can be protected by a small lead shield.
4. Use 6 to 9 MV electrons to treat the entire thickness of the ear.
5. Place a 0.5 cm bolus over the lesion for maximal dose on the skin.
6. Dose schedules are the same as for radiation therapy for skin cancer in general.

The treatment results are shown in Table 4-7.

## Carcinoma of the Skin Overlying the Pre- or Postauricular Sites

Carcinomas arising from the pre- or postauricular sites should not be treated by external beam alone, since excessive radiation dose to the temporomandibular joint or temporal bone may result in radiation complications such as TMJ ankylosis or temporal bone necrosis.

**TABLE 4-7   Local Control of Carcinoma of the Skin: Over the Nose and Ear**

| | |
|---|---|
| Regato[11] | 53/56-95% |
| Fitzpatrick[17] | Nose: 285/320-89% |
| | Ear: 672/743-90 |

Such lesions are best managed by a combination of low energy electron beam and interstitial implant.

### Technical Pointers

1. Use 6 to 9 MV electrons for treatment 1 to 1.5 cm below the surface.
2. Vary the thickness of the bolus to determine the depth dose desired.
3. For moderate-sized lesions, plan 30 Gy electrons in 2 weeks to be followed by a 30 to 35 Gy interstitial implant.
4. For a preauricular implant, insert sources horizontally (i.e., AP direction). For postauricular lesions, insert sources vertically, suture the auricle, and fold it forward over the preauricular area.
5. Be certain the auriculomastoid sulcus is adequately covered.

## MISCELLANEOUS SKIN TUMORS OF RADIOTHERAPEUTIC INTEREST

To illustrate salient features of different kinds of skin cancer and their treatment techniques and results, a series of cases is presented in Figures 4-7 through 4-14.

## Skin Appendage Carcinomas[18,19]

Carcinomas of the sebaceous glands, eccrine sweat glands, and apocrine glands may occur on the head and neck region. Sebaceous gland carcinoma occurs most frequently on the eyelids as a malignant lesion of the meibomian gland. Widespread aggressive metastatic disease is often seen with the eyelid lesions. Carcinomas of the eccrine sweat glands and apocrine glands are locally invasive and tend not to metastasize. For the most part, treatment of these malignant appendage tumors is by radical resection. The role of radiation therapy is not well recognized. Our experience however indicates that these lesions respond well to high dose (i.e., 70–75 Gy irradiation), with good local control. If the lesions remain localized, yet unresectable, a trial

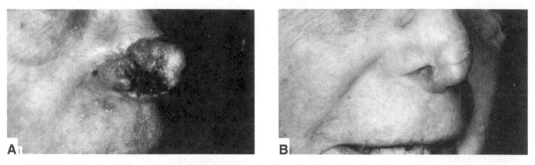

**FIGURE 4-7**    An 83-year-old male had a recurrent basal cell carcinoma on the right nasal ala **(A)**, previously treated by excision and skin graft. The recurrent lesion was treated with 12 MV electrons for 30 Gy in 10 daily fractions, followed by interstitial implant of 30 Gy in 60 hours. The patient was NED 2.5 years after implant **(B)**.

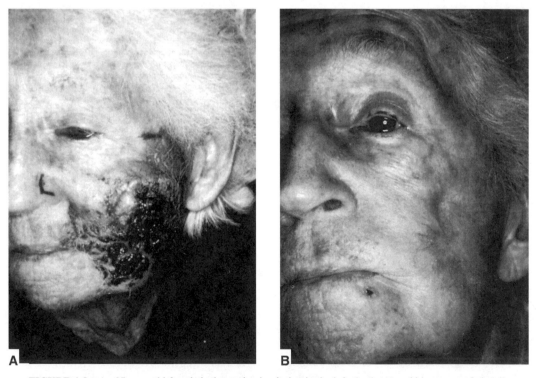

**FIGURE 4-8**    An 87-year-old female had an enlarging lesion in the left cheek **(A)** and biopsy revealed well-differentiated squamous cell carcinoma with no regional adenopathy. Radiation therapy was given using combination of 12 and 15 MV electrons for 30 Gy and lateral wedge pair $^{60}$Co x-rays for 40 Gy in 45 days. The total TDF value was 136. The patient was NED one year after treatment **(B)**.

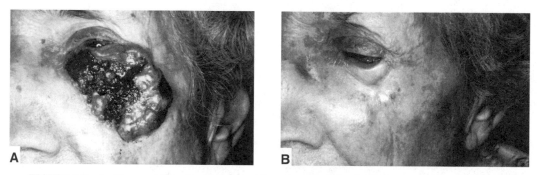

**FIGURE 4-9**   An 83-year-old female with large mobile and exophytic basal cell carcinoma of the left malar region involving the lower eyelid **(A)**. Radiation therapy consisted of 45 Gy using 9 MV electrons with 0.5 cm bolus in nine daily fractions, with eye protection. Three weeks later, an additional 10 Gy in a single treatment was given, using a 6 MV electron beam. TDF was 145. The patient was NED 1.5 years later **(B)**.

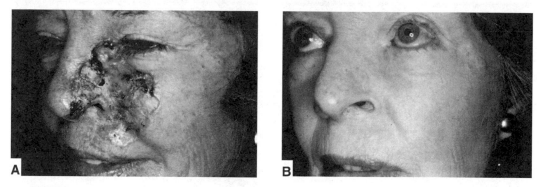

**FIGURE 4-10**   A 63-year-old female noticed a scaly, eczematoid squamous cell carcinoma on the left side of her face and nose **(A)** for 5 years. The $7 \times 7$ cm$^2$ lesion was freely mobile from the underlying structures, and there was no parotid or cervical adenopathy. The lesion was treated with 64 Gy in 25 fractions over 35 elapsed days with good response. Five years after radiation therapy the patient showed excellent response with good cosmesis **(B)**.

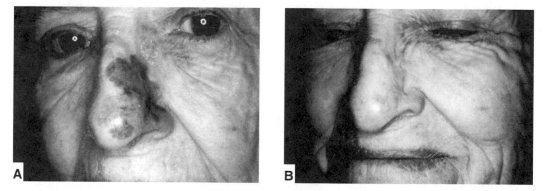

**FIGURE 4-11**   An 81-year-old female with lentigo malignum in the left side of the nose **(A)**. After 10 years, the lesion was treated using 6 MV electrons, 5 Gy per fraction per day, for 45 Gy in 13 elapsed days. Three weeks later, in the absence of severe reaction, an additional 10 Gy was given in a single fraction. The patient was last seen 2 years after radiation therapy, and the pigmented lesion had completely disappeared **(B)**, with good skin and subcutaneous tissue.

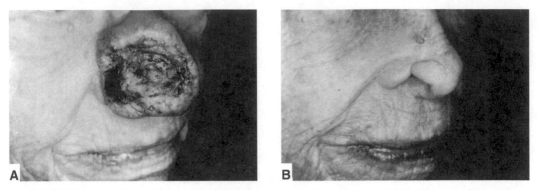

**FIGURE 4-12** An 85-year-old female with rapidly enlarging keratoacanthoma on the tip of the nose of 6 weeks' duration (**A**). Radiation therapy of 12 Gy, using 4 Gy per fraction was given. Five weeks later, owing to persistence of disease, additional 5 Gy given. The patient was NED 3.5 years after radiation therapy (**B**).

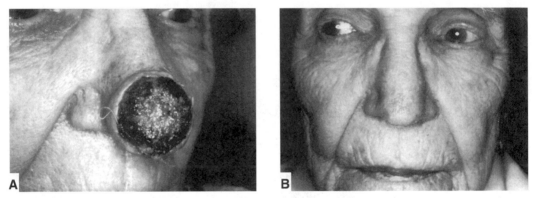

**FIGURE 4-13** A 93-year-old female noted a rapidly enlarging mass on the nose for 3 months. Biopsy results showed well-differentiated squamous cell carcinoma. The clinical course was that of Keratoacanthoma. The lesion (**A**) was treated for 32 Gy in 10 days with 4 Gy per fraction of 12 MV electron. The tumor completely vanished (**B**) leaving a relatively normal-looking nose.

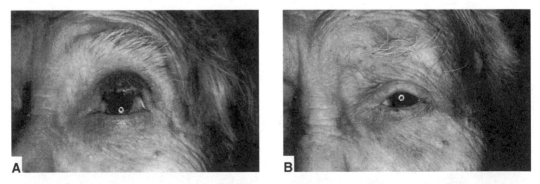

**FIGURE 4-14** A 98-year-old woman had a small lump in the left upper eyelid with a preauricular lymph node (**A**). The eyelid lesion was biopsied showing a Merkel cell tumor and was treated with 51 Gy in 16 days, with eye protection, and the left parotid node was treated with a separate field to 60 Gy in 29 days, using a combination of electrons and $^{60}$Co radiation, twice a day, with 2 Gy per fraction. There was complete disappearance of both lesions after the treatment (**B**). The patient developed fulminating cervical and supraclavicular metastatic lesions and received chemotherapy for palliation.

course of radiation therapy is worthwhile.[16] A 5-year survival after treatment is estimated to be approximately 70%.[11]

## Merkel Cell Tumor[20-23]

Merkel cell tumors are small-cell neuroendocrine undifferentiated neoplasms of the skin that occurs on sun-exposed areas, especially on the face and arms of elderly men and women. Not infrequently such a tumor will run a fulminating clinical course with regional and distant metastases. Merkel cell tumor is quite radiosensitive and responds to a modest dose of radiation therapy. Generally a dose of 45 to 50 Gy in 3 to 4 weeks is sufficient for local control. Because of the propensity to distant metastases, the eventual outcome of these patients is extremely poor. The 5-year survival is estimated to be 50%.[11] Chemotherapy has been used, but its efficacy remains primarily palliative.[21]

## Keratoacanthoma (KA)[24,25]

A benign lesion, histologically similar to well-differentiated carcinoma, Keratoacanthoma can grow to 1 to 2 cm in a few weeks. The lesions are often umbilicated and covered with a central keratin plug. The diagnosis can often be made on clinical grounds. Although biologically the lesion may undergo spontaneous resolution, leaving a depressed scar, Keratoacanthomata occurring on the eyelid, nose, and lip may cause significant loss of soft tissue, with resultant facial and functional deformity. Therefore radiation therapy is required for local control.

A dose of 25 Gy in one week or its equivalent is sufficient for most lesions (Figure 4-8). If the tumor fails to show good regression in 2 weeks with such doses, additional higher radiation dose (i.e., 60–65 Gy) should be given, as if the lesion were a genuine squamous cell carcinoma (see Figure 4-9).

## Lentigo Malignum

Circumscribed precancerous melanosis or melanotic freckle of Hutchinson is a noninvasive melanotic lesion occurring primarily in elderly persons, on the face. It is usually a flat, tan lesion with irregular borders and areas of lighter pigmentation. Treatment of choice is surgical excision. In areas of cosmetic and functional importance such as eyelid, pinna of the ear, and bridge and ala of the nose, radiation therapy is employed in lieu of surgery and can achieve satisfactory local control.[26] Doses similar to those for treatment of carcinoma of the skin are recommended, that is, 45 Gy in nine daily fractions or its equivalent (Figure 4-10).

## Kaposi Sarcoma[27,28]

Kaposi sarcoma is a multicentric, incurable lesion. The tumors are extremely radiosensitive, and for small, symptomatic lesions, a single dose of 10 or 15 Gy in three fractions should produce lasting regression. Kaposi sarcoma associated with AIDS can also be irradiated with good local control. A dose of 25 to 30 Gy in one week or its biological equivalent should suffice. Unfortunately the survival of AIDS patients is short, in terms of months.

## SUMMARY

Cancers of the skin of the head and neck are very common. BCC and squamous cell carcinoma, the common histologic types, are curable in the early stage in about 90% to 95% of patients. The selection of various methods is highly important in their management, and depends on such considerations as the availability and skill of specialists, the location and size of the lesion, the cosmetic and functional results anticipated after treatment, the cost, and the effects on and convenience to the patient. Many small accessible basal cell carcinomas of the face can be expediently treated by excisional biopsy, electrodesiccation, and curettage. Large and superficial lesions arising in the difficult sites for which surgery might result in significant cosmetic mutilation are best dealt with by radiation therapy. Surgical excision may be used for large, deeply infiltrative lesions with bone involvement in accessible locations. The time-consuming, laboratory-taxing, and tissue-destroying Mohs procedure is generally reserved for the treatment of recurrent carcinoma.

The use of radiation therapy for Merkel cell tumor, keratoacanthoma, lentigo malignum, and Kaposi sarcoma has been gradually recognized and in selected cases may be rewarding.

Radiation therapy for carcinoma of the skin requires careful planning and the use of techniques with various energies of photons and electrons intermixed with brachytherapy, calling for greater professional skills, ingenuity, and individuality. Proper selection of quality and quantity of irradiations and fraction size, with careful protection of adjacent and underlying structures, can result in extremely high cure rates and excellent cosmesis without complications. Success at this level requires personal interest and enthusiasm on the part of the radiation oncologist.

## REFERENCES

1. American Joint Cancer Committee, *AJCC Cancer Staging Manual*, 5th ed. Philadelphia, Lippincott Raven, 1997.

2. McGavran MH: Skin tumors, in LV Ackerman, J Rosai (eds): *Surgical Pathology,* 5th ed. St. Louis, CV Mosby, 1974.

3. Moss WT, Bran WN, Battifora H: Metastasis of squamous cell carcinoma of the skin by region and frequency of surgical control of metastasis, in WR Moss, WN Brand, and AH Battifora (eds): *Radiation Oncology,* 5th ed. St Louis, CV Mosby, 1979.

4. del Regato JA, Vuksanovic M: Radiotherapy of carcinomas of the skin overlying the cartilages of the nose and ear. *Radiology* 1962;79:203–208.

5. Parker RG, Wildermuth O: Radiation therapy of lesions overlying cartilage. *Cancer* 1962;15: 57–65.

6. Zacarian S (ed): *Cryosurgical Advances in Dermatology and Tumors of Head and Neck. Dermatology.* Springfield, IL, Charles C Thomas, 1977.

7. Mohs EE: Chemosurgery: Microscopically controlled surgery for skin cancer—Past, present and future. *J Dermatol Surg Oncol* 1978;4:41.

8. Klein E, Helen F, Milgram H, et al: Tumors of the skin, effects of local use of cytostatic agents. *Skin* 1962;1:89.

9. Strandquist M: Time–dose relationship. *Acta Radiol* 1977; suppl 55:1.

10. Fitzpatrick PJ, Jamieson DM, Thompson GA, et al: Tumors of the eyelids and their treatment by radiotherapy. *Radiology* 1972;104:661–665.

11. del Regato JA, Spjut J, Cox JD: *Ackerman & del Regato's Cancer—Diagnosis, Treatment and Prognosis,* 6th ed. St Louis, CV Mosby, 1985, pp 203–206.

12. Lauritzen RE, Johnson RE, Spratt JS Jr: Pattern of recurrences in basal cell carcinoma. *Surgery* 1965;57:813–816.

13. Freeman RG, Duncan WC: Recurrent skin cancer. *Arch Dermatol* 1973;107:395–399.

14. del Regato, JA: Roentgen therapy of carcinoma of the eyelids. *Radiology* 1949;52:564–573.

15. Wildermuth O, Evans JC: The special problem of cancer of the eyelid. *Cancer* 1956;9: 837–841.

16. Pardo F, Wang CC, Albert D, et al: Sebaceous carcinoma of the ocular adnexae: A role of radiotherapy. *Int J Radiat Oncol Biol Phys* 1988;15:167.

17. Fitzpatrick, PJ: Radiation therapy of tumors of the skin of the head and neck, in SE Thawley, WR Panje, JG Batsakis, and RD Lindberg (eds): *Comprehensive Management of Head and Neck Tumors.* Philadelphia, Saunders, 1987, pp 1208–1220.

18. Miller WL: Sweat gland carcinoma. *Am J Clin Pathol* 1967;47:767.

19. Wertkin MG, Bauer JJ: Sweat gland carcinoma. *Arch Surg* 1976;111:884–885.

20. Sibley RK, Dehner LP, Rosai J: Primary neuroendocrine (Merkel cell?) carcinoma of the skin. *Am J Surg Pathol* 1985;9:2–95.

21. George TK, Santagnese A, Bennett JM: Chemotherapy for metastatic Merkel cell carcinoma. *Cancer* 1985;56:1034–1038.

22. Goepfert H, Remmier D, Silva E, Wheeler B: Merkel cell carcinoma (endocrine carcinoma of the skin) of the head and neck. *Arch Otolaryngol* 1984;110:707–712.

23. Warner TF, Uno H, Hafez GR, et al: Merkel cells and Merkel cell tumors: Ultrastructure, immunocytochemistry and review of the literature. *Cancer* 1983;52:238–245.

24. Finley AG: Keratoacanthoma. *Aust J Dermatol* 1954;2:144.

25. Shimm D, Duttenhaver J, Doucette J, et al: Radiation therapy of keratoacanthomas. *Int J Radiat Oncol Biol Phys* 1983;9:759–761.

26. Harwood AR: Conventional radiotherapy in the treatment of lentigo maligna and lentigo melanoma. *J Am Acad Dermatol* 1982;6:310.

27. O'Brien PH, Brasfield RD: Kaposi's sarcoma. *Cancer* 1966;19:1497.

28. Holecek MJ, Harwood AR: Radiotherapy of Kaposi's sarcoma. *Cancer* 1978;41:1733.

# CHAPTER 5

# CANCERS OF THE HEAD AND NECK

C. C. WANG

## GENERAL COMMENTS

The head and neck regions, such as oral cavity, pharynx and larynx, (Figure 5-1) are common sites of many malignant neoplasms. These include lesions arising from the mucous membranes, salivary and mucous glands, the lymphatic system, and the mesenchymal and other supporting tissues. Among these, squamous cell carcinoma, adenocarcinoma, and lymphoma are of common occurrence and account for a great majority of cancers of the head and neck. It is estimated that in 1998 approximately 58,600 persons in the United States were afflicted, and of these about one-quarter to one-third died of such malignancies.[1]

A voluminous literature and a few good textbooks have been devoted solely to the understanding and treatment of malignancies arising from this region of the human body. Discussion in this chapter is limited to the common neoplasms seen in daily practice at a general hospital (Massachusetts General Hospital-MGH). For more detailed information on various head and neck malignancies, readers are referred to special textbooks available in most medical libraries.

Carcinomas originating from the mucous membrane of the upper aerodigestive tract are predominately squamous cell carcinomas of varying degrees of differentiation, ranging from in situ carcinoma and verrucous carci-

noma to poorly differentiated carcinomas, including lymphoepithelioma. The early mucosal lesion may appear as an indurated nodule or as a shallow ulcer with poorly defined margins. Most patients present with unilateral sore throat or canker sore in the mouth, or unilateral otitis media, frequently of several weeks' or months' duration, odynophagia, or hoarseness as their only symptoms of the presence of the extensive disease. These tumors may be exophytic or infiltrative and may extend rapidly into the underlying muscle and cause fixation, with resultant hoarseness, or difficulty in speech or swallowing; in the advanced stage, there may be impairment of hearing, trismus of the jaw, cranial nerve paralysis, and difficulty in breathing. The metastatic disease usually occurs in the homolateral cervical lymph nodes although bilateral or contralateral metastases commonly develop from midline lesions. Distant metastases below the clavicles are not common, but they may occur late in the disease or with extensive cervical metastases.

For evaluation of the extent of the lesion, careful inspection and palpation of the primary site and neck areas is mandatory whenever possible. Indirect laryngoscopy and/or fiberopticscopy are extremely informative in evaluating the extent of the lesion as well as the mobility of the involved parts. Direct laryngoscopy and multiple biopsies to define mucosal and submucosal extension of tumor or to rule out a

*Clinical Radiation Oncology: Indications, Techniques, and Results, 2nd ed.* Edited by C.C. Wang.
ISBN: 0-471-23803-1 Copyright © 2000 Wiley-Liss, Inc.

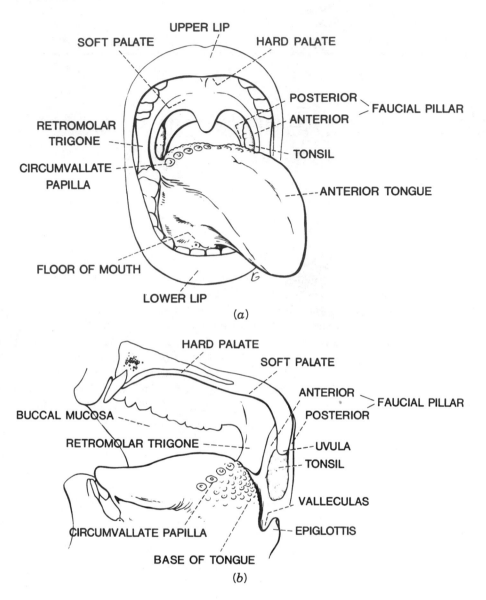

**FIGURE 5-1**    Diagrams showing various anatomic sites of the oral cavity: (**a**) anterior view and (**b**) lateral view.

second primary cancer should be carried out prior to any definitive therapeutic program. Appropriate x-ray imaging examinations are used to assess the extent of the lesion as well as bone and muscle invasion. Most of the conventional radiographic examinations, except polytomes of the larynx and barium swallow for the esophageal lesion, have been largely replaced by CT and MR scans for evaluation of most of the head and neck tumors. As part of the medical workup, a general physical examination, chest radiographs, and a basic liver profile are necessary to assess the medical condition of the patient. Since the hemoglobin level may affect local control of head and neck tumors, anemia found to be present should be corrected.

A variety of therapeutic measures is available for the management of localized carcinomas of the head and neck. These include surgical resection, radiation therapy, laser beam excision, and a combination of these methods. The choice of treatment depends on the site and size of the primary lesion, the presence or absence of metastatic disease in the neck, the general medical health and age of the patient, the morbidity after the treatment program, the experience and skill of both the surgeon and the radiation oncologist, and last, but not least, the wishes of the patient.

## Radiation Modalities

The radiotherapeutic modalities used for treatment of carcinomas of the head and neck are primarily megavoltage radiations with energies of several million volts, such as x-rays generated from 4 to 10 MV linear accelerators with interplay of electron beam.

Brachytherapy using iridium-192 afterloading interstitial implants for treatment of lesions of the oral cavity and skin, and intracavitary implant using cesium-137 or high dose rate (HDR) iridium 192 source for carcinoma of the nasopharynx, serve primarily to boost the primary site with additional radiation after external beam comprehensive radiation therapy.

Intraoral cone (IOC) or peroral route radiation therapy using electrons or low energy x-rays spares the jaw and salivary glands, thus reducing the magnitude of radiation xerostomia and injuries to the mandible and teeth, and is commonly used in cooperative patients to boost the primary site to a higher dosage for small tumors (T1 and T2) of the oral tongue, floor of the mouth, soft palate, and retromolar trigone.

The radiation dosage is determined by the tumor site, size of the lesion, irradiated volume, number of fractions of treatment, and total elapsed time of the treatment course, as well as by various techniques of delivery of radiation, and also by the tolerance of the patient and the response of the tumor to irradiation. In general, a dose of 50 to 55 Gy in 5 to 6 weeks is considered to be adequate for sterilization of microscopic or occult disease, and 65 to 70 Gy in 7 weeks for control of gross squamous cell carcinoma. Such a dosage is usually given initially with 45 to 50 Gy wide-field irradiation, including the primary lesion and the regional nodal areas as a comprehensive procedure, with a further boost to the primary site by reduced portal toward completion. However, although dose–response curves demonstrate the importance of adequate dosage for tumor control, these same curves cannot show convincingly that higher doses (>75 Gy) produce a substantial further improvement in local control rates. Also, such high doses carry a substantially higher risk of severe complications such as painful fibrosis of the subcutaneous tissues of the neck, osteoradionecrosis of the mandible, orocutaneous fistulas, and severe wound healing problems, should salvage surgery be performed for radiation failures.

The physical aspects of radiation therapy are discussed in detail in Chapter 3.

For staging carcinomas of the head and neck, the TNM system, as adopted by the American Joint Committee will be used.[2]

The T stage is defined by the size of the lesions, mobility of the involved part, and number of the involved anatomic subsites. For the N and M extent of the disease, the definition is identical among all sites of the head and neck and is as follows:

N0    No regional lymph node node metastasis

N1    Metastasis in a single ipsilateral lymph node, 3 cm or less in greatest dimension

N2    Metastasis in a single ipsilateral lymph node, more than 3 cm but not more than 6 cm in greatest dimension; or in multiple ipsilateral lymph nodes, none more than 6 cm in greatest dimension; or in bilateral or contralateral lymph nodes, none more tham 6 cm in greatest dimension

N2a    Metastasis in single ipsilateral lymph node more than 3 cm but not more than 6 cm in dimension

N2b    Metastasis in multiple ipsilateral lymph nodes none more then 6 cm in great dimension

N2c    Metastasis in bilateral or contralateral lymph nodes, none more than 6 cm in greatest dimension

N3    Metastasis in a lymph node more than 6 cm in greatest dimension

## REFERENCES

1. Cancer statistics: *CA Cancer J Clin* 1998; 48:1.
2. American Joint Committee on Cancer: *Cancer Staging Manual,* 5th ed. Philadelphia, Lippincott-Raven, 1997.

# A. CARCINOMA OF THE ORAL CAVITY

The oral cancers can be arbitrarily subdivided as follows: lip, anterior two-thirds of the tongue (mobile tongue), floor of the mouth, anterior faucial pillar and retromolar trigone, buccal mucosa, gum (alveolar ridge), and palate (soft and hard). In contrast to oropharyngeal cancer, the majority of oral cancers are well to moderately well differentiated squamous carcinomas.

AJCC staging for lip and oral cavity cancers is as follows:

T1    Tumor 2 cm or less in greatest diameter

T2    Tumor more than 2 cm but not more than 4 cm in greatest diameter

T3    Tumor more than 4 cm in greatest diameter

T4    Lip: tumor invades adjacent structures (e.g., through cortical bone, inferior alveolar nerve, floor of mouth, skin of face)

T4    Oral cavity: tumor invades adjacent structures (e.g., through cortical bone, into deep [extrinsic] muscle of tongue, maxillary sinus, skin). Superficial erosion alone of bone/tooth socket by gingival primary is not sufficient to classify as T4

## THE LIP

Squamous cell carcinomas of the lip occur in the older males (90%), usually situated in the lower lip (90%), well differentiated, and less than 1 cm in size (90%). The incidence of regional lymph node metastasis is low. Upper lip carcinomas are generally more aggressive and virulent than their lower lip counterparts in their clinical behavior and in their ability to metastasize more often.[1-3] The nodal involvements of lip carcinoma are shown in Figures 5-2 and 5-3.

A small carcinoma of the lip can be dealt with expediently by V excision if the procedure will not result in cosmetic and functional deformity. Radiation therapy is best suited for superficial cancers involving more than one-third of the lip, for tumors involving the lip commissure and recurrent tumors after excision, and for patients who refuse surgery. Surgical excision is used for radiation failures and for extensive lesions that involve the mandible or are associated with significant loss of soft tissue requiring major reconstruction after the disease has been controlled by radiation therapy. Since radiation therapy or surgery has yielded extremely high cure rates for small limited cancers, the selection of treatment modality must depend on the cosmetic result that follows the procedure. Radiation therapy for superficial, small tumors (T1) consists of radiation of superficial penetration or low megavoltage electrons. For extensive tumors (T2 and T3), combined external beam therapy and interstitial isotope implant yields excellent cure rates and cosmetic results. For the far advanced tumors, high energy x-rays are used to include the primary site as well as the regional metastatic nodes.

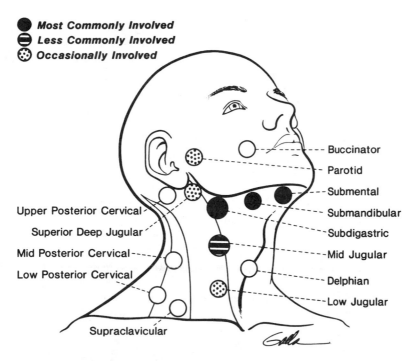

**FIGURE 5-2**   Lymph node involvement from carcinoma of the lower lip.

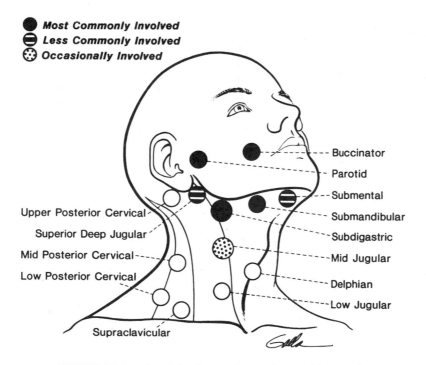

**FIGURE 5-3**  Lymph node involvement from carcinoma of the upper lip.

Although radical neck dissection with adjuvant radiation therapy is necessary for metastatic nodes, that is, N2 and N3 disease, prophylactic or elective neck dissection or irradiation for N0 neck in patients with lip cancer is not indicated.[4]

## Radiotherapeutic Management

For early and well-differentiated lesions lacking in palpable nodes, radiation therapy is directed to the primary site. For superficial, small tumors (T1), 6 to 9 MeV electrons beams are employed with a dose of 45 to 50 Gy in 3 weeks, similar to dosages for treatment of skin cancer. For larger tumors (T2 and T3) involving more than half the lip, or a tumor extending below the bucco gingival sulcus that makes shielding of the underlying mandible impossible, a combination of 30 Gy in 2 weeks by electrons and 35 to 40 Gy in 4 days by interstitial implant offers the best local control and cosmesis. For far advanced tumors with metastatic nodes or recurrent tumors after previous surgical procedures, 4 to 6 MV x-rays are used to include the primary site and the first echelon of lymph nodes; total dose up to 50 Gy in 5 weeks is followed by a localized boost to the primary site with an interstitial implant for an additional 15 to 20 Gy. Any residual nodes in the neck will be dealt with by neck dissection after the primary lip disease has been controlled.

## Radiotherapeutic Results

Control of lip lesions by radiation therapy or surgery is extremely good and for T1 and T2 lesions local control (no evidence of disease) rates range from 80% to 90%.[5–7] In general, however, radiation therapy produces superior cosmetic and functional results. Survival is much better for tumors of the lower lip than for the upper lip,[3] and in patients having small primary lesions without nodes. The presence of metastases reduces the survival rate to approximately 50%.[8,9] Recurrent carcinomas of the lip after radiation therapy may be salvaged by surgery with good local control. On the other hand, recurrences af-

ter surgery tend to be massive, with a higher incidence of nodal metastases, and the results of salvage by radiation therapy are generally poor.

## MGH Experience

Although carcinoma of the lip is a common cancer of the oral cavity, most lesions are traditionally treated by surgery and the number of patients referred for radiation therapy is infinitely small. Up to 1994, a total of 123 patients received radiation therapy, 118 patients with previously untreated carcinoma of the lip and 7 patients with gross postoperative recurrence. Of the former group, 105 lesions occurred in the lower lip, 6 in the upper lip, and 7 in the lip commissure. The male-to-female ratio was 10:1 for the lower lip lesions. The treatment results are shown in Table 5-1.

## Discussion and Summary

Squamous cell carcinoma of the lip is a highly curable malignancy. Surgery and radiation therapy produce similarly high cure rates. For the larger tumors involving more than one-third of the lip and lip commissure, radiation therapy produces better cosmetic and functional results. Radiation therapy failures can still be salvaged by surgery with high success, but the reverse is

**TABLE 5-1   3-Year Local Control of Squamous Cell Carcinoma of the Lip after Radiation Therapy (MGH Experience)**

| Area | Patients Receiving Local Control/Patients Treat (%) | |
|---|---|---|
| | By Area | Total |
| Lower Lip | | |
| T1-2 N0 | 88/92 (96) | |
| T3 N0 | 13/15 (87) | |
| | | 101/107 (94) |
| T1-3 N1-3 | 1/7 (14) | |
| Upper lip | 1/3 (33) | |
| T1-2 N0 | 3/7 (43) | |
| | | 4/10 (40) |
| T1-3 N1-3 | 0/2 (0) | |

seldom true. Treatment must be tailored to the cell type, grade, and location of the lesions, as well as the presence or absence of metastatic nodes. Since the substance of the lip generally can tolerate a very high dose of radiation therapy, thus resulting in favorable "therapeutic ratio," localized tumor can be expected to be highly curable by radiation therapy. To avoid osteoradionecrosis, the mandible should be spared from high doses of radiations; this can be achieved by means of combined low megavoltage electron beam and interstitial implant. Careful treatment planning for this disease is rewarding.

## References

1. Wurman LH, Adams GL, Meyerhoff WL: Carcinoma of the lip. *Am J Surg* 1975;130:470.

2. Lund C, Sogaard H, Elbrond O, et al: Epidermoid carcinoma of the lip. Histologic grading in the clinical evaluation. *Acta Radiol Ther Phys Biol* 1975;14:465–474.

3. Jorgensen K, Elbron O, Anderson AP: Carcinoma of the lip: A series of 869 cases. *Acta Radiol* 1973; 12:177–190.

4. Wilson JSP, Kemble JVH: Cancer of the lip at brisk. *Br J Oral Surg* 1972; 9:186.

5. Petrovich Z, Kuisk H, Tobochnik N, et al: Carcinoma of the lip. *Arch Otolaryngol* 1979;105:187–191.

6. Dick D: Clinical and cosmetic results in squamous cancer of the lip treated by 140 kV radiation therapy. *Clin Radiol* 1962;13:304–312.

7. Cerezo L, Liu FF, Tsang R, Payne: Squamous cell carcinoma of the lip: analysis of the Princess Margaret Hospital experience. *Radio Oncol* 1993; 29:142–147.

8. del Regato JA, Sala JM: The treatment of carcinoma of the lip. *Radiol* 1959;73:839.

9. Modlin J: Neck dissections in cancer of the lower lip. *Surgery* 1950; 28:404–412.

## THE ANTERIOR TWO THIRDS OF TONGUE (MOBILE TONGUE)

Carcinoma of the anterior two thirds or the mobile portion of the tongue is a common type of oral cancer and includes the lesions arising from anterior to the circumvallate papillae. It frequently invades the underlying muscle, causing fixation of the organ, and is attended by a high incidence of cervical lymph node metastasis (Figure 5-4). Surgical resection is often indicated for lesions limited to the tip of the tongue or small lesions suitable for simple excision in aged, feeble patients, or recurrences or residual disease following unsuccessful radiation therapy. Small tumors (T1) arising from the anterior lateral border of the tongue respond equally well to partial glossectomy or radiation therapy. If such primary lesions are treated by simple surgical excision alone with the neck untreated, the primary site and neck nodes should be carefully followed because of the high incidence of local recurrence and/or nodal metastases as high as 40%.[1,2] In such circumstances, postoperative adjuvant radiation therapy should be considered in order to improve local control rates.[3,4] For superficial, medium sized tumors (T2) involving the adjacent floor of the mouth, or situated posteriorly near the faucial pillar, which are not suitable for excision via the peroral route, surgical treatment would have to include procedures of partial glossectomy with partial or marginal mandibulectomy, and radical neck dissection. For such lesions, therefore, comprehensive radiation therapy is preferred owing to its superior cosmetic and functional results and high cure rate. Advanced disease (T3 and T4) with deep muscle invasion often associated with cervical lymph node metastases is unlikely to be cured by radiation therapy alone and is therefore managed by combined radical surgery and postoperative radiation therapy if possible.[5–8]

## Radiotherapeutic Management

Comprehensive irradiation to the primary site and the first echelon nodes is essential for treatment of carcinoma of the oral tongue (Figure 5-5) and is carried out with a dose of 45 to 50 Gy in 5 weeks. The primary lesion is boosted either by interstitial implant or by intraoral cone to bring the total dose to approximately 72 to 75

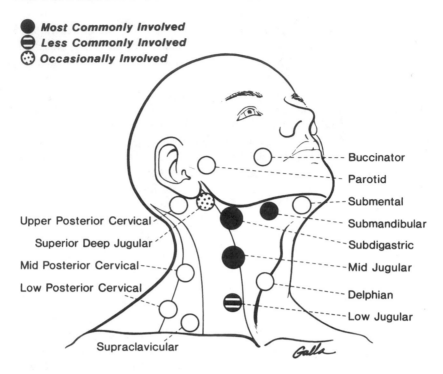

**FIGURE 5-4** Diagrams showing lymph node involvement from carcinoma of the oral tongue.

Gy in 6 to 7 weeks. Such an approach can deliver a very high dose to the primary tumor in the tongue and yet avoid excessive irradiation to the mandible. For advanced disease (T3 and T4), interstitial implantation or IOC is ineffective, and therefore surgical resection must be followed by external beam therapy.

For interstitial implant for carcinoma of the oral tongue, a single plane and double planes are commonly used to irradiate slabs of tissue 1 and 2 cm thick, respectively.[9–11] Except for treatment of a tumor arising from the dorsum of the tongue volume, implant is rarely used. To obtain good geometric distribution of the implant, an afterloading technique angiocaths inserted percutaneously through the submental route is practical and effective.

Irradiation delivered through an intraoral cone employing 6 or 9 MeV electrons from the linear accelerator is highly effective for local control of the small primary lesions.[12,13] Generally peroral radiation therapy is carried out

in the early phase of the treatment program as a boost technique. In a well-situated carcinoma without involvement of the gingival ridge, a boost dose of 24 Gy in eight daily fractions can be given. In addition to the comprehensive radiation therapy of 50 Gy, this program has resulted in high cure rates and has practically replaced the use of interstitial implant for treatment of carcinoma of the oral tongue at the MGH.

## Radiotherapeutic Results

The results of radiation therapy for carcinoma of the oral tongue are as good as surgery and are related to the size and location of the primary lesion and the presence or absence of metastatic nodes. For T1 and T2 lesions, the 5-year local control rates after radiation therapy are 80% and 60%, respectively. The results for T3 and T4 lesions are generally poor, being in the neighborhood of 25% to 30%. Survival rates decrease as the primary site moves toward the posterior third: 80% versus 30% for anterior and posterior tongue lesions, respectively. The survival rates are considerably better, by approximately a factor of 2, in patients without nodes than in patients with nodes.

## MGH Experience

From 1970 through 1994 a total of 291 patients with carcinoma of the oral tongue were treated definitively with curative radiation therapy. The 5-year actuarial local control (LC) rates for the entire group of patients after radiation therapy alone was 60%, and disease specific survival (DSS) rate was 66% (Table 5-2). For T1 and T2 lesions the corresponding LC rates were 86% and 64%, and DSS rates were 96% and 67%, respectively. Large tumors (T3 and T4) generally responded poorly to radiation therapy, with local control rate of 33% and disease-specific survival rate of 42%. The disease in the neck indicated very poor local control and survival. Patients with N1 disease had only half the local control and survival of those without nodes. Patients with extensive neck disease (N2 and N3) had approximately 15% local control and survival, as shown in Table 5-2.

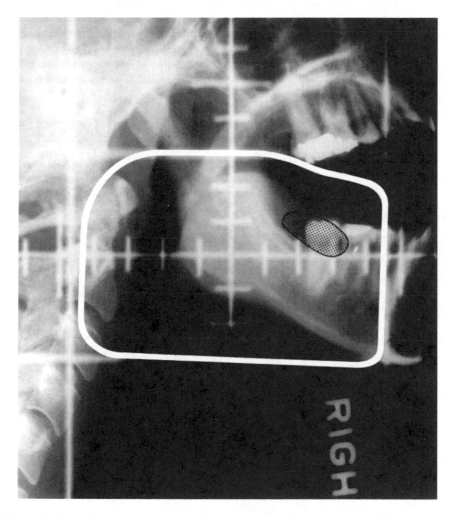

**FIGURE 5-5**   Simulation film showing placement of portal in lateral projection for T1N0 carcinoma of the oral tongue.

**TABLE 5-2   5-Year Actuarial Local Control and Survival of Oral Tongue Carcinoma after Radiation Therapy**

| Stage | n | LC | DSS(%)* |
|-------|-----|-----|---------|
| T1 | 62 | 86 | 96 |
| T2 | 139 | 64 | 67 |
| T3 | 63 | 42 | 55 |
| T4 | 28 | 9 | 9 |
| T3-4 | 90 | 33 | 42 |
| Total | 291 | 60 | 66 |
| N0 | 222 | 67 | 77 |
| N1 | 36 | 39 | 36 |
| N2-3 | 13 | 13 | 16 |

*$p = 0.0001$.

Metastatic disease in the neck from carcinoma of the oral tongue presents a difficult management problem. The incidence of neck failure in patients with early lesions is high. For T1 N0 and T2 N0 lesions, 4 of 31 patients (13%) and 30 of 64 patients (47%) respectively, developed metastatic lymph nodes when the neck received partial or no elective radiation therapy prior to 1978 at the MGH (Table 5-3).

## Discussion and Summary

Squamous cell carcinoma of the oral tongue is a common cancer of the head and neck. Its therapeutic management is extremely complex. The small, mucosal tumors can be treated successfully with either radiation therapy or surgical excision with equally good results. When the tumors become large or extend to the underlying muscle, the incidence of metastatic lymph nodes is high. For T1 N0 and T2 N0 lesions, if the neck is not treated though clinically normal, approximately one-fourth to one-third of patients will develop lymph node disease. When the disease becomes advanced (T3 and T4), the incidence of occult and overt neck disease ranges from 50% to 70%.

Except for small, mucosal lesions, radiation therapy therefore must consist of comprehensive external beam therapy to the primary site and the first echelon lymph nodes with approximately 50 to 60 Gy, with local boost to the primary lesion either via interstitial implant or IOC to a total tumor dose of approximately 72 to 75 Gy in 6 weeks. Occasionally, in lieu of radiation boost, limited surgical excision of the residual disease or nidusectomy at the primary site is effective.

When the primary lesion is treated only by simple excision, the neck must be considered at risk for relapse due to occult metastases and should be closely observed. Other options are to perform a functional neck dissection for sampling purposes or postoperative radiation therapy to the neck electively.

The program of combined IOC boost and comprehensive external beam radiation therapy has resulted in approximately 80% to 90% local control of T1 N0 and T2 N0 carcinoma of

**TABLE 5-3   Incidence of Nodal Recurrence from Occult Metastasis in Patients with T1 N0 and T2 N0 Lesions and No Elective Neck Irradiation: 1960–1980**

| Stage | Number of Patients | | | |
|-------|-------|-------|-------|-------|
| | Total | | With Radical Neck Dissection | Total |
| T1 N0 | 31 | 1 | 3/6 (33%) | 4/31 (13%) |
| T2 N0 | 64 | 23 | 7/30 (23%) | 30/64 (47%) |
| | 95 | 24 | 10/36 (28) | 30/95 (36%) |

*$p = 0.0001$.
**$p = 0.0002$.

the oral tongue, and at the MGH it is the procedure of choice.

Extensive tumors (large T3 and T4 lesions) with or without nodes are rarely curable with radiation therapy. At present, combined surgery and radiation therapy is preferred. Accelerated hyperfractionation radiation therapy has resulted in some improvement of local control, particularly for the T2 and T3 lesions.

The role of chemotherapy for these advanced tumors is controversial, and the duration of response is usually measured in terms of weeks or months. The use of chemotherapy before radiation therapy or surgery does not appear to increase patient survival.

## REFERENCES

1. Johnson JT, Leipzig B, Cummings CW: Management of T1 carcinoma of the anterior aspect of the tongue. *Arch Otolarygnol* 1980;106, 249–251.

2. Odell EW, Jani P, Sherriff M, Ahluwalia SM, Hibbert J, Levison DA, Morgan PR: The prognostic value of individual histologic grading parameters in small lingual squamous cell carcinomas. The importance of the pattern of invasion. *Cancer* 1994;74,789–794.

3. Million RR: Elective neck irradiation for Tx N0 squamous cell carcinoma of the oral tongue and floor of mouth. *Cancer* 1971;34:149–155.

4. Leborgne F, Leborgne JH, Barlocci L, Ortega B: Elective neck irradiation in the treatment of cancer of the oral tongue. *Int J Radiat Oncol Biol Phys* 1987;13:1149–1153.

5. Saxena VS: Cancer of the tongue: Local control of the primary. *Cancer* 1970;26:788.

6. Ange DW, Lindberg RD, Guillamondegui OM: Management of squamous cell carcinoma of the oral tongue and floor of mouth after excisional biopsy. *Radiology* 1975;116:143–146.

7. Spiro RH, Strong EW: Epidermoid carcinoma of the mobile tongue, treatment by partial glossectomy alone. *Am J Surg* 1971;122:707.

8. Spiro RH, Strong EW: Surgical treatment of cancer of the tongue. *Surg Clin North Am* 1974; 4:759.

9. (a) Pierquin B, Chassagne D, Baillet F, et al: The placement of implantation in tongue and floor of mouth cancer. *JAMA* 1971:215:961. (b) Botstein C, Silver C, Ariaratnam L: Treatment of carcinoma of the oral tongue by radium needle implantation. *Am J Surg* 1976;132:523.

10. Decroix Y, Ghossein N: Experience of the Curie Institute in the treatment of cancer of the mobile tongue. *Cancer* 1981;47:496–502.

11. Horiuchi J, Okuyama T, Shibuya H, Takeda M: Results of brachytherapy for cancer of the tongue with special emphasis on local prognosis. *Int J Radiat Oncol Biol Phys* 1982; 8:829–835.

12. Wang CC, Doppke KP, Biggs PJ: Intra-oral cone radiation therapy for selected carcinomas of the oral cavity. *Int J Radiat Oncol Biol Phys* 1983;9:1185–1189.

13. Wang CC: Radiotherapeutic management and results of T1 N0, T2 N0 carcinoma of the oral tongue: Evaluation of boost technique. *Int J Radiat Oncol Biol Phys* 1989;17:287–291.

## THE FLOOR OF THE MOUTH

Carcinoma of the floor of the mouth is often located in the anterior portion of the floor adjacent to the orifice of Wharton's duct and frequently spreads along the directional course of the submaxillary duct. The early lesions are seldom symptomatic and are commonly diagnosed by a dentist during ordinary dental work. In extensive lesions the tumor may extend deeply into the muscle of the adjacent tongue and the alveolar ridge, presenting as a continuous mass extending from the floor of the mouth onto the submandibular triangle. Far advanced lesions may invade the neighboring mandible. Figure 5-6 shows the nodal involvement of floor-of-mouth carcinoma.

### Selection of Therapy

When the tumor is small or limited to the mucosa, it is highly curable by radiation therapy[1–3] alone, and therefore radiation therapy should be the treatment of choice. For the moderately advanced lesion (T2 or early exophytic T3), a trial course of radiation therapy may be given first with radical resection as a salvage for failure. For extensive infiltrative lesions with fixation or

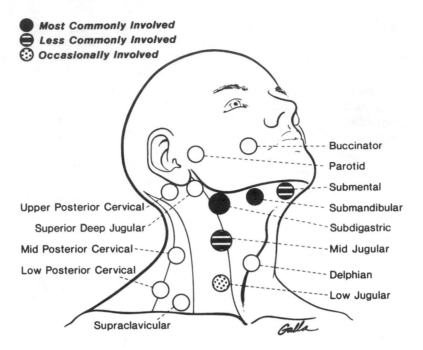

FIGURE 5-6 Diagram showing lymph node involvement in carcinoma of the floor of the mouth.

tethering to the adjacent mandible, though the surface size is still small and categorized as T1-2, surgical excision with a rim of normal inner border of the mandible (marginal mandibulectomy: Figure 5-7)[4] is the treatment of choice. This is followed by postoperative radiation therapy to sterilize any microscopic disease at the previous tumor site. For large, extensive, infiltrative lesions (T3 and T4) with marked involvement of the adjacent muscle of the tongue and mandible, combined surgery in the form of composite resection and plastic repair followed by postoperative radiation therapy is the procedure of choice.

## Radiotherapeutic Management

Radiation therapy for early lesions (T1 and T2) consists of external beam therapy with interplay of interstitial implant or IOC. For the small, well-defined lesions, IOC may be given at the very onset for approximately 21 Gy in seven daily fractions. Additional external radiation therapy is given to bring the total dose to the primary site up to 70 Gy in 6 to 7 weeks.

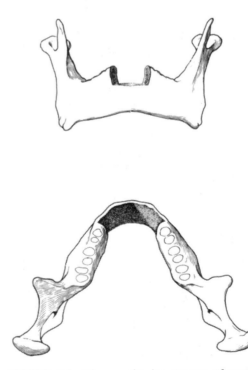

FIGURE 5-7 Diagram showing concept of partial mandibulectomy or rim resection for treatment of carcinoma of the floor of the mouth.

Because of the extremely low incidence of occult metastases or developing sequential nodal disease in the T1 N0 and early T2 N0 lesions, elective neck irradiation or radical neck dissection is not indicated.

For T3 and T4 lesions, combined surgery and external beam radiation therapy is the procedure of choice. Postoperative external beam therapy is given through opposing laterals with equal load-ing, covering the primary lesion as well as the nodal areas, generally commencing 3 to 4 weeks after surgery and continuing up to approximately 50 to 55 Gy in 5 weeks (Figure 5-8).

## Radiotherapeutic Results

The results of treatment by radiation therapy are comparable to those achieved with radical

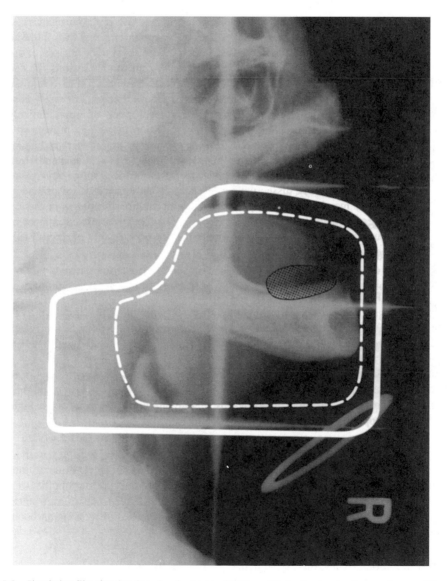

**FIGURE 5-8** Simulation film showing Cerrobend cutout to shield parotid glands when treating carcinoma of the anterior floor of the mouth.

surgery. The early mucosal lesions, T1 and T2, are controlled satisfactorily by combination of external radiation therapy intermixed with intraoral cone electron beam therapy or interstitial implant. The local control rates are approximately 80% and 60%, respectively.[3,5,6] Extensive infiltrative lesions (T3 and T4) with involvement of the gum and the mandible or deeply infiltrative into the adjacent musculature, often with cervical lymph node metastases, are rarely controlled by radiation therapy alone; local control rates are approximately 20% to 30%.[1,5,7] The tolerance of the mandible to radiation is low and prevents the use of high dose of external beam therapy alone. Likewise, the use of brachytherapy has resulted in an extremely high incidence of osteoradionecrosis of the mandible. Therapeutic neck dissection for nodal metastases does not jeopardize survival as compared to elective neck dissection for N0 neck. Carcinomas of the floor of the mouth are frequently associated with multiple primaries in the upper aerodigestive tract, ranging from 25% to 33% after successful treatment of the previous tumors. This certainly accounts the poor results of overall survival of the patients.

## MGH Experience

From 1970 through 1994, 309 patients with carcinoma of the floor of the mouth were treated by radiation therapy. Of these, 154 patients were treated with accelerated (i.e., administered twice a day) radiation therapy.

The incidence of nodal metastases at the time of diagnosis for early lesions is remarkably low, being 10% for T1 and 18% for T2 lesions. When the lesions become large and extensive, invading adjacent musculature and bone, the incidence is high, averaging approximately 70%, (Table 5-4).

### Results of Combined Radiation Therapy and Surgery    Of 33 patients with T3 and T4 lesions who underwent planned combined surgery and radiation therapy, the 5-year actuarial local control and disease specific survival rates were as shown in Table 5-5.

**TABLE 5-4    5-Year Actuarial Local Control and Disease-Specific Survival after Radiation Therapy for Floor-of-Mouth Carcinomas 1970–1994**

| Stage | n | LC % | DSS (%) | Ultimate Local Control |
|---|---|---|---|---|
| T1 | 92 | 90 | 95 | 95 |
| T2 | 159 | 71 | 75 | 81 |
| T1-2 | 251 | 79 | 82 | |
| T3 | 31 | 9 | 23 | 29 |
| T4 | 27 | 26 | 36 | 30 |
| T3-4 | 58 | 28 | 27 | |
| Total | 309 | 69 | 72 | |
| N0 | 260 | 74 | 77 | |
| N1 | 27 | 53 | 52 | |
| N2-3 | 71 | 4 | 28 | |

*$p = 0.0001$.

**TABLE 5-5    5-Year Actuarial Local Control and Disease-Specific Survival for Floor-of-Mouth Cancers after Combined Surgery and Radiation Therapy: 1970–1994**

| Stage | n | LC (%) | DDS (%) |
|---|---|---|---|
| T3-4 | 33 | 80 | 62 |

### Results of Bid Radiation Therapy Twice a Day    From 1979 through 1994, 154 patients with carcinoma of the floor of the mouth received radiation therapy twice a day. The results of treatment compared to daily radiation therapy are shown in Table 5-6.

## Discussion and Summary

Carcinoma of the floor of the mouth is a readily recognizable cancer and can be diagnosed early. It is quite dissimilar to carcinoma of the oral tongue from the standpoints of pattern of spread, incidence of nodal metastases, and radiation tolerance of its adjacent tissues. Early lesions tend to develop nodal metastases much less often than oral tongue carcinoma. The T1 N0 and T2 N0 lesions can be successfully treated by radiation therapy alone, with satisfactory cosmetic and functional results.

**TABLE 5-6    5 Year Actuarial Local Control and Disease-Specific Survival after Twice-Daily Radiation Therapy: 1970–1994**

| Stage | n | LC (%) | DSS (%) |
|-------|-----|-----------|-----------|
| T1 | | | |
| BID | 22 | 94 | 93 |
| QD | 69 | 89 | 95 |
| | | $p = 0.52$ | $p = 0.97$ |
| T2 | | | |
| BID | 83 | 81 | 88 |
| QD | 167 | 77 | 80 |
| | | $p = 0.48$ | $p = 0.15$ |
| T3-4 | | | |
| BID | 49 | 62 | 59 |
| QD | 100 | 68 | 71 |
| | | $p = 0.40$ | $p = 0.43$ |

Advanced disease (T3 and T4 with nodes) is better treated by combined surgery and radiation therapy. In certain large, exophytic tumors, a trial course of radiation therapy is justified, with salvage surgery being reserved for failures.

External beam therapy to the primary site is a major portion of the radiation treatment, with the dose to the lesion is boosted by reduced portals or by IOC if feasible. Interstitial implant has been found to be associated with a high incidence of soft tissue ulceration or osteoradionecrosis. At the present time, if the primary site cannot be boosted by IOC, electron beam radiation therapy through submental approach has been used with good results.

## REFERENCES

1. Pierquin B, Chassagne D, Baillet F, et al: The place of implantation in tongue and floor of mouth cancer. *JAMA* 1971;215:961.
2. Campos JL, Lampe I, Fayos JV: Radiotherapy of carcinoma of the floor of the mouth. *Radiol* 1971;99:677–682.
3. Harold CC: Management of cancer of the floor of the mouth. *Am J Surg* 1971;122:487.
4. Guillamondegui OM, Jesse RH: Surgical treatment of advanced carcinoma of the floor of the mouth. *Am J Radiol* 1976;126:1256.
5. Fu KK, Lichter A, Galante M: Carcinoma of the floor of the mouth: An analysis of treatment results and the sites and causes of failures. *Int J Radiat Oncol Biol Phys* 1976;1:829–837.
6. Fayos JV, Lampe I: Treatment of squamous cell carcinoma of the oral cavity. *Am J Surg* 1972; 124:493.

## THE RETROMOLAR TRIGONE AND ANTERIOR POLLAR

The retromolar trigone is a triangular area that covers the anterior aspect of the ascending ramus of the mandible posterior to and between the upper and lower third molars. The mucous membranes of this site blend medially with the anterior tonsillar pillar. Squamous cell carcinomas arising from the retromolar trigone and anterior faucial pillar may therefore be included under one heading for purposes of discussion. The lesions may spread to the posterior gingival ridge, buccal mucosa, floor of the mouth, tonsillar fossa, base of the tongue, and the adjacent soft and hard palates. Advanced lesions may extend to the pterygoid fossa, resulting in trismus. Most of these tumors are well differentiated. The lymphatic drainage of the retromolar trigone is the submandibular and subdigastric nodes, commonly ipsilateral. Figure 5-9 illustrates lymph node involvement. Approximately one-third of patients with this disease have ipsilateral lymph node metastases when the diagnosis is initially made. For the early T1 and T2 lesions, the incidence of nodal metastases is low, less than 20%.[1] However, for advanced lesions (T3 and T4) the incidence is high, approximately 50%, and of these, 10% are bilateral. When the soft palate or tonsillar fossa is extensively involved, the superior deep jugular nodes are at risk of involvement (Figure 5-10).

### Selection of Therapy

For superficial T1 and T2 lesions, radiation therapy employing external beam radiation is considered the treatment of choice. The large infiltrating lesions (T3 and T4), with or without

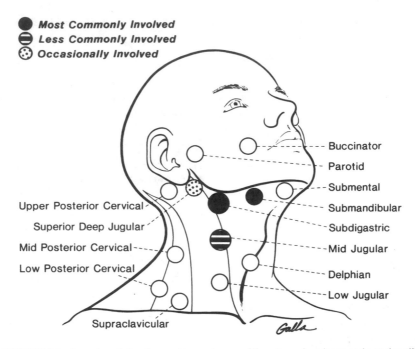

● *Most Commonly Involved*
⊖ *Less Commonly Involved*
⊙ *Occasionally Involved*

Buccinator

Parotid

Submental

Upper Posterior Cervical

Superior Deep Jugular

Mid Posterior Cervical

Low Posterior Cervical

Submandibular

Subdigastric

Mid Jugular

Delphian

Low Jugular

Supraclavicular

**FIGURE 5-9**   Lymph node involvement in carcinoma of the retromolar trigone and anterior pillar.

metastatic nodes, are best treated by a combination of surgical resection and postoperative irradiation. The most common sites of failure after radiation therapy alone are the base of the tongue and adjacent mandible infiltrated by tumor. Such residual disease after high dose radiotherapy may be man-aged by limited surgical resection, that is, nidusectomy.[2]

## Radiotherapeutic Management

For early lesions (T1 N0 and T2 N0), not associated with involvement of the base of the tongue or soft palate, the initial dose of 20 Gy may be given through opposed lateral portals as a mouth bath to evaluate the extent of the tumor margins by the development of tumoritis, followed by 45 Gy by ipsilateral wedge pair technique in 4 to 5 weeks if the lesion is eccentrically situated. Some small, well defined, superficial tumors in cooperative patients may be effectively dealt with as a part of the treatment program through intraoral cone electron beam therapy. For the large (T3 and T4) lesions, particularly those as-

sociated with marked involvement of the base of the tongue, combined surgery and radiation therapy is planned. For Nl, N2, and N3, and/or extensive T2, T3, and T4 disease, comprehensive neck irradiation with 50 Gy to the lower neck and supraclavicular area is planned. Figure 5-10 shows placements of portal and shrinking field for extensive carcinoma.

## Radiotherapeutic Results

For early lesions, local control rates by radiation therapy alone are high, ranging from 70% to 80%[3] with excellent cosmesis. The results for advanced tumors are poor with local control rates ranging from 30% to 40%,[4] and the rates may be improved by combined surgical resection and postoperative radiation therapy.

## MGH Experience

From 1970 through 1994, a total of 246 patients with carcinoma of the retromolar trigone and anterior pillar were treated by radiation therapy. Of these, 120 patients received once-daily radiation therapy and 126 patients were treated by irradiation twice a day. Only 2 patients with T3 and T4 lesions had planned combined surgery and radiation therapy. Tables 5-7 and 5-8 show the results for radiation therapy daily and twice-daily, respectively.

In comparison to the daily radiation therapy, there was a significant increase of local control in T3 and T4 lesions in favor of radiation therapy twice a day ($p = .0005$), as shown in Table 5-9.

## Discussion and Summary

Squamous cell carcinoma of the retromolar trigone is a relatively common cancer of the oral cavity. Early lesions are highly curable by irradiation therapy alone, with local control rates of 86% and 68% for T1 and T2 lesions, respectively. Large, infiltrative lesions, T3 and T4 with or without nodes, are best treated by planned combination of composite resection with plastic closure and postoperative radiation therapy. Most inoperable T3 and T4 lesions are managed by a program of twice-daily irradiation, with some improvement in local control rates and patients survival.

Primary radical surgery is attended by significant facial deformity and impairment of speech and swallowing function, and often results in a high incidence of marginal recurrence but may be reserved for the extensive carcinoma. Since metastatic disease in the neck in patients with early lesions is low, elective

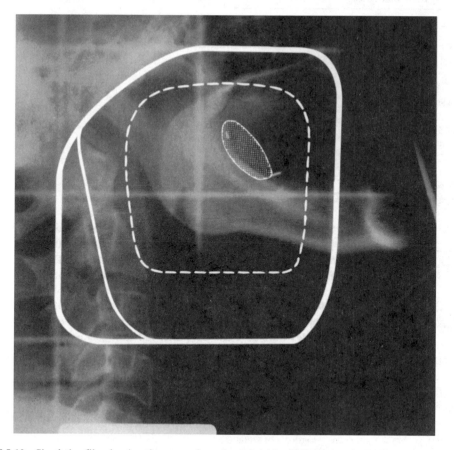

**FIGURE 5-10**   Simulation film showing placement of portal and shrinking field for extensive RMT carcinoma with neck node involvement. Anterior and posterior borders of lesion are marked with gold seeds.

**TABLE 5-7   5-Year Actuarial Local Control and Disease-Specific Survival Rates after Daily Radiation Therapy: 1970–1994**

| Stage | n | LC (%) | DSS (%) |
|-------|-----|--------|---------|
| T1 | 34 | 86 | 86 |
| T2 | 117 | 68 | 70 |
| T3-4 | 95 | 36 | 45 |
| T3 | 66 | 35 | 44 |
| T4 | 29 | 38 | 46 |
| Total | 246 | 58 | 62 |
| N0 | 186 | 63 | 67 |
| N1 | 33 | 46 | 67 |
| N2-3 | 9 | 41 | 11 |

**TABLE 5-8   5-Year Actuarial Local Control and Disease Specific Survival Rates after Twice-Daily Radiation Therapy: 1970–1994**

| Stage | n | LC (%) | DSS (%) |
|-------|-----|--------|---------|
| T1 | 13 | 92 | 76 |
| T2 | 60 | 78 | 79 |
| T3-4 | 53 | 64 | 58 |

**TABLE 5-9   Comparison of Twice-Daily and Daily Radiation Therapy Results**

| Stage | $\mathcal{P}$ LC (%) | DSS (%) |
|-------|--------|---------|
| T1 | 0.67 | 0.07 |
| T2 | 0.28 | 0.45 |
| T3 | 0.0005 | 0.22 |

neck treatment for T1 N0 and T2 N0 lesions, either surgical or radiotherapeutic, is seldom warranted.

## REFERENCES

1. Byers RM, Anderson B, Schwartz EA, et al: Treatment of squamous carcinoma of the retromolar trigone. *Am J Clin Oncol* 1984;7:647–652.
2. Wang CC: Management and prognosis of squamous cell carcinoma of the tonsillar region. *Radiology* 1972;104:667–671.
3. Lo K, Fletcher GH, Byers RM, et al: Results of irradiation in the squamous cell carcinomas of the anterior faucial pillar–retromolar trigone. *Int J Radiat Oncol Biol Phys* 1987;13:969–974.

## THE BUCCAL MUCOSA

Anatomically, the buccal mucosa is composed of the inner lining of the cheeks and lips. Under the mucosa lies the buccinator muscle, which is covered on the outside by the skin of the face. Squamous cell carcinomas arising from this area are usually well differentiated and are frequently associated with areas of leukoplakia. This disease occurs most commonly in older patients and is rarely seen before age 40. There is a higher incidence in persons who chew tobacco.[1,2] Because the mucous membranes adhere closely to the underlying muscle, early invasion of the buccinator muscle by the ulcerative lesions is likely to occur, resulting in trismus. The tumors may also spread to the deep lobe of the parotid gland, the pterygoid fossa and the buccogingival sulcus, and the commissure of the lip; in advanced stages the skin of the cheek may be perforated. The incidence of metastases for T1 and T2 lesions is 10% to 20%. The ulcerative advanced tumors have a propensity for lymph node metastases as high as 60%.[3,4] The lymph nodes commonly involved include the submandibular and subdigastric and occasionally the submental and parotid nodes (Figure 5-11).

### Selection of Therapy

For small, superficial T1 lesions with well defined margins, primary surgical removal is effective. The procedure not only provides expedient ridding of the malignancy but also eradicates any adjacent leukoplakia. For intermediate lesions (T2), radiotherapy may result in a high cure rate with good functional and cosmetic results and therefore is preferred. For advanced tumors (T3 and T4), en bloc excision of the primary lesion and its regional lymph

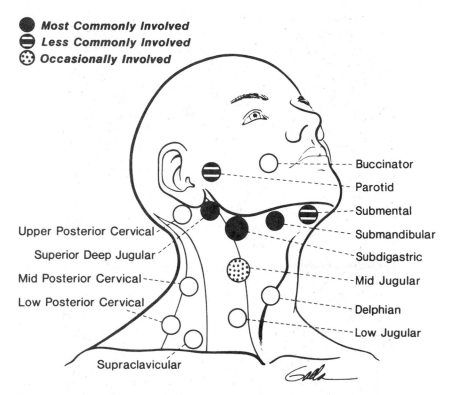

● *Most Commonly Involved*
⊜ *Less Commonly Involved*
⊙ *Occasionally Involved*

- - - Buccinator
- - - Parotid
- - - Submental
- - - Submandibular
- - - Subdigastric
- - - Mid Jugular
- - - Delphian
- - - Low Jugular

Upper Posterior Cervical
Superior Deep Jugular
Mid Posterior Cervical
Low Posterior Cervical

Supraclavicular

**FIGURE 5-11**    Diagram showing lymph node involvement in carcinoma of the buccal mucosa.

node metastases followed by plastic closure[4,5] and postoperative radiation therapy is the treatment of choice. The management of verrucous carcinoma of the buccal mucosa is often controversial. The concept of potential malignant degeneration after radiation therapy as reported in the literature[5,6] is debatable. It is true that such well differentiated lesions are difficult to control with homeopathic doses of radiation therapy and the recurrences may be more aggressive and hard to manage. Also, some cases of so-called verrucous carcinoma, diagnosed by small biopsy, undergoing malignant changes after radiation therapy are in fact due to sampling error, because the entire specimen is not available for pathologic examination prior to radiation therapy. A few patients with a diagnosis of verrucous carcinoma were treated by radiation therapy at the MGH and were NED for 10 or more years without malignant degeneration.

## Radiotherapeutic Management

Generally, the early lesions (T1 and most of T2) without nodes can be managed by external photon or electron beam therapy and/or interstitial implant. In moderately advanced lesions, the radiotherapeutic management of the disease must include treatment of the primary site and the regional lymph nodes. This is best achieved with external beam radiation therapy through ipsilateral and anterior wedge pair fields for a basic tumor dose of 50 to 55 Gy in 5 weeks (Figure 5-12). This should be followed by boost radiation therapy, sparing the mandible by interstitial implant for an additional 15 to 20 Gy. The tissues of the buccal cheek can tolerate such high dose of radiation therapy without significant radiation sequelae. For early lesions with well-differentiated histology, elective neck radiation therapy generally is not indicated. For large tumors, ipsilateral nodal coverage by elective

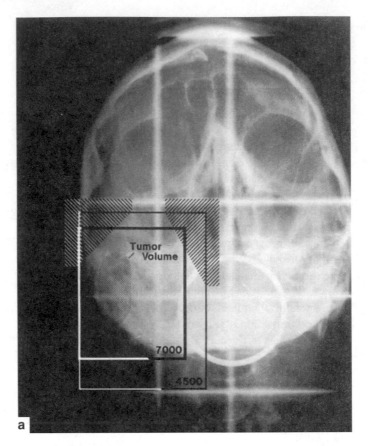

**FIGURE 5-12a** Simulation films showing placement of radiation therapy portals for 45 Gy followed by appositional electron boost to 65 Gy or interstitial implant for T2N0 carcinoma of the buccal mucosa in (a) Anteroposterior (AP).

radiation is advised. Any residual nodes are dealt with by neck dissection.

## Radiotherapeutic Results

Results of treatment of carcinoma of the buccal mucosa are rather sparse. The published results from New York Memorial Hospital indicated a 5-year survival rate of 42%. For the small and intermediate lesions (T1 and T2), the rates were 77% and 65% respectively, and the salvage rates were 27% and 18% for T3 and T4, respectively.[7] The local control rates following radiation therapy ranged from one half to two thirds, depending on the stage of the primary lesions as well as the presence or absence of nodal metastases.[8–10] Large advanced tumors

are rarely curable, and survival rates are approximately one in five. Fixed cervical nodes generally did poorly, with local control rates of less than 10%. The most significant prognostic factor is tumor thickness. For the lesions less than 6 mm, the prognosis is excellent regardless of the tumor size.[11] Neck failures occurred in less than 10% of the patients treated, and elective neck radiation therapy is not indicated.

Fletcher[12] reported 97 patients with T1-4 lesions treated by radiation therapy. For T1 and T2 lesions, the local control rate was 79% (31/39) and for T3 and T4 lesions the rate was 66% (37/56). Ash[13] reported 5-year absolute survival of 35% in 374 patients, with most treated by radiation therapy. The local control rate for early lesions was 54% (T1N0) and for

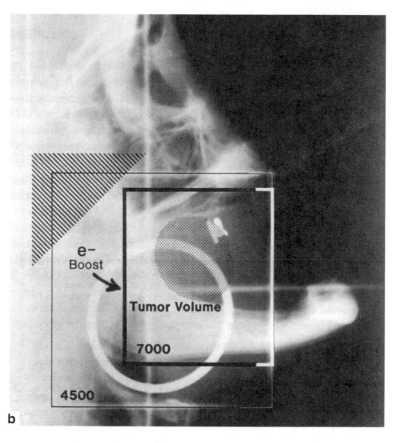

**FIGURE 5-12b**    Lateral projection, using wedge pair techniques.

advanced lesions (T3) 30%; only 5% of patients with T4 were salvaged. Lampe[9] reported on 50 patients with buccal mucosa carcinoma and the 5-year NED survivval was 50% after radiation therapy. These results were comparable to those achievable by surgery.[1,3,14,15]

## MGH Experience

At the MGH, most of the early and superficial carcinomas of the buccal mucosa were traditionally treated by surgical excision. The patients referred for radiation therapy therefore, had relatively large and advanced lesions. From 1970 through 1994, a total of 33 patients were treated by radiation therapy. The 5-year actuarial local control and disease specific survival rates are shown in Table 5-10.

## Discussion and Summary

Squamous cell carcinoma of the buccal mucosa is a relatively uncommon cancer. The small T1 lesion with well-defined borders can be successfully managed by simple excision or localized radiation therapy (either external

**TABLE 5-10    5-Year Actuarial Local Control and Disease-Specific Survival after Radiation Therapy: 1970–1994**

| Stage | $n$ | LC (%) | DSS (%) |
|---|---|---|---|
| T1 | 5 | 66 | 75 |
| T2 | 22 | 60 | 78 |
| T1-2 | 27 | 68 | 77 |
| T3-4 | 6 | 30 | 0 |
| Total | 33 | 55 | 69 |

radiation therapy, interstitial implant, or combination of these modalities). For moderately advanced carcinomas (T2), comprehensive external beam radiation therapy encompassing the primary lesion and nodal drainage areas is advised. This is to be followed by radiation boost to the primary site by interstitial implant or electron beam, to bring the total dose to 75 to 80 Gy in 8 weeks. The dose to the mandible is limited to 65 to 70 Gy in 7 weeks. The residual nodes in the neck after partial or whole neck irradiation are treated by neck dissection. Extensive T3 and T4 infiltrative disease with or without nodes is rarely curable by radiation therapy alone. If operable, these lesions are currently managed by combined therapies (i.e., surgery, radiation therapy, and adjuvant chemotherapy).

## REFERENCES

1. O'Brien JH, Catlin D: Cancer of the cheek (mucosa). *Cancer* 1965;18:1392–1398.
2. Conley J, Sadoyama JA: Squamous cell cancer of the buccal mucosa. *Arch Otolaryngol* 1973; 94:330–333.
3. Modlin J, Johnson RE: The surgical treatment of cancer of the buccal mucosa and lower gingiva. *AJR Am J Roentgenol* 1955;73:620–627.
4. Skolnik EM, Campbell JM, Meyers RM: Carcinoma of the buccal mucosa and retromolar area. *Otolaryngol Clin North Am* 1972;5:327–331.
5. Fonts EA, Greenlaw RH, Rush BF, et al: Verrucous squamous cell carcinoma of the oral cavity. *Cancer* 1969;23:152–160.
6. Kraus FT, Perez-Mesa C: Verrucous carcinoma: clinical and pathologic study of 105 cases involving oral cavity, larynx and gingiva. *Cancer* 1996;19:26–38.
7. Bloom ND, Siro RH: Carcinoma of the cheek mucosa: a retrospective analysis. *Am J Surg* 1980;140:556–559.
8. MacComb WS, Fletcher GH: *Cancer of the head and neck.* Baltimore: Williams & Wilkins, 1967;147.
9. Lampe I: Radiation therapy of cancer of the buccal mucosa and lower gingiva. *AJR Am J Roentgenol* 1955;73:628–638.
10. Nair MK, Sankaranarayanan R, Padamnabhan K: Evaluation of the role of radiotherapy in the management of carcinoma of the buccal mucosa. *Cancer* 1988;61:1326–1331.
11. Urist MM, O'Brien CJ, Soong SJ et al: Squamous carcinoma of the buccal mucosa; analysis of prognostic factors. *Am J Surg* 1987;154: 411–414.
12. Fletcher GH: *Textbook of radiotherapy*, 2nd ed. Philadelphia: Lea & Febiger, 1973;240.
13. Ash CL: Oral cancer: a twenty-five year study. *AJR AM J Roentgenol* 1962;27:417–430.
14. Bakamjian VY: The surgical management of cancers of the cheek. *J Surg Oncol* 1974;6: 255–267.
15. Paymaster JC: Cancer of the buccal mucosa. *Cancer* 1956;9:431.

## THE ALVEOLAR RIDGE

Squamous cell carcinoma of the alveolar ridge usually arises in the posterior portion of the lower dental arch and is associated with leukoplakia. Most of these tumors are well differentiated. Carcinoma of the upper alveolar ridge is an uncommon disease and should not be confused with neoplasm arising in the maxillary sinus secondarily extending to the gum. Radiographic examination of the paranasal sinuses is helpful in differentiating between these two, as well as in evaluating the extent of the bony involvement.

Approximately 80% of the gingival carcinomas arise from the lower gingiva, and of these 60% occur posterior to the bicuspid.[1] Lymphatic spread depends on whether the lesion arises from the buccal surface or the lingual surface of the alveolar ridge. From the buccal side, metastases occur in the submandibular, submental, and subdigastric nodes. From the lingual side, metastases occur in the subdigastric, deep superior jugular, and retropharyngeal nodes. Both upper and lower gingival lesions follow similar patterns of spread (Figure 5-13).

Nodal metastases are found in about one third of patients at the time of diagnosis. The incidence is slightly higher in lower gingival

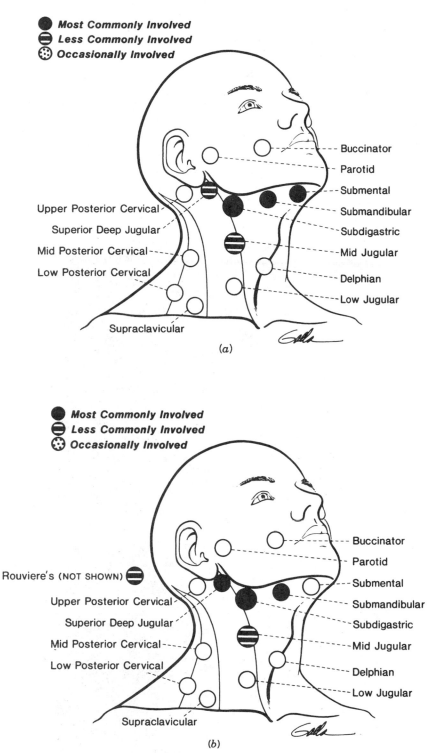

**FIGURE 5-13**  Diagrams showing lymph node involvement from carcinoma of the gingiva: (**a**) tumor arising from the buccal aspect. (**b**) Tumor arising from the lingual aspect.

lesions than in the upper lesions. Radiographic examination of the mandible includes Panorex photographs and CT scans of the mandible. At time, intraoral dental radiographs may better reveal minimal bone involvement of the mandible. Special note should be made between the smooth saucer-shaped pressure defect, which results from a slowly pushing tumor, and the moth-eaten type of bone destruction, which is caused by tumor infiltration with aggressive character. The former can be successfully treated by radiation therapy, whereas the latter cannot.

## Selection of Therapy

Small (T1) exophytic lesions without bone involvement may be managed by external beam therapy alone and/or marginal mandibulectomy and radiation therapy. For advanced lesions with bone destruction of the mandible with or without metastases, radical surgery and mandi-

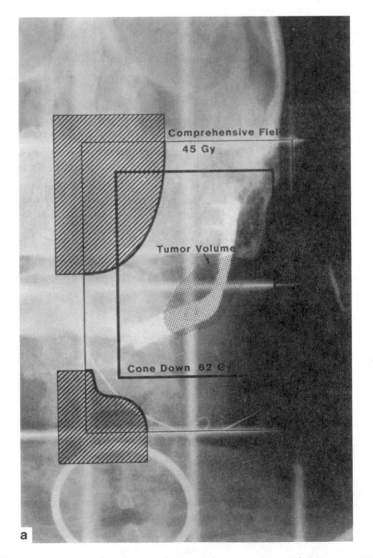

**FIGURE 5-14a**    Simulation film showing placement of postoperative portal: **(a)** anteroposterior view.

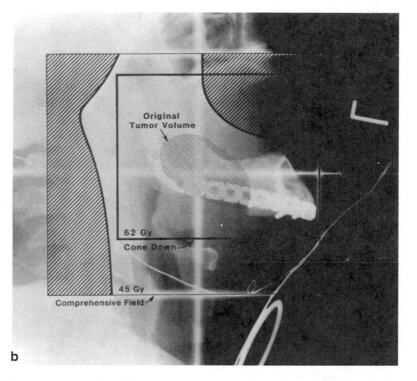

**FIGURE 5-14b**   Simulation film showing placement of postoperatve portal: (**b**) lateral projection.

bular resection[2] is preferred, followed by postoperative radiation therapy.

## Radiation Therapy Management

Because of the eccentric location of both the primary lesion and its regional nodes, radiation therapy is delivered by external photon beam with lateral and anterior wedge pair combining electron beam technique. Radiation portals include the entire resected segment of the hemimandible from the mental symphysis to the temporomandibular joint. Concurrently, the ipsilateral neck is irradiated if nodes are present or lesions are advanced. For postoperative radiation therapy, doses of 55 Gy may be given (Figure 5-14).

## Results of Treatment

Combined mandibular resection and neck dissection can produce good local control and sur-
vival. Cady and Catlin[1] indicated that the most significant factors influencing survival rates were tumor size, evidence of mandibular invasion, and metastases in the neck. Of 557 patients treated for cure, the absolute survival rate was about 50%. The patients with nodeless tumors smaller than 3 cm had survival rate of 82%. Patients with large tumors, (i.e., > 5 cm) and metastases did very poorly. Adjuvant radiation therapy was recommended for large, advanced lesions. Similarly good results in patients with T1 and T2 lesions were reported by Byers et al.,[3] with satisfactory local control and survival. A few scattered reports indicate that the 5-year survival rates after radiation therapy varied from 30% to 50%,[1,4,5] particularly for patients with small mucosal tumors without bone invasions.

## MGH Experience

From 1970 to 1994, a total of 50 patients were managed by radiation therapy alone. The 5-year actuarial local control and disease-specific survival for the entire group of patients are shown in Table 5-11.

Seventeen patients received combined surgery and radiation therapy, mostly partial mandibulectomy; their local control and disease-specific survival rates are shown in Table 5-12.

## Discussion and Summary

Squamous cell carcinoma of the gingiva is a relatively uncommon cancer. Surgical resection is generally considered to be the treatment of choice. However, in a small subset of patients in whom the T1 and T2 lesions are small, exophytic, and nodeless, combined marginal mandibulectomy and radiation therapy may play a curative role in the management of this disease, with satisfactory cure rate and with the integrity of the mandible maintained. For the extensive lesions, T3 and T4, with bone destruction and/or nodal metastases, the treatment of choice is planned segmental mandibulectomy, reconstructive procedure, and postoperative radiation therapy.

**TABLE 5-11    5-Year Actuarial Local Control and Disease-Specific Survival after Radiation Therapy: 1970–1994**

| Stage | n | LC (%) | DSS (%) |
|-------|-----|--------|---------|
| T1 | 15 | 65 | 72 |
| T2 | 15 | 67 | 38 |
| T1-2 | 30 | 65 | 57 |
| T3-4 | 20 | 64 | 70 |
| Total | 50 | 64 | 62 |

**TABLE 5-12    5-Year Actuarial Local Control and Disease-Specific Survival for T3-4 Carcinoma of the Gingival Ridge after Combined Surgery and Postoperative Radiation Therapy: 1970–1994**

| Stage | n | LC (%) | DSS (%) |
|-------|-----|--------|---------|
| T1-2 | 6 | 83 | 83 |
| T3-4 | 11 | 55 | 75 |

· Large, far advanced tumors (T4 N1–3), with extensive bone destruction of the mandible and maxilla are rarely curable by either surgery or radiation therapy or combination of the two. High dose radiation therapy or chemotherapy may offer some degree of palliation.

## REFERENCES

1.  Cady B, Catlin D: Epidermoid carcinoma of the gum: A 20-year survey. *Cancer* 1969;23:551–569.

2.  Barttelbort S, Ariyan S: Mandible preservation with oral cavity carcinoma: Rim mandibulectomy versus sagittal mandibulectomy. *Am J Surg* 1987;154:423–428.

3.  Byers RM, Newman R, Russell N, Yue A: Results of treatment for squamous carcinoma of the lower gum. *Cancer* 1981;47:2236–2238.

4.  Lampe I: Radiation therapy of cancer of the buccal mucosa and lower gingiva. *Am J Surg Radiol* 1955;73:628–635.

5.  Fayos JV, Lampe I: Treatment of squamous cell carcinoma of the oral cavity. *Am J Surg* 1972; 124:493–500.

## THE SOFT PALATE

The palate forms the roof of the oral cavity and is divided into the hard and soft palates. The soft palate is attached anteriorly to the posterior border of the hard palate. Posteriorly its border is free and begins at the junction of the anterior and posterior pillars, both of which contribute to the formation of the central mass called the uvula. These structures, together with the anterior and posterior tonsillar pillars and the tonsillar fossae, are often collectively referred to as the faucial arch.[1]

Squamous cell carcinomas arising from the faucial arch are quite dissimilar from the standpoint of histopathology, mode of spread, and therapeutic management. In this section an attempt is made to discuss lesions of the soft palate and uvula only as oral cancers. Lesions arising from the faucial tonsil and posterior pillars are included with oropharyngeal cancers.

The anterior pillar tumors were discussed in the section on retromolar trigone lesions.

Most tumors of the soft palate and uvula are well differentiated squamous cell carcinomas; they tend to be superficial and ulcerative, with poorly defined borders. Sore throat and odynophagia are common initial symptoms of this disease. Carcinomas arising from the soft palate often are associated with widespread erythroplasia and in situ carcinomas, and multiple primaries either in the adjacent soft palate, the pillars, or the hypopharynx or floor of the mouth are common. Therefore a careful examination of the head and neck region should be carried out to exclude multiple primary carcinomas.

The subdigastric, upper, midjugular, and submandibular nodes are commonly involved. For T1 and T2 mucosal lesions, the incidence of metastases is low (20%). Advanced T3 and T4 lesions are often associated with cervical lymph node metastases, ranging from 65% or higher and are often (20–50%) bilateral (Figure 5-15).

## Selection of Treatment Options

Surgical resection of carcinoma of the soft palate is unsatisfactory and often results in marginal recurrences.[2] Even when surgery is successful, the swallowing and speech functions are severely impaired. Both T1 and T2 exophytic mucosal tumors should be treated by radiation therapy. For advanced T2 and T3 lesions, often associated with lymph node metastases, radiation therapy is given first with curative intent, and any residual disease at the primary site may be dealt with by nidusectomy. Surgical resection is indicated for metastatic nodes, even if bilateral, if the primary lesion is controlled by radiation therapy. At present, massive squamous cell carcinoma of the soft palate, with involvement of the entire oropharynx, the base of the tongue, and the tonsil (often associated with bilateral lymph node metastases) is by any means. High dose radiation therapy with or without chemotherapy may offer some degree of palliation. Attempts to eradicate such advanced

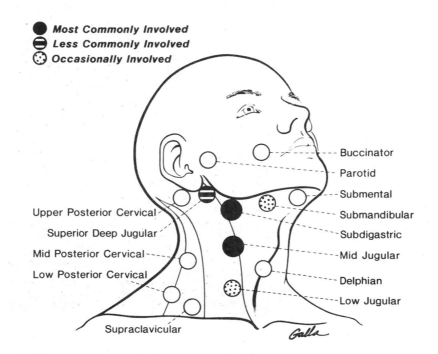

**FIGURE 5-15**  Diagram showing lymph node involvement in carcinoma of the soft palate.

tumors by primary surgery rarely are successful because of the high incidence of marginal recurrence and uncontrolled metastatic neck disease.

## Radiotherapeutic Management

Squamous cell carcinomas of the soft palate tend to spread diffusely along the mucosal surface; their borders are frequently poorly defined and escape detection by the naked eye. Although the Toluidine blue stain may occasonally delineate the tumor's extent, the development of tumoritis following initial doses of 15 to 20 Gy in 2 weeks in the form of mouth bath has been found extremely useful for deter-

minining tumor margins prior to further radiation therapy.

For small, superficial T1 lesions, IOC electron beam radiation therapy is highly effective, without significant radiation sequelae such as dental caries and xerostomia. For T2 and T3 lesions, opposing lateral portals with equal loading are used (Figure 5-16). After 45 Gy the spinal cord is removed from the treatment field and the primary disease is treated to 65 to 70 Gy in 7 weeks. The residual palpable nodes in the posterior cervical triangle are boosted by electrons. Lower neck and supraclavicular irradiation will also be given for 50 Gy in 5 weeks for patients with extensive primary or nodal disease.

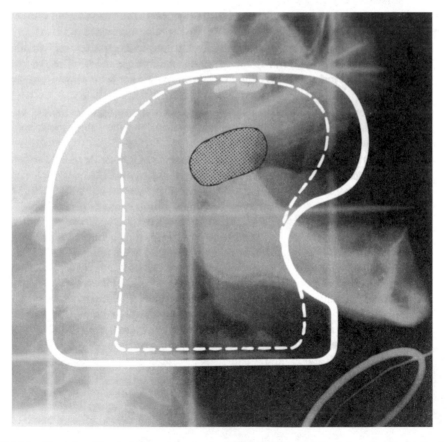

**FIGURE 5-16**   Simulation film showing portal arrangement and shrinking field technique for RT of soft palate carcinoma. The final boost may be given by IOC if feasible after 65 Gy up to 72 Gy to the primary.

## Radiotherapeutic Results

For small T1 and T2 tumors, very good control rates (80–90%) have been achieved with radiation therapy, with excellent functional results.[3,4] The local control of advanced (T3) disease by radiation therapy is poor, approximately 10% to 20%. Far advanced (T4) lesions, which are inoperable and rarely curable, are treated with radiation therapy for palliation and/or with chemotherapy.

## MGH Experience

From 1970 through 1994 a total of 144 patients with squamous cell carcinoma of the soft palate and uvula were treated by radiation therapy. The 5-year actuarial local control and disease specific survival rates are shown in Table 5-13.

### *Results of Bid Radiation Therapy Twice a Day*

From 1979 through 1994, 99 patients received twice-daily radiation therapy. The 5-year actuarial local control rates and DSS are shown in Table 5-14.

## Discussion and Summary

Squamous cell carcinoma of the soft palate is a relatively less common cancer of the oral cavity. The early superficial mucosal lesions (T1 N0 and T2 N0) are highly amenable to treatment with radiation therapy, with extremely high cure rates and preservation of speech and swallowing mechanisms. For advanced disease, cure rates with radiation therapy are poor. The presence of lymph node metastasis reduces survival to about half that without affected nodes. Elective lower neck irradiation does not seem to be indicated in patients with early superficial (T1 N0) lesions; however, in advanced disease and in patients with affected lymph nodes, aggressive radiation treatment to the primary site and neck may produce good local control and higher survival rates. Radical neck dissection for residual lymph nodes is efficacious for controlling neck disease. Primary surgery for carcinoma of the soft palate is not rewarding and often is unsuccessful because of the high incidence of tumor recurrence at the margins after surgery.

Squamous cell carcinoma of the soft palate tends to be associated with cancerous field diathesis and often with multiple primary lesions of the head and neck. Close follow-up of all patients treated is required. A few so-called local recurrences at the irradiated site or adjacent area may in fact be second or third primary carcinomas. Because of high tolerance of the mucomuscular structures of the soft palate, a fact rarely appreciated, repeat irradiation of small recurrences or second primary lesions is feasible and occasionally successful with careful technique (i.e., IOC electron beam radiation therapy).

**TABLE 5-14   5-Year Actuarial Local Control and Disease-Specific Survival after Twice-Daily Radiation: 1979–1994**

| Stage | n | LC (%) | DSS (%) |
|-------|-----|--------|---------|
| T1 | 14 | 91 | 81 |
| T2 | 51 | 79 | 82 |
| T3-4 | 34 | 68 | 54 |

**TABLE 15-13   5-Year Actuarial Local Control and Disease-Specific Survival after Radiation Therapy: 1970–1994**

| Stage | n | LC (%)* | DSS (%)* |
|-------|-----|---------|----------|
| T1 | 39 | 96 | 86 |
| T2 | 65 | 81 | 82 |
| T3 | 27 | 55 | 40 |
| T4 | 13 | 24 | 24 |
| T3-4 | 40 | 45 | 34 |
| Total | 144 | 75 | 70 |
| N0 | 107 | 85 | 81 |
| N1 | 5 | 20 | 40 |
| N2-3 | 32 | 55 | 41 |

*$p = 0.0001$.

## REFERENCES

1. Gelinas M, Fletcher GH: Incidence and causes of local failure of irradiation in squamous cell

carcinoma of the faucial arch, tonsillar fossa and base of tongue. *Radiology* 1973;108: 383–387.

2. Strong E: Sites of treatment failure in head and neck cancer. *Cancer Treat Symp* 1987;2:5–20.

3. Lindberg RD, Fletcher GH; The role of irradiation in the management of head and neck cancer. Analysis of results and causes of failure. *Tumori* 1978;64:313–325.

4. Chung CK, Constable WC: Treatment of squamous cell carcinoma of the soft palate and uvula. *Int J Radiat Oncol Biol Phys* 1979;5: 845–850.

## THE HARD PALATE

The hard palate is the most common site for occurrence of minor salivary gland tumors in the oral cavity. Squamous cell carcinomas arising from the hard palate are quite rare; they are usually ulcerative and generally invade the underlying bone in the early stage of disease.[1] Appropriate x-ray examinations, including CT scans, should be obtained to evaluate the extent of bone involvement. Most carcinomas are well differentiated, with a low incidence of lymph node metastases (15–20%). The submandibular upper jugular and subdigastric nodes are commonly involved.[2]

### Selection of Therapy

Early lesions without bony involvement can be treated satisfactorily by radiation therapy alone. Advanced, deeply ulcerative, infiltrative lesions with bone destruction are better treated by combined surgery and radiation therapy[2]; the resulting bony defect can be corrected by an obturator. Malignant salivary gland tumors are treated by surgery and postoperative radiation therapy. Some inoperable malignancies of the minor salivary glands can be palliated well by high dose radiation therapy.

### Radiotherapeutic Management

Radiation therapy for early carcinoma of the hard palate is generally directed to the treatment of the primary site if the neck is free from metastases. Parallel opposing lateral portals are used to cover the entire palate for approximately 60 Gy in 6 weeks. The primary lesion may be boosted with IOC electron beam therapy if possible.

For advanced disease with bone destruction and nodes, postoperative radiation therapy includes the primary site as well as the regional nodes for approximately 60 Gy in 6 weeks.

### Radiotherapeutic Results

Radiotherapeutic results for carcinoma of the hard palate are sparse owing to the rarity of this disease. Scattered case reports suggest that local control rates can be achieved in approximately one-third to one-half of the patients treated.[3] Patients with nodes and bone destruction are unlikely to be cured by radiation therapy alone. Combined surgery and radiation therapy have provided some improvement in survival.

### REFERENCES

1. Ratzcr ER, Schweitzer RJ, Frazell EL: Epidermoid carcinoma of the palate. *Am J Surg* 1970; 119:294–297.

2. Konrad HR, Canalis RF, Calcaterra TC: Epidermoid carcinoma of the palate. *Arch Otolaryngol* 1978;104:208–212.

3. Schotlenfeld D: Cancer of the buccal cavity and pharynx: a review of end results of primary treatment of 2877 cases: 1948–1964. *Clin Bull* 1972;2:51–57.

# B. CARCINOMA OF THE OROPHARYNX

The oropharynx includes the base of the tongue, the posterior tonsillar pillars, the glossotonsillar sulci, the faucial tonsils, and the oropharyngeal walls. The important anatomic structures of the oropharynx were shown in Figure 5-1.The TNM staging system for this disease is similar to that for carcinoma of the oral cavity according to the size of the lesions as following:

T1   Tumor 2 cm or less in greatest diameter
T2   Tumor more than 2 cm but not more than 4 cm in greatest diameter
T3   Tumor more than 4 cm in greatest diameter
T4   Tumor invades adjacent structures [e.g., pterygoid (muscles) mandible, hard palate, deep muscle of tongue, larynx]

Discussions in this section are limited to the lesions commonly seen in a general hospital, that is, faucial tonsil and base of tongue.

## THE TONSIL

Squamous cell carcinoma of the faucial tonsil is prone to spread posteriorly to the lateral pharyngeal wall, inferiorly to the base of the tongue, and superiorly to the soft palate. Approximately 60% to 70% of patients on admis-sion and during their clinical course have nodal metastases. Once the disease has extended to a major portion of the base of the tongue or soft palate, bilateral lymph node metastases are found in 15% to 20% of patients. The principal groups of lymph nodes involved in this disease (Figure 5-17) are the subdigastric node, commonly called the tonsil node, the superior deep jugular, and Rouviere nodes. The submandibular nodes are rarely involved.[1]

## Selection of Therapy

Squamous cell carcinoma of the faucial tonsil can be treated by surgery or radiation therapy.[2] Primary surgical resection is effective for early carcinoma, but the procedure is attended by high functional and cosmetic morbidity. Since most of the carcinomas of the tonsil are radiosensitive and in early stages highly radiocurable, radiation therapy is the treatment of choice for T1 and T2 lesions. Advanced tumors of the tonsil (T3 and T4) with invasion of the base of the tongue are managed by combined radical resection and

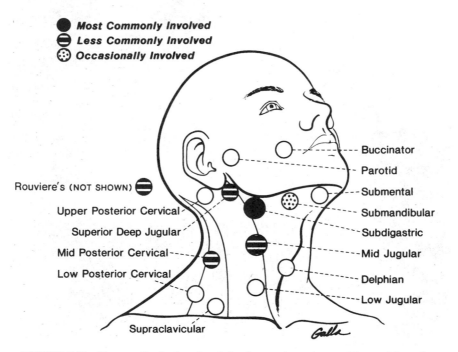

**FIGURE 5-17**   Diagram showing lymph node involvement in carcinoma of the vaucial tonsil.

postoperative radiation therapy.[3,4] Another option consists of high dose external beam therapy through the shrinking field technique, followed by limited surgery with removal of residual disease commonly present in the base of the tongue or adjacent mandible. Any residual nodal disease in the neck following radiation therapy is dealt with by neck dissection.

## Radiation Therapy Management

Radiation therapy for carcinoma of the faucial tonsil is primarily by external beam radiation with large portals to include the primary site and adjacent structures, that is, the base of tongue and lower nasopharynx and hypopharynx as well as the regional nodes (Figure 5-18). For the early lesions (T1 and T2) without involvement of the base of the tongue, the initial 20 Gy is given through opposing lateral portals to evaluate the extent of tumor by the development of tumoritis. If the lesion remains eccentric, further radiation therapy consisting of 45 Gy is given by lateral wedge pair technique. This will result in sparing of the contralateral salivary glands and will avoid excessive xerostomia. On the other hand, if the base of the tongue or soft palate is significantly involved, the contralateral lymph nodes are at risk; therefore most of the radiation therapy is given through opposed lateral portals after the initial radiation therapy of 20 Gy for additional 40 to 45 Gy for the remaining radiotherapy. For the massive tumors (T3 and T4), high dose BID radiotherapy for approximately 65 to 70 Gy in 7 weeks is given; for occult disease, ipsilateral or bilateral elective low neck irradiation of 50 Gy is given in 5 weeks.

## Radiotherapeutic Results

The results of treatment of carcinoma of the tonsil varied. In general, early carcinoma of the

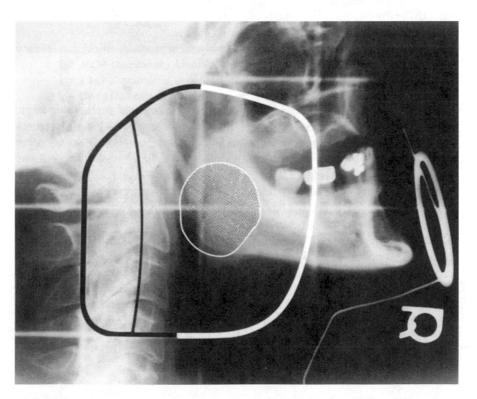

**FIGURE 5-18**  Simulation film illustrating portal arrangement and shrinking field off cord technique.

tonsil carried a highly favorable prognosis, with local control rate better than 80%.[5-10] When the disease becomes massive, the results are poor, ranging from 15% to 20%. Interstitial brachytherapy boost after external beam radiation therapy did not improve the local control rates particularly for the T3 and T4 lesions.[11] The N2a-N3 disease may require neck dissection for residual nodes after a full course of radiation therapy. Since 80% of the clinical N1 and N2b necks can be controlled by radiation therapy alone, routine planned neck dissection is not warranted.

## MGH Experience

From 1970 through 1994, a total of 269 patients with squamous cell carcinoma of the faucial tonsil received radiation therapy: 143 patients were treated with QD radiation therapy and 119 patients received BID and 19 patients had planned combined radical surgery and radiation therapy. The 5-year actuarial rates of the entire

**TABLE 5-15  5-Year Actuarial Local Control and Disease-Specific Survival for Tonsillar Carcinoma Related to T Stage after Radiation Therapy: 1970–1994**

| T-Stage | n | LC (%)* | DSS (%)** |
| --- | --- | --- | --- |
| T1 | 27 | 81 | 87 |
| T2 | 111 | 79 | 75 |
| T3 | 103 | 60 | 48 |
| T4 | 28 | 23 | 22 |

*p = 0.001.

**p = 0.0001.

**TABLE 5-16  5-Year Actuarial Local Control and Disease-Specific Survival Tonsillar Carcinoma after Radiation Therapy: 1970–1994**

| Stage | n | LC (%) | DSS (%) |
| --- | --- | --- | --- |
| T1 | 13 | 81 | 71 |
| T2 | 65 | 73 | 68 |
| T1-2 | 78 | 75 | 69 |
| T3 | 51 | 45 | 32 |
| T4 | 14 | 17 | 14 |

**TABLE 5-17  5-Year Actuarial Rates for Tonsillar Carcinoma after Twice-Daily Radiation Therapy Therapy: 1970–1994**

| Stage | n | LC (%) | DSS (%) |
| --- | --- | --- | --- |
| T1 | 13 | 80 | 100 |
| T2 | 43 | 88 | 83 |
| T1-2 | 56 | 86 | 87 |
| T3 | 52 | 78 | 41 |
| T4 | 11 | 39 | 47 |

**TABLE 5-18  Comparision of Twice-Daily and Daily Radiation Therapy Related to Local Control and Disease-Free Survival**

| Stage | $\mathcal{V}$ | |
| --- | --- | --- |
| | LC (%) | DSS (%) |
| T1 | NS | 0.06 |
| T2 | 0.02 | 0.01 |
| T1-2 | 0.02 | 0.002 |
| T3 | 0.01 | 0.03 |
| T4 | NS | 0.07 |

group are shown in Table 5-15, and Table 5-16 shows results after daily radiation therapy.

The results after BID radiation therapy are shown in Table 5-17, and Table 5-18 compares daily and twice-daily rates of local control and disease-free survival.

Table 5-18 compares BID and QD rates of LC and DSS.

## Discussion and Summary

Squamous cell carcinoma of the tonsil is a fairly common malignant tumor of the head and neck. It should not be confused with squamous cell carcinoma of the retromolar trigone and anterior pillar. The latter would be best grouped with carcinoma of the oral cavity because of their similarity in terms of tumor growth, spread, and prognosis and therapeutic management.[7]

Early carcinoma of the tonsil is highly radiocurable. The presence of early nodal disease (N1) did not affect survival—a typical feature of carcinoma of the oropharynx compared with the carcinomas of the oral cavity. The lymph node disease can be sterilized by radiation therapy with a high degree of success. Most of the radiation failures were due to inability to control the primary sites with or without neck disease, particularly the T3 and T4 lesions. Distant metastases alone occurred in 7% who died of the disease.

Planned combined radiation therapy and surgery plays an important role for the treatment of advanced T3 and T4 lesions. With the advent of techniques of reconstructive surgery, more patients are subjected to radical resection first followed by external beam postoperative radiation therapy without significant complications. Massive disease, often associated with nodal metastases, is currently managed by twice-daily radiation therapy and/or chemotherapy.

## THE BASE OF TONGUE

The base of the tongue is the fixed portion or the posterior third of the tongue starting anteriorly from the circumvallate papillae toward the epiglotticopharyngeal folds and valleculae posteriorly. Squamous cell carcinomas arising from this site in the early stages are often asymptomatic, and therefore the disease can be diagnosed early only in rare cases. Moderately advanced tumors may be accompanied by pain and unilateral sore throat. Odynophagia, dysphagia, otalgia, hemorrhage, and hot potato voice may be associated with large tumors of this region. Most tumors tend to be aggressive, deeply infiltrative, and moderately to poorly differentiated. The base of the tongue is supplied with rich lymphatics with multiple crossings, and some of the squamous cell carcinomas in the neck with so-called unknown primaries may have their primary lesions originating in this region. Metastases occur in the upper deep cervical, subdigastric, and midjugular nodes (Figure 5-19).

### Selection of Therapy

Most of the carcinomas of the base of the tongue are so situated that appropriate surgery

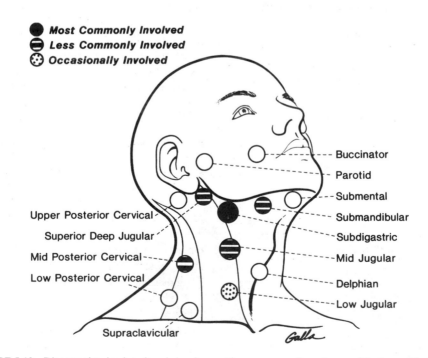

FIGURE 5-19   Diagram showing lymph node involvement in squamous cell carcinoma of the base of the tongue.

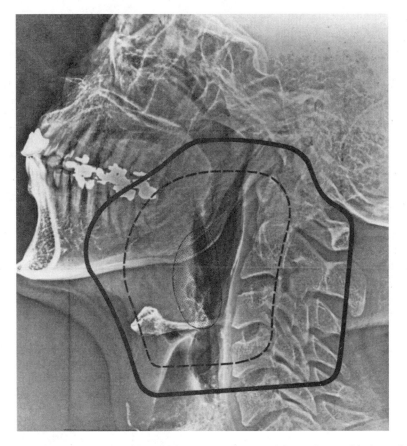

**FIGURE 5-20**   Radiograph showing radiation therapy portal arrangement for carcinoma of the base of the tongue.

would have to include excision of the entire tongue and laryngectomy. Such aggressive primary surgery is extremely mutilating, and often is followed by marginal recurrence at the primary site and by nodal disease in the neck. In spite of improvement of technique, treatment of carcinoma of the base of the tongue by radical surgery is unrewarding owing to dismal cure rates and is seldom practiced in our institution.

The exophytic and superficial T1 and T2 carcinomas are radiosensitive and radiocurable by radiation therapy alone, and the results are comparable to those obtained by surgery. The large infiltrative T3 and T4 lesions are rarely operable or curable by either radiation therapy or surgery. Currently combined high dose radiation therapy and limited surgery (i.e., nidusectomy), are being utilized increasingly in an attempt to improve results. Palliative radiation therapy or chemotherapy is all that can be offered for totally inoperable lesions.

## Radiotherapeutic Management

Since most of the tumors in the base of the tongue are poorly differentiated carcinomas and deeply infiltrative with ill-defined borders and often associated with lymph node metastases, radiation therapy must be comprehensive. Generally, opposing lateral portals with equal loading are used for a minimum tumor dose of 65 to 70 Gy in 7 to 8 weeks (Figure 5-20). Concurrently the lower necks are irradiated electively for 50 Gy for microscopic disease. Gross disease is boosted for an additional 5 to 10 Gy. The spinal cord dose is limited to 45 Gy in 5 weeks. Currently most tongue base lesions are treated by means of a twice-daily program.[5]

## Radiotherapeutic Results

The results of treatment of carcinoma of the base of the tongue by either radiation therapy or surgery generally were considered to be unsatisfactory. Most reported series often consisted of extensive T3 and T4 lesions with the reputed poor local control and survival rates. Interstitial implant was used to boost the dose to the tumors but was not found to be essential.[11] Whicker et al.[12] reported no evidence of disease (NED) in 57% of 102 patients after surgery. Dalley[13] indicated that 12% of 102 patients were NED at 5 years, and 28% in 28 patients without nodes. Most of the surgical patients failed from marginal recurrence.[14] The recent series of Spanos et al.[15] showed NED

Table 5-19   5-Year Actuarial Local Control and Disease-Specific Survival for Carcinoma of the Base of Tongue after Radiation Therapy: 1970–1994

| Stage | n | LC (%) | DSS (%) |
|-------|-----|--------|---------|
| T1 | 40 | 89 | 78 |
| T2 | 69 | 79 | 76 |
| T3 | 78 | 48 | 40 |
| T4 | 37 | 21 | 16 |
| T3-4 | 11 | 53 | 932 |

*$p = 0.0001.$
**$p = 0.0001.$

TABLE 5-20   5-Year Actuarial Local Control and Disease-Specific Survival for Carcinoma of the Base of Tongue after Daily Radiation Therapy: 1970–1994

| Stage | n | LC (%) | DSS (%) |
|-------|-----|--------|---------|
| T1 | 17 | 87 | 70 |
| T2 | 30 | 72 | 68 |
| T1-2 | 50 | 78 | 58 |
| T3 | 29 | 26 | 15 |
| T4 | 23 | 16 | 13 |

TABLE 5-21   5-Year Actuarial Local Control and Disease-Specific Survival for Carcinoma of the Base of Tongue after Twice-Daily Radiation Therapy: 1970–1994

| Stage | n | LC (%) | DSS (%) |
|-------|-----|--------|---------|
| T1 | 23 | 90 | 85 |
| T2 | 33 | 84 | 84 |
| T1-2 | 56 | 87 | 84 |
| T3 | 46 | 63 | 54 |
| T4 | 14 | 27 | 16 |

TABLE 5-22   Comparision of Twice-Daily and Daily Radiation Therapy Related to Local Control and Disease-Specific Survival

| Stage | $\mathcal{V}$ | |
|-------|--------|---------|
|  | LC (%) | DSS (%) |
| T1 | NS | NS |
| T2 | NS | NS |
| T1-2 | NS | NS |
| T3 | 0.0003 | 0.004 |
| T4 | 0.0002 | 0.005 |

rates of 91% for T1, 71% for T2, and 78% for T3 after radiation therapy at 2 years. It is apparent that the local control of the small T1 and T2 lesions of the tongue can be achieved satisfactorily. Similarly good local control resulted after hyperefractionated radiation therapy.[5]

## MGH Experience

From 1970 to 1994, a total of 224 patients with squamous cell carcinoma of the base of tongue received radiation therapy. Of these, 99 patients received once-daily radiation therapy and 116 received it twice daily. The 5-year actuarial rates are shown in Tables 5-19 to 5-22.

## DISCUSSION AND SUMMARY

Squamous cell carcinoma of the base of the tongue is not accessible for causal clinical examination and tends to be advanced when the diagnosis is initially made. Traditionally, the prognosis of this disease was known to be notoriously poor after either radiation therapy or surgery. Primary surgery is rarely successful because of the extensive primary lesions and high incidence of marginal recurrence and nodal metastases, often bilateral. For the early tumors (T1-2) the treatment of choice is comprehensive radiation therapy, with surgery being reserved for salvage. For the extensive disease (T3-4, N2-3), chemotherapy may be used first, followed by radiation therapy and surgery. Our experience, however, indicates that stage for stage, the therapeutic results for carcinoma arising from the base of the tongue compare favorably with those of carcinoma of the oral tongue. Currently most cancers of the base of the tongue are managed by a twice-daily program at the MGH.

## REFERENCES

1. Lindberg R: Distribution of cervical lymph node metastases from squamous cell carcinoma of the upper respiratory and digestive tracts. *Cancer* 1972;29:1446.

2. Perez CA, Mills WB, Ogura JH, et al: Carcinoma of the tonsil: Sequential comparison of four treatment modalities. *Radiology* 1970;94: 649.

3. Maltz R, Shumrick DA, Aron BS, et al: Carcinoma of the tonsil: Results of combined therapy. *Laryngoscope* 1974;84:2172.

4. Rolandier LL, Everts EC, Shumrick DA: Carcinoma of the tonsils: A planned combined therapy approach. *Laryngoscope* 1971;81:1199.

5. Wang CC, Montgomery W, Efird J: Local control of oropharyngeal carcinoma by irradiation alone. *Laryngoscope* 1995;105:5, 529–533.

6. Weller SA, Goffinet DR, Goode RL, et al: Carcinoma of the oropharynx: Results of megavoltage radiation therapy in 305 patients. *Am J Roentgenol Radium Ther Nucl Med* 1976; 126:236.

7. Wang CC: Management and prognosis of squamous cell carcinoma of the tonsillar region. *Radiology* 1972;104:667.

8. Shukovsky LJ, Fletcher GH: Time–dose and tumor volume relationships in the irradiation of squamous cell carcinoma of the tonsillar fossa. *Radiology* 1973;107:621–626.

9. Mendenhall WM, Parsons JT, Cassisi NJ, Million RR: Squamous cell carcinoma of the tonsillar area treated with radical irradiation. *Radiother Oncol* 1987;10, 23–30.

10. Wong CS, Ang KK, Fletcher GH, Thames HD, Peters LJ, Byers RM, Oswald MJ: Definitive radiotherapy for squamous cell carcinoma of the tonsillar fossa. *Int J Radiat Oncol Biol Phys* 1989;16: 657–662.

11. Foote RL, Parsons JT, Mendenhall WW, et al: Is interstitial implantation essential for successful radotherapeutic treatment of base of tongue carcinoma? *Int J Radiat Oncol Biol Phys* 1990;18: 1293–1298.

12. Whicker JH, DeSanto IW, Devine KD: Surgical treatment of squamous cell carcinoma of the base of the tongue. *Laryngoscope* 1972;82: 1853–1860.

13. Dalley VM: Cancer of the laryngopharynx. *J Laryngol Otol* 1968;82:407–419.

14. Strong E: Sites of treatment failure in head and neck cancer. *Cancer Treat Symp* 1987;2:5–20.

15. Spanos WT, Shukovsky LJ, Fletcher GH: Time, dose and tumor volume relationships in irradiation of squamous cell carcinomas of the base of the tongue. *Cancer* 1976;37:2591–2599.

# C.  CARCINOMA OF THE HYPOPHARYNX

The hypopharynx includes the posterior pharyngeal wall, pyriform sinus, and postcricoid area, as shown in Figure 5-21. Most tumors tend to be extensive, frequently with extensive cervical lymph node metastases, often bilateral.[1-3] The principal nodes of involvement are the subdigastric, superior deep jugular, midjugular, and retropharyngeal nodes (Rouviere

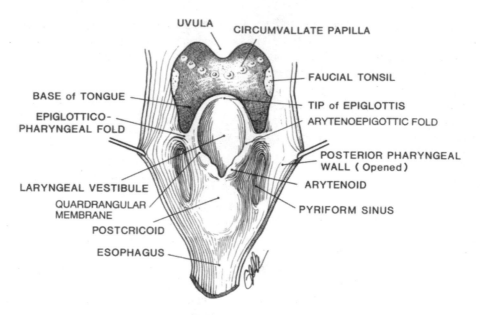

**FIGURE 5-21**   Diagram showing the interior anatomic sites of the hypopharynx.

nodes). Involvement of the posterior cervical triangle is uncommon.[4]

The majority of tumors (60–70%), arise from the pyriform sinus, and approximately one-quarter arise from the posterior pharyngeal wall. The postcricoid tumors are in fact tumors of the upper cervical esophagus, and in the United States are the least common.

The T staging is as follows:

T1   Tumor limited to to one subsite of hypopharynx and 2 cm or less in greatest dimension

T2   Tumor involves more than one subsite of hyphparnyx, or as adjacent site, or measures more than 2 cm but not more than 4 cm in greatest diameter without fixation of hemilarynx

T3   Tumor measures more than 4 cm in greatest dimension or with fixation of hemilarynx

T4   Tumor invades adjacent structure (e.g., thyroid/cricoid cartilage, carotid artery, soft tissue of neck, prevertebral fascia/muscles, thyroid, and /or esophagus)

## THE PYRIFORM SINUS

Carcinomas originating from the apex of the pyriform sinus tend to be aggressive, infiltrative, and extensive. The true tumor extent may be deceiving, since the iceberg presentation of the lesion often involves the adjacent cartilage, larynx, and upper trachea. To the contrary, the lesions arising from the upper membranous lateral wall of the pyriform sinus tend to be exophytic and less aggressive, with lesser incidence of nodal involvement. Figure 5-22 shows the nodal involvement of pyriform carcinoma.

### Selection of Therapy

For T1 N0 and T2 N0 exophytic carcinomas arising from the membranous portion of the pyriform sinus, radiation therapy may be considered as a curative procedure, reserving surgery for salvage. For the extensive (T3 and T4 lesions) but medically operable tumors arising from the apex of the pyriform sinus with or without nodes, the combination of surgery and radiation therapy has yielded higher local control and survival and is the treatment of choice.

## Radiotherapeutic Management

Radiation therapy for carcinoma of the pyriform sinus requires large portal high dose technique, including the primary site as well as the superior, midjugular, and Rouviere nodes (Figure 5-23). Since the apex of the pyriform sinus lies below the level of the true cords, the inferior border of the portal must include the lower border of the cricoid cartilage and upper trachea, with a total dose of 65 to 70 Gy in 7 weeks. For postoperative radiation therapy, following laryngopharyngectomy and reconstruction, a total dose of 55 Gy may be given in 6 weeks and generally is well tolerated. Frequently, if the tumor is found to extend close to the resection margins, an additional 10 Gy to the tracheal stoma is given with electron beam as a boost.

## Results of Treatment

For squamous cell carcinoma of the pyriform sinus, the local control rate after radiation therapy is approximately 20%.[5,6,7,10,11] Combined surgery and radiation therapy[9,12,13] has improved the rates more than double in the T3 group, and triple in lesions with metastatic nodes. The majority of therapeutic failures are due to uncontrolled nodal disease in the neck, recurrence in the base of the tongue, tracheal stoma, or tumor extension into the cervical esophagus or into the base of the skull. A small number of patients die with distant metastases.

## MGH Experience

From 1970 through 1994, a total of 186 patients with carcinoma of the pyriform sinus were treated by radiation therapy at the MGH. The 5-year actuarial rates of the entire group are shown in Tables 5-23 and 5-24.

### Planned Combined Surgery and Radiation Therapy

Sixty-six patients with carcinoma of the pyriform sinus were treated by planned combined therapies. For the T1 and T2 lesions, the local control at the primary sites and DSS rates were 91% and 100%. For the

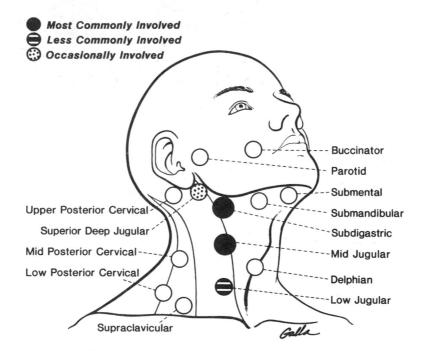

**FIGURE 5-22**   Diagram showing lymph node involvement in carcinoma of the pyriform sinus.

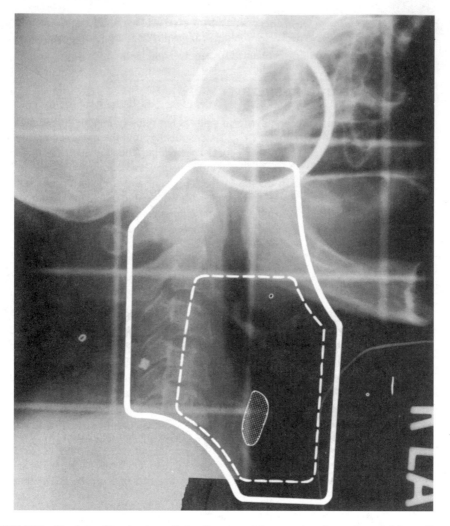

**FIGURE 5-23** Simulation film showing radiation therapy portal arrangement for carcinoma of the pyriform sinus.

advanced tumors (T3-T4), the corresponding rates were 45% and 33%, respectively. The difference is statistically significant ($p = 0.005$).

## THE POSTERIOR PHARYNGEAL WALL

Carcinoma of the posterior pharyngeal wall is a rather unusual tumor. Most lesions are quite large and exophytic and may extend laterally to involve the lateral pharyngeal wall and to infiltrate inferiorly toward the esophagus. The prevertebral fascia hinders tumor extension pos-

teriorly, and therefore the muscles or vertebral bodies are rarely involved. Approximately one of two patients when first seen presents with cervical lymph node metastases, and these are often bilateral. The retropharyngeal or Rouviere nodes are frequently affected, the incidence as high as 44%.[1–3] Figure 5-24 shows nodal involvement of the posterior pharyngeal wall.

### Selection of Therapy

Because of the close proximity of the primary lesion to the adjacent fascia and muscles, sur-

**TABLE 5-23  5-Year Actuarial Local Control and Disease-Specific Survival Rates after Radiation Therapy: 1970–1994**

| Stage | $n$ | LC (%) | DSS (%) |
|-------|-----|--------|---------|
| T1 | 29 | 73 | 68 |
| T2 | 58 | 80 | 64 |
| T3-4 | 99 | 29 | 24 |
|  |  | $p = 0.0001$ | $p = 0.0001$ |
| N0 | 63 | 65 | 68 |
| N1 | 32 | 46 | 41 |
| N2-3 | 69 | 39 | 28 |
|  |  | $p = 0.04$ | $p = 0.0001$ |

gical resection frequently is associated with local recurrence due to "dirty" resection margins. Therefore, like carcinoma of the nasopharynx, carcinoma of the posterior pharyngeal wall is often considered inoperable and is best treated by radiation therapy.

## Radiotherapeutic Management

Because of the axial submucosal spread of the lesion along the prevertebral fascia, which may involve the posterior faucial pillar and, in advanced cases, the nasopharynx and soft palate, radiation therapy calls for large portals including the entire pharynx and upper cervical esophagus, and superiorly to the nasopharyngeal vault, and the superior deep jugular and Rouviere nodes. Figure 5-25 shows the radiation therapy portal arrangement for this disease. The dose to the prevertebral tumor should be 65 to 70 Gy in 6 to 7 weeks and the spinal cord dose limited to 45 Gy in 5 weeks.

**TABLE 5-24  5-Year Actuarial Local Control and Disease-Specific Survival Rates after Twice-Daily and Daily Radiation Therapy: 1970–1994**

| Stage | $n$ | LC (%) | DSS (%) |
|-------|-----|--------|---------|
| T1-2 |  |  |  |
|   BID | 52 | 74 | 71 |
|   QD | 23 | 76 | 72 |
|  |  | $p = 0.85$ | $p = 0.67$ |
| T3-4 |  |  |  |
|   BID | 45 | 51 | 44 |
|   QD | 44 | 17 | 15 |
|  |  | $p = 0.05$ | $p = 0.09$ |

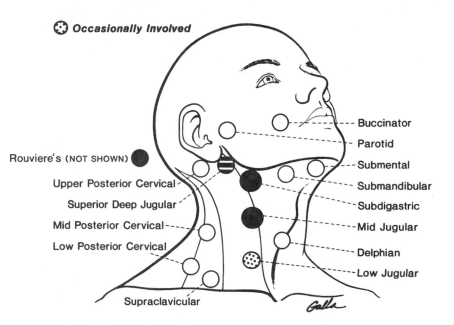

**FIGURE 5-24**  Diagram showing lymph node involvement in carcinoma of the posterior pharyngeal wall.

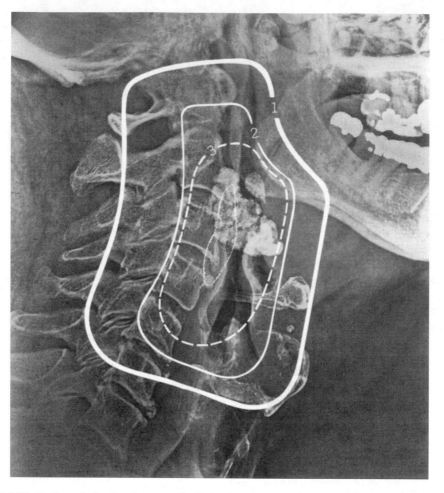

**FIGURE 5-25** Radiograph showing placement of radiation therapy portal for carcinoma of the posterior pharyngeal wall with multiple shrinking fields: (1) comprehensive, (2) intermediate off-cord, and (3) final boost. (Position of calcified subdigastric node is seen.)

## Results of Therapy

The results following treatment of posterior pharyngeal carcinoma generally are poor. The reported local control rates ranged from 15% to 30% by radiation therapy alone. For the early T1 and T2 lesions, the radiotherapeutic results are approximately 50%. Advanced tumors carry approximately 10% cure rate after radiation therapy. Patients without nodes generally do better than patients with nodes. Far-advanced lesions and/or massive bilateral cervical metastases are rarely curable by radiation therapy or surgery and currently are treated for palliation.

## MGH Experience

From 1970 to 1994, 135 patients with carcinoma of the posterior pharyngeal wall were treated at the MGH. The results of treatment are shown in following Tables 5-25 and 5-26.

## DISCUSSION AND SUMMARY

Carcinoma of the hypopharynx is a silent disease, and the tumors frequently are advanced and bulky, with extensive lymph node metastases. For the early T1 and T2 lesions arising

**TABLE 5-25   5-Year Acturial Rates of Local Control and Survival Rates for Carcinoma of the Posterior Pharyngeal Wall after Radiation Therapy: 1970–1994**

| Stage | n | LC (%)* | DSS (%)** |
|-------|-----|---------|-----------|
| T1 | 29 | 81 | 74 |
| T2 | 54 | 55 | 57 |
| T3-4 | 52 | 40 | 35 |

*$p = 0.0008$.
**$p = 0.0007$.

**TABLE 5-26   5-Year Actuarial Local Control and Disease-Specific Survival Rates for Carcinoma of the Posterior Pharyngeal Wall after Twice-Daily and Daily Radiation Therapy: 1970–1994**

| Stage | n | LC (%) | DSS (%) |
|-------|-----|--------|---------|
| BID | 37 | 74 | 71 |
| QD | 27 | 55 | 60 |
|  |  | $p = 0.08$ | $p = 0.53$ |
| T3-4 |  |  |  |
| BID | 19 | 70 | 53 |
| QD | 22 | 33 | 35 |
|  |  | $p = 0.010$ | $p = 0.16$ |
| Total |  |  |  |
| BID | 56 | 72 | 64 |
| QD | 49 | 45 | 49 |
|  |  | $p = 0.001$ | $p = 0.13$ |

from the membranous portion of the pyriform sinus, a trial course of high dose radiation therapy is worthwhile, with surgery being reserved for salvage. For the bulky lesions arising from the apex of the pyriform sinus, planned combined radiation therapy and surgery is preferred.

For early (T1-2) posterior pharyngeal wall lesions, radiation therapy is the treatment of choice. Far-advanced lesions with extensive nodal disease are rarely curable by radiation therapy, and perhaps combined therapies including chemotherapy, radical surgery, and postoperative radiation therapy at the expense of functional and anatomic mutilation, may offer a glimpse of hope of improved results.

# REFERENCES

1. American Joint Committee on cancer: *A manual for staging of cancer*, 4th ed. Philadelphia: Lippincott, 1992.

2. McGavran MH, Bauer WC, Spjut HJ, et al: Carcinoma of the pyriform sinus: the results of radical surgery. *Arch Otolaryngol* 1963;78:826.

3. Byers RM, Wolf PF, Ballantyne AJ: Rationale for elective modified neck dissection. *Head Neck Surg* 1988;10:160–167.

4. Balley VM: Cancer of the laryngohparynx. *J Laryngol Otol* 1968;82:407–419.

5. Krischner JA: Pyriform sinus cancer: a clinical and laboratory study. *Ann Otol Rhinol Laryngol* 1975;84:793–803.

6. Wang CC, Schulz MD, Miller D: Combined radiation therapy and surgery for carcinoma of the supraglottis and pyriform sinus. *Laryngoscope* 1970;82:1883–1890.

7. Ballantyne AJ: Principles of surgical management of cancer of the pharyngeal walls. *Cancer* 1967;20:663–667.

8. Briant TD, Bryce DP, Smith TJ: Carcinoma of the hypopharynx—a five year follow-up. *J Otolaryngol* 1977;6:353–362.

9. Mancuso AA, Harnsberger HR, Muraki AS, Stevens MH: Computed tomography of cervical and retropharyngeal lymph nodes: normal antatomy variants of normal, and applications in staging head & neck cancer. Part II: Pathology. *Radiology* 1983;148:715–723.

10. Ballantyne AJ: Significance of retropharyngeal nodes in cancer of the head and neck. *Am J Surg* 1964:108:500.

11. Guillamondegui OM, Meoz R, Jesse RH: Surgical treatment of squamous cell carcinoma of the pharyngeal walls. *Am J Surg* 1978;136:474–576.

12. Wang CC: Radiotherapeutic management of carcinoma of the posterior pharyngeal wall. *Cancer* 1971;27:894–896.

13. Meoz-Mendez RT, Fletcher GH, Guillamondegui OM, Peters LJ: Analysis of the results of irradiation in the treatment of squamous cell carcinomas of the pharyngeal walls. *Int J Radiat Oncol Biol Phys* 1978;4:579–585.

14. Marks JE, Freeman RF, Lee F, et al: Pharyngeal wall cancer: an analysis of treatment results, complications and patterns of failure. *Int J Radiat Oncol Biol Phys* 1978;4:587–593.

# D. CARCINOMA OF THE LARYNX

Anatomically and therapeutically, the larynx can be divided into three separate portions, the supraglottis, the glottis, and the subglottis, as shown in Figure 5-26. Subglottic cancers, which are extremely rare and uncommonly seen in general hospitals, are not discussed in this section.

The TNM staging system for squamous cell carcinoma of the larynx is as follows:

Glottis

Tis   Carcinoma in situ

T1   Tumor limited to vocal cord(s) (may involve anterior or posterior commisissure) with normal mobility

T2   Tumor extends to supraglottis and/or subglottis, and/or with impaired cord mobility

T3   Tumor limited to the larynx with vocal cord fixation

T4   Tumor invades through the thyroid cartilage and/or other tissues beyond he larynx (e.g., trachea, soft tissues of the neck, including thyroid, pharynx)

Supraglottis

Tis   Carcinoma in situ

T1   Tumor limited to one subsite of supraglottis with normal vocal cord mobility

T2   Tumor invades mucosa of more than one adjacent subsite of supraglottis or glottis or region outside of the supraglottis (e.g., mucosa of base of tongue, vallecula, medial wall of pyriform sinus) without fixation of the larynx

T3   Tumor limited to larynx with vocal cord fixation and/or invades any of the following: postcricoid area, pre-epiglottic tissues

T4   Tumor invades through the thyroid cartilage, and/or extends into soft tissues of the neck, thyroid, and/or esophagus

## LYMPH NODE METASTASES

The lymphatic network of the larynx varies with different anatomical sites.[1-4] The true vocal cords are void of lymphatics. Therefore the

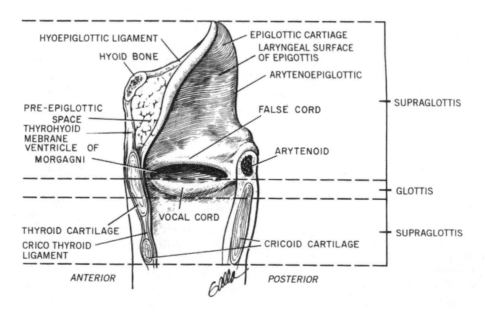

**FIGURE 5-26**   Anatomic subdivisions of the larynx: supraglottis, glottis, and subglottis.

incidence of lymph node metastases generally is low. With tumor confined to the cord with normal mobility (T1), the incidence ranges from 0% to 2%. For the T2 lesion with impaired cord mobility and for T3 lesions, the incidence increases to 10% and 15% respectively. Carcinomas arising from the supraglottic region tend to develop lymph node metastases frequently. As a rule of thumb, as the lesions arise further from the glottis superiorly toward the base of the tongue, or further posteriorly toward the esophagus, there is a higher incidence of lymph node metastases. The difference in incidence may vary from 30% to 75%, depending on the stage of the primary lesions. Bilateral cervical lymph node metastases are common and occur in one-fourth to one-third of patients. The principal group of lymph nodes involved by supraglottic carcinoma includes the subdigastric, the superior deep jugular, and the midjugular nodes. The Rouviere nodes are occasionally involved.

## THE GLOTTIS

### Selection of Therapies

*T1 Carcinomas*   Treatment of early glottic carcinomas (T1) can be by either radiation therapy or surgery. Radiation therapy provides excellent local control. If radiation therapy fails, the success of salvage surgery is extremely high. Conservation surgery such as cordectomy or partial laryngectomy can control early glottic lesions, but the functional results are inferior because of the permanent residual hoarseness. Partial laryngectomy is not suitable for patients of advanced age for patients with chronic obstructive pulmonary disease.

*T2 Carcinomas with Normal Cord Mobility (T2a)*   Lesions of the cords extending into the extracordal area with preservation of cord mobility are generally highly amenable to treatment by radiation therapy, with high cure rates. Failures after radation therapy can often be salvaged by surgery.

*T2 Carcinomas with Impaired Cord Mobility (T2b)*   The cure rates for this stage of disease are not entirely favorable. If the extent of the lesion precludes partial laryngectomy, it is justified to proceed with curative radiation therapy, reserving surgery in form of total laryngectomy for salvage.

*T3 Carcinomas*   Fixation of the vocal cord is a grave prognostic sign. The local control rates for such advanced lesions are low by radiation therapy alone, and such lesions are often treated by planned combined surgery and radiation therapy. If the lesion is limited to the cord and its adjacent supraglottic structures, vertical hemilaryngectomy may be considered with total laryngectomy being reserved for salvage.

*T4 Carcinomas*   Far advanced glottic lesions are unusual and most likely represent extensive supraglottic or pyriform sinus carcinomas with secondary involvement of the glottis. Treatment comprises combined therapies with surgery and radiation.

*Radiotherapeutic Management*   Radiation therapy for early T1 glottic lesions is directed treatment to the glottis with portal sizes of 5/5 cm or 6/5 cm for a total dose of 67 to 70 Gy in 7 weeks. The radiation therapy techniques vary according to the contour and thickness of the anterior neck using either opposing or laterals and anterior oblique wedge pair as shown in Figure 5-27. For most of the advanced T2 and T3 lesions, the portals include the entire larynx with shrinking field techniques for 70 Gy and currently are treated with the twice-daily radiation therapy program at the MGH (Figure 5-28).

### Radiotherapeutic Results

The results of treatment of early T1 glottic carcinoma by irradiation as reported in the literature showed excellent local control, ranging from 80% to 90%[5-9] and including surgical salvage 95% to 98%. This is comparable to the control achievable by hemilaryngectomy, laser excision,[4,10] or laryngofissure and cordectomy.[11]

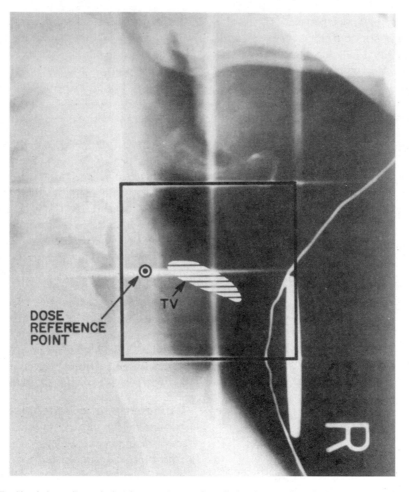

**FIGURE 5-27**   Simulation radiograph showing arrangement for radiation therapy of T1 glottic carcinoma in lateral projection.

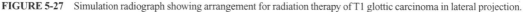

For the T2 lesions, the results are still quite high, approximately 70% to 80%, or approximately 90% when surgical salvage is included. For the T3 lesion, the results following radiation therapy are not entirely satisfactory, being approximately 30% to 65%[5–9]; when surgical salvage is included, the rates ranged from 40% to 70%.

### MGH Experience

From 1970 through 1994, a total of 970 patients with glottic carcinoma were treated by radiation therapy at the MGH. There were 665 patients with T1, 145 with T2a, 92 with T2b, 65

with T3, and 3 with T4. The incidence of nodal metastases at diagnosis was less than 1% for T1, 4% for T2a, and 5% to 10% for T2b and T3 lesions.

The treatment results and differences between the twice-daily and daily programs are presented in Tables 5-27 to 5-30.

Salvage surgery was carried out for the radiation failures at the primary sites. The rate of success was 82% for T1 lesions, 63% for T2a, and 50% for T2b and T3.

***Combined Therapies for Glottic Carcinoma***   A small number of patients were treated by combined surgery and irradiation re-

**TABLE 5-27  5-Year Actuarial Local Control and Disease-Specific Survival of Carcinoma of the Glottis after Radiation Therapy: 1970–1994**

| Stage | n | LC (%)* | DSS (%)** |
|-------|-----|---------|-----------|
| T1 | 665 | 93 | 98 |
| T2a | 145 | 77 | 92 |
| T2b | 92 | 71 | 84 |
| T3 | 65 | 57 | 75 |
| T4 | 3 | 67 | 33 |

*$p = 0.0001$.

**$p = 0001$.

**TABLE 5-28  5-Year Actuarial Local Control and Disease-Specific Survival after Twice-Daily Radiation Therapy for Glottic Carcinoma: 1979–1994**

| Stage | n | LC (%) | DSS(%) |
|-------|-----|--------|--------|
| T2a | 76 | 83 | 93 |
| T2b | 61 | 72 | 87 |
| T3 | 41 | 67 | 85 |

**TABLE 5-29  5-Year Actuarial Local Control and Disease-Specific Survival after Twice-Daily and Daily Radiation Therapy for Glottic Carcinoma**

| Stage | $\mathcal{V}$ |
|-------|------|
| T2a | 0.07 |
| T2b | 0.66 |
| T3 | 0.03 |

**TABLE 5-30  5-Year Actuarial Rates for Tis of the Glottis after Radiation Therapy:1970–1995**

| n | LC (%) | DSS (%) |
|-----|--------|---------|
| 60 | 92 | 98 |

**TABLE 5-31  5-Year Actuarial Rates after Planned Combined Surgery and Radiation Therapy for Glottic Carcinoma**

| Stage | n | LC (%) | DSS (%) |
|-------|-----|--------|---------|
| T2 | 9 | 78 | 89 |
| T3 | 25 | 73 | 72 |
| T4 | 1 | 100 | 100 |

lated to various stages of glottic carcinoma, and the results of combined therapies did not show any significant improvement versus those after primary radiation therapy with surgical salvage, as shown in Table 5-29.

## THE SUPRAGLOTTIS

Carcinoma of the supraglottis ranks second to glottic carcinoma in incidence and generally is associated with a poorer prognosis. Most of these tumors are moderately well to poorly differentiated, with a propensity for regional lymph node metastases. Figure 5-29 shows nodal involvement of supraglottic carcinoma.

### Selection of Therapy

Management of supraglottic carcinoma is extremely controversial. Some advocate total laryngectomy, others call for radiation therapy alone, and still others recommend supraglottic laryngectomy. The selection of methods of treatment depends on the extent, anatomical location, and growth pattern of the primary lesion, its nodal status, the skill of the surgeon and the radiation oncologist, and last but not least the wishes of the patient.

In general, for a superficial early lesion (T1 N0 or T2 N0), radiation therapy may be considered as the initial method of treatment. This is particularly true for the exophytic tumors arising from the tip of the epiglottis and free margins of the aryepiglottic fold. For extensive deeply ulcerative lesions and/or cervical lymph node metastases (i.e., T3-4 N1 or N2) the treatment of choice is surgery followed by postoperative radiotherapy to the entire neck, tracheal stoma, and upper mediastinum.

### Radiotherapeutic Management

Radiation therapy for supraglottic carcinomas must include treatment of the primary lesions and regional nodes in the neck even in T1 N0

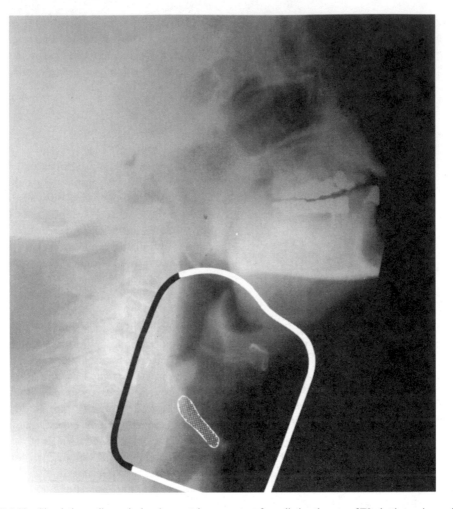

**FIGURE 5-28**    Simulation radiograph showing portal arrangement for radiation therapy of T2 glottic carcinoma in lateral projection.

lesions because of the propensity for nodal metastases. Generally large opposing lateral portals are employed for the initial 45 Gy. After this has been achieved, the spinal cord is excluded from the portals by means of the shrinking field technique, and additional radiation therapy is delivered to the primary site to bring the total dose to 65 to 70 Gy in 7 weeks (Figure 5-29). For extensive disease with nodal metastases, laryngectomy and neck dissection may be considered, followed by postoperative radiation therapy through large lateral portals or minimantle technique

for 55 to 60 Gy, followed by electron stomal boost high risk neck nodes. Most patients with advanced lesions are currently treated by the twice-daily radiation therapy program at the MGH.

### Radiotherapeutic Results

The 5-year NED rates following radiation therapy vary depending on the extent of the primary tumor and the status of the cervical nodes. For T1 N0 and T2 N0 lesions, the 5-year NED rates range from 65% to 80% following

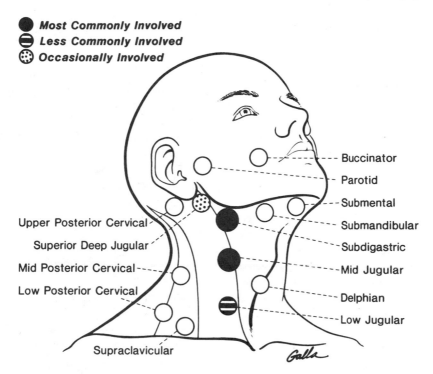

● **Most Commonly Involved**
⊜ **Less Commonly Involved**
⊛ **Occasionally Involved**

Buccinator
Parotid
Submental
Submandibular
Subdigastric
Mid Jugular
Delphian
Low Jugular

Upper Posterior Cervical
Superior Deep Jugular
Mid Posterior Cervical
Low Posterior Cervical

Supraclavicular

**FIGURE 5-29**   Principal lymph node involvement in supraglottic carcinoma.

radiation therapy alone.[9-12] For T3 and T4 lesions, survivals range from 20% to 35% by radiation therapy alone, when treatment consists of combined therapies, that is, laryngectomy and irradiation, the rates are considerably higher, approximately 50% to 60%.[13-18]

The results of once-daily radiation therapy for advanced supraglottic carcinoma have not been highly satisfactory. At the present time, hyperfractionated radiation therapy programs are extensively used with considerable promise, especially for the T3 and T4 tumors.[19,20]

## MGH Experience

From 1970 through 1994 a total of 566 patients with supraglottic carcinoma were treated at the MGH. Of these, 244 patients received once daily radiation therapy and 322 patient received radiation therapy twice a day. The results of treatment after radiation therapy are shown in Table 5-32.

***Results of Bid Radiation Therapy***   From 1979 through 1994, a total of 322 patients with supraglottic carcinoma received BID radiation therapy. The results are shown in Table 5-33.

Comparison of QD and BID results indicated significant improvement related to T2-3-4 ($p = 0.005$) and N0 ($p = 0.008$) and N2-3 ($p = 0.0001$)

***Planned Combined Radiation Therapy***
Up to 1994, a total of 187 patient with advanced supraglottic carcinoma were treated at the

**TABLE 5-32   5-Year Actuarial Local Control and Disease-Specific Survival of Supraglottic Carcinoma after Daily Radiation Therapy: 1970–1994**

| Stage | $n$ | LC (%) | DSS (%) |
| --- | --- | --- | --- |
| T1 | 72 | 74 | 76 |
| T2 | 85 | 61 | 70 |
| T3 | 47 | 56 | 56 |
| T4 | 40 | 29 | 21 |
| T1-4 | 244 | 58 | 60 |

**TABLE 5-33   5-Year Actuarial Local Control and Disease-Specific Survival of Supraglottic Carcinoma after Twice-Daily Radiation Therapy: 1979–1994**

| Stage | n | LC (%) | DSS (%) |
|-------|-----|--------|---------|
| T1 | 42 | 84 | 90 |
| T2 | 126 | 83 | 88 |
| T3 | 136 | 71 | 70 |
| T4 | 18 | 84 | 74 |
| T1-4 | 322 | 78 | 80 |

MGH by combined surgery and radiation therapy. The 5-year actuarial rates are compared with QD radiation therapy alone in Table 5-34.

Failures after combined therapies were mostly due to regional recurrent disease at the resection margins and stomal site, and nodal disease in the neck. Distant metastases occurred in one in five failures. These data indicated higher local control for the T3 lesions by combined surgery and radiation therapy, but the DSS rates showed no significant difference. More than half the patients treated by radiation therapy only retained their voice.

### Tracheal Stoma Recurrence: Importance of Neck and Stomal Irradiation

Tracheal stoma recurrence following laryngectomy is an ominous complication of treatment of laryngeal carcinoma. The incidence averages approximately 5%. The occurrence is often due to extensiveness of the lesion, with submucosal extension or lymphatic spread, paratracheal nodal metastases (most commonly found with advanced glottic and supraglottic tumors extending to the subglottic area), subglottic carcinoma, or extensive carcinoma of the pyriform sinus.

The most important concept for treatment of stomal recurrence is prevention. Patients with high risk for stomal recurrence would benefit from a course of postoperative radiation therapy to the neck and stoma with a dose of 55 Gy electively. For the past 25 years very few patients have developed this complication after laryngectomy at the MGH and Massachusetts Eye and Ear Infirmary (MEEI).

### REFERENCES

1. Ogura JH, Sessions DG, Spector GJ: Conservation surgery for epidermoid carcinoma of the supraglottic larynx. *Laryngoscope* 1975;85:1808.

2. McGavran MH, Bauer WC, Ogura JH: The incidence of cervical lymph node metastases from epidermoid carcinoma of the larynx and their relationship to certain characteristics of the primary tumor. A study based on the clinical and pathological findings for 96 patients treated by primary en bloc laryngectomy and radical neck dissection. *Cancer* 1961;14:55.

3. Skolnik EM, Yee KF, Friedman M, Golden TA: The posterior triangle in radical neck surgery. *Arch Otolaryngol* 1976;102:1–4.

4. Hawkins NV: The treatment of glottic carcinoma: An analysis of 800 cases. *Laryngoscope* 1975;85:1485.

**TABLE 5-34   5-Year Actuarial Local Control and Disease-Specific Survival of Supraglottic Carcinoma after Radiation Therapy and Combined RT And Surgery (SR): 1950–1994**

| Stage | Method | n | LC (%) | DSS (%) |
|-------|--------|-----|--------|---------|
| T2 | RT | 252 | 72 | 76 |
|    | SR | 47 | 79 | 77 |
|    |    | $p = 0.13$ | $p = 0.76$ | |
| T3 | RT | 230 | 60 | 60 |
|    | SR | 140 | 95 | 66 |
|    |    | $p = 0.0001$ | $p = 0.24$ | |

5. Wang CC: Treatment of glottic carcinoma by megavoltage radiation therapy and results. *Am J Roentgenol Radium Ther Nucl Med* 1974;120: 157.

6. Mendenhall WM, Parson JT, Million RR, et al: T1-2 squamous cell carcinoma of the glottic larynx treated with radiation therapy: Relationship of dose-fractionation factors to local control and complications. *Int J Radiat Oncol Biol Phys* 1988;15:1267–1273.

7. Woodhouse RJ, Quivey JM, Fu KK, et al: Treatment of carcinoma of the vocal cord: A review of 20 years experience. *Laryngoscope* 1981;91: 1155.

8. Fletcher GH, Jesse RH, Lindberg RD, et al: The place of radiotherapy in the management of the squamous cell carcinoma of the supraglottic larynx. *Am J Roentgenol* 1970;108:19.

9. Harwood AR, Beale FA, Cumming BJ, et al: T3 glottic cancer: An analysis of dose–time–volume factors. *Int J Radiat Oncol Biol Phys* 1980;6:675.

10. Wetmore S, Key M, Suen J: Laser therapy for T1 glottic carcinoma of the larynx. *Arch Otolaryngol Head Neck Surg* 1986;112:853–855.

11. Kirchner JA, Owen JR: Five hundred cancers of the larynx and pyriform sinus. Results of treatment of radiation and surgery. *Laryngoscope* 1977;87:1288.

12. Wang CC: Megavoltage radiation therapy for supraglottic carcinoma result of treatment. *Radiology* 1973;109:183–186.

13. Fu KK, Eisenberg L, Dedo HH, et al: Results of integrated managements of supraglottic carcinoma. *Cancer* 1977;40:2874–2881.

14. Reddi RP, Mercado R Jr: Low-dose preoperative radiation therapy in carcinoma of the supraglottic larynx. *Radiology* 1979;130:469.

15. Biller HF, Ogura JJ, Pratt L: Hemilaryngectomy for T2 glottic cancers. *Arch Otolaryngol* 1971; 93:128.

16. Coates HL, DeSanto LW, Devine KD, et al: Carcinoma of the supraglottic larynx. A review of 221 cases. *Arch Otolaryngol* 1976;102:686.

17. Shah JP, Tollefsen HR: Epidermoid carcinoma of the supraglottic larynx. Role of neck dissection in initial surgical treatment. *Am J Surg* 1974;128:494.

18. (a) Wang CC, Schulz MD, Miller D: Combined radiation therapy and surgery for carcinoma of the supraglottis and pyriform sinus. *Am J Surg* 1972;124:551. (b) Rothman KJ: Epidemiology of head and neck cancer. *Laryngoscope* 1978; 88:435.

19. Wang, CC, Suit HD, Blitzer PH: Twice-a-day radiation therapy for supraglottic carcinoma. *Int J Radiat Oncol Biol Phys* 1986;12:3–7.

20. Wendt CD, Peters LJ, Ang KK, et al: Hyperfractionated radiotherapy in the treatment of squamous cell carcinomas of the supraglottic larynx. *Int J Radiation Oncology Biol Phys.* 1989;17: 1057–1062.

# E. CARCINOMA OF THE NASOPHARYNX

The nasopharynx consists of the vault, the lateral walls (including the fossae of Rosenmuller and the mucosa covering the torus tubarius forming the eustachian tube orifice), and the posterior wall. The floor is the superior surface of the soft palate. Figure 5-29 shows the relative position of various structures of the nasopharynx as seen in the lateral view. Figure 5-30 demonstrates the important parts as seen by CT scans in horizontal and coronal projections. Pathologically, the nasopharyngeal carcinoma consists of various cell types, including lymphoepithelioma, transitional cell carcinoma, and undifferentiated carcinoma.[1] An asymptomatic mass in the neck, unilateral impairment of hearing or otitis media, nasal obstruction, epistaxis, and diplopia due to sixth cranial nerve involvement are the common manifestations of this disease and should arouse suspicion of nasopharyngeal carcinoma. Evaluation of the extent of the lesion should include nasopharyngoscopy by fiberoptiscope, as well as CT and MR scans for evidence of bone destruction, pterygoid space involvement, and/or intracranial tumor extension and cervical lymph node involvement.

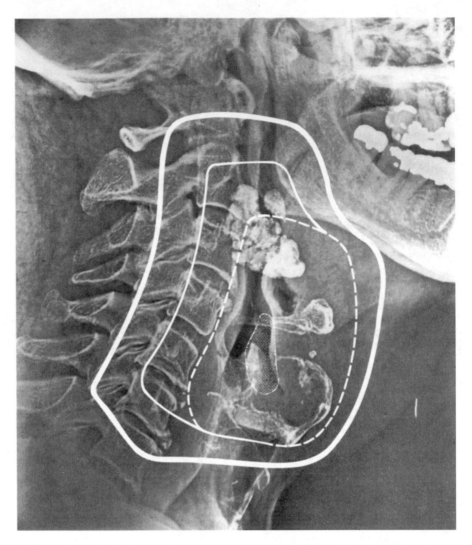

**FIGURE 5-30**   Radiograph showing portal arrangements with shrinking field technique for radiation therapy of supra-glottic carcinoma. (Calcified subdigastric node is shown.)

The latest AJCC staging of carcinoma of the nasopharynx is as follows[2]:

T1   Tumor confined to the nasopharynx
T2   Tumor extends to soft tissues of oro-pharynx and/or nasal cavity
    T2a   without parapharyngeal extension
    T2b   with parapharyngeal extension
T3   Tumor invades bony structures and/or paranasal sinuses

T4   Tumor with intracranial extension and/or involvement of cranial nerves, infra-temporal fossa, hypopharynx, or orbit
N0   No regional lymph node metastasis
N1   Unilateral metastasis in lymph node(s), 6 cm or less in greatest dimension, above the supraclavicular fossa
N2   Bilateral metastsis in lymph node(s), 6 cm or less in greatest dimension, above the supraclavicular fossa

N3 Metastasis in a lymph node(s)
- N3a greater than 6 cm in dimension
- N3b extension to the supraclavicular fossa

This staging system, published by the American Joint Committee on Cancer in 1997, is markedly different from the staging system of 1992. The discussions of treatment results in this section, follow the 1992 version.[3]

## Selection of Therapy

Owing to the rich lymphatic supply, carcinoma of the nasopharynx has a notoriously high incidence of regional cervical lymph node metastases (Figure 5-32), ranging from 60% to 80% irrespective of T stage. Therefore, in the management of carcinoma of the nasopharynx, similar to carcinomas of the oropharyrx and supraglottis, treatment must be directed to both the primary site and the neck, even in patients with N0 neck. Surgery has played an insignificant role in the treatment of the primary lesions but may be used for the management of residual metastic nodes in the neck.

## Radiotherapeutic Management

Primary lesions including those located in the base of the skull and middle ear and the upper neck, are treated in continuity first through opposed lateral portals, as shown in Figure 5-33a. When a dose of 45 Gy is reached, the primary lesion is treated separately by either rotational technique, or two anterior infraorbital oblique portals for an additional 20 Gy in 2 weeks. The neck nodes, including the subdigastric and submastoid nodes, are treated through anterior and posterior tangential portals for a total dose of approximately 60 to 65 Gy. The lower neck and supraclavicular areas

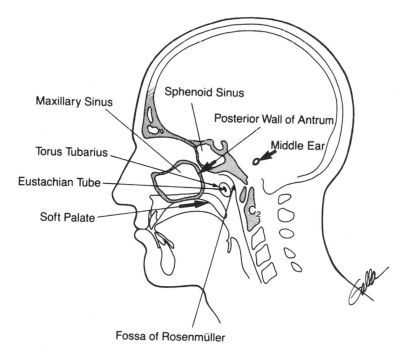

**FIGURE 5-31** Diagram showing various anatomic structures adjacent to the nasopharynx. Note position of fossa of Rosenmüller, torus tubarius, and eustachian tube.

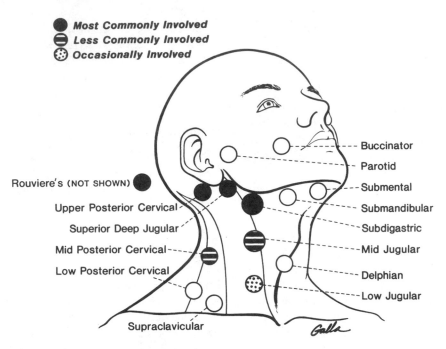

● *Most Commonly Involved*
⊜ *Less Commonly Involved*
⊛ *Occasionally Involved*

Rouviere's (NOT SHOWN)
Upper Posterior Cervical
Superior Deep Jugular
Mid Posterior Cervical
Low Posterior Cervical
Supraclavicular

Buccinator
Parotid
Submental
Submandibular
Subdigastric
Mid Jugular
Delphian
Low Jugular

**FIGURE 5-32**    Diagram showing important group of lymph nodes involved by nasopharyngeal carcinoma.

are irradiated electively for 50 Gy for occult metastases. After this procedure has been completed, the primary lesion in the nasopharynx is boosted by intracavitary implant for an additional 7 Gy. This program is suitable for most early superficial lesions, that is, T1 and T2.

For lesions invading the base of the skull or extending into the intracranial cavity, intracavitary implant is not advisable; the only effective treatment is external beam radiation therapy delivering a total dose to the nasopharynx of up to 70 to 75 Gy in 8 weeks. The dose to the temporal lobe, spinal cord, and temporomandibular joint is limited to 50 to 55 Gy in 5 weeks. Since lymphoepithelioma or transitional cell carcinoma represents a variant of undifferentiated carcinoma, there is no allowance for adjustment of tumor dose among various cell types of carcinoma, although their radiation response may vary. Most of the nasopharyngeal carcinoma patients are currently treated with the twice-daily program at the MGH.[4]

Carcinoma of the nasopharynx has a propensity for local recurrence at the primary site 5 or more years after initial radiation therapy.[5] Retreatment for recurrence at the primary site by a second course of radiation therapy is feasible with meticulous technique. Radiation therapy for most of the recurrent lesions if small T1 or early T2, relies greatly on the use of intracavitary implants in combination with external beam therapy.[6] In general, approximately 40 Gy in 5 weeks is given through relatively small portals followed by one or two intracavitary implants to deliver an additional 20 Gy. Recurrent disease in the neck following radiation therapy should be dealt with by neck dissection, if operable.

## Radiotherapeutic Results

For the T1 and T2 lesions, the local control rates ranged from 70% to 90%; for the T3 and T4 tumors the rates were 50% to 65% and 30% to 40% respectively.[7,8] The survival rates ranged from 40% to 60%, and the disease-free rate was approximately 55%.[6,8,9,10] The local control rates of metastatic nodes in the neck by radiation therapy were remarkably satisfactory. For the N0-1 nodes, the local control rates were over 90%. For the N2 neck the rates ranged from 80% to 90%, and for N3 disease, about 50%.

Although the local control rates in the neck were high, the presence of extensive disease in the neck affected the patients' survival. For the N0-1 disease, the 5-year survival rates ranged 60% to 75%, and for the patients with N2-3 nodes, the survival rates dropped to 40% to 50%.[11–13]

The results of reirradiation for recurrent nasopharyngeal carcinoma varied, and generally were not entirely satisfactory. For T1 and T2 locally recurrent carcinoma, the 5-year local control and survival rates ranged from 30% to 50%;[4,14,15] For extensive recurrence with invasion of the base of the skull and cranial nerve

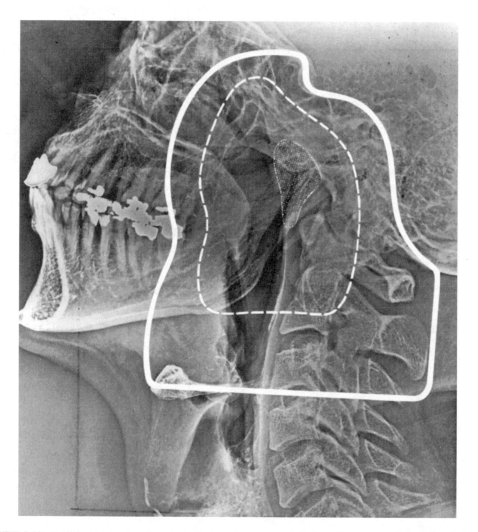

**FIGURE 5-33** Radiograph showing placement of comprehensive portal for the primary site and bilateral neck for treatment of carcinoma of the nasopharynx. Dashed-line circle identifies "off cord" portal for boosting dose to the primary site.

deficits, the rates were approximately 20% to 25%. Far advanced recurrences after high dose radiation therapy were rarely salvageable by reirradiation.

## MGH Experience

From 1970 through 1994, 261 patients with squamous cell carcinoma of the nasopharynx received radical radiation therapy. Of this group, 125 received daily and 134 twice-daily radiation therapy; 171 were male, 88 were female, for a M:F ratio of 2:1. The 5-year actuarial rates are shown in Tables 5-35 to 5-38.

Carcinoma of the nasopharynx tends to develop distant metastasis.[16,17] Its incidence is related to the extent of the primary lesion and the status of the neck nodes, with increasing T and N status, as shown in Table 5-39.

**TABLE 5-35  5-Year Actuarial Rates of Local Control and Disease-Specific Survival of Nasopharyngeal Carcinoma after Radiation Therapy: 1970–1994**

| Stage | n | LC (%) | DSS (%) |
|---|---|---|---|
| T1-2 | 148 | 72 | 65 |
| T3 | 46 | 66 | 58 |
| T4 | 65 | 49 | 42 |
| T3-4 | 111 | 56 | 50 |
| | | $p = 0.006$ | $p = 0.02$ |
| T1-4 | 261 | 65 | 59 |
| N0 | 92 | 62 | 63 |
| N1 | 24 | 63 | 63 |
| N2-3 | 144 | 67 | 56 |
| | | $p = 0.58$ | $p = 0.20$ |

**TABLE 5-36  5-Year Actuarial Rates after Daily Radiation Therapy for Nasopharyngeal Carcinoma: 1970–1994**

| Stage | n | LC (%) | DSS (%) |
|---|---|---|---|
| T1-2 | 71 | 71 | 60 |
| T3-4 | 54 | 47 | 35 |
| T1-4 | 125 | 60 | 49 |
| N0-1 | 58 | 57 | 52 |
| N2-3 | 67 | 64 | 47 |

**TABLE 5-37  5-Year Actuarial Rates after Twice-Daily Radiation Therapy for Nasopharyngeal Carcinoma: 1979–1994**

| Stage | n | LC (%) | DSS (%) |
|---|---|---|---|
| T1-2 | 78 | 72 | 70 |
| T3-4 | 57 | 65 | 70 |
| T1-4 | 134 | 69 | 69 |
| N0-1 | 57 | 68 | 76 |
| N2-3 | 77 | 68 | 63 |

**TABLE 5-38  Comparison of Daily and Twice Daily Radiation Therapy of the Primary Lesion and Nodal Status**

| Stage | $\mathcal{P}$ | |
|---|---|---|
| | LC (%) | DSS (%) |
| T1-2 | NS | 0.09 |
| T3-4 | 0.0009 | 0.0002 |
| T1-4 | 0.008 | 0.0001 |
| N0-1 | NS | 0.01 |
| N2-3 | 0.04 | 0.003 |

**TABLE 5-39  Incidence of Distant Metastases Related to Primary Lesions and Nodal Status: 1970–1994**

| Stage | Patients with DM | |
|---|---|---|
| | Number | Percent |
| T1 | 46 | 6 | 13 |
| T2 | 102 | 20 | 19.6 |
| T3 | 46 | 9 | 19.5 |
| T4 | 65 | 15 | 23 |
| T1-4 | 259 | 50 | 19.3 |
| N0 | 92 | 16 | 17.3 |
| N1 | 23 | 0 | 0 |
| N2 | 128 | 29 | 22.6 |
| N3 | 16 | 5 | 31 |
| N0-3 | 259 | 50 | 19.3 |

## DISCUSSION AND SUMMARY

Carcinoma of the nasopharynx is uncommon in the United States. Its management is primarily with high dose radiation therapy. Because of the adjacent vital structures, such as the pituitary gland, brain stem, temporal lobes, eyes, optic nerves, and temporomandibular joint, radiation therapy calls for careful treatment planning with multiportal techniques through the use of high energy radiation and/or intracavitary implant.

All cervical lymph nodes, including the Rouviere node, should be irradiated electively, even in patients without palpable nodes. Although neck failure alone is uncommon, occasionally residual node disease after radiation therapy can be treated with neck dissection if the primary lesion is controlled.

Recurrent carcinoma of the nasopharynx is one of the few malignant lesions in the head and neck in which reirradiation can be carried out, with careful technique, with occasional success. Reirradiation dosage must be radical if lasting control is the aim; low dose retreatment generally is ineffective.

Of the entire group of patients treated primarily with radiation therapy de novo, none developed serious radiation therapy complications. With careful treatment techniques and moderation of doses, the incidence of transverse myelitis, brain necrosis, or pituitary dysfunction can be reduced to minimum. Minor sequelae of radiation therapy, such as xerostomia and dental caries, were common but generally well tolerated by most patients.

# REFERENCES

1. Shanmugaratnam K: Histopathology of nasopharyngeal carcinoma. Correlations with epidemiology, survival rates and other biological characteristics. *Cancer* 1979;44(3):1029–1044. (b) Reference to histopathology and the possibility of earlier recognition. *Acta Psychiatr Scand (suppl)* 1944;34:1–323.

2. American Joint Committee on Cancer: *Manual for Staging of Cancer*, 5th ed. Philadelphia, Lippincott, 1997.

3. American Joint Committee on Cancer: *Manual for Staging of Cancer*, 4th ed. Philadelphia, Lippincott, 1992.

4. Wang CC: Accelerated hyperfractionation radiation therapy for carcinoma of the nasopharynx. Technique and results. *Cancer* 1989;63:2461–2467.

5. Wang CC: Re-irradiation of recurrent nasopharyngeal carcinoma—Treatment techniques and results. *Int J Radiat Oncol Biol Phys* 1987; 13(7):953–956.

6. Wang CC: Improved local control of nasopharyngeal carcinoma after intracavitary brachytherapy boost. *Am J Clin Oncol* 1991;14(1):5–8.

7. Bedwinek JM, Perez CA, Keys DJ: Analysis of failures after definitive irradiation for epidermoid carcinoma of the nasopharynx. *Cancer* 1980;45:2725–2829.

8. Mesic JB, Fletcher GH, Goepfert H: Megavoltage irradiation of epithelial tumors of the nasopharynx. *Int J Radiat Oncol Biol Phys* 1981; 7(4):447–453.

9. Moench HC, Phillips TL: Carcinoma of the nasopharynx: Review of 146 patients with emphasis on radiation dose and time factors. *Am J Surg* 1972;124:515–518.

10. Bailet JW, Mark RJ, Abemayor E, et al: Nasopharyngeal carcinoma: Treatment results with primary radiation therapy. *Laryngoscope* 1992; 102(9):965–972.

11. Neel HBI: Nasopharyngeal carcinoma: Diagnosis, staging, and management. *Oncology* 1992;6(2):87–95.

12. Frezza G, Barbieri E, Emiliani E, Silvano M, Babini L: Patterns of failure in nasopharyngeal cancer treated with megavoltage irradiation. *Radiother Oncol* 1986;5:287–294.

13. Fandi A, Altun M, Azli N, Armand JP, Cvitkovic E: Nasopharyngeal cancer: Epidemiology, staging, and treatment. *Semin Oncol* 1994;21: 382–397.

14. Fu KK, Newman H, Phillips TL: Treatment of locally recurrent carcinoma of the nasopharynx. *Radiology* 1975;117(2):425–431.

15. Pryzant RM, Wendt CD, Delclos L, Peters LJ: Re-treatment of nasopharyngeal carcinoma in 53 patients. *Int J Radiat Oncol Biol Phys* 1992; 22(5):941–947.

16. Ahmad A, Stefani S: Distant metastases of nasopharyngeal carcinoma: A study of 256 male patients. *J Surg Oncol* 1986;33(3):194–197.

17. Al-Sarraf M, Pajak TF, Cooper JS, Mohiuddin M, Herskovic A, Ager PJ: Chemo-radiotherapy in patients with locally advanced nasopharyngeal carcinoma: A radiation therapy oncology group study. *J Clin Oncol* 1990;8(8):1342–1351.

# F. THE NASO-SINUSES CARCINOMAS

## PARANASAL SINUS

Carcinoma arising from the paranasal sinuses generally is a silent tumor. The maxillary and ethmoid sinuses are commonly involved. Tumor arising from the sphenoid or frontal sinuses alone is rare. Figure 5-34 shows the paranasal sinuses, the nasal cavity, and the vestibule.

The 1997 AJCC staging of squamous cell carcinoma of the maxillary and ethmoid sinuses is as follows:

### For Maxillary Sinus

T1  Tumor limited to the antral mucosa with no bone erosion or destruction

T2  Tumor causing bone erosion or destruction, except for the posterior antral wall, including extension into the hard palate and/or the middle nasal meatus

T3  Tumor invades any of the following: bone of the posterior wall of maxillary sinus, subcutanous tissues, skin of cheek, floor or medial wall of orbit, infratemporal fossa, pterygoid plate, ethmoid sinus

T4  Tumor invades orbital contents beyond the floor or medial wall including any of the following: orbit apex, cribriform plate, base of skull, nasopharynx, sphenoid, frontal sinuses

### For Ethmoid Sinus

T1  Tumor confined to the ethmoid with or without bone erosion

T2  Tumor extends into the nasal cavity

T3  Tumor extends to the anterior orbit and/or maxillary sinus

T4  Tumor with intracranial extension, orbital extension including apex, involving sphenoid, and/or frontal sinus and/or skin of external nose

*Note*: Nonepithelial tumors such as those of lymphoid tissue, soft tissue, bone, and cartilage are not included.

Squamous cell carcinoma of varying degree of aggressiveness is the predominant cell type, constituting over 80% of the group. The overall incidence of nodal metastases is low, even in the late stage of the disease. The first echelon of lymphatic drainage of paranasal sinuses is the deep superior jugular and subdigastric nodes as well as the retropharyngeal nodes (Rouviere nodes). Other cell types include adenocarcinoma or adenoid cystic carcinoma, malignant lymphoma, melanoma, and malignant mesenchymal tumors. Inverted papilloma is a histologically benign but biologically aggressive tumor. In approximately 10% to 15% of patients, the tumor is associated with invasive squamous cell carcinoma or adenocarcinoma, concurrently or sequentially during the course of the disease.

## Selection of Therapy

Treatment of this group of lesions is combination of surgery and radiation therapy. Since the incidence of lymph node metastases is quite low in carcinomas, being approximately 20% of all cases, routine radical neck dissection or elective neck irradiation is not recommended in patients without nodes. For most operable cases, radical surgery is performed first. Radiation therapy is used as an adjuvent procedure, given postoperatively with boost technique to the tumor-involved site or to any area of residual disease. For inverted papilloma, wide local resection is the treatment of choice. If the resection margins are free from disease, no adjuvant therapy is considered. On the other hand, local recurrences after previous multiple resections call for high dose radiation therapy because of their malignant potential. Therefore the lesions are managed in a fashion similar to invasive carcinomas.

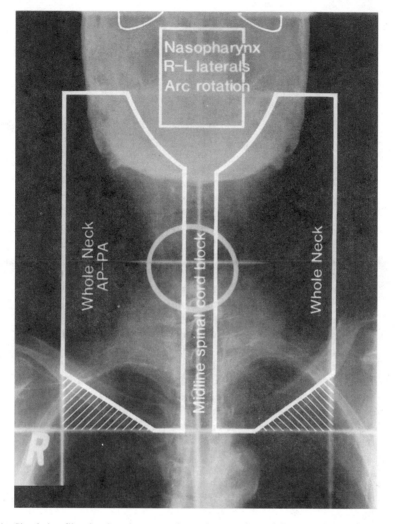

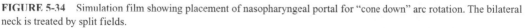

**FIGURE 5-34** Simulation film showing placement of nasopharyngeal portal for "cone down" arc rotation. The bilateral neck is treated by split fields.

## Radiotherapeutic Management

For the advanced lesions, often with extensive bone involvement, the treatment of choice is combined surgery and postoperative radiation therapy, which is given to the hemiparanasal sinuses with 55 Gy in 6 weeks. If neck disease is present, radical neck dissection and ipsilateral neck radiation therapy is given as an adjuvant procedure.

For the inoperable lesions, a dose of 60 Gy in 6 weeks is given, as either a preoperative or a palliative procedure. Generally a three-field technique is used to deliver a relatively uniform dose to the maxillary sinus, nasal cavity, and ethmoid and sphenoid sinuses, as shown in Figure 5-35. Figure 5-36 shows the isodose distribution to the hemiparanasal sinuses with the three-field technique megavoltage radiations.

## Radiotherapeutic Results

Owing to the locally advanced stages of carcinoma of the paranasal sinuses, the therapeutic

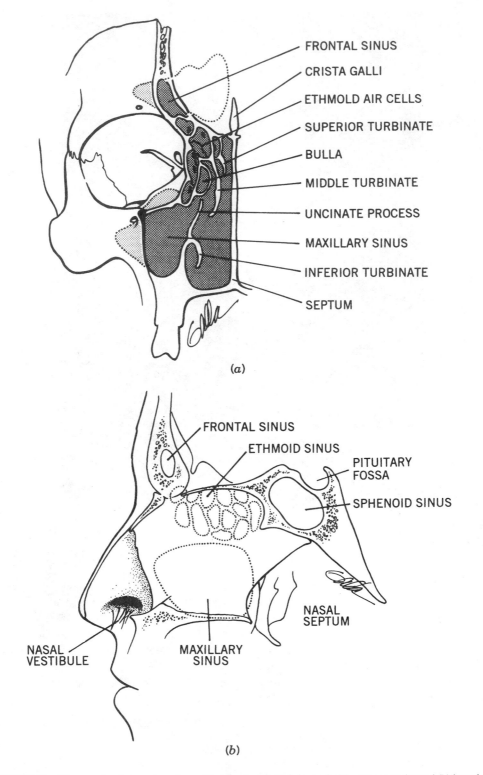

FRONTAL SINUS

CRISTA GALLI

ETHMOLD AIR CELLS

SUPERIOR TURBINATE

BULLA

MIDDLE TURBINATE

UNCINATE PROCESS

MAXILLARY SINUS

INFERIOR TURBINATE

SEPTUM

(a)

FRONTAL SINUS

ETHMOID SINUS

PITUITARY FOSSA

SPHENOID SINUS

NASAL SEPTUM

NASAL VESTIBULE

MAXILLARY SINUS

(b)

**FIGURE 5-35**   Diagram showing nasal cavity, vestibule, and paranasal sinuses in (**a**) anteroposterior and (**b**) lateral view.

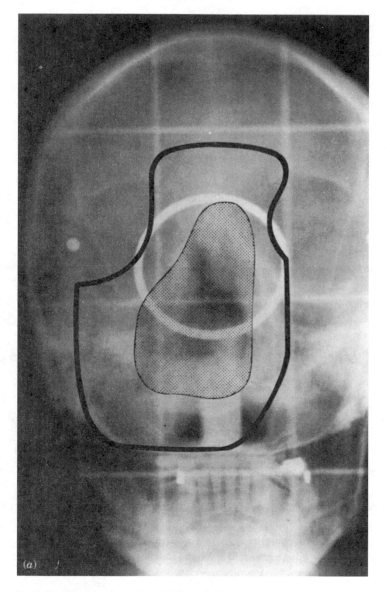

**FIGURE 5-36a**    Simulation films showing a three-field portal arrangement (**a**) anteroposterior and (**b**) opposing lateral wedge portals for treatment of carcinoma of the paranasal sinus. The bulk of the treatment is given through the anterior portal and the laterals are used to boost the posterior volume. (Keep in mind the postoperative cavity effect in determining dosage, and be careful to shield the optic nerve.)

results following either radiation therapy alone or combined surgery and radiation therapy are not outstanding. In series of unselected cases, the combined therapies yielded survival rates of about 25% and in operable cases the rate is nearly 45% to 50%.[1-4] Generally, carcinomas of the antrum arising from the infrastructures have somewhat higher survivorship than suprastructure lesions. In carcinoma of the ethmoid sinuses, the survival data following various forms of therapy are scarce and vary considerably. The crude overall survival is about 20% to 25%. Because of the rarity of the disease, no meaningful data are available for

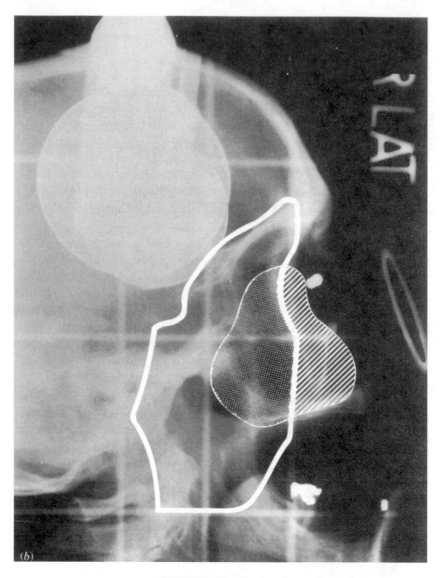

**FIGURE 5-36b** *Continued*

carcinoma of the sphenoid or frontal sinuses. Radical neck dissection is indicated only when metastatic nodes in the neck are present or apparent, although the survival of the patients with cervical metastatic disease is poor owing to propensity for distant metastases.

## MGH Experience

From 1970 to 1994, a total of 74 patients with squamous cell carcinoma of the paranasal si-

nuses received radiation therapy. Of these, 66 patients had lesions arising from the maxillary and/or ethmoid sinuses, 8 from the sphenoid and/or frontal sinus.

Of 66 patients with carcinoma of the maxillary/ethmoid sinus, 27, or 40%, were treated by definitive irradiation; 39, or 60%, received combined surgery and radiation therapy. Most of these patients had advanced disease (T3-4) or inoperable lesions. The treatment results after radiation therapy are shown in Tables 5-40 and 5-41.

**TABLE 5-40   5-Year Actuarial Local Control and Disease-Specific Survival after Radiation Therapy Only (RT) and Combined Surgery and Radiation Therapy (SR)**

| Treatment Method | n | LC (%)* | DSS (%)** |
|---|---|---|---|
| RT | 27 | 49 | 42 |
| SR | 39 | 57 | 67 |

*p = 0.5

**p = 0.05.

**TABLE 5-41   5-Year Actuarial Rates after Bid and QD Radiation Therapy for Squamous Carcinoma of the Paranasal Sinuses: 1970–1994**

| Treatment Program | n | LC (%)* | DSS (%)** |
|---|---|---|---|
| BID | 42 | 52 | 69 |
| QD | 32 | 67 | 54 |

*p = 0.3.

**p = 0.2.

## THE NASAL CAVITY

Carcinomas arising from the nasal cavity are identifiable with their origin in the nasal septum, turbinate, or roof of the nasal cavity. Squamous cell carcinomas arising from the high nasal septum generally are more aggressive than those of the nasal vestibule, and the lesions arising from the posterior nasal cavity have a pattern of lymphatic spread similar to that of the antro–ethmoid complex. Occasionally, spread is to the retropharyngeal, deep superior jugular, and subdigastric nodes (Figure 5-37). Other tumors include salivary gland malignancies, inverted papillomas, plasmacytomas, melanomas, lymphomas, olfactory neuroblastomas, and, rarely, basal cell carcinomas.

### Selection of Therapy

Treatment of malignant epithelial lesions including the esthesioneuriblastomas arising from the roof of the nasal cavity, turbinates, and high nasal septum, is planned combined surgery through lateral rhinotomy and postoperative radiation therapy. For the inoperable lesions, external beam radiation therapy is given first, followed by resection if made operable by radiation therapy. For the radioresponsive tumors, such as the lymphomas and plasmacytomas, primary radiation therapy is the treatment of choice, with good local control with or without chemotherapy, although the radiotherapeutic failures are frequently due to distant metastases.

## Radiotherapeutic Results

Since squamous cell carcinomas of the nasal septum and turbinates are uncommon malignancies, reports of results of radiotherapy are scarce. Most reports[5–7] indicate local control rates ranging from 40% to 60%. Bosch and associates[8] showed 49% 5-year control rates in a group of 40 patients treated by radiation therapy alone.

### MGH Experience

Results of radiation therapy for carcinomas of the nasal cavity are sparse. From 1960 to 1985, a total of 19 patients with "localized" squamous cell carcinoma arising from the nasal septum and/or turbinates received radiation therapy or combined radiotherapy and surgery. Of 10 patients who were treated by radiation therapy alone after biopsy of the lesion or for recurrences, 5, or 50%, were NED. Nine patients were treated by combined surgery and radiation therapy, and of these, seven, or 78%, were NED at 3 years. All treatment failures were due to uncontrolled primary lesions with or without disease in the neck. Three patients with adenoid cystic carcinoma were treated, and all were NED after combined surgery and postoperative radiotherapy. One patient with malignant melanoma was managed by combined approach and was NED at 5 years (Figure 5-38).

Of a total 18 patients with estheioneuroblastoma, the 5-year LC and DSS were 56% and 68%, respectively.

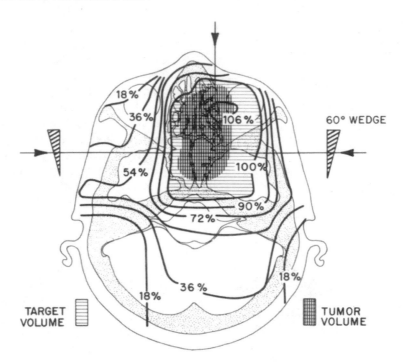

**FIGURE 5-37**   Diagram showing distribution in the target volume using a three-field technique. Loading: ANT:R:L = 7:2:1

## THE NASAL VESTIBULE

Malignant tumors arising from the nasal vestibule, often referred to as "nose picker's cancer," are quite uncommon. Squamous cell carcinoma is the most common cell type. The lymphatic drainage of the nasal vestibule is predominantly to the submandibular, subdigastric, and occasionally to the submental, buccinator, and preauricular nodes (Figure 5-39). Bilateral involvement is not unusual.

### Classification

There is no official staging system for carcinoma of the nasal vestibule. For the purpose of review of the radiation therapy results, the following staging has been proposed:[9]

T1   Lesion is limited to the nasal vestibule, and is relatively superficial, involving one or more sites within the vestibule

T2   The lesion extends from the nasal vestibule to its adjacent structures such as the upper nasal septum, upper lip, philtrum, and skin of the nose and/or nasolabial fold, but is not fixed to the underlying bone

T3   The lesion becomes massive with extension to the hard palate, buccogingival sulcus, large portion of the upper lip, upper nasal septum, and turbinate and/or adjacent paranasal sinuses, and is fixed with deep muscle and bone involvement

### Selection of Therapy

The small (T1) squamous cell carcinomas can be treated either by surgery or by radiation therapy alone with a satisfactory cure rate.[10,11] The choice of treatment modality for such lesions depends on the cosmetic result following the procedure. If significant defor-

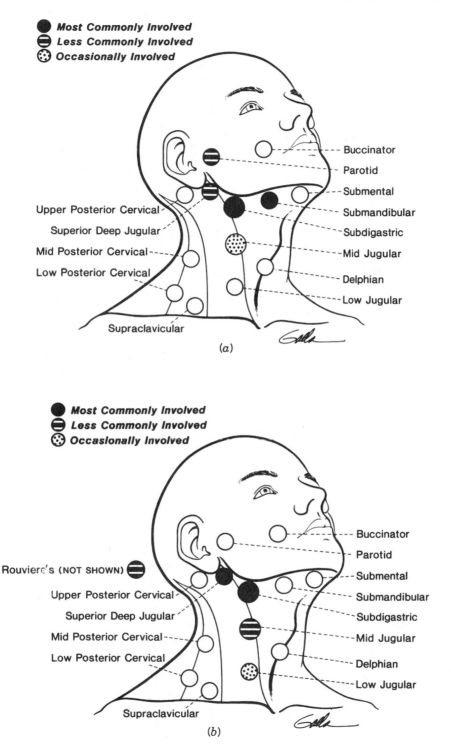

**FIGURE 5-38**   Diagram showing involvement of lymph nodes by squamous cell carcinoma of (**a**) anterior and (**b**) posterior nasal cavities.

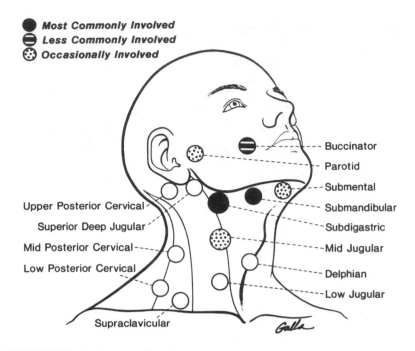

**FIGURE 5-39**   Involvement of lymph nodes in squamous cell carcinoma of the nasal vestibule.

mity or mutilation results following surgery, radiation therapy should be the treatment of choice. For the extensive (T3) lesions with bone involvement, radical surgery with postoperative radiation therapy is preferred. Because of the relatively low incidence of occult metastasis (<10%) for T1 N0 and T2 N0 lesions, elective neck dissection or irradiation is not warranted.

## Radiotherapeutic Management

Because most of the lesions are relatively superficially situated, low energy photons or

electron beam irradiation is employed with a dose of approximately 30 Gy in 2 weeks followed by interstitial implants delivering a dose of approximately 30 Gy. Most of the extensive lesions (T3) are treated by external beam therapy alone employing anterior oblique wedge pair technique with a total dose of approximately 65 Gy in 5 to 6 weeks.

## Radiotherapeutic Results

The radiation therapy results for early lesions generally are extremely satisfactory with local control rates ranging from 80% to 90%.[9–11] For advanced disease often associated with lymph node metastases the local control rate is approximately 40%.[5]

## MGH Experience

From 1960 to 1995, a total of 54 patients with squamous cell carcinoma of the nasal vestibule were treated by radiation therapy alone. The treatment results are shown in Table 5-42.

**TABLE 5-42   5-Year Actuarial Local Control and Disease-Specific Survival after Radiation Therapy for Carcinoma of the Nasal Vestibule: 1960–1994**

| Stage | n | LC (%) | DSS (%) |
| --- | --- | --- | --- |
| T1 | 34 | 81 | 93 |
| T2 | 16 | 79 | 92 |
| T3 | 4 | 53 | 40 |

## DISCUSSION AND SUMMARY

1. Carcinomas of the naso-paranasal sinus are relatively uncommon lesions of the head and neck. The tumors tend to involve the antro–ethmoid complex and to spread locally to the adjacent sinuses, orbit or the neighboring soft tissues. Except for the rare mucosal tumors, the treatment of choice is the combination of surgery and radiation therapy.

2. Squamous cell carcinoma arising from the nasal vestibule is relatively rare and is often referred to as "nose picker's cancer." The small lesions (T1 and T2) are highly curable by radiation therapy alone with good functional and cosmetic results. The advanced lesions (T3) with bone destruction and/or metastases are best treated by combined therapies, that is, radical surgery in the form of nosectomy and/or palatectomy and postoperative irradiation, if the lesions are resectable. For the inoperable tumors, high dose irradiation may offer palliation and occasionally an unexpected cure.

## REFERENCES

1. Hamberger CA, Martensson G: Carcinoma of the paranasal sinuses, combined approach. *Front Radiat Ther Oncol* 1970;5:130–146. (b) Ash JE, Beck MR, Wilkes IJD: Tumors of the upper respiratory tract and ear, in *Atlas of Tumor Pathology*, Sect IV, Fasc 12 and 13. Washington, DC, Armed Forces Institute of Pathology, 1964, p 79.

2. Jesse RH: Pre-operative versus post-operative radiation in the treatment of squamous carcinoma of the paranasal sinuses. *Am J Surg* 1965;110:552–556.

3. Cheng VST, Wang CC: Carcinomas of the paranasal sinuses. A study of sixty-six cases. *Cancer* 1977;40:3038–3041.

4. Pezner RD, Moss WT, Tong D, et al: Cervical lymph node metastases in patients with squamous cell carcinoma of the maxillary antrum. *Int J Radiat Oncol Biol Phys* 1979;55:1977.

5. Yarington CT, Jaquiss GW, Sprinkle PM: Carcinoma of the nose and nasal septum: Treatment and reconstruction. *Trans Am Acad Ophthalmol Otolaryngol* 1969;73:1178–1183.

6. Young JR: Malignant tumors of nasal septum. *J Laryngol Otol* 1979;93:817–832.

7. Lewis JS, Castro EB: Cancer of the nasal cavity and paranasal sinuses. *J Laryngol Otol* 1972;86:255–262.

8. Bosch V, Vallecillo L, Frias Z: Cancer of the nasal cavity. *Cancer* 1976;37:1458.

9. Wang CC: Treatment of carcinoma of the nasal vestibule by irradiation. *Cancer* 1976;3X:100–106.

10. Goepfert H, Guillamondegui OM, Jesse RH, et al: Squamous cell carcinomas of the nasal vestibule. *Arch Otolaryngol* 1974;100:8–10.

11. Haynes WD, Tapley NV: Radiation treatment of carcinoma of the nasal vestibule. *Am J Roentgenol* 1974;120:595–602.

# G. THE SALIVARY GLANDS

Malignant tumors of the salivary glands comprise mucoepidermoid carcinoma, adenoid cystic carcinoma, malignant pleomorphic adenoma, undifferentiated carcinoma, squamous cell carcinoma, adenocarcinoma, and others including lymphoma, melanoma, and some soft tissue sarcomas. Most of the tumors occur in the parotid gland submandibular and sublingual glands, and minor salivary glands, in decreasing order of frequency. Figure 5-40 shows the location of parotoid gland related to the mandible and base of skull the minor salivary glands are least commonly affected. The growth usually manifests as a painless swelling or a nodule. In the advanced stage, these lesions may rapidly increase in size and become associated with pain or ulceration in the parotid region, as well as facial nerve paralysis. These tumors are marked by their unpredictable clinical course and are characterized by chronicity and a tendency to multiple recurrences.

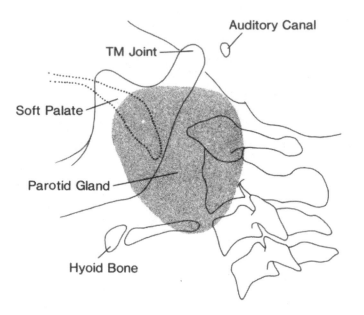

**FIGURE 5-40**    Diagram showing anatomic position of a normal parotid gland from a sialogram related to the bony landmarks of the mandible and skull base. The contralateral normal parotid gland should be spared if possible during irradiation.

The spread of most malignant salivary gland tumors is by local infiltration, perineural extension, and by hematogenous and, less commonly, lymphatic routes. The incidence of regional lymph node metastases depends on the cell type of the tumors and their stage at presentation. Pulmonary metastases are common in patients with adenoid cystic carcinoma and sometimes late in the course of the disease. Patients may survive for an extended period of time, relatively symptom free.

The staging for salivary gland cancer is as follows:

T1    Tumor 2 cm or less in greatest dimension without extraparenchymal extension
T2    Tumor more than 2 cm but not more than 4 cm in greatest dimension without extraparenchymal extension
T3    Tumor having extraparenchymal extension without seventh nerve involvement and/or more than 4 cm but not more than 6 cm in greatest dimension without significant local extension

T4    umor invades base of skull, invades seventh nerve, and/or exceeds 6 cm in greatest dimension

The first therapeutic approach is surgical removal, if the lesions are operable. Postoperative radiation therapy is often given as a curative, adjuvant, or palliative procedure and is indicated in the following condition.[1–5]

1. Incomplete surgical removal with known residual disease and/or difficulty with clearance of resection margins
2. Tumor extension beyond the capsule found during histologic examination
3. Adenoid cystic carcinoma with extensive perineural involvement
4. High grade malignant tumors and/or lymph node metastases
5. Facial nerve sparing procedure with close tumor margins
6. Most patients with large tumors requiring radical resection (of facial nerve, mandible, temporal bone, etc.)

7. Parotid tumors of deep lobe origin with inadequate resection margins
8. Tumors with one or more local recurrences after previous surgical procedures
9. Inoperable lesions
10. Patients who refuse surgery

## Radiotherapeutic Management

The incidence of nodal metastases in patients with low grade localized lesions is low; the management of these lesions generally does not include treatment of cervical disease. Generally, a dose of 65 to 70 Gy in 7 weeks is given for lesions with known residual disease or inoperable lesions. For microscopic disease, a dose of 55 to 60 Gy in 6 weeks is given. For parotid tumors, radiation therapy is often deliver by a combination of external beam photon therapy with wedge pair technique for about 45 Gy with electron beam boost for an additional 10 to 15 Gy (Figure 5-41).

For the undifferentiated carcinoma of the salivary glands, elective neck irradiation may

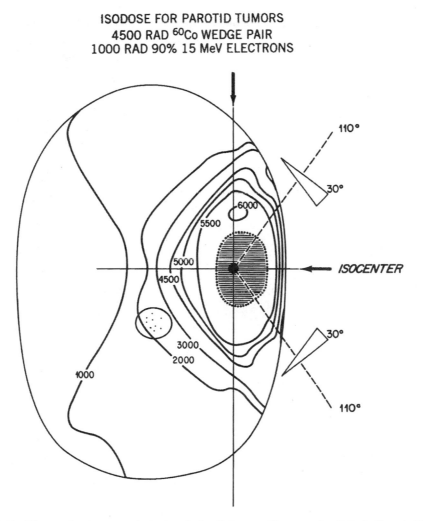

ISODOSE FOR PAROTID TUMORS
4500 RAD $^{60}$Co WEDGE PAIR
1000 RAD 90% 15 MeV ELECTRONS

**FIGURE 5-41**  Diagram showing composite isodose for irradiating parotid tumor, using 45 Gy ipsilateral oblique wedge pair and 10 Gy appositional 15 MeV electron beam boost (90% isodose line).

be carried out with a dose of 50 Gy in 5 weeks, but its value is uncertain. Although radical neck dissection is not indicated in patients with N0 neck, it is often employed for palpable metastatic disease in the neck, followed by postoperative radiation therapy.

In the large inoperable parotid tumors for which ipsilateral oblique wedge pair technique may not be feasible, radiation therapy may be given through large AP and PA portals sparing the eye for the initial 40 Gy, followed by electron beam therapy to bring the total dose up to 65 Gy in 6 weeks.

For the past decade, neutron therapy has been used for extensive and /or inoperable salivary gland malignancies. The local control appeared to be improved with somewhat higher radiation complications.

The management of the minor salivary gland lesions varies according to the location and the stage of the disease as the head and neck lesions in general.[6,7]

### Radiotherapeutic Results

The results after surgery are quite satisfactory with 5-year survival rates of 85%, 67%, and 10% for T1, T2, and T3 lesions, respectively. The prognosis of malignant salivary gland tumors is closely related to tumor size, cell type and grade, site of origin, status of nodal disease, and resectability. In general, acinic cell tumors, low grade mucoepidermoid carcinoma, and pleomorphic adenoma have favorable biologic behavior. On the other hand, adenocarcinoma, adenoid cystic carcinoma, high grade mucoepidermoid carcinoma, poorly differentiated carcinoma, and squamous cell carcinoma are generally aggressive with poor prognosis. If the lesion is totally resected, the patient's survival prospects are reasonably good. The patients with tumors in the parotid gland have a better outlook than those with tumors in the submaxillary or sublingual glands.

Information regarding the results of radiation therapy for minor salivary gland malignancies in the oral cavity and oropharynx is sparse. Approximately two thirds of patients were alive and well at 3 years. The patients with adenocarcinoma and adenoid cystic carcinoma had somewhat higher survival.[8]

### MGH Experience

Our experience in treatment of major salivary glands is shown in Table 5-43.

***BID Radiation Therapy***  For the past 15 years, accelerated hyperfractionated radiation therapy with two daily fractions of 1.6 Gy each has been used at the MGH for treatment of inoperable or advanced salivary gland malignant tumors and the short-term local control has been quite satisfactory. The results indicated good local control of some of the unresectable carcinomas.[9,10]

**TABLE 5.43  Actuarial Rates of Parotid Carcinoma after Combined Surgery and Radiation Therapy: 1975–1994**

| Actuarial Rates | T1-2 ($n = 64$) | T3-4 ($n = 37$) |
|---|---|---|
| Local control | | |
| 5 years | 92 | 90 |
| 10 years | 87 | 90 |
| Disease-specific survival** | | |
| 5 years | 89 | 82 |
| 10 years | 68 | 60 |

*$p$ NS.
**$p = 0.007$.

## DISCUSSION AND SUMMARY

Malignant tumors arising from the salivary glands are uncommon lesions. These tumors have varied biologic courses and clinical unpredictability. Their primary treatment is surgical resection with or without radiation therapy. Radiation therapy is used as adjuvant, either before or after surgery, or sandwich for unresectable tumors. The radiation techniques should be individualized according to the size and site of the lesions. For small lesion, arising from the oral cavity, local control can be achieved by combined external radiation and interstitial implant with good functional and cosmetic results. Recurrent pleomorphic adenomas are treated by debulking surgery and postoperative radiation. These tumors tend to late recurrences. Therefore long-term follow-up is required.

## REFERENCES

1. Johns ME, Kaplan MJ: Surgical therapy of tumors of the salivary gland. In S Thawley, W Panje, JG Batsakis, and R Lindberg (eds.), *Comprehensive Management of Head and Neck Tumors*, 1987, p 1122.

2. Fu KK, Leibel SA, Levine ML, et al: Carcinoma of the major and minor salivary glands. *Cancer* 1977;40:2882–2890.

3. Shidnia H, Hornbsek NB, Hamaker R, et al: Carcinoma of the major salivary glands. *Cancer* 1980;45:693–697.

4. McNaney D, McNeese MD, Guillamondegui OM, et al: Postoperative irradiation in malignant epithelial tumors of the parotid. *Int J Radiat Oncol Biol Phys* 1983;9:1289–1295.

5. Borthne A, Kjellevold K, Kaalhus O, et al: Salivary gland malignant neoplasms: Treatment and prognosis. *Int J Radiat Oncol Biol Phys* 1986;12:747–754.

6. Griffin TW, Pajak, Laramore LE, et al: Neutron versus photon irradiation of inoperable salivary gland tumors: Results of an RTOG-MRC cooperative randomized study. *Int J Radiat Oncol Biol Phys* 1988;15:1085–1090.

7. Duncan W, Orr JA, Amott SJ, et al: Neutron therapy for malignant tumors of the salivary gland. *Radiother Oncol* 1987;8:97–104.

8. Gates GA: Current concepts in otolaryngology: Malignant neoplasms of the minor salivary glands. *New Engl J Med* 1982;306:718–722.

9. Spiro IJ, Wang CC, Montgomery WW: Carcinoma of the parotid gland. *Cancer* 1993;71:2699–2705.

10. Wang CC, Goodman M: Photon irradiation of unresectable carcinomas of salivary glands. *Int J Radiat Oncol Biol Phys* 1991;21:569–576.

# H.  THE CERVICAL NODES WITH UNKNOWN PRIMARY

A lump in the neck or an enlarged cancerous cervical node in an adult presents a challenge to diagnostic acumen and therapeutic skills. Squamous cell carcinoma arising primarily from a branchial cleft is extremely rare. Therefore, any carcinoma in the cervical node must be considered to represent a metastasis.

## ENLARGED NODE

An enlarged cervical node calls for careful general and head and neck evaluation before a biopsy is performed. The head and neck examination includes fiberoptiscopy of the nasopharynx, oropharynx, and larynx to exclude the possibility of primary carcinoma arising from the upper air and food passages with cervical metastases. Radiographic evaluation by CT and MR scans may indicate abnormalities in the head and neck regions for biopsy. If no primary lesion is found clinically, incisional or preferably excisional biopsy of the node may yield invaluable information regarding the histologic cell type (i.e., epithelial v. lymphomatous cancers and grade of the lesions).

## Selection of Therapy

The therapeutic options include primary neck dissection followed by a "wait and see" policy for the manifestation of primary lesions. Although reports showed approximately one-third to one-half of patients with unknown primary have been cured by surgical treatment to the neck alone,[1] Patients who later developed primary lesions have poorer survival rates than with patients whose primary lesions remained occult: 30% versus 60%.[1-3]

## Therapeutic Options

For high neck N1 lesions, it is recommended that the node be treated by excisional biopsy followed hy comprehensive radiation therapy to the entire Waldeyer's ring.

For large N2 lesions, incisional or excisional biopsy of one of the smaller nodes is followed by radiation therapy to Waldeyer's ring and both sides of the neck, and postradiation neck dissection for residual nodes.

For N3 disease, high dose radiation therapy to the whole neck is followed by limited resection for residual disease.

## Radiotherapeutic Management

Generally, a dose of 60 Gy in 7 weeks through opposed laterals is planned. After the initial 20 Gy, the patient must be carefully examined for evidence of "tumoritis," which may indicate the occult primary lesion and call for alteration of treatment portal or an additional radiation boost to the suspicious area. After comprehensive radiation therapy of 60 Gy is given, the residual nodes are managed by neck dissection. The spinal cord dose is limited to 45 Gy in 5 weeks, and therefore the disease lying within the posterior cervical triangle is boosted by electrons (Figure 5-42, 5-43).

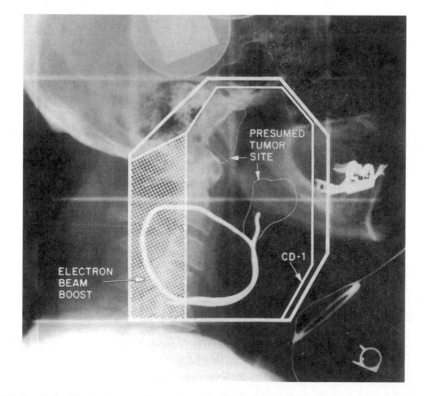

**FIGURE 5-42** Simulation film showing portal arrangement for large squamous cell carcinoma in the neck with an occult primary, presumably in Waldeyer's ring. The patient is NED 25 years after treatment but developed a second primary in the lung.

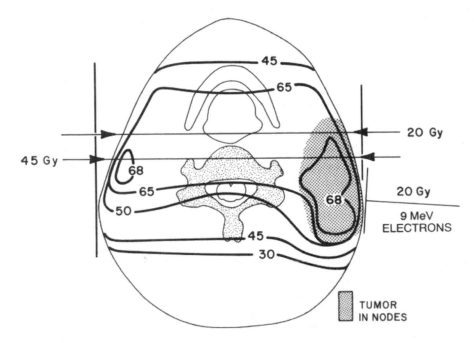

**FIGURE 5-43**   Composite isodoses of external photons through opposing lateral portals and electron boost to the node.

## Results of Therapy

Most reported series indicate that surgery or radiation therapy yielded 3-year survival of 40% to 50% and 5-year survival of 25% to 50%.[4,5] Results after combined therapies (i.e., surgery and radiation therapy) generally showed somewhat higher survival rates. Recent publications indicated that the local control rates ranged from 70% to 80% at 5 years, and corresponding survival rates of 30% to 60%. The prognosis is influenced by the N-stage,

number of positive nodes, fixation of node, and extracapsular tumor spread, probably cell types, and level of the nodes in the neck.[1,6-8] The incidence of development of primaries ranged from 20% to 30% without irradiation. For contralateral neck metastases,15% developed primaries if the contralateral neck did not receive either irradiation or surgical treatment.[3]

## MGH Experience

From 1970 through 1994, 88 patients received radiation therapy for squamous cell carcinoma in the neck with unknown primary. The treatment results are shown in Table 5-44.

## DISCUSSION AND SUMMARY

Squamous cell carcinoma in the cervical lymph nodes is not a disease per se but represents a variety of malignancies arising from different anatomic sites of the head and neck. The most common sites of the occult primary lesions are within Waldeyer's ring, the hypopharynx, and

**TABLE 5-44   5-Year Actuarial Rates of Local Control and Disease-Specific Survival after Treatment of Occult Primary with or without Radical Neck Dissection: 1970–1994**

| Stage | $n$ | LC (%) | DSS (%) |
|-------|-----|--------|---------|
| N1    | 20  | 88     | 89      |
| N2    | 47  | 58     | 57      |
| N3    | 21  | 81     | 65      |
| Total | 88  | 74     | 68      |

the supraglottis; the least common sites are the oral cavity and the nasosinuses.

The prognosis depends on the radiosensitivity of the lymph nodes and the extent of neck involvement. Most therapeutic failures are due to inability to control the disease in the neck and/or development of contralateral neck nodes if only one side of the diseased neck is treated either by surgery or radiation therapy in favorable patients. Generally a dose of 60 Gy to the occult sites can sterilize the microscopic primary lesion satisfactorily.

For N1 lesions diagnosed with either lumpectomy or incisional biopsy, neck dissection alone may be adquate in highly selected patients, and the presumed primary sites will be easily observed. Since radiation therapy to the suspected primary site and the neck can achieve a high cure rate without the necessity of neck dissection, radiation therapy is a good alternative treatment method. For N2 and N3 lesions, the management should be combined therapies, that is, neck dissection with postoperative radiation therapy to both sides of the neck.

## REFERENCES

1. Coster JR, Foote RL, Olsen KD, et al: Cervical nodal metastases of squamous cell carcinoma of unknown origin: Indications for withholding radiation therapy. *Int J Radiat Oncology Bio Phys* 1992;23:(4)742–749.

2. Glynne-Jones RGT, Anand AK, Young TE, Berry RJ: Metastasic carcinoma in the cervical lymph nodes from an occult primary: A conservative approach to the role of radiotherapy. *Int J Radiot Oncol Biol Phys* 1990;18:289.

3. Carlson LS, Fletcher GH, Oswald MJ: Guidelines for radiotherapeutic techniques for cervical metastases from an unknown primary. *Int J Radiot Oncol Biol Phys* 1984;12:2101.

4. Coker DD, Casterline PF, Chambers RG, et al: Metastases to lymph nodes of the head and neck from an unknown primary site. *Am J Surg* 1977;134:517–522.

5. Barrie JR, Knapper, WH, Strong EW: Cervical nodal metastases of unknown origin. *Cancer* 1971;21:112–119.

6. Stell PM, Mortin RP, Singh SD: Cervical lymph node metastases: The significance of the level of the lymph node. *Clin Oncology* 1983;9:101–106.

7. Maulard C, Hoisset M, Brunel P, et al: Postoperative radiation therapy for cervical lymph node metastases from an occult squamous cell carcinoma. *Laryngoscope* 1992;102.

8. Dickson R, Vargas DR: Occult primary of the head and neck. *J Otolaryngol* 1979;8:427.

# I. THE TEMPORAL BONE TUMORS

## MALIGNANT TUMORS

Malignant tumors arising from the temporal bone (i.e., external auditory canal, middle ear, or mastoid) are extremely rare. Incidence is estimated to be one case in 10,000 to 20,000 otologic pathologic conditions.[1] Chronic otitis externa and otorrhea are often associated with carcinoma of the external auditory canal. About one-quarter of carcinomas of the middle ear and mastoid are superimposed with cholesteatoma formation.[2] Various cell types are diagnosed, including squamous cell carcinoma, adenoid cystic carcinoma, myoepithelioma, adenocarcinoma, and poorly differentiated carcinoma.[3–5] Benign tumors adjacent temporal area includes paraglangioma and vascular tumors.

Evaluation of the extent of the disease includes includes CT and MR scans with or without contrasts. Angiography may be supplemented for the vascular lesions. If the site is accessible, biopsy should be done for histologic confirmation of nature of the disease prior to definitive therapies.

### Selection of Therapy

Because of the rarity of these tumors, treatments vary greatly in various institutions. For example, radical surgery and radiation therapy are used, alone or in combination.

The data that follow, however, suggest that most malignant lesions would benefit from a combination of surgery and postoperative radiation therapy with local control of 10% to 50%.[5–7] Except in early lesions without evidence of bone destruction, primary radiation therapy for this disease is rarely successful and therefore is not advised.

For the benign tumors such as paragangliomas limited to the middle ear, surgical removal may be possible, but it is often incomplete

and followed by local recurrence or persistence of the tumor.[8–12] Large tumors extending intracranially are rarely amenable to curative treatment by surgical removal. Radiation therapy is often used as a growth restraint procedure. It may be applied to patients with residual or recurrent disease after radical mastoidectomy and/or temporal bone resection or for inoperable lesions.

### Radiotherapeutic Management

Radiation therapy calls for meticulous technique. Ipsilateral wedge-paired or Ap-PA

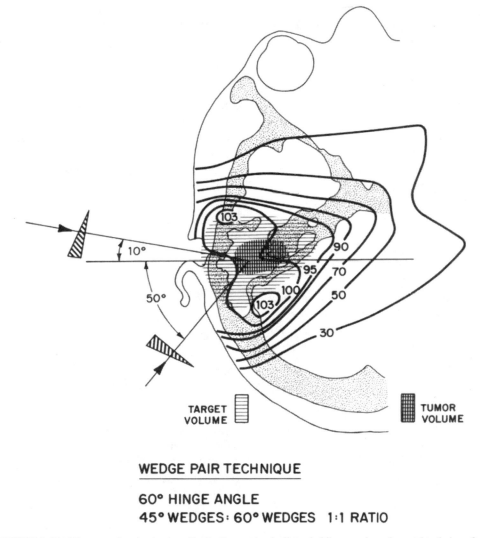

**WEDGE PAIR TECHNIQUE**

**60° HINGE ANGLE**
**45° WEDGES : 60° WEDGES  1:1 RATIO**

**FIGURE 5-44**  Diagrams showing isodose distributions: using ipsilateral oblique wedge pair portal technique for tumors arising within the temporal bone for 50 Gy and supplemented by electron beam to higher dose as needed.

portals with megavoltage radiations and appositional electron boost are found to be satisfactory in delivering a uniform dosage throughout the entire tumor-bearing volume in the temporal bone. The radiation dosage is limited to 60 Gy in 6 weeks (Figure 5-44).

## MGH and MEEI Experience

From 1956 through 1994 inclusive, of a total of 63 patients with carcinoma of the temporal bone region received radiation therapy, 59 had combined surgery and radiation therapy, and 4, who had inoperable lesions, had radiation therapy alone. Of the latter group, 34 had carcinoma arising from the external auditory canal, and 29 had tumors involving the middle ear and mastoid.

Of the 34 patients with carcinoma of the external auditory canal, the local control rates for 5 and 10 years were 64% and 60%, respectively. For the 29 patients with middle ear and mastoid carcinomas, the corresponding rates were 48% and 48%.

Six patients with adenoid cystic carcinoma and two with adenocarcinoma had 100% survival, except for one whose tumor recurred at the sixth year after treatment. One patient with myoepithelioma was free of disease 5 years after combined therapies. Four patients received radiation therapy alone because of inoperability of the lesion and died within 2 years.

Fifty-eight patients with paragangliomas were treated by radiation therapy. Of these, 23 received postoperative radiation therapy for residual disease preceded by radical mastoidectomy and/or temporal bone resection; 26 received radiation therapy alone for inoperable tumors. Nine patients with gross recurrence after previous surgery had radiation therapy as a salvage procedure. The 5- and 10-year actuarial progression free-survival of the entire group of patients, ranging from 1 to 25 years, was 98% and 87%, respectively.

## DISCUSSION AND SUMMARY

Carcinoma arising from or adjacent to the temporal bone is rare. The treatment of choice of this disease is combined surgery and radiation therapy. More than half the patients so treated had survivorship of 5 or more years. Except in extremely early lesions without bony involvement, treatment by radiation therapy alone is rarely successful and therefore is not recommended.

Paragangliomas near the temporal bone or the skull base are treated by combined surgical resection and postoperative radiation therapy, if the lesions are operable. For the inoperable glomus tumors, radiation therapy alone is the preferred treatment modality with satisfactory local control and can provide the patients with tumor progression–free survival. For the patients in poor health with prospect of short-term survival only, no treatment of a benign growth is probably appropriate.

The most serious complication, osteoradionecrosis of the temporal bone, is often due to excessively high dose of radiation therapy. It can be minimized, however, by improvement of radiotherapeutic and surgical techniques. Treatment of benign paraganglioma tumor, either surgical or radiotherapeutic, must be tempered with conservatism. Aggressive radiation therapy with excessively high dose resulting osteonecrosis is a disservice to patients with this disease[13,14]

## REFERENCES

1. Lewis JS: Cancer of the external auditory canal, middle ear and mastoid, in JY Suen and EN Myers (eds): *Cancer of the Head and Neck.* New York, Churchill-Livingston, 1981, pp 561–562.

2. Lewis JS: Squamous cell carcinoma of the ear. *Arch Otolaryngol* 1973;97:41–42.

3. Johns ME, Headington JT: Squamous cell carcinoma of the external auditory canal. A clinicopathologic study of 20 cases. *Arch Otolaryngol* 1974;100:45–49.

4. Sinha PP, Aziz HI: Treatment of carcinoma of the middle ear. *Radiology* 1978;126:485–487.

5. Sorenson H: Cancer of the middle ear and mastoid. *Acta Radiol* 1960;54:460–468.

6. Wang CC: Radiation therapy in the management of carcinoma of the external auditory

canal, middle ear or mastoid. *Radiology* 1975;116:713–715.

7. Kinney SE: Squamous cell carcinoma of the external auditory canal. *Am J Otol* 1989;10:111–116.

8. Fuller AM, Brown HA, Harrison EG, et al: Chemodectomas of the glomus jugulare tumors. *Laryngoscope* 1967;77:218–238.

9. Hatfield PM, James AE, Schulz MD: Chemodectomas of the glomus jugulare. *Cancer* 1972;30:1164–1168.

10. Bradshaw JD: Radiotherapy in glomus jugulare tumors. *Clin Radiol* 1961;12:227–234.

11. Hudgins PT: Radiotherapy for extensive glomus jugulare tumors. *Radiology* 1972;103:427–429.

12. Simko TG, Griffin TW, Gerdes AJ, et al: The role of radiation therapy in the treatment of glomus jugulare tumors. *Cancer* 1978;42:104–106.

13. Schuknecht HF, Karmody CS: Radionecrosis of the temporal bone. *Laryngoscope* 1966;76:1416–1428.

14. Wang CC, Doppke K: Osteoradionecrosis of the temporal bone: Consideration of nominal standard dose. *Int J Radiol Oncol Biol Phys* 1976;1:881–883.

# J. RADIATION THERAPY SEQUELAE AND COMPLICATIONS

The sequelae of radiation therapy for head and neck cancer including xerostomia, loss of taste, and epilation of the irradiated skin, are relatively common. These are unfortunate but unavoidable and can be managed by supportive measures. Most of the unpleasant side effects relative to taste and dry mouth are temporary, although in some instances the side effects are long lasting.

Although carious teeth should be extracted prior to radiation therapy to minimize infection of the alveolar bone and later osteitis, sound teeth and teeth in good repair can survive radiation therapy well and need not be extracted if the radiation dosages are kept within the limits of tolerance of the mandible and a dental hygiene program such as fluoridation of teeth is maintained after radiation therapy.

Major complications include soft tissue ulceration, orocutaneous fistulas of the mandible and hard palate. These invariably follow curative irradiation but may be coincidental to unusually aggressive radiation therapy or faulty treatment technique. Important factors in the occurrence of such complications include the treatment modalities employed, the time–dose–fractionation (TDF) program and the size of the irradiated portals and magnitude of radiation dosages, the extent of the disease and its location, as well as the patient's age and nutritional status.[1] Incidence is further exaggerated following combined radiation therapy and surgery, owing to excessive impairment of local blood supply and secondary infection. This is particularly true when curative doses of radiation therapy are given to tumors first, followed by radical surgical procedure. In such an environment, the postoperative morbidity, including delayed wound healing and occasionally carotid blowout and mortality, could be exceptionally high and, at times, unacceptable in the practice of modern oncology.

Osteoradionecrosis is often the result of an excessive dose of radiation therapy and may occur even in the edentulous jaw. A dose in excess of 70 Gy or TDF of 120 carries a high risk of osteoradionecrosis,[2] which may occur many years after radiation therapy following slight trauma. Treatment should be conservative and palliative. Small necroses can be managed with meticulous oral hygiene, frequent irrigation with a mild solution of mixed salt, and soda rinses. An extensive area may take months to heal. Small areas of osteoradionecrosis may heal after conservative measures, including oral hygiene and analgesics. The sequestrum may work its way out of the jaw and be removed, whereupon the vitalized bone may heal. In severe cases with intractable pain and infection, surgical removal of the necrotic bone or partial mandibulectomy or hyperbaric oxygen therapy[3] may be necessary to effect a cure.

Temporal bone necrosis is one of the most serious complications after radiation therapy for carcinoma arising from the middle and inner ear or for glomus jugulare tumors.[4] It is rarely amenable to treatment by surgical resection and may lead to the death of the patient. To control cancers permanently, high dose radiation therapy is justified with a risk of major complications. On the other hand, the development of osteoradionecrosis of the temporal bone after radiation therapy for glomus jugulare tumors, which are benign, is seldom warranted and should be avoided. Studies[5] show that a biologic dose of 72 Gy in 7.5 weeks or a TDF value of 120 should be considered the upper limits of tolerance of the temporal bone.

Radiation necrosis of the larynx, or functionless larynx, is also related to high dose and large fraction size radiation therapy with large irradiated portals. The condition is likewise exaggerated by the presence of large infected tumors within the larynx. For prevention of such complications, the logical approach is surgical resection followed by postoperative radiation therapy with modest doses.

Radiation injuries to the visual apparatus occur following radiation therapy to the lesions within or adjacent to the orbit or the ethmoidal and spheroidal sinuses.[6] These include radiation keratitis, cataract, retinal degeneration, retinopathy, or ophthalmitis with loss of vision. The incidence of radiation therapy injuries to the optic nerve and chiasm is related to the total dose and, more importantly, the increased fraction size (2.5 Gy per fraction), which leads to blindness.[7] Diabetic retinopathy may mimic changes of the retina after radiation therapy.

Radiation neuritis of the twelfth cranial nerve following curative radiation therapy for oropharyngeal cancer[5] is fortunately infrequent, and its incidence can be markedly reduced if the radiation therapy dosage is kept below 70 Gy in 7 weeks.

Other uncommon radiotherapeutic sequelae are radiation-induced carotid artery disease,[8] hypopituitarism,[9,10] and hypothyroidism.[11] These complications and unpleasant sequelae of treatment should be accepted as risks in the management of extensive head and neck tumors, but they may be minimized by observing careful radiotherapeutic and surgical techniques and principles. Radiation-induced transverse myelitis is fortunately extremely rare and should be avoided at all costs by limiting the dose to the cord below 45 Gy in 4.5 to 5 weeks.[12,13]

Long-term effects such as abnormal facial growth or radiation-induced malignancy,[14] particularly in childhood, have been observed, but the incidence of malignant transformation is extremely low and should not be taken seriously into consideration in the selection of radiation therapy for life-threatening malignant tumors.

With the use of megavoltage radiation, careful radiation therapy planning and techniques with the aid of dedicated computers, better understanding of radiobiology, tolerance of normal tissues and organs—most importantly the patterns of radiation treatment schedules and fractionation (i.e., fraction sizes, total doses, etc.)—and improvement of surgical techniques, major complications occur less frequently in the modern practice of radiation therapy.

## RERERENCES

1. Grant BP, Fletcher GH: Analysis of complications following megavoltage therapy for squamous cell carcinomas of the tonsillar area. *Am J Roentgenol Radium Ther Nucl Med* 1966,96: 28–36.

2. Cheng VST, Wang CC: Osteoradionecrosis of the mandible resulting from external megavoltage radiation therapy. *Radiology* 1974;112: 685–689.

3. Mainour EG, Hart GB: Osteoradionecrosis of the mandible: Treatment and hyperbaric oxygen. *Arch Otolaryngol* 1975;101:173–177.

4. Wang CC, Doppke K: Osteoradionecrosis of the temporal bone—Consideration of nominal standard dose. *Int J Radiat Oncol Biol Phys* 1976; 1:881–883.

5. Cheng VST, Schulz MD: Unilateral hypoglossal nerve atrophy as a late complication of radia-

tion therapy of head and neck carcinoma: A report of four cases and a review of the literature on peripheral and cranial nerve damages after radiation therapy. *Cancer* 1975;35:1537–1544.

6. Shukovsky LJ. Fleteher GH: Retinal and optic nerve complications in a high dose irradiation technique of ethmoid sinus and nasal cavity. *Radiology* 1972;104:629–634.

7. Harris JR, Levene MB: Visual complications following irradiation for pituitary adenomas and cardiopharyngiomas. *Radiology* 1976;120:167–171.

8. Silverberg GD, Britt RH, Goffinet DR: Radiation induced carotid artery disease. *Cancer* 1978;41:130–137.

9. Aristizibal S, Caldwell WL, Avilla J: Relationship of time dose factors to tumor control and complications in the treatment of Cushing's disease by irradiation. *Int J Radiat Oncol Biol Phys* 1977;2:47–54.

10. Samaan NA, Bakdash MM, Caderao IB, et al: Hypopituitarism after external irradiation: Evidence for both hypothalamic and pituitary origin. *Ann Intern Med* 1975;83:771–777.

11. Shafer RB, Nuttall FO, Pollack K, et al: Thyroid function after radiation and surgery for head and neck cancer. *Arch Intern Med* 1975;135:843–846.

12. Abbatucci JS, Delozier T, Quint R, et al: Radiation myelopathy of the cervical spinal cord. Time, dose and volume factors. *Int J Radiat Oncol Biol Phys* 1978;4:239–248.

13. Wara W, Phillips RL, Sheline GE, et al: Radiation tolerance of the spinal cord. *Cancer* 1975;35:1558–1562.

14. Southwick HW: Radiation-associated head and neck tumors. *Am J Surg* 1977;134:438–443. *Radiology* 1959;72:68–74.

# THYROID CARCINOMAS

JAMES R. WONG and C. C. WANG

## INTRODUCTION

Thyroid cancers are relatively rare and account for 1.2% of nonskin malignancies and 0.2% of cancer deaths in the United States. There are about 16,000 new cases of thyroid cancer diagnosed each year, with 1200 deaths resulting from this disease.[1] However, presence of a nodule near the thyroid or in the thyroid is not uncommon. Thus, a series of clinical and diagnostic measures, including careful history, physical examination, blood work, and imaging studies, is needed to evaluate these nodules to rule out malignancies either in the thyroid or in the upper aerodigestive tract. In general, most thyroid nodules are asymptomatic, and pain is usually not an early symptom of thyroid cancers. As the cancer increases in size, pain near the nodule, dysphagia, dyspnea, hoarseness, or the development of Horner syndrome may occur. Other associated signs may include fixation of the mass to the structures under the skin, or presence of cervical lymphadenopathy. Thyroid function test and radioactive iodine-131 may be used to identify underlying thyroid pathology and to assess the functional capacity of the thyroid nodule but will not establish whether the lesion is benign or malignant with complete reliability. High resolution ultrasound, computerized tomography (CT), and/or magnetic resonance imagining (MRI) may yield extremely useful information regarding the size, extent, and involvement of the thyroid lesion, and fine-needle aspiration or incisional biopsy is needed to establish the exact nature of the thyroid nodule.[2,3]

The thyroid gland is composed of right and left lobes connecting at the isthmus, which crosses the upper trachea. The average weight of the thyroid is 20 g. The recurrent laryngeal nerves lie medial to the lateral aspect of both lobes. The lymphatic pathways follow the superior and inferior thyroid blood vessels and thus drain in the superior, lateral, and inferior directions. Regional lymph node spread from thyroid cancer is common. The first echelon of lymph node drainage is the paralaryngeal, paratracheal, and prelaryngeal (Delphian) nodes. The next echelon of nodal metastasis may involve the mid- and lower cervical, supraclavicular nodes. Superior mediastinal node involvement is not infrequent, especially in the presence of extensive cervical metastasis. Other lymph node involvement may include the submandibular, submental, and retropharyngeal lymph nodes. Distant metastasis spread occurs hematogenously and may involve the lung, bone, and other sites.

Thyroid cancers are divided into four major histopathologic types[4]:

1. Papillary carcinoma (including those with follicular foci)
2. Follicular carcinoma
3. Medullary carcinoma
4. Anaplastic or undifferentiated carcinoma

The TNM staging of thyroid cancers according to the American Joint Committee on Cancer (AJCC, 1997) is as follows[4]:

### Primary Tumor (T)

| | |
|---|---|
| Tx | Primary tumor cannot be assessed |
| T1 | Tumor ≤ 1 cm or less, limited to the thyroid |
| T2 | Tumor less than 1 cm but no greater than 4 cm, limited to the thyroid |
| T3 | Tumor greater than 4 cm, limited to the thyroid |
| T4 | Tumor any size but extending beyond the thyroid capsule |

Regional Lymph Nodes (N)

Nx   Regional lymph nodes cannot be
     assessed
N0   No regional lymph node metastasis
     N1a   Metastasis in ipsilateral cervical
           lymph node(s)
     N1b   Metastasis in bilateral, midline,
           or contralateral cervical or
           mediastinal lymph nodes

Distant Metastasis (M)

Mx   Distant metastasis cannot be assessed
M0   No distant metastasis
M1   Distant metastasis

## THERAPEUTIC CONSIDERATIONS

Four therapeutic modalities are commonly
considered, either singly or in combination.
These are surgery, radioactive iodine (RaI),
external beam radiotherapy, and chemotherapy. For the differentiated carcinoma (papillary or follicular) and medullary carcinoma,
surgical removal plays the dominant role, with
external beam irradiation used as an adjuvant
procedure. Radioactive iodine is used in postoperative settings when appropriate. For the
anaplastic carcinoma, external beam irradiation and chemotherapy are generally employed. In this section, efforts are limited to
external beam radiation; consult subspecialty
books as well.[5–8]

In general, surgical resection is the most
effective treatment for most of the thyroid
malignancies. When the surgical resection is
incomplete, radiation therapy may be considered. Since, however, the indication for external beam radiation therapy is controversial in
many circumstances, it must be highly individualized according to cell type, extent of
the lesion after surgery, presence or absence
of distant metastasis, and whether the lesions
can be treated with radioactive iodine or
medically with thyroid hormone or
chemotherapy.

## TREATMENT OF THYROID CANCERS BY RADIATION THERAPY

### Papillary and Follicular Carcinoma

Papillary and follicular carcinomas of the thyroid are generally considered to be differentiated
thyroid carcinomas. The use of external beam
radiation therapy for these carcinomas is controversial, and the indication varies from center to
center. In general, if a complete resection is
achieved, adjuvant external beam radiation is
not indicated. In patients with definite or possible (close surgical margin) microscopic residual
disease, radioactive iodine-131 is the treatment
of choice if the lesions are found to concentrate
iodine. The presence of lymph node metastases
in the neck does not constitute a strong indication for postoperative radiation therapy because
differentiated thyroid carcinomas grow slowly,
and thus these patients may survive for a long
time without significant symptoms. However,
external beam irradiation is probably indicated
in patients with high risk for local recurrence in
the following circumstances: (1) there is high
risk for local recurrence evidence of tumor extension beyond the thyroid capsule into the adjacent organs[8–11]; (2) there is gross bulky disease
that is unresectable (for these patients, [131]I is unlikely to eradicate the residual tumor unless an
extremely high absorbed dose is achieved)[12];
and (3) the surgical resection is incomplete and
the tumor does not take up [131]I.[13]

### Medullary Carcinoma

Medullary carcinoma is similar to differentiated thyroid carcinoma in that in both cases the
indication for external beam irradiation after
surgery is controversial. Most reported series
are retrospective and small, and conclusion for
the role of radiation therapy is contradictory.[13]
There is no definitive evidence that postoperative radiation improves survival, although it appears that local control is improved with the
addition of radiation.[14–17] Because these lesions
generally do not concentrate radioactive [131]I
well, and local recurrence may impact on the

quality of life of these patients, we recommend postoperative radiation therapy if there is extrathyroid invasion, widespread lymph node metastasis, or residual disease after resection.

### Anaplastic Thyroid Carcinoma

Curative surgery is usually performed for a small number of patients. The surgical procedure is often used to maintain the airway and to prevent obstruction prior to initiation of radiation therapy. Radiation therapy, alone or in combination with chemotherapy (often Adriamycin based), is used in an attempt to control this disease locally, although the beneficial effects are usually short-lived.[18]

## RADIATION THERAPY TECHNIQUES

External radiation therapy is given in the form of minimantle technique [19] with 6 to 10 MV photons. The portals should cover the whole neck and upper mediastinum through opposing anterior–posterior (AP-PA) portals with posterior cord block, 4:1 loading in favor of the AP portal. After approaching cord tolerance, one applies anterior right and left oblique wedge pair boost to the tumor site for the desired dose. For small, superficial lesions, the boost can be accomplished with en face electrons. Figures 5-45 and 5-46 show the portal arrangement with the minimantle and the composite isodose distribution employing the

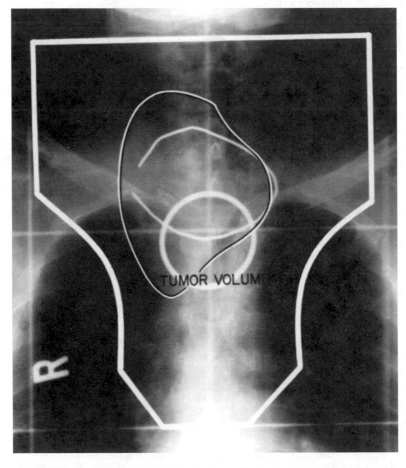

**FIGURE 5-45**    Portal arrangement for treatment of patients with cancer of the thyroid.

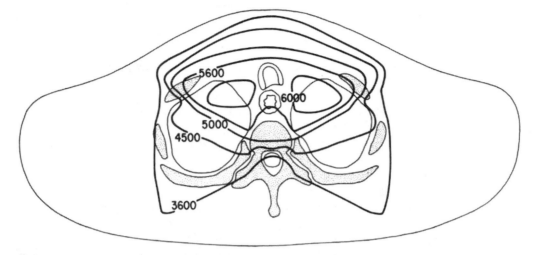

**FIGURE 5-46**   Composite isodose distribution employing minimantle and left and right oblique wedge pair boost technique.

minimantle and oblique wedge pair technique, respectively. With the increasing common availability of computerized assistance conformal of three-dimensional planning, the isodose distribution can be improved by adjusting the weighting of the portals, depending on the situation.

For differentiated carcinoma or medullary carcinoma, the total tumor dose should be around 60 to 66 Gy, with the spinal cord dose limited to less than 45 Gy during the entire course of radiation therapy.

For anaplastic carcinoma, if curative radiation is intended, we recommend radiation alone or in combination with chemotherapy. For patients who receive chemotherapy, the technique and final total dosage of radiation is similar to that described as for differentiated or medullary carcinoma. If irradiation alone is employed, we recommend a multi fraction-per-day regimen, with fraction dose of 1.5 Gy per fraction, given twice a day to a dosage of 36–39 Gy through the minimantle field, followed by oblique wedge pair boost for another 21 to 24 Gy, and then electron boost if possible, bringing the final total dosage to 65 to 70 Gy. The total spinal cord dose is limited to less than 40 Gy. We schedule a 1- to 2-week break after 36 to 39 Gy to allow the acute side effects of radiation to subside, if necessary.

## RADIATION THERAPY RESULTS

### Differentiated Thyroid Carcinoma

The reported series of radiation therapy for well-differentiated carcinoma of the thyroid are generally retrospective. Moreover, these tumors usually follow an indolent clinical course, with an average time to local relapse after radiation as long as 8.5 years.[20] Thus, the data regarding survival results are difficult to assess. Nevertheless, several reports have shown a decrease in local recurrence rate with adjuvant radiation therapy, especially in the presence of gross local disease.[20–23] The survival rate, however, does not seem to be affected by beam radiation therapy.[11,12]

One of the largest studies of well-differentiated thyroid cancer was reported from France by Tubiana et al.[20] In this study, 539 patients had initial clinical disease confined to the neck. After surgical resection, 61 patients received prophylactic [131]I for extensive lymph node involvement, upper mediastinal involvement, invasion of neighboring muscles, or difficult surgical resection. A similar group of 66 patients received postoperative external beam radiation. The 5- and 10-year relapse-free survival rates were 67 and 44% for the [131]I group, compared with 70 and 53% for the external beam group. Another group of 97 patients received external beam radiation because of gross incomplete resection. The 5- and 15-year relapse-free survival rates were 58 and 39%, respectively. In total, 180 patients received postoperative external beam radiation for prophylactic, gross residual, or unknown reasons. These patients had a statistically significant lower local recurrence rate (14%) compared to 336 patients who did not receive postoperative external beam (21%)

Simpson et al.[24] from Canada summarized the experience of 1578 patients with well-differentiated thyroid cancer: 201 patients had postoperative external beam radiation therapy, 214 patients had [131]I, and 107 patients had both. These treatments were used more often in patients with a poor prognosis than in those with good prognostic factors. In patients with no residual disease, the addition of postoperative treatments offered no advantage to those treated with surgery alone. For those with microscopic disease, the addition of postoperative radiation ([131]I or external beam) had a statistical advantage over surgical resection alone for both local recurrence or survival. There was, however, no significant difference among the [131]I, external beam, or [131]I and external beam groups with regard to local recurrence or survival.

## Medullary Carcinoma

External radiation is effective in treating medullary carcinoma of the thyroid despite slow shrinkage. Mak et al.[15] reported an actuarial local–regional control rate of 84% with surgery and postoperatively radiation therapy, compared with 13% for patients treated with surgery alone. The survival rate, however, was not improved with radiation. Similarly, Brierley and Tsang[12] of the Princess Margaret Hospital reported a 10-year local control rate of 86% for patients with presumed or definite microscopic residual disease or lymph node involvements who received postoperative radiation versus 52% who did not receive radiation.

## Anaplastic Thyroid Carcinoma

Anaplastic thyroid tumors usually are unresectable and respond poorly to radiation. Various treatment modalities including standard fractionation, hyperfractionation, and combined modalities with chemotherapy and radiation have been attempted. The results are uniformly poor, with 2-year survival rates ranging from 11% to 20% and a median survival rate in the order of months.[12,18,25] Most patients succumb to local–regional relapses and/or distant metastasis.

## REFERENCES

1. Parker SL, Tong T, Bolden, et al: Cancer statistics. *Calif Cancer J Clin* 1997;47(1):5.

2. Wang CA, Vickery AL, Maloof F: Needle biopsy of the thyroid: Technique, clinical applications and limitation. *Surg Gynecol Obstet* 1976;143:365–368.

3. Wang CA, Guyton SP, Vickery AL: A further note on the large needle biopsy of the thyroid. *Surg Gyecol Obstet* 1983;156:508–510.

4. American Cancer Society, *AJCC Cancer Staging Manual*, 5th ed. Lippincott-Raven, Philadelphia, 1997.

5. Wang CA: Thyroid cancer—General concepts in management, in *Clinical Radiation Oncology, Indications, Techniques and Results*, 1st ed, in CC Wang (ed): PSG Publishing Company, Littleton, MA, 1988.

6. Singer PA, Cooper DS, Daniels GH, et al: Treatment guidelines for patients with thyroid nodules and well-differentiated thyroid cancer. *Arch Intern Med* 1996;156:2165–2172.

7. Baverman LE, Utiger RD (eds): *Werner and Ingbar's The Thyroid: a Fundamental and Clinical Text*, 7th ed. Lippincott-Raven, Philadelphia, 1996.

8. Mazzaferri E: *Radioiodine and Other Treatments and Outcomes*. Philadelphia, Lippincott, 1991, pp 1138–1165.

9. Cady B, Rossi R: An expanded view of risk-group definition in differentiated thyroid carcinoma. *Surgery* 1988;160:947–953.

10. Cunningham M, Duda R, Recant W, et al: Survival discriminants for differentiated thyroid cancer. *Surgery* 1990;160:344–347.

11. Samman NA, Schultz PN, Hickey RC, et al: The results of various modalities of treatment of well-differentiated thyroid carcinoma: A retrospective review of 1599 patients. *J Clin Endocrinol Metab* 1992;75:714–720.

12. Brierley JD, Tsang RW: External radiation therapy in the treatment of thyroid malignancy. *Endocrin Metabol Clin North Am* 1996;25:141–157.

13. Schlumberger MJ: Papillary and follicular thyroid carcinoma. *N Engl J Med* 1998;338:297–306.

14. Jensen MH, Davis RK, Derrick L: Thyroid cancer: A computer-assisted review of 5287 cases. *Otolaryngol Head Neck Surg* 1990;102;51–65.

15. Mak A, Morrison W, Garden A, et al: The value of postoperative radiotherapy for regional medullary carcinoma of the thyroid. *Int J Radiat Oncol Biol Phys* 1994;30:234.

16. Nguyen T, Chassord J, Lagarede P: Results of postoperative radiation therapy in medullary carcinoma of the thyroid. *Radiother Oncol* 1992; 23:1.

17. Samaan N, Schultz P, Hickey R: Medullary thyroid carcinoma: Prognosis of familial versus sporadic disease and the role of radiotherapy. *Medicine* 1988;67:801 805.

18. Tennvall J, Lundell G: Combined doxorubicin, hyperfractionated radiotherapy, and surgery in anaplastic thyroid carcinoma. *Cancer* 1994;74:1348–1354.

19. Doppke K, Novack D, Wang CC: Physical considerations in the treatment of advanced carcinomas of the larynx and pyriform sinuses using 10 MV x-rays. *Int J Radiat Oncol Biol Phys* 1980;6:1251–1255.

20. Tubiana M, Haddad E, Schlumberger M, et al: External radiotherapy in thyroid cancers. *Cancers* 1985;55:2062–2071.

21. Sheline GE, Galante M, Lindsay S: Radiation therapy in the control of persistent thyroid cancer. *Am J Roentgenol Radium Ther Nucl Med* 1966;97:923–930.

22. Phlips P, Hanzen C, Andry G, et al: Postoperative irradiation for thyroid cancer. *Eur J Surg Oncol* 1993;19:399–404.

23. Simpson W, McKinney S, Carruthers J, et al: Papillary and follicular thyroid cancer: Prognostic factors in 1578 patients. *Am J Med* 1987;83:479–488.

24. Simpson WJ, Panzarella T, Carruthers JS, et al: Pappillary and follicular thyroid cancer: Impact of treatment in 1578 patients. *Int J Radiat Oncol Biol Phys* 1988;14:1063–1075.

25. Junor E, Paul J, Reed N: Anaplastic thyroid carcinoma: 91 patients treated by surgery and radiotherapy. *Eur J Surg* 1992;18:83–88.

# CHAPTER 6

# CANCER OF THE BREAST

BARBARA FOWBLE and GARY FREEDMAN

## INTRODUCTION

Breast cancer is the most common malignancy in women in the United States. It accounts for 30% of all female cancers,[1] with approximately 178,700 new invasive cancers diagnosed in 1998.[1] The lifetime risk of developing breast cancer was 12.52% (one in eight) for the years 1992–94. Wingo et al.[2] recently reported a leveling of breast cancer incidence rates for the period from 1990 to 1995. Breast cancer accounts for 16% of all cancer deaths in women, second only to lung cancer.[1] Fortunately, the mortality rates for breast cancer in the United States in the 1990s have begun to decline.[2–4] This decline has been attributed to earlier detection through screening mammography and improvements in treatment strategies.[3] The 1980s witnessed the implementation of adjuvant chemotherapy and/or hormonal therapy for axillary node negative and positive women, and multiple randomized clinical trials have confirmed a survival benefit with systemic therapy in these patients.[5] Dose–intense chemotherapy regimens with autologous bone marrow transplantation or peripheral stem cell rescue are currently being evaluated in clinical trials.

Breast cancer treatment calls for a multidisciplinary approach involving physicians from diagnostic radiology, pathology, surgery, reconstructive surgery, medical oncology, and radiation oncology. This approach ensures the individual patient of a balanced presentation of treatment options and exposure to the expertise of all the specialties.

Radiotherapy has played an integral role in the treatment of breast cancer. It is routinely employed in breast conservation therapy. Its role as adjuvant therapy in selected patients undergoing mastectomy for stages I and II disease is currently evolving, and it has become an essential component of the combined modality approach for stage III disease. This chapter focuses on the role of radiation in breast cancer treatment, the technical aspects of its delivery, and its potential complications. The discussion of treatment recommendations emphasizes a review of the available literature to support clinical management decisions. Since our presentation is confined to treatment-related issues, we have purposely omitted sections related to epidemiology, natural history, detection, and basic pathology. In addition, rather than providing a detailed review of the role of adjuvant or neoadjuvant chemotherapy or hormonal therapy in breast cancer treatment, we discuss the interaction of these modalities with radiation.

*Clinical Radiation Oncology: Indications, Techniques, and Results, 2nd ed.* Edited by C.C. Wang.
ISBN: 0-471-23803-1   Copyright © 2000 Wiley-Liss, Inc.

## STAGING

The staging for breast cancer of the American Joint Committee Staging on Cancer is as follows[6]:

PRIMARY TUMOR (T)

TX    Primary tumor cannot be assessed

T0    No evidence of primary tumor

Tis   Carcinoma in situ: intraductal carcinoma, lobular carcinoma *in situ*, or Paget disease of the nipple with no tumor

T1    Tumor 2 cm or less in greatest dimension

    T1mic   Microinvasion 0.1 cm or less in greatest dimension

    T1a     Tumor more than 0.1 but not more than 0.5 cm in greatest dimension

    T1b     Tumor more than 0.5 cm but not more than 1 cm in greatest dimension

    T1c     Tumor more than 1 cm but not more than 2 cm in greatest dimension

T2    Tumor more than 2 cm but not more than 5 cm in greatest dimension

T3    Tumor more than 5 cm in greatest dimension

T4    Tumor of any size with direct extension to (a) chest wall or (b) skin, only as described below:

    T4a     Extension to chest wall

    T4b     Edema (including peau d'orange) or ulceration of the skin of the breast or satellite skin nodules confined to the same breast

    T4c     Both (T4a and T4b)

    T4d     Inflammatory carcinoma (see definition of inflammatory carcinoma in the introduction)

*Note:* Paget disease associated with a tumor is classified according to the size of tumor.

REGIONAL LYMPH NODES (N)

NX    Regional lymph nodes cannot be assessed (e.g., previously removed)

N0    No regional lymph node metastasis

N1    Metastasis to movable ipsilateral axillary lymph node(s)

N2    Metastasis to ipsilateral axillary lymph node(s) fixed to one another or to other structures

N3    Metastasis to ipsilateral internal mammary lymph node(s)

PATHOLOGIC<br>CLASSIFICATION (pN)

pNX   Regional lymph nodes cannot be assessed (e.g., previously removed, or not removed for pathologic study)

pN0   No regional lymph node metastasis

pN1   Metastasis to movable ipsilateral axillary lymph node(s)

    pN1a    Only micrometastasis (none larger than 0.2 cm)

    pN1b    Metastasis to lymph node(s), any larger than 0.2 cm

        pN1bi    Metastasis in 1 to 3 lymph nodes, any more than 0.2 cm and all less than 2 cm in greatest dimension

        pN1bii   Metastasis to 4 or more lymph nodes, any more than 0.2 cm and all less than 2 cm in greatest dimension

        pN1biii  Extension to tumor beyond the capsule of a lymph node metastasis less than 2 cm in greatest dimension

        pN1biv   Metastasis to a lymph node 2 cm or more in greatest dimension

pN2   Metastasis to ipsilateral axillary lymph nodes that are fixed to one another or to other structures

pN3   Metastasis to ipsilateral internal mammary lymph node(s)

DISTANT METASTASIS (M)

MX  Distant metastasis cannot be assessed
M0  No distant metastasis
M1  Distant metastasis [includes metastasis to ipsilateral supraclavicular lymph node(s)]

STAGE GROUPING

| Stage 0 | Tis | N0 | M0 |
|---|---|---|---|
| Stage I | T1* | N0 | M0 |
| Stage IIA | T0 | N1 | M0 |
| | T1* | N1** | M0 |
| | T2 | N0 | M0 |
| Stage IIB | T2 | N1 | M0 |
| | T3 | N0 | M0 |
| Stage IIIA | T0 | N2 | M0 |
| | T1* | N2 | M0 |
| | T2 | N2 | M0 |
| | T3 | N1 | M0 |
| | T3 | N2 | M0 |
| Stage IIIB | T4 | Any N | M0 |
| | Any T | N3 | M0 |
| Stage IV | Any T | Any N | M1 |

*Note:* T1 includes T1mic
**Note:* The prognosis of patients with N1a is similar to that of patients with pN0.

The clinical primary tumor size may be determined by physical examination findings and/or size measurements from the mammographic abnormality (microcalcifications, mass, or both, or architectural distortion). The pathologic tumor size includes only the size of the invasive cancer. Microinvasive cancer is defined as a focus of invasion not larger than 1 mm. Macroscopic multiple simultaneous cancers in a single breast are recorded by the largest individual tumor size and not the summation of each of the cancers. Localized erythema or nipple or skin retraction may occur with T1, T2, or T3 cancers and should not result in a T4 classification unless other factors are present. The chest wall does not include the pectoral muscle but does include ribs or the serratus anterior or intercostal muscles. Paget disease of the nipple without an invasive cancer is Tis. Positive intramammary nodes (within breast tissue) are considered regional metastases.

## LOBULAR CARCINOMA IN SITU

The term "lobular carcinoma in situ" (LCIS) was first used by Foote and Stewart to describe a distinct pathologic entity arising in lobules and terminal ducts.[7,8] The authors concluded that the lesion was precancerous and recommended simple mastectomy as treatment. Subsequent studies, however, have demonstrated that LCIS is probably not a precursor lesion and may be best viewed as a pathologic marker for an increased risk of breast cancer.[9]

LCIS is usually detected as an incidental finding at the time of biopsy of a benign clinical or mammographic abnormality.[7,10] The clinical finding prompting biopsy is usually a mass,[7,10] and the mammographic finding is usually the appearance of clustered calcifications, which are not usually associated with LCIS.[11,12] The majority of women with LCIS are premenopausal,[10,13,14] and 15% to 20% will have a positive family history of breast cancer.[10]

Prior to 1970, the predominant treatment of LCIS was ipsilateral simple mastectomy with or without a contralateral breast biopsy. This approach was based on the observation that LCIS was frequently multifocal and/or bilateral.[7,11,15–21] Long-term follow-up studies of patients whose sole treatment for LCIS was excision alone have demonstrated that 20% to 30% of these patients will develop an invasive breast cancer[10,14,21–25] that has almost the same probability of occurring in the breast with LCIS as the contralateral breast.[10,14,21–23,15] The mean interval to the development of an invasive cancer ranges from 8 to 20 years.[10,23] The risk appears to increase with time. Bodian et al.[14] in a series of 236 patients with LCIS and a median follow-up of 18 years reported a 13% probability of cancer 10 years after a diagnosis of LCIS, a 26% probability at 20 years, and a 35% probability by 35 years. The extent of LCIS in the biopsy specimen as measured by the number of involved lobules or number of slides does not significantly correlate with the subsequent risk of an invasive cancer[10,12,14,25] in most studies; in one study, however, there was a correlation.[26] A positive family history of breast cancer also does not appear to increase the risk of subsequent cancer[10,14,25] in women with LCIS. The majority of invasive cancers developing after a diagnosis of LCIS are ductal cancers.[8,10,21,27] This observation, as well as the development of cancer in either breast, provides support for the interpretation of LCIS as a pathologic marker for an increased risk for breast cancer rather than as a precursor lesion. Unilateral treatment strategies (i.e., simple mastectomy) do not address the potential for contralateral breast cancer. Contralateral breast biopsy may be associated with a sampling error and, when negative, provides no assurance that a future cancer will not develop in that breast.[15]

The current recommended treatment approach following a biopsy demonstrating LCIS is careful observation. There is no role for radiation directed to one or both breasts. It is uncertain whether negative resection margins will reduce the subsequent incidence of breast cancer. A recent study of 182 women with LCIS registered in the National Surgical Adjuvant Breast Project (NSABP) protocol B-17 reported only seven ipsilateral cancers (invasive or DCIS) and four contralateral cancers with a mean follow-up of 5 years.[12] The authors favored the interpretation of LCIS as a precursor lesion and argued that the lower incidence of a subsequent cancer in their study could be attributed to negative resection margins. However, longer follow-up is needed to confirm these results. When the goal is maximum prevention, bilateral mastectomy may be considered in the individual patient in whom any risk of a subsequent invasive breast cancer is unacceptable. Axillary dissection is not indicated, since the incidence of positive nodes secondary to an occult invasive cancer ranges from 0% to 4%.[16–18,27,28] Women with LCIS are candidates for cancer prevention trials. The results of the NSABP prevention trial employing tamoxifen

for 5 years in these women will provide information regarding the potential effectiveness of this strategy.

## DUCTAL CARCINOMA IN SITU

### Introduction

Ductal carcinoma in situ (DCIS) by definition represents carcinoma confined to the preexisting duct system of the breast without evidence discernible by light microscopy of penetration of the basement membrane. Ductal carcinoma in situ comprises 10% to 15% of all breast cancers and 20% to 30% of those that are mammographically detected.[29] The reported incidence of ductal carcinoma in situ in the United States has increased since 1983, and this increase has paralleled the increased use of screening mammography in asymptomatic individuals.[30,31] In 1998 approximately 36,900 women will be diagnosed with in situ breast cancer, with the majority of cancers ductal carcinoma in situ.[1] Approximately 85% of all ductal carcinomas in situ are detected by mammographic screening, with the most common finding being microcalcifications with or without a mass.[30,31] Approximately 20% of the DCIS detected solely by mammography presents as a mammographic mass.[32,33]

DCIS demonstrates heterogeneity not only in terms of its clinical presentation and mammographic appearance but with respect to its distribution in the breast, pathologic features, and the presence or absence of various biologic markers. Ductal carcinoma in situ has been classified into subtypes based on architectural pattern, the presence or absence of necrosis, or nuclear grade. These subdivisions serve to establish prognostic factors for recurrence and survival in patients undergoing breast conservation therapy. In addition, they identify pathologic factors that may correlate with the biologic potential for multicentricity, occult invasion, positive axillary nodes, and progression to an invasive breast cancer. An appreciation of these factors has influenced treatment recommendations for patients with ductal carcinoma in situ. DCIS has been divided into five architectural patterns: comedo, cribriform, papillary, micropapillary, and solid DCIS. There are three categories for nuclear grade (low grade, intermediate, and high grade). Necrosis must be distinguished from secretory material and is classified as comedo necrosis (central zone of necrosis with a linear pattern on longitudinal sections) or punctate (nonzonal).[34] The relative importance of each of these pathologic factors in predicting recurrence following breast conservation therapy or progression to an invasive cancer remains to be determined. Additional factors that have an impact on clinical outcome include the age of the patient, the size and extent of DCIS, and the resection margin status.

Treatment options for ductal carcinoma in situ include wide excision with or without radiation and mastectomy. Ernster et al.[30] reported that of the 2145 cases of ductal carcinoma in situ in the National Cancer Institute's Surveillance and Epidemiology and End Results (SEER) program, 43.8% underwent mastectomy, 23.3% lumpectomy and radiation, and 30.2% lumpectomy alone. From 1983 to 1992, the use of mastectomy decreased from 71% to 43.8%, while lumpectomy and radiation increased from 6.2% to 23.3% and lumpectomy alone from 19.4% to 30.2%. Winchester et al.[35] reported an increase in the use of breast conservation therapy from 1985 to 1993 from 31% to 54% in the 39,010 patients with ductal carcinoma in situ in the National Cancer Data Base. In 1993, 54% of the patients undergoing breast conservation therapy received postoperative radiation and 48.9% of the patients were treated with mastectomy.

## Rationale for Treatment

The rationale for treatment directed to the entire breast with either radiation or mastectomy is related to the potential for multicentric foci of DCIS and/or the presence of an occult invasive cancer. The reported incidence of multicentricity varies from 0% to 47%.[16,36–41]

However, in these series, assessment of multicentricity was performed by obtaining only random sections from quadrants beyond that of the index cancer. When the serial subgross and correlated mammographic technique is issued for analysis of mastectomy specimens, the incidence of multicentricity ranges from 1% to 32%.[42–44] Holland et al.[4,3] employing the Egans serial subgross method noted only 1 of 82 patients with ductal carcinoma in situ to have a true multicentric distribution (i.e., separate and discrete areas of ductal carcinoma in situ). Stereoscopic and three-dimensional sampling of tissue blocks revealed that the great majority of patients had contiguous extension of their disease, which in earlier series could have been interpreted as multicentric disease. Multifocal disease in the same quadrant, however, is not an uncommon finding for patients with DCIS. Following wide excision with negative margins, 24% to 43% of the patients have been found to have residual ductal carcinoma in situ in the same quadrant.[36,37,45] Faverly et al.[44] analyzed the distribution and growth pattern of DCIS in 60 patients who underwent mastectomy. The authors examined three-dimensional views of the ductal network and reported that 48% of these patients had multifocal involvement (defined as ≥ 2 foci separated by an uninvolved portion of the duct of ≤ 4 cm). Multifocality correlated with nuclear grade, with 70% of the low grade lesions having multifocal involvement versus only 10% of the high grade lesions. Only 17% of the patients with multifocality had a distance of uninvolved ducts between foci of 1 cm or more, and 75% of these occurred in the low-grade lesions.

The incidence of multicentricity or multifocality has also been correlated with tumor size, method of detection, and architectural pattern. Micropapillary DCIS has been reported as having the highest incidence of multicentricity,[46] and Holland et al.[43,47] reported that with this histologic subtype, the extent of the DCIS was frequently underestimated on mammograms by 2 cm or greater. Multicentricity is more common for tumors exceeding 2.5 cm in diameter and those presenting as a palpable mass or mammographic abnormality, compared to those detected as an incidental finding at the time of biopsy of an abnormality that proves to be benign.[39,41,46,48] The incidence of occult invasion ranges from 2% to 21%[16,38,39,42] and is more common in patients presenting with a palpable mass, tumors exceeding 5 cm, and comedo histologic subtype.[39,49]

## Conservative Surgery and Radiation

Mastectomy has been the traditional treatment for ductal carcinoma in situ with or without a low axillary dissection. Its role in the treatment of DCIS has been challenged by the reported success of breast conservation therapy for early stage invasive breast cancer. The results of conservative surgery and radiation for ductal carcinoma in situ are presented in Table 6-1. The crude incidence of breast recurrence ranges from 0% to 18%, and deaths due to breast cancer have been reported in 0% to 2% of the pa-

tients treated. The long-term results of conservative surgery and radiation for ductal carcinoma in situ were reported by Solin et al.[50] This collaborative study from nine institutions in the United States and Europe analyzed outcome for 259 patients with a median follow-up of 10.3 years. The 15-year actuarial breast recurrence rate was 19% and the 15-year actuarial cause-specific survival was 96%. However, only 40% of these patients had DCIS detected solely by mammography.

A recurrence in the breast following conservative surgery and radiation may be related to the persistence of the original primary, which was inadequately excised, to persistence of an occult invasive cancer, or to the development of a new primary, either invasive or noninvasive. A number of factors have been analyzed for their ability to predict for a breast recurrence in patients undergoing conservative surgery and radiation for ductal carcinoma in situ. These include clinical fac-

**TABLE 6-1    Results of Retrospective Series of Conservative Surgery and Radiation for Ductal Carcinoma In Situ (DCIS)**

| Study | Number of Patients | Median Follow-Up (years) | Crude Breast Recurrence (%) | Deaths Due to Disease (%) |
|---|---|---|---|---|
| Warneke et al.[564] | 21 | 3 | 0 | 0 |
| McCormick et al.[51] | 54 | 3 | 18 | 0 |
| Haffty et al.[565] | 60 | 3.6 | 7 | 0 |
| Kuske et al.[60] | 70 | 4 | 4 | 0 |
| Bullock et al.[67] | 43 | 5 | 7 | 0 |
| Kurtz et al.[566] | 47 | 5 | 4 | 2 |
| Ray et al.[567] | 56 | 5 | 9 | 0 |
| Fowble et al.[32] | 110 | 5.3 | 3 | 0 |
| Ciatto et al.[568] | 37 | 5.5 | 5 | |
| Solin et al.[57] | 51 | 5.7 | 10 | 0 |
| Hiramatsu et al.[56] | 76 | 6.2 | 9 | 1 |
| Vicini et al.[55] | 105 | 6.5 | 9 | 1 |
| Fisher et al.[45] | 27 | 7.1 | 7 | 0 |
| Sneige et al.[52] | 49 | 7.2 | 10 | 2 |
| Silverstein et al.[61] | 185 | 7.5 | 16 | 1 |
| Gallagher et al.[569] | 4 | 8 | 0 | 0 |
| Fourquet et al.[570,571] | 67 | 8.7 | 10 | 0 |
| Collaborative Group[50] | 268 | 10.3 | 17 | 1 |
| Delouche et al.[572] | 18 | 11 | 5 | |

tors such as age, menopausal status, tumor location, method of detection, the presence of a bloody nipple discharge, and a positive family history. Pathologic factors include histologic subtype, nuclear grade, necrosis, and margins of resection. Treatment–related factors include the role of reexcision and the total radiation dose. Several factors have been associated with an increased risk of breast recurrence in patients undergoing conservative surgery and radiation for DCIS. The presence of residual microcalcifications on a post-biopsy mammogram has been associated with a 100% incidence of breast recurrence in the five patients reported, in whom all malignant–appearing calcifications were not removed prior to radiation.[51,52] A postbiopsy mammogram that demonstrates excision of all malignant-appearing calcifications is essential prior to the initiation of radiation. Young age has been associated with an increased risk of breast recurrence. In the collaborative study,[53] the breast recurrence rate was 25% for women under 50 years of age with DCIS treated with radiation, versus 2% for those over 50 years of age. The median follow-up was 9.3 years. Van Zee et al.[54] reported a 40%, 6-year actuarial breast recurrence rate in women under 40 years of age treated with wide excision and radiation versus 9% for women 40 to 69 years of age and 0% for women over 70 years of age. Fowble et al.[32] reported a 5-year actuarial breast recurrence of 25% in women 40 years of age or younger who were treated with conservative surgery and radiation versus 0% in women over 40 years of age. Vicini et al.[55] reported a 17% crude breast recurrence rate in 36 women 50 years of age or under who were treated with conservative surgery and radiation for DCIS versus 6% for women over 50 years, with a median follow-up of 6.5 years. Two series, however, have found no correlation between young age and breast recurrence rates.[52,56] The presence of a bloody nipple discharge has also been associated with an increased risk of breast recurrence in two series.[57,58] In the collaborative group

study, the breast recurrence rate was 25% in patients presenting with a bloody nipple discharge versus 15% for those not presenting with bloody nipple discharge.[50] Two series have suggested that women with a positive family history with DCIS have a higher risk of breast recurrence than women with a negative family history.[51,56] However, Fowble et al.[32] and Szelei-Stevens et al.[59] reported no increased incidence of breast recurrence in women with a positive family history and mammographically detected DCIS. The impact of a positive family history on the treatment of DCIS will require further evaluation.

The contributions of certain pathologic factors to the risk of a breast recurrence following conservative surgery and radiation have varied (Table 6-2). Several series have suggested that comedo DCIS or DCIS with high nuclear grade may have a higher risk of breast recurrence.[60,61] In the collaborative group study, neither of these factors alone predicted for an increased risk of breast recurrence at 8 years; however, the combination of the two factors was significant (8-year breast recurrence rate 20% for comedo and nuclear grade III vs. 5% for absence of these two features).[62] However in a subsequent update, the 10-year actuarial breast recurrence rate was 18% for comedo and nuclear grade III tumors versus 15% when these factors were absent ($p = 0.15$).[50] The median interval to recurrence for the comedo DCIS was 3.1 years, versus 6.5 years for non-comedo DCIS. Thus it is seen that series with more limited follow-up will underestimate the number of recurrences for low grade or non-comedo DCIS.

The method of detection of DCIS has changed significantly over the last 10 years. Currently, 85% of all DCIS is detected solely as a mammographic finding, which is most often characterized by the presence of micro-calcifications. The results of conservative surgery and radiation presented in Table 6-1 include data from a number of patients whose DCIS was clinically evident (i.e., palpable mass or bloody nipple discharge). The treatment of these patients not infrequently paralleled that of an invasive cancer (i.e., axillary node dissection or regional node irradiation and the use of adjuvant systemic therapy). There is limited information regarding the long-term results of conservative surgery and radiation for mammographically detected DCIS (Table 6-3). The collaborative group study[53] reported a 14% 10-year actuarial breast recurrence rate in 110 patients with mammographically detected DCIS, with a median follow-up of 9.3 years. For patients with negative margins of resection, the 10-year actuarial breast recurrence rate was 8%.

The differences in the reported breast recurrence rates for mammographically detected DCIS reflect variations in patient selection, surgical technique, and the extent of the mammographic and pathologic correlation. There is increasing evidence (Table 6-4) that positive and close margins result in an increased breast recurrence rate compared to negative margins. Silverstein et al.[61] reported a 25% breast recurrence rate for margins less than 1 mm versus 15% for 1 to 9 mm margins, and 3% for margins of 1 cm or more. Breast recurrence rates have ranged from 0%

**TABLE 6-2  Breast Recurrence Following Conservative Surgery and Radiation DCIS Related to Pathologic Features**

| | Breast Recurrence (%) | | | |
|---|---|---|---|---|
| Study | Comedo | High Grade | Noncomedo | Low Grade |
| Collaborative Group[50] | 7 | 21 | 15 | 13 |
| Kuske et al.[60] | 12 | | 0 | |
| Silverstein et al.[61] | 35 | 24 | 16 | 12 |
| White et al.[68] | 6 | 13 | 6 | 0 |
| Solin et al.[57] | 7 | 7 | 4 | 0 |
| Bornstein et al.[58] | 22 | 20 | 20 | 100 |
| Sneige et al.[52] | 11 | 4 | 10 | 0 |
| Fowble et al.[32] | 0 | | 0 | |

**TABLE 6-3  Results of Conservative Surgery and Radiation for Mammographically Detected DCIS**

| | | Breast Recurrence Rate (Invasive) (%)[a] | | | | |
|---|---|---|---|---|---|---|
| | Number of Patients | Actuarial | | | | Median Follow-Up (years) |
| Study | | 5 yr | 8 yr | 10 yr | Crude % | |
| Kuske et al.[60] | 44 | 7 | | | 7 (7) | 4 |
| Fowble et al.[32] | 110 | 1 (1) | | 15 (15) | 3 (3) | 5.3 |
| Hiramatsu et al.[56] | 54 | 2 | | 23 | 7 (2) | 6.2 |
| Vicini et al.[55] | 105 | 9 | | 10 | 10 (7) | 6.5 |
| Sneige et al.[52] | 31 | 0 | | 8 | 3 (0) | 7.2 |
| Silverstein et al.[61] | 185[b] | 13 | | 22 | 16 (9) | 7.5 |
| NSABP B17[33] | 411[c] | 10 | 12 (4) | | 11 (4) | 7.5 mean |
| Collaborative Group[53] | 110 | 7 | | 14 | 14 (5) | 9.3 |

[a]Number of patents in parentheses.

[b]Mammographically detected: 89%.

[c]Mammographically detected: 81%.

**TABLE 6-4    Results of Conservative Surgery and Radiation DCIS Related to Resection Margin Status**

| Study | Breast Recurrence (%)[a] Margin Status | | Median Follow-Up (years) |
| | Negative | Positive/Close | |
| --- | --- | --- | --- |
| McCormick et al.[51] | 19 (16) | 100 (3) | 3 |
| Kuske et al.[60] | 6 (16) | 0 (2) | 4 |
| NSABP B-17[36] | 4 (249) | 10 (50) | 4 |
| Ray et al.[567] | 8 (13) | 37 (8) | 5 |
| Fowble et al.[32] | 0 (68) | 8 (20) | 5.3 |
| Hiramatsu et al.[56] | 6 (34) | 4 (22) | 6.2 |
| Vicini et al.[55] | 6 (82) | 17 (24) | 6.5 |
| Sneige et al.[52] | 4 (25) | | 7.2 |
| Silverstein et al.[61] | 12 (124) | 25 (61) | 7.5 |
| Collaborative Group | | | |
| All patients[50] | 10 (95) | 17 (47) | 10 actuarial |
| Mammographically detected[53] | 7 (42) | 29 (17) | 9.3 |

[a]Number of patients in parentheses.

**TABLE 6-5    Breast Recurrence Rates in Patients with Mammographically Detected DCIS and Negative Margins Treated with Conservative Surgery and Radiation**

| Study | Definition Negative Margin | Crude Breast Recurrence Rate (%)[a] | Follow-Up (years) |
| --- | --- | --- | --- |
| Collaborative Group[53] | ≥ 2 mm | 7 (42) | 9.3 median |
| Silverstein et al.[61] | ≥ 1 mm | 12 (124) | 7.5 median |
| Fowble et al.[32] | ≥ 2 mm | 0 (68) | 5.3 median |
| NSABP B-17[36] | 1 cell | 4 (249) | 4 mean |
| Sneige et al.[52] | NS | 4 (25) | 10 actuarial |
| Vicini et al.[55] | ≥ 2 mm | 6 (82) | 6.5 median |

[a]Number of patients in parentheses.

to 12% for patients with mammographically detected DCIS and negative resection margins (Table 6-5).

An additional concern is the overall size or extent of DCIS that is acceptable for breast conservation therapy with radiation. Methods for assessing size or extent of DCIS include measuring the area of calcification on the mammogram, measuring the area on a given slide, or reporting the percentage of slides containing ductal carcinoma in situ. As noted earlier, the area of calcifications on a mammo-gram may underestimate the pathologic extent of DCIS[43,47]; therefore, determinations of size made solely by mammographic measurements may not be accurate. A single series[61] with mammographic and pathologic correlation reported increasing breast recurrence rates as the extent of DCIS increases. The crude breast recurrence rates were 7% for patients with DCIS of 1.5 cm or less, 24% for those of 1.6 to 4 cm, and 55% for DCIS of 4.1 cm or more. The median follow-up in this series was 7.5 years. These data would suggest that the maximum size of DCIS acceptable for breast conservation therapy with radiation is probably no greater than 4 cm.

Silverstein et al.[63] proposed the Van Nuys classification based on tumor size, margin status, and nuclear grade to predict breast recurrence rates for ductal carcinoma in situ following breast conservation treatment with or without radiation. There are three categories for each of the factors with an assigned score of 1 to 3. The size categories are as follows: ≤1.5 cm, 1.6 to 4 cm, and ≥4.1 cm. The margin categories are as follows: ≤1 cm, 1 to 9 mm, and >1 mm. The pathologic categories are low grade without necrosis, low grade with necrosis, and high grade with or without necrosis. For patients treated with conservative surgery and radiation, the 10-year actuarial disease-free survival was 100% for scores of 3–4, 77% for scores of 5–7, and 37% for scores of 8–9.[64] The general applicability of this prognostic score has been questioned,[65] since the precise measurement of some of the factors is difficult. In particular, the pathologic determination of the extent of DCIS requires complete and sequential sectioning of all tissue. Representative sections will not accurately determine the full extent of DCIS, although the area on a given slide may be assessed. The index has also been questioned in regard to the reproducibility of the pathologic classification as well as the difficulty in assessing resection margins.[65] The index weighs all three factors equally, but the assumption behind this practice may not be accurate. Patient age is not a consideration. The Van Nuys prognostic index, therefore, represents an attempt to assess treatment outcome based on three pathologic characteristics and does provide a framework for the comparison of treatment options. Its validity will require longer follow-up and confirmation by other groups.

The majority of breast recurrences in patients undergoing conservative surgery and radiation for ductal carcinoma in situ occur in the vicinity of the original tumor, and approximately 50% are invasive (Table 6-6). Therefore, the overall risk of a subsequent ipsilateral invasive breast cancer is approximately 5% (Table 6-3). The primary surgical

**TABLE 6-6   Patterns of Breast Recurrence and Results of Salvage Treatment DCIS Treated with Conservative Surgery and Radiation**

| Study | Total Number of Patients | Pathology Recurrence (% invasive) | Recurrence Among Those Who Died of Disease (%) | |
|---|---|---|---|---|
| | | | Noninvasive | Invasive |
| Ray et al.[567] | 5 | 20 | 0 | 0 |
| Haffty et al.[565] | 4 | 25 | 0 | 0 |
| McCormick et al.[51] | 8 | 37 | 0 | 0 |
| Howard et al.[573] | 3 | 33 | 0 | 0 |
| Solin et al.[57] | 5 | 40 | 0 | 0 |
| Silverstein et al.[61] | 30 | 53 | 0 | 19 |
| Collaborative Group[574] | 42 | 55 | 0 | 17 |
| Hiramatsu et al.[56] | 7 | 57 | 0 | 25 |
| Sneige et al.[52] | 5 | 60 | 0 | 33 |
| Vicini et al.[55] | 10 | 70 | 0 | 14 |
| Fourquet et al.[570] | 7 | 71 | 0 | 0 |
| Kurtz et al.[566] | 3 | 100 | | 33 |
| Kuske et al.[60] | 3 | 100 | | 0 |
| Fowble et al.[32] | 3 | 100 | | 0 |
| NSABP B-17[36] | 47 | 36 | 3 | 6 |

TABLE 6-7  Results of Conservative Surgery Alone for Mammographically Detected DCIS

| | | Breast Recurrence Rate (%) (Invasive)[a] | | | | |
|---|---|---|---|---|---|---|
| | | Actuarial | | | | Median Follow-Up (years) |
| Study | Number of Patients | 5 yr | 8 yr | 10 yr | Crude | |
| Dixon et al[575] | 36 | | | | 6 (3) | 3 |
| Silverstein[66] | 130 | 21 | | | 14 (5) | 3.8 |
| Hughes et al.[576] | 60 | 18 | | | 12 (7) | 3.8 |
| Schwartz[577] | 194 | 14 | | 25 | 14 (3) | 4.4 |
| Schreer[578] | 102 | | | | 24 (10) | 4.7 |
| Sibbering and Blarney[579] | 48 | | | | 6 (2) | 4.8 |
| Arnesson and Olsen[580] | 169 | 16 | | 22 | 15 (5) | 6.7 |
| NSABP B-17[33] | 403 | 21 (10) | 27 (14) | | 26 (13) | 7.5 mean |
| Lagios et al.[70] | 79 | 12 | | 19 | 19 (10) | 10.3 mean |

[a]Percent of invasive recurrences.

treatment for a recurrence following conservative surgery and radiation has been mastectomy. The results of salvage treatment in these patients are presented in Table 6-6. Virtually all patients who develop a noninvasive recurrence are salvaged, and approximately 75% of those with an invasive recurrence are salvaged. The 10- and 15-year cause-specific survival for patients with DCIS treated with conservative surgery and radiation ranges from 96% to 100%.[50,56,61,66–68]

Radiation for ductal carcinoma in situ should include tangential breast irradiation to total dose of 4600 to 5000 cGy delivered over a period of 4.5 to 5 weeks. For patients with negative resection margins in whom no boost is planned, the total breast dose should be 5000 cGy delivered at 200 cGy per fraction over a period of 5 weeks based on the NSABP B-17 trial.[33] The role of a localized boost in patients with ductal carcinoma in situ has not been evaluated. However, the general principles for the use of a boost in invasive breast cancer apply. A number of series have employed boost doses in the range of 1000 to 1600 cGy for total doses of 6000-6600 cGy to the biopsy site for patients with DCIS.[50] For patients with negative resection margins, the total dose to the biopsy site has ranged from 6000 to 6400 cGy, and for those with close or positive margins it

has ranged from 6400 to 7000 cGy. Neither axillary dissection not radiation of the regional nodes is indicated in ductal carcinoma in situ, since the risk of positive axillary nodes is 4% or less.[69]

## Conservative Surgery Alone

The rationale for treatment directed to less than the entire breast for DCIS is the observation that not all patients with ductal carcinoma in situ have multicentric disease, occult invasion, or recurrence following excision alone. Lagios[70] proposed the following criteria for selection of patients with DCIS for wide excision alone: mammographically detected DCIS presenting as microcalcifications (size $\leq$ 2.5 cm), negative resection margins, negative postbiopsy mammogram, and a patient capable of understanding the risk of subsequent recurrence and amenable to careful follow-up. With a mean follow-up of 10.3 years, 15 of the 79 (19%) patients in his study experienced a recurrence in the index breast. Fifty-three percent of the recurrences were an invasive cancer. A number of additional series using similar criteria have reported breast recurrence rates in patients whose sole treatment has been wide excision alone (Table 6-7). The actuarial breast recurrence rates have ranged from 12% to 21% at 5 years, and from 19% to 25% at 10 years.

The patterns of breast recurrence following conservative surgery alone for ductal carcinoma in situ are presented in Table 6-8. Similar to patients undergoing conservative surgery and radiation, the majority of recurrences occur in the vicinity of the primary tumor, and approximately 50% recur as an invasive tumor and 50% as a noninvasive tumor. The risk of a subsequent ipsilateral invasive breast recurrence (Table 6-7) ranges from 2% to 13% depending on the period of follow-up. Pathologic features that correlate with the risk of a breast recurrence following wide excision alone include the architectural pattern, nuclear grade, tumor size, and resection margins. Patients with comedo DCIS or high nuclear grade have been reported to have a higher ipsilateral breast tumor recurrence rate following wide excision alone compared to patients with noncomedo DCIS or low nuclear grade (Table 6-9). Lagios[70] reported a 15% crude breast recurrence rate for patients whose DCIS was less than 1.5 cm and 50% for those with DCIS of 1.6 to 4 cm treated with wide excision alone. The mean follow-up was 10 years. Silverstein[71] reported a 45% breast recurrence rate for patients with DCIS of 1.6 to 4 cm treated with wide excision alone with a median follow-up of 3.8 years. Hetelekidis et al.[72] reported a 25% 5-year actuarial breast recurrence rate for patients with margins less than 1 mm, 100% for positive margins, and 8% for margins exceeding 1 mm. Silverstein reported crude breast recurrence rates of 63% for patients undergoing conservative surgery alone with margins less than 1 mm and 16% for margins 1 to 9 mm and 5% for those over 1 cm.[66] The median follow-up in this group of patients was 3.8 years. The 10-year actuarial breast recurrence rates were 3% for women with a Van Nuys prognostic score of 3–4, 37% for 5–7, and 100% for 8–9.[64] Therefore, similar to patients undergoing conservative surgery and radiation, the extent of DCIS and margin width correlate with the risk of a breast recurrence in patients undergoing conservative surgery alone. Van Zee et al.[54] also reported increased breast recurrence rates for women under 40 years of age treated with wide excision alone. The 6-year actuarial breast recurrence rate was 54% for women under 40 years of age, 18% for those 40 to 69 years of age, and 12% for those 70 years of age or older.

The results of salvage treatment for a breast recurrence following wide excision alone in

TABLE 6-8  Results of Salvage Treatment in Patients with DCIS Initially Treated with Limited Surgery

| Study | Total Number of Patients | Recurrence, Invasive (%) | Recurrence Among Those Who Died of Disease (%) | |
| --- | --- | --- | --- | --- |
| | | | Noninvasive | Invasive |
| Gallagher et al.[569] | 5 | 60 | 0 | 100 |
| Lagios et al.[70] | 15 | 53 | 0 | 0 |
| Arnesson and Olsen[580] | 24 | 33 | 0 | 0 |
| Fisher et al.[73] | 9 | 56 | 0 | 40 |
| Rosen et al.[581] | 10 | 80 | 0 | 37 |
| Page et al.[582] | 7 | 100 | | 43 |
| Silverstein[66] | 18 | 33 | 0 | 0 |
| Price et al.[583] | 22 | 54 | 0 | 17 |
| Schwartz[577] | 28 | 18 | 0 | 0 |
| Sibbering and Blarney[579] | 3 | 33 | 0 | 0 |
| Schreer[578] | 24 | 42 | 0 | 10 |
| NSABP B-17[36] | 104 | 50 | 0 | 2 |

TABLE 6-9    Breast Recurrence Following Conservative Surgery Alone—DCIS Related to Pathologic Features

| | Breast Recurrence (%) | | | |
| Study | Comedo | High Grade | Noncomedo | Low Grade |
|---|---|---|---|---|
| Bellamy et al.[584] | 42 | 40 | 18 | 0 |
| Lagios et al.[42] | 32 | 32 | 6 | 3 |
| Schwartz[577] | 32 | | 2 | |
| Ottensen et al.[585] | 48 | 31 | 14 | 6 |
| Kuske et al.[60] | 100 | | | |
| NSABP B-17[36] | | 17 | | 11 |
| Warneke et al.[564] | 27 | | 0 | |
| Silverstein[66,71] | | 64 | | 10 |
| Schreer[578] | 26 | | 20 | |

patients with DCIS are presented in Table 6-8. All the noninvasive recurrences have been salvaged, with approximately 75% of invasive recurrences salvaged.

## Comparisons of Treatment Options

As noted earlier, treatment options for ductal carcinoma in situ include wide excision with or without radiation or mastectomy. A single prospective randomized trial reported the results of these three treatment options.[45,73] While the NSABP B-06 trial was designed for early stage invasive breast cancer, 76 patients with ductal carcinoma in situ were inadvertently randomized. The majority of these patients presented with a palpable mass. In the 21 patients who underwent excision with negative margins, breast recurrence developed in 43%, and 10% of these patients died of their disease. Of the 27 patients randomized to conservative surgery and radiation, 7% developed a breast recurrence and none have died of their disease. Twenty-eight patients underwent mastectomy; none experienced a chest wall recurrence, and 4% died of their disease. The NSABP B-17 trial randomized patients with ductal carcinoma in situ to wide excision with or without radiation.[33,74] Eighty-one percent of these patients had DCIS detected solely by mammography, and negative margins of resec-

tion were required for entry into the trial. The 8-year actuarial risk of a breast recurrence in patients undergoing wide excision alone was 27% versus 12% in patients undergoing wide excision and radiation. The 8-year actuarial risk of an ipsilateral invasive cancer was 4% in patients undergoing conservative surgery and radiation versus 13% for those undergoing wide excision alone. These two trials demonstrate a significant decrease in breast recurrence rates following wide excision alone with the addition of radiation. The B-17 trial suggested that this decrease was most evident for the subsequent development of an ipsilateral invasive cancer.

The primary issue in the selection of treatment options for patients with DCIS is to identify women who will not develop a breast recurrence (either noninvasive or invasive) after wide excision alone and for whom radiation may be omitted. In the NSABP B-17 trial, significant factors for breast recurrence were margin status and the presence of moderate to marked comedo necrosis.[36] Table 6-10 presents clinical outcome related to treatment for this trial.

In each of the subgroups shown in Table 6-10, radiation diminished the risk of a breast recurrence; for patients with negative margins of resection, however, the crude breast recurrence rate for lesions with absent to slight necrosis was 7% without radiation versus 4% with radiation. For patients with negative margins and moderate to marked necrosis, radiation decreased the crude breast recurrence rate from 16% to 4%. This trial suggests that patients who benefit least from radiation are those with negative margins and absent to slight necrosis.

Table 6-11 presents preliminary results of trial 10853 of the European Organization for Research and Treatment of Cancer (EORTC). There appears to be no significant difference in breast recurrence rates when patients who did receive radiation are compared with those who did not; however, the median follow-up reported by the Milan group is only 2.7 years. Retrospective comparisons of conservative surgery alone versus conservative surgery and radiation based on the Van Nuys prognostic index, Lagios's criteria, patient age, tumor size, and margin width are presented in Table 6-12. The addition of radiation to conservative surgery alone resulted in a statistically significant decrease in ipsilateral breast tumor recurrence rates for the Van Nuys prognostic index scores of 5–7 and 8–9 but not 3 and 4.[64] Radiation diminishes the risk of a breast recurrence in patients of all ages, those with larger tumors, or margin width less than 1 mm. Its role in the treatment of small, adequately excised (margin $\geq$ 1 cm), low grade DCIS requires further evaluation.

## The Role of Tamoxifen in the Treatment of Ductal Carcinoma In Situ

Approximately 50% of all DCIS lesions are estrogen receptor positive, and estrogen receptor positivity has been correlated with low nuclear grade and noncomedo DCIS.[75] If the inhibition of progression of DCIS by tamoxifen is dependent on the estrogen receptor, patients who would be expected to benefit most from tamoxifen would be those with low nuclear grade DCIS or noncomedo DCIS.[76,77] Two prospective randomized trials have evaluated the role of tamoxifen in the treatment of ductal carcinoma in situ. The United Kingdom randomized trial began in 1990 and randomized women 50 to 64 years of age with mammographically detected DCIS to no further therapy, radiation, tamoxifen for 5 years, or both radiotherapy and tamoxifen for 5 years, following wide excision. The end point

**TABLE 6-10   Breast Recurrence Related to Pathologic Findings from the NSABP B-17 Randomized Trial[36]: Conservative Surgery (CS) Versus CS Plus Radiation Therapy (XRT)**

| Finding | Crude Breast Recurrence (%)[a] | |
|---|---|---|
| | CS | CS & XRT |
| Nuclear grade | | |
| Poor | 17 (128) | 7 (147) |
| Good | 11 (146) | 3 (152) |
| Necrosis | | |
| Moderate/marked | 19 (123) | 5 (131) |
| Absent/slight | 9 (151) | 5 (168) |
| Histologic subtype | | |
| Pure solid | 17 (69) | 8 (53) |
| Pure cribriform | 9 (33) | 0 (69) |
| Mixed | 13 (172) | 2 (177) |
| Mean follow-up, 4 years | | |

[a]Total number of patients in parentheses.

**TABLE 6-11** **Results of Prospective Randomized Trials Evaluating Conservative Surgery with and Without Radiation DCIS**

| Study | Number of Patients | Breast Recurrence (Invasive)[a] (%) | | | Interval Reported (years) |
|---|---|---|---|---|---|
| | | No XRT | XRT | All Patients | |
| NSABP B-17[33] | 790 | 27 (13) | 12 (4) | | 7.5 mean |
| EORTC 10853[586] | 1010 | | | 15 (5) | 4.5 median |
| Milan[587] | 151 | 13 (8) | 12 (5) | 12 (7) | 2.7 median |

[a]Percent of invasive recurrences in parentheses.

of the study is the subsequent development of an ipsilateral invasive breast cancer. The NSABP B-24 trial randomized patients from 1992 to 1994 with ductal carcinoma in situ to wide excision and radiation or wide excision, radiation, and tamoxifen for 5 years. The trial broadened the criteria for conservative surgery and radiation and included patients with grossly negative margins, unifocal or gross multicentric disease, and focal or diffuse microcalcifications. Microscopically negative margins were not required. The end point of the study is ipsilateral breast tumor recurrence. The trial has accrued 1804 patients.

## Summary

Standards for the evaluation and treatment of DCIS developed by the American College of Radiology, the American College of Surgeons, the Society of Surgical Oncology, and the College of American Pathologists were reported in 1998 by Winchester and Strom.[78] Mastectomy is the preferred surgical treatment for patients with ductal carcinoma in situ whose primary tumor extent is greater than 4 cm, determined either pathologically or clinically, for those in whom negative margins of resection cannot be achieved after a reasonable attempt at surgical excision, and for those in whom there is clinical evidence of more than one area of ductal carcinoma in situ in the breast or for whom mastectomy is the chosen treatment. Patients who are candidates for conservative surgery and radiation include those with ductal carcinoma in situ 4 cm or less in extent, determined either clinically or pathologically, those for whom the DCIS clinically is confined to one area of the breast, and those for whom negative margins of resection can be achieved following a reasonable surgical excision. The risk of an ipsilateral breast tumor recurrence is minimized in patients undergoing conservative surgery and radiation when margins of resection are 2 mm or more. Patients with low to intermediate grade DCIS ($\leq$ 2.5 cm measured pathologically) with negative resection margins ($>$ 2 mm) and a negative postbiopsy mammogram may be candidates for wide excision alone.

The Eastern Cooperative Oncology Group has initiated a prospective study of local excision alone for selected patients with ductal carcinoma in situ. Patients eligible for this study include those with low or intermediate grade DCIS ($\leq$ 2.5 cm measured pathologically) and high grade DCIS ($\leq$ 1 cm measured pathologically). The DCIS must be mammographically detected and margins must be 3 mm or more. The end points of this study are ipsilateral breast tumor recurrence rates at 5 years (invasive or noninvasive cancer). Early stopping rules for this study include an ipsilateral breast tumor recurrence rate of exceeding 10% at 5 years, pathology discordance on central review of more than 15% for the diagnosis of DCIS, or more than 25% discordance for nuclear grade. The results of this study will

**TABLE 6-12   Retrospective Comparisons of Conservative Surgery with and Without Radiation DCIS**

| | Breast Recurrence (%)[a] | | Follow-Up |
|---|---|---|---|
| | No XRT | XRT | (years) |
| Lagios's criteria | | | |
| Lagios et al.[70] | 19 (79) | | 10 actuarial |
| Fowble et al.[32] | | 0 (16) | 4.9 median |
| Collaborative Group[53] | | 0 (21) | 9.3 median |
| Silverstein[66] | 14 (64) | 10 (98) | 5 actuarial |
| Van Nuys Prognostic Score[64] | | | 10 actuarial |
| 3–4 | 3 (81) {>0.05} | 0 (35) | |
| 5–7 | 37 (115) {0.03} | 23 (130) | |
| 8–9 | 100 (13) {0.03} | 63 (20) | |
| Age[54] | | | |
| < 40 years | 54 | 40 | 6 actuarial |
| 40–69 years | 18 | 9 | |
| ≥ 70 years | 12 | 0 | |
| Tumor size | | | |
| ≤ 1.5 cm | | | |
| Lagios et al.[70] | 15 (71) | | 10 mean |
| Silverstein[66] | | 7 (108) | 7.5 median |
| 1.6–4 cm | | | |
| Lagios et al.[70] | 50 (8) | | 10 mean |
| Silverstein[66] | 45 (48)[b] | 24 (66)[c] | 3.8 mean[b] |
| | | | 7.5 median[c] |
| Margin width[66] | | | |
| < 1 mm | 63 (28)[b] | 25 (61)[c] | 3.8 mean[b] |
| 1–9 mm | 16 (49)[c] | 15 (95)[c] | 7.5 median[c] |
| ≥ 1 cm | 5 (53)[b] | 3 (29)[c] | |

[a] Number of patients in parentheses.
[b]
[c]

provide further information regarding the role of wide excision alone in selected patients with DCIS.

## STAGE I AND II INVASIVE BREAST CANCER

### Breast Conservation Therapy

*Introduction*   The traditional surgical approach throughout most of the twentieth century for early stage invasive breast cancer has been the radical or modified radical mastectomy. With the published results of conservative surgery and radiation from single institutions followed by the demonstration that breast con-servation therapy was equal to mastectomy in six prospective randomized trials, the 1980s began to witness a slow but gradual transition from an almost exclusively mastectomy-based pattern of care to a more balanced one including breast conservation. Despite initial progress, recent studies indicate that in the United States only 40% to 45% of patients with early stage breast cancer undergo breast preserving surgery with or without radiation.[79–81] Geographic variations have been documented,[82,83] and the passage of legislation requiring a discussion of treatment options has not significantly altered practice patterns.[84] The underutilization of breast-conserving surgery has been attributed in part to surgical recommendations based on individual physician preference rather than clinical or pathologic factors necessitating a mastectomy.[85–89] The standards for breast conservation therapy were reported in 1998 by Winchester and Cox.[90]

### Results of Prospective Randomized Trials Comparing Mastectomy with Conservative Surgery and Radiation for Early Stage Invasive Breast Cancer

The first prospective randomized trials to compare breast conservation therapy with mastectomy were initiated by the Institut Gustave-Roussy (IGR) in 1972 and the Milan Cancer Institute in 1973. These trials were followed by four additional ones in the United States and Europe (Table 6-13). These latter trials expanded patient eligibility to include primary tumors up to 4 to 5 cm and clinically positive nonfixed axillary nodes. The trials have varied in the degree of surgical resection, technical aspects of radiation, and the use of adjuvant systemic therapy. Despite these variations, the results have been consistent (Tables 6-13 and 6-14). The trials have demonstrated no significant difference in terms of local regional recurrence, distant metastases, or long-term survival for the two treatments. In particular, two of the trials reported no improvement in survival in axillary node positive patients treated with mastectomy.[91,92] In the NSABP B-06 trial, the 8-year actuarial overall survival was 60% for patients undergoing mastectomy versus 68% for those undergoing conservative surgery and radiation.[91] In the Milan I trial, the 10- and 18-year overall survival rates were 77% and 58% for patients undergoing quadrantectomy, axillary dissection, and radiation, and 66% and 55% for those undergoing radical mastectomy.[92] Morris et al.[93] performed a meta-analysis of these trials with updated patient data from the National Cancer Institute, the European Organization for Research and Treatment of Cancer, and Institut Gustave-Roussy trials. The pooled odds ratio at 10 years favored breast conservation therapy over mastectomy for overall survival. Some of the trials employed postmastectomy irradiation in axillary node positive patients, and in these trials the results appeared equal. The Early Breast Cancer Trialists' Cooperative Group[94] also performed a meta-analysis of nine prospective randomized trials comparing breast conservation surgery and mastectomy. There were no survival differences in seven of the trials, and local recurrences were reported in 6.2% of the mastectomy patients and 5.9% of the patients treated with conservative surgery and radiation. In summary, six randomized trials have found no disadvantage for the use of conservative surgery and radiation in appropriately selected patients with stage I-II breast cancer in terms of local–regional recurrence, distant metastases, or overall survival.

**TABLE 6-13** **Prospective Randomized Trials Comparing Conservative Surgery[a] and Radiation with Mastectomy for Early Stage Breast Cancer**

| Study[b] | Treatment Period | Number of Patients | Primary Tumor Size | Stage | Surgery for Primary Tumor | Adjuvant Treatment |
|---|---|---|---|---|---|---|
| Milan I[92,441] | 1973–80 | 701 | ≤ 2 cm | I | Q, RM | CMF |
| IGR[546] | 1972–80 | 179 | ≤ 2 cm | I | WE, MRM | None |
| NSABP B-06[129] | 1976–84 | 1219 | ≤ 4 cm | I-II | WE, MRM | Melphalan, F |
| NCI[127] | 1979–87 | 237 | ≤ 5 cm | I-II | LE, MRM | AC |
| EORTC[128] | 1980–86 | 874 | ≤ 5 cm | I-II | LE, MRM | CMF |
| DBCG[588] | 1983–89 | 904 | T1-T3 | I-III | WE, Q, MRM | CMF, T |

[a]Q, quadrantectomy; RM, radical mastectomy; WE, wide excision; MRM, modified radical mastectomy; LE, local excision; C, cyclophosphamide; A, doxorubicin; M, methotrexate; T, tamoxifen; F, 5-fluorouracil.

[b]IGR Institut Gustave-Roussy; NSABP, National Surgical Adjuvant Breast and Bowel Project; NCI, National Cancer Institute; EORTC, European Organization for Research and Treatment of Cancer; DBCG, Danish Breast Cancer Group.

*Patient Selection* The majority of patients with stage I-II breast cancer are candidates for breast conservation therapy. Surgery consists of an excision of the primary tumor, which ideally achieves pathologically negative resection margins, and a level I-II axillary dissection. Various clinical and pathologic factors should be considered before breast conservation therapy is recommended. The clinical factors include past medical history, patient age, family history, the clinical presentation, tumor size and location, and breast size. The pathologic factors include the presence or absence of ductal carcinoma in situ and its extent, histology, lymphatic invasion, axillary nodal status, and resection margin status. The potential for an unacceptable cosmetic result, a significant risk of complications, or a substantial risk of ipsilateral breast tumor recurrence may favor a recommendation for mastectomy.

*Clinical Factors* Women with breast cancer and a history of preexisting collagen vascular disease (lupus, scleroderma, or mixed connective tissue disease) have developed severe fibrosis or soft tissue or bone necrosis after receiving conventional doses of radiation.[95-99] A history of lupus or scleroderma is considered by most investigators to be an absolute contraindication to conservative surgery and radiation. Conservative surgery and radiation may be considered in patients with rheumatoid arthritis.[100] One series,[97] however, reported late complications in two patients with rheumatoid arthritis who received radiation for breast cancer. These complications, however, were not representative of the severe fibrosis or soft tissue necrosis reported with lupus or scleroderma.[97] Patients who have received prior chest or mantle irradiation are generally not considered to be candidates for conservative surgery and radiation for breast cancer. The potential for severe complications from reirradiation of the soft tissues and ribs as well as the possibility of a late radiation-induced sarcoma warrants a recommendation for mastectomy. Pregnant women should not receive breast irradiation during their pregnancy because of the scattered dose to the fetus. Therefore, it is important to evaluate the medical history in all patients to determine whether there is a history of scleroderma or lupus, mantle or chest irradiation, or the possibility of pregnancy.

A number of series have evaluated the role of conservative surgery and radiation in young women ($< 35$ years of age) with early stage invasive breast cancer (Table 6-15). The majority of these series have demonstrated an increased risk of ipsilateral breast tumor recurrence in young women undergoing conservative surgery and radiation in comparison to older women. However, the magnitude of this risk has varied, ranging in some from 10% to 15% at 5 years to 20% to 25% in others. It has been suggested that some of this increased risk of breast recurrence may be due to a greater prevalence of tumors with an extensive

**TABLE 6-14  Results of Prospective Randomized Trials Comparing Conservative Surgery and Radiation (BCT) with Mastectomy**

| Study | Local Recurrence (%) | | Overall Survival (%) | | Interval Results Reported (years) |
|---|---|---|---|---|---|
| | BCT | M | BCT | M | |
| Milan I[92] | 7 | 4 | 65 | 65 | 18 |
| IGR[546] | 9 | 14 | 73 | 65 | 15 |
| NSABP B-06[129] | 10 | 8 | 63 | 59 | 12 |
| NCI[127] | 16 | 6 | 77 | 75 | 10 |
| EORTC[128] | 13 | 9 | 54 | 61 | 8 |
| DBCG[588] | 5 | 6 | 79 | 82 | 6 |

**TABLE 6-15    Breast Recurrence Following Conservative Surgery and Radiation Related to Young Age (≤ 35 years)**

| Study | Breast Recurrence (%) at Younger/Older Age[a] | | Follow-up (years) |
| | ≤ 35 years | ≥ 35 years | |
| --- | --- | --- | --- |
| Burke et al.[113] | 0 (45) | 5 (467) | 5 actuarial |
| Clarke et al.[130] | 9 (32) | 5 (424) | 5 mean |
| Halverson et al.[589] | 9 (37) | 12 (474) | 7 actuarial |
| Vicini et al.[104] | 12 (44) | 7 (554) | 5 actuarial |
| Veronesi et al.[92] | 13 (168) | 6 (2065) | 8.5 median |
| Dewar et al.[166,b] | 14 (105) | 7 (652) | 9 median |
| Haffty et al.[590] | 15 (34) | 11 (349) | 8.2 median |
| Matthews et al.[108] | 15 (72) | 5 (306) | ≥ 2 |
| Pierce et al.[116] | 15 (20) | 6 (135) | 5 actuarial |
| Kurtz et al.[103] | 16 (91) | 10 (1291) | 11 mean |
| Vicini et al.[104] | 21 (65) | 9 (721) | 5 actuarial |
| Cabanes et al.[187] | 24 (35) | 7 (623) | 5 actuarial |
| Fisher et al.[153] | 24 (38) | 7 (450) | 8 median |
| Fowble et al.[106] | 24 (64) | 13 (916) | 8 actuarial |
| Kini et al.[591] | 25 (20) | 7 (380) | 10 actuarial |
| Fourquet et al.[105,c] | 34 (35) | 9 (483) | 8.6 median |

[a]Total number of patients in parentheses.

[b]< 32 years.

[c]< 40 years.

intraductal component in young women or to the presence of adverse histopathologic factors, including high nuclear and histologic grade or the presence of necrosis.[101-103] Inadequate surgery of the primary tumor has been associated with an increased risk of breast recurrence in young women.[104,105] Vicini et al.[104] reported a decrease in the 5-year actuarial risk of breast recurrence in young women from 20% to 12% with the use of reexcision. However, in the series reported by Fowble et al.,[106] reexcision did not appear to diminish the risk of a breast recurrence in young women. The use of adjuvant systemic chemotherapy has been reported to decrease the risk of breast recurrence in young women undergoing conservative surgery and radiation.[106,107] Young women undergoing mastectomy have been reported to have an increased risk of local–regional recurrence over older women, and this risk appears to be similar to the risk of an ipsilateral breast tumor recurrence.[108-110] There is no evidence to suggest that young women

treated by mastectomy have a survival or disease-free survival benefit compared with those receiving conservative surgery and radiation.[108] Therefore, young age is not a contraindication to breast conservation therapy. However, the use of adjuvant systemic chemotherapy and an excision that achieves negative resection margins will diminish the risk of a subsequent ipsilateral breast tumor recurrence.

It is estimated that 5% to 10% of women with breast cancer have hereditary breast cancer (autosomal dominant Mendelian pattern of inheritance), and 20% have familial breast cancer (one or more first- or second-degree relatives without an autosomal dominant pattern).[111] The identification of the *BRCA1* and *BRCA2* breast cancer susceptibility genes has directed increasing attention to the hereditary form of breast cancer and its treatment. Some authors have recommended mastectomy as the preferred surgical treatment for these women. There is little information regarding the efficacy of conservative surgery and radiation in women with hereditary breast cancer. However, several series have reported the outcome of breast conservation therapy in women with a positive family history of breast cancer.[112–117] There is no evidence that women with a positive family history of breast cancer have a higher risk of ipsilateral breast tumor recurrence versus those with a negative family history. However, patients with hereditary breast cancer have not been distinguished from those with familial breast cancer. The frequency of *BRCA1* mutations increases as the number of affected relatives increases.[118,119]

Peterson et al.,[114] in a series from the University of Pennsylvania and Fox Chase Cancer Center, reported a decrease in breast recurrence rates as the number of affected relatives with breast cancer increased. In this series, there were no breast recurrences in the 14 patients with three or more affected relatives. The 5-year actuarial breast recurrence rate was 8% for the 47 patients with two affected relatives and 6% for the 203 patients with one affected relative. For the 517 patients without a family history of breast cancer, the 5-year actuarial rate of breast recurrence was 9%. The role of conservative surgery in young women ($\leq$ 35 years of age) with a positive family history has been evaluated by two series.[114,117] In both series, women with a positive family history had a lower 5-year actuarial breast recurrence rate than young women with a negative family history. Therefore, based on the available information, a positive family history of breast cancer is not a contraindication to conservative surgery and radiation. Further studies are needed for women with proven hereditary breast cancer.

The clinical presentation of more than one area of malignancy in a single breast demonstrated by physical examination and/or mammogram is a relative contraindication to breast conservation therapy. This presentation has been termed "clinically apparent gross multicentric or multifocal disease," with the distinction between multifocal and multicentric based on whether the lesions are confined to a single quadrant or are present in separate quadrants. Three series have reported breast recurrence rates of 35% to 40% in patients with clinical evidence of more than one malignancy in a single breast treated with conservative surgery and radiation.[120–122] The increased risk is similar for both gross multifocal and multicentric disease and does not appear to be diminished for lesions in the same quadrant.[121] The increased risk of breast recurrence in patients with clinical gross multicentric or multifocal disease is related to a significant residual tumor burden, as demonstrated by pathologic studies at the University of Pennsylvania and Fox Chase Cancer Center.[123] In 57 patients with gross multifocal or multicentric disease who underwent mastectomy, residual tumor was identified in 46% of the patients in two or more quadrants of the breast. Multifocal disease may also be identified grossly by the surgeon intraoperatively or by the pathologist on gross examination of the biopsy specimen. Breast recurrence rates in patients with pathologic gross multifocal disease have ranged from 4% to 50%.[120–122,124] Wilson et al.[122] reported no breast recurrences in four patients with gross multifocal disease detected intraoperatively by the surgeon. For patients undergoing mastectomy for gross multiple focal or multicentric disease, local–regional recurrence rates are under 10%.[123] Therefore, for patients with clinical evidence of more than one cancer in a single breast, mastectomy is the recommended surgical procedure.

Five of the six prospective randomized trials, and the majority of the retrospective single institution studies, have limited consideration of breast conservation therapy to tumors no larger than 4 to 5 cm. The rationale for this size limitation is based on mastectomy series that have demonstrated a significant risk of multicentricity for tumors 5 cm or greater in size.[125,126] There appears to be no significant difference in breast recurrence rates when T1 and T2 tumors are compared, provided an adequate excision has been performed.[127–134] The role of breast conservation therapy in T3 tumors is being evaluated in studies employing neoadjuvant chemotherapy to reduce the size of the primary tumor prior to radiation. The results of these studies are discussed later in the chapter.

The location of the primary tumor in the breast may impact on cosmetic results. Approximately 10% of patients with subareolar tumors require resection of the nipple–areolar complex to achieve negative margins.[135,136] The subsequent appearance of the breast may be unacceptable to some patients. However, the cosmetic result is likely to be as good as that of the reconstructed breast following mastectomy. Patients with subareolar tumors have not been found to have a risk of ipsilateral breast tumor recurrence that is increased in comparison to those with tumors in the outer or inner quadrants.[112,135–137]

In patients with very small breasts, a complete excision of the primary tumor may result in an unacceptable cosmetic defect. Patients with large, pendulous breasts or obese patients are less likely to receive a good to excellent cosmetic result because of dose inhomogeneity, resulting in an increased incidence of breast fibrosis and retraction.[138–141] However, reconstruction following mastectomy in these patients may be more complex and may require reduction mammoplasty of the contralateral breast. Breast size is becoming less important in the selection of patients for conservative surgery and radiation with improved radiotherapy technique and the use of high energy photon beams with beam spoilers.[142] Experience with conservative surgery and radiation in the prosthetically augmented breast is limited. The primary concern is cosmesis and is related to the development of capsular contracture. Fair to poor cosmetic results have been reported in a significant percentage of these patients.[143–147] Mark et al.[143] reported capsular contracture and fair to poor cosmetic results in 12 of 21 patients (57%) with augmentation mammoplasty treated with conservative surgery and radiation. The median follow-up was 1.8 years, and the results were not correlated with the location or type of implant or radiation dose. Victor et al.,[147] however, reported excellent or good cosmetic results in all eight patients with augmented breasts treated with radiation, with a median follow-up of 2.7 years.

*Pathologic Factors*  A number of pathologic factors have been evaluated for their ability to identify patients with an increased risk of ipsilateral breast tumor recurrence following conservative surgery and radiation.

Approximately 70% to 80% of all invasive breast cancers are of ductal histology, and 50% of these have ductal carcinoma in situ (DCIS) associated with the invasive cancer.[148] Schnitt et al.[149] first described the pathologic entity of an extensive intraductal component (EIC). By their criteria, EIC-positive tumors were characterized by the simultaneous presence of ductal carcinoma in situ comprising 25% or more of the primary tumor and its presence in the normal surrounding breast tissue. The definition also included microinvasive ductal cancer (i.e., DCIS with focal areas of invasion). Women with EIC-positive tumors have been reported to have a higher rate of breast recurrence than EIC-negative women in the majority of series (Table 6-16). This increased risk of breast recurrence appears to be related to the presence of a significant residual tumor burden following simple gross excision. Studies of mastectomy specimens have demonstrated that at a distance of 2 cm from the edge of the primary tumor, 59% of EIC-positive tumors had residual disease (primarily DCIS) versus 29% of EIC-negative tumors.[150] Residual carcinoma was found at a distance of 6 cm from the primary tumor in 21% of the EIC-positive tumors and 8% of the EIC-negative tumors. Negative pathologic resection margins (i.e., 1–2 mm) are important to diminish the risk of a breast recurrence in EIC-positive tumors.[113,151–154] Patients with EIC-positive tumors with close or positive resection margins have had breast recurrence rates in the range of 20% to 40%,[113,151,154] versus 11% or less with negative margins.[113,151,153–155] Gage et al.[154] divided margin involvement into focal ($\leq$ 3 low power fields) and diffuse ($> 3$ low power fields). Diffuse margin involvement for EIC-positive tumors resulted in a 42% 5-year crude breast recurrence rate. In contrast, women with EIC-positive tumors with focally positive margins had a 7% 5-year crude breast recurrence rate. Therefore, pathologic assessment of resection margin status is important in determining treatment options for EIC-positive tumors. If a reasonable attempt at surgical excision cannot achieve negative margins, mastectomy is the preferred surgical treatment.

Approximately 20% to 30% of all invasive breast cancers are lobular or special histologic subtypes of ductal cancer (i.e., medullary, colloid, or mucinous and tubular cancers). These patients are candidates for breast conservation therapy, provided the presence of other clinical or pathologic factors does not exclude them (Table 6-17). Invasive lobular cancers may be diffuse in the breast, and not infrequently demonstrate a pathologic extent which is not clinically appreciated. Negative resection margins are important to assure that these patients can be offered conservative surgery and radiation with an acceptable breast recurrence rate.[156] Approximately one-third of tubular cancers have an extensive intraductal cancer, and the foregoing discussion of EIC-positive tumors is applicable to these patients.[157]

In contrast to an extensive intraductal component, the presence of lobular carcinoma in situ (LCIS) in association with an invasive ductal or lobular cancer does not increase the risk of an ipsilateral breast tumor recurrence. Schnitt et al.[158] reported 10-year crude breast recurrence rates of 12% and 0% for invasive lobular cancers with or without LCIS, respectively, 10% and 14% for invasive ductal cancers with or without LCIS, and 16% and 15% for mixed invasive ductal and lobular cancers with or without LCIS. The extent of the LCIS did not correlate with the risk of an ipsilateral breast recurrence. Moran and Haffty[159] reported a 23% 10-year actuarial breast recurrence rate for patients with an invasive ductal or lobular cancer and LCIS, compared with 16% for those without LCIS. LCIS as previously discussed is considered a pathologic marker that identifies patients at increased risk for the subsequent development of a cancer. A similar pathologic marker is atypical ductal hyperplasia. When found in

**TABLE 6-16    Breast Recurrence Related to the Presence of an Extensive Intraductal Component (EIC)**

| Study | Breast Recurrence (%)[a] | | Follow-up (years) |
| --- | --- | --- | --- |
| | EIC Negative | EIC Positive | |
| Bartelink et al.[152] | 2 (208) | 9 (79) | 5 |
| Krishnan et al.[592] | 5 (189) | 9 (61) | 5 |
| Burke et al.[113] | 2 (369) | 10 (69) | 5 |
| Paterson et al.[593] | 3 (190) | 11 (46) | 4 |
| Fisher et al.[153] | 9 (366) | 11 (56) | 8 median |
| Zafrani et al.[594] | 6 (361) | 11 (63) | 5 |
| Salvadori et al.[595,b] | 8 (1751) | 16 (152) | 11 median |
| Jacquemier et al.[596] | 8 (390) | 18 (105) | 5 |
| Fowble et al.[597] | 4 (252) | 22 (23) | 5 |
| Harris et al.[598] | 6 (418) | 23 (166) | 5 |
| Leborgne et al.[134] | 8 (769) | 23 (48) | 6 median |
| Veronesi et al.[92,441,c] | 8 (307) | 30 (38) | 5 |

[a]Number of patients in parentheses.

[b]Quadrantectomy.

[c]Tumorectomy.

**TABLE 6-17   Breast Recurrence Following Conservative Surgery and Radiation Related to Histology**

| | Breast Recurrence (%)[a] | | | | |
|---|---|---|---|---|---|
| Study | Invasive Ductal | Invasive Lobular | Medullary | Colloid | Tubular |
| Mate et al.[599] | 13 (108) | 25 (12) | | | |
| Calle et al.[463] | 8 (193) | 0 (4) | | | |
| Peiro et al.[600] | 16 (930) | 18 (77) | | | |
| Bouvet et al.[156] | | 10 (74) | | | |
| Poen et al.[601] | | 2 (60) | | | |
| White et al.[602] | 4 (346) | 3 (30) | | | |
| Silverstein et al.[603] | 5 (534) | 5 (65) | | | |
| Salvadori et al.[595] | 7 (1903) | 7 (286) | | | |
| Burke et al.[113] | 4 (448) | 10 (14) | | | |
| Bornstein et al.[604] | 13 (682) | 15 (54) | | | |
| Leborgne et al.[134] | 9 (791) | 9 (35) | 13 (15) | 23 (13) | |
| Kurtz et al.[566] | 9 (709) | 14 (67) | 4 (27) | 0 (11) | |
| Weiss et al.[605] | 8 (757) | 9 (41) | 4 (28) | 18 (12) | 14 (18) |
| Haffty et al.[606] | 15 (761) | 17 (54) | 25 (17) | 0 (16) | 0 (21) |
| Vicini et al.[607] | 9 (343) | 3 (31) | 0 (3) | 0 (13) | 0 (13) |

[a]Number of patients in parentheses.

the normal background breast tissue of an invasive cancer, atypical ductal hyperplasia also does not seem to be a predictor for an increased risk of ipsilateral breast tumor recurrence in patients treated with conservative surgery and radiation.[32]

The presence of lymphatic vascular invasion has been correlated with an increased risk of ipsilateral breast tumor recurrence as well as distant metastases in patients undergoing quadrantectomy and axillary dissection.[160] Veronesi et al.[160] reported a 21% 8-year cumulative incidence of breast recurrence in patients with lymphatic/vascular invasion versus 6% in the absence of this feature.

Patients with histologically positive axillary nodes do not have an increased risk of ipsilateral breast tumor recurrence (Table 6-18). The diminished risk of a breast recurrence in these patients may be related to the combined effects of chemotherapy and/or hormonal therapy (see discussion integration systemic therapy).

As noted earlier, negative resection margins are important to minimize the risk of an ipsilateral breast tumor recurrence in patients with EIC-positive tumors. Assessment and signifi-

cance of resection margins in other clinical scenarios remain controversial, however. Part of the controversy relates to differences of opinion on how to best assess the resection margin and to the lack of a consensus on what constitutes a negative margin. Currently, the most commonly used pathologic method for

**TABLE 6-18   Breast Recurrence Following Conservative Surgery and Radiation Related to Pathologic Nodal Status**

| | Breast Recurrence (%) | |
|---|---|---|
| Study | Node Negative | Node Positive[a] |
| Clarke et al.[130] | 4 | 7 |
| Fowble et al.[131] | 8 | 7 |
| Boyages et al.[137] | 14 | 9 |
| Haffty et al.[446] | 12 | 4 |
| Leborgne et al.[134] | 9 | 8 |
| Veronesi et al.[454] | 7 | 5 |
| NSABP B-06[129] | 12 | 5 |
| NCI[127] | 13 | 7 |
| Milan I[92,441] | 10 | 3 |
| EORTC[128] | 10 | 19 |

[a]With chemotherapy, 15; without chemotherapy, 23.

assessing microscopic margins involves the inking of the breast specimen with sections taken perpendicular to the inked surface. The distance between the cancer cells and the inked margin determines the margin status. An alternative pathologic method consists of shaving some or all of the surface of the specimen in a tangential manner. Cancer cells anywhere on these histologic sections indicate a positive margin. The shaved-margin technique may be more accurate than the use of perpendicular sections of the margins for identifying microscopically positive margins.[161] Some surgeons initially excise the biopsy cavity and then take an additional rim of tissue from all the margins. Cancer found in this additional rim of tissue implies a positive margin. With this technique, the identification of the location of the positive margin allows for a more directed reexcision if indicated. There appears to be general agreement on the definition of a positive margin: namely, cancer cells (invasive or DCIS) at the resection margin. Margin positivity can be focal ($\leq$ 3 low power fields) or diffuse ($>$ 3 low power fields), single or multiple.[154] The definition of a negative margin has ranged from no cancer cells at the margin to a distance of greater than 1 to 2 mm. Some series have used the term "close margin" for cancer cells within 1 to 2 mm but not at the margin.[131,154,162]

The influence of resection margin status on breast recurrence rates has varied (Table 6-19). The majority of the series demonstrate an increased risk of breast recurrence in patients with positive margins. This risk is most evident at 10 years[163–167] and appears to be related to the fact that patients with positive margins more often have larger primary tumors, positive axillary nodes, and receive adjuvant systemic therapy.[168–170] Adjuvant chemotherapy and/or hormonal therapy has delayed the median interval to a breast recurrence from 3 years to 6 to 7 years, and at least initially, appears to decrease the risk of a breast recurrence in patients with positive margins.[168] Patients for whom positive margin(s) have resulted in a significant risk of ipsilateral breast

tumor recurrence include young women, those with EIC-positive tumors, and those who do not receive adjuvant chemotherapy and/or hormonal therapy.[154,166,168] Diffuse margin involvement or involvement of two or more margins has resulted in breast recurrence rates of 40% in some series.[154,164] Ideally, negative margins of resection should be achieved in all patients undergoing breast conservation therapy to minimize the risk of ipsilateral breast tumor recurrence.

## Radiotherapy Considerations for Breast Conservation Therapy

Following surgical excision of the primary and an axillary node dissection, radiation is directed to the entire breast via tangential fields to a total dose of 4500 to 5000 cGy in a period of 4.5 to 5.5 weeks. Prolongation of the overall treatment time with less than 800 cGy delivered per week has resulted in breast recurrence rates of 25% to 30%.[171,172] Following treatment to the entire breast, a supplemental dose of radiation (i.e., boost) may be given to the excisional biopsy site via radioactive implant, electrons, or photons. There has been no correlation between the type of boost selected and the subsequent risk of a breast recurrence.[165,167,173] The routine use of a boost in patients with negative resection margins has been questioned by the findings from the NSABP B-06 randomized trial.[129] In this trial patients with negative margins received 5000 cGy (200 cGy/day) in 5 weeks to the entire breast with a boost. The 10-year cumulative incidence of a recurrence was 12% and was comparable to that reported by series employing a boost[151,163,165–167] in similar patients. [Institutions that employ a boost in patients with negative margins often use a lower total dose to the entire breast (4500–4600 cGy) than the NSABP B-06 guidelines. The boost dose then achieves $\geq$ 6000 cGy to the biopsy site. Romestaing et al.[174] reported the results of a prospective randomized trial comparing 5000 cGy to the breast with or without a 1000 cGy

**TABLE 6-19  Breast Recurrence Related to Microscopic Resection Margin**

| | Breast Recurrence (%)[a] | | |
| --- | --- | --- | --- |
| | Node Positive | Node Negative | Interval Reported (years) |
| Fein et al.[168] | 5 (106) | 4 (554) | 5 actuarial |
| Anthony et al.[608] | 5 (251) | 4 (651) | 5 actuarial |
| Clarke et al.[130] | 9 (88) | 4 (274) | 5 mean |
| Smitt et al.[151] | 9 (14) | 2 (157) | 5 actuarial |
| Pierce et al.[116] | 10 (33) | 3 (363) | 5 actuarial |
| Anscher et al.[609] | 10 (32) | 2 (132) | 5 actuarial |
| Slotman et al.[610] | 10 (31) | 3 (459) | 5.7 mean |
| Heiman et al.[611] | 11 (82) | 2 (762) | 5 actuarial |
| Dewar et al.[166] | 14 (149) | 6 (514) | 10 actuarial |
| Gage et al.[154] | 16 (131) | 3 (107) | 5 crude |
| Mansfield et al.[165] | 16 (143) | 8 (561) | 10 actuarial |
| Veronesi et al.[441] | 17 (46) | 9 (243) | |
| Fowble et al.[163] | 17 (157) | 8 (973) | 10 actuarial |
| Kini et al.[591] | 17 (30) | 6 (300) | 10 actuarial |
| Spivak et al.[612] | 18 (44) | 4 (214) | 4 mean |
| Van Donegan et al.[613] | 20 | 9 | 8 actuarial |
| Kurtz et al.[103] | 24 (49) | 8 (283) | 5.9 median |
| Pittinger et al.[614] | 25 (4) | 3 (122) | 4.5 median |
| Komarnicky et al.[164] | 33 (92) | 15 (371) | 10 actuarial |

[a]Number of patients in parentheses.

boost in patients with primary tumors of 3 cm or less and negative margins. The 5-year actuarial breast recurrence rate was 4.5% for no boost versus 3.6% for the boost arm. However, the 8-year actuarial rate was 21% for patients who did not receive a boost versus 5% for those who did. The results of the EORTC randomized trial of boost versus no boost in a similar group of patients will provide further information. The use of a boost in patients with positive or unknown margins has resulted in decreased breast recurrence rates in comparison to no boost.[130,175,176]]

The role of regional node irradiation in patients with early stage invasive breast cancer remains controversial. There is general agreement that treatment of the axillary, supraclavicular, and internal mammary nodes is not indicated in women with histologically negative axillary nodes who have had an adequate axillary dissection. The role of regional node irradiation in axillary node positive patients undergoing conservative surgery and radiation

has been evaluated by two prospective randomized trials.[177,178]

In the first 2 years of the Milan I trial, patients with positive axillary nodes were randomized to regional node irradiation (33 patients) versus none (23 patients).[177] At 10 years, the disease-free survival was better in the group who did not receive regional node irradiation (68% vs. 40%).[177] In the Institut Gustave-Roussy trial, patients with positive axillary nodes randomized to regional node irradiation (41 patients) had a 5-year relapse-free survival of 62% versus 66% for 31 patients who did not receive this treatment.[178] Regional node recurrences, however, were fewer in the women who received radiation (19% vs. 35%). The Milan I trial subsequently omitted regional node irradiation in axillary node positive patients based on the initial findings.

In the NSABP B-06 trial, radiation was directed to the breast only in axillary node negative and positive patients. The median follow-up was 11 years, and the regional node recurrence rates was 5.1% for all patients.[129] Regional node recurrence rates from retrospective series as correlated with the number of positive nodes are presented in Table 6-20. There appears to be little benefit from regional node irradiation in patients with one to three positive axillary nodes. However, supraclavicular recurrences are diminished in patients with four or more positive nodes receiving radiation to this region.[179–182] The supraclavicular field also includes level III axillary nodes, and is also indicated in patients whose highest dissected axillary node is positive. Level I and a portion of the level II axillary nodes are included within the tangential fields.

Extracapsular extension used to be an indication for axillary irradiation. However, several recent studies have failed to demonstrate an increased risk of axillary failure in these patients without axillary radiation following an adequate axillary dissection.[183–186] Axillary radiation in patients with clinically negative axillary nodes results in regional control rates comparable to those of an axillary dissection.[187,188] Therefore, in patients not undergoing an axillary dissection, regional radiation may be employed. The extent of the radiation required for control in the axilla has been questioned. Several recent series have demonstrated low axillary recurrence rates in elderly women with small primary invasive cancers ($\leq$ 1–2 cm) whose axillary nodes were included solely in the tangential breast fields.[189–194] These women have a relatively low risk of positive axillary nodes and may not require treatment to the supraclavicular field with or without a posterior axillary field. Treatment directed to the internal mammary nodes has not resulted in a significant decrease in the clinical incidence of internal mammary node recurrences in patients undergoing breast conservation therapy.[195,196]

If a decision is made to treat the regional nodes, the total dose is 4500 to 5000 cGy over 4.5 to 5.5 weeks (180–200 cGy per fraction). Match line techniques for the supraclavicular and tangential fields are discussed later in the chapter. For treatment of the internal mammary nodes, the use of electrons or a combination of electrons and photons minimizes the dose to the lung, heart, and thoracic spine and decreases the incidence of symptomatic pneumonitis in comparison to photons alone.[197–199] The use of deep tangents to treat the internal mammary nodes may result in irradiation of a significant amount of heart and/or lung.[197,199] There is increasing evidence that the posterior axillary field may not be required to treat the

**TABLE 6-20  Regional Node Recurrence in Axillary Node Positive Patients Related to the Number of Positive Nodes and the Region(s) Treated**

| Region Treated | Regional Node Recurrence (%)[a] | |
| --- | --- | --- |
| | 1–3 Positive Nodes | $\geq$ 4 Positive Nodes |
| Breast | | |
| Recht et al.[200,203] | 2 (47) | 0 (10) |
| Fowble et al.[196] | 2 (44) | |
| Halverson et al.[202] | 0 (28) | 0 (2) |
| Vicini et al.[181] | 6 (38) | 17 (13) |
| Breast and regional nodes | | |
| Recht et al.[200,203] | 1 (276) | 2 (98) |
| Fowble et al.[196] | 3 (180) | 5 (64) |
| Halverson et al.[202] | 2 (65) | 15 (20) |
| Vicini et al.[181] | 7 (31) | 0 (24) |

[a] Total number of patients in parentheses.

axilla and does not decrease axillary recurrence rates over use of tangents and a supraclavicular field.[200–203]

## The Role of Radiation Following Conservative Surgery in Women with Early Stage Invasive Breast Cancer

As the equivalence of breast conservation therapy and mastectomy became evident through the published results of randomized trials, the role of radiation following conservative surgery was questioned. The rationale for treatment directed to the entire breast either by mastectomy or radiation is based on the potential for microscopic foci of tumor in areas separate from the index cancer. Approximately 25% to 30% of patients who undergo excision of the primary tumor that achieves negative margins will have residual tumor at the time of reexcision or mastectomy despite negative margins.[151,204–209] Factors that have been associated with a low risk of residual tumor at a distance 2 to 3 cm beyond the index cancer include small primary tumor size (≤ 2 cm), noncentral tumor location, older age, absence of an extensive intraductal component, lymphatic invasion or invasive lobular cancer, low histologic grade, and negative axillary nodes.[125,210,211]

The role of radiation following partial mastectomy or quadrantectomy has been evaluated in six prospective randomized trials (Table 6-21). Four of the trials included axillary node positive patients who also received adjuvant systemic therapy. The results of the trials are presented in Table 6-22. All these trials have demonstrated a significant reduction in the incidence of breast recurrence with the addition of radiation in both axillary node negative and axillary node positive patients. Without radiation, ipsilateral breast tumor recurrence rates have ranged from 12% to 40% in the axillary node negative patients and 27% to 41% in the axillary node positive patients.

A number of clinical and pathologic factors have been evaluated for their correlation with an increased risk of ipsilateral breast tumor recurrence in patients undergoing conservative surgery alone both in the prospective randomized trials and in retrospective series. Clinical factors associated with an increased risk of ipsilateral breast tumor recurrence include primary tumor size and young age.[212–218] Pathologic factors include the presence of an extensive intraductal component, lymphatic invasion, positive margins, and positive axillary nodes.[212,214,215,218–221] The presence of one or more of these factors results in a 30% to 40% risk of breast recurrence. Table 6-23 summarizes factors from the various series that have been identified as having a low risk of ipsilateral breast tumor recurrence. In these selected patients, the risk of an ipsilateral breast tumor recurrence ranges from 0% to 18%.

Table 6-24 presents the results of conservative surgery with or without radiation for T1, pathologic node-negative patients from the retrospective series and prospective randomized trials. Even in this select group of patients, radiation appears to decrease the risk of a breast recurrence, although the magnitude of the benefits varies. Schnitt et al.[222] reported the results of a single-arm prospective clinical trial of conservative surgery only for 87 patients with T1 pathologic node-negative breast cancer. With a median follow-up of 4.7 years, the breast recurrence rate was 16%. An increased risk of early recurrence (i.e., within 3 years) was observed for high histologic grade tumors, patients with a positive family history of breast cancer, and pathologic tumor size exceeding 1 cm. The authors concluded that despite careful patient selection (primary tumor size ≤ 2 cm, no extensive intraductal component, no lymphatic–vascular invasion, negative margins, and a negative postbiopsy mammogram), the risk of a breast recurrence was unacceptably high.

Four ongoing prospective randomized trials are evaluating conservative surgery with or without radiation in the treatment of early stage invasive breast cancer. The Cancer and Leukemia Group B (CALGB) trial randomizes to breast irradiation and tamoxifen or ramoxifen alone women 70 years of age and older with primary tumors of 2 cm or less, negative

TABLE 6-21   Prospective Randomized Trials Comparing Conservative Surgery with and Without Radiation

| | | | Study | | | |
|---|---|---|---|---|---|---|
| | Swedish[225] | Milan[92,213,441] | OCOG[226] | NSABP B-06[129] | Scottish[354,615] | British[221] |
| Treatment period | 1981–88 | 1987–89 | 1984–89 | 1976–84 | 1983–89 | 1981–90 |
| Number of patients | 381 | 601 | 837 | 1265 | 584 | 399 |
| Tumor size | < 2 cm | < 2.5 cm | < 4 cm | < 4 cm | < 4 cm | ≤ 5 cm |
| 1° surgery | Q | Q | WE | WE | WE | WE |
| Margins | Negative | | Negative | Negative | | |
| Axillary nodes | Negative | Positive, negative | Negative | Positive/Negative | Positive/Negative | Positive–Negative |
| Adjuvant treatment | None | CMF TAM | None | L-PAM[a] 5FU | CMF TAM | CMF TAM |
| Follow-up, years | 5.3 mean | 3.2 mean | 7.6 median | 12.5 mean | 5.7 median | > 5 |

[a]L-Phenylalanine mustard.

resection margins, and a clinically negative axilla. Axillary node dissection is optional. The accrual goal is 572 patients over 38 months to detect a 50% reduction (20% to 10%) in the risk of a breast recurrence with radiation. The Princess Margaret trial randomizes women 50 years of age and older with primary tumors of 4 cm or less, negative margins of resection, and pathologically negative axillary nodes to tamoxifen with or without breast irradiation. Women 65 years of age and older with clinically negative axillary nodes are eligible without an axillary dissection. The accrual goal is 900 patients over 5 years to detect a 7% difference in the 4-year disease-free survival. The EORTC trial randomizes pathologic node negative women 50 years of age and older with primary tumors of 2 cm or less and negative margins of resection to radiation versus no radiation. Tamoxifen is optional, and the accrual goal is 874 women. The NSABP B-21 trial randomizes patients with invasive cancers under 1 cm and negative axillary nodes to radiation with or without tamoxifen or tamoxifen alone. The accrual goal is 1350 patients.

The role of tamoxifen as a substitute for breast irradiation has been evaluated in several series. Breast recurrence rates of 5% to 20% have been reported in elderly women with T1-T2 tumors treated with wide excision and tamoxifen.[223,224] Lee et al.[223] reported a 4% crude breast recurrence rate at 8 years in women above 70 years of age with T1 tumors treated with wide excision and tamoxifen. This was similar to the 5% rate for those treated with wide excision and radiation. However for T2 or T3 tumors, wide excision and radiation resulted in a decreased risk of breast recurrence when compared to wide excision and tamoxifen (10% vs. 32%). Cooke et al.[224] compared wide excision and tamoxifen to wide excision, radiation, and tamoxifen in axillary node positive, estrogen receptor positive patients. The addition of radiation diminished the risk of a breast recurrence in all patients, as well as in those with negative margins of resection. It is unknown at present whether tamoxifen will significantly decrease the risk of a breast recurrence in selected elderly women with early stage breast cancer and obviate the need for

**TABLE 6-22  Results of Prospective Randomized Trials Comparing Conservative Surgery (CS) with and Without Radiation (XRT)**

| Study | Primary Tumor Size (cm) | Breast Recurrence | | Overall Survival (%) | | Interval Results Reported (years) |
|---|---|---|---|---|---|---|
| | | CS | CS & XRT | CS | CS & XRT | |
| Swedish, node negative[225] | ≤2 | 18 | 2 | 90 | 91 | 5 actuarial |
| Milan III[92,213,441] | <2.5 | 18 | 2 | 92 | 92 | 5 actuarial |
| Node negative | | 12 | 2 | 95 | 98 | 3 actuarial |
| Node positive | | 27 | 4 | | | |
| NSABP B-06[129] | <4 | 35 | 10 | 58 | 62 | 12 actuarial |
| Node negative | | 32 | 12 | 74 | 78 | 10 actuarial |
| Node positive | | 41 | 5 | 62 | 70 | 8 actuarial |
| Ontario, node negative[226] | <4 | 40 | 18 | 72 | 74 | 10 actuarial |
| Scottish[354,a] | <4 | 28 | 6 | 85 | 88 | 5 actuarial |
| ER positive | | 25 | 3 | | | 5.1 median |
| ER negative | | 44 | 14 | | | 5.5 median |
| British[221] | ≤5 | 35 | 13 | | | 5 |
| Node negative | | 32 | 9 | | | |
| Node positive | | 39 | 20 | | | |

[a]ER, estrogen receptor.

radiation. The results of these ongoing trials will help to clarify this issue. In addition, the Joint Center for Radiotherapy (JCRT) has initiated a single-arm prospective study of wide excision and tamoxifen for women with T1 invasive ductal cancers without an extensive intraductal component or lymphatic invasion and with negative axillary nodes.

Even though radiation has demonstrated a significant decrease in the risk of an ipsilateral breast tumor recurrence in almost all patients evaluated, a significant survival benefit has yet to be demonstrated. Three of the prospective randomized trials evaluating radiation following breast conservation surgery have reported distant metastasis for pathologic node-negative patients.[129,225,226] In all three of these trials, patients treated with conservative surgery only had a higher incidence of distant metastasis than those who received radiation. In the Ontario Clinical Oncology Group trial, the radiation patients had a higher incidence of distant metastasis as first site of failure, while the conservative surgery alone group had a higher incidence of distant metastases occurring after an ipsilateral breast tumor recurrence, resulting in higher total incidence of distant metastasis in patients who did not receive radiation.[226] Fisher et al.[129] reported a statistically significant or nearly significant improvement in disease–free and distant disease-free survival with the addition of radiation to wide excision and axillary node-negative patients in the NSABP B-06 trial. Unfortunately, distant metastases were not reported for axillary node positive patients, and only one of the trials has reported survival results for axillary node positive women.[91] As presented in Table 6-22 the survival benefit for radiation for axillary node negative patients ranges from 1% to 4%. Radiation resulted in an 8% survival benefit in axillary node positive patients in the NSABP B-06 trial at 8 years.[91] None of these differences was statistically significant because of the low number of patients in the trials. For patients with the lowest risk of breast recurrence without radiation (i.e., elderly, pathologically node negative, no extensive intraductal component or lymphatic invasion, primary tumor size ≤ 1 cm, negative margins, estrogen receptor positive), a survival benefit of 1% to 4% could be expected with the addition of radiation.

In summary, breast conservation therapy for early stage invasive breast cancer currently includes radiation in almost all patients. For axillary node negative patients, the addition of radiation decreases the risk of an ipsilateral breast tumor recurrence from 20% to 30% to 5% to 10%, resulting in a 1% to 4% improvement in overall survival. For axillary node posi-

TABLE 6-23   Identification of Low Risk Patients with Invasive Breast Cancer and Negative Margins for Conservative Surgery Alone

| Study | Low Risk | Breast Recurrence (%) | Follow-Up (years) |
|---|---|---|---|
| Schnitt et al.[222] | Pathology N0, ≤ 2 cm, tubular, mucinous | 0 | 4.7 median |
| Swedish[225] | Pathology N0, ≤ 2 cm, > 60 years | 6 | 5 actuarial |
| McCready et al.[215] | Pathology N0, ≥ 50 years, EIC and LVI negative, ER positive | 6 | 10 actuarial |
| Moffat et al.[616] | Pathology N0, ≤ 2.5 cm, LVI and EIC negative | 9 | 7.2 median |
| Milan III[213] | EIC negative, age > 55 years | 9 | 8 actuarial |
| Dalberg et al.[214] | Pathology N0, age ≥ 50 years | 9 | 10 actuarial |
| Clark et al.[226] | ≥ 50 years ≤ 1 cm | 18 | 7.6 median |

**TABLE 6-24    Results of Conservative Surgery with and Without Radiation: T1, Pathology N0, Invasive Breast Cancer**

| Study | No XRT | XRT | Follow-up (years) |
|---|---|---|---|
| Schnitt et al.[222] | 16 | 0 | 4.7 median |
| Moffat et al.[616] | 9 | 0 | 7.2 median |
| Milan III[92,441] | 12 | 2 | 5 actuarial |
| Swedish[225] | 18 | 2 | 5 actuarial |
| NSABP B-06[212] | | | 8 actuarial |
| < 1 cm | 24 | 15 | |
| 1–2 cm | 34 | 18 | |
| Ontario[226,a] | | | 7 median |
| 1 cm | 28 | 10 | |
| 1–2 cm | 33 | 9 | |
| Silvestrini et al.[617] | | | 6 actuarial |
| ≤ 1 cm | 21 | 14 | |
| > 1 cm | 19 | 10 | |

[a]Age > 50 years.

tive patients, the addition of radiation decreases the risk of an ipsilateral breast tumor recurrence from 30% to 50% to 10% and, in one of the prospective randomized trials, resulted in an 8% improvement in overall survival.[91]

## Postmastectomy Radiation for Early Stage Invasive Breast Cancer

**Background**    As discussed earlier in this chapter, approximately 50% or more of patients with early stage invasive breast cancer in the United States are treated by mastectomy. Some of the earliest prospective randomized trials evaluated the role of postmastectomy radiation in patients who did not receive adjuvant systemic therapy. Surgery for the primary tumor consisted of radical mastectomy, modified radical mastectomy, or simple mastectomy, with or without radiation. The results of the trials are presented in Table 6-25. These early trials have been criticized for lack of a consistent randomization process and inadequate stratification,[227–229] unequal patient distribution among the treatment arms,[227] the use of confounding adjuvant therapy including oophorectomy[227,230] and chemotherapy,[227] and inadequate radiation in terms of the total dose employed[227–232] and/or the regions treated.[227–230] Irrespective of the

variations in the patient population and radiotherapy technique, the results from the trials are similar. All have demonstrated a decrease in the incidence of local–regional recurrence with radiation. Four of the five trials that reported the incidence of distant metastasis demonstrated an initial increase in this site of failure in patients who received radiation.[188,230,233–235] A significant improvement in disease-free survival was reported by four of the trials.[188,230,235,236] Five of the trials demonstrated an improvement in survival,[188,230,235–237] with an absolute benefit ranging from 1% to 8%. The benefit was greatest for axillary node positive patients (3–8%). However, this benefit was not statistically significant in any of the trials.

A combined analysis of the long-term results of the Oslo and Stockholm trials[235] reported a significant improvement in the 10-year disease-free and distant disease–free survival in axillary node positive patients who received radiation. A meta-analysis of the mortality results from eight of these randomized trials was first published in 1987 by Cuzick et al.[238] and updated in 1994.[239] In the initial analysis, there was no survival benefit with radiation for the first 10 years of follow-up. However, in patients who survived more than 10 years, radiation was associated with increased mortality. Subsequent

**TABLE 6-25  Prospective Randomized Trials Comparing Radical Mastectomy (RM), Modified Radical Mastectomy (MRM), and Simple Mastectomy (SM), with and Without Radiation (R)**

| Conditions | Treatment Period | Number of Patients | Stage | Local–Regional Recurrence (%) | | Overall Survival (%) | | Follow-Up (years) |
|---|---|---|---|---|---|---|---|---|
| | | | | M | M & R | M | M & R | |
| RADICAL MASTECTOMY | | | | | | | | |
| Manchester[228,229] | | | | | | | | |
| I | 1948–52 | 720 | I-II | | | | | 30 |
| Node neg. | | | | | | 24 (0.05) | 12 | |
| Node pos. | | | | | | 9 (0.9) | 9 | |
| II | 1953–55 | 741 | I-II | | | | | 30 |
| Node neg. | | | | | | 25 (0.13) | 16 | |
| Node pos. | | | | | | 10 (0.7) | 10 | |
| NSABP B-02[227] | 1961–68 | 787 | I-III | 19 | 8 | 62 | 56 | 5 |
| MODIFIED RADICAL MASTECTOMY | | | | | | | | |
| Oslo[230] | | | | | | | | |
| I | 1964–67 | 546 | I-II | | | | | 14 |
| Stage I | | | | | | 69 | 70 | |
| Stage II | | | | | | 35 | 56 | |
| II | 1968–72 | 542 | I-II | | | | | |
| Stage I | | | | | | 76 (0.12) | 63 | |
| Stage II | | | | | | 45 | 48 | |
| Stockholm[235] | 1964–67 | 644 | I-III | 33 (<0.001) | 9 | 51 (0.09) | 59 | 15 |
| Node negative | | | | 23 (<0.001) | 5 | 64 | 69 | |
| Node positive | | | | 48 (<0.001) | 15 | 31 | 40 | |
| SIMPLE MASTECTOMY | | | | | | | | |
| Cancer Research Campaign[233,234] | 1970–75 | 2800 | I-II | 39 (<0.001) | 17 | 55 (0.88) | 55 | 10 |
| Southampton[237] | 1973–76 | 150 | I-II | 28 (<0.05) | 9 | 78 | 81 | 3 |
| Manchester Regional[236] | 1970–75 | 714 | I | 42 (<0.0001) | 22 | 55 (0.20) | 62 | 10 |
| Edinburgh I[261] | 1974–79 | 342 | I-II | 24 | 14 | 80 | 73 | 4 |

reports from the individual trials[230,240–242] indicated that the increase in mortality was related to cardiovascular disease. In the 1994 update,[239] the significant increase in mortality for the 10-year survivors was no longer evident. However, an increase in cardiac deaths was observed in patients who received radiation, but this was offset by a decrease in the number of breast cancer–related deaths. After 15 years, cardiac-related causes of death increased in patients who had undergone a radical or modified radical mastectomy followed by radiation. It was most apparent in women who were 50 years of age or older and clinically node negative. The increased incidence of cardiac deaths was seen in the trials that employed orthovoltage radiation[241,243] or cobalt-60 radiation to the internal mammary nodes.[230,242]

In 1995 the Early Breast Cancer Trialists' Cooperative Group (EBCTCG) published a second meta-analysis of prospective randomized trials of radiation and surgery for operable breast cancer.[94] This analysis included 36 trials initiated before 1985, 32 of which evaluated the role of postmastectomy irradiation with or without chemotherapy. The cause of death was available from 28 of the trials. Overall mortality was not increased in the patients who received radiation. Radiation resulted in a decrease in the number of breast cancer deaths but an increase in the number of non–breast cancer deaths, which for the first two decades after treatment was more evident in women 60 years of age or older. These meta-analyses suggest improvements in radiation technique could diminish the risk of cardiac morbidity and non–breast cancer related deaths.

### Risk Factors for Local–Regional Recurrence

Perhaps the most substantial criticism of these early prospective randomized trials is that the majority of patients did not have a significant risk for postmastectomy local–regional recurrence, and therefore, the expected benefit from radiation would be minimal. Several clinical and pathologic factors have been correlated with the risk of a local (chest wall) or regional (axilla, supraclavicular, or internal mammary node) recurrence following radical or modified radical mastectomy. The two most important factors appear to be the axillary nodal status and the size of the primary tumor. Patients with primary tumors 5 cm or more in diameter as well as those with four or more positive axillary nodes have been reported to have a 25% to 30% incidence of local–regional recurrence.[227,244–251] Patients with primary tumors 2 cm or less and/or negative axillary nodes have a much lower risk of local–regional recurrence ($\leq$ 10%).[227,244–246,249–251] For patients with one to three positive axillary nodes and/or primary tumor between 2 and 5 cm, the risk of a local–regional recurrence is approximately 15%.[227,244–246,249–251] Additional factors that may contribute to an increased risk of local–regional recurrence in otherwise low risk patients include high histologic grade and young age.[108,152,244,252–254] Pectoral fascia involvement has also been reported to result in a 30% risk of local–regional recurrence.[244,255]

The correlation between the status of the mastectomy resection margin and chest wall recurrence is controversial. In axillary node negative patients with primary tumors of 5 cm or less and a close margin ($\leq$ 4 mm), the reported incidence of local–regional recurrence is 6%.[256] Mentzer et al.[257] were unable to correlate the incidence of local–regional recurrence with margin status in 100 women with stage II breast cancer. Margin status, however, was assessed grossly in 67% of these patients. A recent study from Fox Chase Cancer Center[258] reported a 28% 8-year actuarial rate of local–regional recurrence in women 50 years of age or under with primary tumor size of 5 cm or more and zero to three positive nodes with close ($\leq$ 5 mm) or positive mastectomy margins. In contrast, none of the patients over 50 years of age with similar features experienced a local–regional recurrence. The risk of an axillary recurrence is related to the extent of the axillary surgery as well as the number of axillary nodes removed. Axillary recurrence rates range from 17% to 37% in patients with a clinically negative undissected axilla.[188,245,259–262] Forty percent of patients with clinically positive nodes who do not undergo an axillary node dissection will experience progression within 2 years.[259] Fisher et al.[263] correlated the risk of an axillary recurrence with the number of axillary nodes removed. Axillary recurrence occurred in 27% of the patients who had no nodes removed, 11% with fewer than 6 nodes, 5% with 6 to 10 nodes, and <1% for more than 10 nodes. Fowble et al.[255] reported a 15% incidence of local–regional recurrence at 3 years for patients with 10 or fewer axillary nodes examined versus 10% for those with more than 10 nodes examined. Supraclavicular recurrences have been correlated with positive axillary nodes. The incidence of a supraclavicular recurrence ranges from 10% to 26% for patients with positive axillary nodes to 5% or less for those with negative axillary nodes.[227,264] The majority of supraclavicular recurrences are associated with positive nodes at multiple levels or extensive axillary node involvement.[265] Clinical internal mammary node recurrences have been reported in fewer than 10% of all patients undergoing modified radical or radical mastectomy.[188,227,255,264,266–269] There appears to be some correlation between the location of the primary tumor and positive axillary nodes and the clinical incidence of internal mammary recurrence.[270]

The most common location of an isolated local–regional recurrence following mastectomy is the chest wall.[195,235,271–274] The second most common site is the supraclavicular nodes.[195,235,271–273] Axillary recurrences are uncommon in patients who have had an adequate axillary dissection, and clinical internal mammary recurrences, as just noted, occur in fewer than 10% of all patients undergoing mastectomy for early stage invasive breast cancer.

There is little evidence to suggest that adjuvant systemic chemotherapy significantly impacts on the overall incidence or pattern of local–regional recurrence following mastectomy. Similar to the findings of studies of patients treated without adjuvant systemic therapy, axillary node negative patients have a low risk of recurrence (i.e., ≤ 10%).[275–279] In patients with primary tumors of 5 cm or

more and four or more positive axillary nodes, the incidence of local–regional recurrence is 20% to 30%.[251,255,280–287] Patients with one to three positive axillary nodes have a 10% to 15% incidence of local–regional recurrence.[11,13,50,56,61,69,76,97,122,243,282] Young age has also been correlated with an increased incidence of local–regional recurrence in patients receiving postmastectomy adjuvant chemotherapy.[281,288]

Adjuvant systemic therapy may also delay the interval to local–regional recurrence. For patients not receiving adjuvant therapy, the majority of postmastectomy local–regional recurrences occur within 5 years of surgery,[271,289–293] with a peak incidence in the second year.[290] For patients receiving adjuvant systemic therapy, 30% to 40% of the local–regional recurrences occur after 3 years.[285,294] Pisansky et al.[285] reported a 3- and 8-year cumulative incidence of isolated local–regional recurrence of 12% and 20%, respectively, in axillary node positive patients entered into prospective randomized trials evaluating cyclophosphamide, 5-fluorouracil, and prednisone with or without radiation. In a more recent review,[295] the incidence of isolated local–regional recurrence following mastectomy in axillary node positive patients did not appear to be influenced by the use of multiagent chemotherapy versus single agent,[296] long versus shorter duration of therapy,[297–301] modifications of cyclophosphamide, methotrexate, and 5-fluorouracil,[302–305] the use of doxorubicin-based regimens,[306–309] or sequential versus alternating regimens.[284,310–312] There are minimal data on the incidence of postmastectomy local–regional recurrence in patients receiving dose-intensive chemotherapy with or without autologous bone marrow transplant or peripheral stem cell reinfusion.[201,313–317] In the Cancer and Leukemia Group B trial,[315] low dose, low intensity CAF (cyclophosphamide, doxorubicin, 5-fluorouracil) resulted in a higher incidence of local–regional recurrence. However, dose-intensive CAF was not associated with a lower incidence of local–regional recurrence than the same total dose of CAF given in a moderately dose-intensive regimen. Peters et al.[317] reported local–regional recurrences at the first site of failure in three of nine patients with 10 or more axillary nodes who received standard dose CAF followed by high dose chemotherapy (cyclophosphamide, cisplatin, carmustine), and autologous bone marrow transplant. This observation prompted the routine use of postmastectomy radiation in patients with 10 or more positive nodes in two prospective ongoing randomized trials evaluating high dose chemotherapy with autologous bone marrow transplantation (CALGB 9082 and Intergroup 0121).

The effect of tamoxifen on postmastectomy local–regional recurrence has varied. The addition of oophorectomy or tamoxifen to chemotherapy in axillary node positive premenopausal women has not significantly decreased the incidence of local–regional failures or altered the proportion of failures that are local–regional.[255,294,318,319] In postmenopausal women, the addition of tamoxifen to chemotherapy,[255,296,320–322] or the addition of chemotherapy to tamoxifen,[302,321,323–326] has decreased the incidence of a local–regional recurrence by a modest amount. The NSABP B-14 trial demonstrated a decrease in the incidence of local recurrence with tamoxifen versus observation alone for estrogen receptor positive axillary node negative women.[284]

### Relative Effectiveness of Radiation Versus Systemic Therapy
Two prospective randomized trials have suggested that postmastectomy radiation is more effective than chemotherapy in the prevention of a local–regional recurrence.[327–329] In the Stockholm Breast Cancer Group trial, premenopausal and postmenopausal women with positive axillary nodes and primary tumor size exceeding 3 cm were randomized to postmastectomy radiation or CMF (cyclophophamide, methotrexate, 5-fluorouracil). With a median follow-up of 6.5 years, the local–regional recurrence rate was 12% in the radiation group and 22% in the chemotherapy group ($p = 0.001$). In the Glasgow randomized trial comparing postmastec-

tomy radiation, CMF, and radiation plus CMF, the local–regional recurrence rate was 31% for patients receiving CMF versus 16% for those receiving radiation with or without CMF.[328,329]

The relative effectiveness of tamoxifen over radiation in the prevention of postmastectomy local–regional recurrence was evaluated in the South Sweden Breast trial.[330] The patients (719 postmenopausal women) were randomized to radiation alone, radiation plus tamoxifen, or tamoxifen alone. With a median follow-up of 8 years, the incidence of local–regional recurrence was 8%, 6%, and 18%, respectively. Two prospective randomized trials have evaluated the addition of tamoxifen to postmastectomy radiation. In the Stockholm trial, 427 postmenopausal women with positive axillary nodes or primary tumor size exceeding 3 cm were randomized to radiation alone, radiation plus tamoxifen, CMF alone, or CMF plus tamoxifen.[322] Local–regional recurrence rates were 13% in the patients who received radiation, and 12% in those who received radiation plus tamoxifen with a median follow-up of 6.5 years. In the Danish Breast Cancer Cooperative Group study 77C, 1716 postmenopausal women were randomized to radiation alone or radiation plus tamoxifen.[331,332] The 9-year local–regional recurrence rate was 17% with radiation and 12% with radiation and tamoxifen. Therefore, the addition of tamoxifen to radiation appears to decrease the risk of local–regional recurrence.

### Prospective Randomized Trials Evaluating Postmastectomy Radiation in Patients Receiving Adjuvant Systemic Therapy
Ten prospective randomized trials have evaluated the role of postmastectomy irradiation and adjuvant chemotherapy in axillary node positive patients. The trials and their results are presented in Tables 6-26 and 6-27. All the trials except the University of Arizona Cancer Center trial[333] demonstrated a decrease in the incidence of local–regional recurrence with the addition of radiation. In the Arizona trial, randomization to radiation was not strict, and the dose of radiation employed has been

questioned. Two prospective randomized trials have evaluated postmastectomy radiation in axillary node positive patients receiving adjuvant tamoxifen.[325,330,334,335] Postmastectomy radiation decreased the incidence of local–regional recurrence in both these trials. In the Danish Breast Cancer Group trial 82C, the 7-year actuarial local–regional recurrence rate was 40% in patients who received tamoxifen versus 9% in those who received tamoxifen and radiation ($p = < 0.0001$).[325,334,335] In the South Sweden trial, the 8-year actuarial local–regional recurrence was 18% in patients who received tamoxifen versus 6% who received tamoxifen and radiation.[330]

While these trials have demonstrated the ability of postmastectomy irradiation to decrease the incidence of local–regional recurrence, the majority have failed to demonstrate a survival benefit. The absence of such a benefit has led some investigators to question the role of postmastectomy irradiation even in patients who are at high risk for local–regional recurrence without such treatment. However, the recent publication of two prospective randomized trials of postmastectomy radiation in premenopausal axillary node positive women receiving CMF chemotherapy has provided support for a survival benefit from postmastectomy radiation. In the British Columbia trial,

postmastectomy radiation decreased local–regional recurrence rates from 33% to 13% at 15 years and resulted in a significant improvement in the 15-year breast-cancer-specific survival (47% vs. 57%, $p = 0.05$).[336] In the Danish Breast Cooperative Group trial, the 10-year local–regional recurrence rate was 26% without radiation and 5% with; the 10-year actuarial overall survival was 45% for CMF alone and 54% for CMF and radiation ($p = < 0.001$).[337]

As previously noted, patients receiving adjuvant systemic therapy at greatest risk for local–regional recurrence following mastectomy are those with four or more positive axillary nodes and/or a primary tumor size ($\geq 5$ cm). Four of the six trials reporting results for patients with four or more positive nodes have demonstrated an absolute overall survival benefit of 6% to 12% with the addition of radiation (Table 6-27).[329,336-338] However, none of these trials had enough patients to demonstrate that this modest benefit was statistically significant. An unexpected finding in the British Columbia trial and in Danish Breast Cancer Group trial 82B was the local–regional recurrence and survival benefit with the addition of radiation in patients with one to three positive nodes. In the British Columbia trial, the 15-year local–regional recurrence rate was 33% for patients with one to three positive nodes receiving CMF

**TABLE 6-26    Prospective Randomized Trials Comparing Adjuvant Chemotherapy with and Without Postmastectomy Radiation in Axillary Node Positive Patients with Stage I-II Breast Cancer**

| Study[a] | Accrual Period | Number of Patients | Chemotherapy[b] |
|---|---|---|---|
| Mayo Clinic[618,619] | 1973–80 | 313 | Melphalan, CFp |
| Piedmont[620] | | 159 | Melphalan, CMF |
| Glasgow[329] | 1972–82 | 322 | CMF |
| British Columbia[336] | 1979–86 | 318 | CMF |
| DBCG[318,337] | 1982–89 | 1708 | CMF ±T |
| Southeastern Group[338] | 1976–81 | 331 | CMF |
| Dana Farber[282] | 1974–84 | 83 | CMF/MF |
| | | 123 | CA |
| University of Arizona[333] | 1974–80 | 159 | AC |
| M.D. Anderson[283,621] | 1977–80 | 238 | FAC |
| Helsinki[622] | 1981–84 | 200 | CAFft ±T |

[a]DBCG, Danish Breast Cancer Cooperative Group; ECOG, Eastern Cooperative Oncology Group.

[b]A, Adriamycin; C, cyclophosphamide; F, Fluorouracil; ft, Ftorafur; H, Halotestin; m, Methotrexate; T, tamoxifen; V, vincristine.

**TABLE 6-27    Results of Prospective Randomized Trials Evaluating Postmastectomy Radiation (RT) in Axillary Node Positive Breast Cancer Patients Receiving Adjuvant Chemotherapy**[a]

| | Number of Patients | Local–Regional Recurrence (%) | | Survival (%) | | | Follow-Up (years) |
|---|---|---|---|---|---|---|---|
| | | Chemo | Chemo + RT | Chemo | | Chemo + RT | |
| *All Patients* | | | | | | | |
| CMF | | | | | | | |
| British Columbia (pre)[336,341] | 318 | 23 (0.003) | 13 | 46 | (0.07) | 54 | 15 actuarial |
| | | | | 47Δ | (0.05) | 57Δ | 15 actuarial |
| DBCG (pre)[318,337] | 1708 | 26 | 5 | 45 | (0.001) | 54 | 10 actuarial |
| Piedmont[620] | 159 | 14 | 5 | 58 | | 46 | 10 actuarial |
| Mayo Clinic[618,619] | 313 | 18 | 4 | 66 | | 68 | 5 actuarial |
| Glasgow[329] | 322 | 25 | 12 | 63Δ | (0.24) | 68Δ | 5 actuarial |
| ADRIAMYCIN-BASED | | | | | | | |
| Helsinki[622] | 200 | 24[b] | 7[b] | 69 | | 65 | 8 actuarial |
| M.D. Anderson[283,621] | 238 | 13 | 7 | 71 | (0.71) | 70 | 5 actuarial |
| University of Arizona[333] | 159 | 11 | 11 | 67 | (0.92 | 62 | 5 actuarial |
| *1–3 Positive Nodes* | | | | | | | |
| CMF | | | | | | | |
| British Columbia (pre)[336,341] | 183 | 33 | 10 | (48) | (0.06) | (64) | 15 actuarial |
| DBCG (pre)[318,337] | 1061 | 30 | 7 | 54 | | 62 | 10 actuarial |
| Glasgow[329] | 141 | | | 68 | (0.76) | 76 | 5 actuarial |
| Pre | | | | 84 | (0.40) | 78 | |
| Post | | | | 61 | (0.86) | 73 | |
| Dana Farber[282] | 83 | 5 | 2 | 85 | (>0.05) | 77 | 4.4 median |
| ADRIAMYCIN-BASED | | | | | | | |
| University of Arizona[333] | 87 | 11 | 0 | {71} | (<0.05) | {88} | 5 actuarial |
| *4 or More Positive Nodes* | | | | | | | |
| CMF | | | | | | | |
| British Columbia (pre)[336,341] | 112 | 46 (0.04) | 21 | 41 | (0.7) | 47 | 10 actuarial |
| Southeastern Group[338] | 331 | 20 (0.09) | 10 | 34 | (0.33) | 46 | 10 actuarial |
| DBCG (pre)[318,337] | 510 | 42 | 14 | 20 | | 32 | 10 actuarial |
| Glasgow[329] | 72 | | | 46Δ | (0.01) | 54Δ | 5 actuarial |
| Pre | | | | 54Δ | (0.04) | 49Δ | |
| Post | | | | 43Δ | (0.09) | 58Δ | |
| ADRIAMYCIN-BASED | | | | | | | |
| University of Arizona[333] | 72 | 12 | 18 | {58} | (0.95) | {46} | 5 actuarial |
| Dana Farber[282] | 123 | 20 (0.03) | 6 | 63 | (0.27) | 59 | 3.7 median |

[a]( ), survival free of systemic disease; { }, relapse-free survival; Δ, cause-specific survival; pre, premenopausal; post, postmenopausal.

and 10% for those receiving CMF and radiation.[336] In the Danish trial the 10-year rates were 30% for CMF alone and 7% for CMF and radiation.[337] The 30% rate of local–regional recurrence in premenopausal patients with one to three positive nodes in these two trials is higher than the rate reported by other studies (Table 6-27).[251,255,256,281,282,287,302,310,339] In the Southeastern Cancer Group study, the 10-year actuarial rate of local–regional recurrence for premenopausal women with one to three positive nodes receiving CMF and no radiation was 9%.[338] In the Danish trial, 45% of the local–regional recurrences were axillary, suggesting inadequate initial surgery.[326] If these axillary recurrences were eliminated by adequate axillary surgery, a diminished benefit from radiation would be seen in patients with one to three positive nodes, and the local–regional recurrence rate would be similar to that reported by earlier studies. In addition, the extent of nodal positivity increases with the number of axillary nodes examined (up to approximately 10 nodes).[263] The median number of nodes removed in the Danish trial was seven. It is possible that a significant number of patients with one to three positive nodes who had seven or fewer nodes removed actually had four or more positive nodes and, therefore, would have experienced a significant benefit from radiation. Therefore, the Danish trial suggests that premenopausal women with one to three positive axillary nodes who have had an inadequate axillary dissection may be at substantial risk for an axillary recurrence, and postmastectomy radiation may be indicated on this basis.

The British Columbia trial also demonstrated that the benefit from postmastectomy radiation becomes more evident with longer follow-up (i.e., allowing for the manifestation of distant metastasis subsequent to local–regional failure). Initially, the 8-year overall survival was 60% for patients who did not receive radiation versus 57% for those who did.[340] However, the 15-year actuarial overall survival rates were 46% for the chemotherapy patients and 54% for the chemotherapy and radiation patients.[336] The two prospective randomized trials that reported a decreased survival in patients with four or more positive nodes receiving postmastectomy radiation reported results at relatively short intervals (i.e., 3.7 years median follow-up and 5-year actuarial).[282,333] These findings are not too dissimilar from the 3% decrement in overall survival reported at 8 years by the British Columbia study. Therefore with longer follow-up, these trials may also demonstrate a survival benefit.

In summary, the randomized trials of postmastectomy irradiation in axillary node positive patients receiving adjuvant systemic therapy have demonstrated for the most part a decreased incidence in isolated local–regional failure and an improvement in overall survival in five of ten trials, and these benefits were statistically significant in two. The survival benefit from postmastectomy irradiation in these patients ranges from 5% to 10% and is of a magnitude similar to that of the survival benefit seen with adjuvant chemotherapy and/or tamoxifen in axillary node positive patients.[5] Attention to radiation technique has the potential for diminishing cardiac morbidity and the subsequent increased risk of non–breast cancer related deaths in patients receiving radiation.

***Indications for Postmastectomy Radiation***    Indications for postmastectomy radiation include four or more positive axillary nodes and/or primary tumor diameter of at least 5 cm, pectoral fascia involvement, and a close or positive inked mastectomy margin in women under 50 years of age who would otherwise be deemed at low to intermediate risk. As demonstrated by the Danish Breast Cancer Group study of premenopausal women, inadequate axillary surgery in patients with positive axillary nodes may be an additional indication for postmastectomy irradiation.[318,337] Multiple studies have failed to demonstrate an increased risk of axillary recurrence in patients with extracapsular extension who did not receive axillary radiation.[186,275–277] However, in the British Columbia trial, postmastectomy radiation resulted in a significant improvement in the 10-year actuarial overall and disease-free survival in patients with extensive extracapsular spread.[341] This study, however, does not specifically address the role of axillary radiation in the presence of extracapsular extension. While the definition of inadequate axillary surgery based on the number of nodes removed can be questioned, the removal of 10 or more axillary nodes has been associated with decreased axillary recurrence rates and an improved ability to adequately assess the extent of axillary nodal positivity.[263] The presence of gross multifocal or multicentric disease is not an indication for postmastectomy irradiation in the absence of other factors (i.e., primary tumor size $\geq$ 5 cm or four or more positive axillary nodes).[123] The role of postmastectomy radiation in the treatment of operable T3 pathologically node-negative breast cancer is controversial. Mignano et al.[342] reported a 12% crude local–regional recurrence rate in 101 patients with negative microscopic margins with a median follow-up of 93 months. Only 9% of these patients received adjuvant systemic therapy. However, the majority of patients in this series underwent a radical mastectomy. Two prospective randomized trials have addressed the issue of postmastectomy irradiation in operable T3 node negative breast cancer.[337,343] In the Helsinki trial,[343] local–regional recurrence was reported in 2 of the 27 patients with T3 pathologic node-negative breast cancer who received postmastectomy radiation versus 5 of the 13 patients who did not. In the Danish Breast Cancer Cooperative Group trial 82B, local–regional recurrence rates were 17% in the 77 premenopausal women randomized to CMF and 3% in the 58 women randomized to CMF and radiation.[337] The 10-year actuarial overall survival was 82% for patients who received CMF and radiation compared to 70% for CMF alone.[337] Survival results were not reported for the Helsinki trial. Therefore, at least one prospective randomized trial would support a recommendation for postmastectomy irradiation in operable T3 node-negative breast cancer.

***Radiotherapy Considerations*** Since the most common sites of local–regional recurrence following mastectomy are the chest wall and the supraclavicular region, postmastectomy radiation should include at a minimum the chest wall and the supraclavicular region in axillary node positive patients. In general, the chest wall is treated via tangential fields to a total dose of 5000 cGy over period of 5 to 5.5 weeks at 180 to 200 cGy per fraction. The dose to the supraclavicular region is 4600 to 5000 cGy over a period of 4.5 to 5 weeks. For photon beam energies of 6 MV or greater, bolus tissue equivalent material is employed over the chest wall on an every-other-day basis. A single study has demonstrated that daily bolus or a boost to the surgical scar following treatment to the entire chest wall does not decrease the incidence of chest wall recurrence.[344] Level III axillary nodes are included within the supraclavicular field, and level I and the majority of level II axillary nodes are included within the tangential fields. A posterior axillary field has frequently been used to supplement the midplane dose to the axilla for the level II axillary nodes. However, recent studies have demonstrated that the use of the posterior axillary field does not decrease the risk of an axillary recurrence compared to the use of the supraclavicular field alone.[200–203] As well, recent studies have demonstrated that if an adequate axillary dissection has been performed, extracapsular extension is not an indication for the use of a posterior axillary field.[186,275–277]

The role of internal mammary node irradiation in early stage invasive breast cancer remains controversial, with advocates both for[320,345] and against.[295,346] Approximately 25% of the lymphatic channels of the breast drain primarily to the internal mammary nodes.[347] Metastasis to the internal mammary nodes occurs most frequently in the second inner space, followed by the third and first.[347] The fourth and fifth inner spaces are least often involved. The incidence of histologically positive internal mammary nodes is related to the pathologic status of the axilla and the location of the primary tumor in the breast. For patients with outer quadrant lesions and negative axillary nodes, the incidence of positive internal mammary nodes is 10% or less.[264,266–268,348–350] For patients with inner or central primary tumors and negative axillary nodes, the incidence of positive internal mammary nodes is 10% to 15%.[264,266–268,348–350] For patients with positive axillary nodes and outer quadrant tumors, the reported incidence of positive internal mammary nodes ranges from 17% to 64%.[264,266–268,348–350] However, for inner or central quadrant lesions with positive axillary nodes, the incidence ranges from 29% to 59%.[264,266–268,348–350] Veronesi et al.[351] also reported a higher incidence of positive internal mammary nodes in women under 40 years of age with positive axillary nodes and primary tumor size exceeding 2 cm.

Despite the high incidence of occult metastasis to the internal mammary nodes in patients with inner or central quadrant tumors and positive axillary nodes, the incidence of clinical internal mammary recurrence is extremely low.[188,227,264,266–269] Internal mammary node recurrences are infrequent in patients with positive axillary nodes who receive adjuvant chemotherapy.[255] Donegan reported a 10% incidence of clinical internal mammary node recurrence in patients with histologically positive internal mammary nodes versus a 6% incidence in patients with histologically negative internal mammary nodes.[268]

Treatment of the internal mammary nodes with radiation has not resulted in a significant decrease in the incidence of clinical internal mammary node recurrences but has resulted in an increased incidence of complications, including symptomatic pneumonitis, and increased mortality from cardiovascular disease.[201,202,230,242] Therefore, elective radiation of the internal mammary nodes does not significantly decrease this clinical pattern of failure and may contribute to the observed complications. Some have argued that microscopic involvement of the internal mammary nodes may be a source of distant metastases and, therefore, treatment of these nodes may decrease the incidence of distant metastases and improve survival.[345,352] Several prospective randomized trials have been cited as studies that support the role of internal mammary node treatment in axillary node positive patients, especially those with medial tumors.[230,235,318,336,337,341] However, in these trials, radiation was directed to the chest wall and regional nodes, and therefore it is difficult to ascertain the specific contribution of treatment to the internal mammary nodes to any survival benefit. In the Stockholm trial, there was no significant difference in the reduction of distant metastasis between medial and central lesions versus lateral lesions, suggesting no preferential benefit to radiation for a medial or central primary tumor.[235]

Three prospective randomized trials have specifically evaluated the role of regional node irradiation following mastectomy.[227–230] In these trials, radiation was not delivered to the chest wall, and therefore any improvement in survival may be attributed to treatment to the regional nodes (i.e., internal mammary nodes, supraclavicular nodes, and apical axillary nodes). In the Manchester II trial, patients with negative axillary nodes who received radiation had a decreased 30-year survival, and patients with positive axillary nodes who received radiation had a survival identical to those who did not.[228,229] Similarly in the Oslo II trial, regional node irradiation in stage I patients resulted in a decreased 14-year survival, and for stage II patients, there was a 3% survival benefit with radiation.[230] The NSABP B-02 trial demonstrated a 6% reduction in the overall survival in patients who received regional node irradiation at 5 years.[227] Arriagada et al.[353] reported on a retrospective series of patients treated at the Institut Gustave-Roussy with either surgical resection or radiation or both to the internal mammary nodes; these patients had histologically positive axillary nodes and primary tumors up to 7 cm in diameter; there was a 10-year overall survival of 50% for patients treated by radical or modified radical mastectomy, versus 52% for those who underwent extended radical mastectomy. The incidence of distant metastasis was 46% in patients who did not have surgical dissection of the internal mammary nodes versus 44% in those who did.

At the present time, there is no agreement on the role of internal mammary node irradiation in the treatment of operable breast cancer. If a decision is made to treat the internal mammary nodes, modifications of the treatment technique must be employed to limit the dose to the heart and the lung. Marks et al.[345] have suggested irradiating only the upper internal mammary nodes, since these are the most commonly involved nodes. Another technique includes the use of the electrons to treat the medial aspect of the chest wall and internal mammary nodes to avoid dose to the underlying heart and lungs. (See discussion of radiation technique.)

## Integration of Adjuvant Systemic Therapy with Conservative Surgery and Radiation or Postmastectomy Radiation

The sequencing of adjuvant systemic therapy and radiation either as part of breast conservation therapy or following mastectomy has generated considerable debate. As noted earlier, chemotherapy and/or tamoxifen do not significantly decrease the incidence of local–regional recurrence following mastectomy in high risk patients; similarly, CMF or modifications thereof or tamoxifen in patients undergoing breast conservation therapy have been associated with a 30% to 40% incidence of ipsilateral breast tumor recurrence in the absence of radiation.[129,213,221,226,354] However, the addition of radiation to adjuvant systemic chemotherapy and/or tamoxifen decreases the incidence of local–regional recurrence in patients undergoing breast conservation surgery as well as mastectomy.[127,129,131,134,137,355,356]

The options for the sequencing of radiation and chemotherapy include the delivery of all chemotherapy prior to radiation, the delivery of radiation prior to chemotherapy (sequential regimens), the simultaneous initiation of chemotherapy and radiation (concurrent regimen),[127,134,137] and the initiation of radiotherapy in the midst of the chemotherapy program (sandwich regimen). Concurrent regimens have the theoretical advantage of initiating local–regional treatment and systemic therapy at the same time without a delay in either modality, but they are limited by the drugs that can be given concurrently with radiation. The simultaneous use of methotrexate in patients receiving regional node irradiation has resulted in a significant incidence of symptomatic pneumonitis.[357] For sequential regimens, delaying initiation of radiotherapy may result in an increased risk of local–regional recurrence, and

similarly, delays to the initiation of systemic therapy may result in an increased risk of distant metastasis.

*Postmastectomy Radiation* In clinical practice, postmastectomy irradiation is often initiated after the completion of all adjuvant systemic chemotherapy. Three studies have reported an increased incidence of local–regional recurrence in patients whose radiation was delayed until the completion of all chemotherapy.[358-360] Buchholz et al.[358] reported a 23% 5-year actuarial local–regional recurrence rate in the 35 patients who received radiation 6 months or longer after mastectomy. In contrast, for the 19 patients who received radiation within 6 months, the local–regional recurrence rate was 5%. The two groups, however, were not comparable: doxorubicin-based regimens were more commonly used in the delayed radiation group, and a greater percentage of patients in the early radiation group had close or positive margins or four or more positive nodes. Buzdar et al.[359] reported a 16% 10-year actuarial local–regional recurrence rate in patients who received chemotherapy first following mastectomy versus 8% who received radiation first. Local–regional recurrences occur infrequently during chemotherapy. Stefanik et al.[280] observed a single postmastectomy local–regional recurrence during chemotherapy. Griem et al.[282] reported two local–regional recurrences during chemotherapy in 100 women with four or more positive axillary nodes. The impact of the sequencing of postmastectomy radiation and adjuvant systemic chemotherapy on survival is limited.[282] Buchholz et al.[358] reported no significant differences in survival when patients who received postmastectomy radiation within 6 months of surgery were compared with those whose treatment was delayed for more than 6 months (5-year actuarial survival 78% vs. 73%, $p = 0.32$). Brufman et al.[361] reported a 42% 7-year relapse-free survival in patients who received radiation prior to chemotherapy versus 77% for those who received concurrent chemotherapy and radiation or chemotherapy first. Two prospective randomized trials have demonstrated no adverse effect on survival with delays to the initiation of chemotherapy for the completion of postmastectomy radiation.[306,338] In the Oncofrance trial of doxorubicin, vincristine, cyclophosphamide, and 5-fluorouracil (AVCF) versus CMF for axillary node positive breast cancer patients, 55% of the patients received postmastectomy radiation.[306] No difference in outcome was observed when patients who received radiation first were compared with those who received chemotherapy first. In the Southeastern Cancer Group study,[338] the 10-year actuarial overall survival was 46% when radiation was given first followed by six cycles of CMF chemotherapy versus 34% in patients who received 6 cycles of CMF without radiation. Lara Jimenez et al.[362] reported a statistically significant improvement in 10-year disease-free survival in patients who received three cycles of CMF, followed by radiation, followed by an additional three cycles of CMF, versus patients who received radiation first or chemotherapy first (57% vs. 46%, $p = 0.05$). At present, postmastectomy radiation is commonly delayed until after completion of all chemotherapy in high

risk axillary node positive patients. In the ongoing prospective randomized trials evaluating dose-intense chemotherapy with autologous bone marrow transplantation or peripheral stem cell rescue, postmastectomy radiation is initiated after the completion of standard chemotherapy or the dose-intensive regimen.

***Breast Conservation Therapy*** The integration of adjuvant systemic chemotherapy with conservative surgery and radiation is more controversial. Breast recurrence rates related to delays in the initiation of radiation for adjuvant systemic chemotherapy are presented in Table 6-28. The results are variable, with some series demonstrating an increased risk of ipsilateral breast tumor recurrence with delays to the initiation of radiation of 4 to 6 months,[358,363–365] and others demonstrating no adverse effect.[365] The first evidence of an increased risk of ipsilateral breast tumor recurrence with delays to the initiation of radiation appeared in a report from the Joint Center for Radiotherapy.[365] In a subsequent update,[366] the authors reported a 5% 5-year actuarial breast recurrence rate in 252 patients who began ra-

**TABLE 6-28 Effect of Sequencing of Radiation and Adjuvant Chemotherapy on Ipsilateral Breast Tumor Recurrence**

| Study | Interval to XRT (months) | Breast Recurrence (%)[a] Early | Delayed | Follow-up (years) |
|---|---|---|---|---|
| Leonard et al.[372] | 4 | 6 (17) | 3 (88) | 3.5 mean |
| Buzdar et al.[359] | 5–6 | 5 (46) | 3 (39) | 5 actuarial |
| NSABP B-16[324] | 3 | | 4 (112) | 8 |
| Heiman et al.[623] | | 5 (67) | 7 (166) | 6 actuarial |
| Willers et al.[624] | 5–6 | 6 (22) | 8 (52) | 4 crude |
| Dabrow et al.[625] | 6 | | 9 (23) | 4 median |
| IBCSG[626,b] | 7 | 8 (213) | 9 (220) | 4 actuarial |
| NSABP B-15[308] | 3 | 10 (204) | 10 (420) | 8 |
| Hartsell et al.[363] | 4 | 2 (42) | 14 (43) | 5 actuarial |
| McCormick et al.[364] | 4 | 5 (86) | 14 (53) | 5 actuarial |
| | 6 | | 40 | 5 crude |
| Buchholz et al.[358] | 6 | 0 (26) | 20 (22) | 8 actuarial |
| Recht et al.[365] | 4 | 5 (252) | 28 (34) | 5 actuarial |

[a]Number of patients in parentheses.

[b]IBCSG, International Breast Cancer Study Group.

TABLE 6-29    Distant Failure and Survival Related to the Sequencing of Chemotherapy and Radiation

| | | | | 5-Year Actuarial | | | |
| | | | | Metastases XRT | | Survival (%) XRT | |
| Study | Number of Patients | 1–3 Positive Nodes (%) | Chemo[a] | Early | Delayed | Early | Delayed |
|---|---|---|---|---|---|---|---|
| Markiewicz et al.[544] | 157 | 78 | CMF, CAF | 18 | | 86 | |
| Overmoyer et al.[627] | 209 | 65 | CMF | 23 | | 87 | |
| Hartsell et al.[363] | 84 | 50 | CMF, CAF, AC | 15 | 19 | 87 | 82 |
| Buchholz et al.[358] | 48 | | CMF (VP) | | | 96[b] | 48[b] |
| Leonard et al.[372] | 105 | 17 | CMF (VP) | | | 94 | 95 |
| IBCSG[626,c] | | | | | | | |
|    Premenopausal | 433 | 76 | CMF | 18 | 23 | 90[c] | 84[c] |
|    Postmenopausal | 285 | 73 | CMF, T | 18 | 15 | 89[c] | 89[c] |
| Buzdar et al.[359] | 85 | 70 | FAC | 19 | 28 | | |
| Recht et al.[365] | 127 | 100 | CMF | 24 | 50 | | |
| Recht et al. randomized trial[367] | 244 | 60 | CAMF | 36 | 25 | 73 | 81 |

[a]C, cyclophosphamide; M, methotrexate; F, 5-fluorouracil; A, doxorubicin; V, vincristine; P, prednisone; T, tamoxifen.

[b]8-year actuarial.

[c]4-year actuarial.

diation within 4 months versus 28% for 34 patients in whom the initiation of radiation was delayed for more than 16 weeks. A single prospective randomized trial has evaluated the sequencing of conservative surgery and radiation and adjuvant systemic chemotherapy for early stage invasive breast cancer.[367] In 1984 the Dana Farber Cancer Institute initiated a trial in which 244 patients were randomized to receive four cycles of cyclophosphamide, doxorubicin, methotrexate, 5-fluorouracil, and prednisone (CAMFP) every 3 weeks prior to or following radiation. The trial was completed in 1992 and the results were reported in 1996.[367] Recalling the retrospective series, delays to the initiation of radiation resulted in an increased risk of ipsilateral breast tumor recurrence. The 5-year crude rate of a breast recurrence was 5% for the patients who received radiation first versus 14% for the patients who received chemotherapy first. Factors that correlated with an increased risk of ipsilateral breast tumor recurrence in patients whose radiation was delayed included primary tumor size, the presence of an extensive intraductal

component, the absence of a reexcision, and a close, positive, or unknown margin. For patients with negative resection margins, there was no increased incidence of ipsilateral breast tumor recurrence with delays to the initiation of radiation. Hartsell et al.[363] also demonstrated no significant increase in ipsilateral breast tumor recurrence in patients with negative margins in whom radiation was delayed. Therefore, at the present time, patients with positive, close, or unknown margins should undergo a reexcision to achieve negative margins if they have had chemotherapy prior to radiation in connection with conservation therapy.

An unexpected finding in the Dana Farber Cancer Institute trial was that delays in the initiation of chemotherapy resulted in an increased incidence of distant–regional failure and a nonstatistically significant decrease in survival. This is the only prospective randomized trial to address this question in patients undergoing conservative surgery and radiation and also the only study in which this potential adverse effect has been identified. The 5-year crude distant–regional recurrence rates were 32% for patients who received radiation first and 20% for those receiving chemotherapy first. The majority of the patients in this trial had one to three positive nodes, and for them the sequencing of radiation and chemotherapy had no impact on breast recurrence or distant–regional failure.[367] For the 35 patients with negative axillary nodes and the 60 patients with four or more positive axillary nodes, radiation first was associated with an increased risk of distant–regional failure. The results from retrospective series reporting distant failure and survival related to sequencing of chemotherapy and radiation in patients undergoing conservative surgery and radiation are presented in Table 6-29. The 5-year actuarial distant metastases are highest, and the overall survival the lowest, in the Dana Farber Cancer Institute randomized trial for patients who received radiation first, despite a not dissimilar incidence of one to three positive nodes, compared to other series. The Joint Center for Radiotherapy recently completed a phase II study evaluating concurrent chemotherapy (CMF) and radiation.[368] Based on this study, a prospective randomized trial comparing concurrent chemotherapy (CMF) and radiation with CMF for six cycles followed by radiation in patients with no to three positive nodes and negative margins has been initiated.

The integration of adjuvant tamoxifen with conservative surgery and radiation has also been questioned. In vitro studies have demonstrated that tamoxifen delays or blocks the progression of cells from early $G_1$ to mid-$G_1$.[369] Cells delayed in $G_1$ may exhibit radiation resistance.[370] Therefore, concern has been raised regarding the concurrent administration of tamoxifen and radiation and the potential for an increased risk of ipsilateral breast recurrence. However, in the NSABP B-14 trial,[371] tamoxifen was begun prior to initiation of radiation. With a mean follow-up of 4.4 years, the ipsilateral breast tumor recurrence was 2% in the patients receiving tamoxifen and 3% in the patients who did not receive tamoxifen. All patients had negative axillary nodes. A number of retrospective series have also demonstrated the ability of tamoxifen to decrease ipsilateral breast tumor recurrence, especially in axillary node positive patients.[134,167,364,372–375] However, the simultaneous administration of tamoxifen and radiation has been noted to increase the incidence of breast edema and breast hyperemia.[375] The initiation of tamoxifen after completion of radiation may decrease this effect. For the impact of adjuvant systemic therapy on cosmesis and on the development of complications, see the complications section.

## NEOADJUVANT CHEMOTHERAPY FOR EARLY STAGE BREAST CANCER

### Rationale for Treatment

The most commonly employed sequencing of adjuvant systemic therapy and local therapy for early stage invasive breast cancer is initial surgery followed by systemic therapy.[376] The rationale for using chemotherapy (i.e., neoadjuvant chemotherapy) prior to surgery for clinically operable T1 and T2 tumors includes the following: the early initiation of systemic therapy to improve treatment of occult micrometastatic disease, the use of the response of the primary tumor as an indicator of chemosensitivity, the use of the tumor response as an early surrogate end point for subsequent risk of recurrence, and the possibility of increasing rates of breast conservation for large T2 tumors.[377–384]

### Response Rates and Survival

There is a high rate of clinical response for operable primary tumors in the breast after induction chemotherapy (Table 6-30). The clinical complete response rates for T1 and T2 tumors ranges from 19% to 57%, with objective responses of 50% or more reduction in size from 72% to 85%.[377–379,382,384,385] The rate of clinical complete response has been reported to be higher for smaller tumors and additional cycles

**TABLE 6-30    Response Rates of the Primary Tumor to Induction Chemotherapy for Clinically Operable Stage I–III Breast Cancer**

| Series | Number of Patients | Tumor Size (cm) | Induction Chemotherapy[a] | Cycles | Clinical Complete Response (+ Clinical Partial Response) (%)[b] | Pathological Clinical Response (%) |
|---|---|---|---|---|---|---|
| Rilke et al.[385] | 31 | ≤ 2.5 | A or FNC | 3 | 19 (—) | 3 |
| Powles et al.[382] | 101 | ≤ 5 cm in 97% | McNM ±T | 3 | 19 (85) | 10 |
| Calais et al.[384] | 82 | 3.1–5 | N (or E) +VCF | 3 | 27 (72) | |
| | 76 | > 5 | | | 19 (58) | |
| Hortobagyi et al.[412] | 48 | Stage IIIA | FAC | 3 | 29 (89) | |
| Bonadonna et al.[377] | 292 | 2.5–4 | CMF, FAC, | 3–4 | — (76) | 3 |
| | 160 | 4.1–5 | FEC, FNC, | | — (79) | 3 |
| | 84 | > 5 | A, or E | | — (67) | 1 |
| Jacquillat et al.[379] | 23 | ≤ 2 | VbThMFPr ±AT | 3–4 | 48 (44)[c] | |
| | 112 | 2.1–5 | | | 27 (40) | |
| | 57 | > 5 | | | 23 (47) | |
| Fisher et al.[378] | 131 | ≤ 2 | AC | 4 | 57 (79) | 14 |
| | 445 | 2.1–5 | | | 35 (81) | 9 |
| | 117 | > 5 | | | 17 (75) | 3v |
| Scholl et al.[380] | 191 | 4.7 mean; range 3–7 | CAF | 4 | 24 (65) | |
| Danforth et al.[628] | 22 | ≤ 5 | FLAC-GMCSF | 5 | 50 (92) | 36 |
| Pierce et al.[421] | 48 | Stage IIIA | CAMF ±PT | 5 (median) | 33 (73) | 29 |
| Mauriac et al.[381] | 134 | 4.3 mean; range 3–8 | EVM and McThVi | 6 | | |
| Ellis et al.[392] | 185 | 5.5 median; range 1–12 | CMF, McMN, ECiF, or FEC | 6–8 | 36 (82) | 9[d] |
| Schwartz[408] | 119 | Stage II-IIIA | CMF or CAF | 7 | — (91)[e] | |
| Merajver et al.[406] | 43 | Stage IIIA | CAMFPT | 9 | 65 (98) | 29 |

[a]Chemotherapy: C, cyclophosphamide; M, methotrexate; F, fluorouracil; A, doxorubicin; E, epirubicin; N, mitoxantrone; L, leucovorin; Ci, cisplatin; V, vincristine; Vb, vinblastine; Mc, mitomycin C; Th, Thiotepa; Vi, vindesine; P, Premarin; Pr, prednisone; T, tamoxifen; GMCSF, granulocyte–macrophage colony stimulating factor.

[b]Numbers in parentheses, % partial response.

[c]Partial response defined as over 75% regression.

[d]Percentage in patients undergoing surgery.

[e]Partial response defined as over 25% regression.

of induction therapy.[378–380,384] Despite these high clinical response rates, the pathologic complete response rates are low in these series, ranging from only 3% to 14%. There is also a low but significant risk of lack of response (5%–17%) or local tumor progression (2%–3%) for T1 and T2 tumors during neoadjuvant chemotherapy.

The National Surgical Breast and Bowel Project (NSABP) conducted the largest prospective randomized trial (B-18) testing the benefit of neoadjuvant chemotherapy for operable breast cancer.[378] Between 1988 and 1993, 1523 patients were randomized to receive local therapy and adjuvant systemic chemotherapy or the same chemotherapy as induction prior to surgery. The clinical tumor size was T1 or T2 in 87% of patients. The results after 5 years showed no difference in the rates of initial distant metastases, actuarial disease-free survival, or overall survival between patients receiving neoadjuvant chemotherapy and those who had postoperative chemotherapy.[386] There have been four smaller randomized trials testing neoadjuvant versus adjuvant chemotherapy in predominantly T2 tumors (Table 6-31). Small trends toward improved survival with earlier chemotherapy were reported after short follow-up in three of the series, but this lost significance in two of them with their 5-year updates.[380–382,387–390]

Induction chemotherapy significantly downstages the pathologic status of the axilla at time of surgery. In the NSABP B-18 trial, 59% of patients randomized to preoperative chemotherapy had negative nodes versus 43% in the postoperative group.[378] There were also reductions in the numbers of patients having 4 to 9 or 10 or more nodes in the induction chemotherapy arm compared to controls. However, the patients treated with neoadjuvant chemotherapy did not have reduced distant metastases or death from disease despite this pathologic downstaging of the axilla. Thus the axillary response after chemotherapy may not be a reliable early marker of outcome, because the behavior of these patients was the same as that of their initial presumed nodal status in the control group. This raises concern about the potential loss of information useful in determining prognosis and selection for more aggressive therapies in patients treated by induction chemotherapy.

## Breast Conservation Therapy

The rate of breast conservation is another potential end point for studying the efficacy of neoadjuvant chemotherapy. In the NSABP B-18 trial, the frequency of lumpectomy and radiation actually performed was modestly increased for T2 tumors receiving preoperative chemotherapy. In the control group, the performance of lumpectomy was 79% for T1 tumors and 63% for T2 tumors, versus 81% for T1 tumors and 71% for T2 tumors treated with neoadjuvant chemotherapy.[378] Powles et al.[382] reported performance of mastectomy in only 13% of patients randomized to induction chemotherapy before surgery versus 28% of controls who received standard adjuvant therapy. Mauriac et al.[381] reported mastectomy in 37% of tumors treated by induction chemotherapy that were initially greater than 3 cm (80% T2) and felt to require mastectomy. Calais et al.[384] reported that 77 of 158 patients (52% T2, 48% T3) had tumor size less than 3 cm after induction chemotherapy and were able to avoid mastectomy. Bonadonna et al.[377] reported breast-conserving surgery and radiation after induction chemotherapy in 85% of patients with tumors 2.5 cm or greater (84% T2). Jacquillat et al.[379] reported breast conservation after a complete response to induction chemotherapy and radiation without surgery in all 135 patients with T1-T2 tumors.

The mechanism by which induction chemotherapy may increase the ability to perform wide local excision and radiation has not been well characterized. The choice was not a part of a randomization process in any of these trials; rather, it was a function of the response to chemotherapy and the surgeon's preference. The likely factor in most of these trials has been a decrease in clinical size of the primary tumor below an institution's

**TABLE 6-31 Comparisons of 5-Year Survival Results in Prospective Randomized Trials of Neoadjuvant Chemotherapy Versus Initial Local Therapy and Adjuvant Chemotherapy[a]**

| Series | Arms | Number of Patients | T1 or T2 (%) | Metastasis-Free (%) | Disease-Free Survival (%) | Overall Survival (%) |
|---|---|---|---|---|---|---|
| Fisher et al.[378,386] | CTX + local | 747 | 87 | 84[b] | 67 | 80 |
| | Local + CTX | 759 | 87 | 84[b] | 67 | 80 |
| Mauriac et al.[381,387] | CTX + local | 134 | 79 | 66 | 62 | 78 |
| | Local +/− CTX | 138 | 86 | 66 | 60 | 82 |
| Powles et al.[382,389] | CTX + local + CTX | 101 | 97 | No significant difference | | No significant difference[c] |
| | Local + CTX | 99 | 92 | | | |
| Scholl et al.[390] | CTX + local + CTX | 95 | 45 | | No significant difference | No significant difference |
| | Local + CTX | 86 | 34 | | | |
| Scholl et al.[380,388] | CTX + local | 200 | 70 | 72 | | 84 |
| | Local + CTX | 190 | 76 | 65[d] | | 78[e] |

[a]CTX, chemotherapy; local, local therapy consisting of surgery and/or radiation.

[b]Considering distant metastases as site of first treatment failure.

[c]Median follow-up of 36 months.

[d]$p = 0.09$.

[e]$p = 0.18$.

threshold for recommending mastectomy. For example, a T2 tumor that is already considered a candidate for wide excision in the United States could be downstaged to below a 2 to 2.5 cm threshold for breast conservation in Europe by even a modest partial response to induction chemotherapy. A postchemotherapy tumor volume may be more amenable to breast conservation if the ratio of tumor to breast size is more favorable or the extent of wide local excision needed to obtain negative margins is reduced.

However, questions remain regarding the technique of conservative surgery after induction chemotherapy. A surgeon may be unable to determine the original location of the primary if it becomes nonpalpable after downstaging by chemotherapy. It is not known whether chemotherapy causes gross regression of tumor toward a central volume, or leaves microscopic nests scattered throughout the original tumor volume. In the latter case, resecting the postchemotherapy volume would leave significant residual disease in the breast. In the randomized study published by Powles et al.,[382] there was a nonsignificant increase in the rate of positive margins at wide local excision after neoadjuvant chemotherapy compared to adjuvant chemotherapy controls. After induction chemotherapy, whether pathologic assessment of the excision margins remains predictive of breast recurrence after conservative surgery and radiation is also unknown. For all these reasons, some surgeons have recommended tattooing the initial tumor volume to guide the postchemotherapy extent of resection.[391] Malignant calcifications are unlikely to disappear after induction chemotherapy, and should be completely excised because of the high association with persistent tumor.[391]

The breast recurrence rates after induction chemotherapy, conservative surgery, and radiation for operable T1 and T2 tumors appear to be similar or slightly increased over those for adjuvant chemotherapy. In the NSABP B-18 trial, the incidence of first recurrence in the treated breast after 5 years was 6% after wide

local excision, radiation, and postoperative chemotherapy and 8% after preoperative chemotherapy.[386] The hazard rates for first failure were also higher in the neoadjuvant chemotherapy group (1.8 vs. 1.3 events per 100 person-years). In the series by Bonadonna et al.,[377] the rate of local recurrence as a first event after neoadjuvant chemotherapy, quadrantectomy, and radiation was only 6.8% at 8 years. Calais et al.[384] selected breast conservation when there was a residual tumor smaller than 3 cm after induction chemotherapy in a series of 82 T2 and 76 T3 patients. After a median follow-up of 38 months, the local recurrence was 2 of 32 (6%) after radiotherapy alone in complete responders, the majority of whom initially had T2 tumors. The local recurrence was 4 of 45 (9%) after tumorectomy and radiation in partial responders, and 5 of 81 (6%) after mastectomy.

Breast conservation without surgery has in other series been associated with a higher rate of local failure even after a good response to induction chemotherapy. Jacquillat et al.[379] reported no breast failures in 23 patients with T1 tumors, and a 5-year actuarial local–regional recurrence rate of 13% in 112 T2 tumors that had a complete response after neoadjuvant chemotherapy and radiotherapy alone. In a randomized trial updated by Avril et al.,[387] the crude 5-year isolated local recurrence was 27% in complete responders to chemotherapy treated by radiotherapy alone. The 5-year isolated rate of local recurrence was 10% in patients with a residual tumor under 2 cm after induction chemotherapy who were treated by conservative surgery and radiation, and only 5% for those randomized to mastectomy and adjuvant chemotherapy. Ellis et al.[392] reported on 71 patients with operable stage I or II breast cancer treated with induction chemotherapy followed by radiotherapy, mastectomy, or conservative surgery and radiation based on response. Patients treated without surgery tended to have complete or near-complete responses to chemotherapy. The crude local recurrence after a median follow-up of 41 months was already

19% in those having a complete response to induction chemotherapy, versus only 6% after a partial response and 10% after no response. The 5-year local recurrence-free survival was only 75% in patients with stage I or II disease achieving a complete response to induction chemotherapy.

After neoadjuvant chemotherapy and conservative surgery for early stage breast cancer, the whole breast has been treated with tangential fields to a dose of 50 Gy, with a range of 45 to 54 Gy in the reported series.[377,378,381,382,384] The largest of these series treated the breast alone without regional nodal irradiation,[377,378,381] while others have recommended treatment of the supraclavicular and axillary nodes in all[384] or only node-positive[382] patients. The NSABP protocol called for treatment of the whole breast without a boost to the tumor bed, while most other series have employed a boost to the tumor bed after conservative surgery of 10 to 15 Gy.[381,382,384] In series using radiation and chemotherapy without conservative surgery, higher (20–35 Gy) boosts to the tumor bed have been employed.[379–381,384] Whether this boost should encompass the initial tumor volume or the postchemotherapy volume has not been addressed by these series. In addition to higher boost doses for the primary tumor, series employing radiation without conservative surgery have consistently also included treatment of the axillary, supraclavicular, and internal mammary lymph nodes.[379–381,384]

In summary, induction chemotherapy has not produced improvements in patient disease-free or overall survival as opposed to standard adjuvant chemotherapy. Some patients who do not require adjuvant chemotherapy thus may be overtreated by routine use prior to definitive local–regional staging. Downstaging by induction chemotherapy may cause a loss of important prognostic information about nodal status, as well as uncertainty during conservative surgery about the location and extent of the primary tumor in the breast. The use of neoadjuvant chemotherapy in early stage T1 and T2 disease remains in-vestigational until these questions concerning patient selection and ultimate local failure rates after breast conservation have been answered by clinical trials.

## LOCALLY ADVANCED BREAST CANCER

### T3 Operable Breast Cancer

Category T3 operable breast cancer corresponds to stages IIB (T3 N0) and IIIA (T1-2 N2 and T3 N1-2) in the 1997 UICC-AJCC staging classification[6] and includes tumors that are clinically greater than 5 cm (T3) and/or have axillary lymph nodes fixed to each other (N2), yet at presentation are judged to be resectable by modified radical mastectomy.

The standard management of patients presenting with operable locally advanced tumors is by initial modified radical mastectomy.[376] Systemic therapy is also an integral part of the treatment of these tumors because of the high risk for distant metastases.[343,393] Postmastectomy radiation is indicated for operable T3 patients to decrease the high risk (20%–40%) of local–regional failure even after adjuvant systemic therapy.[246,255,285,337,343,394,395] This benefit also extends to patients with axillary node negative tumors greater than 5 cm.[337,343] Postmastectomy radiation may safely be delayed until after the completion of adjuvant systemic chemotherapy.[344] Local–regional control rates range from 85% to 95% with 10-year survivals of 40% to 45%[337,343,344,393,395–397] for operable stage III breast cancer treated with modified radical mastectomy, adjuvant systemic chemotherapy, and postmastectomy radiation.

The results of four prospective randomized trials evaluating postmastectomy radiation for operable stage IIIA tumors are shown in Table 6-32. Postmastectomy radiation significantly decreased the risk of a local–regional recurrence to 12% to 15% in all four trials versus 23% to 58% after mastectomy and adjuvant systemic chemotherapy alone. Of the four trials, three have reported an absolute survival benefit of 7%, 7%, and 25% respectively with radiation.[337,394,398] This was statistically significant in only the Danish and Helsinki trials.[337,343,398] With only 131 patients, the South African trial had insufficient power for the 7% improvement in survival to reach statistical significance. The failure of the Eastern Cooperative Oncology Group[395] randomized trial of postmastectomy radiation in patients with T3-T4 operable breast cancer to demonstrate a survival benefit has been attributed in part to the reporting of the trial as well as the analysis.[295] Eighteen percent of the 164 patients randomized to radiation never received the treatment, and 30% of the patients who received radiation had major protocol variations. The results were reported in terms of intent to treat and included in the group assigned to radiation 30 patients who actually never received it. For patients receiving radiation, the isolated local–regional recurrence rate as the first site of failure was 4% versus 21% for those who did not receive radiation. The median survival for the patients who actually received radiation was 9.6 years versus 8.1 years for those randomized to observation. The authors unfortunately did not report overall survival for the group of patients who actually received radiation versus those who did not.

Experience with radiation alone for locally advanced tumors comes from the era prior to the advent of effective systemic chemotherapy. Because of the high rate of distant metastases and poor survival after radical or extended rad-

ical mastectomy that were the standard treatments of that era, primary irradiation was used to improve local–regional tumor control while avoiding the deformity and morbidity of radical surgery. The rates of local failure for operable locally advanced tumors treated by primary radiation were reported from 30% to 55% even after doses of 70 to 90 Gy.[399–402] The complications and frequent fair to poor cosmesis resulting from treatment also limited the applicability of this technique.[399,403] The advent of effective systemic chemotherapy has relegated primary radiation to historic interest only. There is little information on the breast recurrence rates for operable T3 breast cancers treated with conservative surgery and radiation with or without adjuvant systemic therapy. Toonkel et al.[402] reported that out of a series of 470 patients with operable stage III disease and a mean follow-up of 8 years, only two local recurrences were seen in 34 patients treated by breast-conserving surgery and radiation. Khanna et al.[404] also reported the results of conservative surgery and radiation in 36 patients with operable T3 tumors. Their local–regional recurrence was 3 of 36 (8%) patients within a median follow-up of 46 months.

Neoadjuvant chemotherapy has been used for operable T3 tumors to downstage the primary tumor and permit attempts at breast conservation. Although there is a high rate of clinical response to induction therapy, few patients overall will have a pathologic complete response (Table 6-30). Many series have inves-

**TABLE 6-32    Results of Randomized Trials of Postmastectomy Radiation Using Adjuvant Systemic Chemotherapy in Operable Stage IIIA Tumors**

| | | No Radiation | | | Radiation | |
|---|---|---|---|---|---|---|
| Trial | Number of Patients | Local–Regional Failure (%) | Overall Survival (%) | Number of Patients | Local–Regional Failure (%) | Overall Survival (%) |
| Helsinki[343,398] | 40 | 58 | 70 | 39 | 13 | 95 |
| Eastern Cooperative Oncology Group[395] | 148 | 24 | 47 | 164 | 15 | 46 |
| South Africa[394] | 64 | 23 | 56 | 67 | 12 | 63 |
| Danish[337] | 135 | 42 | 33 | 99 | 12 | 40 |

tigated a combined modality approach to treatment that tailors the selection of breast conservation to the response to induction chemotherapy. Danforth et al.[405] updated the results of a prospective trial by the National Cancer Institute in 126 patients, of whom 45% had clinical IIIA, 10% IIIB inoperable, and 45% IIIB inflammatory disease. All patients were treated to maximal clinical response with induction chemotherapy followed by repeat biopsies of the breast. Of 57 stage IIIA patients, only 18 had a clinical and pathologic complete response permitting local treatment by radiotherapy alone. The remaining patients underwent mastectomy and postoperative radiation. The overall local–regional failure rate for stage IIIA disease was 18% after a median potential follow-up of 8.3 years. Of the 18 patients treated with breast conservation, there were no in-breast recurrences. Three of 39 patients (8%) treated with mastectomy and radiation had a component of failure in the chest wall. A similar protocol was conducted in 89 patients at the University of Michigan.[406] Of 43 stage IIIA patients, only 12 were clinical and pathologic complete responders to induction. After a median follow-up of 4 to 4.5 years, the local–regional failure as an isolated component of first failure was 23% for stage IIIA disease. The result by choice of local treatment was reported for stage IIIA and B patients combined, but the local failure rate was 18% after radiotherapy alone and 30% after radiotherapy and mastectomy ($p = 0.5$).

Other series have also shown rates of local failure after breast conservation for operable T3 disease higher than those expected after conservative surgery and radiation in T1 and T2 disease or mastectomy and radiation in T3 disease. Jacquillat et al.[379] reported a 5-year actuarial breast recurrence of 18% for 57 T3 tumors having a complete response to induction chemotherapy and radiation alone. Buzdar et al.[407] reported that 15 of 60 T3 tumors were treated by conservative surgery and radiation after four cycles of induction chemotherapy and 3 (20%) had a breast recurrence after a median follow-up of only 43 months. Ellis et

al.[392] reported a series of patients with operable (62% stage III) breast cancer treated with induction chemotherapy followed by radiotherapy, mastectomy, or conservative surgery and radiation based on response. Patients treated without surgery tended to have complete or near-complete responses to chemotherapy. The crude local recurrence after a median of 41 months was 21% in those treated without surgery, and only 7% in those treated with mastectomy or conservative surgery ($p = 0.02$).

A few series have reported more favorable results when patients were selected for conservative surgery and radiation after induction chemotherapy. Bonadonna et al.[377] treated 52 of 84 (62%) women with tumors initially greater than 5 cm with quadrantectomy and radiation after induction chemotherapy, and reported an 8-year 4.3% risk of local recurrence. Schwartz[408] reported 160 patients with stage IIB-IIIB breast cancer who had a partial or complete response after induction chemotherapy. After patient selection based on the initial tumor characteristics and response to chemotherapy, the mastectomy group had a crude isolated local recurrence of 6% after a median of 53 months, while those treated with breast conservation had a crude local recurrence of only 2% after a median of 29 months.

Postmastectomy radiation for operable T3 breast cancers has been discussed elsewhere in this chapter. After neoadjuvant chemotherapy for operable T3 tumors, the radiation technique is similar to that described for T1 and T2 tumors. The whole breast has been treated with photon tangential fields to a dose of 50 Gy, with a range in reported series of 45 to 54 Gy.[377,378,380,381,384,392,409] Most series have employed a boost for an additional 10 to 20 Gy[377,381,384,392,410] after conservative surgery, and higher boosts for treatment with radiation alone.[379–381,384,405,406,409,410] Only the National Cancer Institute specified the boost volume after neoadjuvant chemotherapy in relation to the original prechemotherapy tumor volume.[405] Many series after conservative surgery have treated the breast alone without regional nodal irradiation.[377,378,381] Most others with or without conservative surgery have included treatment of the supraclavicular and axillary nodes,[379–381,384,409,410] while others have added a posterior axillary boost only if the axilla was undissected.[392,405,406] No specific attempt was made to treat clinically uninvolved internal mammary nodes in most series,[377,378,381,392,406] but some series treated them variably[405,409] or in all patients.[379,380,384]

## Inoperable Locally Advanced Breast Cancer

Patients with inoperable disease have tumors that are unresectable at presentation by modified radical or radical mastectomy. This corresponds to stage IIIB (T4 N1-3 or T1-3 N3) in the 1997 UICC-AJCC staging classification.[6] Inoperable locally advanced breast cancer includes tumors with ulceration of the skin, edema, satellite skin nodules or chest wall fixation (T4), or unresectable axillary nodes (N2). Internal mammary node disease (N3) is also considered in this category, although it is rarely diagnosed at presentation.

Induction doxorubicin-based neoadjuvant chemotherapy is the standard approach for inoperable stage III patients.[376] The response rates of stage IIIB noninflammatory breast cancer to induction chemotherapy are high, but complete responses are seen less often than in operable stage III tumors or inflammatory disease. After three to four cycles of doxorubicin and vincristine, Valagussa et al.[411] reported a complete clinical regression in only 7% and partial regression in 62%. After three cycles of fluorouracil, doxorubicin, and cyclophosphamide, Hortobagyi et al.[412] reported a clinical complete response in only 8% and partial response in 79%. With a median number of seven cycles of induction cyclophosphamide, doxorubicin, and fluorouracil, Schwartz[408] reported a higher overall response rate of 80%. Induction chemotherapy is successful in rendering these tumors resectable in most cases.[411–413]

The response of inoperable tumors to induction chemotherapy has been shown to be prognostic for subsequent disease-free and overall survival.[379,410,412] For example, Hortobagyi et al.[412] reported a 5-year survival of 88% for patients having a complete clinical response to three cycles of induction chemotherapy versus 44% after a partial response and 24% after no response ($p = 0.01$). A higher local–regional recurrence also was seen after a less than complete clinical response to induction chemotherapy. Second-line chemotherapy should be considered for the few patients remaining unresectable after first-line induction. Alternatively, radiation therapy may be used for patients not rendered resectable by chemotherapy.[414] Preoperative radiation in inoperable disease increases the response rates and resectability after less than a complete response to induction chemotherapy.[379,410,415,416] Because of the significant toxicity with concurrent radiation and chemotherapy, the need for dose reductions or avoidance of doxorubicin with previous or concurrent radiation, and increase in perioperative morbidity after chemoradiation, the sequential delivery of radiation after chemotherapy and mastectomy is preferable.[414,415,417]

Treatment after chemotherapy, mastectomy, and radiation is associated with local–regional control rates of 80% to 95%.[409–411,415] The rates of local recurrence after mastectomy are consistently lower than the results after radiation alone in retrospective series (Table 6-33). Valagussa et al.[411] reported that high dose irradiation after induction chemotherapy for inoperable tumors was associated with local recurrence rates of 30% to 40%. The incorporation of mastectomy into their regimen decreased the local failure rate to only 15%. Perloff et al.[413] reported a series of 112 stage III patients with T3 (36), T4 (62), or T4 (14) inflammatory tumors. After induction chemotherapy, only 87 patients were eligible for randomization to local treatment by either mastectomy or radiotherapy. The crude rate of first local relapse was 19% after mastectomy and 27% after radiotherapy, although this did not reach statistical significance.

The subset of patients with a complete response to induction chemotherapy may have an

**TABLE 6-33  Local-Regional Failure in Patients with Locally Advanced Breast Cancer Completing Combined Modality Treatment with Induction Chemotherapy Followed by Radiation with or Without Mastectomy**

| Study | Number of Patients | Stage | Induction Chemotherapy[a] | Local–Regional Failure (%) XRT Alone | XRT + Mastectomy | Follow-up (years) |
|---|---|---|---|---|---|---|
| Touboul et al.[410] | 97 | IIIA-B | AVFC23 | 5 | | 10 actuarial |
| Merajver et al.[406] | 75 | IIIA-B | CAMFPT | 18 | 30 | 5 actuarial |
| Perez et al.[409] | 165 | IIIA-B | CAF or CMF | 85 | 17 | 10 actuarial |
| Danforth et al.[405] | 57 | IIIA | CAMFPT | $0^b$ | $8^b$ | 8 median |
| | 12 | IIIB | | $20^b$ | $0^b$ | |
| | 55 | T4d | | $39^b$ | $22^b$ | |
| Valagussa et al.[411] | 206 | IIIB | AV  35 | 15 | | 10 crude |
| Brun et al.[427] | 22 | T4d | AVCF45 | 18 | | 4 minimum |
| Fleming et al.[422] | 172 | T4d | FAC ±VPr | 36 | 16 | 7 median |
| Perez et al.[419] | 121 | T4d | CAF or CMF | 63 | 21 | 4 median |

[a]Chemotherapy: C, cyclophosphamide; M, methotrexate; F, fluorouracil; A, doxorubicin; E, epirubicin; N, mitoxantrone; L, leucovorin; Ci, cisplatin; V, vincristine; Vb, vinblastine; Mc, mitomycin C; Th, Thiotepa; Vi, vindesine; P, Premarin; Pr, prednisone; T, tamoxifen; GMCSF, granulocyte–macrophage colony stimulating factor.

[b]Crude rate of local failure (breast or chest wall).

improved rate of local control with breast conservation, but still higher than that seen after mastectomy. Touboul et al.[410] reported after induction chemotherapy that 5- and 10-year local failure rates were 16% and 23% in patients treated by breast radiation alone after a complete response, and 16% and 30% after wide excision and radiation after a partial response. The corresponding rates were only 5% at 5 and 10 years after mastectomy. Schaake-Koning et al.[416] reported a 28% local recurrence rate for inoperable tumors after radiation with or without chemotherapy, even when there was a complete clinical response to therapy. Buzdar et al.[407] reported that only 6% of T4 tumors were able to be treated with breast conservation on their protocol after four cycles of induction chemotherapy, and 1 of 5 (20%) had a breast recurrence after a median follow-up of 43 months. Danforth et al.[405] reported that 5 of 12 patients (42%) with stage IIIB noninflammatory tumors had a clinical and pathologic complete response after neoadjuvant chemotherapy, permitting local treatment by radiotherapy alone. One of 5 patients (20%) treated with breast conservation had a breast recurrence, and none of the 7 patients treated with mastec-

tomy and radiation had a component of failure in the chest wall.

After neoadjuvant chemotherapy and mastectomy for initially inoperable tumors, the chest wall has been treated using tangents with doses in the range of 45 to 54 Gy.[405,506,409] Bolus is applied every other day. For patients treated preoperatively, the whole breast should be treated using tangent fields to 45 to 50 Gy.[379,406,409,410,413,414] For patients not undergoing surgery, a breast boost can be employed for an additional 20 to 30 Gy.[379,405,406,409–411,413] Most series have also employed treatment of the supraclavicular and axillary nodes for inoperable tumors,[379,409–411,413,414,416] while some have used a posterior axillary field only if the nodes had not been dissected.[405,406] Internal mammary nodes have been treated in most series of patients with inoperable tumors,[379,410,411,413,416] but variably or not at all in others.[405,406,409,414]

## Inflammatory Breast Cancer

Inflammatory carcinoma is a distinct clinical entity within stage IIIB, staged by the UICC-AJCC as T4d.[6] Inflammatory carcinomas present with clinical findings of diffuse erythema, warmth, skin edema, and induration of greater than one-third of the breast. Regardless of the resectability at time of presentation, inflammatory breast cancers are characterized as inoperable because of the high rates of recurrence after initial local–regional therapy. Dermal lymphatic invasion, a pathologic hallmark of inflammatory disease, is not required for the diagnosis in the presence of clinical findings.[418,419] The diagnosis should not be based on secondary inflammatory changes immediately associated with neglected locally advanced tumors or dermal lymphatic invasion alone.

Induction chemotherapy is the primary treatment of inflammatory tumors.[376] The response rates to induction chemotherapy are comparable to or even higher than inoperable tumors and range from 46% to 97%.[406,408,419–423] Complete responses are seen in 11% to 58%.[406,419–423] Over one-half to two-thirds of these patients with a complete clinical response to induction chemotherapy are found to have microscopic residual disease.[406,420,421] The degree of response to induction chemotherapy, and the subsequent finding of a pathologic complete response, are prognostic for local–regional control and survival for inflammatory breast cancers.[420,422–425] Therefore, such measures as sequential administration of second-line chemotherapy or radiation to improve response are not infrequently employed prior to surgery for those not initially achieving a complete clinical response. The 5-year survival for patients with inflammatory disease after combined modality therapy incorporating systemic chemotherapy with local treatment is 36% to 59%.[420–423,425] In patients obtaining a complete response to induction chemotherapy prior to local therapy, 5-year disease-free survivals of over 60% have been reported.[420,422,425]

The importance of obtaining a complete clinical response prior to surgery, the recognition of the need for aggressive combined modality therapy, and the promising use of high dose chemotherapy for locally advanced disease,[424,426] are all reflected in a current Philadelphia Bone Marrow Transplant protocol. This study enrolls patients with inoperable or inflammatory stage IIIB disease and is designed to maximize the chance that a patient will reach a complete clinical response prior to undergoing mastectomy. The induction chemotherapy phase involves doxorubicin for four cycles and tamoxifen. Patients having a complete response go on to mastectomy, while those with only a partial response receive taxol. After mastectomy, all patients have postmastectomy radiation. The favorable subgroup with a complete pathologic response at mastectomy undergoes additional adjuvant conventional dose chemotherapy. High dose chemotherapy with bone marrow transplant or peripheral stem cell support is used in all other patients with residual disease in the mastectomy specimen, or preoperatively for those still not achieving a complete response after taxol.

The highest local–regional control rates for inflammatory breast cancers are achieved by using mastectomy in addition to radiation and chemotherapy (Table 6-33). Fowble and Glover[420] reported a 5-year 8% rate of local–regional failure in 38 patients with inflammatory carcinoma treated by induction chemotherapy, radiation, and mastectomy. The rate of local–regional failure after induction chemotherapy and radiation alone has exceeded 30% to 40% in other series.[423,425] Fleming et al.[422] reported a statistically significant decrease in local–regional relapse from 36% to 16% ($p = 0.016$) when mastectomy was added to the combined modality regimen of chemotherapy and radiation. Mastectomy decreased the rate of local–regional recurrence and improved disease-free survival in this series even in the subsets of patients with a clinical complete or partial response to induction therapy. A significant decrease in local–regional failures when mastectomy was added to combined modality regimens incorporating chemotherapy and radiation has been reported in several other retrospective studies.[419,427]

Some series have used a selective approach to breast conservation versus mastectomy based on response to induction chemotherapy. Jacquillat et al.[379] reported a 19% 5-year actuarial breast recurrence for 58 patients with T4 tumors (mostly inflammatory) with a complete response after induction chemotherapy and radiation without mastectomy. Danforth et al.[405] updated the results of a prospective trial by the National Cancer Institute in which patients with locally advanced disease were treated to maximal clinical response with induction chemotherapy followed by a rebiopsy of the breast. Of 55 patients with inflammatory carcinoma, only 18 had a clinical and pathologic complete response, permitting local treatment by radiotherapy alone. The remaining patients underwent mastectomy and postoperative radiation. The overall local–regional failure rate was 36% after a median potential follow-up of 8.3 years. Of the 18 patients treated with breast conservation, 39% experienced an in-breast recurrence. Eight of 37 patients (22%) treated with mastectomy and radiation had a component of failure in the chest wall. A similar protocol was conducted in 89 patients at the University of Michigan.[406] Of 36 inflammatory patients, only 8 were clinical and pathologic complete responders to induction. After a median follow-up of 4 to 4.5 years, the local–regional failure as an isolated or component of first failure was 28% for inflammatory disease. The result by choice of local treatment was reported for stage IIIA and B patients combined, but the local failure rate was 18% in complete pathologic responders treated by radiotherapy alone and 30% after radiotherapy and mastectomy ($p = 0.5$).

After a mastectomy for inflammatory breast cancer, the entire chest wall has been treated to 50 Gy with a range of 50 to 54 Gy in most series.[405,506,419,428] Bolus is applied every other day. For preoperative treatment of inflammatory breast cancer, 50 to 54 Gy to the whole breast has been given.[405,406,419,420,423,428] Bolus of the intact breast is decreased to every third day to avoid severe moist desquamation.[420] For patients treated with neoadjuvant chemotherapy and radiation alone, boost doses to the tumor bed are employed up to 60 to 75 Gy.[405,406,419,423,425] The supraclavicular nodes should also be treated in all patients.[405,406,419,420,423,428] Axillary recurrence has been reported to be an uncommon (< 10%) component of failure after an adequate dissection, obviating the need for a posterior axillary boost in those patients.[405,406,419,428] Internal mammary node recurrence is extremely rare with[405,419,421–423,428] or without[405,406,419,420] specifically directed internal mammary irradiation, with no reported differences in regional failure rates or survival. Caution is needed after high dose chemotherapy before postmastectomy radiation is begun, particularly if the internal mammary nodes are to be included, because of the high risks of pulmonary or hematologic toxicity.[201] Blood counts should be allowed to reach levels above 100,000 platelets and 3000 white cells before starting, even if a prolonged interval between transplant and radiation is necessary.

## RADIATION TECHNIQUES FOR THE TREATMENT OF BREAST CANCER

Patients are simulated in the supine position. An alpha-cradle cast is used for immobilization to improve daily setup accuracy. The cast also will improve comfort and support of the arms and shoulders. An angle board of 10°–20° levels the curvature of the chest wall in the horizontal plane and prevents shift of breast tissue superiorly.

### Tangent Fields for Treatment of the Intact Breast

The clinical target volume to be treated after wide excision includes the surgical cavity as defined by radiopaque clips, the entire remaining breast tissue down to the pectoralis muscles, the axillary tail, and chest wall lymphatics beneath the breast. Opposed tangential fields are used with a gantry rotation to create a non-diverging posterior edge

The clinical landmarks used during simulation to set up the tangents are as follows: superiorly 2 cm beyond the most cephalad extent of palpable breast tissue, inferiorly 2 cm below the most inferior aspect of the breast, laterally 2 cm beyond palpable breast tissue, and medially at midline. The radiographic borders of the tangent fields are as follows (Figure 6-1): inferiorly 2 cm below the breast, anteriorly to include 1.5 to 2 cm of air beyond the breast, and posteriorly to include 1.5 to 2 cm of lung tissue. More lung may be required posteriorly to have at least 1 cm margin around clips in far medial or lateral tumor beds. The superior border as determined clinically will usually extend at or higher than the clavicular head but should be inferior to the glenoid fossa and the humeral head. Collimator rotation is used to optimize the position of both the upper and lower posterior corners within the chest wall. For left-sided tangents, excess collimator rotation could result in excessive heart volume within the field. The edges of the tangents should always be checked clinically at simulation to ensure proper coverage of the breast and surgical scars.

Das et al.[429] have analyzed the simulation films from over 100 women treated with conventionally designed breast tangents and correlated them with the resulting volume of irradiated heart and lung determined by CT simulation. There was a direct linear correlation of the central lung distance on the simulator film with the volume of lung irradiated: 0.6%/mm on the left and 0.5%/mm on the right. A typical tangent field with 1.5 to 2 cm of lung would therefore treat approximately 8% to 12% of the ipsilateral lung volume. The percentage of heart irradiated from left-sided tangents was inversely related to the gantry angle, reflecting increasing heart dose with deeper tangents, and only weakly correlated with the central lung distance. Eighty percent of patients had less than 3% of the heart volume irradiated; fewer than 3% of patients had 10% or more.

A single transverse contour of the breast through the isocenter of the tangent fields is taken during simulation. Dosimetric calcula-

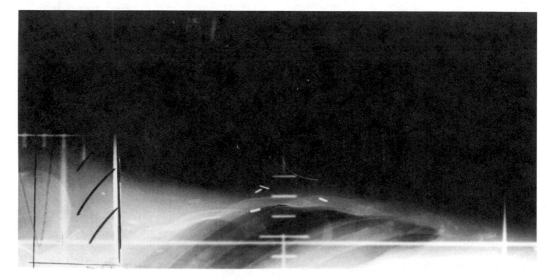

**FIGURE 6-1** Simulation film of a breast tangent field. This patient was treated with a three-field technique, so a block was placed over the image of the rod and chain superiorly to create the match plane with the supraclavicular field shown later (see Figure 6-3).

tions are then commonly performed without lung inhomogeneity corrections. Wedges are used in the tangent fields to improve homogeneity of the isodose distribution. The point to which the prescribed dose is delivered, or the normalization point, varies by convention among institutions.[430] Selection of a point 1.5 cm from the nondivergent posterior beam edge guarantees treatment of all breast tissue to a minimum of the prescribed dose. The ICRU 50 convention is to a point on the central axis midway on a perpendicular line between the breast apex and the posterior field edge.[431] The dose variability by choice of prescription points is generally within an average of 5% except for large breast separations and prescribing to the maximum dose point.[430]

Three-dimensional treatment planning of breast tangent radiation is possible when CT-based technology is used. The potential advantages over conventional dosimetry lie in the ability to correct the dose inhomogeneity within the breast due to changes in contour away from the central axis and to the decreased photon attenuation by low density lung tissue. The use of three-dimensional treatment planning and custom tissue compensators has been proposed but rarely used in clinical practice because of the considerable time, expense, and complexities of design and use.[432,433] The potential benefit of three-dimensional planning is small for most patients because of the excellent results and low complications already seen with conventional dosimetry. Lung density corrections will generally increase the calculated hot spots within the breast and result in a prescription that reduces the actual dose delivered to the breast compared to conventional dose calculations. The clinical impact on breast recurrence rates caused by lung density corrections is uncertain. Lung density corrections have been routinely employed for conservative surgery and radiation at the National Cancer Institute and University of Michigan.[116,127] The NCI reported a high 10-year actuarial first ipsilateral breast recurrence rate of 18% in 121 patients. In contrast, the University of Michigan re-

ported an actuarial recurrence rate of 4% at 5 years in 429 women.

Women with large breast size and separations greater than 22 cm often have an unacceptable (> 10%) inhomogeneity in the central axis when 6 MV photons are used.[430] A Lucite beam spoiler can be placed in a higher energy beam to improve dose homogeneity.[142] The beam spoiler will increase the subcutaneous dose in the buildup region of the 10 or 18 MV beams. The advantage of a beam spoiler over bolus is that the skin-sparing effect of the megavoltage energies is maintained. A support bra may also be used for large or pendulous breasts during simulation and daily treatment. The bra improves consistency of daily setup, and also decreases desquamation of the inframammary fold during treatment. The use of a breast-positioning ring for large-breasted women has been associated with a high rate of acute moist desquamation and resulting treatment interruptions.[434]

The usual dose of the tangent fields used for invasive disease is 46 Gy in 23 fractions over 4.5 weeks. A slightly higher dose of 50 Gy in 25 fractions over 5 weeks is recommended for microinvasive or noninvasive disease because of the higher risk of multicentric disease. When no boost is planned for invasive disease, the total dose of the tangents should also be increased to 50 Gy.

## Intact Breast Boost

A boost to the biopsy site after tangential irradiation is frequently employed. The clinical target volume is the tumor bed as defined by surgical clips, the lumpectomy cavity, or architectural distortion seen on CT images. An additional margin is allowed for daily setup error and constriction of the higher isodose curves with depth. The entire surgical scar should be included, but the practice of drawing a simple field on the skin around the scar without regard to the internal anatomy should be avoided. Conventional methods of creating the electron boost field using fluoroscopy or CT have been described.[435]

CT simulation provides accurate localization in the intact breast of the surgical tumor bed, and greater ability to optimize the parameters of the electron beam than are possible with conventional simulation.[436,437] The patient should undergo the CT scan in the same treatment position, cast, and angle board as the tangent fields. Virtual simulation permits the optimization of field size, treatment depth, gantry angle, and couch position for the electron boost (Figure 6-2). The volume of breast irradiated is minimized by positioning the surgical scar over the clips or imaged biopsy cavity. A perpendicular incidence of the electron beam will also result in maximum skin sparing. A digitally reconstructed radiograph includes visual information about the orientation of the beam, position of the scar and surgical clips, and treatment depth. This provides reliable setup information for accurate daily reproducibility, and permanent documentation of the electron boost field for the medical record.

The dose for the electron boost varies according to the extent of surgery and final margin status: 14 Gy for a reexcision with no

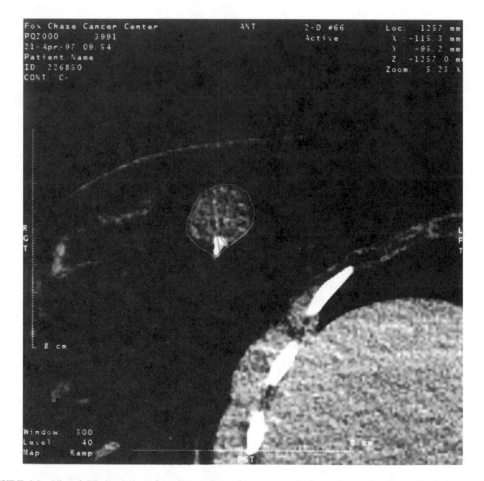

**FIGURE 6-2**   Virtual CT simulation of an electron breast boost. (a) A single axial CT slice through the breast. The clips and biopsy cavity can be contoured separately. The depth to the deepest clip is easily determined during the virtual simulation. (b) An optimized beam's-eye view of the electron boost that overlaps the scar and the clips within the smallest boost field possible.

residual tumor, 18 Gy for either a single excision or a reexcision with residual tumor, and 20 Gy for a focally positive margin. For noninvasive disease, the same guidelines are used less 4 Gy because of the higher dose given with the tangents.

### Tangent Fields for the Treatment of the Chest Wall

The chest wall is treated postmastectomy with opposed tangential photon fields with a gantry rotation to create a nondiverging poste-

rior edge. The clinical and radiographic borders of the tangent fields are modified from those for the intact breast to encompass the entire chest wall and surgical scar, which are at risk for failure. Partial chest wall treatment is inadequate. The most common dose employed is 50 Gy in 25 fractions of 2 Gy over 5 weeks. Both fields should be treated daily, 5 days a week. Wedge filters and/or high energy beams with a spoiler may be used to improve dose homogeneity as in the intact breast. A bolus material of 1 cm thickness should be placed over the entire chest wall daily when

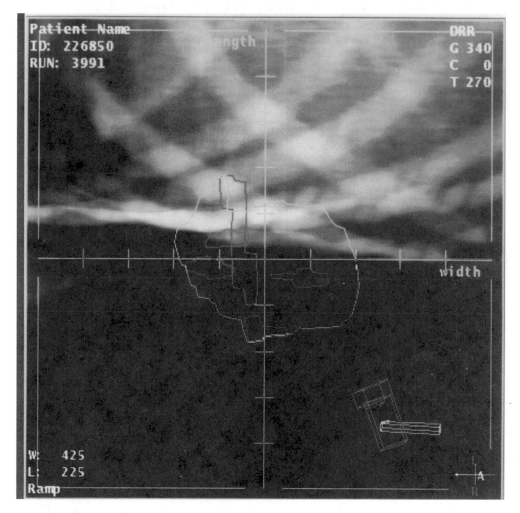

**FIGURE 6-2**   *(Continued)*

beam energies of 6 MV or higher are used. There is no additional local control benefit to a boost of the scar or increased use of bolus material daily.[344]

## Supraclavicular Nodes

The borders of the supraclavicular field are inferiorly at the inferior aspect of the clavicular head, superiorly at the cricothyroid notch, medially 1 cm across midline at the sternal notch, and laterally at the medial border of humeral head (Figure 6-3). When a posterior axillary boost is planned, the lateral border of the supraclavicular field is the midhumeral head. The gantry is angled 11°–12° to shield the spinal cord. A block is placed medial to the sternocleidomastoid muscle to shield the larynx. A half-beam block creates a nondivergent inferior beam edge. The dose is 46 Gy in 23 fractions of 2 Gy over 4.5 weeks. The anterior photon field is prescribed to a depth of 3 cm.

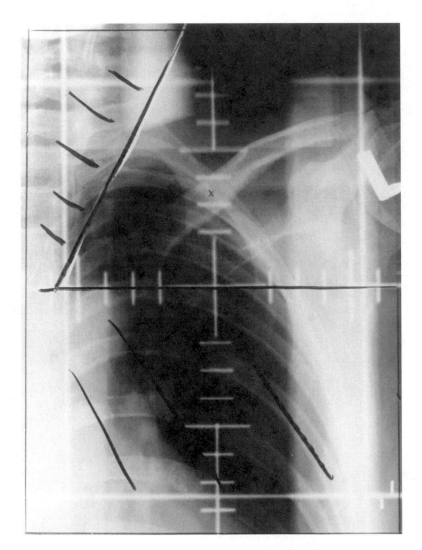

**FIGURE 6-3** Simulation film of a supraclavicular field when a posterior axillary field was not used. A half-beam block has been used to create a nondiverging inferior match to the tangent field shown in Figure 6-1.

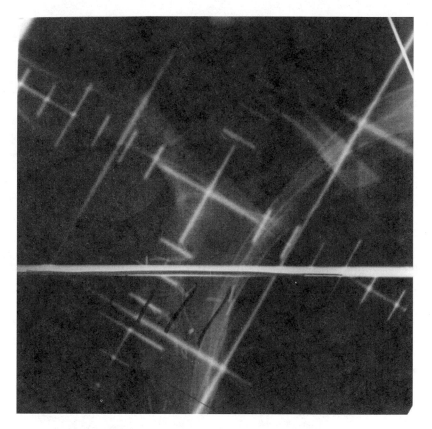

**FIGURE 6-4**    Simulation film of a posterior axillary boost field.

A geometrically nondivergent match plane between the supraclavicular field and tangent fields is created by means of a metal rod and chain.[438] The advantages of this technique include simplicity, low cost, a sensitivity to errors in couch position of as little as half a degree, and the absence of a requirement for half-beam blocks for tangent fields. In addition, the patient surface tattoos can be used for reliable repositioning of rod and chain to recreate the match plane, and the rod and chain are visible on simulation and portal films for reliable verification of match plane. The metal rod is placed on the skin along inferior border of the supraclavicular field with chains hanging by gravity at 90° angles to the rod. The superior border of the tangents is extended to 2 to 3 cm within the supraclavicular field. The couch is rotated until the rod and chain images overlap on fluoroscopy. This match plane defined by rod and chain on simulation film indicates position for the Cerrobend block covering the portions of the tangent fields that overlap the supraclavicular field.

## Axilla

When a decision has been made to boost the midaxillary lymph nodes, a single posterior field delivering 1 Gy per day, 2 to 3 days per week, will bring the total dose to the midaxillary nodes to 46 Gy. A dose calculation at the prescription point and depth of the brachial plexus should account for the contribution from the supraclavicular and posterior axillary fields to avoid exceeding peripheral nerve tolerance.

The posterior axillary field is set up radiographically (Figure 6-4). The collimator is rotated to create a border superiorly that is parallel to and just above the midclavical, medially 1 cm within and parallel to the chest wall, and laterally at the midhumeral head. A block is placed to create the border inferiorly at the match plane with the tangent fields.

## Internal Mammary Nodes

When a decision has been made to treat the internal mammary lymph nodes, the technique chosen should not only result in good anatomical coverage but also give minimum irradiation of normal tissues (heart and lung). Significant acute hematologic complications and symptomatic pneumonitis have been reported with internal mammary irradiation given after systemic chemotherapy.[201] Radiation has been associated with increased cardiac mortality when

techniques are used that irradiate a significant volume of the heart.[239,439] The internal mammary field should be individualized to each patient's anatomy with CT-based planning. This will help to optimize a technique that treats to an appropriate depth for nodal coverage and allows three-dimensional dosimetry of the dose homogeneity and dose to the normal tissue. The dose to the nodes at risk should be 50 Gy in 25 fractions, daily over 5 weeks.

A direct anterior or angled photon field matched medially to shallow tangents should be avoided because this arrangement will result in a high cardiac dose and irradiated volume.[197,440] For increased coverage of the internal mammary nodes compared to standard tangents, the medial border of the tangent fields can be moved to 3 cm across midline on the contralateral side. This deep

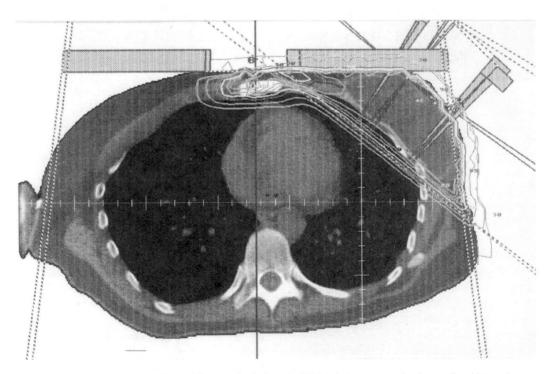

**FIGURE 6-5**   Dosimetry in the plane of the central axis for a six-field technique to treat the chest wall and internal mammary lymph nodes. Two separate three-field arrangements, an anterior electron field matched to shallow tangents, are given on alternating days with feathering of the match line. The result shown is full dose coverage to the nodes at risk with minimization of the cold region beneath the match line that would result from a single three-field arrangement. This technique also preserves skin cosmesis and irradiates a minimum volume of heart and lung.

tangent technique is suboptimal because of the large volume of irradiated lung and subsequent risk of symptomatic pneumonitis.[197] This technique will also treat a significant volume of heart for left-sided tumors and complicate any additional contralateral radiation. Marks et al.[345] have reported a modification of this technique that uses CT planning to treat only the superior internal mammary nodes at highest risk for disease with this deep tangent technique, yet shallower fields more inferiorly to protect the heart.

A single anterior electron field can be matched medially to shallow tangent fields to treat the internal mammary nodes. This setup has the advantage of minimizing dose to the heart and lung compared to the previous techniques. When deeper coverage of the nodes is needed based on the patient's anatomy, a photon beam can be mixed with the electrons to increase the dose at depth yet minimize dose to the skin and heart in comparison to electrons alone. The anterior electron beam technique will result in a volume beneath the match line that is underdosed.[440] A rotation of the electron field parallel to the photon tangents to eliminate this cold spot will cause significantly more lung to be irradiated.[197] Overlapping the photon tangents and anterior electrons increases the skin dose and creates a hot spot under the match. Electron arc therapy or matching electron beams alone[440] for treating the chest wall and internal mammary nodes have been employed.

One arrangement that treats the internal mammary nodes and addresses all these concerns is shown in Figure 6-5. This technique involves feathering the match line of an anterior electron beam and shallow tangents during treatment to spread out and minimize the cold spot under the match, preserve the skin cosmesis, and avoid increased heart or lung irradiation. At simulation, two separate three-field arrangements of matching anterior electron beams to shallow tangents can be created, with the match lines 0.5 to 1 cm apart on skin. The two separate arrangements are alternated every other day.

## TREATMENT OF LOCAL–REGIONAL RECURRENCE FOLLOWING BREAST CONSERVATION THERAPY

Approximately 10% of patients with stage I-II invasive breast cancer with negative resection margins will develop an ipsilateral breast tumor recurrence at 10 years.[92,129,131,151,441] The majority of breast recurrences are detected by physical examination, with approximately one-third being detected by mammography alone.[442–448] The mammographic finding of microcalcifications associated with a mass is virtually always indicative of a recurrence.[445] Approximately two-thirds of patients whose sole mammographic finding is the appearance of microcalcifications have biopsy-proven recurrence.[442–445] The finding of a mass on mammogram only is associated with biopsy-proven recurrence in 30% to 60% of patients.[442–445] The majority of recurrences following conservative surgery and radiation are in the vicinity of original primary tumor, with 20% to 30% of recurrences occurring in a quadrant separate from the original cancer.[448–453] The incidence of recurrences in a separate quadrant increases as the time interval to recurrence increases, as well as extensiveness of the surgical procedure. Approximately 50% of breast recurrences following quadrantectomy occur in a separate quadrant,[454] and the majority of recurrences after 10 years are in a separate quadrant.[449] The median interval to a breast recurrence is approximately 4 years, and the risk of a breast recurrence in 5 years has been estimated to be 1.5% to 2.5% per year, diminishing to 1% per year after 8 to 10 years.[453,455] Approximately 10% of patients with an ipsilateral breast tumor recurrence following conservative surgery and radiation will present with simultaneous or antecedent distant metastasis.[449–452] Most (85–90%) of those without distant metastasis are surgically operable. Ninety percent of breast recurrences are invasive cancer, with only 10% being ductal carcinoma in situ.[448,452] Approximately one-third of patients with an invasive breast cancer at the time of salvage mastectomy and axillary dissection have positive axillary nodes.[448,449] The standard treatment of an ipsilateral breast tumor recurrence following conservative surgery and radiation in the absence of distant metastasis is mastectomy. Five-year survival rates following salvage mastectomy range from 55% to 85%.[130,447,448,454,456–462] Salvage mastectomy has resulted in subsequent local–regional control rates of 90%.[448,449,461] The impact of a breast recurrence on ultimate survival has been evaluated by several series. An ipsilateral breast tumor recurrence within 5 years of initial diagnosis is associated with an increased risk of distant metastasis.[455,460] Two series[463,464] have demonstrated no difference in 10-year survival when patients who developed an isolated breast recurrence and underwent salvage mastectomy are compared with those who did not. Kurtz et al.[457] reported that recurrences occurring after 5 years had no adverse effect on prognosis up to 15 years after initial treatment. However, recurrences within 5 years were associated with a decreased survival at 5, 10, and 15 years. Stotter et al.[459] reported a 5-year survival of 78% following initial treatment of patients with a local failure, versus 88% for those who did not develop a recurrence. Chauvet et al.[465] also reported a decreased survival at 5 years in patients who developed ipsilateral breast tumor recurrence versus those who did not.

The role of surgical procedures less than mastectomy in the treatment of an isolated breast recurrence following conservative surgery and radiation has been evaluated by Kurtz et al.[466] Fifty patients with an isolated breast recurrence were treated with wide excision alone, and the subsequent 5-year actuarial breast recurrence rate was 37%. The only group of patients in whom the subsequent risk of an ipsilateral breast tumor recurrence was less than 10% consisted of those in whom the disease-free interval exceeded 5 years. Second recurrences occurred in 24% of patients with negative margins of resection versus 47% in those with positive or unknown margins. Supplemental local radiotherapy to the region of recurrence did not result in a further decrease in the risk of a breast recurrence (i.e., 36%

with supplemental radiotherapy vs. 39% without). A second recurrence was associated with a significant decrease in 5-year survival. Therefore, at the present time mastectomy represents the standard treatment for an ipsilateral breast tumor recurrence following conservative surgery and radiation in the absence of distant metastasis.

The incidence of regional node recurrence following conservative surgery and radiation is less than 5%.[196,202,203] The most common site for a regional recurrence is the axilla with or without a simultaneous breast failure, and the most second common site is the supraclavicular nodes. The treatment of a regional node relapse following conservative surgery and radiation is related to the site of failure and to prior treatment. Isolated axillary failures may be treated successfully with repeat axillary dissection,[196,449] to maximize regional control. Mastectomy is not indicated in patients with an isolated axillary recurrence who have no clinical or mammographic evidence of a simultaneous breast recurrence. Supraclavicular recurrences, where possible, should be treated by excisional biopsy followed by regional radiation, provided this area has not been treated previously. Approximately 50% of patients are alive without evidence of disease following salvage therapy for an axillary recurrence,[196,203,449] whereas supraclavicular failures are associated with a poor prognosis and a high risk of distant metastasis.[196,203,454]

## Local–Regional Recurrence Following Mastectomy

Overall, 10% of patients who undergo a modified radical mastectomy for stage I-II breast cancer will experience a local–regional recurrence. This pattern of failure represents approximately 30% of all first recurrences.[194,250,255,280,302,467] The chest wall is the most common site of failure, either as the only site or as a component of multiple sites.[195,271,272,274,468–473] The second most common site of failure is the supraclavicular region, followed by the axilla. Clinical internal mammary recurrences are infrequent. Ten to 30% of patients will have involvement of multiple sites.[195,271,274,468,469,471,473] At the time of a postmastectomy local–regional recurrence, 30% of patients will have had antecedent distant metastasis, and 25% will develop distant metastasis within several months of the diagnosis of recurrent disease.[470,474,475]

In general, the treatment of an isolated local–regional recurrence following mastectomy involves surgical excision where possible, radiation, and systemic therapy. Complete excision prior to radiation has resulted in an improvement in local control as well as overall survival.[274,476,477] Aberizk et al.[274] reported local control rates of 57% at 5 years in patients who had undergone total gross excision versus 24% without excision. Beck et al.[476] reported a 5-year survival rate of 63% for recurrences that were excised versus 24% for those not excised. Since the extent of disease is related to resectability as well as to overall prognosis, the improvement in overall survival may not be solely related to the surgical procedure. However, the use of an excisional biopsy prior to radiation results in improved local control and permits the use of lower doses of radiation. Several series have reported the results of excision alone as the sole treatment for a local recurrence. Sixty to 70% of patients who undergo excision alone will subsequently develop a second local recurrence.[244,470,472,476,478] Radical resections of the chest wall have also been employed for selected patients. The resection may include the full thickness of the chest wall, skin, subcutaneous tissue, muscle, and ribs or sternum. Local control rates range from 60% to 80%, with major complications occurring in 0% to 33%.[479–481] Five-year survival rates range from 31% to 58%.[479,481]

Radiotherapy has been the primary treatment for local–regional recurrence following mastectomy. The results achieved in this heterogeneous group of patients have varied owing to differences in surgical and radiotherapy techniques. For patients with an isolated chest wall recurrence, treatment is initially directed to the entire chest wall and supraclavicular region.

The use of small fields to treat only the clinical area of recurrence has resulted in significant failure rates.[273,468,477,482,483] Omission of elective treatment of the supraclavicular region has resulted in supraclavicular failure rates of 16% to 28%.[195,470] Treatment of the entire chest wall and elective treatment of the supraclavicular region has resulted in improved local control as well as 5-year survival rates.[195,471,484] Elective treatment of the axilla and internal mammary node regions has not been associated with improved local–regional control or survival for an isolated chest wall recurrence.[195,470] Elective treatment of the chest wall is indicated for a supraclavicular or internal mammary recurrence but not for an axillary recurrence.[195] The recommended dose of radiation is dependent on the extent of the disease as well as the extent of surgical resection. For electively treated sites, a dose of 4500 to 5000 cGy results in 90% control.[485] For patients who have undergone complete excision of their recurrent disease, doses in the range of 4500 to 5000 cGy result in control rates of 90%.[195,271,468–470] A boost dose of an additional 1000 to 1500 cGy may be considered in patients with positive or unknown margins of resection. For gross residual tumor, local control is related to the size of the residual disease as well as radiation dose. For tumors in the range of 1 to 3 cm, Halverson et al.[195] reported local–regional control with doses greater than 6000 cGy in 100% versus 76% with doses less than 6000 cGy. For larger recurrences, doses in the range of 6000 to 7000 cGy result in control in 50% of the patients, and this rate does not appear to increase with doses in excess of 7000 cGy.[195] For patients presenting with regional node recurrences, surgical excision prior to radiation should be considered. Halverson et al.[195] reported regional control rates in 82% of patients who underwent excision prior to radiation and 66% for those with gross residual tumor in a regional node site. Fletcher and Montague[486] reported an 87% regional control rate in patients with palpable axillary disease and 98% in patients with supraclavicular adenopathy who received 6000 to 7000 cGy. Complications related to treatment were reported in 26% of the patients and included arm edema and brachial plexopathy. Therefore excision prior to radiation results in improved regional control and allows for the use of lower doses of radiation. For patients with gross residual disease, complete response rates to radiation range from 40% to 97%.[271,274,468,469,473,476,477,482,487] Despite a complete clinical response, recurrences following radiation are common and occur in approximately 50% of the patients treated.[271,272,274,473,482] Local–regional control rates in patients with gross residual disease who achieve a complete clinical response with radiation are similar to those achieved in patients who have had an excisional biopsy followed by radiation.[274,470,477] A CT scan of the chest prior to the initiation of radiation will help to determine the extent of local–regional disease and may detect an unsuspected parasternal recurrence. Approximately 50% of patients undergoing computerized tomography of the chest have been found to have unsuspected local–regional disease, and 25% have been found to have unsuspected distant metastasis, with these findings leading to a change in treatment in 30% to 70% of patients.[488–491]

The role of adjuvant systemic therapy in the treatment of an isolated local–regional recurrence following mastectomy remains controversial. Several studies have demonstrated an improvement in local–regional control and overall survival with the addition of chemotherapy compared to radiation alone.[271,473,476,487,492,493] Olson et al.[492] reported the results of a randomized trial of radiation and actinomycin D versus radiation alone. The rate of local control was 80% in the chemotherapy and radiation group (15 patients) and 59% in the radiation alone group (17 patients). Halverson et al.[494] in a retrospective series with matched pair analysis noted no significant differences between patients treated with radiation alone versus radiation and chemotherapy in terms of local control, freedom from distant metastasis, disease-free survival, or overall survival. In practice, chemotherapy and/or hormonal therapy is often administered to patients with an isolated local–regional re-

currence, and these patients are now eligible for dose-intense chemotherapy regimens employing peripheral stem cell rescue or autologous marrow transplant. A single prospective randomized trial has evaluated the addition of tamoxifen to radiation for isolated local–regional recurrences.[495] Eligibility criteria included positive or unknown estrogen receptor status, disease-free interval greater than 1 year, complete excision of three or fewer nodules no larger than 3 cm in diameter. Patients received 5000 cGy in 5 weeks to the involved region and were randomly assigned to tamoxifen or observation. The 5-year relapse-free survival rate was 59% for tamoxifen and radiation versus 36% for radiation alone, and the difference was statistically significant. Tamoxifen appeared to reduce the risk of subsequent local treatment failure from 33% to 12% but did not impact on the rate of distant metastasis; by 8 to 9 years, the difference in relapse-free survival had disappeared. In their retrospective series with matched pair analysis, Halverson et al.[494] reported a statistically significant improvement in freedom from distant metastasis, disease-free survival, and overall survival for 59 patients treated with hormonal therapy and radiation with those treated with radiation alone. There was no improvement in local control.

Survival following a postmastectomy isolated local–regional recurrence at 5 years ranges from 10% to 50%,[195,272–274,292,293,468,469,471,473–477,482,496,497] with 10-year survival rates ranging from 5% to 26%. The prognosis of a patient with an isolated local–regional recurrence following mastectomy is related to the disease-free interval, the initial nodal status, the initial tumor size, hormone receptor status, the size of the recurrence, the number of sites involved, the use of surgery, and adequate radiation. The most important factors are the disease-free interval between primary treatment and the recurrence, the initial disease extent as reflected by initial tumor size and histologic nodal status, and the extent of recurrence. The 5-year survival for a disease-free interval of less than 2 years ranges from 10% to 30% versus 40% to 70% for a disease-free interval greater than 2 years.[271–274,292,472,473,482,484] The 5-year survival rate for initially node-negative patients range from 5% to 60% versus 30% to 40% for node-positive patients, and only 20% for those with four or more positive nodes.[292,468,472,476,482] Disease-free interval and stage of disease appear to be related in that patients with stage I or II disease have a longer disease-free interval than those with stage III disease.[474,476] Survival is also influenced by the extent of the recurrent disease. A single nodule on the chest wall has an improved survival over multiple nodules.[273,475,477,482,487,498] The size of the largest recurrence is also a predictor for survival.[273,482] Patients with an isolated chest wall recurrence have better survival than those with a chest wall and a nodal recurrence.[473,498] Patients who have locally controlled disease have better 5-year survival than those with uncontrolled disease.[195,271,272,468,469,477,482,487,499] Schwaibold et al.[271] identified a favorable subgroup of patients with an isolated local–regional recurrence treated with radiation with or without systemic therapy. This favorable subgroup comprised only 18% of the entire group of patients and was characterized by a disease-free interval of 24 months or more, an excisional biopsy prior to radiation, and local–regional control. In this group of patients, the 5-year survival was 61% and the relapse-free survival was 59%. Willner et al.[483] also identified a favorable subgroup of patients among those with a postmastectomy local–regional recurrence. The group comprised 10% of the patients and was characterized by a single chest wall or axillary recurrence, age greater than 50 years, disease-free interval of 1 year or more, initial T1 or T2 tumor without necrosis, and control of the recurrence. The 5- and 10-year survival rates were 100% and 69%, respectively.

Treatment options for patients who develop a second local–regional recurrence after treatment with radiation for an initial local–regional recurrence include surgical resection, reirradiation, radiation combined with hyperthermia, and photodynamic therapy. For patients with a small localized recurrence, wide excision alone may be employed. Radical chest wall resections were discussed earlier. The role of reirradiation for a chest wall recurrence is not well established. The second course of radiation not infrequently consists of electrons, and doses of 4000 to 5000 cGy have resulted in stable or controlled disease in approximately 60% of patients.[500,501] The role of low dose reirradiation in combination with hyperthermia has been evaluated by a number of investigators.

In a randomized phase III trial comparing radiation and hyperthermia with the radiation alone for superficial tumors, hyperthermia appeared to provide no additional benefit over radiation alone.[502] Complete response rates range from 35% to 74% for hyperthermia and radiation for recurrent chest wall disease.[503–508] Following radiation and hyperthermia, further infield recurrence rates range from 15% to 39%.[503–508] Lee et al.[503] reported actuarial local tumor control rates of 33% at 3 years. These results were similar to those reported by Kapp et al.[509]

The response to hyperthermia and radiation is influenced by tumor size, volume, surface area, and depth, with larger lesions having lower complete response rates.[503,505,508] Complications following hyperthermia and radiation include severe thermal blisters and necrosis, or skin ulcers. In the RTOG study, 16% of the patients experienced a complication.[502] Kapp et al.[509] reported complications in 35% of the patients treated at Stanford. Bornstein et al.[510] evaluated concomitant chemotherapy, radiation, and hyperthermia for patients with postmastectomy local–regional recurrence. The authors reported no improvement in response rates in comparison to studies using radiation alone or radiation and hyperthermia. However, significant toxicity was encountered.

The technical aspects of the delivery of hyperthermia have also been reported to influence outcome. Lee et al.[503] demonstrated via multivariate analysis that the specific absorption rate was the most important factor correlating with local tumor control. Photodynamic therapy employs hematoporphyrin derivatives as a photosensitizing agent for high intensity xenon arc lamps or lasers. Several studies have evaluated the role of photodynamic therapy in the treatment of locally recurrent breast cancer.[511–513] These studies have demonstrated complete responses in the minority of patients with transient improvement. Studies are ongoing to evaluate the role of photodynamic therapy in these patients.

## COMPLICATIONS OF RADIATION THERAPY

The potential complications of radiation after either breast-conserving surgery or mastectomy include arm edema, symptomatic pneumonitis, rib fracture, radiation-related heart disease, brachial plexopathy, marked fibrosis, or soft tissue necrosis, and second malignancy. The incidence of these complications is related to surgical and radiation technique and to the use of adjuvant systemic therapy.

### Lymphedema

The incidence of lymphedema with postoperative radiation ranges from 2% to 37%[187,514] and is related to the extent of the axillary surgery and the regions treated with radiation. The incidence of arm edema for patients treated without axillary surgery is 5% or less,[187,514] and in the Institut Curie prospective randomized trial comparing axillary dissection and axillary radiation, there was no significant difference between the two groups in terms of arm edema.[187] Larson et al.[514] reported a 37% risk of arm edema at 6 years in patients who had complete axillary dissection and axillary radiation and a 7% risk of arm edema in patients who had a limited axillary dissection and axillary radiation. For patients receiving postmastectomy radiation and adjuvant chemotherapy, the incidence of severe lymphedema ranges from 9% to 13%.[336,397,515] The radiation factor that appears to contribute most to the development of lymphedema is the use of a supraclavicular field.[202] The use of a posterior axillary field

does not increase the risk in comparison to a supraclavicular field only.[202] The risk of lymphedema is also increased by the development of infection in the ipsilateral arm, by obesity, or by significant weight gain after breast cancer treatment.

### Symptomatic Pneumonitis

Symptomatic pneumonitis is characterized by the development of a dry cough, dyspnea, and low grade fever within 6 to 12 weeks of postoperative radiation for breast cancer. The incidence of symptomatic pneumonitis ($\leq 5\%$) is related to the number of fields treated and the use of adjuvant systemic therapy. For patients receiving tangential breast or chest wall irradiation without adjuvant therapy, the incidence of symptomatic pneumonitis is less than 1%.[517] In contrast, Lingos et al.[517] reported a 9% incidence of symptomatic pneumonitis in patients who received treatment to the breast and regional nodes with concurrent chemotherapy including methotrexate. In the prospective randomized trial reported by Recht et al.,[367] patients who received chemotherapy following radiation to the breast and regional nodes also had a 9% incidence of symptomatic pneumonitis, in contrast to 0% for those who received their chemotherapy first.

Symptomatic pneumonitis has been reported in 5% or less of patients receiving postmastectomy radiation and standard chemotherapy.[367,397] Marks et al.[201] reported a 16% incidence of symptomatic pneumonitis in 32 patients who received dose-intensive chemotherapy (cyclophosphamide, cisplatin, carmustine) with autologous bone marrow support and postmastectomy radiation that included the internal mammary nodes. Symptomatic pneumonitis was not observed in the six patients in whom the internal mammary nodes were excluded from the treatment fields. Gianni et al.[313] reported a 15% incidence of pulmonary fibrosis in patients with 10 or more positive axillary nodes who received high dose sequential adjuvant chemotherapy and radiation. However, only one of these patients was symptomatic.

## Cardiac Morbidity

Potential cardiac events related to radiation for breast cancer include the development of coronary artery disease and ischemic heart disease. An initial meta-analysis of mortality results from eight prospective randomized trials evaluating postmastectomy radiation[238] reported an increased mortality in patients who survived more than 10 years after receiving postmastectomy radiation. Subsequent reports from the individual trials indicated that the increased mortality was related to cardiovascular disease in patients with left-sided tumor, and those who received orthovoltage or cobalt-60 radiation of the regional nodes were at greatest risk.[230,240–243] In an update of the meta-analysis,[239] an increase in cardiac deaths was observed in patients who received radiation, but this was offset by the decrease in the number of breast cancer related deaths. The increased mortality from a cardiac event was most apparent in women 50 years of age or older with clinically negative nodes.

The meta-analysis just described suggested that improvements in radiotherapy technique could diminish the risk of cardiac morbidity and mortality. Subsequent studies have reported a decreased incidence of cardiac toxicity in patients receiving postmastectomy radiation or breast conservation therapy. Fowble et al.[397] reported no radiation-related cardiac toxicity in 63 high risk patients who received postmastectomy radiation and chemotherapy consisting of cyclophosphamide, methotrexate, or 5-fluorouracil, or cyclophosphamide, doxorubicin, and 5-fluorouracil. None of these patients had radiation specifically directed to the internal mammary nodes. Ragaz et al.[336] reported no cardiac events in premenopausal patients receiving radiation and CMF in the British Columbia trial despite the use of a direct photon beam to treat the internal mammary nodes. Harrigan et al.[518] reported a 3.6% incidence of cardiac events in patients who received cumulative dose of doxorubicin of 450 mg and radiation directed to the internal mammary nodes, and a 3.7% incidence in patients who received a similar cumulative dose of doxorubicin but radiation to the left side limited to tangents only. In contrast, cardiac events were reported in only 1% of patients whose cumulative dose of doxorubicin was 225 mg with or without radiation.

Valagussa et al.[519] reported a 2.6% incidence of congestive heart failure and 6% incidence of electrocardiographic changes indicative of ischemic heart disease in 114 patients who received doxorubicin and radiation to the left side with tangents only. In contrast, there was no incidence of congestive heart failure and a 4% incidence of EKG changes suggestive of ischemic heart disease in 71 patients who received non-doxorubicin-based chemotherapy and radiation to the left side. EKG evidence of ischemic heart disease occurred in 1 of the 175 patients who received radiation to the right side and none of these patients experienced congestive heart failure.

The risk of cardiac events was increased in obese patients, those older than 55 years of age, and those with a history of hypertension or diabetes. These events, however, occurred relatively early, unlike the late cardiac morbidity reported in the meta-analysis, which was evident only in the 10-year survivors. In the study of Valagussa et al.,[519] the median interval to congestive heart failure was 6 months after surgery, and the median interval to ischemic heart disease was 2 months after all treatment. Rutqvist et al.[520] reported no increased risk of myocardial infarction in 684 women with early stage breast cancer treated with conservative surgery and tangential field irradiation of the breast versus 4996 women treated with mastectomy without radiation. The median follow-up period was 9 years. Nixon et al.[521] reported no increase in cardiac mortality when they compared 365 patients who received left breast irradiation with 380 patients who received radiation to the right breast with a minimum follow-up of 12 years. Tangential field irradiation of the left chest wall or breast may include up to 10% of the left ventricle.[199,522–526] The left circumflex and right coronary arteries are spared with tangential radiation alone; however, a segment of the left anterior descending artery may be included.[524,525] The late effects of combined modality therapy on cardiac morbidity require further evaluation.

### Brachial Plexopathy

Brachial plexopathy is an uncommon event following radiation for breast cancer. It is usually characterized by pain in the ipsilateral shoulder and arm, paresthesias, and subsequent weakness in the arm and hand.[527,528] Radiation brachial plexopathy is related to the region(s) treated, the total dose, and the fraction size. Pierce et al.[527] reported no instance of radiation-induced brachial plexopathy in patients receiving tangential breast radiation only. The addition of the supraclavicular field resulted in a 0.6% incidence of brachial plexopathy in patients who did not receive chemotherapy versus a 4.5% incidence in those who received chemotherapy and radiation to the breast and supraclavicular region. Doses up to 5000 cGy to the supraclavicular field resulted in a 0.4% incidence of brachial plexopathy in patients who did not receive chemotherapy and a 3.7% incidence in patients who received chemotherapy. For doses exceeding 5000 cGy, the incidence of brachial plexopathy was 3.2% in the absence of chemotherapy and 7.9% in patients who also received chemotherapy. Olsen et al.[528] also reported an increased incidence of brachial plexopathy in patients receiving chemotherapy. Powell et al.[529] reported a 5.9% incidence of brachial plexopathy at 6 years in patients who received 5600 cGy in 15 fractions to the axilla and a 1% incidence for patients who received 5400 cGy in 30 fractions.

### Rib Fractures

Rib fractures occur in less than 5% of patients receiving radiation for breast cancer. The incidence of rib fracture is related to the photon beam energy employed to treat breast or chest wall, total radiation dose, and the use of adjuvant chemotherapy. Rib fractures are more common in patients treated with cobalt-60 or 4 MV photons, presumably related to the increased dose in the peripheral aspects of the chest wall or breast with these beam energies.[527] Pierce et al.[527] reported a 5.7% incidence of rib fracture in patients treated with 4 MV photons with a total breast dose 5000 cGy or more. Chemotherapy has also been reported to increase the incidence of rib fracture in some series.[527,530–532]

### Cosmesis

Several factors influence the cosmetic result following conservative surgery and radiation for early stage invasive breast cancer. The most commonly employed scoring system for cosmesis is that described by the Joint Center for Radiation Therapy.[533] Harris et al.[533] assigned a score of "excellent" when the appearance of the treated breast was almost identical to that of the untreated breast, a score of "good" when there was minimal difference between the two breasts, "fair" when there was an obvious difference, and "poor" when there were marked changes in the treated breast. The changes in the treated breast may include volume loss related to surgery or fibrosis secondary to radiation, retraction, and telangiectasia.

The majority of patients undergoing conservative surgery and radiation for early stage invasive breast cancer have a good to excellent cosmetic result.[131,534,535] The cosmetic result is primarily influenced by the extent of the surgical procedure for the primary tumor. The use of quadrantectomy has resulted in a greater difference between the treated and untreated breast in comparison to gross tumor excision.[534,536–538] Increasing breast size has been correlated with a somewhat worse cosmetic result. Clarke et al.[138] reported excellent cosmesis in only 50% of patients with a D cup versus 100% of patients with an A cup, 84% of patients with a B cup, and 78% of patients with a C cup. Gray et al.[139] reported a decreased mean cosmetic score in patients whose weight was 80 kg or more, bra size 40 or larger, cup size D or larger, or tangential separation 23 cm or more. At 3 and 5 years, these patients had increased incidence of asymmetry and retraction. The use of high energy beams with a beam spoiler may result in improved cosmetic results in women with large breasts.[142]

Radiotherapy technique may also impact on cosmetic results, and an adverse cosmetic result has been associated with the use of daily fractions of 250 cGy or more, a total dose to the breast exceeding 5000 cGy, the use of a large volume boost, and the use of lower photon beam energies (cobalt-60 or 4 MV) and a higher total breast dose.[138,533,539–541] The use of a supraclavicular field has also been associated with adverse cosmetic results in comparison to tangential fields alone.[138,542] The use of concurrent chemotherapy with cyclophosphamide, methotrexate, and 5-fluorouracil has been reported to result in worse cosmesis.[530,535,543] The omission of methotrexate during radiation has not been associated with an adverse cosmetic outcome.[531] Patients treated with sequential chemotherapy have been reported to have increased good to excellent cosmetic results in some series,[534,544] but not in others.[545]

Tamoxifen has also been reported to diminish the incidence of good to excellent cosmesis in one series.[538] However, in an update, Wazer et al.[373] found no adverse effect of tamoxifen on cosmesis. Two additional series have reported similar findings.[375,545] Tamoxifen may induce radiation recall and may result in a more prolonged breast erythema or hyperemia after completion of treatment.[375]

## Second Malignancies

Second malignancies following radiation for breast cancer include contralateral breast cancer, second non–breast cancer malignancies,

and bone or soft tissue sarcomas. Four of the prospective randomized trials comparing conservative surgery and radiation to mastectomy[92,127,129,441,546] and two of the prospective randomized trials evaluating postmastectomy radiation[336,547] reported the incidence of contralateral breast cancer and second non–breast cancer malignancy. None of these prospective randomized trials reported an increased risk of contralateral breast cancer or second non–breast cancer malignancy in patients who received radiation. A review of the NSABP trials reported by Fisher et al.[548] suggested that breast cancer patients treated with regional radiotherapy have a 10-fold risk of acute leukemia. The cumulative risk of leukemia was 1.37% in patients receiving regional radiation who had no evidence of disease for greater than or equal to 10 years versus 0.06% for those undergoing surgery alone. Further analysis revealed that this risk was primarily seen in patients who received postmastectomy radiation to the chest wall and regional nodes and was not observed in patients receiving tangential breast radiation in the NSABP B-06 protocol.

Curtis et al.[549] reported a relative risk of 1.6 for leukemia following radiation for breast cancer in a population-based, case-controlled study from the Connecticut Tumor Registry. In a subsequent report by the same authors,[550] a significantly elevated risk of nonlymphatic leukemia was related to regional radiation following mastectomy. The relative risk was 2.4 for patients receiving radiation alone and 17.4 for those receiving radiation and chemotherapy with an alkalating agent. The risk for chemotherapy alone employing an alkalating agent was 10.0. The risk from radiation was greatest for patients receiving 900 cGy or more to the total active bone marrow. Similar risks were noted for the use of cyclophosphamide. The authors concluded that approximately 5 of 10,000 patients treated for 6 months with a cyclophosphamide-based adjuvant chemotherapy regimen might be expected to develop leukemia within 10 years of the diagnosis of breast cancer. A similar incidence might be associated with radiotherapy alone especially when the active bone marrow received 900 cGy or more. Hahn et al.[551] in a case-controlled study reported a relative risk of 12 for leukemia in women receiving chemotherapy for breast cancer. There was no increased risk for those receiving radiation.

While six prospective randomized trials have demonstrated no increased risk of contralateral breast cancer in patients receiving radiation either following conservative surgery or mastectomy,[92,127,129,336,441,546,597] Boice et al.[552] reported a small but marginally significant elevated risk of contralateral breast cancer with radiation in a case control study from the Connecticut Tumor Registry. This risk was primarily seen in women under the age of 45 and was not observed among older women. The relative risk of women under the age of 45 was 1.59. Of all second breast cancers after radical mastectomy, 2.7% were attributed to radiotherapy. Factors that have been correlated with the risk of contralateral breast cancer include young age, lobular histology, and positive family history. Unfortunately, this study lacked information on family history in approximately 40% of the patients, and the histologic subtype was not specified. Therefore, two important factors that contribute to the incidence of contralateral breast cancer were not evaluated.

In an earlier case control study[553] from the Connecticut Tumor Registry, radiation was not associated with an increased risk of a contralateral breast cancer, and an increased risk was associated with lobular histology and positive progesterone receptor. Boice et al.[552] concluded that the risk of radiation-induced contralateral breast cancers is small and should not be a factor in selection of treatment options. The cumulative incidence of sarcoma following radiation for breast cancer has been reported to be 0.2% at 10 years.[554] Kurtz et al.[555] estimated that two radiation-induced sarcomas will be observed for every thousand 5-year survivors for each decade of follow-up. A total of three cases of soft tissue sarcoma have been reported in 3295 patients treated in the first four Milan

randomized trials.[556] The risk, therefore, remains small.

The median interval to a radiation-induced sarcoma is approximately 10 years. The most frequent site of a soft tissue sarcoma is the treated breast or chest wall, and the most common histology is angiosarcoma, fibrosarcoma, or malignant fibrous histiocytoma. Bone sarcomas most commonly affect the scapula and humerus, and the most frequent histology is osteosarcoma. Several studies have reported an increased risk of lung cancer in women receiving radiation for breast cancer.[557-561] The increased risk does not appear until 10 years after treatment, and the relative risk ranges from 1.8 to 3.2. The risk appears to be greatest for ipsilateral lung cancer, and there appears to be no increased risk for contralateral lung cancer. Neugut et al.[559] reported a 33-fold increased risk of lung cancer in 10-year survivors of breast cancer who both are smokers and receive radiation. The risk for 10-year survivors who are nonsmokers and receive radiation was 3.2. These studies were population based on information from the Connecticut Tumor Registry and are limited by small sample size, the reliance on registry data for a history of radiation and smoking, as well as missing information regarding smoking history and radiation details.

Travis et al.[557] reported a relative risk of lung cancer of 1.93 in 5923 10-year survivors of breast cancer treatment who received postmastectomy radiation. The increased risk was noted for small-cell carcinomas, squamous cell carcinomas, and adenocarcinomas. The authors did not identify an increased risk for women treated with radiation following conservative surgery. Inskip et al.[561] estimated the absolute risk of a radiation-induced lung cancer to be 9 cases per year among 10,000 women who survived at least 10 years and received an average lung dose of 1000 cGy. Practical recommendations to diminish the risk of lung cancer include minimizing the volume of lung within the treatment field and advising current smokers to stop smoking. Scanlon et al.[562] also reported an increased risk of pulmonary metastasis in women smokers who developed breast cancer. In the British Columbia prospective randomized trial of postmastectomy radiation in premenopausal patients with positive axillary nodes receiving CMF, none of the radiation patients developed a primary lung cancer.[336] Malignant pleural mesotheliomas have also been reported following radiation for breast cancer.[563]

In summary, complications following radiation for breast cancer include arm edema, symptomatic pneumonitis, brachial plexopathy, rib fracture, cardiac events, altered cosmesis, and secondary cancers. Overall, the incidence of these complications is relatively small and is influenced by surgical and radiotherapy technique as well as the use of adjuvant systemic therapy.

## REFERENCES

1. Landis SH, Murray T, Bolden S, Wingo PA: Cancer statistics 1998. *CA Cancer J Clin* 1998; 48:6–29.

2. Wingo P, Ries LAG, Rosenberg HM, Miller DS, Edwards BK: Cancer incidence and mortality 1973–1995. A report card for the U.S. *Cancer* 1998; 82:1197–1207.

3. Chu KC, Tarone RE, Kessler LG, Ries LAG, Hankey BF, Miller BA, Edwards BK: Recent trends in U.S. breast cancer incidence survival and mortality rates. *J Natl Cancer Inst* 1996; 88:1571–1579.

4. Cole P, Rodu B: Declining cancer mortality in the United States. *Cancer* 1996; 78:2045–2048.

5. Early Breast Cancer Trialists' Collaborative Group: Systemic treatment of early breast cancer by hormonal, cytotoxic or immune therapy: 133 randomized trials involving 31,000 recurrences and 24,000 deaths among 75,000 women. *Lancet* 1992; 339:1–15, 71–85.

6. American Joint Committee on Cancer. *AJCC Cancer Staging Manual,* 5th ed. Philadelphia, Lippincott-Raven, 1997, pp 173–174.

7. McDivitt RW, Hutter RVP, Foote FW, Stewart FW: In situ lobular carcinoma. A prospective follow-up study indicating cumulative patient risks. *JAMA* 1967; 201:82–96.

8. Foote FWJ, Stewart FW: Lobular carcinoma in situ. A rare form of mammary cancer. *Am J Pathol* 1941; 17:491–495.

9. Rosen PP: Proliferative breast "disease." An unresolved diagnostic dilemma. *Cancer* 1993; 71:3798–3807.

10. Rosen PP, Kosloff C, Lieberman PH, Adair F, Braum DWJ: Lobular carcinoma in situ of the breast. Detailed analysis of 99 patients with average follow-up of 24 years. *Am J Surg Pathol* 1978; 2:225–251.

11. Schwartz GF, Feig SA, Patchefsky AS: Significance and staging of nonpalpable carcinomas of the breast. *Surg Gynecol Obstet* 1988; 166: 6–10.

12. Fisher ER, Costantino J, Fisher B, Palekar AS, Paik SM, Suarez CM, Wolmark N, for the National Surgical Adjuvant Breast and Bowel Project Collaborating Investigators: Pathologic findings from the National Surgical Adjuvant Breast Project (NSABP) Protocol B-17. Five-year observations concerning lobular carcinoma in situ. *Cancer* 1996; 78:1403–1416.

13. Rosen PP, Senie RT, Farr GH, Schottenfeld D, Ashikari R: Epidemiology of breast carcinoma: Age, menstrual status, and exogenous hormone usage in patients with lobular carcinoma in situ. *Surgery* 1979; 85:219–224.

14. Bodian CA, Perzin KH, Lattes R: Lobular neoplasia long term risk of breast cancer and relation to other factors. *Cancer* 1996; 78: 1024–1034.

15. Rosen PP, Braun DW Jr, Lyngholm B, Urban JA, Kinne DW: Lobular carcinoma in situ of the breast: Preliminary results of treatment by ipsilateral mastectomy and contralateral breast biopsy. *Cancer* 1981; 47:813–910.

16. Rosen PP, Senie R, Schottenfeld D, Ashikari R: Noninvasive breast carcinoma. Frequency of unsuspected invasion and implications for treatment. *Ann Surg* 1989; 189:377–383.

17. Carter D, Smith RR: Carcinoma in situ of the breast. *Cancer* 1977; 40:1189–1193.

18. Wanebo HJ, Huvos AG, Urban JA: Treatment of minimal breast cancer. *Cancer* 1974; 33:349–357.

19. Andersen JA: Multicentric and bilateral appearance of lobular carcinoma in situ of the breast. *Acta Pathol Microbiol Scand A* 1974; 82:730–734.

20. Shah JA, Rosen PP, Robins GF: Pitfalls of local excision in the treatment of carcinoma of the breast. *Surg Gynecol Obstet* 1973; 136: 721–725.

21. Wheeler JE, Enterline HT, Roseman JM, Tomasulo JP, McIlvaine CH: Lobular carcinoma in situ of the breast. Long-term followup. *Cancer* 1974; 34:554–563.

22. Haagensen CD, Lane N, Lattes R, Bodian C: Lobular neoplasia (so-called lobular carcinoma in situ) of the breast. *Cancer* 1978; 42:737–769.

23. Hutter RVP, Foote FWJ: Lobular carcinoma in situ. Long term follow-up. *Cancer* 1969; 24:1081–1085.

24. Andersen JA: Lobular carcinoma in situ of the breast. An approach to rational treatment. *Cancer* 1977; 39:2597–2602.

25. Page DL, Kidd TEJ, Dupont WD, Simpson JF, Rogers LW: Lobular neoplasia of the breast: Higher risk for subsequent invasive cancer predicted by more extensive disease. *Hum Pathol* 1991; 22:1232–1239.

26. Ottensen GL, Graversen HP, Blichert-Toft M, Zedeler K, Andersen JA: Lobular carcinoma in situ of the female breast: Short-term results of a prospective nationwide study. *Am J Surg Pathol* 1993; 17:14–21.

27. Dall'Olmo CA, Ponka JL, Hern RC, Riu R: Lobular carcinoma of the breast in situ. Are we too radical in its treatment? *Arch Sug* 1975; 110:537–542.

28. Benfield JR, Jacobson M, Warner NE: In situ lobular carcinoma of the breast. *Arch Surg* 1965; 91:130–135.

29. Rebner M: Noninvasive breast cancer. *Radiology* 1994; 190:623–631.

30. Ernster VL, Barclay J, Kerlikowske K, Grady D, Henderson C: Incidence and treatment for ductal carcinoma in situ of the breast. *JAMA* 1996; 275:913–918.

31. Ernster VL: Epidemiology and natural history of ductal carcinoma in situ, in MJ Silverstein (ed): *Ductal Carcinoma In Situ of the Breast.* Philadelphia, Williams & Wilkins, 1997, pp 23–33.

32. Fowble B, Hanlon AL, Fein DA, Hoffman JP, Sigurdson ER, Patchefsky A, Kessler H: Results of conservative surgery and radiation for mammographically detected ductal carcinoma

in-situ (DCIS). *Int J Radiat Oncol Biol Phys* 1997; 38:949–957.

33. Fisher B, Dignam J, Wolmark N, Mamounas E, Costantino J, Poller W, Fisher ER, Wickerham DL, Deutsch M, Margolese R, Dimitrov N, Kavanah M: Lumpectomy and radiation therapy for the treatment of intraductal breast cancer: Findings from the National Surgical Adjuvant Breast and Bowel Project B-17. *J Clin Oncol* 1998; 16:441–452.

34. Consensus Conference Committee: Consensus conference on classification of ductal carcinoma in situ. *Cancer* 1997; 80:1798–1802.

35. Winchester DJ, Menck HR, Winchester DP: National treatment trends for ductal carcinoma in situ of the breast. *Arch Surg* 1997; 132:660–665.

36. Fisher ER, Costantino J, Fisher B, Palekar AS, Redmond C, Mamounas E: Pathologic findings from the National Surgical Adjuvant Breast Project (NSABP) protocol B-17 Intraductal carcinoma (ductal carcinoma in situ). *Cancer* 1995; 75:1310–1319.

37. Silverstein MJ, Gierson ED, Colburn WJ, Cope LM, Furmanski M, Senofsky GM, Gamagami P, Waisman JR: Can intraductal breast carcinoma be excised completely by local excision? Clinical and pathologic predictors. *Cancer* 1994; 73:2985–2989.

38. Schuh ME, Nemoto T, Penetrante RB, Rosner D, Dao TL: Intraductal carcinoma. Analysis of presentation, pathologic findings and outcome of disease. *Arch Surg* 1986; 121:1303–1307.

39. Fentiman IS, Fagg N, Millis RR, Hayward JL: In situ ductal carcinoma of the breast: Implications of disease pattern and treatment. *Eur J Surg Oncol* 1986; 12:261–266.

40. Brown PW, Silverman J, Owens E, Tabor DC, Terz JJ, Lawrence W Jr: Intraductal "non-infiltrating" carcinoma of the breast. *Arch Surg* 1976; 111:1063–1067.

41. Schwartz GF, Feig SA, Rosenberg AL, Patchefsky AS, Schwartz AB: Staging and treatment of clinically occult breast cancer. *Cancer* 1984; 53:1379–1384.

42. Lagios MD, Westdahl PR, Margolin FR, Rose MR: Duct carcinoma in situ: Relationship of extent of noninvasive disease to the frequency of occult invasion multicentricity lymph node metastases and short term treatment failures. *Cancer* 1982; 50:1309–1314.

43. Holland R, Hendriks JHCL, Verbeek ALM, Mravunac M, Stekhoven JHS: Extent distribution and mammographic/histologic correlations of breast ductal carcinoma in situ. *Lancet* 1990; 335:519–522.

44. Faverly DRG, Burgers L, Bult P, Holland R: Three dimensional imaging of mammary ductal carcinoma in situ: Clinical implications. *Semin Diagn Pathol* 1994; 11:193–198.

45. Fisher ER, Sass R, Fisher B, Wicherham L, Paik SM: Pathologic findings from the National Surgical Adjuvant Breast Project (Protocol 6). I. Intraductal carcinoma (DCIS). *Cancer* 1986; 57:197–208.

46. Patchefsky AS, Schwartz GF, Finkelstein SD, Prestipino A, Sohn SE, Singer JS, Feig SA: Heterogeneity of intraductal carcinoma of the breast. *Cancer* 1989; 63:731–741.

47. Holland R, Hendricks JHCL: Microcalcifications associated with ductal carcinoma in situ: Mammographic–pathologic correlation. *Semin Diagn Pathol* 1994; 11:181–192.

48. Gump FE, Jicha DL, Ozello L: Ductal carcinoma in situ (DCIS): A revised concept. *Surgery* 1987; 102:790–795.

49. Lagios MD, Margolin FR, Westdahl PR, Rose MR: Mammographically detected duct carcinoma in situ: Frequency of local recurrence following tylectomy and prognostic effect of nuclear grade on local recurrence. *Cancer* 1989; 63:618–624.

50. Solin LJ, Kurtz J, Fourquet A, Amalric R, Recht A, Bornstein BA, Kuske R, Taylor M, Barrett W, Fowble B, Haffty B, Schultz DJ, Yeh I-T, McCormick B, McNeese M: Fifteen-year results of breast conserving surgery and definitive breast irradiation for the treatment of ductal carcinoma in situ (intraductal carcinoma of the breast). *J Clin Oncol* 1996; 14:754–763.

51. McCormick B, Rosen PP, Kinne D, Cox L, Yahalom J: Duct carcinoma in situ of the breast: An analysis of local control after conservative surgery and radiotherapy. *Int J Radiat Oncol Biol Phys* 1991; 21:289–292.

52. Sneige N, McNeese MD, Atkinson EN, Ames FC, Kemp B, Sahin A, Ayala AG: Ductal carcinoma in situ treated with lumpectomy and irradiation: Histopathologic analysis of 49 specimens with emphasis on risk factors and long term results. *Hum Pathol* 1995; 26:642–649.

53. Solin LJ, McCormick B, Recht A, Haffty B, Taylor M, Kuske R, Bornstein B, McNeese M, Schultz DJ, Fowble BL, Barrett W, Yeh I-T, Kurtz J, Amalric R, Fourquet A: Mammographically detected clinically occult ductal carcinoma in situ (intraductal carcinoma) treated with breast-conserving surgery and definitive breast irradiation. *Cancer J Sci Am* 1996; 2:158–165.

54. Van Zee KJ, Borgen PI: Memorial Sloan-Kettering Cancer Center, in MJ Silverstein (ed): *Ductal Carcinoma In Situ of the Breast.* Baltimore, Williams & Wilkins, 1997, pp 455–462.

55. Vicini FA, Lacerna MD, Goldstein NS, Horwitz EM, Dmuchowski CF, White JR, Gustafson GS, Ingold JA, Martinez AA: Ductal carcinoma in situ detected in the mammographic era: An analysis of clinical, pathologic, and treatment-related factors affecting outcome with breast-conserving therapy. *Int J Radiat Oncol Biol Phys* 1997; 39:627–635.

56. Hiramatsu H, Bornstein BA, Recht A, Schnitt SJ, Baum JK, Connolly JL, Duda RB, Guidi AJ, Kaelin CM, Silver B, Harris JR: Local recurrence after conservative surgery and radiation therapy for ductal carcinoma in situ Possible importance of family history. *Cancer J Sci Am* 1995; 10:55–61.

57. Solin LJ, Fowble BL, Schultz DJ, Yeh I-T, Kowalyshyn MJ, Goodman RL: Definitive irradiation for intraductal carcinoma of the breast. *Int J Radiat Oncol Biol Phys* 1990; 19:843–850.

58. Bornstein BA, Recht A, Connolly JL, Scnitt SJ, Lady B, Koufman C, Love S, Osteen RT, Harris JR: Results of treating ductal carcinoma in situ of the breast with conservative surgery and radiation therapy. *Cancer* 1991; 67:7–13.

59. Szelei-Stevens KA, Kuske RR, Bolton JS, Bowen JC, Fuhrman GM, Fineberg BB: The influence of young age and positive family history on local recurrence after three treatment strategies for ductal carcinoma in situ. *Int J Radiat Oncol Biol Phys* 1997; 39:264 (abstr).

60. Kuske RR, Bean JM, Garcia DM, Perez CA, Andriole D, Philpott G, Fineberg B: Breast conservation therapy for intraductal carci-

noma of the breast. *Int J Radiat Oncol Biol Phys* 1993; 26:391–396.

61. Silverstein MJ, Beron P, Lewinsky BS: Breast-conserving therapy for ductal carcinoma in situ: The Van Nuys experience with excisional plus radiation therapy. *Breast J* 1997; 3:36–41.

62. Solin LF, Yeh I-T, Kurtz J, Fourquet A, Recht A, Kuske R, McCormick B, Cross MA, Schultz DJ, Amalric R, Livolsi VA, Kowalyshyn MJ, Torhorst J, Jacquemier J, Westermann CD, Mazeujian G, Zafrani B, Rosen PP, Goodman RL, Fowble BL: Ductal carcinoma in situ (intraductal carcinoma) of the breast treated with breast-conserving surgery and definitive irradiation: Correlation of pathologic parameters with outcome of treatment. *Cancer* 1993; 71:2532–2542.

63. Silverstein MJ, Poller DN: Van Nuys ductal carcinoma in situ classification, in MJ Silverstein (ed): *Ductal Carcinoma In Situ of the Breast.* Baltimore, Williams & Wilkins, 1997, pp 247–258.

64. Silverstein MJ: Van Nuys prognostic index, in MJ Silverstein (ed): *Ductal Carcinoma In Situ of the Breast.* Baltimore, William & Wilkins, 1997, pp 491–501.

65. Schnitt SJ, Harris JR, Smith BL: Developing a prognostic index for ductal carcinoma in situ of the breast: Are we there yet? *Cancer* 1996; 77:2189–2192.

66. Silverstein MJ: Ductal carcinoma in situ of the breast: The Van Nuys experience by treatment. *Breast J* 1997; 3:232–237.

67. Bullock CG, Magnant C, Ayoob M, Berg CD: The utility of conservative surgery and radiation therapy in ductal carcinoma-in-situ. *Int J Radiat Oncol Biol Phys* 1993; 27:268 (abstr).

68. White J, Levine A, Gustafson G, Wimbish K, Ingold J, Pettinga J, Matter R, Martinez A, Vicini F: Outcome and prognostic factors for local recurrence in mammographically detected ductal carcinoma in-situ of the breast treated with conservative surgery and radiation therapy. *Int J Radiat Oncol Biol Phys* 1995; 31:791–797.

69. Morrow M: Surgical overview of the treatment of ductal carcinoma in situ, in MJ Silverstein (ed): *Ductal Carcinona In Situ of the Breast.* Baltimore, Williams & Wilkins, 1997, pp 469–478.

70. Lagios MD: Lagios experience, in MJ Silverstein (ed): *Ductal Carcinoma In Situ of the Breast.* Baltimore, William & Wilkins, 1997, pp 361–366.

71. Silverstein MJ: Predicting local recurrences in patients with ductal carcinoma in situ, in MJ Silverstein (ed): *Ductal Carcinoma In Situ of the Breast.* Baltimore, William & Wilkins, 1997, pp 271–284.

72. Hetelekidis S, Collins L, Schnitt SJ, Recht A, Nixon AJ, Bornstein BA, Abner A, Silver B, Harris JR: Predictors of local recurrence following excision alone for ductal carcinoma in situ. *Int J Radiat Oncol Biol Phys* 1997; 39:138 (abstr).

73. Fisher ER, Leiming R, Anderson S, Redmond C, Fisher B, and Collaborating NSABP Investigators: Conservative management of intraductal carcinoma (DCIS) of the breast. *J Surg Oncol* 1991; 47:139–147.

74. Fisher B, Constantino J, Redmond C, Fisher E, Margolese R, DiMitrov N, Wolmark N, Wickerham DL, Deutsch M, Ore L, Mamounas E, Poller W, Kavanah M: Lumpectomy compared with lumpectomy and radiation therapy for the treatment of intraductal breast cancer. *N Engl J Med* 1993; 328:1581–1586.

75. Ravdin PM: Biomarkers, in MJ Silverstein (ed): *Ductal Carcinoma In Situ of the Breast.* Baltimore, William & Wilkins, 1997, pp 51–57.

76. Holland PA, Knox WF, Potten CS, Howell A, Anderson E, Baildam AD, Bundred NJ: Assessment of hormone dependence of comedo ductal carcinoma in situ of the breast. *J Natl Cancer Inst* 1997; 89:1059–1065.

77. Kendra K, Love RR: Systemic therapy for ductal carcinoma in situ, in MJ Silverstein (ed): *Ductal Carcinoma In Situ of the Breast.* Baltimore, Williams & Wilkins, 1997, pp 585–592.

78. Winchester DP, Strom EA: Standards for diagnosis and management of ductal carcinoma in situ (DCIS) of the breast. *CA Cancer J Clin* 1998; 48:108–128.

79. Johantgen ME, Coffey RM, Harris DR, Levy H, Clinton JJ: Treating early stage breast cancer: Hospital characteristics associated with breast-conserving surgery. *Am J Public Health* 1995; 85:1432–1434.

80. Albain KS, Green SR, Lichter AS, Hutchins LF, Wood WC, Henderson IC, Ingle JN, O'Sullivan J, Osborne CK, Martino S: Influence of patient characteristics, socioeconomic factors, geography and systemic risk on the use of breast-sparing treatment in women enrolled in adjuvant breast cancer studies: An analysis of two intergroup trials. *J Clin Oncol* 1996; 14:3009–3017.

81. Winchester DJ, Menck HR, Winchester DP: The National Cancer Data Base Report on the results of a large nonrandomized comparison of breast preservation and modified radical mastectomy. *Cancer* 1997; 80:162–167.

82. Farrow DC, Hunt WC, Samet JM: Geographic variation in the treatment of localized breast cancer. *N Engl J Med* 1992; 326:1097–1101.

83. Nattinger AB, Gottlieb MS, Veum J, Yahnke D, Goodwin JS: Geographic variation in the use of breast-conserving treatment for breast cancer. *N Engl J Med* 1992; 326:1102–1107.

84. Nattinger AB, Hoffman RG, Shapiro R, Gottlieb MS, Goodwin JS: The effect of legislative requirements on the use of breast conserving surgery. *New Engl J Med* 1996; 335:1035–1040.

85. Morrow M, Schmidt R: Are medical contraindications a major factor in the underutilization of breast conserving therapy? *Breast Cancer Res Treat* 1996; 41:221 (abstr).

86. Kotwall CA, Maxwell JG, Covington DL, Churchill P, Smith SE, Covan EK: Clinicopathologic factors and patient perceptions associated with surgical breast-conserving treatment. *Ann Surg Oncol* 1996; 3:169–175.

87. Foster RS, Farwell ME, Costanza MC: Breast-conserving surgery for breast cancer: Patterns of care in a geographic region and estimation of potential applicability. *Ann Surg Oncol* 1995; 2:275–280.

88. Wei JP, Sherry RM, Baisden BL, Peckel J, Lala G: Prospective hospital-based survey of attitudes of southern women toward surgical treatment of breast cancer. *Ann Surg Oncol* 1995; 2:360–364.

89. Polednak AP: Predictors of breast-conserving surgery in Connecticut 1990–92. *Ann Surg Oncol* 1997; 4:259–263.

90. Winchester DP, Cox JD: Standards for diagnosis and management of invasive breast carcinoma. *CA Cancer J Clin* 1998; 48:83–107.

91. Fisher B, Redmond C, Poisson R, Margolese R, Wolmark N, Wickerham L, Fisher E, Deutsch M, Caplan R, Pilch Y, Glass A, Shibata H, Lerner H, Terz J, Sidorovich L: Eight-year results of a randomized clinical trial comparing total mastectomy and lumpectomy with or without irradiation in the treatment of breast cancer. *N Engl J Med* 1989; 320:822–828.

92. Veronesi U, Salvadori B, Luini A, Greco M, Saccozzi R, del Vecchio M, Mariani L, Zurrida S, Rilke F: Breast conservation is a safe method in patients with small cancer of the breast. Long-term results of three randomized trials on 1973 patients. *Eur J Cancer* 1995; 31A:1574–1579.

93. Morris AD, Morris RD, Wilson JF, White J, Steinberg S, Okunieff P, Lê MG, Blichert-Toft M, van Dongen JA: Breast-conserving therapy vs. mastectomy in early-stage breast cancer: A meta-analysis of 10-year survival. *Cancer J Sci Am* 1997; 3:6–12.

94. Early Breast Cancer Trialists' Collaborative Group: Effects of radiotherapy and surgery in early breast cancer. An overview of the randomized trials. *New Engl J Med* 1995; 333:1444–1455.

95. Abrams JS, Phillips PH, Friedman MA: An appraisal of research results for the local treatment of early stage breast cancer. *J Natl Cancer Inst* 1995; 87:1837–1845.

96. Fleck R, McNeese MD, Ellerbroek NA, Hunter TA, Holmes FA: Consequences of breast irradiation in patients with pre-existing collagen vascular disease. *Int J Radiat Oncol Biol Phys* 1989; 17:829–833.

97. Ross JG, Hussey DH, Mayr NA, Davis CS: Acute and late reactions to radiation therapy in patients with collagen vascular diseases. *Cancer* 1993; 71:3744–3752.

98. Robertson JM, Clarke DH, Pevzner MM, Matter RC: Breast conservation therapy. Severe breast fibrosis after radiation therapy in patients with collagen vascular disease. *Cancer* 1991; 68:502–508.

99. Mayr NA, Riggs CE, Saag KG, Wen B-C, Pennington EC, Hussey DH: Mixed connective tissue disease and radiation toxicity. A case report. *Cancer* 1997; 79:612–618.

100. Morris MM, Powell SN: Irradiation in the setting of collagen vascular disease: Acute and

late complications. *J Clin Oncol* 1997; 15:2728–2735.

101. Nixon AJ, Neuberg D, Hayes DF, Gelman R, Connolly JL, Schnitt S, Abner A, Recht A, Vicini F, Harris JR: Relationship of patient age to pathologic features of the tumor and prognosis for patients with stage I or II breast cancer. *J Clin Oncol* 1994; 12:888–894.

102. Nixon AJ, Schnitt S, Connolly JL, Abner A, Silver B, Recht A, Harris JR: Relationship of patient age to pathologic features of the tumor and the risk of local recurrence for patients with stage I or II breast cancer treated with conservative surgery and radiation therapy. *Int J Radiat Oncol Biol Phys* 1992; 24:221–222 (abstr).

103. Kurtz JM, Jacquemier J, Amalric R, Brandone H, Ayme Y, Hans D, Bressac C, Spitalier JM: Why are local recurrences after breast-conserving therapy more frequent in younger patients? *J Clin Oncol* 1990; 8:591–598.

104. Vicini F, Recht A, Abner A, Silver BA, Harris JR: The association between very young age and recurrence in the breast in patients treated with conservative surgery and radiation therapy. *Int J Radiat Oncol Biol Phys* 1990; 19:132 (abstr).

105. Fourquet A, Campana F, Zafrani B, Mosseri V, Vielh P, Durand JC, Vilcoq JR: Prognostic factors of breast recurrence in the conservative management of early breast cancer: A 25 year follow-up. *Int J Radiat Oncol Biol Phys* 1989; 17:719–725.

106. Fowble B, Schultz DJ, Overmoyer B, Solin LJ, Fox K, Jardines L, Orel S, Glick JH: The influence of young age on outcome in early stage breast cancer. *Int J Radiat Oncol Biol Phys* 1994; 30:23–33.

107. Rose MA, Henderson IC, Gelman R, Boyages J, Gore SM, Come S, Silver B, Recht A, Connolly JL, Schnitt SJ, Coleman CN, Harris JR: Premenopausal breast cancer patients treated with conservative surgery, radiotherapy and adjuvant chemotherapy have a low risk of local failure. *Int J Radiat Oncol Biol Phys* 1989; 17:711–717.

108. Matthews RH, McNeese M, Montague ED, Oswald NJ: Prognostic implications of age in breast cancer patients treated with tumorectomy and irradiation or with mastectomy. *Int J Radiat Oncol Biol Phys* 1988; 14:659–663.

109. Bouvet M, Babiera GV, Tucker SL, McNeese MD, Singletary SE: Does breast conservation therapy in young women with breast cancer adversely affect local disease control and survival rate? The M.D. Anderson Cancer Center experience. *Breast J* 1997; 3:169–175.

110. De la Rouchfordiere A, Asselain B, Campana F, Fenton J, Vilcoq JR, Fourquet A: Breast cancer in premenopausal women: Is young age at diagnosis an independent prognostic factor? *Int J Radiat Oncol Biol Phys* 1992; 24:222 (abstr).

111. Weber BC, Garber JE: Familial breast cancer, in JR Harris, ME Lippman, M Morrow, and S Hellman (eds): *Disease of the Breast.* Philadelphia, Lippincott-Raven, 1996, pp 168–184.

112. Kurtz JM: Factors influencing the risk of local recurrence in the breast. *Eur J Cancer* 1992; 28:660–666.

113. Burke MF, Allison R, Tripcony L: Conservative therapy of breast cancer in Queensland. *Int J Radiat Oncol Biol Phys* 1995; 31: 295–303.

114. Peterson M, Fowble B, Solin LJ, Schultz DJ: Family history status as a prognostic factor for women with early stage breast cancer treated with conservative surgery and radiation. *Breast J* 1995; 1:202–209.

115. Chen LM, Mundt AJ, Powers C, Halpern HJ, Weichselbaum RR: Significance of family history in breast cancer treated with breast conservation therapy. *Breast J* 1996; 2: 238–245.

116. Pierce LJ, Strawderman MH, Douglas K, Lichter AS: Conservative surgery and radiotherapy for early-stage breast cancer using a lung density correction: The University of Michigan experience. *Int J Radiat Oncol Biol Phys* 1997; 39:921–928.

117. Chabner E, Nixon AJ, Garber J, Gelman R, Bornstein B, Connolly J, Hetelekidis S, Recht A, Schnitt S, Silver B, Harris JR: Family history suggestive of an inherited susceptibility to breast cancer and treatment outcome in young women after breast-conserving therapy. *Int J Radiat Oncol Biol Phys* 1997; 39:137 (abstr).

118. Newman B, Mu H, Butler LM, Millikan RC, Moorman PG, King M-C: Frequency of breast cancer attributable to *BRCA1* in a population-

based series of American women. *JAMA* 1998; 279:915–921.

119. Malone KE, Daling JR, Thompson ID, O'Brien CA, Francisco LV, Ostrander EA: *BRCA1* mutations and breast cancer in the general population. *JAMA* 1998; 279:922–929.

120. Leopold KA, Recht A, Schnitt SJ, Connolly JL, Rose MA, Silver B, Harris JR. Results of conservative surgery and radiation therapy for multiple synchronous cancers of one breast. *Int J Radiat Oncol Biol Phys* 1989; 16:11–16.

121. Kurtz JM, Jacquemier J, Amalric R, Brandone H, Ayme Y, Hans D, Bressac C, Spitalier JM: Breast-conserving therapy for macroscopically multiple cancers. *Ann Surg* 1990; 212:38–44.

122. Wilson LD, Beinfield M, McKhann CF, Haffty BG: Conservative surgery and radiation in the treatment of synchronous ipsilateral breast cancers. *Cancer* 1993; 72:137–142.

123. Fowble B, Yeh I-T, Schultz DJ, Solin LJ, Rosato EF, Jardines L, Hoffman J, Eisenberg B, Weiss MC, Hanks G: The role of mastectomy in patients with stage I-II breast cancer presenting with gross multifocal or multicentric disease or diffuse microcalcifications. *Int J Radiat Oncol Biol Phys* 1993; 27:567–573.

124. Hartsell WF, Recine DC, Griem KL, Cobleigh MA, Witt TR, Murthy AK: Should multicentric disease be an absolute contraindication to the use of breast-conserving therapy? *Int J Radiat Oncol Biol Phys* 1994; 30:49–53.

125. Dutt PL, Page DL: Multicentricity of in situ and invasive carcinoma, in KI Bland, and EM Copeland III (eds): *The Breast. Comprehensive Management of Benign and Malignant Diseases.* Philadelphia, Saunders, 1991, pp 299–308.

126. Fisher ER, Gregorio R, Redmond C, Vellios F, Sommers SC, Fisher B: Pathologic findings from the National Surgical Adjuvant Breast Project (Protocol 4). I. Observations concerning the multicentricity of mammary cancer. *Cancer* 1975; 35:247–254.

127. Jacobson JA, Danforth DN, Cowan KH, D'Angelo T, Steinberg SM, Pierce L, Lippman ME, Lichter AS, Glatstein E, Okunieff P: Ten-year results of a comparison of conservation with mastectomy in the treatment of stage I and II breast cancer. *N Engl J Med* 1995; 332:907–911.

128. Van Dongen JA, Bartelink H, Fentiman IS, Lerut T, Mignolet F, Olthus G, van der Schueren E, Sylvester R, Winter J, van Zijl K: Randomized clinical trial to assess the value of breast conserving therapy in stage I and II breast cancer; EORTC trial 10801. *Monogr Natl Cancer Inst* 1992; 11:15–18.

129. Fisher B, Anderson S, Redmond CK, Wolmark N, Wickerham DL, Cronin WM: Reanalysis and results after 12 years of follow-up in a randomized clinical trial comparing total mastectomy with lumpectomy with or without irradiation in the treatment of breast cancer. *N Engl J Med* 1995; 333:1456–1461.

130. Clarke DH, Le MG, Sarrazin D, Lacombe M, Fontaine F, Travagli JP, May-Levin F, Contesso G, Arriagada R: Analysis of local–regional relapse in patients with early breast cancers treated by excision and radiotherapy: Experience of the Institut Gustave-Roussy. *Int J Radiat Oncol Biol Phys* 1985; 11:137–145.

131. Fowble B, Solin LJ, Schultz DJ, Goodman RL: Ten-year results of conservative surgery and irradiation for stage I and II breast cancer. *Int J Radiat Oncol Biol Phys* 1991; 21:269–277.

132. Eberlein TJ, Connolly JL, Schnitt SJ, Recht A, Osteen RT, Harris JR: Predictors of local recurrence following conservative breast surgery and radiation. The influence of tumor size. *Arch Surg* 1990; 125:771–775.

133. Stotter AT, McNeese MD, Ames FC, Oswald MJ, Ellerbroek NA: Predicting the rate and extent of locoregional failure after breast conservation therapy for early breast cancer. *Cancer* 1989; 64:2217–2225.

134. Leborgne F, Leborgne JH, Ortega B, Doldan R, Zubizarreta E: Breast conservation treatment of early stage breast cancer: Patterns of failure. *Int J Radiat Oncol Biol Phys* 1995; 31:765–775.

135. Fowble B, Solin LJ, Schultz DJ, Weiss MC: Breast recurrence and survival related to primary tumor location in patients undergoing conservative surgery and radiation for early-stage breast cancer. *Int J Radiat Oncol Biol Phys* 1992; 23:933–939.

136. Haffty BG, Wilson LD, Smith R, Fischer D, Beinfield M, Ward B, McKhann C: Subareolar breast cancer: Long-term results with conservative surgery and radiation. *Int J Radiat Oncol Biol Phys* 1995; 33:53–57.

137. Boyages J, Recht A, Connolly JL, Schnitt SJ, Gelman R, Kooy H, Love S, Esteen RT, Cady B, Silver B, Harris JR: Early breast cancer: Predictors of breast recurrence for patients treated with conservative surgery and radiation therapy. *Radiother Oncol* 1990; 19:29–41.

138. Clarke D, Martinez A, Cox RS: Analysis of cosmetic results and complications in patients with stage I and II breast cancer treated by biopsy and irradiation. *Int J Radiat Oncol Biol Phys* 1983; 9:1807–1813.

139. Gray JR, McCormick B, Cox L, Yahalom J: Primary breast radiation in large breasted or heavy women: Analysis of cosmetic outcome. *Int J Radiat Oncol Biol Phys* 1991; 21:347–354.

140. Ray GR, Fish VJ: Biopsy and definitive radiation therapy in stage I and II adenocarcinoma of the female breast: Analysis of cosmesis and the role of electron beam supplementation. *Int J Radiat Oncol Biol Phys* 1983; 9:813–818.

141. Moody AM, Mayles WPM, Bliss JM, A'Hern RP, Owen JR, Regan J, Broad B, Yarnold JR: The influence of breast size on late radiation effects and association with radiotherapy dose inhomogeneity. *Radiother Oncol* 1994; 33: 106–112.

142. Klein EE, Michalet-Lorenz M, Taylor ME: Use of a Lucite beam spoiler for high-energy breast irradiation. *Med Dos* 1995; 20:89–94.

143. Mark RJ, Zimmerman RP, Greif JM: Capsular contracture after lumpectomy and radiation therapy in patients who have undergone uncomplicated bilateral augmentation mammoplasty. *Radiology* 1996; 200:621–625.

144. Kuske RR, Schuster R, Klein E, Young L, Perez CA, Fineberg B: Radiotherapy and breast reconstruction: Clinical results and dosimetry. *Int J Radiat Oncol Biol Phys* 1991; 21:339–346.

145. Guenther JM, Tokita KM, Giuliano AE: Breast conserving surgery and radiation after augmentation mammoplasty. *Cancer* 1994; 73:2613–2618.

146. Halpern J, McNeese MD, Kroll SS, Ellerbroek N: Irradiation of prosthetically augmented breasts: A retrospective study on toxicity and cosmetic result. *Int J Radiat Oncol Biol Phys* 1990; 18:189–191.

147. Victor SJ, Brown DM, Horwitz EM, Martinez AA, Kini VR, Pettinga JE, Shaheen KW, Benitez P, Chen PY, Vicini FA: Treatment outcome with radiation therapy after breast augmentation or reconstruction in patients with primary breast carcinoma. *Cancer* 1998; 82:1303–1309.

148. Rosen PP: Invasive mammary carcinoma, in JR Harris, ME Lippman, M Morrow, and S Hellman (eds): *Disease of the Breast.* Philadelphia, Lippincott-Raven, 1996, pp 393–444.

149. Schnitt SJ, Connolly JL, Harris JR, Hellman S, Cohen RB: Pathologic predictors of early local recurrence in stage I and II breast cancer treated by primary radiation therapy. *Cancer* 1984; 53:1049–1057.

150. Holland R, Connolly JL, Gelman R, Mravunac M, Hendriks JH, Verbeek AL, Schnitt SJ, Silver B, Boyages J, Harris JR: The presence of an extensive intraductal component following a limited excision correlates with prominent residual disease in the remainder of the breast. *J Clin Oncol* 1990; 8:113–118.

151. Smitt MC, Nowels KW, Zdeblick MJ, Jeffrey S, Carlson RW, Stockdale FE, Goffinet DR: The importance of the lumpectomy surgical margin status in long term results of breast conservation. *Cancer* 1995; 76:259–267.

152. Bartelink H, Border JH, van Dongen JA, Peterse JL: The impact of tumor size and histology on local control after breast conserving therapy. *Radiother Oncol* 1988; 11:297–303.

153. Fisher ER, Anderson S, Redmond C, Fisher B: Ipsilateral breast tumor recurrence and survival following lumpectomy and irradiation: Pathologic findings from NSABP B06. *Semin Surg Oncol* 1992; 8:161–166.

154. Gage I, Schnitt SJ, Nixon AJ, Silver B, Recht A, Troyan SL, Eberlein T, Love SM, Gelman R, Harris JR, Connelly JL: Pathologic margin involvement and the risk of recurrence in patients treated with breast-conserving therapy. *Cancer* 1996; 78:1921–1928.

155. Solin LJ, Fowble BL, Yeh I-T, Kowalyshyn MJ, Schultz DJ, Weiss MC, Goodman RL: Microinvasive ductal carcinoma of the breast treated with breast conserving surgery and definitive irradiation. *Int J Radiat Oncol Biol Phys* 1992; 23:961–966.

156. Bouvet M, Ollila DW, Hunt KK, Babiera GV, Spitz FR, Giuliano AE, Strom EA, Ames FC, Ross MI, Singletary SE: Role of conservation

therapy for invasive lobular carcinoma of the breast. *Ann Surg Oncol* 1997; 4:650–654.

157. Nixon AJ, Schnitt S, Gelman R, Gage I, Bornstein B, Hetelikidis S, Recht A, Silver B, Harris JR, Connolly JL: Relationship of tumor grade to other pathologic features and to treatment outcome for patients with early-stage breast cancer treated with breast-conserving therapy. *Cancer* 1996; 78:1426–1431.

158. Schnitt S, Connolly J, Recht A, Bornstein B, Nixon A, Hetelikidis S, Silver B, Harris J: Is the presence or extent of lobular carcinoma in situ related to the risk of local recurrence in patients with invasive breast cancer treated with conservative surgery and radiation therapy? *Breast Cancer Res Treat* 1996; 41:224 (abstr).

159. Moran M, Haffty BG: Lobular carcinoma in situ as a component of breast cancer: The long-term outcome in patients treated with breast conservation therapy. *Int J Radiat Oncol Biol Phys* 1998; 40:353–358.

160. Veronesi U, Marubini E, DelVecchio M, Manzari A, Andreola S, Greco M, Luini A, Merson M, Saccozzi R, Rilke F, Salvadori B: Local recurrences and distant metastasis after conservative breast cancer treatments: Partly independent events. *J Natl Cancer Inst* 1995; 87:19–27.

161. Guidi AJ, Connolly JL, Harris JR, Schnitt SJ: The relationship between shaved margin and inked margin status in breast excision specimens. *Cancer* 1997; 79:1568–1573.

162. Solin LJ, Fowble B, Schultz DJ, Goodman RL: The significance of pathology margins of the tumor excision on the outcome of patients treated with definitive irradiation for early-stage breast cancer. *Int J Radiat Oncol Biol Phys* 1991; 21:279–287.

163. Fowble B, Rosser C, Hanlon A: Conservative surgery and radiation for stages I and II breast cancer, in KI Bland, and EM Copeland III (eds): *The Breast: A Comprehensive Textbook for the Management of Benign and Malignant Disease.* Philadephia, Saunders, 1998.

164. Komarnicky LT, Mansfield CM, DiBiase SJ: Prognostic significance of the number of positive margins in breast conserving treatment for early-stage breast cancer. Proceedings of the American Radium Society 79th Annual Meeting. *Cancer J Sci Am* 1997; 3:119 (abstr).

165. Mansfield CM, Komarnicky LT, Schwartz GF, Rosenberg AL, Krishnan L, Jewell WR, Rosato FE, Moses ML, Haghbin M, Taylor J, Barbot D, Cohn HE, Gillum DR, Taylor JT: Ten year results in 1070 patients with stages I and II breast cancer treated by conservative surgery and radiation therapy. *Cancer* 1995; 75:2328–2336.

166. Dewar JA, Arriagada R, Benhamou S, Benhamou E, Bretel J-J, Pellae-Cosset B, Marin J-L, Petit J-Y, Contesso G, Sarrazin D, for the Institut Gustave-Roussy Breast Cancer Group: Local relapse and contralateral tumor rates in patients with breast cancer treated with conservative surgery and radiotherapy (Institut Gustave-Roussy 1970–1982). *Cancer* 1995; 76:2260–2265.

167. Perez CA, Taylor ME, Halverson K, Garcia D, Kuske RR, Lockett MA: Brachytherapy or electron beam boost in conservation therapy of carcinoma of the breast: A nonrandomized comparison. *Int J Radiat Oncol Biol Phys* 1996; 34:995–1007.

168. Fein DA, Fowble BL, Hanlon AL: The influence of pathologic margin status adjuvant treatment and residual tumor within the re-excision specimen on breast recurrence. *Int J Radiat Oncol Biol Phys* 1996; 36:275 (abstr).

169. Fisher B, Bauer M, Margolese R, Poisson R, Pilch Y, Redmond C, Fisher E, Wolmark N, Deutsch M, Montague E, et al: Five year results of a randomized clinical trial comparing total mastectomy and segmental mastectomy with or without radiation in the treatment of breast cancer. *N Engl J Med* 1985; 312:665–673.

170. McCormick B, Kinne D, Petrek J, Osborne M, Cox L, Shank B, Hellman S, Yahalom J, Rosen PP: Limited resection for breast cancer: A study of inked specimen margins before radiotherapy. *Int J Radiat Oncol Biol Phys* 1987; 13:1667–1671.

171. Osborne MP, Ormiston N, Harmer CL, McKinnaa A, Baker J, Greening WP: Breast conservation in the treatment of early breast cancer: A 20-year follow-up. *Cancer* 1984; 53:349–355.

172. Kurtz JM, Amalric R, Brandone H, Ayme Y, Spitalier JM: How important is adequate radiotherapy for the long-term results of breast-conserving treatment? *Radiother Oncol* 1991; 20:84–90.

173. Pezner RD, Lipsett JA, Desai K, Vora N, Terz J, Hill LR, Luk KH: To boost or not to boost: Decreasing radiation therapy in conservative breast cancer treatment when "inked" tumor resection margins are pathologically free of cancer. *Int J Radiat Oncol Biol Phys* 1988; 14:873–877.

174. Romestaing P, Lehingue Y, Carrie C, Coquard R, Montbarbon X, Ardiet J-M, Mamelle N, Gérard J-P: Role of 10-Gy boost in the conservative treatment of early breast cancer: Results of a randomized clinical trial in Lyon, France. *J Clin Oncol* 1997; 15:963–968.

175. Ryoo ME, Kagan AR, Wollin M, Tome MA, Tedeschi MA, Rao AR, Hintz BL, Kuruvilla AM, Nussbaum H, Stretter OE, Tabola BR, Miller MJ: Prognostic factors for recurrence and cosmesis in 393 patients after radiation therapy for early mammary carcinoma. *Radiology* 1989; 172:555–559.

176. Galinsky DL, Sharma M, Hartsell WF, Griem KL, Murthy A: Primary radiation therapy to T1 and T2 breast cancer following conservative surgery. Which patient should be boosted? *Am J Clin Oncol* 1994; 17:60–63.

177. Veronesi U, Zucali R, Luini A: Local control and survival in early breast cancer: The Milan trial. *Int J Radiat Oncol Biol Phys* 1986; 12:717–720.

178. Sarrazin D, Le MG, Fontaine MF, Arriagada R: Conservative treatment versus mastectomy in T1 or small T2 breast cancer: A randomized clinical trial, in J Harris, S Hellman, and W Silen (eds): *Conservative Management of Breast Cancer.* Philadelphia, Lippincott, 1983, pp 101–111.

179. Kuske RR, Hayden D, Bischoff R, Farr GH, Fineberg BB: The impact of extracapsular axillary nodal extension (ECE) with or without irradiation on patterns of recurrence and survival from breast cancer. *Int J Radiat Oncol Biol Phys* 1996; 36:277 (abstr).

180. Korzeniowski S, Dyba T, Skolyszewski J: Classical prognostic factors for survival and loco-regional control in breast cancer patients treated with radical mastectomy alone. *Acta Oncol* 1994; 33:759–765.

181. Vicini FA, Horwitz EM, Lacerna MD, Brown DM, White J, Dmuchowski CF, Kini VR, Martinez A: The role of regional nodal irradiation in the management of patients with early-stage breast cancer treated with breast-conserving therapy. *Int J Radiat Oncol Biol Phys* 1997; 39:1069–1076.

182. Ewers S-B, Attewell R, Baldetorp B, Borg A, Ferno M, Langstrom E, Ryden S, Killander D: Flow cytometry DNA analysis and prediction of loco-regional recurrences after mastectomy in breast cancer. *Acta Oncol* 1992; 31:733–740.

183. Donegan WL, Stine SB, Samter TG: Implications of extracapsular nodal metastases for treatment and prognosis of breast cancer. *Cancer* 1993; 72:778–782.

184. Leonard C, Corkill M, Tompkin J, Zhen B, Waitz D, Norton L, Kinzie J: Are axillary recurrence and overall survival affected by axillary extranodal tumor extension in breast cancer? Implications for radiation therapy. *J Clin Oncol* 1995; 13:47–53.

185. Hetelekidis S, Silver B, Schnitt SJ, Connolly JL, Bornstein BA, Nixon AJ, Recht A, Gelman R, Harris JR: The significance of axillary extracapsular extension in breast cancer. *Int J Radiat Oncol Biol Phys* 1996; 36:275 (abstr).

186. Pierce LJ, Oberman HA, Strawderman MH, Lichter AS: Microscopic extracapsular extension in the axilla: Is this an indication for axillary radiotherapy? *Int J Radiat Oncol Biol Phys* 1995; 33:253–259.

187. Cabanes PA, Salmon RJ, Vilcoq JR, Durand JC, Fourquet A, Gautier C, Asselain B, for the Breast Carcinoma Collaborative Group of the Institut Curie: Value of axillary dissection in addition to lumpectomy and radiotherapy in early breast cancer. *Lancet* 1992; 339:1245–1248.

188. Fisher B, Redmond C, Fisher ER, Bauer M, Wolmark N, Wickerham L, Deutsch M, Montague E, Margolese R, Foster R: Ten year results of a randomized clinical trial comparing radical mastectomy and total mastectomy with or without radiation. *N Engl J Med* 1985; 312:674–681.

189. Wong JS, Recht A, Beard CJ, Busse PM, Cady B, Chaffey JT, Come S, Fam S, Kaelin C, Lingos TI, Nixon AJ, Shulman LN, Troyan S, Silver B, Harris JR: Treatment outcome after tangential radiation therapy without axillary dissection in patients with early-stage breast cancer and clinically negative axillary nodes. *Int J Radiat Oncol Biol Phys* 1997; 39:915–920.

190. Mazeron JJ, Otmezguine Y, Huart J, Pierquin B: Conservative treatment of breast cancer:

Results of management of axillary lymph node area in 3353 patients (letter to the editor). *Lancet* 1985; 1:1387.

191. Ebbs SR, Yarnold JR: Patient and anatomical selectivity in postoperative radiotherapy for early breast cancer: A British perspective. *Semin Surg Oncol* 1992; 8:167–171.

192. Halverson KJ, Taylor ME, Perez CA, Garcia DM, Myerson R, Philpott G, Levy J, Simpson JR, Tucker G, Rush C: Management of the axilla in patients with breast cancers one centimeter or smaller. *Am J Clin Oncol* 1994; 17:461–466.

193. Hoskin PJ, Rajan B, Ebbs S, Tait D, Milan S, Yarnold JR: Selective avoidance of lymphatic radiotherapy in the conservative management of early breast cancer. *Radiother Oncol* 1992; 25:83–88.

194. Bonadonna G, Valagussa P, Rossi A, Tancini G, Brambilla C, Zambetti M, Veronesi U: Ten-year experience with CMF-based adjuvant chemotherapy in resectable breast cancer. *Breast Cancer Res Treat* 1985; 5:95–115.

195. Halverson KJ, Perez CA, Kuske RR, Garcia DM, Simpson JR, Fineberg B: Isolated local–regional recurrence of breast cancer following mastectomy: Radiotherapeutic management. *Int J Radiat Oncol Biol Phys* 1990; 19:851–858.

196. Fowble B, Solin LJ, Schultz DJ, Goodman RL: Frequency, sites of relapse and outcome of regional node failures following conservative surgery and radiation for early breast cancer. *Int J Radiat Oncol Biol Phys* 1989; 17: 703–710.

197. Roberson PL, Lichter AS, Bodner A, Fredrickson HA, Padikal TN, Kelly BA, van de Geijn J: Dose to lung in primary breast irradiation. *Int J Radiat Oncol Biol Phys* 1983; 9:97–102.

198. Romsdahl MM, Montague ED, Ames FC, Richards PC, Schell SR: Conservation surgery and irradiation as treatment for early breast cancer. *Arch Surg* 1983; 118:521–528.

199. Danoff BF, Galvin JM, Cheng E, Brookland RK, Powlis WD, Goodman RL: The clinical application of CT scanning in the treatment of primary breast cancer, in FC Ames, GR Blumenschein, and ED Montague (eds): *Current Controversies in Breast Cancer.* Austin, University of Texas Press, 1984, pp 391–397.

200. Recht A, Houlihan MJ: Axillary lymph nodes and breast cancer—A review. *Cancer* 1995; 76:1491–1512.

201. Marks LB, Halperin EC, Prosnitz LR, Ross M, Vredenburgh JJ, Rosner GL, Peters W: Postmastectomy radiotherapy following adjuvant chemotherapy and autologous bone marrow transplantation for breast cancer patients with ≥10 positive axillary nodes. *Int J Radiat Oncol Biol Phys* 1992; 23:1021–1026.

202. Halverson KJ, Taylor ME, Perez CA, Garcia DM, Myerson R, Philpott G, Levy J, Simpson JR, Tucker G, Rush G: Regional nodal management and patterns of failure following conservative surgery and radiation therapy for stage I and II breast cancer. *Int J Radiat Oncol Biol Phys* 1993; 26:593–599.

203. Recht A, Pierce SM, Abner A, Vicini F, Osteen RT, Love SM, Silver B, Harris JR: Regional node failure after conservative surgery and radiotherapy for early-stage breast carcinoma. *J Clin Oncol* 1991; 9:988–996.

204. Jardines L, Fowble B, Schultz D, Mackie J, Buzby G, Torosian M, Daly J, Weiss M, Orel S, Rosato E: Factors associated with a positive reexcision following excisional biopsy for invasive breast cancer. *Surgery* 1995; 118:803–809.

205. Gwin JL, Eisenberg BL, Hoffman JP, Ottery FD, Boraas M, Solin LJ: Incidence of gross and microscopic carcinoma in specimens from patients with breast cancer after reexcision lumpectomy. *Ann Surg* 1993; 218:729–734.

206. Schnitt SJ, Connolly JL, Khettry U, Mazoujian G, Brenner M, Silver B, Recht A, Beadle G, Harris JR: Pathologic findings on re-excision of the primary site in breast cancer patients considered for treatment by primary radiation therapy. *Cancer* 1987; 59:675–681.

207. Frazier TG, Wong RW, Rose D: Implications of accurate pathologic margins in the treatment of breast cancer. *Arch Surg* 1989; 1224: 37–38.

208. Lee CH, Carter D: Detecting residual tumor after excisional biopsy of impalpable breast carcinoma: Efficacy of comparing preoperative mammograms with radiographs of the biopsy specimen. *Am J Radiol* 1995; 164:81–86.

209. Wazer DE, Schmidt-Ullrich RK, Schmid CH, Ruthazer R, Kramer B, Safaii H, Graham R: The value of breast lumpectomy margin as-

sessment as a predictor of residual tumor burden. *Int J Radiat Oncol Biol Phys* 1997; 38: 291–299.

210. Fowble B: Is there a subset of patients with early stage invasive breast cancer for whom irradiation may not be indicated after conservative surgery alone? *Breast J* 1995; 1:79–90.

211. Recht A, Houlihan MJ: Conservative surgery without radiotherapy in the treatment of patients with early-stage invasive breast cancer. A review. *Ann Surg* 1995; 222:9–18.

212. Fisher B, Redmond C, and others for the National Surgical Adjuvant Breast and Bowel Project: Lumpectomy for breast cancer: An update of the NSABP experience. *Monogr Natl Cancer Inst* 1992; 11:7–13.

213. Veronesi U, Luini A, Del Vecchio M, Greco M, Galimberti V, Merson M, Rilke F, Sacchini V, Saccozzi R, Savio T, Zurrida S, Salvadori B: Radiotherapy after breast preserving surgery in women with localized cancer of the breast. *N Engl J Med* 1993; 328:1587–1591.

214. Dalberg K, Mattsson A, Rutqvist LE, Johansson U, Riddez L, Sandelin K: Breast conserving surgery for invasive breast cancer: Risk factors for ipsilateral breast tumor recurrences. *Breast Cancer Res Treat* 1997; 43: 73–86.

215. McCready DR, Hanna W, Kahn H, Chapman J-A, Wall J, Fish EB, Lickley HLA: Factors associated with local breast cancer recurrence after lumpectomy alone. *Ann Surg Oncol* 1996; 3:358–366.

216. Greening WP, Montgomery ACV, Gordon AB, Gowing NFC: Quadrantic excision and axillary node dissection without radiation therapy: The long-term results of a selective policy in the treatment of stage I breast cancer. *Eur J Surg Oncol* 1998; 14:221–225.

217. Sauer R, Tulusan AH, Lang N, Dunst J: Can breast irradiation be omitted in low risk breast cancer patients after segmentectomy? First results of Erlangen protocol. *Int J Radiat Oncol Biol Phys* 1993; 27:146–147 (abstr).

218. Nemoto T, Patel JK, Rosner D, Dao TL, Schuh M, Penetrante R: Factors affecting recurrence in lumpectomy without irradiation for breast cancer. *Cancer* 1991; 67:2079–2082.

219. Butler JA, Bretsky S, Menendez-Botet C, Kinne DW: Estrogen receptor protein of breast cancer as a predictor of recurrence. *Cancer* 1985; 55:1178–1181.

220. Lagios MD, Richard UE, Rose MR, Yee E: Segmental mastectomy without radiotherapy: Short-term follow-up. *Cancer* 1983; 52: 2173–2179.

221. Renton SC, Gazet J-C, Ford HT, Corbishley C, Sutcliffe R: The importance of the resection margin in conservative surgery for breast cancer. *Eur J Surg Oncol* 1996; 22:17–22.

222. Schnitt SJ, Hayman J, Gelman R, Eberlein TJ, Love SM, Mayzel K, Osteen RT, Nixon AJ, Pierce S, Recht A, Harris JR: A prospective study of conservative surgery alone in the treatment of selected patients with stage I breast cancer. *Cancer* 1996; 77:1094–1100.

223. Lee KS, Plowman PN, Gilmore OJ, Gray R: Breast conservation therapy: How safe is postoperative tamoxifen only in the elderly and frail? *Proc Am Soc Clin Oncol* 1992; 11:50 (abstr).

224. Cooke AL, Perera F, Fisher B, Opeitum A, Yu N: Tamoxifen with and without radiation after partial mastectomy in patients with involved nodes. *Int J Radiat Oncol Biol Phys* 1995; 31:771–778.

225. Liljegren G, Holmberg L, Adami HO, Westman G, Graffman S, Bergh J, Uppsala–Orebro Breast Cancer Study Group: Sector resection with or without postoperative radiotherapy for stage I breast cancer: 5 year results of a randomized trial. *J Natl Cancer Inst* 1994; 86:717–722.

226. Clark RM, Whelan T, Levine M, Roberts R, Willan A, McCullock P, Lipa M, Wilkinson RH, Mahoney LJ: Randomized clinical trial of breast irradiation following lumpectomy and axillary dissection for node-negative breast cancer: An update. *J Natl Cancer Inst* 1996; 88:1659–1664.

227. Fisher B, Slack NH, Cavanaugh PJ, Gardner B, Ravdin RG: Post-operative radiotherapy in the treatment of breast cancer: Results of the NSABP clinical trial. *Ann Surg* 1970; 172: 711–732.

228. Easson EC: Post-operative radiotherapy in breast cancer, in APM Forrest, and PB Kunkler (eds): *Prognostic Factors in Breast Cancer.* Edinburgh, E & S Livingstone, 1968, pp 118–135.

229. Palmer MK, Ribeiro GG: Thirty-four year follow-up of patients with breast cancer in clinical trial of postoperative radiotherapy. *Br Med J* 1985; 291:1088–1091.

230. Host H, Brennhoud IO, Loeb M: Post-operative radiotherapy in breast cancer: Long-term results from the Oslo study. *Int J Radiat Oncol Biol Phys* 1986; 12:727–732.

231. Brinkley D, Haybittle JL, Houghton J: The Cancer Research Campaign (King's/Cambridge) trial for early breast cancer: An analysis of the radiotherapy data. *Br J Radiol* 1984; 57:309–316.

232. Lythgoe JP, Leck I, Swindell R: Manchester regional breast study. Preliminary results. *Lancet* 1978; i:744–747.

233. Berstock DA, Houghton J, Haybittle J, Baum M: The role of radiotherapy following total mastectomy for patients with early breast cancer. *World J Surg* 1985; 9:667–670.

234. Cancer Research Campaign Working Party: Cancer Research Campaign (King's/Cambridge) trial for early breast cancer: A detailed update at the tenth year. *Lancet* 1980; ii:55–60.

235. Rutqvist LE, Pettersson D, Johansson H: Adjuvant radiation therapy versus surgery alone in operable breast cancer: Long-term follow-up at a randomized clinical trial. *Radiother Oncol* 1993; 26:104–110.

236. Lythgoe JP, Palmer MK: Manchester regional breast study: 5 and 10 year results. *Br J Surg* 1982; 69:693–696.

237. Turnbull AR, Turner DT, Chant AD, Shepherd JM, Buchanan RB, Fraser JD: Treatment of early breast cancer. *Lancet* 1978; ii:7–9.

238. Cuzick J, Stewart H, Peto H, Baum M, Fisher B, Host H, Lythgoe JP, Ribeiro G, Scheurlen H, Wallgren A: Overview of randomized trials of postoperative adjuvant radiotherapy in breast cancer. *Cancer Treat Rep* 1987; 71:15–29.

239. Cuzick J, Stewart H, Rutqvist L, Houghton J, Edwards R, Redmond C, Peto R, Baum M, Fisher B, Host H, Lythgoe JP, Ribeiro G, Scheurlen H: Cause-specific mortality in long-term survivors of breast cancer who participated in trials of radiotherapy. *J Clin Oncol* 1994; 12:447–453.

240. Gyenes G, Fornander T, Carlens P, Rutqvist LE: Morbidity of ischemic heart disease in early breast cancer 15–20 years after adjuvant radiotherapy. *Int J Radiat Oncol Biol Phys* 1994; 28:1235–1241.

241. Haybittle JL, Brinkley D, Houghton J, A'Hern RP, Baum M: Postoperative radiotherapy and late mortality: Evidence from the Cancer Research Campaign trial for early breast cancer. *Br Med J* 1989; 298:1611–1614.

242. Rutqvist LE, Lat I, Fornander MD: Cardiovascular mortality in a randomized trial of adjuvant radiation therapy versus surgery alone in primary breast cancer. *Int J Radiat Oncol Biol Phys* 1992; 22:887–896.

243. Jones JM, Ribeiro GG: Mortality patterns over 34 years of breast cancer patients in a clinical trial of post-operative radiotherapy. *Clin Radiol* 1989; 40:204–208.

244. Donegan WL, Perez-Mesa CM, Watson FR: A biostatistical study of locally recurrent breast carcinoma. *Surg Gynecol Obstet* 1966; 122: 529–540.

245. Dao TL, Nemoto T: The clinical significance of skin recurrence after radical mastectomy in women with cancer of the breast. *Surg Gynecol Obstet* 1963; 117:447–453.

246. Rosenman J, Bernard S, Kober C, Leland W, Varia M, Newsome J: Local recurrences in patients with breast cancer treated at the North Carolina Memorial Hospital. *Cancer* 1986; 57:1421–1425.

247. Baker RR, Montague AC, Childs JN: A comparison of modified radical mastectomy to radical mastectomy in the treatment of operable breast cancer. *Ann Surg* 1979; 189:553–559.

248. Maddox WA, Carpenter JT, Laws HT, Soong SJ, Cloud G, Urist MM, Balch CM: A randomized prospective trial of radical (Halsted) mastectomy versus modified radical mastectomy in 311 breast cancer patients. *Ann Surg* 1983; 198:207–212.

249. Haagensen CD: *Diseases of the Breast,* 3rd ed. Philadelphia, Saunders, 1986, pp 924–929.

250. Valagussa P, Bonadonna G, Veronesi U: Patterns of relapse and survival following radical mastectomy: Analysis of 716 consecutive patients. *Cancer* 1978; 41:1170–1178.

251. Lee YN: Breast carcinoma: Pattern of recurrence and metastasis after mastectomy. *Am J Clin Oncol* 1984; 7:443–448.

252. Donegan WL: Cancer of the breast, in WL Donegan, and JS Spratt (eds): *Cancer of the*

*Breast,* 3rd ed. Philadelphia, Saunders, 1998, pp 648–663.

253. Hopton DS, Thorogood J, Clayden AD, MacKinnon D: Histologic grading of breast cancer: Significance of grade on recurrence and mortality. *Eur J Surg Oncol* 1989; 15:25–31.

254. Williams MR, Hinton CP, Todd JH, Morgan DA, Elston CW, Blamey RW: The prediction of local or regional recurrence after simple mastectomy for operable breast cancery. *Br J Surg* 1985; 72:721–723.

255. Fowble B, Gray R, Gilchrist K, Goodman RL, Taylor S, Tormey DC: Identification of a subgroup of patients with breast cancer and histologically positive nodes receiving adjuvant chemotherapy who may benefit from postoperative radiotherapy. *J Clin Oncol* 1988; 6: 1107–1117.

256. Ahlborn TN, Gump FE, Bodain C, Habif DV, Kister S: Tumor to fascia margin as a factor in local recurrence after modified radical mastectomy. *Surg Gynecol Obstet* 1988; 166:523–526.

257. Mentzer SJ, Osteen RT, Wilson RE: Local recurrence and the deep resection margin in carcinoma of the breast. *Surg Gynecol Obstet* 1986; 16:513–517.

258. Freedman GM, Fowble BL, Hanlon AL, Myint MA, Hoffman JP, Sigurdson ER, Eisenberg BL, Goldstein LJ, Fein DA: A close or positive margin after mastectomy is not an indication for chest wall irradiation except in women aged fifty or younger. *Int J Radiat Oncol Biol Phys* 1997; 39:266 (abstr).

259. Baum M, Coyle PJ: Simple mastectomy for early breast cancer and the behavior of the untreated axillary nodes. *Bull. Cancer* 1977; 64:603–610.

260. Crile G: Results of simplified treatment of breast cancer. *Surg Gynecol Obstet* 1964; 118:517–523.

261. Forrest APM, Stewart JH, Roberts MM, Steele RJC: Simple mastectomy and axillary node sampling (pectoral node biopsy) in the management of primary breast cancer. *Ann Surg* 1982; 196:371–378.

262. Cancer Research Campaign: Management of early cancer of the breast: Report of an international multicenter trial supported by the Cancer Research Campaign. *Br Med J* 1976; 1:1035–1038.

263. Fisher B, Wolmark N, Bauer M, Redmond C, Gebhardt MR: The accuracy of clinical nodal staging and of limited axillary dissection as a determinant of histologic nodal status in carcinoma of the breast. *Surg Gynecol Obstet* 1981; 152:765–772.

264. Veronesi U, Valagussa P: Inefficacy of internal mammary node dissection in breast cancer surgery. *Cancer* 1981; 47:170–175.

265. Smith JA 3rd, Gamez-Araujo JK, Gallagher HS, White EC, McBride CM: Carcinoma of the breast: Analysis of total lymph node involvement versus level of metastases. *Cancer* 1977; 39:527–532.

266. Urban JA, Marjani MA: Significance of internal mammary lymph node metastases in breast cancer. *Am J Roentgenol Radium Ther Nucl Med* 1971; 111:130–136.

267. Handley RS: The conservative radical mastectomy of Patey: 10 year results in 425 patients. *Breast* 1976; 2:16–21.

268. Donegan WL: The influence of untreated internal mammary metastases upon the course of mammary cancer. *Cancer* 1977; 39: 533–538.

269. Meier P, Ferguson DJ, Karrison T: A controlled trial of extended radical versus radical mastectomy: Ten-year results. *Cancer* 1989; 63:188–195.

270. Urban JA: Management of operable breast cancer: The surgeon's view. *Cancer* 1978; 42: 2066–2077.

271. Schwaibold F, Fowble BL, Solin LJ, Schultz DJ, Goodman RL: The results of radiation therapy for isolated local–regional recurrence after mastectomy. *Int J Radiat Oncol Biol Phys* 1991; 21:299–310.

272. Danoff BF, Coia LR, Cantor RI, Pajak TF, Kramer S: Locally recurrent breast carcinoma: The effect of adjuvant chemotherapy on prognosis. *Radiology* 1983; 147:849–852.

273. Bedwinek JM, Lee J, Fineberg B, Ocwieza M: Prognostic indicators in patients with isolated local–regional recurrence of breast cancer. *Cancer* 1981; 47:2232–2235.

274. Aberizk WJ, Silver B, Henderson IC, Kady B, Harris JR: The use of radiotherapy for treatment of isolated locoregional recurrence of breast carcinoma after mastectomy. *Cancer* 1986; 58:1214–1218.

275. Fisher B, Redmond C, Others for the National Surgical Adjuvant Breast and Bowel Project: Systemic therapy in node-negative patients: Updated findings from NSABP clinical trials. *Monogr Natl Cancer Inst* 1992; 11:105–116.

276. Mansour EG, Eudey L, Termey DC, Shatilo AH, Osborne CK, Gilchrist KW, Cooper MR, Falkson G: Chemotherapy versus observation in high risk node negative breast cancer patients. *Monogr Natl Cancer Inst* 1992; 11:97–104.

277. Goldhirsch A, Castiglione M, Gelber (for the International Breast Cancer Study Group, formerly Ludwig Group), RD: A single perioperative adjuvant chemotherapy course for node-negative breast cancer: Five year results of Trial V. *Monogr Natl Cancer Inst* 1992; 11:89–96.

278. Zambetti M, Bonadonno G, Valagusso P, Daidone MG, Coradini D, Bignami P, Contesso G, Silvestrini R: Adjuvant CMF for node-negative and estrogen receptor–negative breast cancer patients. *Monogr Natl Cancer Inst* 1992; 11:77–83.

279. Morrison JM, Howell A, Kelly KA, Grieve RJ, Monypenny IJ, Walker RA, Waterhouse JAH: West Midlands Onocology Association trials of adjuvant chemotherapy in operable breast cancer: Results after a median follow-up of 7 years. I. Patients with involved axillary nodes. *Br J Cancer* 1989; 60:911–918.

280. Stefanik D, Goldberg R, Bryne P, Smith F, Uneo W, Smith L, Harter K, Bachenheimer L, Beizer C, Dritschilo A: Local–regional failure in patients treated with adjuvant chemotherapy for breast cancer. *J Clin Oncol* 1985; 3:660–665.

281. Rao AF, Murthy AK, Hendrickson FR, Rossof A, Bonomi P, Shorey W: Analysis of risk factors for loco-regional failure in stage II breast carcinoma treated with mastectomy and adjunctive chemotherapy. *Int J Radiat Oncol Biol Phys* 1985; 11:151 (abstr).

282. Griem KL, Henderson IC, Gelman R, Ascoli D, Silver B, Recht A, Goodman RL, Hellman S, Harris JR: The 5-year results of a randomized trial of adjuvant radiation therapy after chemotherapy in breast cancer patients treated with mastectomy. *J Clin Oncol* 1987; 5: 1546–1555.

283. Buzdar AU, Blumenshein GR, Smith TL, Powell KC, Hortobagyi GN, Yap HY, Schell FC, Barnes BC, Ames FC, Martin RG, et al: Adjuvant chemotherapy with fluorouracil, doxorubicin and cyclophosphamide, with or without irradiation in operable breast cancer. A prospective randomized trial. *Cancer* 1984; 53:384–389.

284. Buzzoni R, Bonadonna G, Valagussa P, Zambetti M: Adjuvant chemotherapy with doxorubicin plus cyclophosphamide, methotrexate, and fluorouracil in the treatment of resectable breast cancer with more than three positive axillary nodes. *J Clin Oncol* 1991; 9:2134–2140.

285. Pisansky TM, Ingle JN, Schaid DJ, Hass AC, Krook JE, Donohue JH, Witzig TE, Wold LE: Patterns of tumor relapse following mastectomy and adjuvant systemic therapy in patients with axillary lymph node-positive breast cancer. Impact on clinical, histopathologic and flow cytometric factors. *Cancer* 1993; 72: 1247–1260.

286. Kaufmann M, Jonat W, Abel U, Hilfrich J, Caffier H, Kreienberg R, Trams G, Brunnert K, Schermann J, Kleine W, Mahlke M, Neises M, Stosiek U, Stiglmayer R, Seeger F, Langnickel D, Nagel G, Gampe M, Maas H, Kubli F: Adjuvant randomized trials of doxorubicin/cyclophosphamide versus doxorubicin/cyclophosphamide/tamoxifen and CMF chemotherapy versus tamoxifen in women with node-positive breast cancer. *J Clin Oncol* 1993; 11:454–460.

287. Sykes HF, Sim DA, Wong CJ, Cassady JR, Salmon SE: Local–regional recurrences in breast cancer after mastectomy and Adriamycin-based adjuvant chemotherapy: Evaluation of the role of postoperative radiotherapy. *Int J Radiat Oncol Biol Phys* 1989; 16: 641–647.

288. Pritchard KJ, Paterson AHG, Fine S, Paul N, Pater J, Zee B, Warr D, Knowling M, Abu-Zahra H, Levine M, Bramwell V, Norris B, Poljiack M, Perrault D, Ragaz J, Verme S, Bowman D: A randomized trial of CMF chemotherapy added to tamoxifen as adjuvant therapy in post-menopausal women with node positive estrogen and/or progesterone receptor positive breast cancer. *Proc Am Soc Clin Oncol* 1992; 11:60 (abstr).

289. Fowble B: Local–regional treatment options for early invasive breast cancer, in B Fowble, RL Goodman, JH Glick, and EF Rosato (eds): *Breast Cancer Treatment: A Comprehensive*

*Guide to Management.* St Louis, Mosby, 1991, pp 25–88.

290. Donegan WL: Local and regional recurrence, in Donegan WL, and Spratt JS (eds): *Cancer of the Breast.* Philadelphia, Saunders, 1988, pp 648–663.

291. Pawlias KT, Dockerty MB, Ellis FH: Late locally recurrent carcinoma of the breast. *Ann Surg* 1958; 148:192–196.

292. Di Pietro S, Bertario L, Piva L: Prognosis and treatment of loco-regional breast cancer recurrences: Critical considerations on 120 cases. *Tumori* 1980; 66:331–336.

293. Shimkin MB, Lucia EL, Low-Beer VA, Bell HG: Recurrent cancer of the breast: Analysis of frequency distribution and mortality at the University of California Hospital, 1918 to 1947, inclusive. *Cancer* 1954; 7:29–34.

294. Crowe JP, Gordon NH, Antunez AR, Shenk RR, Hubay CA, Shuck JM: Local–regional breast cancer recurrence following mastectomy. *Arch Surg* 1991; 126:429–432.

295. Fowble B: Postmastectomy radiation: Then and now. *Oncology* 1997; 11:213–239.

296. Rivkin SE, Green S, Metch B, Glucksberg H, God-el-Mawla N, Constanzi JJ, Hoogstraten B, Athens J, Maloney T, Osborne CK, Vaughn CB: Adjuvant CMFVP versus melphalan for operable breast cancer with positive axillary nodes: 10 year results of a Southwest Oncology Group study. *J Clin Oncol* 1989; 7:1229–1238.

297. Tancini G, Bonadonna G, Valagussa P, Marchini S, Veronesi U: Adjuvant CMF in breast cancer: Comparative 5-year results of 12 versus 6 cycles. *J Clin Oncol* 1983; 1:2–10.

298. Falkson HE, Gray RG, Wolberg WH, Gilchrist KW, Harris JE, Tormey DC, Falkson G: Adjuvant trial of 12 cycles of CMFPT followed by observation or continuous tamoxifen versus 4 cycles of CMFPT in postmenopausal women with breast cancer: An Eastern Cooperative Oncology Group Phase III study. *J Clin Oncol* 1990; 8:599–607.

299. Levine MN, Gent M, Hyrniuk WM, Bramwell V, Abu-Zahra H, DePauw S, Arnold A, Findlay B, Levin L, Skillings J, Bush H, Goodyear MD, Roberts R: A randomized trial comparing 12 weeks versus 36 weeks of adjuvant chemotherapy in stage II breast cancer. *J Clin Oncol* 1990; 8:1217–1225.

300. Rivkin SE, Gree S, Metch B, Jewell WR, Costanzi JJ, Altman SJ, Minton JP, O'Bryan RM, Osborne CK: One versus 2 years of CM-FVP adjuvant chemotherapy in axillary node-positive and estrogen receptor–negative patients: A Southwest Oncology Group study. *J Clin Oncol* 1993; 11:1710–1716.

301. Ludwig Breast Cancer Group: Combination adjuvant chemotherapy for node-positive breast cancer: Inadequacy of a single perioperative cycle. *N Engl J Med* 1988; 319:677–683.

302. Goldhirsch A, Gelber R: Adjuvant treatment for early breast cancer: The Ludwig Breast Cancer studies. *Natl Cancer Inst Monogr* 1986; 1:55–70.

303. Castiglione-Gertsch M, Johnsen C, Goldhirsch A, Gelber RD, Rudenstam CM, Collins J, Lindtner J, Hacking A, Cortes-Funes H, Forbes J, et al: The International (Ludwig) Breast Cancer Study Group trials I–IV: 15 years follow-up. *Ann Oncol,* 1994; 5:717–724.

304. Tormey DC, Weinberg VE, Holland JF, Weiss RB, Glidewell OJ, Perloff M, Falkson G, Falkson HC, Henry PH, Leone LA, et al: A randomized trial of five and three drug chemotherapy and chemoimmunotherapy regimens in women with operable node positive breast cancer. *J Clin Oncol* 1983; 1:138–145.

305. Wood WC, Weiss RB, Tormey DC, Holland JF, Henry PH, Leone LA, Rafla S, Silver RT, Carey RW, Lesnick GJ, et al: A randomized trial of CMF versus CMFVP as adjuvant chemotherapy in women with node-positive stage II breast cancer. A CALGB study. *World J Surg* 1985; 9:714–718.

306. Misset J-L, diPalma M, Delgado M, Plagne R, Chollet P, Fumoleau P, Le Mevel B, Belpomme D, Guerrin J, Fargeot P, Metz R, Ithzaki M, Hill C, Mathé G, for the Groupe Oncofrance: Adjuvant treatment of node-positive breast cancer with cyclophosphamide, doxorubicin, fluorouracil and vincristine versus cyclophosphamide, methotrexate, and fluorouracil: Final report after a 16-year median follow-up duration. *J Clin Oncol* 1996; 14:1136–1145.

307. Fisher B, Redmond C, Wickerham DL, Bowman D, Schipper H, Wolmark N, Sass R, Fisher ER, Jochimsen P, Legault-Poisson S, Dimitrov N, Wolter J, Bornstein R, Elias EG, LiCalzi N, Patersen AHG, Sutherland CM: Doxorubicin-

containing regimens for the treatment of stage II breast cancer: The National Surgical Adjuvant Breast and Bowel Project experience. *J Clin Oncol* 1989; 7:572–582.

308. Fisher B, Brown A, Dimitrov NV, Poisson R, Redmond C, Margolese RG, Bowman D, Wolmark N, Wickerham DL, Kardinal CG, Shibata H, Paterson AHG, Sutherland CM, Rohert NJ, Ager PJ, Levy L, Wolter J, Wozniak T, Fisher ER, Deutsch M: Two months of doxorubicin–cyclophosphamide with and without interval reinduction therapy compared with 6 months of cyclophosphamid, methotrexate, and fluorouracil in positive-node breast cancer patients with tamoxifen-nonresponsive tumors: Results from the National Surgical Adjuvant Breast and Bowel Project B-15. *J Clin Oncol* 1990; 8:1483–1496.

309. Budd GT, Green S, O'Bryan RM, Martino S, Abeloff MD, Rinehart JJ, Hahn R, Harris J, Tormey D, O'Sullivan J, Osborne CK: Short course FAC-M versus 1 year of CMFVP in node-positive hormone receptor–negative breast cancer: An intergroup study. *J Clin Oncol* 1995; 13:831–839.

310. Moliterni A, Bonadonna G, Valagussa P, Ferrari L, Zambetti M: Cyclophosphamide, methotrexate, and fluorouracil with and without doxorubicin in the adjuvant treatment of resectable breast cancer with one to three positive axillary nodes. *J Clin Oncol* 1991; 91:1124–1130.

311. Bonadonna G, Zambetti M, Valagussa P: Sequential or alternating doxorubicin and CMF regimens in breast cancer with more than three positive nodes. Ten-year results. *JAMA* 1995; 273:542–547.

312. Tormey DC, Gray R, Abeloff MD, Roseman DL, Gilchrist KW, Barylak EI, Stott P, Falkson G: Adjuvant therapy with a doxorubicin regimen and long-term tamoxifen in premenopausal breast cancer patients: An Eastern Cooperative Oncology Group trial. *J Clin Oncol* 1992; 10:1848–1856.

313. Gianni AM, Siena S, Bregni M, DiNicole M, Dodero A, Zambetti M, Orefice S, Salvadori B, Luini A, Greco M, Zucali R, Valagusse P, Bonadonna G: 5-Year results of high-dose sequential adjuvant chemotherapy in breast cancer with ≥ 10 positive nodes. *Proc Am Soc Clin Oncol* 1995; 14:90 (abstr).

314. Dimitrov N, Anderson S, Fisher B, Redmond C, Wickerham DL, Pugh R, Spurr C, Goodnight JJ, Abramson N, Walter J: Dose intensification and increased total dose of adjuvant chemotherapy for breast cancer: Findings from NSABP B-22. *Proc Am Soc Clin Oncol* 1994; 13:64 (abstr).

315. Wood WC, Budman DR, Korzun AH, Cooper MR, Younger J, Hart RD, Moore A, Ellerton JA, Norton L, Ferree CR, Ballow AC, Frei E, Henderson IC: Dose and dose intensity of adjuvant chemotherapy for stage II node positive breast carcinoma. *N Engl J Med* 1994; 330:1253–1259.

316. Marks LB, Rosner GL, Prosnitz LR, Ross M, Vredenburgh JJ, Peters WP: The impact of conventional plus high dose chemotherapy with autologous bone marrow transplantation on hematologic toxicity during subsequent local–regional radiotherapy for breast cancer. *Cancer* 1994; 74:2964–2971.

317. Peters WP, Ross M, Vredenburgh JJ, Meisenberg B, Jones R, Shpall E, Wu K, Rosner G, Gilbert C, Mathias B, Coniglio D, Petros W, Henderson IC, Norton L, Weiss RB, Budman D, Hurd D: High-dose chemotherapy and autologous bone marrow support as consolidation after standard-dose adjuvant therapy for high-risk primary breast cancer. *J Clin Oncol* 1993; 11:1132–1143.

318. Dombernowsky P, Hansen PS, Mouridsen HT, Overgaard M, Rose C, Zedeler K: Randomized trial of adjuvant CMF and radiotherapy vs. CMF alone vs. CMF and tamoxifen in pre- and menopausal stage II breast cancer. *Eur J Cancer* 1994; 30A:S28 (abstr).

319. Rubens RD, Knight RK, Fentiman IS, Howell A, Crowther D, George WD, Hayward JL, Bulbrook RD, Chaudary M, Bush H, Sellwood RA, Howat JMT: Controlled trial of adjuvant chemotherapy with melphalan for breast cancer. *Lancet* 1983; i:839–843.

320. Ingle JN, Everson LK, Wieand HS, Martin JK, Votava HJ, Wold LE, Krook JE, Cullinan SA, Paulsen JK, Twito DI, Ahmann DL, Foley JF, Green SJ: Randomized trial of observation versus adjuvant therapy with cyclophosphamide, fluorouracil, prednisone with or without tamoxifen following mastectomy in postmenopausal women with node-positive breast cancer. *J Clin Oncol* 1988; 6:1388–1396.

321. Boccardo F, Rubagotti A, Amoroso D, Sismondi P, Genta F, Nenci I, Piffanelli A, Farris A, Castagnetta L, Traina A, Cappellini M, Pacini P, Sassi M, Malacarne P, Donati D, Mustacchi G, Galletto L, Schleppati G, Villa E, Bolognesi A, Gallo L, and other participants in the GROCTA: Chemotherapy versus tamoxifen versus chemotherapy plus tamoxifen in node-positive, oestrogen–receptor positive breast cancer patients. An update at 7 years of the 1st GROCTA (Breast Cancer Adjuvant Chemo-hormone Therapy Cooperative Group) trial. *Eur J Cancer* 1992; 28:673–680.

322. Rutqvist LE, Cedermark B, Glas U, Johansson H, Rotstein S, Skoog L, Somell A, Theve T, Wilking N, Askergren J, Hjalmar M-L: Randomized trial of adjuvant tamoxifen combined with post-operative radiotherapy or adjuvant chemotherapy in postmenopausal breast cancer. *Cancer* 1990; 66:89–96.

323. Rivkin SE, Green S, Metch B, Cruz AB, Abeloff MD, Jewell WR, Costanzi JJ, Farrar WB, Minton JP, Osborne CK: Adjuvant CMFVP versus tamoxifen versus concurrent CMFVP and tamoxifen for postmenopausal, node positive, and estrogen receptor–positive breast cancer patients: A Southwest Oncology Group Study. *J Clin Oncol* 1994; 12:2078–2085.

324. Fisher B, Redmond C, Legault-Poisson S, Dimitrov NV, Brown AM, Wickerham DL, Wolmark N, Margolese RG, Bowman D, Glass AG, Kardinal CG, Robideux A, Jochimsen P, Cronin W, Deutsch M, Fisher ER, Myers DB, Hoehn JL: Post-operative chemotherapy and tamoxifen compared with tamoxifen alone in the treatment of positive-node breast cancer patients aged 50 years and older with tumors responsive to tamoxifen: Results from the National Surgical Breast and Bowel Project B16. *J Clin Oncol* 1990; 8:1005–1018.

325. Rose C, Anderson J, Axelsson M, Blichert-Toft M, Dombernowsky P, Hansen M, Krag C, Kristensen B, Mouridsen H, Overgaard M, Rasmussen B, Zedeler K: A randomized DBCG trial of adjuvant tamoxifen and radiotherapy vs. tam alone vs. tam and CMF in postmenopausal breast cancer patients with high risk of recurrence. *Proc Am Soc Clin Oncol* 1992; 11:58 (abstr).

326. Overgaard M, Christensen JJ, Johansen H, Nybo-Rasmussen A, Roe C, Van der Kooy P, Panduro J, Laursen F, Kjaer M, Srensen NE, Gadeberg CC, Hjelm-Hansen M, Overgaard J, Andersen KW, Zedeler K: Evaluation of radiotherapy in high-risk breast cancer patients: Report from the Danish Breast Cancer Cooperative Group (BBCG 82) trial. *Int J Radiat Oncol Biol Phys* 1990; 19:1121–1124.

327. Rutqvist LE, Cedermark B, Glas U, Johansson H, Rotstein S, Skoog L, Somell A, Theve T, Askergren J, Friberg S, Bergstrom J, Blomstedt B, Rat L, Silfversward C, Einhorn J: Radiotherapy, chemotherapy and tamoxifen as adjuncts to surgery in early breast cancer: A summary of three randomized trials. *Int J Radiat Oncol Biol Phys* 1989; 15:629–639.

328. Smith DC, Crawford D, Dykes EH, Calman KC, Russell AR, McArdle CS: Adjuvant radiotherapy and chemotherapy in breast cancer, in SE Jones, and SE Salmon (eds): *Adjuvant Therapy of Cancer IV.* Orlando, FL: Grune & Stratton, 1984, pp 283–289.

329. McArdle CS, Crawford D, Dykes EH, Colman KC, Hole D, Russell AR, Smith DC: Adjuvant radiotherapy and chemotherapy in breast cancer. *Br J Surg* 1986; 73:264–266.

330. Tennrall-Nittby L, Tengrup J, Landberg T: The total incidence of loco-regional recurrence in a randomized trial of breast cancer TNM stage II. The South Sweden Breast Cancer Trial. *Acta Oncol* 1993; 32:641–646.

331. Mouridsen HT, Rose C, Overgaard M, Dombernowsky P, Panduro J, Thorpe S, Rasmussen BB, Blichert-Toft M, Andersen VW: Adjuvant treatment of postmenopausal patients with high risk primary breast cancer. Results from the Danish adjuvant trials DBCG 77C and DBCG 82C. *Acta Oncol* 1988; 27: 699–705.

332. Overgaard M, Christensen JJ, Johansen H, Nybo-Rasmussen A, Brincker H, van der Kooy P, Frederiksen PL, Gadeberg CC, Hjelm-Hansen M, Overgaard J, Andersen KW, Zedelor K: Post-mastectomy irradiation in high risk breast cancer patients. Present status of the Danish Breast Cancer Cooperative Group trials. *Acta Oncol* 1988; 27:707–714.

333. Allen H, Brooks R, Jones SE, Chase E, Heusinkveld RS, Giordano GF, Ketchel SJ, Jackson RA, Davis S, Moorn TE, Salmon SE: Adjuvant treatment for stage II (node positive) breast cancer with Adriamycin–cyclophos-

phamide (AC) and radiotherapy (XRT), in SE Salmon, and SE Jones (eds): *Adjuvant Therapy for Cancer III.* New York, Grune & Stratton, 1981, pp 453–562.

334. Rose C, Hansen M, Dombernowsky P, Mouridsen H, Overgaard M, Rasmussen B, Zedeler K: A randomized DBCG trial of adjuvant tamoxifen and radiotherapy vs. tamoxifen alone vs. tamoxifen and CMF in postmenopausal breast cancer patients with high risk of recurrence. *Eur J Cancer* 1994; 30A:S28 (abstr).

335. Overgaard M, Hansen S, Rose C, Engelholm S, Bach F, Kjaer M, Gadeberg C, Overgaards J, West Andersen K, Zedeler J: Postmastectomy radiotherapy and adjuvant systemic treatment in high risk breast cancer patients. *Eur J Cancer* 1994; 30A:S28 (abstr).

336. Ragaz J, Jackson SM, Nhu L, Plenderleith IH, Spinelli JJ, Baso VE, Wilson KS, Knowling MA, Coppin CML, Paradis M, Coldman AJ, Olivotto IA: Adjuvant radiotherapy and chemotherapy in node-positive premenopausal women with breast cancer. *N Engl J Med* 1997; 337:956–962.

337. Overgaard M, Hansen PS, Overgaard J, Rose C, Andersson M, Bach F, Kjaer M, Gadeberg CC, Mouridsen HT, Jensen MB, Zedeler K: Postoperative radiotherapy in high-risk premenopausal women with breast cancer who receive adjuvant chemotherapy. *N Engl J Med* 1997; 337:949–955.

338. Velez-Garcia E, Carpenter JT Jr, Moore M, Vogel CL, Marcial V, Ketcham A, Singh KP, Bass D, Bartolucci AA, Smalley R: Postsurgical adjuvant chemotherapy with or without radiotherapy in women with breast cancer and positive axillary nodes: A Southeastern Cancer Study Group (SEG) trial. *Eur J Cancer Clin Oncol* 1992; 28A:1833–1837.

339. Bonadonna G, Valagussa P, Tancini G, Rossi A, Brambilla C, Zambetti M, Bignami P, DiFronzo G, Silvestrini R: Current status of Milan adjuvant chemotherapy trials for node-positive and node-negative breast cancer. *Natl Cancer Inst Monogr* 1986; 1:45–491.

340. Ragaz J, Jackson S, Wilson K, Plenderleith IH, Knowling M, Basco V, Ng V: Randomized study of locoregional radiotherapy (XRT) and ovarian ablation in premenopausal patients with breast cancer treated with adjuvant

chemotherapy. *Proc Am Soc Clin Oncol* 1988; 7:12 (abstr).

341. Ragaz J, Jackson S, Le N, Plenderleith IH, Spinelli J, Wilson K, Knowling M, Olivotto I, Coldman A: Can adjuvant locoregional therapy reduce systemic recurrences in stage I-II breast cancer patients? Recurrence analysis of the British Columbia randomized trial. *Proc Am Soc Clin Oncol* 1996; 15:121 (abstr).

342. Mignano JE, Gage I, Piantadosi S, Chakravarthy A, Dooley WM. Local recurrence after mastectomy in patients with T3 N0 breast carcinoma treated without postoperative irradiation. *Breast Cancer Res Treat* 1996; 41:255 (abstr).

343. Klefström P, Grohn P, Heinonen E, Holsti L, Holsti P: Adjuvant postoperative radiotherapy, chemotherapy and immunotherapy in stage III breast cancer. *Cancer* 1987; 60:936–942.

344. Freedman GM, Fowble BL, Hanlon AL, Fein DA, Hoffman JP, Sigurdson ER, Goldstein LJ: Postmastectomy radiation and adjuvant systemic therapy. Outcome in high risk women with stage II-III breast cancer and assessment of clinical pathologic and treatment related factors influencing local–regional control. *Breast J* 1997; 3:337–344.

345. Marks LB, Hebert ME, Bentel G, Spencer DP, Sherouse GW, Prosnitz LR: To treat or not to treat the internal mammary nodes: A possible compromise. *Int J Radiat Oncol Biol Phys* 1994; 29:903–909.

346. Singletary SE: Postmastectomy radiation. *Oncology* 1997; 11:243.

347. Turner-Warnick RT: Lymphatics of the breast. *Br J Surg* 1959; 46:524–529.

348. Livingston SF, Arlen M: The extended extrapleural radical mastectomy: Its role in the treatment of carcinoma of the breast. *Ann Surg* 1974; 179:260–265.

349. Caceres E: An evaluation of radical mastectomy and extended radical mastectomy for cancer of the breast. *Surg Gynecol Obstet* 1967:125:337–341.

350. Lacour J, Bucalossi P, Caceres E, Jacobelli G, Koszarowski T, Le M, Rumeau-Rouquette C, Veronesi U: Radical mastectomy vs. radical mastectomy plus internal mammary dissection: Five-year results of an international cooperative study. *Cancer* 1976; 37:206–214.

351. Veronesi U, Cascinelli N, Greco M, Bufalino R, Morabito A, Galluzzo D, Conti R, DeLellis R, DelleDonne V, Piotti P, et al: Prognosis of breast cancer patients after mastectomy and dissection of internal mammary nodes. *Ann Surg* 1985; 202:702–707.

352. Lichter A: Postmastectomy radiation. *Oncology* 1997; 11:239–240.

353. Arriagada A, Le MG, Mouriesse H, Fontaine F, Dewar J, Rochard F, Spielmann M, Lacour J, Tubiana M, Sarrazin D: Long-term effect of internal mammary chain treatment: Results of a multivariate analysis of 1195 patients with operable breast cancer and positive axillary nodes. *Radiother Oncol* 1988; 11:213–222.

354. Forrest AP, Stewart HJ, Everington D, Prescott RJ, McArdle CS, Harnett AN, Smith DC, George WD, on behalf of Scottish Cancer Trials Breast Group: Randomized controlled trial of conservation therapy for breast cancer: 6 year analysis of the Scottish trial. *Lancet* 1996; 348:708–713.

355. Fisher B, Dignam J, Mamounas EP, Costantino JP, Wickerham DL, Redmond C, Wolmark N, Dimitrov NV, Bowman DM, Glass AG, Atkins JN, Abramson N, Sutherland CM, Aron BS, Margolese RG: Sequential methotrexate and fluorouracil for the treatment of node-negative breast cancer patients with estrogen receptor–negative tumors: Eight year results from National Surgical Adjuvant Breast and Bowel Project (NSABP) B-13 and first report of findings from NSABP B-19 comparing methotrexate and fluorouracil with conventional cyclophosphamide methotrexate and fluorouracil. *J Clin Oncol* 1996; 14:1982–1992.

356. Haffty BG, Wilmarth L, Wilson L, Fischer D, Beinfield M, McKhann C: Adjuvant systemic chemotherapy and hormonal therapy. Effect on local recurrence in the conservatively treated breast cancer patient. *Cancer* 1994; 73:2543–2548.

357. Botnick L, Come S, Rose C, Goldstein M, Lange R, Tishler S, Schnippler L: Primary breast irradiation and concomitant adjuvant chemotherapy, in J Harris, S Hellman, and W Silen (eds): *Conservative Management of Breast Cancer.* Philadelphia, Lippincott, 1983, pp 321–328.

358. Buchholz TA, Austin-Seymour MM, Moe RE, Ellis GK, Livingston RB, Pelton JG, Griffin TW: Effect of delay in radiation in the combined modality treatment of breast cancer. *Int J Radiat Oncol Biol Phys* 1993; 26:23–35.

359. Buzdar AU, Kau SW, Smith TL, Ames F, Singletary E, Strom E, McNeese M, Hortobagyi GN: The order of administration of chemotherapy and radiation and its effect on the local control of operable breast cancer. *Cancer* 1993; 71:3680–3684.

360. Klefstrom P, Nuortio L, Taskinen E: Postoperative radiation therapy and adjuvant chemoimmunotherapy in breast cancer. Aspects of timing and immune competence. *Acta Radiol* 1986; 25:161–166.

361. Brufman G, Sulkes ASB: Effect of timing of onset of chemotherapy on relapse-free survival in stage II breast cancer. *Proc Am Soc Clin Oncol* 1986; 5:62 (abstr).

362. Lara Jimenez P, Garcia Puche J, Pedraza V: Adjuvant combined modality treatment in high risk breast cancer patients: Ten year results. Presentation at the Fifth EORTC Breast Cancer Working Conference, Leuven, Belgium, 1991 (abstr), A293.

363. Hartsell WF, Recine DC, Griem KL, Murthy AK: Delaying the initiation of intact breast irradiation for patients with lymph node positive breast cancer increases the risk of local recurrence. *Cancer* 1995; 76:2497–2503.

364. McCormick B, Norton L, Yao TJ, Yahalom J, Petrek JA: The impact of the sequence of radiation and chemotherapy on local control after breast-conserving surgery. *Cancer J Sci Am* 1996; 2:39–457.

365. Recht A, Come SE, Gelman RS, Goldstein M, Tishler S, Gore SM, Abner AL, Vicini FA, Silver B, Connolly JL, Schnitt SJ, Coleman CN, Harris JR: Integration of conservative surgery, radiotherapy, and chemotherapy for the treatment of early-stage node-positive breast cancer: Sequencing timing and outcome. *J Clin Oncol* 1991; 9:1662–1667.

366. Recht A, Coleman C, Harris J, Come SE, Gelman RS: Timing of radiotherapy in the treatment of early-stage breast cancer (letter). *J Clin Oncol* 1993; 11:191–192.

367. Recht A, Come SE, Henderson IC, Gelman RS, Silver B, Hayes DF, Shulman LN, Harris JM: The sequencing of chemotherapy and radiation therapy after conservative surgery for

early-stage breast cancer. *N Engl J Med* 1996; 334:1356–1361.

368. Dubey AK, Recht A, Shulman L, Come S, Gelman R, Silver B, Harris JR: Outcome following concurrent chemotherapy (CT) and reduced-dose radiation therapy for patients with early stage breast cancer. *Int J Radiat Oncol Biol Phys* 1997; 39:267 (abstr).

369. Osborne CK, Boldt DH, Clark GM, Trent JM: Effects of tamoxifen on human breast cancer cell cycle kinetics: Accumulation of cells in early G1 phase. *Cancer Res* 1983; 43: 3583–3585.

370. Sinclair WK: Cyclic x-ray responses in the mammalian cells in vitro. *Radiat Res* 1968; 33:620–643.

371. Fisher B, Anderson S: Conservative surgery for the management of invasive and noninvasive carcinoma of the breast: NSABP trials. *World J Surg* 1994; 18:63–69.

372. Leonard CE, Wood ME, Zhen B, Rankin J, Waitz DA, Norton L, Howell K, Sedlacek S: Does administration of chemotherapy before radiotherapy in breast cancer patients treated with conservative surgery negatively impact local control? *J Clin Oncol* 1995; 13:2906–2915.

373. Wazer DE, Morr J, Erban JK, Schmid CH, Ruthazer R, Schmidt-Ullrich RK: The effects of postradiation treatment with tamoxifen on local control and cosmetic outcome in the conservatively treated breast. *Cancer* 1997; 80:732–740.

374. Rutqvist LE, Cedermark B, Glas U, Johansson H, Rotstein S, Skoog L, Somell A, Theve T, Wilking N, Askergren J, Hjalmar M-L, Ringborg U: Randomized trial of adjuvant tamoxifen in node negative postmenopausal breast cancer. *Acta Oncol* 1992; 31:265–270.

375. Fowble B, Fein DA, Hanlon AL, Eisenberg BL, Hoffman JP, Sigurdson ER, Daly MB, Goldstein LJ: The impact of tamoxifen on breast recurrence, cosmesis, complications, and survival in estrogen receptor positive early stage breast cancer. *Int J Radiat Oncol Biol Phys* 1996; 35:669–677.

376. National Comprehensive Cancer Network: Update of the NCCN guidelines for treatment of breast cancer. *Oncology* 1997; 11:199–220.

377. Bonadonna G, Valagussa P, Brambilla C, Ferrari L, Moliterni A, Terenziani M, Zambetti M: Primary chemotherapy in operable breast cancer: Eight-year experience at the Milan Cancer Institute. *J Clin Oncol* 1998; 16:93–100.

378. Fisher B, Brown A, Mamounas E, Wieand S, Robidoux A, Margolese RG, Cruz AB Jr, Fisher ER, Wickerham DL, Wolmark, N, DeCillis A, Hoehn JL, Lees AW, Dimitrov NV: Effect of preoperative chemotherapy on local–reginal disease in women with operable breast cancer: Findings from National Surgical Adjuvant Breast and Bowel Project B-18. *J Clin Oncol* 1997; 15:2483–2493.

379. Jacquillat C, Weil M, Baillet F, Borel C, Auclerc G, de Maublanc MA, Housset M, Forget G, Thill L, Soubrane C, Khayat D: Results of neoadjuvant chemotherapy and radiation therapy in the breast-conserving treatment of 250 patients with all stages of infiltrative breast cancer. *Cancer* 1990; 66:119–129.

380. Scholl SM, Fourquet A, Asselain B, Pierga JY, Vilcoq JR, Durand JC, Dorval T, Palangié T, Jouve M, Beuzeboc P, Gracio-Giralt E, Salmon RJ, de la Rochefordière A, Campana F, Pouillart P: Neoadjuvant versus adjuvant chemotherapy in premenopausal patients with tumours considered too large for breast conserving surgery: Preliminary results of a randomised trial: S6. *Eur J Cancer* 1994; 30A:645–652.

381. Mauriac L, Durand M, Avril A, Dilhuydy J: Efffects of primary chemotherapy in conservative treatment of breast cancer patients with operable tumors larger than 3 cm. *Ann Oncol* 1991; 2:347–354.

382. Powles TJ, Hickish TF, Makris A, Ashley SE, O'Brien MER, Tidy VA, Casey S, Nash AG, Sacks N, Cosgrove D, MacVicar D, Fernando I, Ford HT: Randomized trial of chemoendocrine therapy started before or after surgery for treatment of primary breast cancer. *J Clin Oncol* 1995; 13:547–552.

383. Legler CM, Shapiro CL, Harris JR, Hayes DF: Primary chemotherapy of resectable breast cancer. *Breast J* 1995; 1:42–51.

384. Calais G, Berger C, Descamps P, Chapet S, Reynaud-Bougnoux A, Body G, Bougnoux P, Lansac J, LeFloch O: Conservative treatment feasibility with induction chemotherapy, surgery, and radiotherapy for patients with breast carcinoma larger than 3 cm. *Cancer* 1994; 74:1283–1288.

385. Rilke F, Veronesi U, Luini A, Brambilla C, Galimberti V, Zurrida S, Pilotti S, Di Palma S, Zucali R, Lozza L: Preoperative chemotherapy alone and combined with preoperative radiotherapy in small-size breast cancer. *Breast J* 1996; 2:176–180.

386. Fisher B, Brown A, Mamounas E, Wieand S, Fisher E, Robidoux A, Margolese R, Cruz A, Wickerham DL, Wolmark N: Effect of preoperative therapy for primary breast cancer (BC) on local–regional disease, disease-free survival (DFS) and survival (S); results from NSABP B-18. *Proc Am Soc Clin Oncol* 1997; 16:127a (abstr).

387. Avril A, Faucher A, Bussières E, Stöckle E, Durand M, Mauriac L, Dilhuydy JM, Bonichon F, Campo ML: Operable breast cancer greater than 3 cm: Results of a randomized study comparing immediate mastectomy versus neoadjuvant chemotherapy and attempt at conservative treatment. *Lyon Chir* 1993; 89: 191–197.

388. Scholl SM, Asselain B, Beuzeboc P, Pierga JY, Dorval T, Garcia-Giralt E, Jouve M, Palangié T, Fourquet A, Durand JC, Pouillart P: Neoadjuvant versus adjuvant chemotherapy in premenopausal patients with tumours considered too large for breast conserving surgery. An update. *Proc Am Soc Clin Oncol* 1995; 14:125.

389. Makris A, Powles TJ, Ashley SE, Dowsett M, Allred DC, Trott PA, Osborne CK, Chang J, Gregory K, Nash AG, Querci della Rovere U: A randomized trial of neoadjuvant chemoendocrine therapy in operable breast cancer. *Proc Am Soc Clin Oncol* 1996; 15:A51 (abstr).

390. Sholl SM, Asselain B, Palangie T, Dorval T, Jouve M, Garcia Giralt E, Vilcoq J, Durand JC, Pouillart P: Neoadjuvant chemotherapy in operable breast cancer. *Eur J Cancer* 1991; 27:1668–1671.

391. Veronesi U, Bonadonna G, Zurrida S, Galimberti V, Greco M, Brambilla C, Luini A, Andreola S, Rilke F, Raselli R, Merson M, Sacchini V, Agresti R: Conservation surgery after primary chemotherapy in large carcinomas of the breast. *Ann Surg* 1995; 222:612–618.

392. Ellis P, Smith I, Ashley S, Walsh G, Ebbs S, Baum M, Sacks N, McKinna J: Clinical prognostic and predictive factors for primary chemotherapy in operable breast cancer. *J Clin Oncol* 1998; 16:107–114.

393. Buzdar AU, Kau SW, Smith TL, Hortobagyi GN: Ten-year results of FAC adjuvant chemotherapy trial in breast cancer. *Am J Clin Oncol* 1989; 12:123–128.

394. Spangenberg JP, Nel CJC, Anderson ID, Doman MJ: A prospective study of the treatment of stage III breast cancer. *S Afr J Surg* 1986; 24:57–60.

395. Olson JE, Neuberg D, Pandya KJ, Richter MP, Solin LJ, Gilchrist KW, Tormey DC, Veeder M, Faulkson G: The role of radiotherapy in the management of operable locally advanced breast cancer. *Cancer* 1997; 79:1138–1149.

396. Uematsu M, Bornstein BA, Recht A, Abner A, Come SE, Shulman LN, Silver B, Harris JR: Long-term results of post-operative radiation therapy following mastectomy with or without chemotherapy in stage I-III breast cancer. *Int J Radiat Oncol Biol Phys* 1993; 25:765–770.

397. Fowble B, Glick J, Goodman R: Radiotherapy for the prevention of local–regional recurrence in high risk patients post mastectomy receiving adjuvant chemotherapy. *Int J Radiat Oncol Biol Phys* 1988; 15:627–631.

398. Gröhn P, Heinonen E, Klefström P, Tarkkanen J: Adjuvant postoperative radiotherapy, chemotherapy, and immunotherapy in stage III breast cancer. *Cancer* 1984; 54:670–674.

399. Sheldon T, Hayes DF, Cady B, Parker L, Osteen R, Silver B, Recht A, Come S, Henderson IC, Harris JR: Primary radiation therapy for locally advanced breast cancer. *Cancer* 1987; 60:1219–1225.

400. Amalric R, Santamaria F, Robert F, Siegle J, Altschuler C, Kurtz JM, Spitalier JM, Brandone H, Ayme Y, Pollet JF, Burmeister R, Abed R: Radiation therapy with or without primary limited surgery for operable breast cancer: A 20-year experience at the Marseilles Cancer Institute. *Cancer* 1982; 49:30–34.

401. Van Limbergen E, Van der Schueren E, Van den Bogaert W, Van Wing J: Local control of operable breast cancer after radiotherapy alone. *Eur J Cancer* 1990; 26:674–679.

402. Toonkel LM, Fix I, Jacobson LH, Bamberg N, Wallach CB: Locally advanced breast carcinoma: Results with combined regional therapy. *Int J Radiat Oncol Biol Phys* 1986; 12: 1583–1587.

403. Spanos WJ, Montague ED, Fletcher GH: Late complications of radiation only for advanced

breast cancer. *Int J Radiat Oncol Biol Phys* 1980; 6:1473–1476.

404. Khanna MM, Mark RJ, Silverstein MJ, Juillard G, Lewinsky B, Giuliano AE: Breast conservation management of breast tumors 4 cm or larger. *Arch Surg* 1992; 127:1038–1041.

405. Danforth DN Jr, Zujewski J, O'Shaughnessy J, Riseberg D, Steinberg SM, McAtee N, Noone M, Chow C, Chaudhry U, Lippman M, Jacobson J, Okunieff P, Cowan KH: Selection of local therapy after neoadjuvant chemotherapy in patients with stage IIIA,B breast cancer. *Ann Surg Oncol* 1998; 5:150–158.

406. Merajver SD, Weber BL, Cody R, Zhang D, Strawderman M, Calzone KA, LeClaire V, Levin A, Irani J, Halvie M, August D, Wicha M, Lichter A, Pierce LJ: Breast conservation and prolonged chemotherapy for locally advanced breast cancer: The University of Michigan experience. *J Clin Oncol* 1997; 15:2873–2881.

407. Buzdar AU, Singletary SE, Booser DJ, Frye DK, Wasaff B, Hortobagyi GN: Combined modality treatment of stage III and inflammatory breast cancer. *Surg Oncol Clin North Am* 1995; 4:715–734.

408. Schwartz GF: Breast conservation following induction chemotherapy for locally advanced breast cancer: A personal experience. *Breast J* 1996; 2:78–82.

409. Perez CA, Graham ML, Taylor ME, Levy JF, Mortimer JE, Philpott GW, Kucik NA: Management of locally advanced carcinoma of the breast. I. Noninflammatory. *Cancer* 1994; 74: 453–465.

410. Touboul E, Buffat L, Lefranc J, Blondon J, Deniaud E, Mammar H, Laugier A, Schlienger M: Possibility of conservative local treatment after combined chemotherapy and preoperative irradiation for locally advanced noninflammatory breast cancer. *Int J Radiat Oncol Biol Phys* 1996; 34:1019–1028.

411. Valagussa P, Zambetti M, Bonadonna G, Zucali R, Mezzanotte G, Veronesi U: Prognostic factors in locally advanced noninflammatory breast cancer. Long-term results following primary chemotherapy. *Breast Cancer Res Treat* 1990; 15:137–147.

412. Hortobagyi GN, Ames FC, Buzdar AU, Kau SW, McNeese MD, Paulus D, Hug V, Holmes FA, Romsdahl MM, Fraschini G, McBride CM, Martin RG, Montague E: Management of stage III primary breast cancer with primary chemotherapy, surgery, and radiation therapy. *Cancer* 1988; 62:2507–2516.

413. Perloff M, Lesnick GJ, Korzun A, Chu F, Holland JF, Thirlwell MP, Ellison RR, Carey RW, Leone L, Weinberg V, Rice MA, Wood WC: Combination chemotherapy with mastectomy or radiotherapy for stage III breast carcinoma: A Cancer and Leukemia Group B study. *J Clin Oncol* 1988; 6:261–269.

414. Sauter ER, Eisenberg BL, Hoffman JP, Ottery FD, Boraas MC, Goldstein LJ, Solin LJ: Postmastectomy morbidity after combination preoperative irradiation and chemotherapy for locally advanced breast cancer. *World J Surg* 1993; 17:237–242.

415. Piccard MJ, de Valeriola D, Paridaens R, Balikdjian D, Mattheiem WH, Loriaux C, Arrigo C, Cantraine F, Heuson J: Six-year results of a multimodality treatment strategy for locally advanced breast cancer. *Cancer* 1988; 62: 2501–2506.

416. Schaake-Koning C, van der Linden EH, Hart G, Engelsman E: Adjuvant chemo- and hormonal therapy in locally advanced breast cancer: A randomized clinical study. *Int J Radiat Oncol Biol Phys* 1985; 11:1759–1763.

417. Rubens RD, Sexton S, Tong D, Winter PJ, Knight RK, Hayward JL: Combined chemotherapy and radiotherapy for locally advanced breast cancer. *Eur J Cancer* 1980; 16: 351–356.

418. Lucas FV, Perez-Mesa C: Inflammatory carcinoma of the breast. *Cancer* 1978; 41: 1595–1605.

419. Perez CA, Fields JN, Fracasso PM, Philpott G, Soares RL Jr, Taylor ME, Lockett MA, Rush C: Management of locally advanced carcinoma of the breast. II. Inflammatory carcinoma. *Cancer* 1994; 74:466–476.

420. Fowble B, Glover D: Locally advanced breast cancer, in B Fowble, RL Goodman, JH Glick, and EF Rosato (eds): *Breast Cancer Treatment. A Comprehensive Guide to Management.* St. Louis, Mosby-Year Book, 1991, pp 345–372.

421. Pierce LJ, Lippman M, Ben-Baruch N, Swain S, O'Shaughnessy J, Bader JL, Danforth D, Venzon D, Cowan KH: The effect of systemic therapy on local–regional control in locally

advanced breast cancer. *Int J Radiat Oncol Biol Phys* 1992; 23:949–960.

422. Fleming RYD, Asmar L, Buzdar AU, McNeese MD, Ames FC, Ross MI, Singletary SE: Effectiveness of mastectomy by response to induction chemotherapy for control in inflammatory breast carcinoma. *Ann Surg Oncol* 1997; 4:452–461.

423. Palangie T, Mosseri V, Mihura J, Campana F, Beuzeboc P, Dorval T, Garcia-Giralt E, Jouve M, Scholl S, Asselain B, Pouillart P: Prognostic factors in inflammatory breast cancer and therapeutic implications. *Eur J Cancer* 1994; 30A:921–927.

424. Ayash LJ, Elias A, Ibrahim J, Schwartz G, Wheeler C, Reich E, Lynch C, Warren D, Shapiro C, Richardson P, Hurd D, Schnipper L, Frei E III, Antman K: High-dose multimodality therapy with autologous stem-cell support for stage IIIB breast carcinoma. *J Clin Oncol* 1998; 16:1000–1007.

425. Rouëssé J, Friedman S, Sarrazin D, Moureisse H, Le Chevalier T, Arriagada R, Spielmann M, Papacharalambous A, May-Levin F: Primary chemotherapy in the treatment of inflammatory breast carcinoma: A study of 230 cases from the Institut Gustave-Roussy. *J Clin Oncol* 1986; 4:1765–1771.

426. Neidhart JA, Morris DM, Herman TS: Dose-intensification chemotherapy for patients with advanced breast cancer. *Semin Radiat Oncol* 1994; 4:236–241.

427. Brun B, Otmezguine Y, Feuilhade F, Julien M, Lebourgeois JP, Calitchi E, Roucayrol AM, Ganem G, Huart J, Pierquin B: Treatment of inflammatory breast cancer with combination chemotherapy and mastectomy versus breast conservation. *Cancer* 1988; 61:1096–1103.

428. Thoms WW Jr, McNeese MD, Fletcher GH, Buzdar AU, Singletary SE, Oswald MJ: Multimodal treatment for inflammatory breast cancer. *Int J Radiat Oncol Biol Phys* 1989; 17:739–745.

429. Das IJ, Cheng EC, Freedman G, Fowble B: Lung and heart dose volume analyses with CT simulator in tangential field irradiation of breast cancer. *Int J Radiat Oncol Biol Phys* 1998; 42:11–19.

430. Das IJ, Cheng C, Fein DA, Fowble B: Patterns of dose variability in radiation prescription of breast cancer. *Radiother Oncol* 1997; 44:83–89.

431. ICRU Report 50, in *Prescribing, Recording, and Reporting Photon Beam Therapy.* International Commission on Radiation Units and Measurements, 1993.

432. Solin LJ, Chu JCH, Sontag MR, Brewster L, Cheng E, Doppke K, Drzymala RE, Hunt M, Kuske R, Manolis JM, McCormick B, Munzenrider JE: Three-dimensional photon treatment planning of the intact breast. *Int J Radiat Oncol Biol Phys* 1991; 21:193–203.

433. Kutcher GJ, Smith AR, Fowble BL, Owen JB, Hanlon A, Wallace M, Hanks GE: Treatment planning for primary breast cancer: A Patterns of Care study. *Int J Radiat Oncol Biol Phys* 1996; 36:731–737.

434. Bentel GC, Marks LB, Whiddon CS: Acute and late morbidity of radiation therapy in women with large pendulous breasts treated with a breast positioning ring. *Int J Radiat Oncol Biol Phys* 1997; 39:267.

435. Solin LJ, Chu, JCH, Larsen R, Fowble B, Galvin JM, Goodman RL: Determination of depth for electron breast boosts. *Int J Radiat Oncol Biol Phys* 1987; 13:1915–1919.

436. McGarvey E: Breast cancer, in L Coia, T Schultheiss, and G Hanks (eds): *A Practical Guide to CT Simulation.* Madison, WI: Advanced Medical Publishing, 1995, pp 187–195.

437. Das IJ, Cheng EC, Wurzer JC, Freedman G, Fowble B: Impact of CT simulation for cone down electron treatment of breast cancer. Personal communication, 1998.

438. Chu JCH, Solin LJ, Hwang CC, Fowble B, Hanks GE, Goodman RL: A nondivergent three field matching technique for breast irradiation. *Int J Radiat Oncol Biol Phys* 1990; 19:1037–1040.

439. Hanks GE, Peters T, Owen J: Seminoma of the testis: Long-term beneficial and deleterious results of radiation. *Int J Radiat Oncol Biol Phys* 1992; 24:913–919.

440. Pierce LJ, Lichter AS, Archer P: Indications, integration, and technical aspects of local–regional irradiation in the management of advanced breast cancer. *Semin Radiat Oncol* 1994; 4:242–253.

441. Veronesi U, Luini A, Galimberti V, Zurrida S: Conservation approaches for the management of stage I/II carcinoma of the breast: Milan

Cancer Institute Trials. *World J Surg* 1994; 18:70–75.

442. Dershaw DD, McCormick B, Osborne MP: Detection of local recurrence after conservative therapy for breast cancer. *Cancer* 1992; 70:493–496.

443. Hassell PR, Olivotto IA, Mueller HA, Kingston GW, Basco VE: Early breast cancer: Detection of recurrence after conservative surgery and radiation therapy. *Radiology* 1990; 176:731–735.

444. Stomper PC, Recht A, Berenberg AL, Jochelson MS, Harris JR: Mammographic detection of recurrent cancer in the irradiated breast. *Am J Radiol* 1987; 148:39–43.

445. Solin LJ, Fowble BF, Schultz DJ, Rubenstein JR, Goodman RL: The detection of local recurrence after definitive irradiation for early stage carcinoma of the breast: An analysis of the results of breast biopsies in the post-irradiated breast. *Cancer* 1990; 65:2497–2502.

446. Haffty BG, Goldberg NB, Fischer D, McKhann C, Bienfield M, Weissberg JB, Carter D, Gerald W: Conservative surgery and radiation therapy in breast carcinoma: Local recurrence and prognostic implications. *Int J Radiat Oncol Biol Phys* 1989; 17:727–732.

447. Haffty BG, Fischer D, Beinfield M, McKhann C: Prognosis following local recurrence in the conservatively treated breast cancer patient. *Int J Radiat Oncol Biol Phys* 1991; 21: 293–298.

448. Fowble B, Solin LJ, Schultz DJ, Rubenstein J, Goodman RL: Breast recurrence following conservative surgery and radiation: Patterns of failure prognosis and pathologic findings from mastectomy specimens with implications for treatment. *Int J Radiat Oncol Biol Phys* 1990; 19:833–842.

449. DiPaola RS, Orel SG, Fowble BL: Ipsilateral breast tumor recurrence following conservative surgery and definitive radiation therapy. *Oncology* 1994; 8:59–75.

450. Recht A, Silver B, Schnitt S, Connolly J, Hellman S, Harris JR: Breast relapse following radiation therapy for early breast cancer. I. Classification frequency and salvage. *Int J Radiat Oncol Biol Phys* 1985; 11:1271–1276.

451. Recht A, Silen W, Schnitt SJ, Connolly JL, Gelman RS, Rose MA, Silver B, Harris JR: Time course of local recurrence following conservative surgery and radiotherapy for early stage breast cancer. *Int J Radiat Oncol Biol Phys* 1988; 15:255–261.

452. Recht A, Schnitt SJ, Connolly JL, Rose MA, Silver B, Come S, Henderson IC, Slavin S, Harris JR: Prognosis following local or regional recurrence after conservative surgery and radiotherapy for early stage breast carcinoma. *Int J Radiat Oncol Biol Phys* 1989; 16:3–9.

453. Gage I, Recht A, Nixon AJ, Gelman R, Silver B, Bornstein BA: Long-term outcome following breast-conserving therapy in early-stage disease. *Int J Radiat Oncol Biol Phys* 1995; 33:245–251.

454. Veronesi U, Salvador B, Luini A, Banfi A, Zucali R, DelVecchio M, Saccozzi R, Beretta E, Boracchi P, Farrante G, Galimberti V, Mezzanotte G, Sacchini V, Tane S, Marwopini E: Conservative treatment of early breast cancer. Long-term results of 1232 cases treated with quadrantectomy, axillary dissection and radiotherapy. *Ann Surg* 1990; 211:250–259.

455. Fisher B, Anderson S, Fisher ER, Redmond C, Wickerham DL, Wolmark N, Mamounas EP, Deutsch M, Margolese R: Significance of ipsilateral breast tumor recurrence after lumpectomy. *Lancet* 1991; 338:327–331.

456. Kurtz JM, Amalric R, Brandone H, Ayme Y, Jacquemier J, Pietra JC, Hans D, Pollet JF, Bressac C, Spitalier JM: Local recurrence after breast-conserving surgery and radiotherapy. Frequency, time course, and prognosis. *Cancer* 1989; 63:1912–1917.

457. Kurtz JM, Spitalier JM, Amalric R, Brandone H, Ayme Y, Jacquemier J, Hans D, Bressac C: The prognostic significance of late local recurrence after breast-conserving therapy. *Int J Radiat Oncol Biol Phys* 1990; 18:87–93.

458. Clark RM, Wilkinson RH, Miceli PN, MacDonald WD: Breast cancer: Experiences with conservation therapy. *Am J Clin Oncol* 1987; 10:461–468.

459. Stotter A, Atkinson EN, Fairston BA, McNeese M, Oswald MJ, Balch CM: Survival following local–regional recurrence after breast conservation therapy for cancer. *Ann Surg* 1990; 212:166–172.

460. Haffty BG, Reiss M, Beinfield M, Fischer D, Ward B, McKhann C: Ipsilateral breast tumor

recurrence as a predictor of distant disease: Implications for systemic therapy at the time of relapse. *J Clin Oncol* 1996; 14:52–57.

461. Abner AL, Recht A, Eberlein T, Come S, Schulman L, Hayes D, Connolly JL, Schnitt SJ, Silver B, Harris JR: Prognosis following salvage mastectomy for recurrence in the breast after conservative surgery and radiation therapy for early-stage breast cancer. *J Clin Oncol* 1993; 11:44–48.

462. Grosse A, Schreer I, Frischbier H-J, Maass H, Loening T, Bahnsen J: Results of breast conserving therapy for early breast cancer and the role of mammographic follow-up. *Int J Radiat Oncol Biol Phys* 1997; 38:761–767.

463. Calle R, Vilcoq JR, Zafrani B, Vielh P, Fourquet A: Local control and survival of breast cancer treated by limited surgery followed by irradiation. *Int J Radiat Oncol Biol Phys* 1986; 12:873–878.

464. Clark RM, Wilkinson RH, Mahoney LJ, Reid JG, MacDonald WD: Breast cancer: A 21 year experience with conservative surgery and radiation. *Int J Radiat Oncol Biol Phys* 1982; 8:967–975.

465. Chauvet B, Reynaud-Bougnoux A, Calais G, Panel N, Lansac J, Bougnoux P, Le Floch O: Prognostic significance of breast relapse after conservative treatment in node-negative early breast cancer. *Int J Radiat Oncol Biol Phys* 1990; 19:1125–1130.

466. Kurtz JM, Amalric R, Brandone H, Ayme Y, Spitalier JM: Results of wide excision for mammary recurrence after breast-conserving therapy. *Cancer* 1989; 61:1969–1972.

467. Fisher B, Fisher ER, Redmond C: Ten-year results from the NSABP clinical trial evaluating the use of L-phenylalanine mustard (L-PAM) in the management of primary breast cancer. *J Clin Oncol* 1986; 4:929–935.

468. Chen KKY, Montague ED, Oswald MJ: Results of irradiation in treatment of locoregional breast cancer recurrence. *Cancer* 1985; 56:1269–1273.

469. Chu FCH, Lin FJ, Kim JH, Huh SH, Garmatis CJ: Locally recurrent carcinoma of the breast: Results of radiation therapy. *Cancer* 1976; 37:2677–2681.

470. Bedwinek JM, Fineberg B, Lee J, Ocwieza M: Analysis of failures following local treatment of isolated local regional recurrence of breast cancer. *Int J Radiat Oncol Biol Phys* 1981; 7:581–585.

471. Toonkel LM, Fix I, Jacobson LH, Wallach CB: The significance of local recurrence of carcinoma of the breast. *Int J Radiat Oncol Biol Phys* 1983; 9:33–39.

472. Andry G, Suciu S, Vico P, Faverly D, t'Hooft A, Verhesst A, Nogaret JM, Mattheie MW: Locoregional recurrences after 649 modified radical mastectomies: Incidence and significance. *Eur J Surg Oncol* 1989; 15:476–485.

473. Deutsch M, Parsons JA, Mittal BB: Radiation therapy for local regional recurrent breast carcinoma. *Int J Radiat Oncol Biol Phys* 1986; 12:2061–2065.

474. Gilliand MD, Barton RM, Copeland EM: The implications of local recurrence of breast cancer as the first site of therapeutic failure. *Ann Surg* 1983; 197:284–287.

475. Fentiman IS, Mathews PN, Davison OW, Millis RR, Hayward JL: Survival following local skin recurrence after mastectomy. *Br J Surg* 1985; 72:14–16.

476. Beck TM, Hart NE, Woodward DA, Smith CE: Local or regionally recurrent carcinoma of the breast: Results of therapy in 121 patients. *J Clin Oncol* 1983; 1:400–405.

477. Stadler B, Kogelnik D: Local control and outcome of patients irradiated for isolated chest wall recurrences of breast cancer. *Radiother Oncol* 1987; 8:105–110.

478. Tough ICK: The significance of recurrence in breast cancer. *Br J Surg* 1966; 53:897–901.

479. Shah JP, Urban JA: Full thickness chest wall resection for recurrent breast cancer involving the bony chest wall. *Cancer* 1975; 35:567–573.

480. McKenna RJ Jr, Mountain CF, McMurtrey MJ, Larson D, Stiles QR: Current techniques for chest wall reconstruction: Expanded possibilities for treatment. *Ann Thorac Surg* 1988; 46:508–512.

481. Faneyte IF, Rutgers EJTH, Zoetmulder FAN: Chest wall resection in the treatment of locally recurrent breast carcinoma—Indications and outcome for 44 patients. *Cancer* 1997; 80:896–891.

482. Magno L, Bignardi M, Micheletti E, Bardelli D, Plebani F: Analysis of prognostic factors in

patients with isolated chest wall recurrence of breast cancer. *Cancer* 1987; 60:240–244.

483. Willner J, Kiricuta C, Kölbl O: Local–regional recurrence of breast cancer following mastectomy: Always a fatal event? Results of univariate and multivariate analysis. *Int J Radiat Oncol Biol Phys* 1997; 37:853–863.

484. Patanaphan V, Salazar OM, Poussin-Rosillo H: Prognosticators in recurrent breast cancer: A 15 year experience with irradiation. *Cancer* 1984; 54:228–234.

485. Fletcher GH: Local results of irradiation in the primary management of localized breast cancer. *Cancer* 1972; 29:545–551.

486. Fletcher GH, Montague ED: Radical irradiation of advanced breast cancer. *Am J Radiol* 1965; 93:573–578.

487. Janjan NA, McNeese MD, Buzdar AU, Montague ED, Osward MJ: Management of locoregional recurrence of breast cancer. *Cancer* 1986; 58:1552–1556.

488. Rosenman J, Churchill CA, Mauro MA, Parker LA, Newsome J: The role of computed tomography in the evaluation of postmastectomy locally recurrent breast cancer. *Int J Radiat Oncol Biol Phys* 1988; 14:57–62.

489. Villari R, Fargnoli R, Mungai R: CT evaluation of chest wall recurrences of breast cancer. *Eur J Radiol* 1985; 5:206–208.

490. Lindfors KK, Meyer JE, Busse PM, Kopans DB, Munzenrider JE, Sawicka JM: CT evaluation of local and regional breast cancer recurrence. *Am J Radiol* 1985; 145:833–837.

491. Meyer JE, Munzenrider JE: Computed tomographic demonstration of internal mammary lymph node metastasis in patients with locally recurrent breast carcinoma. *Radiology* 1981; 139:661–663.

492. Olson CE, Ansfield FJ, Richards MJ, Ramirez G, Davis HL: Review of soft tissue recurrence of breast cancer irradiated with and without actinomycin D. *Cancer* 1977; 39:1981–1986.

493. Janjan NA, McNeese MD, Buzdar AU, Montague ED: Locoregional recurrent breast cancer treated with radiation or a combination of radiation and chemotherapy. *Int J Radiat Oncol Biol Phys* 1985; 11:152 (abstr).

494. Halverson KJ, Perez CA, Kuske RR, Garcia DM, Simpson JR, Fineberg R: Locoregional recurrence of breast cancer: A retrospective comparison of irradiation alone versus irradiation and systemic therapy. *Am J Clin Oncol* 1992; 12:177–185.

495. Borner M, Bacchi M, Goldhirsch A, Greiner R, Harder F, Castiglione M, Jung WF, Thurlimann B, Cavalli F, Obrecht JP, Layvraz T, Senn HJ, Metzger U, Brunner K, for the Swiss Group for Clinical Cancer Research: First isolated locoregional recurrence following mastectomy for breast cancer: Results of a phase III multicenter study comparing systemic treatment with observation after excision and radiation. *J Clin Oncol* 1994; 12:2071–2077.

496. Tartter PI, Bleiweiss IJ, Levchenko S: Factors associated with clear biopsy margins and clear reexcision margins in breast cancer specimens from candidates for breast conservation. *J Am Coll Surg* 1997; 185:268–273.

497. Karabali-Dalomaga S, Souhami RL, O'Higgins NJ, Soumilas A, Clark CG: Natural history and prognosis of recurrent breast cancer. *Br Med J* 1978; 2:730–734.

498. Halverson KJ, Perez CA, Kuske RR, Garcia DM, Simpson JR, Fineberg B: Survival following locoregional recurrence of breast cancer: Univariate and multivariate analysis. *Int J Radiat Oncol Biol Phys* 1992; 23:285–291.

499. Mora EM, Singletary E, Buzdar AU, Johnston DA: Aggressive therapy for locoregional recurrence after mastectomy in stage II and III breast cancer patients. *Ann Surg Oncol* 1996; 3:162–168.

500. Elkort RJ, Kelly W, Mozden PJ, Feldman MI: A combined treatment program for the management of locally recurrent breast cancer following chest wall irradiation. *Cancer* 1980; 46:647–653.

501. Laramore GE, Griffin TW, Parker RG, Gerdes AJ: The use of electron beams in treating local recurrence of breast cancer in previously irradiated fields. *Cancer* 1978; 41:991–995.

502. Perez CA, Pajak T, Emami B, Hornback NB, Tupchong L, Rubin P: Randomized phase III study comparing radiation and hyperthermia with radiation alone in superficial measurable tumors. Final report by the radiation oncology group. *Am J Clin Oncol (CCT)* 1991; 14:133–141.

503. Lee HK, Antell AG, Perez CA, Straube WL, Ramachandran G, Myerson RJ, Emami B,

Molmenti EP, Buckner A, Lockett MA: Superficial hyperthermia and radiation for recurrent breast carcinoma of the chest wall: Prognostic factors in 196 tumors. *Int J Radiat Oncol Biol Phys* 1998; 40:365–375.

504. Dragovic J, Seydel HG, Sandhu T, Kolosvary A, Blough J: Local superficial hyperthermia in combination with low dose radiation therapy for palliation of locally recurrent breast carcinoma. *J Clin Oncol* 1989; 7:30–35.

505. Graverson HP, Blichert-Toft M, Andersen JA, Zelder K, and the Danish Breast Cancer Cooperative Group: Breast cancer: Risk of axillary recurrence in node negative patients following partial dissection of the axilla. *Eur J Surg Oncol* 1988; 14:407–412.

506. Lindholm CE, Kjellen E, Nilsson P, Hertzman S: Microwave-induced hyperthermia and radiotherapy in human superficial tumors: Clinical results with a comparative study of combined treatment versus radiotherapy alone. *Int J Hyperthermia* 1987; 3:393–411.

507. Seegenschmiedt MH, Brady LW, Rossmeissl G: External microwave hyperthermia combined with radiation therapy for extensive superficial chest wall recurrences. *Recent Results Cancer Res* 1988; 107:147–151.

508. van der Zee J, Treurniet-Donker AD, The SK, Helle PA, Seldenrath JJ, Meerwaldt JH, Wijnmaalen AJ, van den Berg AP, van Rhoon GC, Broekmeyer-Reurink MP, et al: Low dose reirradiation in combination with hyperthermia: A palliative treatment for patients with breast cancer recurring in previously irradiated areas. *Int J Radiat Oncol Biol Phys* 1988; 15:1407–1413.

509. Kapp DS, Barnett TA, Cox RS, Lee ER, Lohrbach A, Fessenden P: Hyperthermia and radiation therapy of local–regional recurrence breast cancer: Prognostic factors for response and local control of diffuse or nodular tumors. *Int J Radiat Oncol Biol Phys* 1991; 20:1147–1164.

510. Bornstein BA, Zouranjian PS, Hansen JL, Fraser SM, Gelwan LA, Teicher BA, Svensson GK: Local hyperthermia, radiation therapy, and chemotherapy in patients with local regional recurrence of breast carcinoma. *Int J Radiat Oncol Biol Phys* 1992; 25:79–85.

511. Schuh M, Nseyo UO, Potter WR, Dao TL, Dougherty TJ: Photodynamic therapy for palliation of locally recurrent breast carcinoma. *J Clin Oncol* 1987; 5:1766–1770.

512. Sperduto PW, Delaney TF, Thomas G, Smith P, Dachowski LJ, Russo A, Bonner R, Glatstein E: Photodynamic therapy for chest wall recurrence in breast cancer. *Int J Radiat Oncol Biol Phys* 1991; 21:441–446.

513. Kahn SA, Dougherty TJ, Mang TS: An evaluation of photodynamic therapy in the management of cutaneous metastasis of breast cancer. *Eur J Cancer* 1993; 29A:1686.

514. Larson P, Weinstein M, Goldberg I, Silver B, Recht A, Cady B, Silen W, Harris JR: Edema of the arm as a function of the extent of axillary surgery in patients with stage I-II carcinoma of the breast treated with primary radiotherapy. *Int J Radiat Oncol Biol Phys* 1986; 12:1575–1582.

515. Ung O, Langlands AO, Barraclough B, Boyajes B: Combined chemotherapy and radiotherapy for patients with breast cancer and extensive nodal involvement. *J Clin Oncol* 1995; 13:435–443.

516. Werner RS, McCormick B, Petrek J, Cox L, Cirrincione C, Gray JR, Yahalom J: Arm edema in conservatively managed breast cancer: Obesity is a major predictive factor. *Radiology* 1991; 180:177–184.

517. Lingos TI, Recht A, Vicini F, Abner A, Silver B, Harris JR: Radiation pneumonitis in breast cancer patients treated with conservative surgery and radiation therapy. *Int J Radiat Oncol Biol Phys* 1991; 21:355–360.

518. Harrigan P, Otis D, Recht A, Gelman R, Hauptman P, Hayes D, Henderson IC, Harris JR, Shapiro C: The effect of adjuvant radiation therapy on cardiac events in breast cancer patients treated with doxorubicin. *Proc Am Soc Clin Oncol* 1995; 14:102 (abstr).

519. Valagussa P, Zambetti M, Biasi S, Moliterni A, Zucali R, Bonadonna G: Cardiac effects following adjuvant chemotherapy and breast irradiation in operable breast cancer. *Ann Oncol* 1994; 5:209–216.

520. Rutqvist LE, Liedberg A, Hammar N, Dalberg K: Myocardial infarction among women with early-stage breast cancer treated with conservative surgery and breast irradiation. *Int J Radiat Oncol Biol Phys* 1998; 40:359–363.

521. Nixon AJ, Manola J, Gelman R, Bornstein B, Abner A, Hetelekidis S, Recht A, Harris JR:

No long-term increase in cardiac-related mortality after breast-conserving surgery and radiation therapy using modern techniques. *J Clin Oncol* 1998; 16:1374–1379.

522. Hughes-Davies L, Sacks D, Rescigno J, Howard S, Harris J: Serum cardiac troponin T levels during treatment of early stage breast cancer. *J Clin Oncol* 1995; 13:2582–2584.

523. Plunkett ME, Bornstein BA, Costello P, Kijewski PK, Harris JR: Use of spiral CT in the assessment of cardiac structures for planning 3D volumetric radiation treatment of the breast. *Radiology* 1993; 189:355 (abstr).

524. Janjan NA, Gillin MT, Prows J, Arnold S, Hassler G, Thorsen MK, Wilson JF: Dose to the cardiac vascular and conduction systems in primary breast irradiation. *Med Dos* 1989; 14:81–87.

525. Fuller SA, Haybittle JL, Smith REA, Dobbs HJ: Cardiac doses in postoperative breast irradiation. *Radiother Oncol* 1992; 25:19–24.

526. Gyenes G, Gagliardi G, Lax I, Fornander T, Rutqvist LE: Evaluation of irradiated heart volumes in stage I breast cancer patients treated with postoperative adjuvant radiotherapy. *J Clin Oncol* 1997; 15:1348–1353.

527. Pierce SM, Recht A, Lingos TI, Abner A, Vicini F, Silver B, Herzog A, Harris JR: Long-term radiation complications following conservative surgery and radiation therapy in early stage breast cancer. *Int J Radiat Oncol Biol Phys* 1992; 23:915–923.

528. Olsen NK, Pfeiffer P, Johannsen L, Schroder H, Rose C: Radiation-induced brachial plexopathy: Neurologic follow-up in 161 recurrence-free breast cancer patients. *Int J Radiat Oncol Biol Phys* 1993; 26:43–49.

529. Powell S, Cooke J, Parsons C: Radiation-induced brachial plexus injury: Follow-up of two different fractionation schedules. *Radiother Oncol* 1990; 18:213–220.

530. Ray GR, Fish VJ, Marmor JB, Rogoway W, Kushlan P, Arnold C, Lee RH, Marzoni F: Impact of adjuvant chemotherapy on cosmesis and complications in stages I and II carcinoma of the breast treated by biopsy and radiation therapy. *Int J Radiat Oncol Biol Phys* 1984; 10:837–841.

531. Danoff BF, Goodman BL, Glick JH, Haller DG, Pajak TF: The effect of adjuvant chemotherapy on cosmesis and complications in patients with breast cancer treated by definitive irradiation. *Int J Radiat Oncol Biol Phys* 1983; 9:1625–1630.

532. Lichter AS, Lippman ME, Gorrell CR, d'Angelo TM, Edwards BK, deMoss EV: Adjuvant chemotherapy in patients treated primarily with irradiation for localized breast cancer, in J Harris, S Hellman, and W Silen (eds): *Conservative Management of Breast Cancer.* Philadelphia, Lippincott, 1983, pp 299–310.

533. Harris JR, Levene MB, Svensson G, Hellman S: Analysis of cosmetic results following primary radiation for stages I and II carcinoma of the breast. *Int J Radiat Oncol Biol Phys* 1979; 5:257–261.

534. de la Rochefordiere A, Abner AL, Silver B, Vicini F, Recht A, Harris JR: Are cosmetic results following conservative surgery and radiation therapy for early breast cancer dependent on technique? *Int J Radiat Oncol Biol Phys* 1992; 23:925–931.

535. Abner AL, Recht A, Vicini FA, Silver B, Hayes D, Come S, Harris JR: Cosmetic results after surgery, chemotherapy and radiation therapy for early breast cancer. *Int J Radiat Oncol Biol Phys* 1991; 21:331–338.

536. Van Limbergen E, Rijnders A, van der Schueren E, Lerut T, Christiaens R: Cosmetic evaluation of breast conserving treatment for mammary cancer. 2. A quantitative analysis of the influence of radiation dose, fractionation schedules and surgical treatment techniques on cosmetic results. *Radiother Oncol* 1989; 16:253–267.

537. Veronesi U, Volterrani F, Luini A, Saccozzi R, Del Vecchio M, Zucali R, Galimberti V, Rasponi A, Di Re E, Squicciarini P, et al: Quadrantectomy versus lumpectomy for small size breast cancer. *Eur J Cancer* 1990; 26:671–673.

538. Wazer DE, DiPetrillo T, Schmidt-Ullrich R, Weld L, Smith TJ, Marchant DJ, Robert NJ: Factors influencing cosmetic outcome and complication risk after conservative surgery and radiotherapy for early-stage breast carcinoma. *J Clin Oncol* 1992; 10:356–363.

539. Apostolikas N, Petraki C, Agnantis NJ: The reliability of histologically negative axillary lymph nodes in breast cancer. Preliminary report. *Pathol Res Pract* 1989; 184:35–38.

540. Biran S, Brufman G, Robinson E, Borovik R, Brenner H, Rath P: Ten-year results of a national cooperative trial of chemotherapy with and without radiotherapy for stage II breast cancer. *Proc Am Soc Clin Oncol* 1988; 7:40 (abstr).

541. Sarin R, Dinshaw KA, Shrivastava SK, Sharma V, Deore SM: Therapeutic factors influencing the cosmetic outcome and late complications in the conservative management in early breast cancer. *Int J Radiat Oncol Biol Phys* 1993; 27:285–292.

542. Olivotto IA, Rose MA, Osteen RT, Love S, Cody B, Silver B, Recht A, Harris JR: Late cosmetic outcome after conservative surgery and radiotherapy: Analysis of causes of cosmetic failure. *Int J Radiat Oncol Biol Phys* 1989; 17:747–753.

543. Gore SM, Come SE, Griem K, Rose MA, Recht A, Botnick LE, Rose C, Beadle G, Silver B, Henderson IC, Harris JR: Influence of the sequencing of chemotherapy and radiation therapy in node-positive breast cancer patients treated by conservative surgery and radiation therapy, in SE Salmon (ed): *Adjuvant Therapy of Cancer V.* Orlando, FL: Grune & Stratton, 1987, pp 365–373.

544. Markiewicz DA, Schultz DJ, Haas JA, Harris EER, Fox KR, Glick JH, Solin LJ: The effects of sequence and type of chemotherapy and radiation therapy on cosmesis and complications after breast conservation therapy. *Int J Radiat Oncol Biol Phys* 1996; 35:661–668.

545. Taylor ME, Perez CA, Halverson KJ, Kuske RR, Philpott GW, Garcia DM, Mortimer JE, Myerson RJ, Radford P, Rush C: Factors influencing cosmetic results after conservation therapy for breast cancer. *Int J Radiat Oncol Biol Phys* 1995; 31:753–764.

546. Arriagada R, Le MG, Rochard F, Contesso G, for the Institut Gustave-Roussy Breast Cancer Group: Conservative treatment versus mastectomy in early breast cancer: Patterns of failure with 15 years of follow-up data. *J Clin Oncol* 1996; 14:1558–1564.

547. Richards MA, O'Reilly SM, Howell A, George WD, Fentiman IS, Chaudary MA, Crowther D, Rubens RD: Adjuvant cyclophosphamide, methotrexate and fluorouracil in patients with axillary node-positive breast cancer: An update of the Guy's/Manchester trial. *J Clin Oncol* 1990; 8:2032–2039.

548. Fisher B, Rockette H, Fisher ER, Wickerham DL, Redmond C, Brown A: Leukemia in breast cancer patients following adjuvant chemotherapy or postoperative radiation: The NSABP experience. *J Clin Oncol* 1985; 3: 1640–1658.

549. Curtis RE, Boice JD, Stovall M, Flannery JT, Moloney WC: Leukemia risk following radiotherapy for breast cancer. *J Clin Oncol* 1989; 7:21–29.

550. Curtis RE, Boice JD, Stovall M, Bernstein L, Greenberg RS, Flannery JT, Schwartz AG, Weyer P, Moloney WC, Hoover RN: Risk of leukemia after chemotherapy and radiation treatment for breast cancer. *N Engl J Med* 1992; 326:1745–1751.

551. Hahn P, Nelson N, Baral E: Leukemia in patients with breast cancer following adjuvant chemotherapy and/or postoperative radiation therapy. *Acta Oncol* 1994; 33:599–602.

552. Boice JD Jr, Harvey EB, Blettner M, Stovall M, Flannery JT: Cancer in the contralateral breast after radiotherapy for breast cancer. *N Engl J Med* 1992; 326:781–785.

553. Horn PL, Thompson D: Risk of contralateral breast cancer: Associations with histologic clinical and therapeutic factors. *Cancer* 1988; 62:412–424.

554. Taghian A, de Vathaire F, Terrier P, Le M, Auquier A, Mouriesse H, Grimaud E, Sarrazin D, Tubiana M: Long-term risk of sarcoma following radiation treatment for breast cancer. *Int J Radiat Oncol Biol Phys* 1991; 21: 361–367.

555. Kurtz JM, Amalric R, Brandone H, Ayme Y, Spitalier JM: Contralateral breast cancer and other second malignancies in patients treated by breast-conserving therapy with radiation. *Int J Radiat Oncol Biol Phys* 1988; 15:277–284.

556. Zucali R, Merson M, Placucci M, Dipalma S, Veronesi U: Soft tissue sarcoma of the breast after conservative surgery and irradiation for early mammary cancer. *Radiother Oncol* 1994; 30:271–273.

557. Travis LB, Curtis RE, Inskip PD, Hankey BF: Lung cancer risk and radiation dose among women treated for breast cancer. *J Natl Cancer Inst* 1995; 87:60–61.

558. Neugut AI, Robinson E, Lee WC, Murray T, Karwoski K, Kutcher GJ: Lung cancer after

radiation therapy for breast cancer. *Cancer* 1993; 71:3054–3057.

559. Neugut AI, Murray T, Santos J, Amols H, Hayes MK, Flannery JT, Robinson E: Increased risk of lung cancer after breast cancer radiation therapy in cigarette smokers. *Cancer* 1994; 73:1615–1620.

560. Inskip PD, Boice JD: Radiotherapy induced lung cancer among women who smoke. *Cancer* 1994; 73:1541–1543.

561. Inskip PD, Stovall M, Flannery JT: Lung cancer risk and radiation dose among women treated for breast cancer. *J Natl Cancer Inst* 1994; 86:983–988.

562. Scanlon EF, Suh O, Murthy SM, Mettlin C, Reid SE, Cummings KM: Influence of smoking on development of lung metastasis from breast cancer. *Cancer* 1995; 75:2693–2699.

563. Shannon VR, Nesbitt JC, Lipshitz HI: Malignant pleural mesothelioma after radiation therapy for breast cancer: A report of two additional patients. *Cancer* 1995; 76:437–441.

564. Warneke J, Grossklaus D, Davis J, Stea B, Bebb G, Taylor C, Hastings R, Villar H: Influence of local treatment on the recurrence rate of ductal carcinoma in situ. *J Am Coll Surg* 1995; 180:683–688.

565. Haffty BG, Peschel RE, Papdopoulis D, Pattare P: Radiation therapy for ductal carcinoma in situ of the breast. *Conn Med* 1990; 54:482–484.

566. Kurtz JM, Jacquemier J, Torhorst J, Spitalier JM, Amalric R, Hunig R, Walther E, Harder F, Almendral A, Brandone H, et al: Conservation therapy for breast cancers other than infiltrating ductal carcinoma. *Cancer* 1989; 63:1630–1635.

567. Ray GR, Adelson J, Hayhurst E, Marzoni A, Gregg D, Bronk M, McClenathan J, Bitar N, Macio I: Ductal carcinoma in situ of the breast: Results of treatment by conservative surgery and definitive irradiation. *Int J Radiat Oncol Biol Phys* 1993; 28:105–111.

568. Ciatto S, Bonardi R, Catalloti L, Cardona G: Intraductal breast carcinoma Review of a multicenter series of 350 cases. *Tumori* 1990; 76:552–554.

569. Gallagher WJ, Koerner FC, Wood WC: Treatment of intraductal carcinoma with limited surgery: Long term follow-up. *J Clin Oncol* 1989; 7:376–380.

570. Fourquet A, Zafrani B, Campana F: Breast conserving treatment of ductal carcinoma in situ. *Semin Radiat Oncol* 1992; 2:116–124.

571. Fourquet A, Zafrani B, Campana F, Clough KB: Institut Curie experience, in MJ Silverstein (ed): *Ductal Carcinoma In Situ of the Breast.* Baltimore, Williams & Wilkins, 1997, pp 391–397.

572. Delouche G, Bachelot F, Premont M, Kurtz JM: Conservation treatment of early breast cancer: Long term results of complications. *Int J Radiat Oncol Biol Phys* 1987; 13:29–34.

573. Howard PW, Locker AP, Dowle CS, Ellis IO, Elston CW, Blamey RW: In situ carcinoma of the breast. *Eur J Surg Oncol* 1989; 15:328–332.

574. Solin LJ, Fourquet A, McCormick B, Haffty B, Recht A, Schultz DJ, Barrett W, Fowble B, Kuske R, Taylor M, McNeese M, Amalric R, Kurtz J: Salvage treatment for recurrent in the breast following breast conserving surgery and definitive radiation for ductal carcinoma in situ (intraductal) of the breast. *Int J Radiat Oncol Biol Phys* 1993; 27:146 (abstr).

575. Dixon JM, Ravisekar O, Cunningham M, Anderson EDC, Anderson TJ, Brown HK: Factors affecting outcome of patients with impalpable breast cancer detected by breast screening. *Br J Surg* 1996; 83:997–1001.

576. Hughes KW, Lee AKC, McLellan R, Mackarem G, Camus M, Joshi M, Walsh JM, Heatley GJ, Rossi RL, Munson JL, Braasch JW, Tsao J, Sanders LE, Barbarisi LJ, Lo TCM, Girschovich L, Healey GA, Buyske J: Breast-conserving therapy for patients with ductal carcinoma in situ. *Breast Dis* 1996; 9:255–268.

577. Schwartz GF: Treatment of subclinical ductal carcinoma in situ by local excision and surveillance: A personal experience, in MJ Silverstein (ed): *Ductal Carcinoma In Situ of the Breast.* Baltimore, Williams & Wilkins, 1997, pp 353–360.

578. Schreer I: Conservation therapy for DCIS without irradiation. *Breast Dis* 1996; 9:27–36.

579. Sibbering DM, Blamey RW: Nottingham experience, in MJ Silverstein (ed): *Ductal Carcinoma In Situ of the Breast.* Baltimore, Williams & Wilkins, 1997, pp 367–372.

580. Arnesson LG, Olsen K: Linkoping experience, in MJ Silverstein (ed): *Ductal Carci-*

*noma In Situ of the Breast.* Baltimore, Williams & Wilkins, 1997, pp 373–377.

581. Rosen PP, Braun DW, Kinne DW: The clinical significance of preinvasive breast carcinoma. *Cancer* 1980; 46:919–925.

582. Page DL, Dupont WD, Rogers LW, Jensen RA, Schuyler PA: Continued local recurrence of carcinoma 15–25 years after a diagnosis of low grade ductal carcinoma in situ of the breast treated only by biopsy. *Cancer* 1995; 76:1197–1200.

583. Price P, Sinnett HD, Gusterson B, Gusterson B, Walsh G, A'Hern RP, McKinna JA: Duct carcinoma in-situ: Can we predict recurrence after surgery? *Lancet* 1989; ii:671–672.

584. Bellamy COC, McDonald C, Salter DM, Chetty U, Anderson TJ: Noninvasive ductal carcinoma of the breast. The relevance of histologic categorization. *Hum Pathol* 1993; 24:16–23.

585. Ottensen GL, Graversen HP, Blichert-Toft M, Zedeler K, Andersen JA: Ductal carcinoma in situ of the female breast. Short-term results of a prospective nationwide study. *Am J Surg Pathol* 1992; 16:1183–1196.

586. Fentiman IS: European Organization for Research and Treatment of Cancer (EORTC) trial 10853: Treatment options for ductal carcinoma in situ of the breast in MJ Silverstein (ed): *Ductal Carcinoma In Situ of the Breast.* Baltimore, Williams & Wilkins, 1997, pp 421–425.

587. Salvadori B, Delledonne V, Rovini D: National Cancer Institute–Milan experience, in MJ Silverstein (ed): *Ductal Carcinoma In Situ of the Breast.* Baltimore, Williams & Wilkins, 1997, pp 427–431.

588. Blichert-Toft M, Rose C, Andersen JA, Overgaard M, Axelsson CK, Anderson KW, Mouridsen HT: Danish randomized trial comparing breast conservation therapy with mastectomy: Six years of life-table analysis Danish Breast Cancer Cooperative Group. *Monogr Natl Cancer Inst* 1992; 11:19–25.

589. Halverson KJ, Perez CA, Taylor ME, Myerson R, Philpott G, Simpson JR, Tucker G, Rush C: Age is a prognostic factor for breast and regional node recurrence following breast conserving surgery and irradiation in stage I and II breast cancer. *Int J Radiat Oncol Biol Phys* 1993; 27:1045–1050.

590. Haffty BG, Fischer D, Rose M, Beinfield M, McKhann C: Prognostic factors for local recurrence in the conservatively treated breast cancer patient: A cautious interpretation of the data. *J Clin Oncol* 1991; 9:997–1003.

591. Kini VR, White JR, Horwitz EM, Dmuchowski CF, Martinez AA, Vicini FA: Long-term results with breast-conserving therapy for patients with early stage breast carcinoma in a community hospital setting. *Cancer* 1998; 82:127–133.

592. Krishnan L, Jewell WR, Krishnan EC, Cherian R, Lin F: Breast cancer with extensive intraductal component as a risk factor for local recurrence after breast-conserving therapy. *Radiology* 1992; 1837:273–276.

593. Paterson DA, Anderson TJ, Jack WJL, Kerr GR, Rodger A, Chetty U: Pathologic features predictive of local recurrence after management by conservation of invasive breast cancer: Importance of noninvasive carcinoma. *Radiother Oncol* 1992; 25:176–180.

594. Zafrani B, Vielh P, Fourquet A, Mosseri V, Durand JC, Salmon RJ, Vilcoq JR: Conservative treatment of early breast cancer: Prognosis value of ductal in situ component and other pathologic variables on local control and survival. *Eur J Cancer Clin Oncol* 1989; 25:1645–1650.

595. Salvadori B, Biganzoli E, Veronesi P, Saccozzi R, Rilke F: Conservative surgery for infiltrating lobular breast carcinoma. *Br J Surg* 1997; 84:106–109.

596. Jacquemier J, Kurtz JM, Amalric R, Brandone H, Ayme Y, Spitalier JM: An assessment of extensive intraductal component as a risk factor for local recurrence after breast-conserving therapy. *Br J Cancer* 1990; 61:873–876.

597. Fowble B, Solin LJ, Schultz DJ: Conservative surgery and radiation for early breast cancer, in B Fowble, RL Goodman, JH Glick, and EF Rosato (eds): *Breast Cancer Treatment: A Comprehensive Guide to Management.* St Louis, Mosby, 1991, pp 105–150.

598. Harris JR: Breast-conserving therapy as a model for creating new knowledge in clinical oncology. *Int J Radiat Oncol Biol Phys* 1996; 35:641–648.

599. Mate TP, Carter D, Fischer DB, Hartman PV, McKhann C, Merino M, Prosnitz LR, Weissberg JB: A clinical and histopathologic analy-

sis of the results of conservation surgery and radiation therapy in stage I and II breast carcinoma. *Cancer* 1986; 58:1995–2002.

600. Peiro G, Schnitt S, Gage I: Treatment outcome following conservative surgery and radiation therapy for infiltrating carcinoma with mixed ductal and lobular features: Comparison with infiltrating ductal and infiltrating lobular carcinoma. *Mod Pathol* 1995; 8:23A (abstr).

601. Poen JC, Tran L, Juillard G, Selch MT, Giuliano A, Silverstein M, Fingerhut A, Lewinsky B, Parker RG: Conservation therapy for invasive lobular carcinoma of the breast. *Cancer* 1992; 69:2789–2795.

602. White JR, Gustafson GS, Wimbish K, Ingold JA, Lucas RJ, Levine AJ, Matter RA, Martinez A, Vicini FA: Conservative surgery and radiation therapy for infiltrating lobular carcinoma of the breast. The role of preoperative mammograms in guiding treatment. *Cancer* 1994; 74:640–647.

603. Silverstein MJ, Lewinsky BS, Waisman JR, Gierson ED, Colburn WJ, Snofsky GM, Gamagami P: Infiltrating lobular carcinoma. Is it different from infiltrating duct carcinoma? *Cancer* 1994; 73:1673–1677.

604. Bornstein BA, Peiro G, Connolly JL, Gelman R, Schnitt SJ, Hetelekidis S, Nixon AJ, Recht A, Silver B, Harris JR: The influence of infiltrating lobular carcinoma on the outcome of patients treated with breast-conserving surgery and radiation therapy. *Int J Radiat Oncol Biol Phys* 1996; 36:180 (abstr).

605. Weiss MC, Fowble BL, Solin LJ, Yeh I-T, Schultz DJ: Outcome of conservative therapy for invasive breast cancer by histologic subtype. *Int J Radiat Oncol Biol Phys* 1992; 23:941–947.

606. Haffty BG, Perrotta PL, Ward B, Moran M, Beinfield M, McKhann C, Fischer D, Carter D: Conservatively treated breast cancer: Outcome by histologic subtype. *Breast J* 1997; 3:7–14.

607. Vicini FA, Horwitz EM, Lacerna MD, Dmuchowski CF, Brown DM, White J, Chen PY, Edmundson GK, Gustafson GS, Clarke PH, Gustafson GS, Matter RC, Marginez AA: Long-term outcome with interstitial brachytherapy in the management of patients with early-stage breast cancer treated with breast-

conserving therapy. *Int J Radiat Oncol Biol Phys* 1997; 37:842–852.

608. Anthony P, Khan K, Keith T: Positive margins and intraductal cancer does not impact local control in treating early stage breast cancer conservatively: A study of 902 cases. *Int J Radiat Oncol Biol Phys* 1996; 36:274 (abstr).

609. Anscher MS, Jones P, Prosnitz LR, Blackstock W, Hebert M, Reddick R, Tucker A, Dodge R, Leight G, Iglehart JD, Rosenman J: Local failure and margin status in early stage breast carcinoma treated with conservative surgery and radiation. *Ann Oncol* 1993; 218:22–28.

610. Slotman BJ, Meyer OWM, Njo KH, Karim ABMF: Importance of timing of radiotherapy in breast conserving treatment for early stage breast cancer. *Radiother Oncol* 1994; 30: 206–212.

611. Heimann R, Power C, Halpern HJ, Michel AG, Ewing CA, Wyman B, Recant W, Weichselbaum RR: Breast preservation in stage I and II carcinoma of the breast. The University of Chicago experience. *Cancer* 1996; 78: 1722–1730.

612. Spivak B, Khanna MM, Tafra L, Juillard G, Giuliano AE: Margin status and local recurrence after breast conserving surgery. *Arch Surg* 1994; 129:952–957.

613. Van Dongen JA, Bartelink H, Fentiman IS, Lerut T, Mignolet F, Olthius G, van der Schueren E, Sylvester R, Tony D, Winter J, Van Zijl K: Factors influencing local relapse and survival and results of salvage treatment after breast conserving therapy in operable breast cancer: EORTC trial 10801 breast conservation compared with mastectomy in TNM stage I and II breast cancer. *Eur J Cancer* 1992; 28A:801–805.

614. Pittinger TP, Maronian NC, Poulter CA, Peacock JL: Importance of margin status and outcome of breast conserving surgery for carcinoma. *Surgery* 1994; 116:605–609.

615. Stewart HJ, Prescott RJ, Forrest PA: Conservation therapy of breast cancer. *Lancet* 1989; ii:168–169.

616. Moffat FL, Ketcham AS: Breast conserving surgery and selective adjuvant radiation therapy for stage I and II breast cancer. *Semin Surg Oncol* 1992; 8:172–176.

617. Silvestrini R, Veneroni S, Benini E, Daidone MG, Luisi A, Leutner M, Maucione A, Kenda

R, Zucali R, Veronesi U: Expression of p53 glutathione *S*-transferase-π and bcl-2 proteins and benefit from adjuvant radiotherapy in breast cancer. *J Natl Cancer Inst* 1997; 89:639–645.

618. Ahmann DL, O'Fallon JR, Scanlon PW, Payne WS, Bisel HF, Edmonson JH, Frytak S, Hahn RG, Ingle JN, Rubin J, Creagan ET: A preliminary assessment of factors associated with recurrent disease in a surgical adjuvant clinical trial for patients with breast cancer with special emphasis on the aggressiveness of therapy. *Am J Clin Oncol* 1982; 5:371–381.

619. Martinez A, Ahmann D, O'Fallon J, Payne W, Scanlon P, Hahn K, Ingle J, Edmonson J: An interim analysis of the randomized surgical adjuvant trial for patients with unfavorable breast cancer. *Int J Radiat Oncol Biol Phys* 1985; 10:150 (abstr).

620. Muss HB, Cooper MR, Brockschmidt JK, Ferree C, Richards F II, White DR, Jackson DV, Spurr CL: A randomized trial of chemotherapy (L-PAM vs. CMF) and irradiation for node positive breast cancer. Eleven year follow-up of a Piedmont Oncology Association trial. *Breast Cancer Res Treat* 1991; 19:77–84.

621. Buzdar A, Smith T, Blumenschein G, Hortobagyi GN, Marcus CE, Hersh EM, Martin RG, Gehan EA, Freireich EJ: Adjuvant chemotherapy with fluorouracil, doxorubicin, and cyclophosphamide (FAC) for stage II or III breast cancer: 5 year results, in SE Salmon, and SE Jones (eds): *Adjuvant Therapy for Cancer III.* New York, Grune & Stratton, 1981, pp 419–426.

622. Blomqvist C, Tiusanen K, Elomaa I, Rissanen P, Hietanen T, Heinonen E, Gröhn P: The combination of radiotherapy, adjuvant chemotherapy (cyclophosphamide-doxorubicin-ftorafur) and tamoxifen in stage II breast cancer. Long-term follow-up results of a randomized trial. *Br J Cancer* 1992; 66:1171–1176.

623. Heimann R, Powers C, Fleming G, Halpern HJ, Rubin SJ, Ewing C, Weichselbaum RR: Does the sequencing of radiotherapy and chemotherapy affect the outcome in early stage breast cancer: A continuing question. *Int J Radiat Oncol Biol Phys* 1994; 30:243–244 (abstr).

624. Willèrs H, Würschmidt F, Janik I, Bünemann H, Heilmann H-P: Combined conservative surgery, chemotherapy, and radiation therapy in treatment of the breast cancer patients: The influence of the interval between surgery and start of irradiation. *Int J Radiat Oncol Biol Phys* 1996; 36:280 (abstr).

625. Dabrow MB, Antoniades J: Sequential adjuvant CMF chemotherapy followed by radiotherapy in the treatment of early-stage breast cancer: The Lankenau Hospital experience. *Breast J* 1997; 3:15–18.

626. Wallgren A, Bernier J, Gelber RD, Goldhirsch A, Roncadin M, Joseph D, Gastiglione-Gertsch M: Timing of radiotherapy and chemotherapy following breast-conserving surgery for patients with node-positive breast cancer. *Int J Radiat Oncol Biol Phys* 1996; 35:649–659.

627. Overmoyer B, Fowble B, Solin L, Goldstein L, Glick J: The long-term results of conservative surgery and radiation with concurrent chemotherapy for early stage breast cancer. *Proc Am Soc Clin Oncol* 1992; 11:90 (abstr).

628. Danforth DN Jr, Zujewski J, Okunieff P, Shriver C, Merino M, McAtee N, Steinberg S, Cowan K: Dose-intense preoperative chemotherapy for patients with stage II breast cancer? A prospective randomized trial. *Soc Surg Oncol*, 1997.

# CHAPTER 7

# CANCER OF THE INTRATHORAX

NOAH C. CHOI

## A. RADIATION THERAPY FOR CARCINOMA OF THE LUNG

### INTRODUCTION

Lung cancer is one of the major challenges to all professionals involved in health care: the incidence of this disease has risen steadily each year without a breakthrough in prevention or management. It was estimated that almost 171,500 new cases of lung cancer, 91,400 in males and 80,100 in females, would occur in the United States in 1998.[1] Lung cancer, which has been the leading cause of cancer death (32% of all cancer deaths) in men, has also become the leading cause of cancer deaths (25% of all cancer deaths) in women. Breast cancer became the second leading cause of cancer death, with 16% of all cancer deaths in women.

Common pathologic types of lung cancer include squamous cell (epidermoid) carcinoma, adenocarcinoma, small-cell carcinoma (oat cell), and large-cell undifferentiated carcinoma.[2] Squamous cell carcinoma accounts for 35% to 40% of all lung cancers; the majority of squamous cell carcinomas are seen in men and smokers. This tumor tends to be centrally located and frequently produces bronchial obstruction. Adenocarcinoma, which constitutes about 25% of lung cancers, is peripherally located and has papillary and glandular structures. This tumor often arises in the area of fibrosis secondary to previous pulmonary damage and has less association with smoking than have other types of lung cancer. Small-cell carcinoma makes up 20% of lung cancers. It is the most aggressive type of the lung cancers characterized by early lymphatic and hematogenous metastases. This tumor frequently produces circulating polypeptides that are associated with various paraneoplastic syndromes. Large-cell, undifferentiated carcinoma constitutes about 10% of lung cancers; whether this is actually a separate type or one in the spectrum of adenocarcinoma is debatable. Other less common types include bronchioalveolar cell carcinomas, carcinoid tumors, and mucoepidermoid varieties.

Lung cancer progresses with the following behavior: local tumor growth with invasion into adjacent structures; regional growth by metastases to hilar, mediastimal, and supraclavicular lymph nodes via lymphatic spread; growth in distant organs via hematogenous metastases; and paraneoplastic syndromes. Common symptoms include cough, hemoptysis, wheeze, and dyspnea from the bronchial obstruction by the primary tumor. Recurrent pneumonitis, not responding to antibiotics,

*Clinical Radiation Oncology: Indications, Techniques, and Results, 2nd ed.* Edited by C.C. Wang.
ISBN: 0-471-23803-1   Copyright © 2000 Wiley-Liss, Inc.

is also a common presentation of lung cancer with bronchial obstruction. Metastatic growth in the mediastinal lymph nodes at the aortic window can cause hoarseness secondary to paralysis of the left recurrent laryngeal nerve. Homer syndrome, due to paralysis of the cervical sympathetic nerve, and brachial plexus syndrome are caused by Pancoast tumor. The superior vena caval syndrome represents advanced regional tumor growth at the mediastinum causing a vascular obstruction of the superior venae cavae and/or innominate vessels.

## DIAGNOSIS

For patients suspected of having lung cancer, the chest radiograph is the primary tool for diagnosis. The study should include the standard posteroanterior (PA) as well as the lateral views. An almost certain presumptive diagnosis of malignancy can frequently be made from radiologic images alone, but proof of diagnosis is necessary before further workup is undertaken to delineate the extent of the tumor. Endoscopic examination of the tracheobronchial tree by flexible fiber-optic scope or rigid bronchoscope is a direct and productive way to obtain a tissue diagnosis for suspicious lesions seen in radiographic studies. Transthoracic fine-needle aspiration biopsy under a fluoroscopic or computed body tomography (CBT) guide has yielded cytologic diagnosis in over 90%, of patients with suspected small peripheral lesions.[3] Diagnosis of lung cancer can also be established by other simple means such as sputum cytology, cytologic studies of pleural fluid, and biopsy of supraclavicular lymph nodes for suspected metastases and other metastatic lesions readily accessible to a simple biopsy procedure. Exploratory thoracotomy is the last method, to be used only after other diagnostic procedures have been exhausted.

## STAGING WORKUP

The staging workup is the next step to define the anatomical extent of the disease on which the selection of the treatment method and the prognosis depend. Physiologic consideration with regard to the patient's ability to tolerate the treatment and to be functional afterward is also important in this regard. A combination of a TNM staging system by the American Joint Committee (AJCC) for Staging and End-Results Reporting (Table 7-1) and physiologic staging of the patient by means of performance and cardiac and pulmonary function status should be a comprehensive basis for selecting proper treatment and estimating results.[4-7] The extent of the primary tumor (T factor) is evaluated by chest radiographs, CBT scan of the chest, and bronchoscopy. A CBT scan of the chest and upper abdomen has provided information that is critical for lung cancer staging but otherwise unavailable or less than satisfactory from conventional radiographs. The size and shape of the primary lesion and its relationship to the surrounding normal structures are very well defined by this method. The mediastinum can satisfactorily be evaluated for direct tumor invasion and metastases. Additional important information from CBT of the upper part of the abdomen includes a satisfactory screening of metastases to the liver, adrenal glands, and upper para-aortic lymph nodes. Mediastinoscopy provides information on metastases to ipsilateral as well as contralateral mediastinal lymph nodes (N factor).[8] Anterior mediastinotomy (the Chamberlain procedure) provides an access to the left subaortic (A-P window) nodes or hilar regions bilaterally. When mediastinal lymph nodes are enlarged by CBT scan of the chest, mediastinoscopy is still indicated, inasmuch as lymphadenitis is the cause of enlarged lymph nodes in 15% to 28% of patients.[9] If the lymph nodes are within normal limit in size by the definition of less than 1.0 cm in short axis diameter, there may still be a 13% risk for having microscopic metastases in the lymph nodes. Opinions differ regarding whether intraoperative staging alone should be done in such patients rather than mediastinoscopy.[10–13]

Workup for distant metastases (M factor) consists of a careful history and physical examination to look for clues of metastatic involvement of cervical lymph nodes, liver, bone, brain, and other distant organs. Liver function studies should be obtained routinely and, when results are abnormal or when hepatomegaly is present on physical examination, CBT with contrast agent for upper abdomen or MR im-

ages of the liver should be obtained to document metastases. Brain CT scan and bone scan are also part of workup for distant metastases.

For patients with a proven diagnosis of small-cell lung carcinoma, staging proceeds somewhat differently. With the establishment of the diagnosis, no further invasive, local, or regional staging procedures are generally performed, but an evaluation of the brain, liver, and bone for metastases is routinely performed. In addition, bone marrow aspiration

**TABLE 7-1    International System for Staging Lung Cancer**

| *Primary Tumor (T)* | | *Nodal Involvement (N)* | |
|---|---|---|---|
| Tx | Primary tumor cannot be assessed; or tumor proven by the presence of malignant cells in sputum or bronchial washings but not visualized by imaging or bronchoscopy | NX | Regional lymph nodes cannot be assessed |
| | | N0 | No regional lymph node metastasis |
| T0 | No evidence of primary tumor | N1 | Metastasis to ipsilateral peribronchial and/or ipsilateral hilar lymph nodes, and intrapulmonary nodes involved by direct extension of the primary tumor |
| Tis | Carcinoma in situ | | |
| T1 | Tumor ≤ 3.0 cm in greatest dimension, surrounded by lung or visceral pleura, without bronchoscopic evidence of invasion more proximal than the lobar bronchus | N2 | Metastasis to ipsilateral mediastinal and/or subcarinal lymph node(s) |
| T2 | Tumor with any of the following features of size or extent: > 3.0 cm in greatest dimension, involves main bronchus, ≥ 2 cm distal to the carina, invades the visceral pleura, or associated with atelectasis or obstructive pneumonitis that extends to the hilar region but does not involve the entire lung | N3 | Metastasis to contralateral mediastinal, contralateral hilar, ipsilateral or contralateral scalene, or supraclavicular lymph node(s) |
| | | | *Distant Metastasis (M)* |
| T3 | Tumor of any size that directly invades the following: chest wall (including superior sulcus tumors), diaphragm, mediastinal pleura, parietal pericardium; or tumor in the main bronchus < 2 cm distal to the carina, but without involvement of the carina; or associated atelectasis or obstructive pneumonitis of the entire lung | Mx | Presence of distant metastasis cannot be assessed |
| | | M0 | No distant metastasis |
| | | M1 | Distant metastasis present—specific site(s) |
| | | | *Stage Grouping* |
| T4 | Tumor of any size that invades any of the following: mediastinum, heart, great vessels, trachea, esophagus, vertebral body, carina; or tumor with a malignant pleural or pericardial effusion, or with satellite tumor nodule(s) within the ipsilateral primary tumor lobe of the lung | 0 | Carcinoma in situ |
| | | Occult stage | Tx N0 M0 |
| | | IA | T1 N0 M0 |
| | | IB | T2 N0 M0 |
| | | IIA | T1 N1 M0 |
| | | IIB | T2 N1 M0, T3 N0 M0 |
| | | IIIA | T3 N1 M0, T1 N2 M0, T2 N2 M0, T3 N2 M0 |
| | | IIIB | T4 N0-3 M0, T1-3 N3 M0 |
| | | IV | Any T, any N M1 |

*Source:* Ref. 5.

and biopsy are also carried out because 25% to 30% of all patients with small-cell carcinoma of the lung have bone marrow metastases.

## TREATMENT

### Surgery

For therapeutic purposes, lung cancer is divided into two groups: non-small-cell lung cancer (NSCLC) and small-cell lung cancer (SCLC). Surgery is the treatment of choice for stage I (T1-2 N0 M0) and stage II (T1-2 N1 M0, T3 N0 M0) NSCLC.[14,15] The 5-year cure rate for stage I disease is on the order of 50%, and its cell type for NSCLC does not appear to be a significant factor for survival. Unfortunately, only a small proportion of patients with lung cancer have stage I disease. In stage II disease, the results of surgery are much less encouraging, with 5-year survival rates varying from 40% for T1 N1 M0 to 30% for T2 N1 M0 and T3 N0 M0 lesions. Again, stage II disease represents a very small number of the total patients seen with lung cancer. Patients with minimal N2 lesions (ipsilateral, limited nodal metastases) should be carefully reviewed for neoadjuvant therapy followed by surgery. Segmental and wedge resection for a small peripheral lung cancer is more often reserved for patients who cannot tolerate a more extended resection because of poor lung function. Sleeve lobectomy is applicable for salvage of lung tissue either for patients with compromised pulmonary function or when such resection can be done electively without compromising excision of the tumor. Surgery is contraindicated for patients with superior vena caval syndrome, vocal cord paralysis, metastases to the supraclavicular lymph nodes, and lymph node in the contralateral mediastinum. For these patients, chemoradiotherapy should be offered with expectation of cure.

### Radiation Therapy

Radiation therapy alone before the era of modern chemotherapy resulted in 5-year survival rate of 5% to 8% for patients with stage III NSCLC by using a conventional dose schedule of 5600 to 6000 cGy in 28 to 30 fractions (F) over 5.6 to 6 weeks (wk) on a once-a-day (QD) schedule.[16–18] Two classic reports contributed in 1960s are those of Guttmann[19] and Smart.[20] In Guttmann's study, 95 patients, surgical rejects at exploratory thoracotomy, were treated with radiation using a 2 MV van de Graaff machine. Seven patients (7.4%) survived 5 years without evidence of disease. The study by Smart dealt with resectable but medically inoperable lung cancer. Forty patients were treated with radiation, and nine patients (22.5%) survived 5 years.

The patient's general condition should be good enough to tolerate a course of thoracic radiotherapy that lasts for 6 to 7 weeks, ascertained by a performance status of at least 70 on the Karnofsky scale[6] and grade 0-1 on the Zubrod scale.[7] When radiation therapy is carefully designed for each patient, it is feasible that an unresectable cancer of the lung that is still limited within the regional lymphatics can be sterilized by high dose radiation (6000–6400 cGy/30–34 F/6–6.4 wk) administered to the tumor-bearing areas, while adjacent normal vital structures, such as the spinal cord, a large volume of the normal lung tissue, and the heart, are spared excessive dose of radiation.[21–23]

### Chemoradiotherapy

The baseline result of radiation therapy alone was improved when it was combined with cisplatin-based chemotherapy. Dillman et al.[24,25] compared radiation therapy alone (6000 cGy/30 F/6 wk) with a sequential chemoradiotherapy in which two cycles of induction chemotherapy (cisplatin, 100 mg/m$^2$ IV, days 1 and 29; vinblastine, 5 mg/m$^2$ IV, days 1, 8, 15, 22, and 29) were administered first, and radiation therapy (6000 cGy/30 F/6 wk) was administered subsequently starting on day 50. The 5-year survival rate was 7% with radiation therapy alone, versus 16% with chemoradiotherapy. It is surprising to see that the 5-year survival rate of 7% resulting from radiation therapy alone in the 1980s is not different from that of Guttmann's study in the 1960s. Arriagada et al.[26] also compared radiation therapy alone with chemoradiotherapy in which three monthly cycles of VCPC (vindesine, 1.5 mg/m$^2$, days 1, 2; cyclophosphamide, 200 mg/m$^2$, days 2–4; cisplatin, 100 mg/m$^2$, day 2; lomustine, 50 mg/m$^2$, day 2, 25 mg/m$^2$ day 3) were administered before and after radiation therapy (6500 cGy/26 F/6.5 wk) for patients with stage IIIA and IIIB NSCLC. The eligibility criteria in this study were less restrictive than those of Dillman et al. The local–regional failure that was assessed by bronchoscopy and biopsy at 3 months after the completion of the therapies was found to be of the order of 80% for the chemoradiotherapy group and for the group that had radiation therapy alone. However, the distant failure rate at 5 years was reduced from 70% of radiation therapy alone to 49% by the addition of chemotherapy. An update of this study showed that the 5-year survival rates were 6% with sequential chemoradiotherapy versus 3% with radiation therapy alone ($p < 0.02$).[27]

## Chemotherapy Alone

The role of chemotherapy alone with cisplatin-based regimens was tested in patients with stage IIIA and IIIB NSCLC by Kubota et al.[28] In this trial, 92 patients with stage III NSCLC were treated with two cycles of cisplatin-based regimen and restaged. Following the restaging, 63 of 92 patients who were free of tumor progression were selected for randomization to receive either further cisplatin-based chemotherapy or radiation therapy (5000–6000 cGy/25–30 F/5–6 wk). The survival rates at 1, 2, and 3 years were 58%, 36%, and 29% with chemoradiotherapy, and 66%, 9%, and 3% with chemotherapy alone group. Local recurrence was seen in 5 of 16 patients with chemoradiotherapy, compared with 15 of 16 patients with chemotherapy alone respectively.

## ROLE OF RADIATION THERAPY

The role of radiation therapy in lung cancer includes the following five major categories:

I. Radiation therapy in combination with chemotherapy for unresectable stage III non-small-cell lung cancer (NSCLC)

II. Radiation therapy for medically inoperable stage I and II NSCLC

III. Postoperative radiation therapy in stage II and III NSCLC

IV. Superior pulmonary sulcus tumor

V. Radiation therapy in small-cell lung cancer (SCLC)

## I. Radiation Therapy in Combination with Chemotherapy for Unresectable Stage III NSCLC

Local–regional treatment does not provide a comprehensive therapy for patients with stage III NSCLC. The significance of combining radiotherapy with chemotherapy has been demonstrated by the randomized studies discussed earlier.[25,26]

The successful outcome of radiation therapy depends on a clear definition of target volume, the optimal radiation dose and fractionation schedules, and proper radiation portal arrangements to secure the optimal dose distribution within the target volume.

***Target Volume***    The incidence of hilar and mediastinal lymph node involvement by metastatic deposits from cancer of the lung varies from 30% to 50% in surgically treated series.[28–30] In the author's series of 162 patients treated with curative radiation therapy for unresectable lung cancer,[17] 90% of patients (147 of 162) had metastatic involvement of either the mediastinal lymph nodes (131 patients) or the mediastinal lymph nodes plus the supraclavicular lymph nodes (16 patients).

The target volume for curative radiation therapy consists of gross target volume (GTV) for radiographically defined gross tumor and clinical target volume (CTV) for potential microscopic tumor extension. For a locally advanced unresectable lung cancer (T1-3 N2-3 M0, T4 N0-1 M0), GTV includes the primary tumor and involved regional lymph nodes. CTV consists of a 1.0 cm margin of clinically uninvolved lung around the primary lesion and a 2.0 to 2.5 cm margin around the involved hilar lymph nodes. CTV for involved mediastinal lymph nodes includes a 2.0 cm circumferential margin and a 2.5 cm margin for coverage of one sentinel nodal station beyond the involved mediastinal lymph nodes along the cranial–caudal direction. An additional 0.7 cm of margin is added to the CTV of the primary tumor and mediastinal lymph nodes as a planning target volume (PTV), to take into account the setup error and patient motion. The CTV for involved mediastinal nodes at mediastinal nodal stations 7 and 4R includes 4L, 5, 6, 2R, and 2L (Figure 7-1). The inferior border of the mediastinal CTV is at the level of a margin of 2.5 cm beyond the involved nodes at station 7 caudally. The surrounding normal structures such as esophagus, aorta, vertebrae, and heart are excluded from CTV as much as possible.

### Optimal Dose and Fractionation Schedules

Several different fractionation schedules have similar biologic effects on normal and on malignant tissues. A time, dose, and fractionation (TDF) model has been advocated as a means of establishing a reference dose when different fractionation schedules of radiation therapy are compared for their effects on normal and tumor tissues.[31,32] An optimal fractionation schedule for lung cancer is a radiation therapy program that gives the best possible

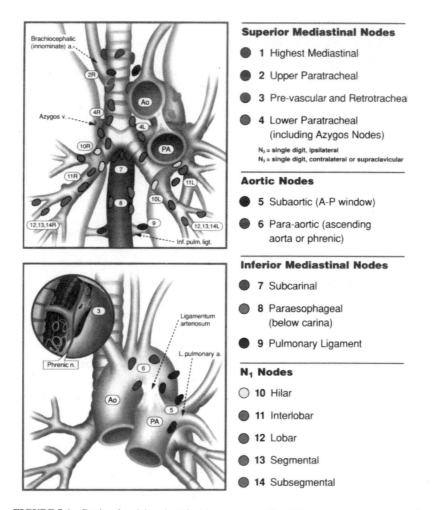

**FIGURE 7-1**   Regional nodal stations for lung cancer staging. (From Mountain and Dressler.[8])
Figure also appears in Color Figure section.

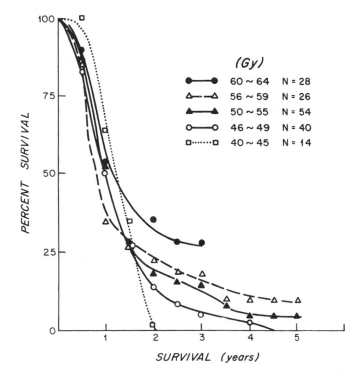

**FIGURE 7-2** Dose–response relation for survival in patients with stage III NSCLC from a sequential dose escalation study.[17]

control of local–regional tumor with the fewest complications. Whereas earlier preoperative radiation therapy studies suggested that radiation dose schedules of 4700 to 6000 cGy given by daily fractions of 180 to 200 cGy, 5 days a week, showed pathologic complete response in 29% to 54% of patients,[33,34] recent studies report a pathologic complete response rate of only 10% to 15% at the primary lesion, although it was 50% to 67% at the involved mediastinal lymph nodes when similar radiation dose schedules were used in preoperative chemoradiotherapy for stage III NSCLC.[35–38] Clinical studies on the relation between radiation dose and local tumor control have demonstrated that there is a reasonable correlation between radiation dose and tumor control in lung cancer (Figure 7-2).[17,18] Other important factors for control of local–regional tumor, in addition to radiation dose, are the tumor size and stage, and the patient's general condition. Radiation therapy administered in a split

course, in which a rest period of 2 to 3 weeks is given at the halfway point of the entire course of treatment (5–6 wk), has been proved to be inferior to the standard fractionation schedule without a break.[22] The current standard dose schedule for definitive radiation therapy is a total dose of 6000 to 6600 cGy, given with daily dose fractions of 180 to 200 cGy, 5 days a week, over a period of 6 to 7 weeks. However, this level of radiation dose schedule is less than the optimum in providing local tumor control to the majority of patients. Ongoing studies are using three-dimensional conformal therapy to search for better and more effective radiation dose schedules.

***Radiation Portal Arrangements*** The arrangement of radiation portals is dependent on the planned total dose, the energy levels of radiation, and the shape of the target volume. Because of the scatter irradiation of low energy beams and the large penumbra of a $^{60}$Co unit, high energy beams (10–25 MV photon) seem to be the choice for curative radiation therapy, with an aimed total dose of 6000 to 6400 cGy. An arrangement of two parallel opposed portals (POP) applied anteroposteriorly (AP) and posteroanteriorly (PA) to the chest is simple and accurate, with the least risk of a geographical miss. The maximum dose that can be administered with this technique is, however, in the range of 4400 cGy because of the tolerance limit of the spinal cord. When a posterior spinal cord block was used to keep the spinal cord dose within the tolerance limit while a total dose of 6000 cGy was administered at the midplane, an increase in local tumor recurrence was noted because of a zone of a low tumor dose at the posterior mediastinum along the vertebral column. An outright three-field arrangement of AP, right posterior oblique (RPO), and left posterior oblique (LPO) has also been used for a small target volume located centrally. Drawbacks to this technique are a relatively higher radiation dose (40–50% of total dose) to the pulmonary tissue in the path of the oblique beams and the difficulty of dealing with a large target volume because of poor pulmonary tolerance. The rotational technique alone is undesirable because of the potential risk of increased pulmonary complications.

A treatment technique the author has used is a combination of AP-PA-POP with a three-field setup of AP-RPO-LPO and oblique opposed boost portals. We have administered a high radiation dose (6000–6400 cGy) to the target volume while normal vital structures are kept below the threshold dose for serious complications (i.e., $\leq$ 4400 cGy to the spinal cord and $\leq$ 1200–1400 cGy to the pulmonary tissue in the path of the oblique beams). For gross tumors involving carina and N3 lesions, a total dose of 6400 to 6600 cGy is administered by a combination of AP-PA-POP for the initial 3600 cGy and AP-RPO-LPO for an additional 2800 to 3000 cGy, using daily fractions of 180 to 200 cGy, 5 days a week.

For metastatic tumors limited to the ipsilateral mediastinum (N2 lesion), GTV is given a supplemental dose of 900 cGy in 5 fractions using oblique opposed portals, for a total dose of 6480 cGy in 36 fractions for 7.2 weeks after 5400 cGy in 30 fraction for 6 weeks by a combination of AP-PA-POP for the initial dose (3600 cGy/20 F/4 wks) and AP-RPO-LPO for an additional dose (1980 cGy/11 F/2.2 wks). Two levels of radiation doses are given: 6400 to 6480 cGy to GTV and 5040 cGy to CTV by reducing the field size at 5040 cGy in 28 fractions of 5.6 weeks. This level of radiation dose is administered in combination with either sequential or concurrent chemotherapy.

With the findings of CBT of the chest, radiation dosimetry is expected to have accurate body contours at different levels of the target volume, improved definition of tumor size and location relative to other normal vital structures, and a precise measurement of the thickness of the pulmonary tissue in the path of the irradiation for which a correction for the increased transmission is made. It is expected that the target volume and the tumor mass will be drawn in a contour with a composite isodose plan from which one can estimate the maximum and minimum tumor doses. Every effort should be made to achieve the ideal treatment plan, which would give the least variation of radiation dose within the target volume with the maximum differential of radiation dose between the tumor and the surrounding normal tissue.

Dose–volume histograms in three-dimensional conformal treatment plans offer a useful means to determine the optimum treatment plan.[39–42] An optimized treatment plan is being studied to achieve the desired balance between normal tissue complication probability (NTCP) and tumor control probability (TCP). To achieve this balance in the most desired form, intensity-modulated photon and proton beams are being studied.

### *Results of High Dose Radiation Therapy*

Cure is the primary goal of high dose radiation therapy for patients with unresectable lung carcinoma. Radiation therapy is, however, a local and regional treatment that cannot alter the course of the disease if there is preexisting distant metastasis. Other goals for high dose radiation therapy include relief of associated symptoms by controlling local–regional tumors. The control rate of the local and the regional tumors is a good criterion for the effectiveness of the dose fractionation schedule tested.

## Results

*Survival Rate*  The actuarial method for computing survival rates is to be favored because it makes use of all the information available without waiting until a specific time has elapsed for the whole group.[43,44] The survival rates at 4 to 5 years are very close to the rates of actual clinical cure, inasmuch as the survival curve for patients with lung cancer treated with curative radiation becomes parallel to that for the normal population of the same age and sex at 4 years. For patients who were subjected to high dose radiation therapy alone for stage III NSCLC, the 5-year survival rate has remained at 5% to 8%.[17,18,23–27] A phase III trial by RTOG compared standard dose of radiation therapy (6000 cGy/30 F/6 wk) with two study regimens:

- a sequential chemoradiotherapy (2 cycles of cisplatin, 100 mg/m$^2$ IV, days 1 and 29; and vinblastine, 5 mg/m$^2$ IV, days 1, 8, 15, 22, and 29) followed by 6000 cGy in 30 fractions for 6 weeks of standard dose of radiation (the study arm of Dillman's trial)
- a twice-daily radiation schedule of 6960 cGy (by a 120 cGy/F, BID, 5 days a week: the best arm from the dose escalation study using a twice-daily schedule of James Cox)[24,45–47]

The median survival time and 5-year survival rates were 11.4 months and 5% for the standard radiation therapy arm, compared with 12.2 months and 6% for the BID radiation arm and 13.7 months and 8% for the combined chemoradiotherapy arm respectively, $p = 0.04$. Therefore, the current data indicate that a sequential combination of two cycles of induc-

tion chemotherapy and radiation therapy can result in a 5-year survival rate ranging from 8% to 16%.

*Local and Regional Tumor Control and Patterns of Failure*  The control rate of local–regional tumors is a function of radiation dose, tumor size, and other less well-understood systemic factors. Clinical work using radiographic studies and a follow-up duration up to 18 months after 5600 to 6000 cGy in 28 to 30 fractions for 5.6 to 6 weeks reported a 50% to 70% rate of progression-free local tumor control (Table 7-2).[17,18] However, according to the study by Arriagada et al.[26] histologic complete response was obtained in only 20% of patients in both sequential chemoradiotherapy and radiation therapy alone (6500 cGy/26 F/45 days) groups when a systematic biopsy of the primary and/or regional lymph nodes was performed as a restaging procedure 3 months after the completion of therapies. A long-term follow-up showed local–regional recurrence to be 85% or greater at 5 years in both groups.[27] In this study, there was a decrease in distant failure rate from 70% of radiation therapy alone to 49% with the sequential combination of chemotherapy and radiotherapy. Frequent sites of distant failure include bone, brain, liver, and the opposite lung. The pattern of failure seems to be related to the histologic type of tumor.[17,18] With squamous cell and large-cell carcinomas there is an association of failure at the local and the regional areas more often than at the distant sites. On the other hand, with

**TABLE 7-2  Local Tumor Control in Relation to Radiation Doses**

| Radiation Dose (Gy) | Local Tumor Control (patients controlled/total patients) | |
|---|---|---|
| | 12 months | 18 months |
| 56–64 | 23/29 (79%) | 13/17 (76%) |
| 50–55 | 23/30 (76%) | 8/16 (50%) |
| 40–49 | 22/32 (69%) | 4/14 (29%) |

*Source:* Reproduced with permission from Choi and Doucette.[17]

adenocarcinoma the association of failure is at the brain or bone more often than at other locations. Therefore, local–regional recurrence remains the major barrier for further improvement in survival with the current combined chemoradiotherapy in stage III NSCLC. Effort is being directed toward a concurrent combination of radiation therapy, systemic chemotherapy, immunotherapy, and antiangiogenic therapy to improve both local and metastatic tumor control.

*Palliation of Distressing Symptoms*   Relief of distressing symptoms is another important goal in addition to cure in thoracic radiation therapy. Hemoptysis, which is alarming to patients and their families, is well relieved in over 90% of patients receiving a moderate dose (3000–4000 cGy) of irradiation.[48,49] Dyspnea associated with obstruction of the trachea, carina, or main stem or lobar bronchi is also well relieved in over 80% of patients with 4500 to 5000 cGy of radiation. Cough associated with a tumor located in the main stem bronchus or carina is more likely to be relieved than cough associated with a peripheral tumor of the lung. Local pain associated with direct spread of the tumor to the surrounding normal structures such as the chest wall, vertebral bodies, brachial plexus, and mediastinum, has also been well relieved with radiation.

SUPERIOR VENA CAVAL SYNDROME   This is a frequent complication of locally advanced lung cancer. The more recent the onset of the symptoms caused by an obstruction of venous drainage, the faster the relief of the distressing symptoms by radiation therapy. For rapid decompression, a very effective regimen, with greater than 80% of relief of the presenting symptoms, has been radiation therapy by either an accelerated schedule, 150 cGy per fraction, twice daily for the first 4 to 5 days followed by a regular schedule of 180 to 200 cGy of daily fractions, 5 days a week, to a total dose of 5000 cGy (an approach we use), or a large fraction, 400 cGy of daily fractions, for the first 3 to 4 days followed by the regular 200 cGy of daily fractions, 5 days a week, to the same total

dose.[50] The former approach, using an accelerated schedule of 150 cGy of dose fractions, twice a day, would be preferable to the latter approach, using the large fraction size, in terms of sparing late-reacting tissues such as the spinal cord and lung. Relief of hoarseness by radiation therapy depends on the degree of injury to the recurrent laryngeal nerve by the tumor and its duration. Hoarseness alone without distant metastases should not preclude high dose radiation therapy, inasmuch as some of these patients can lead normal lives for many years. Complete recovery from hoarseness is, however, rare even with high dose radiation therapy, implying that recovery of the function of a damaged recurrent laryngeal nerve is exceptional.

**Tolerance of Normal Tissue to Radiation**   The response of normal tissue in the thorax to radiation therapy can be categorized as early, intermediate, or late.

*Radiation Esophagitis*   This condition is characterized by a mild to moderate degree of retrosternal discomfort; associated dysphagia usually begins at the third week of irradiation (threshold dose, 2000–2500 cGy) and reaches its peak at the fourth week. Esophagograms taken at the peak of the acute reaction reveal the margins of the barium column to be serrated. Differential diagnosis includes monilial esophagitis and herpes simplex viral esophagitis. Topical analgesics such as lidocaine in a 2% viscous solution provide a good relief of retrosternal discomfort. Antacids such as milk of magnesia or Mylanta [combination product: $Al(OH)_3$, $Mg(OH)_2$, and simethicone] are also very useful in minimizing moderate symptoms. Patients with a history of reflux esophagitis are started on Prilosec, 20 mg twice daily, to minimize the degree of dysphagia.

The course of radiation-induced esophagitis is self-limited, lasting 10 to 14 days after the completion of radiation therapy. Late sequelae such as stenosis, ulceration, and fistula formation of the esophagus are very rare when no direct invasion of the esophagus by the underlying lung cancer is present. There was no incidence of severe late sequelae in our series of 162 cases.[17] The use of certain chemotherapeutic agents (e.g., doxorubicin, daunorubicin, and possibly taxol) has been associated with potentiation and/or recall of radiation-induced esophagitis.[51–53] Even with relatively low radiation doses—for example, 500 to 1500 cGy—which are below the threshold dose for esophagitis, these potentiation and recall phenomena have been observed. Omission of doxorubicin from a few cycles of a combination program of chemotherapy immediately before and after radiation therapy has reduced the frequency and severity of this complication. Frequent recalls of severe radiation-induced esophagitis could lead to a stricture. As more patients are likely to be subjected to doxorubicin because of its effectiveness in small-cell cancer of the lung, it is important to be aware of this potential complication and to plan in advance the use of both radiation therapy and doxorubicin in a way that will minimize this undesirable side effect.

Radiation-induced injuries to normal tissue that appear after an intermediate latent period of 1 to 4 months include radiation pneumonitis and radiation carditis. Radiation-induced myelopathy has a long latent period of 1 to 2 years.

*Radiation Pneumonitis* This is a serious but controllable complication. The threshold dose of radiation pneumonitis is of the order of 2000 to 2500 cGy; thus it is far below the 6000 to 6400 cGy that are being used for control of stage III NSCLC.[54–57] Factors that influence the incidence and the degree of radiation pneumonitis include the volume of lung exposed to irradiation, total radiation dose, fraction size, fractionation schedule, radiation energy, and inhomogeneity factor. Among these factors, the lung volume that will receive radiation dose of 2500 cGy or more is probably the most important and critical factor in curative radiation therapy for lung cancer. The maximum lung volume that can be included in the high dose zone (> 5000 cGy) without the likelihood of significant clinical symptoms has not been well studied.

According to a study by us,[58] loss of pulmonary function as a result of thoracic radiation therapy is closely related to the degree of preexisting pulmonary function before radiation therapy. Patients with $FEV_1$ (forced expiratory volume of air exhaled in 1 second) greater than 50% of that predicted showed a statistically significant 16% to 28% decrease in $FEV_1$, forced vital capacity, maximum breathing capacity, peak expiratory flow rate, arid single-breath diffusing capacity for carbon monoxide. For patients with limited pulmonary reserve, defined as $FEV_1$ less than 50% of that predicted, the pattern of pulmonary function loss after radiation therapy was different. Contrary to the prediction, an improvement in pulmonary function occurred in 52% of patients, and only a small decrease in pulmonary function ($\leq$ 10% of the initial value) occurred in 37% of patients. Radiation therapy to the upper aspect of the chest for upper lobe tumors seems to be associated with a loss of pulmonary function that is much less than that resulting from radiation therapy to other sites, even in patients with poor pulmonary function reserve ($FEV_1$ < 50% of the predicted value). Radiation therapy for a centrally located tumor with associated compromised ventilation or perfusion at the involved side of the lung tends to result in an improvement of pulmonary function. Regional pulmonary function study is useful in predicting postradiotherapy pulmonary function. In our series treated with high dose radiotherapy with individually tailored Cerrobend blocks, a 5% incidence of symptomatic radiation pneumonitis was observed.[17]

With currently available regional pulmonary function studics and a three-dimensional conformal treatment plan, this volume factor can be defined more clearly than before in terms of functioning volume (i.e., ventilation and perfusion). Armstrong et al.[42] reported that the incidence of pulmonary toxicity of grade 3 or higher was 4% (1/23) when the lung volume in the radiation target receiving 2500 cGy or more was 30 or less, compared with 38% (3/8) when the lung volume receiving the same level of radiation dose was more than 30% of whole lung.

This level of pulmonary toxicity (grade $\geq$ 3) was noted in 29% (4/14) of patients when the predicted probability of normal tissue complication probability (NTCP) was at least 12%, whereas it was not observed in any of 17 patients (0/17) when the predicted probability of normal tissue complication probability (NTCP) was less than 12%.

Common presenting symptoms for acute radiation pneumonitis are cough, dyspnea, congestion, fullness of the chest, and a mild to moderate degree of fever (99–101°F). Chest radiographs may be negative at early stages. However, patchy consolidation and diffuse haziness in the area of the previous radiation therapy are the common early diagnostic changes that follow the pattern of radiation portals later. Treatment of acute radiation pneumonitis includes bed rest, bronchodilators, oxygen therapy, and corticosteroids.[59–62] In our experience, the acute symptoms of radiation pneumonitis have been well relieved by prednisone, 20 mg 3 times a day for the first 10 to 14 days. After control of acute symptoms has been achieved, the dose can be tapered over a period of several weeks. One should be aware of the possibility of subclinical radiation injuries in the lung activated by rapid withdrawal of the high dose corticosteroid therapy.[63] Antibiotics are given for positive sputum culture. However, prophylactic use of antibiotics in the absence of positive sputum culture is debatable. The late sequela of acute radiation pneumonitis is pulmonary fibrosis, which usually is asymptomatic and is demonstrable radiographically only along the hilar and paramediastinal areas where the previous radiation therapy was given.

Safety guides for thoracic radiation therapy for the underlying lung cancer include (1) careful selection of patients by exclusion of patients with very large tumors or with severe underlying pulmonary disease, (2) redesign of the radiation portals primarily along the periphery of the primary tumor mass at 2000 to 2500 cGy and again at 3400 to 3600 cGy as either the atelectatic lung reexpands or a significant degree of tumor regression occurs in a patient with a large tumor mass, (3) use of individually tailored Cerrobend blocks or multileaf collimator (MLC) to shield uninvolved pulmonary tissue, (4) use of a regular size of fraction of the order of 180 to 200 cGy, (5) corrections for lung inhomogeneity in the radiation dosimetry, and (6) the use of high energy beams. Split-course radiation therapy is a good and safe approach for patients at high risk for radiation pneumonitis. When total thoracic irradiation is judged necessary for palliation of metastatic tumors, the threshold dose for radiation pneumonitis is in the range of 1800 to 2000 cGy administered at a rate of 150 to 180 cGy daily fractions, 5 days a week, in adults. For young children, a total dose of 1400 to 1500 cGy administered at daily fractions of 150 cGy, 5 days a week, is near the limit of tolerance.[64] When adjuvant chemotherapeutic agents are used, notably actinomycin D, there should be a reduction in the tolerance dose of radiation by at least 10% to 15%.[54] Regional pulmonary function data have been helpful in selecting patients at high risk among those with underlying chronic obstructive pulmonary disease.[58]

*Radiation Pericarditis* Radiation-induced injuries to the heart have been rare in patients treated for lung cancer. An average target volume for high dose curative radiation therapy for lung cancer includes most of both atria and a small portion of the right ventricle at the base. Among 162 patients with lung cancer in our study,[17] there was only one patient whose symptoms were suggestive of pericarditis, and he responded well to conservative measures. A more common cause of pericarditis with pericardial effusion is a direct extension of the tumor from the primary or metastatic disease in the mediastinum to the pericardium. Common presenting symptoms for acute pericarditis induced by irradiation are fever, tachycardia, substernal pain, and dyspnea. Pericardial friction rub and effusion are frequent. Other objective findings include a widened cardiac silhouette and changes on the ECG such as an elevation of the ST segment, decrease in the

QRS voltage, and inversion of T waves. Conservative management with bed rest and other supportive measures usually is adequate. The course is self-limited. However, chronic constrictive pericarditis may occur when a large portion of the heart is included in the target volume. The threshold dose for radiation-induced cardiac damage is 4000 cGy in 20 fractions in 4 weeks to a major portion of the heart.[65] Extreme caution is required when radiation is supplemented by adjuvant chemotherapeutic agents, such as doxorubicin because of the synergistic cardiotoxicity of these drugs.[66] With a well-prepared plan in which doxorubicin is omitted from a few cycles of combination chemotherapy before and after radiation therapy, the risk of synergistic cardiotoxicity can be minimized. Acute exacerbation of subclinical radiation-induced injuries to the heart has also been reported after sudden withdrawal of high doses of corticosteroids.[63]

*Radiation Myelopathy* This is another serious but preventable complication. Two distinct types of radiation injury to the spinal cord are an early transient myelopathy (Lhermitte sign) and a late irreversible injury leading to paresis or paralysis. The early transient myelopathy is characterized by a complaint of electric shock–like sensation radiating down the back and over the extremities on flexion of the neck. It occurs a few months after the completion of radiation therapy and persists for 2 to 3 months without any sequelae. Temporary demyelination of the spinal cord due to the radiation-induced inhibition of myelin production by the oligodendroglia has been postulated as the underlying mechanism for the phenomenon.[67] There is no good correlation between the early transient myelopathy and the late irreversible myelitis. The threshold dose for Lhermitte sign is approximately 4000 cGy in 20 fractions in 4 weeks (TDF 66).

Late irreversible radiation-induced myelitis is a serious complication that should be prevented at all costs because there is no effective treatment for it. It is characterized by a long (10–24 months) latent period and by its resem-blance to a clinical presentation of partial or complete transection of the spinal cord (Brown–Sequard syndrome).[68,69] Diagnosis of this condition is made by exclusion of other conditions such as metastatic tumor compressing the spinal cord. The threshold dose for radiation myelitis is on the order of 4400 to 4600 cGy in 22 to 23 fractions over a period of 4.4 to 4.6 weeks (TDF 73–76) for large-field radiation therapy.[17,68] Careful planning of curative radiation therapy for malignant tumors in the chest is, of course, imperative. The use of a combination of AP-PA-POP with an AP-RPO-LPO (three fields) or multiple fields should prevent this serious late complication.

*New Trends in Prospect* New approaches are being sought to achieve control of local and regional tumors that is better than what the current radiation dose schedule combined with cisplatin-based chemotherapy has been able to attain. Uncontrolled local–regional tumors continue to comprise the major source of distant metastases and eventual failure.

*Altered Fractionation Schedules* Accelerated or hyperfractionated radiation therapy may exploit the radiobiologic advantages of both a reduced fraction size for late-reacting tissues (lung, spinal cord, connective tissue) and a shortened overall treatment time against rapidly proliferating tumors such as lung cancer.[70,71] Repair of sublethal radiation damage in aerobic mammalian cells is essentially complete within 2 to 4 hours.[72,73] When a rapidly proliferating tumor cell population such as lung cancer is growing in normal tissue whose cells are nonproliferative or slowly proliferating, an advantage accrues to the tumor cells if the treatment interval is greater than 4 hours. In such a situation, greater radiotherapeutic efficacy is expected with the use of two or three treatment sessions per day, with an essentially normal dose per fraction, total dose levels, and intervals of at least 4 hours between fractions.

In a clinical study, we compared a once-daily (QD) schedule with twice- and three-times-daily (BID and TID) schedules in the same patients with multiple sites of metastatic carcinoma to evaluate the response of normal human skin to accelerated fractionation schedules using 200 kV deep x-rays. The intertreatment interval was kept at 4 hours. This study showed that the BID or TID dose schedule required an 8% to 10% decrease in the total dose of QD schedule to yield the same level of acute skin response.[74] In Burkitt lymphoma, a complete response was obtained in 74% (25/34) of patients with a hyperfractionation schedule (120 cGy TID), versus 11% (1/9) by a conventional dose schedule (220 cGy QD).[75]

In recent studies, Saunders et al.[76–78] tested a concept of accelerated high dose fractionated radiation administered within a short period of time (12 days) before accelerated tumor proliferation begins in standard QD radiation therapy. Their pilot study with a continuous, hyperfractionated, accelerated radiotherapy (CHART) regimen [54 Gy/36 F/12 days by 1.5 Gy/F, 3 treatments/day (TID), 7 days/wk] showed an encouraging result when it was compared with the historical control at the same institution. The dose-limiting toxicity of this CHART regimen was acute esophagitis. This led to a phase III trial in which the CHART regimen (54 Gy/36 F/12 days by 1.5 Gy/F, 3 F/day, 7 days/wk) was compared with a standard QD radiation schedule (60 Gy/30 F/42 days) in patients with unresectable squamous cell cancer of the lung (stages I–III). The 2-year survival rates were 29% by CHART, compared with 20% by standard QD radiation ($p = 0.006$), and the main difference in survival was seen in T3-4 lesions.[77,78] Even with the total dose and dose intensity of the CHART schedule, the uncontrolled primary tumor was the principal cause of death in 62% of CHART patients, compared with 60% of the standard QD radiation group.[77,78] Therefore, this study seems to suggest that the dose intensity alone at the level of the dose-limiting toxicity of the CHART regimen may not be enough to offer local–regional tumor control to the majority of patients. It is also a concern that this level of dose intensity is most likely to lie beyond the dose-limiting toxicities of the esophageal mucosa for patients with N2 and N3 lesions when this dose is combined with concurrent chemotherapy.[79]

**H**yperfractionated **a**ccelerated **r**adiation **t**herapy (HART), a modified TID schedule of CHART with weekends off (5760 cGy/36 F/15 days), was tested in a phase II study by the Eastern Cooperative Oncology Group (ECOG). Mehta et al.[80] reported that grade 3 acute esophagitis was observed in 21% (6/28) of patients. The overall objective response rate, median survival, and 1-year survival rate were 54%, 13 months, and 57%. A phase III trial is being planned to compare the HART schedule with a conventional one (6000 cGy/30 F/6 wks) in sequential chemoradiotherapy.

*Concurrent Chemoradiotherapy* It has been demonstrated that chemoradiotherapy is better than radiation therapy alone for survival in stage III NSCLC. However, the study by Arriagada et al.[26,27] showed that sequential combination of chemotherapy and radiation therapy was effective in reducing metastatic failure from 70% of radiotherapy alone to 49% by the combined therapy. Even though there was no difference in local control rate, the decrease in distant failure resulted in improved survival. Schaake-Koning et al.[81] showed that radiation therapy combined with daily cisplatin was more effective than radiation therapy alone in achieving local tumor control, and this improved local tumor control was translated into survival gain. Indeed, Furuse et al.[82] conducted a phase III study in which results of concurrent versus sequential radiation therapy in combination with mitomycin, vindesine, and cisplatin were compared in unresectable stage III NSCLC. Preliminary analysis showed that concurrent combination of chemoradiotherapy was more effective than sequential combination in overall response and median survival time. The respective median survival time and 2- and 3-year survival rates were 16.5 months, 37%, and 27% by the concurrent combination, and 13.3 months, 26% and 13% by the sequential combination. More studies are needed to define the optimum chemoradiotherapy schedules.

*Preoperative Chemoradiotherapy Versus Chemotherapy In Stage IIIA And IIIB NSCLC* Fleck et al.[83] conducted a phase III randomized clinical trial in which preoperative concurrent chemoradiotherapy was compared with preoperative chemotherapy alone in patients with stage IIIA (N2) and IIIB (T4) NSCLC. The preoperative chemoradiotherapy consisted of two cycles of cisplatin, 100 mg/m$^2$ IV, on days 1 and 29, 5-fluorouracil (5-FU) in continuous infusion on days 1 to 4 and 29 to 32, and 30 Gy in 15 fractions for 3 weeks of concurrent radiation beginning day 1, and an additional 30 Gy postoperatively for patients with residual disease. Patients in the preoperative chemotherapy alone arm received intravenously three cycles of cisplatin (100 mg/m$^2$) plus mitomycin C (8 mg/m$^2$) on days 1, 29, and 71, and vinblastine (4.5 mg/m$^2$ IV) every 2 weeks for six doses prior to surgery; patients with residual disease received, postoperatively, three additional cycles of intravenous cisplatin (30 mg/m$^2$) plus etoposide (100 mg/m$^2$) every 3 weeks. Surgery was performed 12 weeks after the initiation of the treatment.

The results of this study, all of which favor preoperative concurrent chemoradiotherapy over chemotherapy alone, were as follows: objective response rate, 67% (32/48) versus 44% (21/48), $p = 0.02$; resection rate, 52% (25/48) versus 31% (15/48), $p = 0.03$; and rate of freedom from progression, 40% (19/48) versus 21% (10/48), $p = 0.04$. A high incidence of recurrence in the brain was reported among the patients who relapsed after 18 months. Even though the final report with long-term survival data has not been made, the early results of this study support the hypothesis that preoperative radiotherapy administered concurrently with chemotherapy may result in complete resection rate higher than what preoperative chemotherapy alone can provide. This improved rate of complete resection might have led to the better local tumor control and survival. The preoperative radiation dose schedule (30 Gy/15 F/3 wks) used in this study is judged to be less than optimum dose schedule.

Phase II studies that employed preoperative BID radiation therapy and two cycles of concurrent chemotherapy in patients with mediastinoscopically staged IIIA (N2) and IIIB NSCLC include those of Choi et al.[36] and Grunenwald et al.[37] This BID radiation therapy consisted of 42 Gy in 28 fractions for 4 weeks, broken down as follows: 21 Gy in 14 fractions for 9 days in the first session, a 10-day rest to allow recovery of the esophageal mucosa from mucositis, and another 21 Gy in 14 fractions for 9 days in the second session. The chemotherapy consisted of cisplatin, 100 mg/m$^2$ IV, on days 1 and 29; vinblastine, 4 mg/m$^2$ IV bolus, on days 1 and 29; and 5-FU, 30 mg/kg/day by continuous infusion, on days 1 to 3 and 29 to 31. Postoperative therapy included one more cycle of the same chemotherapy regimen and additional dose of 18 Gy in 12 fractions for 6 treatment days using the BID schedule of 1.5 Gy dose fractions.

The toxicities in the study by Choi et al.[36] included grade 4 neutropenia, 14% (16/113 chemotherapy cycles), hospital admission for febrile neutropenia, 9% (10/113), and grade 4 dysphagia, 14% (6/42 patients). There were three (7%) treatment-associated deaths: one pulmonary embolism during induction therapy, one postoperative death from cardiac failure, and one from aspiration pneumonia.

This study resulted in a complete resection rate of 84%, histopathologic tumor downstaging (from stage IIIA N2 to stages 0, 10%; I, 24%; II, 33%) in 67%, and 5-year survival rate of 37% (Figure 7-3). Patients who attained a tumor downstaging from the initial stage IIIA (N2) to stage 0 or I by the preoperative therapy showed a 5-year survival rate of 60%, whereas it was only 20% for those whose tumor stage remained unchanged (Figure 7-4). The patterns of failure showed overall local–regional failure, 25% (5/20); brain only, 30% (6/20); and systemic in 55% (11/20) of all recurrences.

The results of the study by Grunenwald et al.[37] in patients with stage IIIB NSCLC deserves attention. Thirty patients (T4 lesion, 18; N3, 12) were enrolled into this study between January 1993 and March 1995. Tumor progression occurred in five patients; two patients died, and

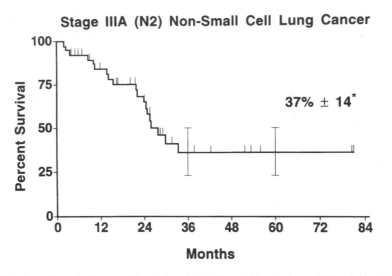

**FIGURE 7-3** Overall survival curve of the study cohort with neoadjuvant chemo-BID radiotherapy; asterisk indicates 95% confidence interval.[36]

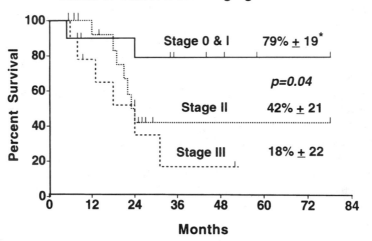

**FIGURE 7-4** Impact of histopathologic tumor downstaging on survival with neoadjuvant chemoradiotherapy; asterisk indicates 95% confidence interval.[36]

one developed intercurrent infection during induction therapy. Complete resection was performed in 57% (17/30) of patients through a midline sternotomy, with bilateral mediastinal lymphadenectomy. There was one postoperative death (6%). Pathologic complete response was obtained in 10% (3/30) of patients. With a median follow-up of 36 months, MST was 15 months and an overall 3-year survival rate was 25% (95% CI: 12–43%). This result is consistent with that of Choi et al.[36] in that the concomitant chemo-BID radiation therapy is effective, with a high resection and survival rate in both stage IIIA and IIIB NSCLC.

In another interesting study, Eberhardt et al.[38] tested preoperative chemo-BID radiotherapy (12 wk course) in patients with stage IIB to IIIB NSCLC. The chemotherapy included four cycles of cisplatin (60 mg/m², days 1 and 7) and etoposide (150 mg/m², days 3–5) every 3 weeks. Three cycles were given before radiation therapy, and the fourth cycle was given with BID radiation (45 Gy, 1.5 Gy/F, BID, in 3 wks). Ninety-four patients (75 men and 19 women) were enrolled into this study. Patient characteristics included the following: median age of 55 (range, 31–71); performance status 1 (range, 0–2) and tumor stages IIB, 6 (T3 N0), IIIA, 46 (T1-2 N2, 29; T3 N2, 17) and IIIB, 42 (T1-3 N3, 23; T4 N0-1, 8; T4 N2-3, 11). Toxicities included grade 3 and 4 leukopenia, 48% and 12%; grade 3 and 4 thrombocytopenia, 18% and 13%; grade 3 infection, 3%; grade 3 and 4 esophagitis, 37% and 3%, and septic death, two patients. Complete resection was obtained in 53% (50/94) of patients, 60% (31/52) of stage IIIA and 45% (19/42) of stage IIIB groups. Pathologic complete response was observed in 29% (15/52) of all stage IIIA, 24% (11/46) of T1-3 N2, 21% (9/42) of all stage IIIB, and 18% (6/34)

of T1-4 N3 groups respectively. The MST and 4-year survival rates were 20 months and 31% for stage IIIA and 18 months and 26% for stage IIIB patients, respectively. The relapse in the brain was observed in 9% (4/47) versus 46% (13/28) of patients with or without elective cranial irradiation. However, this difference in the relapse in the brain was not translated into a gain in survival. The high pathological complete response and 4-year survival rates are very encouraging and may reflect potential achievements in concurrent chemoradiotherapy for an increase in the radiation dose intensity and total dose.

*Innovations in Improving Therapeutic Ratio*
Attempts to improve differential dose distribution between the tumor and the surrounding normal tissue have included interstitial implants of radioactive seeds labeled with iodine-125,[84] the use of intraoperative cobalt 60 or electron beam to either the primary tumor mass or the tumor bed[85] and endobronchial brachytherapy (Figure 7-5). Further studies are necessary to establish

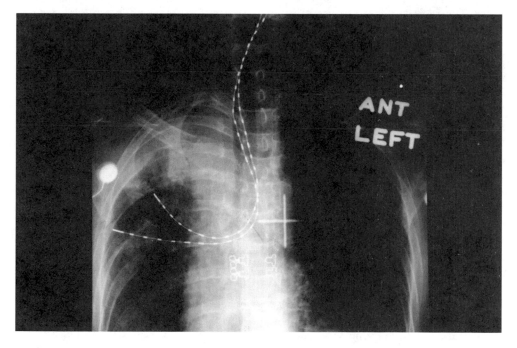

**FIGURE 7-5**   AP film of chest showing two endobronchial catheters placed into the right upper lobe bronchus for endobronchial brachytherapy.

specific roles for these approaches to stage III NSCLC. New approaches that are being developed include intensity-modulated (IM) photon radiotherapy and IM proton radiotherapy optimized to tumor response monitors.

*Measures to Overcome Hypoxic Tumor Cells* Studies aimed at reducing the potential impact of hypoxic tumor cells have included high linear energy transfer (LET) beams such as neutrons,[86] radiation therapy under hyperbaric conditions,[87] hypoxic cell sensitizers such as misonidazole[88] and tirapazamine,[89] and hyperthermia.[90] These studies are still in experimental stages.

## II. Radiation Therapy for Medically Inoperable Stage I NSCLC

*Introduction* Surgery is the treatment of choice for stage I and II NSCLC. However, patients with early-stage NSCLC, even though it is resectable, may not be able to tolerate surgery because of underlying limited pulmonary or cardiac reserve. For such patients, radiation therapy is an acceptable alternative for cure. The radiation dose necessary when the goal is cure is of the order of 6000 to 6600 cGy in 30 to 33 fractions for 6 to 6.6 weeks. High energy photons in the range of 4 to 10 MV from a linear accelerator are suitable for this purpose.

The first report on this subject was made by Hilton[91] and Smart.[20] Nine of 40 patients (22.5%) survived 5 years after radiation therapy alone. Of the many patients for whom curative surgery is not possible, only those with disease still limited to the chest are suitable for curative radiation therapy aimed at eradication of the tumor.

*General Assessment* A patient's general condition, even though not medically suitable for surgery, should be good enough to tolerate a course of thoracic radiotherapy that lasts for 6 to 7 weeks, ascertained by a performance status of at least 70 on the Karnofsky scale and grade 0-1 on the Zubrod scale. Patients who are judged to be potential candidates for curative radiation therapy should be evaluated by complete physical examination and staging workup, as carefully as those for whom curative surgery is contemplated.

Laboratory examination of blood cell counts, blood urea nitrogen, electrolytes, and liver function should be performed. Patients with low hemoglobin concentrations ($\leq$ 10 g/dL) require transfusion of packed red blood cells to increase the hemoglobin level to normal ($\geq$ 12 g/dL). Low hemoglobin concentration was found to be associated with a high rate of local recurrence after radiation therapy in solid tumors. Leukopenia (WBC $\leq$ 2000/mm$^3$) and thrombocytopenia (platelets $\leq$ 100,000/mm$^3$) should be carefully evaluated and corrected before radiation therapy begins. Patients with hepatic or renal failure must be evaluated carefully for their tolerance to high dose radiation therapy. A careful assessment of a patient's cardiopulmonary status is an essential part of the general evaluation for the suitability of curative radiation therapy. It may be necessary to compromise radiation dose and target volume for patients with either poor pulmonary or cardiac reserve. Regional pulmonary function test is useful in assessing pulmonary tolerance in patients with borderline functional reserve inasmuch as it may help predict tolerance to the proposed radiation therapy before it is administered.

*Target Volume* For a peripheral T1-2 N0 M0 lesion, target volume includes the primary lesion (GTV) and a margin of 1.0 cm surrounding normal lung tissue as a CTV. The ipsilateral hilum does not need to be included. For a centrally located T1-2 N0 M0 lesion near the hilum, the ipsilateral hilum is included in CTV because the risk for having microscopic metastasis in the hilar node is higher than that of the peripheral lesion and morbidity added may not be significant. When the ipsilateral hilar lymph nodes are judged to be involved (N1 lesion) by radiographic or histologic examination, target volume includes GTV and CTV of the mediastinal nodal station of 7, 4R, and 4L as a target volume for subclinical disease.

***Radiation Dose and Fractionation Schedules***   There are several different dose fractionation schedules that have similar biologic effects on both normal and malignant tissues. For medically inoperable stages I and II NSCLC, a dose–fractionation schedule of 6000 to 6600 cGy in 30 to 32 fractions for 6 to 6.6 weeks is recommended. The optimal dose schedule for stage I and II NSCLC remains to be determined.

***Radiation Portal Arrangements***   The arrangement of radiation portals depends on the planned total dose, the types of radiation, and the size and location of the target volume. For a peripheral T1-2 lesion, a simple and accurate arrangement, having the least risk of a geographical miss, consists of two parallel opposed portals (POP) applied anteroposteriorly (AP) and posteroanteriorly (PA) or oblique opposed portals to the chest. For a right-sided central lesion near the hilum, a combination of AP-PA-RPO portals may be adequate for high dose radiation therapy with curative intent. CBT of the chest would be useful in determining the angle of oblique beams and portal sizes. Three-dimensional conformal therapy is recommended for radiation dose escalation beyond the dose level of 6600 cGy in 33 fractions for 6.6 weeks.

***Results and Future Directions***   It is very encouraging to note that 5-year cause-specific survival rate can be as high as 32% with contemporary radiotherapy alone, using radiation dose schedules of 6000 to 6600 cGy in 30 to 33 fractions for 6 to 6.6 weeks in stage I medically inoperable NSCLC (Table 7-3).[92–97] However, this level of radiation dose is still associated with a high local failure rate ($\geq$ 50%).[96,97] Distant failure rate was also noted to be high at 40%. Future research should be directed to a radiation dose escalation using three-dimensional conformal therapy to determine the maximum tolerated dose (MTD) of radiation and use of such radiation dose at MTD level for improved local tumor control and survival. It is also desirable to combine weekly chemotherapy (i.e., daily or weekly cisplatin, carboplatin, and taxol regimen) to treat distant microscopic disease as well as to increase local tumor control by chemoradiation interaction.

## III. Postoperative Radiation Therapy in Stage II and III NSCLC

The fate of patients with either unforeseen N2 disease (undetected by mediastinoscopy) or resection margins positive for residual carcinoma (T3-4 lesion) is poor, with a 5-year survival rate ranging from 0% to 20%.[98–101] It has been well demonstrated that radiation therapy is capable of sterilizing carcinoma of the lung at the primary site and the regional lymph nodes when an adequate radiation dose is employed (i.e., 5400 cGy/30 F/6 wks for microscopic tumors and 6400 cGy/32 F/6.4 wk for gross tumors). Therefore carefully planned radiation

**Table 7-3   Radiation Therapy for Medically Inoperable Stage I (T1-2 N0 M0) NSCLC**

| Radiation Dose (cGY) | Stage | Results (%) | | | Ref. |
|---|---|---|---|---|---|
| | | 5-Year Survival | Local Failure | Distant Metastases | |
| 5000–5500 | Limited | 22.5 ($n = 40$) | | | Smart[20] |
| 5400–5900 | T1-2 N0 | 21 ($n = 43$) | 39 | | Haffty et al.[93] |
| 5500–7000 | T1-2 N0 | 32 ($n = 44$) | | | Zhang et al.[94] |
| 5000–6000 | T1 N0 | 29 ($n = 35$) | | | Graham[95] |
| 6000–6500 | T1-2 N0 | 31 ($n = 108$)[a] | 66 | 31 | Krot et al.[96] |
| 6400 | T1-2 N0 | 32 ($n = 141$)[a] | 49 | 38 | Sibley et al.[97] |

[a] Cause-specific survival.

therapy with a moderately high dose (5400–5600 cGy; TDF 89–92) of radiation should be able to convert a surgical resection from incomplete to complete by sterilizing the residual microscopic carcinoma at the tumor bed and regional lymph nodes. When such postoperative radiotherapy is combined with chemotherapy, an improvement in survival may result.

**Review of Previous Studies** Previous studies, including the meta-analysis data by PORT Meta-analysis Trialists Group of individual patient data from nine randomized controlled trials, need a revisit.[102–110]

The meta-analysis data showed that there was no survival advantage to postoperative radiation therapy in stage I disease. This finding is not contrary to expectation. Instead, the survival of these patients was adversely affected by postoperative radiotherapy.[104] Therapeutic factors associated with the adverse outcome included the use of a cobalt-60 unit, postpneumonectomy status, and radiation dose–fractionation schedule using high total dose (6000 cGy/30 F/6 wk) and large fraction sizes (> 200 cGy/F).[102] There was no survival advantage to postoperative radiation therapy in stage II disease as well. The results in stage III NSCLC were inconclusive. A randomized trial by Lung Cancer Study Group (LCSG) also showed that postoperative radiotherapy did not improve survival.[109] However, there was a decrease in local recurrence with postoperative radiotherapy. Dautzenberg et al.[110] conducted a prospective randomized study in which postoperative radiotherapy (n = 129 patients; 6000 cGy/30 F/6 wks) was compared with postoperative sequential chemoradiotherapy (n = 138 patients) in patients with resected stage II and III NSCLC. Chemotherapy consisted of three cycles of cyclophosphamide, doxorubicin, cisplatin, vincristine, and lomustine. There was no difference in overall survival and disease-free survival between the two groups. However, in the N0-1 versus N2 subset analysis, there was a survival gain by sequential chemoradiotherapy over radiation therapy alone in stage III (N2) group (n = 137 pa-

tients). Two- and 5-year survival rates were 22% and 6% for postoperative radiotherapy, compared with 36% and 19% for postoperative sequential chemoradiotherapy group, p = 0.003. In patients with N0-1 lesions (n = 130 patients), the 2- and 5-year survival rates were 54% and 34% for postoperative radiotherapy, respectively, compared with 38% and 17% for chemoradiotherapy groups, p = 0.03.

**Indication for Postoperative Chemoradiotherapy** Postoperative chemoradiotherapy is indicated for the following conditions: T3-4 lesion following an incomplete resection and unforeseen N2 lesion (stage IIIA). The role of postoperative radiotherapy in stage II (N1) NSCLC is less well defined. However, patients with extensive involvement of the lymph nodes at hilar and interlobar nodal stations (≥ 50% of sampled nodes being involved) may have a high risk for regional recurrence, and postoperative radiotherapy combined with chemotherapy may be beneficial in this situation. Patients with stage II (N1) NSCLC by virtue of an involvement of lymph nodes at lobar, segmental, and subsegmental nodal stations may not benefit from postoperative radiotherapy.

**Radiotherapeutic Techniques** The importance of radiotherapeutic techniques cannot be overemphasized, inasmuch as the outcome of the treatment depends heavily on the success or failure of the sterilization of the residual tumor in the target volume and the relative frequency of serious complications associated with the techniques used.[111]

*Target Volume* The target volume for patients with extensively involved lymph nodes at hilar and/or interlobar nodal stations (advanced N1 status) includes the bronchial stump with a 2.0 to 2.5 cm margin of the remaining ipsilateral hilum, and the next sentinel group of mediastinal lymph nodes. The target volume for a right-sided lesion includes the right hilum and the mediastinal sentinel lymph nodes at 7, 4R, and 4L nodal stations (Figure 7-1). For left-sided tumor, the target volume includes bronchial stump, left hilum, and mediastinal sentinel lymph nodes at 7, 4L, 4R, 5, and 6 nodal stations.

When the tumor involves the chest wall or diaphragm, the tumor bed should be treated with a generous margin of 3 to 4 cm. The ipsilateral axilla should be included in the target volume when the upper lateral chest wall is involved by the tumor (T3 lesion). When mediastinal lymph nodes are found to be involved after surgery, the target volume includes the bronchial stump, ipsilateral hilum (after lobectomy), involved nodal station in the mediastinum, and one sentinel nodal station beyond the involved nodal station.

*Optimal Dose and Fractionation Schedule*
The optimal dose schedule for sterilization of microscopic residual carcinoma of the lung at either the tumor bed or the regional lymph nodes is on the order of 5200 to 6000 cGy (TDF 86–99), administered by daily fractions of 180 to 200 cGy, 5 days a week, over a period of 5.5 to 6 weeks. Our previous study showed that a radiation dose schedule of 5400 cGy in 30 fractions for 6 weeks is near optimum in forestalling a relapse of the tumor at the regional lymphatic areas or the tumor bed.[106]

*Radiation Portal Arrangements*   The primary objective for careful selection of radiotherapeutic techniques is to administer a radiation dose of 5400 cGy selectively to the tumor bed and regional lymphatic areas to sterilize residual microscopic carcinoma of the lung, while the remaining pulmonary tissue, the heart, and the spinal cord are spared excessive doses of radiation. In designing the arrangement of radiation portals after lobectomy or pneumonectomy, the author takes into consideration the amount of the remaining pulmonary tissue.[111]

For patients who have had a right upper lobectomy, a total dose of 5400 cGy is administered to the target volume by a combination of AP-PA-RPO portals. With this technique, most of the remaining pulmonary tissue and spinal cord are spared an excessive dose of radiation

while the target volume is adequately treated. For patients who have had a left pneumonectomy, a total dose of 5400 cGy is administered by a combination of AP-PA-LPO portals. With this approach, the bronchial stump and the mediastinal CTV are well covered by an isodose line of greater than 5200 cGy.

*Results*   The ultimate goal of postoperative radiation therapy is to improve the chance of cure for patients with a high risk of local and regional failures. However, postoperative radiation therapy is a local and regional treatment, and if there are preexisting distant metastases, its benefit may not result in a gain in survival.

*Survival in Relation to Stage and Histologic Type*   For patients with early stage of lung cancer (T1 N0 M0, T2 N0 M0 lesions), the cure rate by surgery alone is in the range of 30% to 40%, and the majority of failures are due to the distant metastases. As expected, there has been no significant improvement of survival for patients with early stages of lung cancer after postoperative irradiation.[102]

For patients with locally advanced lung cancer (unforeseen N2, or T3 lesions), carefully administered postoperative radiation therapy has been able to improve survival. As shown in the author's series and others, the cure rate of patients with N2 lesions has been improved from 5% to 10% by surgery alone to 10% to 30% after adjuvant postoperative irradiation.[105–108] Contrary to expectation, the benefit of postoperative radiation therapy for patients with unforeseen N2, or T3 adenocarcinoma seems even better than that for patients with other histologic types.[106,107]

## IV. Superior Pulmonary Sulcus Tumor

Lung cancer occurring at the apex of the lung and invading the superior pulmonary sulcus was first described by Pancoast in 1924.[112] Situated in the narrow confines of the thoracic inlet, this tumor invades the lymphatics in the endothoracic fascia and involves, by direct extensions, the lower routes of the brachial

plexus, the intercostal nerves, the stellate ganglion, the sympathetic chain, and adjacent ribs
and vertebrae, producing severe pain over the
shoulder and along the dermatomes of C-8 and
T-1, and producing Horner syndrome (Pancoast syndrome).[113] Radiographic studies of the
chest show a shadow in the apex of the chest,
and often destruction of the posterior portions
of the second and third ribs and corresponding
transverse processes of the vertebrae. Histologic subtypes include squamous cell carcinoma in 50%, large-cell carcinoma in 30%,
and adenocarcinomas in 20%.

**Workup**    Histologic diagnosis of superior
pulmonary sulcus carcinoma can be made by
needle aspiration biopsy in the majority of patients. CBT scan of the chest provides essential
information in defining the extent of the tumor,
its relationship with the surrounding tissues/
structures, and resectability. MRI of the chest
provides necessary information when the resectability of the tumor is in question because
of its invasion into the spinal canal and/or
brachial plexus. Bone scan is also important in
detecting tumor invasion into the ribs and adjacent vertebrae that may be a subtle finding by
other imaging studies. In addition, mediastinoscopy is also recommended to spare patients
with N2-3 disease from being subjected to radical surgery.

**Treatments and Results**    Radiotherapy
was employed as early as the 1920s for palliation of symptoms, with some benefit.[113] Because of the invasive nature of superior
pulmonary sulcus tumor to the surrounding
important normal structures, surgery alone has
been ineffective in achieving long-term cure.
Paulson and colleagues pioneered a combined
approach of preoperative radiotherapy followed by extended en bloc resection of the tumor, the chest wall, and the involved adjacent
structures.[114–117] The theoretical bases for the
use of preoperative radiation are as follows:

1. The periphery of the tumor is better oxygenated and more sensitive to radiation

than is its core, and inoperable tumors
can be converted operable by a moderate
dose of radiation.

2. Preoperative radiation before surgery
   can reduce the number and mitotic capabilities of tumor cells shed into the operative fields and systemic circulation.

3. More conservative surgery may be used
   with an equal or better chance for cure.

4. Metastatic tumors in the regional lymph
   nodes that are inaccessible to surgery
   can also be controlled.

The results of the combined approach have
been better than those after either radical
surgery or radiation therapy alone.[116,117] The radiation dose schedule used by Mallams et al.
consisted of 3000 cGy in 10 fractions over 12
days to the tumor region, including the adjacent ipsilateral mediastinum.[115] The ipsilateral
hilum was not included in the treatment volume. An extended en bloc resection was carried out 3 to 6 weeks after radiotherapy. The
procedures comprised an extended radical
lobectomy or segmental resection and resection of the posterior portions of the involved
first two or three ribs, the transverse processes
of the upper thoracic vertebrae, the intercostal
nerves, the lower trunk of the brachial plexus,
the stellate ganglion, and a portion of the dorsal sympathetic chain.[114,116] A partial resection
of the upper thoracic vertebrae is also included
if there is a minimal involvement of the vertebrae. Calculated by the actuarial method, Paulson's approach resulted in a 2-, 5-, and 10-year
survival of 39%, 35%, and 26%, respectively,
in carefully selected patients ($n = 68$). When
there was no regional lymph node involvement,
this combined approach resulted in a 5- and 10-
year survival of 44% and 33%, respectively.
There was no 3-year survivor among 15 patients who had involvement of hilar or mediastinal lymph nodes.

The combined approach used by us is somewhat different from that of Paulson and cowork-
ers in two respects, although all the results are
similar.[118,119] In our series, the treatment volume

for preoperative radiation included the ipsilateral hilum and the upper two-thirds of the mediastinum, including the entire thoracic inlet and the subcarinal region. The dose schedule for preoperative radiation consisted of daily fractions of 180 to 200 cGy, 5 days a week, over a period of 5 to 5.6 weeks for a total dose of 4500 to 5000 cGy, followed by an extended en bloc resection 3 to 4 weeks after irradiation. An accelerated dose schedule using a BID radiotherapy was also used in recent patients. This preoperative radiotherapy has also been combined with two cycles of cisplatin-based chemotherapy in the last 2 years. According to the intent-to-treat analysis, preoperative radiotherapy followed by surgery resulted in a 5-year survival rate of 33% ($n = 34$ patients).[120] Radiation therapy alone resulted in a 5-year survival rate of 7% ($n = 39$ patients) in patients who were judged inoperable at the outset (Table 7-4).

Hilaris and Martini reported a 5-year survival of 17% (7 of 41 patients) after use of the combined approach of resection and interstitial implant.[118] For patients who had only a partial resection and implant, the 2-year survival rate was 35%. Of the patients whose condition was considered inoperable, 8% survived for 2 years. The main advantage of an interstitial implant over external irradiation is its ability to

**TABLE 7-4   Results of Therapies for Superior Pulmonary Sulcus Tumor**

| Study | Number of Patients | 5-Year Survival (%) |
|---|---|---|
| *Combined Radiation Therapy and Surgery* | | |
| Paulson[116] | 78 | 35 (44% if N0) |
| Wright et al.[117] | 21 | 27 |
| Hilaris and Manini[118] | 82[a] | 29 |
| Neal et al.[119] | 28 | 21 |
| Hagan et al.[120] | 34 | 33 |
| *Radiation Therapy Alone* | | |
| Van Houtte et al.[121] | 31 | 18 |
| Komaki et al.[122] | 31 | 23 (at 2 years) |
| Hagan et al.[120] | 39 | 7 |

[a]Interstitial brachytherapy was used for patients with incomplete resection.

administer a high radiation dose to the area of the residual tumor while the surrounding normal tissue is spared an excessive radiation dose. However, it is difficult to place the radioactive sources evenly within the complex treatment volume without inducing a hot or cold spot. A combination of external radiation with interstitial implant may improve the dose homogeneity in the target volume.

External radiotherapy alone has also been used for superior pulmonary sulcus tumor if surgery is not to be performed because of the underlying medical condition or extensive invasion of the surrounding structures, that is, the brachial plexus, subclavian arteries, vertebral bodies, and the mediastinum. In definitive radiotherapy, a total dose of 6000 to 6400 cGy is administered in daily fractions of 180 to 200 cGy, 5 days a week. The radiation dose to the CTV is limited to 5000 cGy, and a boost dose of 1600 cGy is given to the GTV. The dose to the spinal cord is limited to 4400 cGy. A reasonable dose distribution within this complex target volume can be achieved by employing a combination of AP-PA-POP for the initial 3600 cGy, AP-RPO-LPO for the next 1800 cGy, and oblique opposed portals for the final 1000 cGy. A long-term cure rate by definitive radiotherapy alone for superior pulmonary sulcus tumor is on the order of 5% to 10%.[121,122] The local failure rate can be as high as 45% to 50% by radiotherapy alone, with tumor spread to the spinal canal being a common final event for tumors located medially along the vertebral bodies.

Since distant metastasis is as frequent as local failure in advanced stage disease, we have used concurrent chemotherapy and radiation therapy with moderate but acceptable esophagitis and leukopenia. The result of this combined approach is expected to be better than that of radiation therapy alone.

## V.   Role of Radiation Therapy in SCLC

***Evolution of Therapeutic Approaches in Limited Stage SCLC***   Therapeutic trials for limited stage SCLC have evolved from local–regional treatments to a combined approach of chemotherapy and radiotherapy. In the early 1960s, the Medical Research Council of Great Britain conducted a prospective randomized trial in which radiation therapy was compared with surgery for patients with operable and resectable SCLC.[123] Radiotherapy resulted in a 5- and 10-year survival of 4% (3 of 73 patients), compared with 0% at 3 years among 34 patients who underwent a complete resection.[123] With the advent of multidrug therapy in the late 1970s came a significant improvement in median survival time (MST) of patients with the limited stage SCLC, from 5 to 6 months with thoracic radiotherapy alone to 10 to 14 months with chemotherapy plus thoracic radiotherapy or chemotherapy alone.[124–126] Even for patients with the extensive stage SCLC, a complete remission was achieved in approximately 20% to 30% of patients, and their survival time could be expected to equal that of patients with the limited stage SCLC.[127] However, despite the earlier optimistic predictions based on short-term experiences with multidrug chemotherapy, the magnitude of improvement in long-term cure by chemotherapy and thoracic radiotherapy seems not to have materialized.[128–131]

Uncontrolled local–regional disease continues to be a major obstacle to efforts to improve survival in patients with limited stage SCLC.[132–135] Cancer and Leukemia Group B (CALGB) conducted a prospective randomized trial in which chemotherapy alone was compared with chemotherapy plus concurrent radiotherapy for local tumor control and survival.[136] The chemotherapy regimen, which was administered every 3 weeks for 18 months, consisted of cyclophosphamide, etoposide, and vincristine, with doxorubicin subsequently replacing etoposide in alternate cycles 7 through 18. The radiotherapy schedule consisted of 5000 cGy in 25 fractions for 5 weeks. Failure-free survival rates at 2 years were 20% for chemotherapy plus radiotherapy, compared with 8% for chemotherapy alone. Local–regional failure rate was 80% for chemotherapy alone, compared with 50% for combined chemotherapy plus radiotherapy.

The current once-a-day (QD) radiotherapy schedules using 4500 to 5000 cGy in 180 to 200 cGy dose fractions, 5 days per week, in concurrent chemoradiotherapy are still associated with a local–regional failure rate of 50% to 70%.[136–138] Therefore, uncontrolled local–regional disease continues to be a major obstacle in an effort to improve survival in patients with limited stage SCLC. An improvement in radiation dose schedules seems necessary for a better local–regional tumor control and survival.

***Radiation Dose–Tumor Response Relationship in SCLC*** Is there a radiation dose–tumor control relationship in SCLC? In a retrospective study, Choi and Carey[132] showed that a reasonable correlation exists between radiation dose and local tumor control. Local–regional tumor control lasting 4 months or more was achieved in 60%, 79%, and 88% at 3000 cGy, 4000 cGy, and 4800 cGy, respectively, using a fractional dose of 200 cGy, 5 fractions per week, in a study that was done prior to the era of cisplatin-based regimens, and median survival time was only 9 months. In a follow-up study,[139] Choi and Carey reported that this same QD radiation schedule of 4500 to 5000 cGy in 25 to 28 fractions for 5.6 weeks, given with concurrent cisplatin-based chemotherapy, was still associated with a local–regional failure rate of 40% (Figure 7-6). As the median survival time was increased from 9 months prior to the era of cisplatin-based chemotherapy to 18 months in the follow-up study, the latent period for local–regional tumor recurrence was increased up to 30 months. Therefore, it was suggested that the effectiveness of a given radiation dose schedule for local–regional tumor control needs to be assessed for a period of 30 months to appreciate the full magnitude of the issue of local failure.

***Significance of Timing Thoracic Radiation Early in Concurrent Chemoradiotherapy*** Murray et al.[140] conducted a randomized trial in which early radiotherapy (with cycle 2 chemotherapy) was compared with late radiotherapy (with cycle 6 chemo-

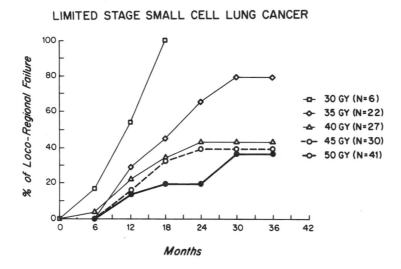

**FIGURE 7-6**  Radiation dose–tumor control relation in limited-stage SCLC.[140]

therapy) in concurrent chemoradiotherapy for patients with limited stage SCLC. The thoracic radiation dose schedule consisted of a total dose of 4000 cGy in 15 fractions for 3 weeks, using a daily dose fractions of 267 cGy. The MST and 3- and 4-year survival rates were 20 months, 32%, and 25% for the early timing group ($n = 155$ patients) of thoracic radiotherapy, compared with 15 months, 22%, and 15% for the late timing group ($n = 153$ patients) of thoracic radiotherapy, $p = 0.016$.

Even though the early timing of thoracic radiotherapy in concurrent chemoradiotherapy resulted in a better survival than that of late timing, the local–regional failure rate was 55% in both early and late radiotherapy groups and was consistent with the dose–response data reported by us.[139] Although the dose intensity of this schedule was higher than that of the standard radiation schedule, the total dose seemed inadequate for achieving a high level of local tumor control.

Arriagada et al. reported results of local tumor control relative to the total radiation dose that was increased from 4500 cGy (1500-1500-1500 cGy of split-course radiation alternating with chemotherapy) to 6500 cGy (2000-2000-2500 cGy) using 250 cGy of dose fractions,

four times per week.[141,142] The rate of local failure varied from 39% to 47% without a significant difference between the radiation schedules. However, the total doses tested in this study were administered in three split radiation sessions over a period of 10.5 to 12 weeks instead of a 5- to 6-week period in the standard once-a-day schedule. Therefore, the dose intensity of these split-course schedules may not have been equivalent to 4500 to 6000 cGy in 25 to 30 fractions for 5 to 6 weeks of the standard QD radiotherapy schedule. In addition, this alternating schedule did not have the advantage of the potentially enhanced cytotoxic effect associated with concurrent chemoradiotherapy. Thus, the absence of a dose–response relationship between the tested dose groups (4500–6500 cGy) in split-course radiotherapy does not preclude the presence of such a relationship in a continuous QD or hyperfractionated–accelerated (HA) BID radiation schedule, especially when the radiation is given concurrently with chemotherapy.

### Gain in Local–Regional Tumor Control Versus Increase in Survival
Will an increase in local–regional tumor control by an improved radiotherapy schedule, that is more

effective than what has been used currently in concurrent chemoradiation, result in a survival gain in patients with limited stage SCLC? Arriagada et al.[143] presented a strong argument for more effort in improving local tumor control that could result in increased survival in limited stage SCLC. By using a competing risk approach, which takes into account local recurrence, distant metastases, and death without cancer as competing events for the same end point, death, Arriagada observed that the 2-year isolated local recurrence rate, 33%, is as high as the 34.1% combined rate of both distant metastases alone (24.6%) and simultaneous distant metastases and local failure (9.5%). When local recurrence alone and local recurrence with simultaneous distant metastases are grouped into one category of local recurrence (42%) and compared with isolated distant metastasis alone (24.6%), the issue of local failure could become even more important. Given the assumption that uncontrolled local–regional tumor remains a persistent source for continuous distant seeding, this latter interpretation may be more appropriate. The negative impact of uncontrolled local disease on survival may have been underestimated by statistical methods that censor or ignore other events.

Meta-analysis data on this subject also support the importance of thoracic radiotherapy in limited stage SCLC.[144,145] Therefore, it is likely that a gain in local–regional tumor control will be translated into an improvement in survival.

### Clinical Experience with Hyperfractionated–Accelerated (HA) BID Radiotherapy in Chemoradiotherapy

Given the rapidly proliferating characteristics of SCLC, BID radiotherapy schedule seems a logical means for an improvement in local tumor control and survival. Repair of sublethal radiation damage in aerobic mammalian cells is essentially complete within 2 to 4 hours.[146] If the interval between radiation fractions is greater than 4 hours, rapidly proliferating tumor cells (i.e., SCLC) can have an advantage in repair and repopulation over nonproliferating or slowly proliferating normal tissue. In such a situation, greater therapeutic efficacy may be expected for any given level of total radiation dose with the administration of two treatment sessions each day, given at least 5 hours apart, using a fraction size of 110 to 160 cGy, which is smaller than that used with conventional schedules (180–200 cGy).[147–149]

HA BID radiotherapy schedules have been studied in SCLC in an attempt to explore the potential benefit of shortened overall treatment time and sparing of late-reacting normal tissues by using the fraction sizes smaller than 200 cGy.[150–154] Choi et al.[150] reported a Cancer Acute Leukemia Group B (CALGB) phase II study in which patients with locally recurrent SCLC after induction chemotherapy (cyclophosphamide, etoposide, and vincristine every 3 wks for six cycles) were treated with an accelerated BID radiation schedule for a total dose of 5010 cGy, using 167 cGy dose fractions, twice daily, 5 days per week, followed by chemotherapy. Complete response was achieved in 73% (8 of 11) of patients. However, marked esophagitis requiring viscous lidocaine was noted in 82% (9 of 11) patients. Two of 11 patients (18%) experienced severe esophagitis requiring intravenous hydration in one and a feeding gastrostomy in another patient. Therefore, acute esophagitis was found to be a dose-limiting toxicity in this BID radiotherapy schedule.

Turrisi et al.[151] treated 23 patients with limited stage SCLC with chemotherapy [cisplatin and etoposide (PE) for 2 cycles] and concurrent BID radiation using 150 cGy dose fractions, twice daily, 5 days a week, for a total dose of 4500 cGy in 30 fractions for 3 weeks, followed by 6 additional cycles of chemotherapy [cyclophosphamide, doxorubicin, vincristine (CAV) for cycles 3, 5, 7, and PE for cycles 4, 6, 8]. Major toxicities included acute esophagitis in 73% (severe in 13%) and grade 4 leukopenia in 17% of patients.

Ihde et al.[154] conducted a similar study in which a combination of chemotherapy (etoposide and cisplatin) and concurrent radiotherapy (150 cGy of dose fractions, twice daily,

5 days/wk, for a total dose of 4500 cGy) was administered to patients with limited stage SCLC. Major toxicities included severe esophagitis requiring hospitalization in 31%, esophageal stricture in 15% of patients, and marked myelosuppression. Although the initial result of this study was remarkable, with complete and partial response rates of 73% and 23%, and MST of over 2 years, 74% of patients relapsed.

Thus, these studies support the finding that acute esophagitis is the main dose-limiting toxicity in HA BID radiotherapy schedule.

### Maximum Tolerated Dose (MTD) of Radiation in Both HA BID and QD Radiotherapy

In searching for radiation dose schedules better than the current one, a radiation dose escalation study was conducted by CALGB (Protocol 8837)[79] to determine the maximum tolerated dose (MTD) of radiation in both QD and HA BID radiation schedules in concurrent chemoradiation. The study design consisted of a sequential dose escalation in both QD and HA BID radiation regimens. Radiation dose to the initial volume was kept at 4000 to 4050 cGy while it was gradually increased to the boost volume by adding a 7% to 11% increment of total dose to subsequent cohorts. MTD was defined as the radiation dose level at one cohort below that which resulted in more than 33% of patients experiencing acute esophagitis of CALGB grade 4 or higher (severe esophagitis that may require IV hydration, nasogastric tube feeding, or total parenteral nutrition) and/or pulmonary toxicity of grade 3 or higher. The study plan included nine cohorts, five in HA BID and four in QD regimens for the dose escalation. Chemotherapy consisted of three cycles of PCE [cisplatin, 33 mg/m$^2$/day, days 1 to 3 over 30 min, cyclophosphamide, 500 mg/m$^2$ IV, over 1 h on day 1, and etoposide, 80 mg/m$^2$/d, on days 1 to 3 over 1 h every 3 wk] and two cycles of PE. Radiotherapy was started at the initiation of the fourth cycle of chemotherapy. MTD of HA BID radiotherapy was determined to be 4500 cGy in 30 fractions for 3 weeks, while it was judged to

be at least 7000 cGy in 35 fractions for 7 weeks for QD radiotherapy.

The overall tumor response for all eligible patients to the combined chemotherapy and radiotherapy included 51% (24 of 47) of complete remission, 38% (18 of 47) of partial remission, and 2% (1 of 47) of stable disease. Median survival time of all patients was 24.4 months, and 2- and 3-year survival rates were 53% and 28%, respectively. With regard to the different radiation schedules, 2- and 3-year survival rates were 52% and 25% for HA BID and 54% and 35% for QD radiotherapy cohorts.

### Clinical Trials Comparing BID with QD Radiation Schedules

A phase III intergroup trial that was reported by Johnson et al.[155] and Turrisi et al.[156] compared a QD radiation schedule of 4500 cGy in 25 fractions for 5 weeks to a HA BID radiation schedule of 4500 cGy in 30 fractions for 3 weeks at the same total dose in patients with limited stage SCLC. All patients received four cycles of chemotherapy (cisplatin, 60 mg/m$^2$, on day 1 and etoposide, 120 mg/m$^2$, on days 1 to 3, every 3 weeks). Radiation therapy was started within 24 hours of cycle 1 chemotherapy. Complete and overall response rates were 48% and 87.1% for QD radiation, compared with 56% and 87.2% for BID radiation schedules, respectively. The median survival time and 2- and 5-year survival rates were 19 months, 41%, and 16% for QD radiation, compared with 22 months, 46%, and 26% for BID radiation schedules, respectively ($p = 0.043$). Local failure was observed in 75% of patients with QD radiation, compared to 42% with BID radiation schedules. These results suggest that radiation dose intensity, which is higher in BID than QD schedules, may account for the difference in local tumor control and survival.

Another phase III study that was reported by Bonner et al.[157] compared a QD radiation schedule (5040 cGy/28 F/5.6 wk) with a BID schedule (4800 cGy/32 F/5.7 wk) by means of a split-course radiation [2400 cGy/16 F/1.6 wk (150 cGy/F, BID, 5 days/wk for 8 days), 2.5 wks of rest, and additional 2400 cGy/16

F/1.6 wk] in concurrent chemoradiotherapy. Chemotherapy consisted of six cycles of etoposide (130 mg/m$^2$, days 1–3 of cycles 1–3, and 100 mg/m$^2$, days 1–3 of cycles 4–6) and cisplatin (30 mg/m$^2$, days 1–3 of cycles 1–6). Patients were randomized into QD versus BID schedules after three cycles of induction therapy. This study was designed to test the significance of radiation fractionation schedule (QD vs. BID) by keeping the total radiation dose and overall duration of radiation therapy at a similar levels. The BID radiation regimen resulted in a higher level of esophagitis of grade 3 or higher (12.7%) than the QD radiation regimen (4.7%). The median survival and 3-year survival rates for the overall group were 21 months and 28.5%, respectively. There was no difference in the therapy outcome up to 3 years between the BID and QD radiation schedules.

The results of these two phase III studies support a premise that both total radiation dose and dose intensity are important factors in local tumor control and survival, and that a resting period during radiation course may adversely affect the therapy result.

### Rationale for Phase III Trial to Compare Standard QD with HA BID Radiotherapy at Their MTD for Gain in Survival

It is very disappointing to note that the control rate of local–regional tumor is only 30% to 50% with the radiation dose schedule (4500–5000 cGy/25 F/5 wk) currently being used in multi-institutional studies.

In searching for an improved radiotherapy schedule in limited stage, small-cell lung cancer, it seems logical to test a regimen of interest at its MTD for tumor control and survival. Since the QD radiotherapy schedule at 4500 cGy in 25 fractions for 5 weeks used in the Intergroup Study is not near the MTD of QD radiotherapy as defined in the CALGB study,[79] it remains to be determined whether standard QD radiotherapy at MTD (7000 cGy/35 F/7 wk) will result in local tumor control and survival equal to or better than that of HA BID radiotherapy at its MTD (4500 cGy/30 F/3 wk).

Since the total radiation dose seems to be as important as the dose intensity for local tumor control and survival, it is reasonable to use one or two dose fractionation schedules in a non-protocol setting. The author recommends the following dose schedules: a QD radiation schedule of 6000 to 6400 cGy in 30 to 32 fractions for 6 to 6.4 weeks, or a BID schedule of 4500 cGy in 30 fractions for 3 weeks.

## Role of Radiotherapy for Extensive Stage SCLC

Routine use of a moderate dose of thoracic radiotherapy to the region of the primary tumor and involved regional lymph nodes in combination with chemotherapy has failed to show any significant improvement in survival because of recurrences at multiple sites.[158] Approximately 20% to 25% of patients with extensive stage disease have shown a complete remission with current multidrug chemotherapy, and their short-term survival is very close to that of patients with limited-stage SCLC.[127,158,159] Common sites of recurrence in this group of patients include the chest and the brain, in addition to the initial sites of bulky tumors.[126] This is the group of patients who may benefit from radiotherapy to the primary site in the chest and elective cranial irradiation (ECI), perhaps with improved survival. For patients who did not achieve complete remission after chemotherapy, the role of radiotherapy is primarily palliation of clinical symptoms, that is, airway obstruction, superior vena caval obstruction, hemoptysis, intractable cough caused by a locally progressive tumor, bone pain, and neurologic deficit caused by metastatic tumors.

### Radiotherapeutic Techniques

*Target Volume for Thoracic Radiotherapy in Limited-Stage SCLC* The most important first step toward successful treatment is a careful assessment of the target volume defined by CBT scan of the chest and upper abdomen.

The optimal clinical target volume (CTV) for limited-stage SCLC has not yet been established. A small treatment volume is inevitably associated with a high rate of marginal failure, owing to geographical miss, although it is better tolerated by patients. However, on the basis of the biologic aggressiveness of the tumor and the data from CBT of the chest, it seems most logical that target volume should include the primary lesion (GTV) with a 1.0 cm margin of radiographically clear pulmonary tissue (CTV), involved nodal station (GTV), and one sentinel nodal group beyond the involved station. For patients with hilar nodal involvement, the mediastinal CTV includes mediastinal nodal stations 7, 4R, and 4L. For patients with an involvement of mediastinal nodal stations 4L and 5, CTV for mediastinal nodal stations includes 7, 6, 4R, 2R, and 2L. For metastatic disease involving mediastinal nodal stations 2R and 2L, CTV includes 1R, 1L, and both supraclavicular regions.

When thoracic radiotherapy is administered after two to three cycles of induction chemotherapy, whether GTV should be determined with the initial CBT scan of the chest prior to the induction chemotherapy or with subsequent restaging CBT scan of the chest after induction chemotherapy remains controversial.

It is of interest to review a randomized trial by the Southwest Oncology Group to assess the clinical and radiological meaning of "complete response."[160] In this study, patients who achieved complete response with induction chemotherapy were randomized to receive either thoracic radiotherapy plus subsequent maintenance chemotherapy or maintenance chemotherapy alone. Local–regional failure (chest failure) as the initial site of failure was noted in 72% (38 of 53) of patients with chemotherapy alone, versus 50% (20 of 40) with chemotherapy plus split-course thoracic radiotherapy. The maintenance chemotherapy alone was unable to prevent local–regional recurrence from microscopic residual disease in the majority of patients who were judged to have achieved complete clinical response. Ian Tannock presented a relationship between clinical remission and cure by using a mathematical model of a 10 g tumor containing $10^{10}$

cells.[161] Three cycles of chemotherapy, each of which inactivates 90% of the tumor cells, may reduce the number of viable tumor cells to less than $10^8$ ($< 0.1$ g), and the patient is judged to be in complete clinical and radiological remission. Furthermore, additional chemotherapy may not be helpful if drug-resistant cells have been selected after three cycles of induction chemotherapy. This model may be pertinent in explaining why the complete response group without thoracic radiotherapy had 72% rate of local failure as the initial site of recurrence. For now, it seems important to include the initial tumor volume determined by imaging studies prior to induction chemotherapy as radiation target volume for thoracic radiotherapy.

*Radiation Portal Arrangements* The arrangement of radiation portals depends on the size and shape of the treatment volume, total radiation dose, and types of radiation. High energy beams, on the order of 4 to 25 MV photons, seem to be the choice, inasmuch as the large penumbra of a $^{60}$Co unit and the scatter radiation of electron or low energy beams are likely to be more harmful to the already-limited pulmonary reserve. Careful selection of radiotherapeutic techniques is essential for delivery of prescribed radiation dose to the primary tumor and the areas of grossly involved regional lymph nodes, while the remaining pulmonary tissue, the heart, and the spinal cord are protected from excessive dose of radiation. The radiotherapeutic technique used by the author consists of a sequential combination of AP-PA-POP for the initial dose (3600 cGy/20 F/4 wk) with a three-field arrangement of AP-RPO-LPO for additional treatment (1800 cGy/10 F/2 wk). A boost dose of 900 cGy in five fractions for 1 week is administered to GTV by oblique opposed portals. With this technique, the target volume is very well covered by an isodose line of 6000 cGy, while the spinal cord, the left ventricle of the heart, and most of the remaining pulmonary tissues are spared an excessive dose of radiation. Any part of the treatment volume away from the main stem bronchus and mediastinum, such as a peripherally located tumor, requires supplemental radiation portals of either AP-PA or oblique opposed portals to secure adequate radiation doses throughout any shape of the target volume. For radiation dose escalation beyond 6600 cGy in 33 fractions for 6.6 weeks, a three-dimensional conformal treatment plan is recommended.

### Elective Cranial Irradiation (ECI) in SCLC

The probability of developing overt metastases in the brain during the course of disease in patients with limited stage SCLC remains as high as 49% by the life table,[138] and radiation therapy for overt metastases in the brain has been ineffective in achieving long-term control.[162] Therefore, ECI continues to be an important component of a comprehensive treatment program in limited-stage SCLC. Arriagada et al.[163] reported a meta-analysis of individual data on 987 patients from seven randomized trials comparing ECI to no ECI in patients with SCLC who achieved complete remission. The primary end point of this study was overall survival, and the analysis was performed on an intention-to-treat basis. The relative risk of death in the ECI group compared to the control group was 0.84 (95% confidence interval = 0.73–0.97, $p = 0.01$), corresponding to a reduction in mortality of 16% in favor of ECI and to a 5.4% increase in the 3-year survival rate (from 15.3% of the control group to 20.7% of the ECI group). This is the first report with a large number of patients showing a survival gain with ECI.

An impairment of cognitive function in patients who are subjected to ECI has been reported. Previous studies using a radiation dose schedule of 3000 cGy in 10 fractions over a period of 2 weeks has been criticized for significant late neurotoxicities such as decreased intellectual function, memory loss, ataxia, and atrophy and ventricular dilatation of the brain by CBT of the brain.[164,165] However, these results were obtained from retrospective and nonrandomized studies, and further studies are necessary to clarify the nature and scope of the neurotoxicities. In a multicenter randomized trial, Gregor et al.[166] conducted an assessment of effects of ECI on cognitive function in patients with SCLC. They reported that an impairment in cognitive function was present in 25% to 40% of patients tested prior to ECI and no sustained or significant deterioration of neuropsychometric performance could be seen with ECI.

Two important factors in obtaining the desired outcome from ECI are timing and dose fractionation schedule. It is recommended that ECI be administered after the completion of all cycles of chemotherapy and to patients who are in complete or near-complete remission after chemoradiotherapy. Even though the optimal fractionation schedule for ECI has not been established, a radiation dose schedule of either 2500 cGy in 10 fractions for 2 weeks or 3000 cGy in 15 fractions for 3 weeks is judged most reasonable.

### Results

Since the advent of effective multidrug therapy in the mid-1970s, the survival of patients with limited-stage SCLC has improved considerably. We have witnessed a significant improvement in MST from 5 to 6 months with thoracic radiotherapy alone to 10 to 14 months with chemotherapy plus thoracic radiotherapy or chemotherapy alone in late 1970s and early 1980s, and to 19 to 22 months with chemoradiotherapy using a cisplatin-based regimen in late 1980s and early 1990s.

Even with extensive stage SCLC, complete remission has been achieved in approximately 20% of patients, and their survival can be expected to be similar to that of those with limited-stage SCLC. The improvement in long-term survival, however, has been far less than expected from the dramatic improvement in short-term survival.

A recent report of an Intergroup study described a 5-year survival rate of 16% with a QD schedule of 4500 cGy in 25 fractions for 5 weeks, compared with 26% with a BID schedule of 4500 cGy in 30 fractions for 3 weeks in concurrent chemoradiotherapy using a cisplatin-based regimen. Even though the 5-year survival rate was improved from 16%

with a QD schedule to 26% with a BID schedule of the same total dose, local failure rates remained high at 75% with QD schedule (4500 cGy/25 F/5 wk) compared with 42% with the BID dose schedule (4500 cGy/30 F/3 wk). To raise the 5-year survival rate beyond the current level, further research is necessary to improve radiation dose schedule and chemotherapy.

## REFERENCES

1. Greenlee RT, Murray T, Bolden S, Wingo PA: Cancer statistics, 2000. *CA Cancer J Clin* 2000;50:7–33.

2. Mark EJ: Pathology of thoracic neoplasms, in NC Choi and HC Grillo (eds): *Thoracic Oncology.* New York, Raven Press, 1983, pp M 23–49.

3. Greene RE: Radiological studies of thoracic neoplasms, in NC Choi and HC Grillo (eds): *Thoracic Oncology.* New York, Raven Press, 1983, pp 59–101.

4. American Joint Committee on Cancer, *Cancer Staging Manual,* 5th ed. AJCC, 1997.

5. Mountain CF: Revisions in the International System for Staging Lung Cancer. *Chest* 1997;111:1710–1717.

6. Karnofsky DA, Golbsy RB, Pool JL: Preliminary studies on the natural history of lung cancer. *Radiology* 1957;69:477–487.

7. Zubrod CG, Schneiderman M, Frei E, et al: Appraisal of methods for study of chemotherapy of cancer in man: Comparative therapeutic trial of nitrogen mustard and triethylene thiophosphoramide. *J Chronic Dis* 1960;11:7–33.

8. Mountain CF, Dresler CM: Regional lymph node classification for lung cancer staging. *Chest* 1997;111:1718–1723.

9. McLoud TC, Bourgouin PM, Greenberg RW, Kosiuk JP, Templeton PA, Shepard JO, Moore EH, Wain JC, Mathisen DJ, Grillo HC: Bronchogenic carcinoma: Analysis of staging in the mediastinum with CT by correlative lymph node mapping and sampling. *Radiology* 1992;182:319–323.

10. Webb WR, Gatsonis C, Zerhouni EA, Heelan RT, Glazer GM, Francis IR, McNeil BJ: CT and MR imaging in staging non–small cell bronchogenic carcinoma: Report of the Radiologic Diagnostic Oncology Group. *Radiology* 1991;178:705–713.

11. Armstrong JD II, Bragg DG: Thoracic neoplasms: Imaging requirements for diagnosis and staging. *Int J Radiat Oncol Biol Phys* 1984;10:109–135.

12. Pearson FG, DeLarue NC, Ilves R, et al: Significance of positive superior mediastinal nodes identified at mediastinoscopy in patients with resectable cancer of the lung. *J Thorac Cardiovasc Surg* 1982;83:1–11.

13. Maassen W: The staging issue—Problems: Accuracy of mediastinoscopy, in NC DeLarue and H Eschapasse (eds): *International Trends in General Thoracic Surgery,* vol 1. Philadelphia, Saunders, 1985, pp 42–53.

14. Wilkins EW Jr, Saita S: Surgery for lung cancer: The Massachusetts General Hospital experience, in NC Choi and HC Grillo (eds): *Thoracic Oncology.* New York, Raven Press, 1983, pp 115–127.

15. Martini N, Flehinger BJ, Zaman MB, et al: Prospective study of 445 lung carcinomas with mediastinal lymph node metastases. *J Thorac Cardiovasc Surg* 1980;80:390–399.

16. Coy P, Kennelly GM: The role of curative radiotherapy in the treatment of lung cancer. *Cancer* 1980;45:698–702.

17. Choi NCH, Doucette JA: Improved survival of patients with unresectable non-small-cell bronchogenic carcinoma by an innovated high-dose en-bloc radiotherapeutic approach. *Cancer* 1981;48:101–109.

18. Perez CA, Stanley K, Grundy G, et al: Impact of irradiation technique and tumor extent in tumor control and survival of patients with unresectable non–oat cell carcinoma of the lung. *Cancer* 1982;50:1091–1099.

19. Guttmann R: Radical supervoltage therapy in inoperable carcinoma of the lung, in TJ Deeley (ed): *Carcinoma of the Bronchus—Modern Radiotherapy.* New York, Appleton-Century-Crofts, 1971, pp 181–195.

20. Smart J: Can lung cancer be cured by irradiation alone? *JAMA* 1966;195:1034–1035.

21. Choi NC: Curative radiation therapy for unresectable non-small-cell carcinoma of the lung: Indications, techniques, results, in NC Choi and HC Grillo (eds): *Thoracic Oncology.* New York, Raven Press, 1983, pp 163–199.

22. Perez CA, Stanley K, Rubin P, et al: A prospective randomized study of various radiation doses and fractionation schedules in the treatment of inoperable non-oat-cell carcinoma of the lung. Preliminary report by the Radiation Therapy Oncology Group. *Cancer* 1980;45:2744–2753.

23. Cox JD, Azarnia N, Byhardt RW, Skin KH, Emami B, Perez CA: N2 (clinical) non–small cell carcinoma of the lung: Prospective trials of radiation therapy with total doses of 60 Gy by the Radiation Therapy Oncology Group. *Int J Radiat Biol Phys* 1991;20:7–12.

24. Dillman RO, Seagren SL, Propert KJ, Guerro J, Eaton WL, Perry MC, Carey RW, Frei E III, Green MR: A randomized trial of induction chemotherapy plus high-dose radiation versus radiation alone in stage III non–small cell lung cancer. *New Engl J Med* 1990;323:940–945.

25. Dillman RO, Herndon J, Seagren SL, Eaton WL, Green MR: Improved survival in stage III non–small cell lung cancer: Seven-year follow-up of Cancer and Leukemia Group B (CALGB) 8433 trial. *J Natl Cancer Inst* 1996;88:1210–1215.

26. Arriagada R, Le Chevalier T, Quoix E, Ruffie P, De Cremoux H, Douillard JY, Tarayre M, Pignon JP, LaPlanche A, for the GETCB, the FNCLCC and the CEBI trialists. ASTRO Plenary: Effect of chemotherapy on locally advanced non–small cell lung carcinoma: A randomized study of 353 patients. *Int J Radiat Oncol Biol Phys* 1991;20:1183–1190.

27. Arriagada R, Le Chevalier T, Rekacewicz C, Quoix E, De Cremoux H, Douillard JY, Tarayre M, for the CEBI-138 trialists and French anticancer centers. Cisplatin-based chemotherapy in patients with locally advanced non–small cell lung cancer: Late analysis of a French randomized trial. *Proc Am Soc Clin Oncol* 1997;16:446a (abstr 1601).

28. Kubota K, Furuse K, Kawahara M, Kodama N, Yamamoto M, Ogawara M, Negoro S, Masuda N, Takada M, Matsui K, Takifuji N, Kudoh S, Kusunoki Y, Fukuoka M: Role of radiotherapy in combined modality treatment of locally advanced non–small cell lung cancer. *J Clin Oncol* 1994;12:1547–1552.

29. Martini N, Flehinger BJ, Bains MS, McCormack P: Management of stage III disease: Alternative approaches to the management of

mediastinal adenopathy, in NC Delarue and H Eschapasse (eds): *International Trends in General Thoracic Surgery,* vol 1, *Lung Cancer.* Philadelphia, Saunders, 1985, pp 108–120.

30. Goldstraw P, Mannam GC, Kaplan DK, Michail P: Surgical management of non–small cell lung cancer with ipsilateral mediastinal node metastases (N2 disease). *J Thorac Cardiovasc Surg* 1994;107:19–28.

31. Orton CG, Ellis F: A simplification in the use of the NSD concept in practical radiotherapy. *Br J Radiol* 1973;46:529–537.

32. Shukovsky LI: Dose, time, volume relationships in squamous cell carcinoma of the supraglottic larynx. *Am J Roentgenol Radium Ther Nucl Med* 1970;108:27–29.

33. Bloedorn FG, Cowley RA, Cuccia CA, et al: Preoperative irradiation in bronchogenic carcinoma. *Am J Roentgenol Radium Ther Nucl Med* 1964;92:77–78.

34. Bromley LL, Szur L: Combined radiotherapy and resection for carcinoma of the bronchus: Experiences with 66 patients. *Cancer* 1955;2: 937–941.

35. Albain KS, Rusch VW, Crowley JJ, Rice TW, Turrisi AT III, Weick JK, Lonchyna VA, Presant CA, McKenna RJ, Gandara DR, Fosmire H, Taylor SA, Stelzer KJ, Beasley KR, Livingston RB: Concurrent cisplatin/etoposide plus chest radiotherapy followed by surgery for stages IIIA (N2) and IIIB non-small-cell lung cancer: Mature results of Southwest Oncology Group Phase II Study 8805. *J Clin Oncol* 1995;13:1880–1892.

36. Choi NC, Carey RW, Daly W, Mathisen D, Wain J, Wright C, Lynch T, Grossbard M, Grillo H: Potential impact on survival of improved tumor downstaging and resection rate by preoperative twice daily radiation and concurrent chemotherapy in stage 111A non–small cell lung carcinoma. *J Clin Oncol* 1997; 15:712–722.

37. Grunenwald D, Le Chevalier T, Arriagada R, Le Pechoux C, Baldeyrou P, Bretel JJ, Le Cesne A, Deenewald G, Girard P, Spaggiari L, Debrosse D, Carde P, Riviere A, Tarayre M, LaPlanche A: Results of surgical resection in stage IIIB non–small cell lung cancer (NSCLC) after concomitant induction chemoradiotherapy. *Lung Cancer* 1997;18 (suppl 1):73 (abstr 280).

38. Eberhardt W, Wilke H, Stamatis G, Stuschke M, Harstrick A, Menker H, Krause B, Muller MR, Stahl M, Flasshove M, Budach V, Greschuchna D, Konietzko N, Sack H, Seeber S: Preoperative chemotherapy followed by concurrent chemoradiotherapy based on hyperfractionated accelerated radiotherapy and definitive surgery in locally advanced non-small-cell lung cancer: Mature results of a phase II trial. *J Clin Oncol* 1998;16:622–634.

39. Emami B, Purdy JA, Manolis J, Barest G, Cheng E, Coia L, Doppke K, Galvin J, LoSasso T, Matthews J, Munzenrider J, Shank B: Three-dimensional treatment planning for lung cancer. *Int J Radiat Oncol Biol Phys* 1991;21:217–227.

40. Graham MV, Purdy JA, Enami B, Matthews JW, Harms WB: Preliminary results of a prospective trial using three dimensional radiotherapy for lung cancer. *Int J Radiat Oncol Biol Phys* 1995;33:993–1000.

41. Martel MK, Strawderman My, Hazuka M, Turrisi, A, Fraass B, Lichter A. Volume and dose parameters for survival of non–small cell lung cancer patients. *Radiother Oncol* 1997; 44:23–29.

42. Armstrong J, Raben A, Zelefsky M, Burt M, Leibel S, Chandra B, Kutcher, Harrison L, Hahn K, Ginsberg R, Rusch V, Kris M, Fuks Z. Promising survival with three-dimensional conformal radiation therapy for non–small cell lung cancer. *Radiother Oncol* 1997;44:17–22.

43. Armitage P: *Statistical Methods in Medical Research.* New York, John Wiley & Sons, 1971, pp 408–414.

44. Colton T: *Statistics in Medicine.* Boston, Little, Brown, 1974, pp 237–250.

45. Cox JD, Azarnia N, Byhardt RW, Shin KH, Emami B, Pajak TF: A randomized phase I/II trial of hyperfractionated radiation therapy with total doses of 60.0 Gy to 79.2 Gy: Possible survival benefit with greater than or equal to 69.6 Gy in favorable patients with Radiation Oncology Group stage III non–small cell lung carcinoma: Report of Radiation Therapy Oncology Group 83-11. *J Clin Oncol* 1990;8: 1543–1555.

46. Sause WT, Scott C, Taylor S, Johnson D, Livingston R, Komaki R, Emami B, Curran WJ, Byhardt RW, Turrisi AT, Dar AR, Cox JD: Radiation Therapy Oncology Group 88-08 and Eastern Cooperative Oncology Group 4588: Preliminary results of a phase III trial in regionally advanced, unresectable non–small-cell lung cancer. *J Natl Cancer Inst* 1995;87: 198–205.

47. Sause WT, Kolesar P, Taylor S, Johnson D, Livingston R, Komaki R, Emami B, Curran WJ, Byhardt RW, Fisher B, Turrisi AT: Five-year results; phase III trial of regionally advanced unresectable non-small-cell lung cancer, RTOG 8808, ECOG 4588, SWOG 8992. *Proc Am Soc Clin Oncol* 1998;17:453 (abstr 1743).

48. Line D, Deeley TJ: Palliative therapy, in TJ Deeley (ed): *Modern Radiotherapy— Carcinoma of the Bronchus.* New York. Appleton-Century-Crofts, 1971, pp 298–306.

49. Schulz MD: Palliation by radiotherapy in bronchogenic carcinoma. *JAMA* 1966;196:850.

50. Rubin P, Ciccio S: High daily dose for rapid decompression in superior mediastinal obstruction, in TJ Deeley (ed): *Modern Radiotherapy—Carcinoma of the Bronchus.* New York, Appleton-Century-Crofts, 1971, pp 276–297.

51. Greco FA, Brereton HD, Kent H, et al: Adriamycin and enhanced radiation reaction in normal esophagus and skin. *Ann Intern Med* 1976;85:294–298.

52. Horwich A, Lokich JJ, Bloomer WD: Doxorubicin, radiotherapy and esophageal stricture. *Lancet* 1975;2:561–562.

53. Newburger PE, Cassady JR, Jaffe N: Esophagitis due to Adriamycin and radiation therapy for childhood malignancy. *Cancer* 1978;42: 417–423.

54. Newton KA, Spittle MF: Analysis of 40 cases treated by total thoracic irradiation. *Clin Radiol* 1969;20:19–22.

55. Phillips T, Margolis L: Radiation pathology and the clinical response of lung and esophagus, in JM Vaeth (ed): *Frontiers of Radiation Therapy and Oncology,* vol 6. Baltimore, University Park Press, 1972, pp 254–273.

56. Roswit B, White DC: Severe radiation injuries of the lung. *Am J Roentgenol Radium Ther Nucl Med* 1977;129:127–136.

57. Rubin P, Casarett GW: *Clinical Radiation Pathology.* Philadelphia, Saunders, 1968, pp 460–461.

58. Choi NC, Karanek DJ, Kazemi H: Physiologic changes in pulmonary function after thoracic radiotherapy for patients with lung cancer and role of regional pulmonary function studies in predicting postradiotherapy pulmonary function before radiotherapy. *Cancer Treat Symp* 1985;2:119–130.

59. Roswit B, White DC: Severe radiation injuries of the lung. *Am J Roentgenol Radium Ther Nucl Med* 1977;129:127–136.

60. Rubin P, Casarett GW: *Clinical Radiation Pathology.* Philadelphia, Saunders, 1968, pp 460–461.

61. Gross NJ: Pulmonary effects of radiation therapy. *Ann Intern Med* 1977;86:81–92.

62. Moss WT, Haddy FJ, Sweany SK: Some factors altering severity of acute radiation pneumonitis: Irradiation with cortisone, heparin and antibiotics. *Radiology* 1960;75:50–54.

63. Castellino RA, Glatstein E, Turbow MM, et al: Latent radiation injury of lungs or heart activated by steroid withdrawal. *Ann Intern Med* 1974;80:593–599.

64. Wohl MEB, Griscom NT, Traggis DG, et al: The effects of therapeutic radiation delivered in early childhood upon subsequent lung function. *Pediatrics* 1975;4:507–516.

65. Stewart JR, Cohn KE, Fajardo LF, et al: Radiation-induced heart disease. *Radiology* 1967;89:302–310.

66. Merrill J, Greco FA, Zimbler H, et al: Adriamycin and radiation: Synergistic cardiotoxicity. *Ann Intern Med* 197S;82:122–123.

67. Jones A: Transient radiation myelopathy (with reference to Lhermitte's sign of electrical paraesthesia). *Br J Radiol* 1964;37:727–744.

68. Boden G: Radiation myelitis of the cervical spinal cord. *Br J Radiol* 1948;21:464–469.

69. Phillips TL, Buschke F: Radiation tolerance of the thoracic spinal cord. *Am J Roentgenol Radium Ther Nucl Med* 1969;104:659–664.

70. Withers HR: Biologic basis for altered fractionation schemes. *Cancer* 1985;55:2086–2095.

71. Thames HD, Peters LJ, Withers HR, et al: Accelerated fractionation vs. hyperfractionation: Rationales for several treatments per day. *Int J Radiat Oncol Biol Phys* 1983;9:127–138.

72. Elkind MM, Sutton H: Radiation response of mammalian cells grown in culture. 1. Repair of x-ray damage in surviving Chinese hamster cells. *Radiat Res* 1960;13:556–593.

73. Suit HD, Urano M: Repair of sublethal radiation injury in hypoxic cells of a C3H mouse mammary carcinoma. *Radiat Res* 1969;37:423–434.

74. Choi CH, Suit HD: Evaluation of rapid radiation treatment schedules utilizing two treatment sessions per day. *Radiology* 1975;116:703–707.

75. Noron T, Onyango I: Radiotherapy in Burkett's lymphoma: Conventional vs. superfractionated regime—Early results. *Int J Radiat Oncol Biol Phys* 1977;2:399–406.

76. Saunders MI, Dische S, Barrett A, Parmar MKB, Harvey A, Gibson D on behalf of the CHART Steering Committee: Randomised multicentre trials of CHART vs conventional radiotherapy in head and neck and non-small-cell lung cancer: An interim report. *Br J Cancer* 1996;73:1455–1462.

77. Saunders MI, Dische S, Barrett A, Harvey A, Gibson D, Parmar MKB, on behalf of the CHART Steering Committee: Continuous hyperfractionated accelerated radiotherapy (CHART) versus conventional radiotherapy in non-small-cell lung cancer: A randomised multicenter trial. *Lancet* 1997;350:161–165.

78. Saunders MI, Dische S, Barrett A, Harvey A, Griffiths G, Parmar M (on behalf of the CHART Steering Committee): Continuous, hyperfractionated, accelerated radiotherapy (CHART) versus conventional radiotherapy in non-small-cell lung cancer: Mature data from the randomised multicenter trial. *Radiother Oncol* 1999;52:137–148.

79. Choi NC, Herndon J, Rosenman J, Carey R, Chung CT, Bernard S, Leone L, Seagren S, Green M: A phase I study to determine the maximum tolerated dose of radiation in standard daily and accelerated twice daily radiation schedules with concurrent chemotherapy for limited stage small cell lung cancer. *J Clin Oncol* 1998;16:3528–3536.

80. Mehta MP, Tannehill SP, Adak S, Martin L, Petereit DG, Wagner H, Fowler JF, Johnson D: Phase II trial of hyperfractionated accelerated radiation therapy for nonresectable non–small-cell lung cancer: Results of Eastern Cooperative Oncology Group 4593. *J Clin Oncol* 1998;16:3518–3523.

81. Schaake-Koning C, Van den Bogaert W, Dalesio O, Fister J, Hoogenhaut J, Van Houtte P, Kirkpatrick A, Koolen M, Moat B, Nijs A, Renaud A, Rodrigus P, Schuster W, Witterhave L, Sculier JP, Vanzandwijk N, Bartelinsk H: Effects of concomitant cisplatin and radiotherapy on inoperable non–small cell lung cancer. *New Engl J Med* 1992;326:524–530.

82. Furuse K, Fukuoka M, Kawahara M, Nishikawa YH, Takada Y, Kudoh S, Katagami N, Ariyoshi Y, for The West Japan Lung Cancer Group: Phase III study of concurrent versus sequential thoracic radiotherapy in combination with mitomycin, vindesine, and cisplatin in unresectable stage III non–small cell lung cancer. *J Clin Oncol* 1999;17:2692–2699.

83. Fleck J, Camargo J, Godoy D, Teixeira P, Braga Filho A, Barletta A, Ferreira P: Chemoradiation therapy alone versus chemotherapy alone as a neoadjuvant treatment for stage III non–small cell lung cancer. Preliminary report of a phase III, randomized trail. *Proc Am Soc Clin Oncol* 1993;12:333 (abstr 1108).

84. Hilaris BS, Martini N: Interstitial brachytherapy in cancer of the lung: A 20 year experience. *Int J Radiat Oncol Biol Phys* 1979;5:1951–1956.

85. Abe M, Takahasi M, Yabumoto E, et al: Clinical experiences with intraoperative radiotherapy of locally advanced cancers. *Cancer* 1980;45:40–48.

86. Eichhorn HJ, Lessel A: A comparison between combined neutron and telecobalt-therapy with telecobalt-therapy alone for cancer of the bronchus. *Br J Radiol* 1976;49:880–882.

87. Cade IS, McEwen JB: Clinical trials of radiotherapy in hyperbaric oxygen at Portsmouth, 1964–1976. *Clin Radiol* 1978;29:333–338.

88. Dische S, Saunders MI. Flockhart IR, et al: Misonidazole—A drug for trial in radiotherapy and oncology. *Int J Radiat Oncol Biol Phys* 1979;5:851–860.

89. Curran WJ, Movsas B, Hancock S, Rosenthal DI, Lockwood G, von Roemeling R, Harvey E: Phase I trial of oral Tirazone (tirapazamine) shows good bioavailability and tolerance. *Abstr Proc ASCO* 1998;17:208 (abstr 802).

90. Sugaar S, LeVeen HH: A histopathologic study on the effects of radiofrequency thermotherapy on malignant tumors of the lung. *Cancer* 1979;43:767–783.

91. Hilton, G. The present position relating to cancer of the lung; results with radiotherapy alone. *Thorax* 1960;15:17–18.

92. Dosoretz DE, Katin MJ, Blitzer PH, Rubenstein JH, Salenius S, Rashid M, Dosani RA, Mestas G, Siegel AD, Chadha TT, Chandrasa T, Hannan SE, Bhat SB, Metke MP: Radiation therapy in the management of medically inoperable carcinoma of the lung: Results and implications for future treatment strategies. *Int J Radiat Oncol Biol Phys* 1992;24:3–9.

93. Haffty BG, Goldberg NB, Gerstley J, Fisher DB, Pesche RE: Results of radical radiation therapy in clinic; 31 stage I and clinically operable non–small lung cancer. *Int J Radiat Biol Phys* 1988;15:69–73.

94. Zhang HX, Yin WB, Zhang LJ, Yang ZY, Zhang ZX, Wang M, Chen DF, Gu XZ: Curative radiotherapy of early operable non-small-cell lung cancer. *Radiother Oncol* 1989;14:89–94.

95. Graham PH, Gebski VJ, Langlands AO: Radical radiotherapy for early non–small cell lung cancer. *Int J Radiat Oncol Biol Phys* 1995;31:261–266.

96. Krol AD, Aussems P, Noordijk EM, Hermans J, Leer JWH: Local irradiation alone for peripheral stage I lung cancer: Could we omit the elective regional nodal irradiation? *Int J Radiat Biol Phys* 1996;34:297–302.

97. Sibley GS, Jamieson TA, Marks LB, Anscher MS, Prosnitz LR: Radiotherapy alone for medically inoperable stage I non–small-cell lung cancer: The Duke experience. *Int J Radiat Biol Phys* 1998;40:149–154.

98. Wilkins EW Jr., Scannell JG, Craver JG: Four decades of experience with resections for bronchogenic carcinoma at the Massachusetts General Hospital. *J Thorac Cardiovasc Surg* 1978;76:364–368.

99. Mountain CF, McMurtrey MJ, Frazier OH: Regional extension of lung cancer. *Int J Radiat Oncol Biol Phys* 1980;6:1013–1020.

100. Paulson DL, Reisch JS: Long-term survival after resection for bronchogenic carcinoma. *Ann Surg* 1976;83:324–332.

101. Shields TW: Classification and prognosis of surgically treated patients with bronchial carcinoma: Analysis of VASOG studies. *Int J Radiat Oncol Biol Phys* 1980;6:1021–1027.

102. PORT Meta-analysis Trialists Group: Postoperative radiotherapy in non–small-cell lung cancer: Systematic review and meta-analysis of individual patient data from nine randomised controlled trials. *Lancet* 1998;352:257–263.

103. Stephens RJ, Girling DJ, Bleehen NM, Moghissi K, Yosef HMA, Machin D: The role of post-operative radiotherapy in non-small-cell lung cancer: A multicenter randomised trial in patients with pathologically staged T1-2, N1-2, M0 disease. *Br J Cancer* 1996;74;632–639.

104. Van Houtte P, Rocmans P, Smets P, et al: Postoperative radiation therapy in lung cancer: A controlled trial after resection of curative design. *Int J Radiat Oncol Biol Phys* 1980:6:983–986.

105. Kirsh MM, Rotman H, Argenta L, et al: Carcinoma of the lung: Results of treatment over 10 years. *Ann Thorac Surg* 1976:21:371–376.

106. Choi NCH, Grillo HC, Gardiello M, et al: Basis for new strategies in postoperative radiotherapy of bronchogenic carcinoma. *Int J Radiat Oncol Biol Phys* 1980;6:31–35.

107. Martini N, Flehinger BJ, Zaman MB, et al: Results of resection in non-oat-cell carcinoma of the lung with mediastinal lymph node metastases. *Ann Surg* 1983;198:386–396.

108. Patterson GA, Ilves R, Ginsberg RJ, et al: The value of adjuvant radiotherapy in pulmonary and chest wall resection for bronchogenic carcinoma. *Ann Thorac Surg* 1982;34:692–697.

109. Lung Cancer Study Group: Effects of postoperative mediastinal radiation on completely resected stage II and stage III epidermoid cancer of the lung. *New Engl J Med* 1986;315:1377–1381.

110. Dautzenberg B, Chastang C, Arriagada R, LeChevalier T, Belpomme D, Hurdebourcq M, Lebeau B, Fabre C, Charvolin P, Guerin R, for the GETCB: Adjuvant radiotherapy versus combined sequential chemotherapy followed by radiotherapy in the treatment of resected nonsmall cell lung carcinoma. *Cancer* 1995;76:779–786.

111. Choi NC, Kazemi H: Evaluation of pulmonary function changes by postoperative radiotherapy in patients with lung cancer. *Int J Radiat Oncol Biol Phys* 1980;6:1339.

112. Pancoast HK: Importance of careful roentgen ray investigations of apical chest tumors. *JAMA* 1924;83:1407–1411.

113. Pancoast HK: Superior pulmonary sulcus tumor: Tumor characterized by pain, Horner's syndrome, destruction of bone, and atrophy of hand muscles. *JAMA* 1932;99:1391–1396.

114. Paulson DL, Shaw RR, Kee JL, et al: Combined preoperative irradiation and resection for bronchogenic carcinoma. *J Thorac Cardiovasc Surg* 1962;44:281–294.

115. Mallams JT, Paulson DL, Collier RE, et al: Presurgical irradiation in bronchogenic carcinoma, superior sulcus type. *Radiology* 1964;82:1050–1054.

116. Paulson DL: Technical considerations in stage III disease: The superior sulcus lesion, in NC Delarue and H Eschapasse (eds): *International Trends in General Thoracic Surgery,* vol 1. Philadelphia, Saunders, 1985, pp 121–131.

117. Wright CD, Moncure AC, Shepard JO, Wilkins EW, Mathisen DJ, Grillo HC: Superior sulcus lung tumors. Results of combined treatment (irradiation and radical resection). *J Thorac Cardiovasc Surg* 1987;94;69–74.

118. Hilaris BS, Manini N: The current state of intraoperative interstitial brachytherapy in lung cancer. *Int J Radiat Oncol Biol Phys* 1988;15:1347–1354.

119. Neal CR, Amdur RJ, Mendenhall WM, Knauf DG, Block AJ, Million RR: Pancoast tumor: Radiation therapy alone versus preoperative radiation therapy and surgery. *Int J Radiat Oncol Biol Phys* 1991;21:651–660.

120. Hagan MP, Choi NC, Mathisen DJ, Wain JC, Wright CD, Grillo HC: Superior sulcus tumors: Impact of local tumor control on survival. *J Thorac Cardiovasc Surg* 1999;117:1086–1094.

121. Van Houtte P, MacLennan I, Poulter C, et al: External radiation in the management of superior sulcus tumor. *Cancer* 1984;54:223–227.

122. Komaki R, Roth J, Cox JD, et al: Superior sulcus tumors: Results of irradiation of 36 patients. *Cancer* 1981;48:1563–1568.

123. Fox W, Scadding JG: Medical Research Council comparative trial of surgery and radiotherapy for primary treatment of small celled or oat celled carcinoma of the bronchus. *Lancet* 1973;2:63–65.

124. Medical Research Council Lung Cancer Working Party: Radiotherapy alone or with chemotherapy in the treatment of small cell carcinoma of the lung. *Br J Cancer* 1979; 40:1–10.

125. Livingston RB, Moore TN, Heilbrun L, et al: Small cell carcinoma of the lung: Combined chemotherapy and radiation. A Southwest Oncology Group study. *Ann Intern Med* 1978;88: 194–199.

126. Maurer LH, Tulloh M, Weiss RB, et al: A randomized combined modality trial in small cell carcinoma of the lung: Comparison of combination chemotherapy–radiation therapy versus cyclophosphamide–radiation therapy effects of maintenance chemotherapy and prophylactic whole brain irradiation. *Cancer* 1980;45: 30–39.

127. Aisner J, Whitacre M, Van Echo DA, et al: Combination chemotherapy for small cell carcinoma of the lung: Continuous versus alternating non-cross-resistant combinations. *Cancer Treat Rep* 1982;66:221–230.

128. Byhardt RW, Cox JD: Is chest radiotherapy necessary in any or all patients with small cell carcinoma of the lung? Yes. *Cancer Treat Rep* 1983;67:209–215.

129. Cohen MH: Is thoracic radiation therapy necessary for patients with limited-stage small cell lung cancer? No. *Cancer Treat Rep* 1983; 67:217–221.

130. Seydel HG, Creech R, Pagano M, et al: Combined modality treatment of regional small cell undifferentiated carcinoma of the lung: A cooperative study of the RTOG and ECOG. *Int J Radiat Oncol Biol Phys* 1983;9:1135–1142.

131. Livingston RB, Stephens RL, Bonnet JD, et al: Long-term survival and toxicity in small cell lung cancer: Southwest Oncology Group study. *Am J Med* 1984;77:415–417.

132. Choi CH, Carey RW: Small-cell anaplastic carcinoma of lung: Reappraisal of current management. *Cancer* 1976;37:2651–2657.

133. Mira JG, Livingston RB: Evaluation and radiotherapy implications of chest relapse patterns in small cell lung carcinoma treated with radiotherapy–chemotherapy. *Cancer* 1980;46: 2557–2565.

134. White JE, Chen T, McCracken J, et al: The influence of radiation therapy quality control on survival, response, and sites of relapse in oat cell carcinoma of the lung. *Cancer* 1982;5 0:1084–1090.

135. Choi NC: Reassessment of the role of radiation therapy relative to other treatments in small cell carcinoma of the lung, in NC Choi and HC Grillo (eds): *Thoracic Oncology.* New York, Raven Press, 1983, pp 233–256.

136. Perry MC, Eaton WL, Propert KJ, et al, for Cancer and Leukemia Group B: Chemotherapy with or without radiation therapy in limited small cell cancer of the lung. *New Engl J Med* 1987;316:912–918.

137. Bunn PA, Jr, Lichter AS, Makuch RW, Cohen MH, Veach SR, Matthews MJ, Anderson AJ, Edison M, Glatstein E, Minna JD, Ihde DC: Chemotherapy alone or chemotherapy with chest radiation therapy in limited stage small-cell lung cancer. *Ann Intern Med* 1987;106: 655–662.

138. Choi NC, Carey RW, Kaufman SD, Grillo HC, Younger J, Wilkins EW Jr.: Small cell carcinoma of the lung: A progress report of 15 years' experience. *Cancer* 1987;59:6–14.

139. Choi NC, Carey RW: Importance of radiation dose in achieving improved locoregional tumor control in limited stage small-cell lung carcinoma: An update. *Int J Radiat Oncol Biol Phys* 1989;17:307–310.

140. Murray N, Coy P, Pater JL, Hodson I, Arnold A, Zee BC, Payne D, Kostashuk EC, Evans WK, Dixon P, Sadura A, Feld R, Levitt M, Wierzbicki R, Ayoub J, Maroun JA, Wilson KS: Importance of timing for thoracic irradiation in the combined modality treatment of limited-stage small-cell lung cancer. *J Clin Oncol* 1993;11:336–344.

141. Arriagada R, Le Chevalier T, Baldeyrou P, Pico JL, Ruffie P, Martin M, El Bakry HM, Duroux P, Bignon J, Lenfant B, Hayat M, Rouesse JG, Sancho-Garnier H, Tubiana M: Alternating radiotherapy and chemotherapy schedules in small-cell lung cancer, limited disease. *Int J Rad Oncol Biol Phys* 1985;11: 1461–1467.

142. Arriagada R, Le Chevalier T, Ruffie P, Chomy P, de Cremoux H, French FNCLCC Lung Cancer Study Group: Alternating radiotherapy and chemotherapy in limited small cell lung cancer: The IGR protocols. *Lung Cancer* 1994:10 suppl S29–S298.

143. Arriagada R, Kramar A, Le Chevalier T, De Cremoux H: Competing events determining relapse-free survival in limited small-cell lung carcinoma. *J Clin Oncol* 1992;10:447–451.

144. Pignon JP, Arriagada R, Ihde DC, Johnson DH, Perry MC, Souhami RL, Brodin O, Joss RA, Kies MS, Lebeau B, Onoshi T, Osterlind K, Tattersall MHN, Wagner H: A Meta-analysis of thoracic radiotherapy for small-cell lung cancer. *New Engl J Med* 1992;327:1618–1624.

145. Warde P, Payne D: Does thoracic irradiation improve survival and local control in limited-stage small-cell carcinoma of the lung? A meta-analysis. *J Clin Oncol* 1992;10:890–895.

146. Elkind MM, Sutton H: Radiation response of mammalian cells grown in culture. I. Repair of x-ray damage in surviving Chinese hamster cells. *Radiat Res* 1960;35:556–593.

147. Noron T, Onyango J: Radiotherapy in Burkitt's lymphoma: Conventional versus superfractionation regime—Early results. *Int J Radiat Oncol Biol Phys* 1977;2:399–406.

148. Suit HD: Superfractionation (editorial). *Int J Radiat Oncol Biol Phys* 1977;2:591–592.

149. Withers HR: Biologic basis for altered fractionation schemes. *Cancer* 1985;55:2086–2095.

150. Choi NC, Propert K, Carey R, Eaton W, Leone LA, Silberfarb P, Green M: Accelerated radiotherapy followed by chemotherapy for locally recurrent small-cell carcinoma of the lung. A phase II study of Cancer and Leukemia Group B. *Int J Radiat Oncol Biol Phys* 1987;13:263–266.

151. Turrisi AT, Glover DJ, Mason BA: A preliminary report: Concurrent twice-daily radiotherapy plus platinum–etoposide chemotherapy for limited small cell lung cancer. *Int J Radiat Oncol Biol Phys* 1988;15:183–187.

152. Mornex F, Trillett V, Chauvin F, Ardiet JM, Schmitt T, Romestaing P, Carrie C, Mahe M, Mornex JF, Fournel P, Souquet PJ, Boniface E, Gerard JP, Groupe Lyonnais d'Oncologie Thoracique: Hyperfractionated radiotherapy alternating with multidrug chemotherapy in the treatment of limited small cell lung cancer (SCLC). *Int J Radiat Oncol Biol Phys* 1990; 19:23–30.

153. Armstrong JG, Rosenstein MM, Kris MG, Shank BM, Scher HI, Fass DE, Harrison LB, Leibel SA, Fuks ZY: Twice daily thoracic irradiation for limited small cell lung cancer. *Int J Radiat Oncol Biol Phys* 1991;21:1269–1274.

154. Ihde DC, Grayson J, Woods E, Gazdar AF, Anderson M, Lesar M, Linnoila I, Minna JD, Glatstein E, Johnson BE: Limited stage small-cell lung cancer treated with concurrent etoposide/cisplatin and twice daily chest irradiation. *Proceedings of Sixth International Conference on the Adjuvant Therapy of Cancer.* Tucson, AZ, 1990, p 37.

155. Johnson DH, Kim K, Sause W, Komaki R, Wagner H, Aisner S, Livingston R, Blum R, Turrisi AT for ECOG: Cisplatin + etoposide + thoracic radiotherapy administered once or twice daily in limited stage small cell lung cancer: Final report of intergroup trial 0096. *Abstr Proc ASCO* 1996;15:374 (abstr 1113).

156. Turrisi AT, Kim K, Blum R, Sause WT, Livingston RB, Komaki R, Wagner H, Aisner S, Johnson DH: Twice-daily compared with once-daily thoracic radiotherapy in limited small-cell lung cancer treated concurrently with cisplatin and etoposide. *New Engl J Med* 1999;340:265–271.

157. Bonner JA, Sloan JA, Shanahan TG, Brooks BJ, Marks RS, Krook JE, Gerstner JB, Maksymiuk A, Levitt R, Mailliard JA, Tazelaar HD, Hillman S, Jett JR: Phase III comparison of twice-daily split-course irradiation versus once-daily irradiation for patients with limited stage small-cell lung carcinoma. *J Clin Oncol* 1999;17:2681–2691.

158. Chahinian AP, Comis RL. Mauter LH, et al: Small cell anaplastic carcinoma of the lung: The Cancer and Leukemia Group B experience. *Bull Cancer* 1982;69:79–82.

159. Markman M, Abeloff MD, Berkman AW, et al: Intensive alternating regimen in small cell carcinoma of the lung. *Cancer Treat Rep* 1985; 69:161–166.

160. Kies MS, Mira JG, Crowley JJ, Chen T, Pazdur R, Grozea PN, Rivkin SE, Coltman CA, Ward JH, Livingston RE: Multimodal therapy for limited small-cell lung cancer: A randomized study of induction combination chemotherapy with or without thoracic radiation in complete responders; and with wide-field versus reduced-field radiation in partial responders: A Southwest Oncology Group study. *J Clin Oncol* 1987;5:592–600.

161. Tannock IF: Combined modality treatment with radiotherapy and chemotherapy. *Radiother Oncol* 1989;16:83–101.

162. Rosenman J, Choi NC: Improved quality of life of patients with small cell carcinoma of the lung by elective irradiation of the brain. *Int J Radiat Oncol Biol Phys* 1982;8:1041–1043.

163. Aupérin A, Arriagada R, Pignon J-P, Le Péchoux C, Gregor A, Stephens RJ, Kristjansen PEG, Johnson BE, Ueoka H, Wagner H, Aisner J: Prophylactic cranial irradiation for patients with small-cell lung cancer in complete remission. *New Engl J Med* 1999;341:476–484.

164. Lee JS, Lee YY, Umsawasdi T, et al: Neurotoxicity in long-term survivors of small cell lung cancer. *Abstr Proc ASCO* 1984;3:220.

165. Craig JB, Jackson DV, Moody D, et al: Perspective evaluation of changes in computed cranial tomography in patients with small cell lung carcinoma treated with chemotherapy and prophylactic cranial irradiation. *J Clin Oncol* 1984;2:1151–1156.

166. Gregor A, Cull A, Stephens RJ, Kirkpatrick JA, Yarnold JR, Girling DJ, Macbeth FR, Stout R, Machin D: Prophylactic cranial irradiation is indicated following complete response to induction therapy in small cell lung cancer: Results of a multicentre randomised trial. *Eur J Cancer* 1997;33:1752–1758.

# B. CARCINOMA OF THE ESOPHAGUS

It remains a difficult task to cure patients with carcinoma of the esophagus, except for a small subset of patients with early stage (T1 N0) tumor by surgery, irradiation, or a combination of both.[1–5] However, recent results with a combined approach of chemoradiotherapy for squamous cell carcinoma, and preoperative chemoradiotherapy and surgery for both squamous cell carcinoma and adenocarcinoma, have been encouraging, and long-term cure for even advanced local–regional carcinoma (stage T2-3 N1) may be attainable in the near future.[6–9] The management of esophageal cancer has undergone a major revision over the past 6 to 10 years, and a review of the role of radiation therapy in multidisciplinary approach for esophageal carcinoma is timely and necessary.[10–14]

In the United States, the incidence of esophageal cancer is low (6/100,000 in men and 1.6/100,000 in women); it represents 1.1% of all cancers in both sexes, excluding skin tumors.[15] The rate of esophageal cancer for males is higher than for females by a ratio of 3:1. Esophageal carcinoma accounts for a higher percentage of all cancers among blacks (3.1%) than among whites (0.9%).[16,17] The average age-adjusted incidence rate for black males is 16.7 per 100,000, 3.6 times that of white males. The American Cancer Society has estimated that 12,300 new cases will be diagnosed in 2000, with approximately 12,100 deaths due to this tumor.[18] There is a great geographical variation in the incidence of esophageal cancer. For example, esophageal cancer poses a major threat to public health on the eastern shore of the Caspian littoral of Iran (the age-adjusted incidence rates are 94–108/100,000 in men and 79–174/100,000 in women[19]), in the Yangcheng, Lin Xian (Shanxi), and Ci Xian regions in northern China (the average age-adjusted mortality rate is 132–169/100,000[20]), and in Sri Lanka, where esophageal cancer is the most common tumor of the gastrointestinal tract.

Etiologic factors and predisposing conditions for esophageal cancer are alcohol and tobacco use, achalasia, Plummer–Vinson syndrome, tylosis, Barrett esophagus, and other less well-defined dietary and soil factors. The epidemiological features of esophageal carcinoma have changed. Squamous cell carcinoma accounted for more than 90% of all esophageal cancers in the past. However, adenocarcinomas that arise in the esophageal gland or in the Barrett esophagus at the lower third of the esophagus, and in the esophagogastric junction have increased in incidence recent years, representing more than 50% of all patients.[21–24] Esophageal cancer presents as a fungating, ulcerative, or infiltrative tumor. The commonest gross appearance of the tumor is a combination of these features with fungating, ulcerated intraluminal tumor infiltrating the esophageal wall and causing concentric narrowing of the central esophageal lumen. Submucosal spread of this tumor can be quite extensive, and skip metastasis along the submucosal lymphatics has been found as far as 8 cm from the site of the gross tumor.[25] The absence of the serosal covering of the esophagus is another significant factor for an early extension of the tumor into the surrounding structures.

## ANATOMICAL CONSIDERATIONS

The esophagus is generally divided into three anatomical regions.[26] The cervical esophagus extends from the cricopharyngeal sphincter at the pharyngoesophageal junction, down to the level of the thoracic inlet, approximately 18 cm from the upper incisor teeth. The middle third extends from the thoracic inlet to a point 10 cm above the gastroesophageal junction, a point usually at the level of the eighth thoracic vertebra and approximately 31 cm from the upper incisors. In the upper two-thirds region, the esophagus is in immediate contact with the tracheobronchus, aorta, the azygous vein, and the vertebral column. The lower third of the esophagus extends from a point 10 cm above the gastroesophageal junction to the cardiac orifice of the stomach a point approximately 40 cm from the upper incisors. The distal thoracic esophagus is also in close contact with the pericardium of the left atrium, the inferior vena cava, and the descending aorta. The relative frequency rate of squamous cell carcinoma in the esophagus is 20% in the upper third, 50% in the middle third, and 30% in the lower third.

## EVALUATION OF THE PATIENT'S GENERAL CONDITION AND TUMOR EXTENT

The esophagogram is the mainstay of radiologic diagnosis. It provides detailed information with regard to the length of the tumor, the degree of obstruction, and its relation to the surrounding normal structure. A fistula between the esophagus and the tracheobronchial tree is best demonstrated by this method. Computed tomography (CT) of the esophagus with barium as a contrast medium is an additional important diagnostic tool in identifying the presence or absence of mediastinal invasion and enlarged mediastinal lymph nodes. Computed tomography of the upper abdomen has also provided very valuable information with regard to the involvement of the liver and upper abdominal lymph nodes. The establishment of a tissue diagnosis of esophageal carcinoma is the first step toward the necessary management. Fiber-optic esophagoscopy with directed biopsy and brush cytology provides a diagnosis of esophageal carcinoma in 90% to 96% of patients. For patients with esophageal cancer involving the upper two-thirds of the esophagus, bronchoscopy should also be performed at the time of esophagoscopy to evaluate the trachea or tracheobronchi for tumor invasion. Endoscopic ultrasound study is also valuable in assessing the depth of invasion, involvement of the surrounding normal tissue and regional lymph node. It is essential to have complete information about the true extent of the tumor to formulate a proper plan of treatment. The patient's general condition should also be carefully evaluated with regard to cardiopulmonary and metabolic status. The TNM staging system by American Joint Committee on Cancer is used to stage carcinoma of the esophagus.[26] The various categories of T, N, and M are grouped into appropriate combinations to categorize five stages of the disease (Table 7-5).

**TABLE 7-5   The 1997 AJCC TNM Staging and Stage Grouping for Esophageal Cancer**

| | *Primary Tumor (T)* | | | | *Distant Metastasis (M)* | | |
|---|---|---|---|---|---|---|---|
| Tx | Primary tumor cannot be assessed | | | MX | Distant metastasis cannot be assessed | | |
| T0 | No evidence of primary tumor | | | M0 | No distant metastasis | | |
| Tis | Carcinoma in situ | | | M1 | Distant metastasis | | |
| T1 | Tumor invades lamina propria or submucosa | | | | Tumors of the lower thoracic esophagus | | |
| T2 | Tumor invades muscularis propria | | | | M1a   Metastasis in celiac lymph nodes | | |
| T3 | Tumor invades adventitia | | | | M1b   Other distant metastasis | | |
| T4 | Tumor invades adjacent structures | | | | Tumors of the midthoracic esophagus | | |

Tumors of the midthoracic esophagus
    M1a  Not applicable
    M1b  Nonregional lymph nodes and/or other distant metastasis
Tumors of the upper thoracic esophagus
    M1a  Metastasis in cervical nodes
    M1b  Other distant metastasis

*Regional Lymph Nodes (N)*

Nx  Regional lymph nodes cannot be assessed
N0  No regional lymph node metastasis
N1  Regional lymph node metastasis

*Stage Grouping*

| | T | N | M |
|---|---|---|---|
| Stage 0 | Tis | N0 | M0 |
| Stage I | T1 | N0 | M0 |
| Stage IIA | T2 | N0 | M0 |
| | T3 | N0 | M0 |
| Stage IIB | T1 | N1 | M0 |
| | T2 | N1 | M0 |
| Stage III | T3 | N1 | M0 |
| | T4 | Any N | M0 |
| Stage IV | Any T | Any N | M1 |
| Stage IVA | Any T | Any N | M1a |
| Stage IVB | Any T | Any N | M1b |

*Regional Lymph Nodes*

Cervical esophagus: scalene, internal jugular, upper cervical, periesophageal, and supraclavicular lymph nodes
Intrathoracic esophagus—upper, middle, and lower: tracheobronchial, superior mediastinal, peritracheal, carinal, hilar, periesophageal, perigastric, paracardial, and mediastinal lymph nodes

*Source:* American Joint Committee on Cancer.[26]

# INDICATION FOR RADIATION THERAPY IN MULTIMODALITY THERAPY FOR CARCINOMA OF THE ESOPHAGUS

The role of radiation therapy in the management of esophageal cancer can be categorized as follows: (1) radiation therapy in combination with multidrug chemotherapy as preoperative therapy for marginally resectable or resectable esophageal cancer, (2) concurrent chemoradiotherapy for locally advanced and/or medically inoperable esophageal cancer, and (3) palliative radiation therapy for obstructive symptoms.

## Radiation Therapy in Combination with Chemotherapy as Preoperative Therapy

The concurrent use of radiation and multidrug chemotherapy is advantageous in achieving the maximum tumor control when the combined antitumor effect from both methods is more than just additive. Leichman et al. at Wayne State University conducted a first study of concurrent chemoradiotherapy in which two cycles of cisplatin plus 5-fluorouracil (5-FU) were given along with 3000 cGy of concurrent radiation at 200 cGy in daily fractions, 5 days per week.[27,28] Cisplatin and 5-FU are known to enhance the effect of irradiation.[29,30] Of 21 patients who were entered into a trial using this approach, two patients refused surgery, leaving 19 patients for survival analysis. Five (26%) of these 19 patients had no tumor at the time of surgery, and all five survived 24 months or longer. Two patients died of apparently unrelated disease, while the other three were alive without evidence of disease. A drawback to concurrent chemotherapy and irradiation may be a potential increase in toxicity. An expanded trial of the same study design by the Southwest Oncology and Radiation Therapy Oncology Groups showed a 9.3% (8/86) operative mortality when patient selection for surgery was limited to those with resectable tumor only. Twenty-two of 86 patients (25%) did not show residual tumor at the time of surgery.[27]

Recent randomized trials compared preoperative chemotherapy and surgery with surgery alone against preoperative chemoradiotherapy and surgery with surgery alone in patients with resectable carcinoma of the esophagus.

1. Kelsen et al.[14] conducted a randomized trial in which surgery alone was compared with three cycles of preoperative chemotherapy (cisplatin, 100 mg/m$^2$, on days 1, 29, and 58; 5-fluorouracil, 1000 mg/m$^2$, as a continuous 24 h infusion on days 1–5 of each cycle) and surgery. Postoperative chemotherapy (two cycles) with a reduced dose of cisplatin (75 mg/m$^2$) was administered to those who had stable or responding disease and had undergone potentially curative resection. The study randomly assigned 467 patients to either surgery alone or preoperative chemotherapy and surgery. Patients with adenocarcinoma accounted for 55% of all patients. After a median possible study time of 55.4 months, there were no differences in resection rates (65% vs. 66%), treatment mortality (6.4% vs. 4.0%), median survival time (14.9 months vs. 16.1 months), and 2-year survival rates (35% vs. 37%), respectively, for preoperative chemotherapy and surgery versus the surgery-alone group. The preoperative chemotherapy used in

this study was not effective in improving resection rate and short-term survival over surgery alone. A further follow-up is necessary to see a potential long-term benefit of this neoadjuvant therapy.

2. Walsh et al.[8] compared preoperative chemoradiotherapy and surgery with surgery alone in 113 patients with esophageal adenocarcinoma. The preoperative therapy included two cycles of chemotherapy in weeks 1 and 6 (5-FU 15 mg/kg, daily for 5 days, and cisplatin, 75 mg/m$^2$, on day 7 of each cycle) and concurrent radiotherapy (4000 cGy/15 F/3 wks). The median survival time was 16 months for the multimodality therapy, compared with 11 months for surgery alone. The survival rates at 1, 2, and 3 years were 52%, 37%, and 32%, respectively, for patients treated with a multimodality regimen, compared with 44%, 26%, and 6% for those assigned to surgery alone, with the survival advantage favoring multimodality therapy ($p = 0.01$).

Urba et al.[9] also reported a randomized study in which the combination of preoperative chemoradiotherapy and surgery was compared with surgery alone. The preoperative therapy consisted of an intensive course of chemotherapy (cisplatin, 20 mg/m$^2$, on days 1–5 and 17–21; vinblastine, 1 mg/m$^2$, days 1–4 and 17–20; 5-FU 300 mg/m$^2$, days 1–21) and radiotherapy (4500 cGy in fractions of 150 cGy, twice daily for 3 wks). Surgery was performed on day 42. Fifty patients were randomized to each arm. Adenocarcinoma accounted for 75% of all patients. The median survival time and 3-year survival rate were 1.41 years and 32% for the combined therapy group, compared with 1.46 years and 15% for the surgery alone group ($p = 0.04$). Local–regional recurrence as the first site of failure was noted in 39% of patients treated with surgery alone, compared with 19% of patients in the combined therapy group ($p = 0.039$). Pathologic complete response was associated with improved survival ($p = 0.006$).

The results of these phase III studies indicate that radiation therapy plays an important role in preoperative therapy for locally advanced, yet resectable, esophageal cancer. Pathologic complete response was also found to be associated with better survival in preoperative chemoradiotherapy.

## Radiation Therapy in Concurrent Chemoradiotherapy for Unresectable Esophageal Cancer

Herskovic et al.[31] compared a concurrent combination of chemotherapy (four cycles of 5-FU, 1000 mg/m$^2$, continuous 24 h IV infusion for the first 4 days of weeks 1, 5, 8, and 11 and cisplatin, 75 mg/m$^2$, on the first day of each cycle) and radiation therapy (5000 cGy/25 F/5 wks) with radiation therapy (6400 cGy/32 F/6.4 wks) alone for patients with carcinoma of the thoracic esophagus. This trial was stopped when the accrual of patients reached 121 and interim analysis showed a significant survival advantage in the chemoradiotherapy arm. An update of this study by Al-sarraf et al. reported median survival times and 5-year survival rates of 14 months and 27% for the combined treatment group, compared with 9.3 months and 0% for the radiation therapy alone group.[7] Squamous cell cancer accounted for 90% of all patients. The results of this study indicate that radiation therapy alone is inadequate in treating patients with inoperable carcinoma of the esophagus.

## Palliative Radiation Therapy for Obstructive Symptoms

Relief of malignant esophageal obstruction is another important goal of therapy. Radiation therapy offers improved quality of life by providing a sustained relief of malignant esophageal obstruction. Radiation dose schedule of 4000 cGy in daily dose fractions of 200 to 250 cGy, five fractions per week, over a period of 3.2 to 4 weeks, has been used with a 60% to 70% rate of relief of obstructive symptoms. Intracavitary brachytherapy has also been used for the goal. Stent can also provide fast relief of dysphagia. However, it is often associated with reflux symptoms.

## RADIATION THERAPY TECHNIQUE

Radiotherapeutic factors important in the achievement of therapeutic goals include a clear definition of target volume, optimal radiation dose and fractionation schedules, and proper radiation portal arrangements to secure adequate dose distribution within the target volume while the surrounding normal tissues are protected.

### Target Volume

The target volume consists of clinical target volume (CTV) and gross tumor volume (GTV). To secure an adequate lateral coverage of the mediastinum, CTV includes margins of at least 5 cm in the cephalad–caudad direction beyond the radiographic extent of the tumor and a lateral margin of 2.5 cm beyond the lateral border of the tumor outlined by the esophagogram. A typical field size for a tumor 6 cm in length is 16 × 9 cm$^2$. For lesions at the lower third of the esophagus and esophagogastric junction, CTV is extended into the lower border of the first lumbar vertebra to include the celiac, gastric, and gastrohepatic lymph nodes. Computed tomography of the upper abdomen is necessary to locate these lymph nodes. Both supraclavicular regions are also included in CTV for lesions involving the upper two-thirds of the thoracic and cervical esophagus.

### Optimal Dose and Fractionation Schedules

Several different fractionation schedules have similar biologic effects on normal and neoplastic tissues. Recent advances in radiation biology indicate that, for the same total dose, the late reaction of the intrathoracic normal tissue can be reduced if small daily fractions (i.e., 180–200 cGy instead of 250–300 cGy) are used.[32,33] A reasonable relation between radiation dose and local tumor control appears to exist in esophageal cancer. Another important factor for local tumor control is tumor size. For an intended cure by concurrent chemoradiotherapy, a total dose of 6000 to 6400 cGy administered at 180 to 200 cGy daily fractions, 5 days a week, would be necessary. A radiation dose higher than this level needs to be tested by means of three-dimensional conformal therapy.

In preoperative chemoradiotherapy for resectable carcinoma of the esophagus, a total dose of 4500 to 5040 cGy administered at 180 cGy daily fractions, 5 days a week, has been used with encouraging results.[34] Altered fractionation schedules such as accelerated schedule (4500 cGy/30 F/3 wks using 150 cGy/F, twice daily treatment schedule) and a hybrid schedule of twice-daily radiation treatment during chemotherapy cycles and once-daily treatment between the chemotherapy cycles (5850 cGy/34 F/5 wk) have been tested for tolerance, tumor response, and survival.[9,35]

Patients judged incurable because of their poor general condition or the presence of distant metastases can be treated by speedy fractionation schedules. A total dose of 4000 to 4500 cGy at 220 to 250 cGy daily fractions, 5 days a week, is a reasonable schedule for palliation of dysphagia.

## Radiation Portal Arrangements

The arrangement of the radiation portals depends on the planned total dose and the region of involvement in the esophagus. An arrangement of two parallel opposed portals (POP), applied anteriorly (AP) and posteriorly (PA) to the mediastinum, is simple and accurate, with the least risk of a geographical miss. However, this approach needs to be combined with oblique and/or lateral portals to spare the spinal cord and heart.[35,36] To deliver a curative dose of radiation to the GTV of esophagus, it is necessary to combine an AP-PA-POP with right posterior oblique (RPO) and left posterior oblique (LPO) portals or with PRO, LPO, and right and left lateral opposing portals.

For cervical and upper thoracic esophageal cancer, the treatment technique used by the author utilizes a sequential combination of AP-PA-POP for the initial dose (3600 cGy/20 F/4

wk) and a three-field (AP-RPO-LPO) arrangement for the subsequent dose (2700 cGy/15 F/3 wk). Radiation dose to CTV is limited to 4500 cGy.

For patients with esophageal carcinoma involving the lower third of the thoracic esophagus and the esophago gastric junction, radiation dose to the heart should be kept below the tolerance limit (i.e., 4000 cGy to the ventricles, especially when this dose is combined with chemotherapy). The arrangement of radiation portals used by the author includes AP-PA-POP for the initial dose (3060 cGy/17 F/3.4 wk), AP-RPO-LPO for a subsequent dose (2520 cGy/14 F/2.8 wk), and right lateral and left lateral POP for an additional (720 cGy/4 F/0.8 wk), for a total dose of 6300 cGy in 35 fractions over 7 weeks. Radiation dose to CTV is again limited to 4500 cGy.

## Results of Radiation Therapy for Squamous Cell Carcinoma of the Esophagus

It has been conventional practice to treat patients with small lesions (T1 N0) surgically, reserving radiation therapy for patients with unresectable (T4 N1) or medically inoperable lesions (Figure 7-7). The study from Edinburgh by Pearson is of interest in that radiation therapy was as effective as surgery at all three anatomical levels of the esophagus, even before the era of effective chemotherapy.[2,37] The long-term cure rate tends to be better for females than for males. Radiation therapy fares better than surgery for lesions at the upper two-thirds of the esophagus, and vice versa for the lower one-third of the esophagus. A wide range of long-term cure rates by radiation therapy has been reported. Pearson et al. reported a cure rate 17% for thoracic and 29% for cervical esophageal carcinoma with radiation therapy alone. A recent report by Al-sarraf et al. described a median survival time of 14 months and 5-year survival rate of 27% with concurrent chemoradiotherapy (5000 cGy/25 F/5 wk), compared with 9.3 months and 0% with radiation therapy alone (6400 cGy/32 F/6.4 wk) for

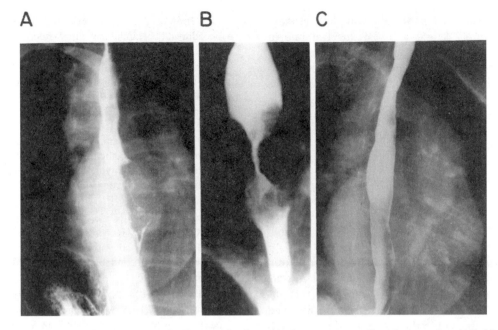

**FIGURE 7-7**    (A, B) Esophagograms of a 53-year-old patient with a large squamous cell carcinoma at the middle third of the esophagus causing a marked obstruction. Operation was not performed because of a severe metabolic disorder. (C) A repeat esophagogram 34 months after 6400 cGy showed a complete remission of the lesion and return of esophageal patency.

patients with locally advanced esophageal carcinoma.[7]

Relief of malignant esophageal obstruction is another important goal of therapy. Radiation therapy offers improved quality of life by providing sustained relief of malignant esophageal obstruction in the majority of patients (60%–70%), even when attempted cure fails. Of 51 patients who received definitive radiation therapy for unresectable tumor at the MGH, 30 (59%) were able to enjoy improved swallowing for two-thirds of the duration of their remaining lifetimes.[4]

## NEW TRENDS

Mass screening for high risk groups by esophageal brushings and washings has led to early detection of esophageal carcinoma and improved cure rates. This approach has achieved a 70% to 80% cure rate by surgery in the northern provinces of China.[20] In addition, preventive measures based on epidemiologic and experimental studies are being instituted in this region.

Innovative approaches are sought to improve the dismal outcome of current treatment for patients with more advanced esophageal cancer (T2-4 or N1). An exploration of concurrent radiation and chemotherapy for potential synergism is an interesting and potentially rewarding approach. Accelerated or hyperfractionated radiation therapy combined with concurrent chemotherapy has a potential for better local tumor and survival.[9]

In a phase II study at the MGH, we combined a three-drug regimen (cisplatin, 5-FU, and taxol) with concurrent radiation using a hybrid schedule of twice-daily radiotherapy during chemotherapy cycles (weeks 1 and 5) and once-a-day radiotherapy between the chemotherapy cycles (weeks 2, 3, and 4). Radiation doses administered consist of 4500 cGy in 25 fractions for 5 weeks for CTV and 5850 cGy in 34 fractions for 5 weeks for GTV by having 1350 cGy in nine fractions as concurrent boost during chemotherapy cycles. This study showed a pathologic complete response rate of 37% and a 3-year survival rate of 50%.[35,38] Further follow-up is necessary to know the impact of increased intensity of radiotherapy in preoperative chemoradiotherapy.

Hypoxic cell sensitizer may have a role in improving local tumor control. Misonidazole has been tried with irradiation in an attempt to improve local tumor control.[39,40] However, the results are not promising. There are other new agents that need to be tested. Particle beam irradiation (neutron, helium ion) has also been tried without positive results.[41,42] Intraluminal therapy by means of intracavitary application of iridium-192 or cobalt-60 has been used either for palliation of esophageal obstruction or for boosting the primary tumor after external beam irradiation.[43–45] However, this approach does not adequately treat the involved areas adjacent to the tumor or regional lymph nodes.

## REFERENCES

1. Wilkins EW Jr: Perspective in esophageal cancer, in NC Delarue, EW Wilkins Jr, and J Wong (eds): *International Trends in General Thoracic Surgery.* St. Louis, CV Mosby, 1988, pp 440–444.

2. Pearson JG: Radiation therapy for carcinoma of the esophagus, in NC Choi and HC Grillo (eds): *Thoracic Oncology.* New York, Raven Press, 1983, pp 303–325.

3. Earlam R, Cunha-Melo JR: Esophageal squamous cell carcinoma: 1. A critical review of surgery. *Br J Surg* 1980;67:381–390.

4. Langer M, Choi NC, Orlow E, et al: Radiation therapy alone or in combination with surgery in the treatment of carcinoma of the esophagus. *Cancer* 1986;58:1208–1213.

5. Choi NC: The role of radiation therapy in the management of malignant neoplasms of the esophagus, in HC Grillo, WG Austen, EW Wilkins Jr, DJ Mathisen, and GJ Vlahakes (eds): *Current Therapy in Cardiothoracic Surgery.* Toronto: BC Decker, l989, pp 197–199.

6. Carey RW, Hilgenberg AD, Wilkins EW, Choi NC, Mathisen DJ, Grillo HC, Wain JC, Logan DL, Bromberg C: Long-term follow-up of neoadjuvant chemotherapy with 5-fluorouracil and cisplatin with surgical resection and possible postoperative radiotherapy and/or chemotherapy in squamous cell carcinoma of the esophagus. *Cancer Invest* 1993;11:99–105.

7. Al-Sarraf M, Martz K, Herskovic A, Leichman L, Brindle JS, Vaitkevicius VK, Cooper J, Byhardt R, Davis L, Emami B: Progress report of combined chemoradiotherapy versus radiotherapy alone in patients with esophageal cancer: An intergroup study. *J Clin Oncol* 1997;15:277–284.

8. Walsh TN, Noonan N, Hollywood D, Kelly A, Stat C, Keeling N, Hennessy PJ: A comparison of multimodality therapy and surgery for esophageal adenocarcinoma. *New Engl J Med* 1996;335:462–467.

9. Urba S, Orringer M, Turrisi A, Whyte R, Iannettoni M, Forastiere A: A randomized trial comparing surgery (S) to preoperative concomitant chemoradiation plus surgery in patients with resectable esophageal cancer: Updated analysis. *Proc ASCO* 1997;16:983 (abstr).

10. Leichman L, Steiger Z, Seydel HG, et al: Combined preoperative chemotherapy and radiation therapy for cancer of the esophagus: The Wayne State University, Southwest Oncology Group, and Radiation Therapy Oncology Group experience. *Semin Oncol* 1984;11:178–185.

11. Kelsen D, Bains M, Hilaris B, et al: Combined modality therapy of esophageal cancer. *Semin Oncol* 1984;11:169–177.

12. Carey RW, Hilgenberg AD, Wilkins EW, et al: Preoperative chemotherapy followed by surgery with possible postoperative radiotherapy in squamous cell carcinoma of the esophagus: Evaluation of the chemotherapy component. *J Clin Oncol* 1986;4:697–701.

13. Forastiere A, Heitmiller R, Ding-Jen L, Zahurak M, Abrams R, Klienberg L, Watkins S, Yeo C, Lillemoe K, Sitzmann J, Sharfman W: Intensive chemoradiation followed by esophagectomy for squamous cell and adenocarcinoma of the esophagus. *Cancer J Sci Am* 1997;3:144–152.

14. Kelsen DP, Ginsberg R, Pajak TF, Sheahan DG, Gunderson L, Mortimer J, Estes N, Haller DG, Ajani J, Kocha W, Minsky BD, Roth JA: Chemotherapy followed by surgery compared with surgery alone for localized esophageal cancer. *New Engl J Med* 1998;339:1979–1984.

15. Cutler SJ, Young JL: Third National Cancer Survey: Incidence data. *Natl Cancer Inst Monogr* 1975;41:12–454.

16. Garfinkel L, Poindexter CE, Silverberg E: Cancer in black Americans. *CA J Cancer Clin* 1980;30:39–44.

17. Rogers EL, Goldkind L, Goldkind SF: Increasing frequency of esophageal cancer among black male veterans. *Cancer* 1982;49:610–617.

18. Greenlee RT, Murray T, Bolden S, Wingo PA: Cancer statistics, 2000. *CA Cancer J Clin* 2000;50:7–33.

19. Kmet J, Mahboubi E: Esophageal cancer in the Caspian littoral of Iran: Initial studies. *Science* 1972;175:846–853.

20. Wu YK, Huang GJ, Shao LF, et al: Progress in the study and surgical treatment of cancer of the esophagus in China, 1940–1980. *J Thorac Cardiovasc Surg* 1982;84:325–333.

21. Naef AP, Savary M, Ozzello L: Columnar-lined lower esophagus: An acquired lesion with malignant predisposition. *J Thorac Cardiovasc Surg* 1975;70:826–835.

22. Poleynard GD, Marty AT, Birnbaum WB, et al: Adenocarcinoma in the columnar-lined (Barrett) esophagus. *Arch Surg* 1977;112:997–1000.

23. Cameron AJ, Ott BJ, Payne WS: The incidence of adenocarcinoma in columnar-lined (Barrett's) esophagus. *New Engl J Med* 1985;313:857–859.

24. Blot WJ, Devesa SS, Kneller RW, Fraumeni JF: Continuing climb in rates of esophageal adenocarcinoma: An update. *JAMA* 1993;270:1320.

25. Watson WL, Goodner JT, Miller TP, et al: Torek esophagectomy: The case against segmental resection for esophageal cancer. *J Thorac Surg* 1956;32:347–357.

26. American Joint Committee on Cancer: *AJCC Cancer Staging Manual,* 5th ed. Philadelphia, Lippincott-Raven, 1997, pp 65–69.

27. Leichman L, Steiger Z, Seydel G, Dindogru A, Kinzie J, Toben S, MacKenzie G, Shell J: Preoperative chemotherapy and radiation therapy for patients with cancer of the esophagus: A potential curative approach. *J Clin Oncol* 1984;2:75–79.

28. Leichman L, Herskovic A, Leichman CG, Steiger LZ, Tapazoglou E, Rosenberg JC, Arbulu A, Asfaw I, Kinzie J: Nonoperative therapy for squamous-cell cancer of the esophagus. *J Clin Oncol* 1987;5:365–370.

29. Douple EB, Richmond RC: Enhancement of the potentiation of radiotherapy by platinum drugs in a mouse tumor. *Int J Radiat Oncol Biol Phys* 1982;8:501–503.

30. Byfield JE, Barone RM, Mendelsohn J, et al: Infusional 5-fluorouracil and x-ray therapy for nonresectable esophageal cancer. *Cancer* 1980;45:703–708.

31. Herskovic A, Martz K, Al-Sarraf, Leichman L, Brindle J, Vaitkevicius, Cooper J, Byhardt R, Davis L, Emami B: Combined chemotherapy and radiotherapy compared with radiotherapy alone in patients with cancer of the esophagus. *New Engl J Med* 1992;326:1593–1598.

32. Thames HD, Peters LJ, Withers HR, et al: Accelerated fractionation vs. hyperfractionation: Rationales for several treatments per day. *Int J Radiat Oncol Biol Phys* 1983;9:127–138.

33. Withers HR: Biologic basis for altered fractionation schemes. *Cancer* 1985;55:2086–2095.

34. Forastiere AA, Heitmiller RF, Lee DJ, Zahurak M, Abrams R, Kleinberg L, Watkins S, Yeo CJ, Lillemoe KD, Sitzmann JV, Sharfman W: Intensive chemoradiation followed by esophagectomy for squamous cell and adenocarcinoma of the esophagus. *Cancer J Sci Am* 1997;3:144–152.

35. Choi N, Lynch T, Mathisen D, Wain J, Wright C, Carey R, Grossbard M, Grillo H: Phase I/II study of preoperative chemo-radiotherapy (CT-RT) using twice daily radiation as concomitant boost during two cycles of taxol, cisplatin, 5-FU in esophageal cancer: Normal tissue tolerance and early results. *Proc Am Soc Ther Radiol Oncol* 1997;39:137 (abstr).

36. Choi NC: The role of radiation therapy in the management of malignant neoplasms of the esophagus, in HC Grillo, WG Austen, EW Wilkins Jr, DJ Mathisen, and GJ Vlahakes (eds): *Current Therapy in Cardiothoracic Surgery.* Toronto, BC Decker, 1989, pp 197–199.

37. Pearson, JG: The value of radiotherapy in the management of squamous esophageal cancer. *Br J Surg* 1971;S8:794.

38. Wright CD, Wain JC, Lynch TJ, Choi NC, Grossbard ML, Carey RW, Moncure AC, Grillo HC, Mathisen DJ: Induction therapy for esophageal cancer with paclitaxel and hyper-

fractionated radiotherapy: A phase I and II study. *J Thorac Cardiovasc Surg* 1997;114:811–816.

39. Schwade JG, Kinsella TJ, Kelly B, et al: Clinical experience with intravenous misonidazole for carcinoma of the esophagus: Results in attempting radiosensitization of each fraction of exposure. *Cancer Invest* 1984;2:91–95.

40. Ydrach AA, Marcial VA, Parsons J, et al: Misonidazole and unconventional irradiation in advanced squamous cell carcinoma of the esophagus: A phase II study of the Radiation Therapy Oncology Group. *Int J Radiat Oncol Biol Phys* 1982;8:357–359.

41. Laramore GE, Davis RB, Olson MH, et al: RTOG phase I study on fast neutron teletherapy for squamous cell carcinoma of the esophagus. *Int J Radiat Oncol Biol Phys* 1983;9:465–473.

42. Castro JR, Saunders WM, Tobias CA, et al: Treatment of cancer with heavy charged parti-

cles. *Int J Radiat Oncol Biol Phys* 1982;8: 2191–2198.

43. Hishikawa Y, Kurisu K, Taniguchi M, Kamikonya N, Miura T: High-dose-rate intraluminal brachytherapy (HDEIBT) for esophageal cancer. *Int J Radiat Oncol Biol Phys* 1991;21: 1133–1135.

44. Pagliero KM, Rowland CG: Brachytherapy for inoperable cancer of the esophagus and cardia, in NC Delarue, EW Wilkins Jr, and J Wong (eds): *International Trends in General Thoracic Surgery.* St. Louis, CV Mosby, 1988, pp 361–367.

45. Rowland CG, Pagliero KM: Intracavity irradiation in palliation of carcinoma of oesophagus and cardia. *Lancet* 1985;2:981.

# CHAPTER 8

# GASTROINTESTINAL MALIGNANCIES

CHRISTOPHER G. WILLETT

## A. PANCREATIC CANCER

### INTRODUCTION

Patients with pancreatic cancer usually present with lesions in the head of the pancreas that either have spread beyond the local area via hematogenous or peritoneal routes or are technically unresectable owing to the local extent of disease.[1] For the latter group, the main surgical options are palliative biliary bypass alone or in combination with elective gastroenterostomy.[1] Until recently, even though a majority of lesions were unresectable and only palliative procedures could be performed, surgery was the only therapy considered in most patients. If gains are to be made with the locally unresectable pancreatic lesions, they will have to be accomplished with radiation, chemotherapy, or both.

### MANAGEMENT

The standard surgical treatment for pancreatic cancer remains the pancreaticoduodenectomy, first described by Whipple et al. in 1935. Initially, high operative morbidity and mortality rates led to technical modifications of the operation that, combined with improvements in anesthesia and critical care, have resulted in current perioperative mortality rates of 2% or less. Surgical resection, as part of a multimodality treatment approach for patients with resectable pancreatic cancer, represents the only potentially curative treatment strategy. Although 5-year survival rates are poor even with resection (5–20%), a significant difference in survival does exist in patients undergoing definitive resection as opposed to palliative bypass or exploration with biopsy alone.[2] Some authors believe that total pancreatectomies can be performed with operative mortality similar to that of less radical "curative" procedures, yielding lymphadenectomy that is nearer to optimal. This approach has not improved survival in most series.

For patients with unresectable tumors or metastatic disease, death often results from hepatic failure due to biliary obstruction by local tumor extension or hepatic replacement by metastases. For the small percentage of patients (10–20%) undergoing a potentially curative pancreaticoduodenectomy, three major sites of disease recurrence dominate: the bed of the resected pancreas (local recurrence), the peritoneal cavity, and the liver. As the data from several patterns of failure studies after resection show, local failure rates are high, ranging from 50% to 86%.[2–4] Pancreatic cancers frequently invade into the retroperitoneal soft tissues, and the high incidence of local failure following pancreaticoduodenectomy reflects the inability to achieve wide retroperitoneal soft tissue margins because of anatomical constraints to further

*Clinical Radiation Oncology: Indications, Techniques, and Results, 2nd ed.* Edited by C.C. Wang.
ISBN: 0-471-23803-1 Copyright © 2000 Wiley-Liss, Inc.

excision of tissue (superior mesenteric artery and vein, portal vein, and inferior vena cava). Furthermore, after a Whipple resection, there is a high incidence of microscopic residual disease remaining in the patient. In a series from the Massachusetts General Hospital, 51% of patients were found to have tumor extension to the surgical margins after Whipple procedure.[4]

## RADIATION TREATMENT PLANNING

The patients should be supine during simulation and treatment by external beam radiation therapy (EBRT).[2] After injection of renal contrast to identify operative clips and renal position relative to the field center, an initial set of anteroposterior (AP) and cross-table lateral films is obtained. Additional films can be ob-

tained with contrast in the stomach and duodenal loop. The intent of treatment is to use multiple-field fractionated external beam techniques with high energy photons to deliver 45 to 50 Gy in 1.80 Gy fractions to unresected or residual tumor, as defined by CT and clips, plus nodal areas at risk. With head-of-pancreas lesions, major node groups include the pancreaticoduodenal, porta hepatis, celiac, and suprapancreatic. The latter node group is included along with the body of pancreas for a 3 to 5 cm margin beyond gross disease, but more than two-thirds of the left kidney is excluded from the AP-PA field, since at least 50% of the right kidney is often in the field because of duodenal inclusion. The entire duodenal loop with margin is included, since head lesions may invade the medial wall of the duodenum and place the entire circumference at risk (Figure 8-1). With

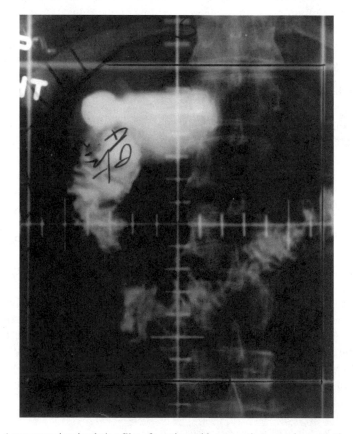

**FIGURE 8-1** Anteroposterior simulation film of a patient with pancreatic cancer demonstrating duodenal sweep.

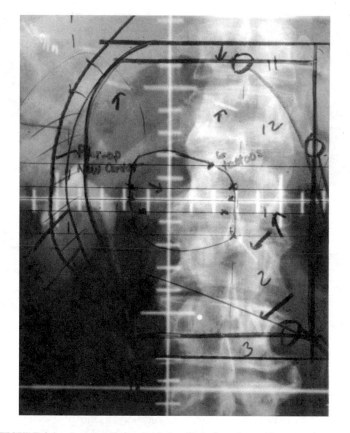

**FIGURE 8-2**    Anteroposterior simulation film of a patient with pancreatic cancer.

body–tail lesions, at least 50% of the left kidney may need to be included to achieve adequate pancreas margins and to include node groups at risk (lateral suprapancreatic and splenic hilum). Since inclusion of the entire duodenal loop is not indicated with body or tail lesions, at least two-thirds of the right kidney can be preserved, but with tailored blocks, one can usually adequately cover pancreaticoduodenal and porta hepatis nodes. For head-of-pancreas lesions, the superior field extent is at mid- or upper-T11 vertebral body for adequate margins on the celiac vessels (T12, L1) (Figure 8-2). The upper field extent is occasionally more superior with body lesions, to obtain adequate margin on the primary lesion. With the lateral fields, the anterior field margin is 1.5 to 2.0 cm beyond gross disease. The posterior margin is at least 1.5 cm behind the anterior

portion of the vertebral body, to allow adequate margins on para-aortic nodes, which are a major node group at risk with posterior tumor extension in either head or body lesions. The lateral contribution is usually limited to 12 to 15 Gy because a moderate volume of kidney or liver may be in the field (Figure 8-3).

## RADIATION THERAPY RESULTS

### Resectable Tumors

In patients who have resectable lesions there is justification for adjuvant treatment on the basis of patterns of failure after resection and the results of a prospective randomized trial from the Gastrointestinal Tumor Study Group.[3] In this study patients were randomized to receive no

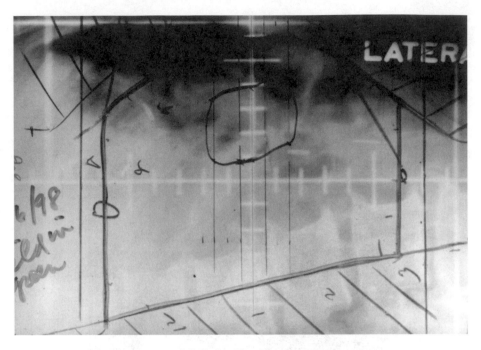

**FIGURE 8-3**   Lateral simulation film of a patient with pancreatic cancer.

further treatment (surgery-alone control arm—22 patients) or irradiation plus 5-fluorouracil (5-FU: 40 Gy in a 6-week split course technique with 5-FU, 500 mg/m$^2$, days 1–3 of each sequence—23 patients). A survival advantage was seen with the combined treatment, with a 2-year survival rate of 42% versus 15% and 5-year survival rate of 14% versus 5% ($p <$ 0.05). Subsequently, the Gastrointestinal Tumor Study Group (GITSG)[6] registered 30 additional patients in the treatment group and replicated and confirmed the improved survival (Table 8-1).[5–10]

It is difficult to interpret the significance of the incidence of local failure in GITSG series. Since the resection-alone group had a median survival of only 10.9 months, many patients were not at risk long enough to develop symptoms of local recurrence. The incidence of local recurrence is excessive with the low doses of irradiation used in this trial (40 Gy in 6 weeks + 5-FU). With the use of multiple shaped fields, it is possible to deliver 45 to 50 Gy in 25 to 28 fractions over 5 to 5.5 weeks, in combination with 5-FU with acceptable tolerance in an adjuvant setting. Prospective nonrandomized data from single-institution studies suggest improved local control and survival for patients receiving postoperative irradiation and 5-FU following resection compared to patients undergoing resection alone (Table 8-1).[7–10] More recently, there has been interest in the use of preoperative chemoirradiation and resection protocols for patients with resectable pancreatic cancer. Data from Japanese and U.S. centers have shown acceptable morbidity and mortality rates with these protocols.[11–13] Preliminary local control and survival results from these studies are summarized in Table 8-2.

Local control results are encouraging, with the incidence of local failure ranging from 9% to 20%. The experience of intraoperative radiation therapy (IORT) as adjuvant therapy in resectable pancreatic cancer is more limited. Investigators at the National Cancer Institute have carried out a controlled prospective trial of adjuvant radiation following curative resection.[14] Patients were randomized to receive 20

Gy IORT immediately after resection, followed by 50 Gy of postoperative external beam irradiation, or 50 Gy postoperative external beam irradiation only. Although overall survival time was the same for the two groups, local control and median survival were improved in patients receiving IORT.

## Unresectable for Cure External Beam Irradiation with or Without Chemotherapy

For unresectable lesions, definite palliation can be obtained by means of external beam irradiation techniques.[2] The duration of pallia-tion appears to increase as the dose of radiation is increased from 40 Gy in 4.5 to 6 weeks to 60 to 65 Gy in 7 to 10 weeks (using a split-course technique with the longer time period). To deliver doses in excess of 45 to 50 Gy with safety, care must be taken to minimize the amount of normal tissue in the irradiated field. This requires an accurate delineation of tumor volume (from CT scan and/or sparsely placed small surgical clips) and the use of multiple-field irradiation techniques. The combination of irradiation and chemotherapy for locally unresectable tumors increases survival compared to radiation alone or chemotherapy alone (Table 8-3).

**TABLE 8-1    Results Following Resection and Postoperative Adjuvant Therapy**

| Study | Number of Patients | EBRT Dose (Gy) | Chemotherapy | Median Survival (months) | 2-Year Survival (%) | Local Failure (%) |
|---|---|---|---|---|---|---|
| GITSG[5,6] | | | | | | |
|   Resection only | 22 | | | 10.9 | 18 | 33 |
|   Resection/EBRT | 19 | 40 Gy | 5-FU | 21 | 46 | 47 |
|   Resection/EBRT | 30 | 40 Gy | 5-FU | 18 | 43 | 55 |
| Whittington et al.[7] | | | | | | |
|   Resection only | 29 | | | 15 | 41 | 85 |
|   Resection/EBRT | 19 | ≤45 Gy | No | 15 | 33 | 55 |
|   Resection/EBRT | 20 | ≥45 Gy | 5-FU/ Mitomycin - C | 16 | 59 | 25 |
| Bossett et al.[8] | 14 | 54 Gy | | 23 | 50 | 50 |
| Foo et al.[9] | 29 | 54 Gy | | 22.7 | 48 | 7 |
| Yeo et al.[10] | | | | | | |
|   Resection | 22 | | | 12 | 0 | Not specified |
|   Resection/EBRT | 56 | Not specified | 5-FU | 20 | 35 | Not specified |

**TABLE 8-2    Results After Preoperative Irradiation with or Without Chemotherapy and Resection for Pancreatic Cancer**

| Study | Number of Patients | EBRT Dose (Gy) | Chemotherapy | Median Survival (months) | 4-Year Actuarial Survival (%) | Local Failure (%) |
|---|---|---|---|---|---|---|
| Ishikawa et al.[13] | 23 | 50 | | 15 | 22 | 20 |
| Hoffman et al.[11] | 11 | 50.4 | 5-FU/Mitomycin-C | 33 | 40 | 9 |
| Staley et al.[12] | 39 | 30–50.4 10 (IORT) | 5-FU | 19 | 19 | 11 |

With the exception of the Eastern Cooperative Oncology Study,[15] this has been shown in randomized studies from the Mayo Clinic[16] and the Gastrointestinal Tumor Study Group[17–20] and in nonrandomized series from Duke[21] and Thomas Jefferson University.[22–24] However, even in the high dose series from Jefferson, local failure was documented in at least two-thirds of patients.

Because of these high local failures, preoperative irradiation has been studied to assess its ability to convert locally unresectable pancreatic cancer to resectable disease. Pilepich and Miller[25] reported a series using preoperative irradiation in 17 patients with unresectable or borderline resectable lesions (16 of 17 were explored, and the main cause of unresectability was vascular adherence or invasion). Lesion size was less than 5 cm in 4 patients and 5 cm or more in 13. Radiation was delivered in 2 Gy fractions to a total of 40 to 50 cGy in 4 to 6 weeks, with reexploration usually in 6 weeks. Eleven of the 17 patients were reexplored. Radical surgery was done in

6, all with lesions in the head (3 of 6, or 50%, were alive at time of publication). Two of six were free of disease at 5 years, and two had known recurrence. In a study from the New England Deaconess Hospital, 16 patients with locally unresectable pancreatic cancer were treated with 45 Gy of external beam irradiation and infusional 5-FU to enhance resectability.[26] Of these 16 patients, only 2 (13%) were able to undergo resection.

## Intraoperative Irradiation (Interstitial Implantation or Electrons)

Specialized radiation therapy techniques that increase the irradiation dose relative to the tumor volume have been used in an attempt to improve local tumor control without increasing normal tissue morbidity. Such measures, which include the use of [125]I implants[27] or intraoperative electrons[28–35] as a boost dose in combination techniques, have resulted in a lower incidence of local failure in most series and improved median survival in some compared with

**TABLE 8-3 Prospective Randomized Studies of Radiation Therapy and Chemotherapy for Unresectable Pancreatic Cancer**

| Study and Treatment[a] | Number of Patients | Median Survival (months) | Local Failure in Evaluable Patients (%) | 2-Year Survival (%) |
|---|---|---|---|---|
| Mayo Clinic[16] | | | | |
| EBRT (35–37.5 Gy/4 wk) only | 32 | 6.3 | | |
| EBRT (35–37.5 Gy/4 wk)/5-FU | 32 | 10.4 | | |
| GITSG[16] | | | | |
| EBRT (60 Gy/10 wk) only | 25 | 5.2 | 24 | 5 |
| EBRT (40 Gy/6 wk)/5-FU | 83 | 9.6 | 26 | 10 |
| EBRT (60 Gy/10 wk)/5-FU | 86 | 9.2 | 27 | 10 |
| GITSG[18] | | | | |
| EBRT (60 Gy/10 wk)/5-FU | 73 | 8.4 | 58 | 12 |
| EBRT (60 Gy/10 wk)/doxorubicin | 72 | 7.5 | 51 | 6 |
| GITSG[19] | | | | |
| EBRT (54 Gy/6 wk)/5-FU/SMF | 31 | 6.5 | 38 | 41 (1 yr) |
| SMF only | 26 | 5.1 | 29 | 19 (1 yr) |
| ECOG[15] | | | | |
| EBRT (40 Gy/4 wk)/5-FU | 47 | 5.1 | 32 | 6 |
| 5-FU only | 44 | 6.5 | 32 | 13 |

[a]EBRT, external beam radiation therapy; GITSG, Gastrointestinal Tumor Study Group; ECOG, Eastern Cooperative Oncology Group; 5-FU, 5-fluorouracil; SMF, streptozotocin, mitomycin-C, and 5-FU.

TABLE 8-4    External Beam Radiation Therapy (EBRT) and Intraoperative Electron Irradiation (IOERT) with and Without Chemotherapy (ChT) for Unresectable Carcinoma of the Pancreas

| Study and Treatment | Number of Patients | Median Survival (months) | 2-Year Actuarial Survival Rate (%) | 2-Year Actuarial Local Failure (%) |
|---|---|---|---|---|
| MGH[27,29,30] | | | | |
| $^{125}$I + EBRT (40–45 Gy/5 wk) ± ChT | 12 | 12 | 20 | 33 |
| EBRT (45–50 Gy/6 wk) ± ChT/IOERT (15–20 Gy) | 22 | 16.5 | 33 | 69 |
| EBRT (45–50 Gy/6 wk) ± ChT/IOERT (20 Gy)/misonidazole | 41 | 12.0 | 20 | 55 |
| Mayo Clinic[28,32] | | | | |
| EBRT (40–60 Gy/6 wk) ± ChT | 122 | 12.6 | 16 | 80 |
| Preoperative EBRT (50.4–54 Gy) ± ChT/IOERT (20 Gy) | 27 | 14.9 | 27 | 32 |
| Postoperative EBRT (45–55) Gy/6 wks ± ChT[a] IOERT (20 Gy) | 56 | 10.5 | 6 | 35 |

[a]In earlier series of 37 patients who received IOERT plus postoperative EBRT at Mayo Clinic, median survival was 13.4 months, 2-year survival was 12%, and liver or peritoneal failure rate was 54%.

conventional external beam irradiation. It is uncertain, however, whether this is due to superior treatment or to case selection (Table 8-4).

A high incidence of distant failure has been reported in several series and may prevent significant improvement in long-term survival. In the Massachusetts General Hospital and Mayo Clinic studies combining external beam and intraoperative irradiation, local tumor control has been improved; median survival is only approximately 12 months however, and the 2-year survival rate varies from 12% to 55% by patient group. Most patients with disease progression have liver metastases, peritoneal seeding, or both. Current protocols are utilizing gemcitabine in combination with 5-FU and external beam irradiation programs.

## CONCLUSIONS

For locally advanced adenocarcinoma of the pancreas, although the use of a combination of intraoperative and external beam irradiation 5-FU has been followed by a decrease in the incidence of local tumor progression in most series

and by an improved median survival in some compared with conventional external beam irradiation, these results may be due to case selection rather than to superior treatment. Although combination methods deliver a much higher effective dose of irradiation than external beam alone, prospective randomized trials are needed to determine whether a therapeutic gain will result from the more aggressive techniques. The use of radiation dose modifiers in conjunction with intraoperative radiation therapy must be investigated in controlled fashion to determine their value. Although slight gains in median survival may be achieved by improving local tumor control, a significant abdominal failure problem prevents significant improvements in long-term survival.

One approach to decreasing the incidence of hepatic metastases is elective hepatic irradiation, but studies employing this technique have shown no clear benefit to this therapy, and significant toxicity has been reported. Another approach to treatment of abdominal failures is the development of effective systemic or intraperitoneal chemotherapy. At present, there is active investigation of gemcitabine in both metastatic and adjuvant settings. If a significant improvement in prevention of abdominal failure does not occur in the next several years, an alternative is to improve or alter patient selection to delete those at high risk for failure outside the pancreas. This could be accomplished by giving intraoperative radiation therapy to those with localized disease.

# B. COLON CANCER

## INTRODUCTION

During the 1970s, studies examining the outcome and patterns of failure of patients undergoing resection of colon and rectal cancer identified subsets of patients at risk for local and/or systemic recurrence (classically by anatomic stage). These investigations determined the frequency and anatomic location of recurrence and served as the basis for the development of adjuvant and neoadjuvant therapies. In the 1970s and 1980s, treatment strategies utilizing external beam irradiation, 5-FU-based chemotherapy, and combinations of these treatments were under way. These initial studies pointed to the possible benefits of these therapies and led to multicenter randomized prospective trials that have assessed their efficacy. For patients with resected high risk colonic cancer, these studies have established the value of adjuvant chemotherapy including 1 year of 5-FU and levamisole or 6 months of 5-FU and leucovorin. Although there is a strong argument for adjuvant irradiation in combination with 5-FU-based chemotherapy for patients with advanced staged colonic cancer, its ultimate efficacy has not been proven with a randomized prospective study. This section reviews the rationale for the use of radiation therapy and 5-FU-based chemotherapy in colonic cancer. Figure 8-4 summarizes the frequently used staging systems of large bowel cancer.

### Adjuvant Therapy

Recent prospective randomized trials have established the value of adjuvant chemotherapy for patients with resected high risk colon cancer. Patients with stage III colon cancer receiving 1 year of 5-FU and levamisole or 6 months of 5-FU and leucovorin have had statistically significant improvements in survival compared to patients receiving no adjuvant therapy or levamisole alone.[36-38] Currently, there is active investigation in defining the optimal sequence, administration, and modulation of 5-FU-based chemotherapy. Because of the documented efficacy of adjuvant chemotherapy and the perception among many oncologists that colonic carcinoma (as opposed to rectal cancer) is

*Staging Systems for Large Bowel Cancer*

| **STAGING SYSTEM** | | | | |
|---|---|---|---|---|
| DUKES[28] | ASTLER-COLLER[4] | MODIFIED ASTLER-COLLER | TNM | DESCRIPTION |
| A | A | A | T1N0 | Nodes negative; limited to mucosa |
| | B1 | B1 | T2N0. | Nodes negative; penetration into submucosa but not through muscularis propria |
| B | B2 | B2 | T3N0 | Nodes negative; penetration through muscularis propria |
| | | B3 | T4N0 | Nodes negative; penetration through muscularis propria with adherence to or invasion of surrounding organs or structures |
| | C1 | C1 | T1–2N1 | Nodes positive; limited to bowel wall |
| C | | C2 | T3N1 | Nodes positive; penetration through muscularis propria |
| | C2 | C3 | T4N1 | Nodes positive; penetration through muscularis propria and adherence to or invasion of surrounding organs or structures |

**FIGURE 8-4**   Staging systems for colon and rectal cancer.

much more likely to recur systemically than lo-cally, there has been little systematic examination of the value of postoperative irradiation with chemotherapy.

The potential indications for postoperative irradiation in patients with colon cancer stem from examinations of the patterns of failure after resection.[39,40] For rectal carcinoma, the most important predictor of local failure is tumor stage, but for colonic carcinoma, both stage and location are important. For lesions in the ascending and descending colon (anatomically immobile bowel), invasion into the retroperitoneum may limit a wide surgical resection. Compromised radial resection margins invite local failure. Unless there is invasion into an adjacent organ, local failure is rare for tumors in the sigmoid and transverse colon (mobile bowel), since a wide resection margin is usually achievable regardless of the extent of invasion into the mesentery. For tumors that arise in the cecum, flexures, or proximal and distal ends of the sigmoid colon, the risk of local failure may be variable depending on the amount of mesentery and the ability to obtain a satisfactory circumferential margin. For any colon tumor adherent to adjacent structures (with and without lymph node involvement), local failure rates exceed 30%. In summary, local failure is an important consideration for large bowel tumors, where there are anatomic constraints on radial resection margins, and for tumors invading adjacent structures. Because of the improved survival seen in patients with node-positive colon carcinoma who receive 5-FU and levamisole or 5-FU and leucovorin, adjuvant radiation therapy for these patients with resected high risk colon cancer will need to be combined with systemic chemotherapy.

Reports on the use of adjuvant postoperative radiation therapy to the tumor bed with and without chemotherapy for colonic carcinoma are limited to single institution retrospective analyses.[41–43] These studies suggest that failure rates in the operative bed are reduced in patients receiving radiation therapy compared with historical controls. Since 1976, patients at the Massachusetts General Hospital (MGH)

with completely resected but high risk colonic carcinoma have been considered for postoperative radiation therapy to the tumor bed.[6] These high risk groups included patients with stage B3 and C3 disease, patients with stage C2 disease except middle sigmoid and transverse colon cancer, and selected patients with stage B2 disease with "tight" margins. In all, 171 patients (1976–1989) received postoperative radiation therapy via a high energy linear accelerator by parallel opposed fields or multifield techniques to irradiate the tumor bed with approximately a 3 to 5 cm margin to a total dose of 45 Gy in 1.8 Gy fractions. This was followed by a shrinking field technique, sparing the small bowel, to 50.4 Gy. Additional treatment above 50.4 Gy was attempted in patients with stage B3 and C3 disease only if the small bowel could be displaced from the field. Fifty-three of 171 patients were treated with adjuvant chemotherapy, usually 5-FU as intravenous bolus for 3 consecutive days (500 mg/m$^2$/day) during the first and last weeks of radiation therapy. These 171 patients receiving postoperative radiation therapy were compared with 395 patients in the MGH series with stage B2, B3, and C3 tumors who underwent surgery only during the period from 1970 to 1977.[39] Table 8-5 shows by stage the 5-year actuarial local control and recurrence-free survival rates for patients undergoing postoperative radiation therapy and patients having surgery alone. Local control and recurrence-free survival was statistically improved for patients with stage B3 and C3 tumors receiving postoperative radiation therapy compared with similarly matched surgical patients. Local control rates for irradiated patients with stage B3 and C3 tumors were 93% and 72%, whereas the rates were 69% and 47%, respectively, in patients having surgery only. Patients with stage B3 and C3 disease receiving postoperative radiotherapy experienced a 16% and 15% point increase in disease-free survival, respectively, compared with the group that had surgery only. In contrast, local control and recurrence-free survival were not improved for B2 and C2 patients receiving postoperative radiation therapy

**TABLE 8-5   Five-Year Actuarial Local Control (LC) and Recurrence-Free Survival (RFS) After Surgery Postoperative Radiotherapy Versus Surgery Alone According to Stage (MGH Experience)**

| | Surgery plus Radiation | | | Surgery Alone | | |
|---|---|---|---|---|---|---|
| Stage | Number of Patients | Local Control (%) | Recurrence-free Survival (%) | Number of Patients | Local Control % | Recurrence-free Survival (%) |
| B2 | 23 | 91 | 72 | 163 | 90 | 78 |
| B3 | 54 | 93 | 79 | 83 | 69 | 63 |
| C2 | 55 | 70 | 47 | 100 | 64 | 48 |
| C3 | 39 | 72 | 53 | 49 | 47 | 38 |

compared with surgery alone. It should be noted, however, that for irradiated patients with stage B2 and C2 lesions, these comparisons may be unfavorably biased against irradiation, since most were referred because of concerns about the adequacy of local control with surgery alone. In this context, to have achieved similar local control and recurrence-free survival in the "high risk" irradiated B2 and C2 patients may actually represent a positive gain.

Other studies have demonstrated improved local control in irradiated patients with high risk colon cancer.[42,43] The results of postoperative radiotherapy at the Mayo Clinic for patients with locally advanced colon cancers were recently analyzed.[42] More than 90% of these had MAC stage B3 and C3 lesions. The 5-year actuarial local failure rate was 10% for patients with no residual disease, 54% for patients with microscopic residual disease, and 79% for patients with gross residual disease ($p$ < 0.0001).

A recent report summarized the results of postoperative radiotherapy at the University of Florida for patients with locally advanced but completely resected colon cancers.[43] This study reported a local control rate of 88%, quite similar to the 90% reported at the Mayo Clinic in patients who had completely resected tumors. In addition, a significant relationship between the radiation dose delivered and the rate of local control was found. The 5-year rate of local control was 96% for those who had received 50 to 55 Gy, compared with 76% for those who had received less than 50 Gy ($p$ = 0.0095).

To assess the merits of postoperative radiation therapy for selected patients with colonic cancer, a randomized prospective intergroup trial combining postoperative irradiation plus 5-FU and levamisole versus 5-FU and levamisole alone was initiated in 1993. Eligible patients included those with stage B3 and C3 lesions and C2 tumors arising in the ascending and descending colon. Unfortunately, this trial was closed in December 1996 because of poor patient accrual. Although the power of the study is reduced by the low number of patients, it is possible that conclusions regarding the efficacy of irradiation with 5-FU and levamisole can be made with respect to the 222 patients entered on this trial.

There are few data evaluating the combined effect of 5-FU and irradiation in colon cancer. In the MGH adjuvant series, 53 patients received 3 days of bolus 5-FU (500 mg/m$^2$/day) for 3 consecutive days during the first and last weeks of irradiation. Local control and recurrence-free survival rates for the adjuvantly treated patients based on 5-FU administration during radiation therapy are listed in Table 8-6. Although no statistically significant differences in local control or recurrence-free survival were observed based on the addition of 5-FU, there was a trend toward improved local control in patients receiving 5-FU. Interestingly, the incidence of acute enteritis in patients receiving irradiation and 5-FU was 16%, versus 4% in patients undergoing irradiation only. No difference in late bowel complications have been observed following 5-FU administration. This higher incidence of acute enteritis is consistent with other reports of combined 5-FU and irradiation in rectal cancer. Our current policy at MGH for patients receiving postoperative irradiation for colon cancer is to utilize continuous infusion 5-FU (225 mg/m$^2$/24 h) 5 days per week, throughout the irradiation. This is followed by 6 months of maintenance 5-FU and leucovorin.

Because of the high incidence of hepatic metastases and peritoneal failures developing in patients with advanced-stage colonic carcinoma, there have been clinical investigations of the efficacy of adjuvant hepatic irradiation as well as whole abdominal radiation therapy. There has only been one randomized prospective trial: the phase III trial of adjuvant hepatic irradiation reported by the Gastrointestinal Tumor Study Group.[44] In this study, 300 patients with completely resected transmural or node-positive colon carcinoma were randomized between two treatment arms: (1) observation or (2) 5-FU and 21 Gy to the liver (1.5 Gy per fraction for 14 treatments). The 5-FU was given as an intravenous bolus during the first 3 days of radiation therapy, as well as maintenance treatment. No statistical differences in survival, recurrence-free survival, or liver recurrence were seen between the control patients and the treated patients.

Several investigators have reported the results and toxicity of whole abdominal irradiation as an adjuvant treatment for patients at risk for hepatic and peritoneal failure.[45–47] None of these studies had concurrent controls. Wang et al. reported the experience at Princess Margaret Hospital of 30 patients receiving whole abdominal irradiation of 14 to 25 Gy over 3 to 5 weeks with or without local tumor boost.[45] The 5-year actuarial survival was 55%. For patients without regional nodal involvement, the survival was 72%, compared with 41% for patients with nodal involvement. After treatment, 4 patients had failure in the peritoneum and 12 had hepatic and extra-abdominal failure. Brenner et al. described 21 patients with Duke C colonic cancer who received whole abdominal radiation therapy to 20 to 30 Gy in 3 weeks to areas at high risk and concurrent weekly 350 mg/m$^2$ doses of 5-FU given intravenously.[46] The patients who underwent radiation therapy were compared with a matched control group of patients who underwent surgery alone, and a statistically significant improvement in the disease-free survival was noted (55% vs. 12%, respectively).

In 1995 the results of a phase I/II Southwestern Oncology Group study (SWOG 8572) utilizing 30 Gy of whole abdominal irradiation and an additional 16 Gy tumor boost with continuous infusional 5-FU (200 mg/m$^2$/24 h) for 41 patients with T3 N1-2 colon cancer were described.[47] In view of the early intolerance, the protocol was amended to insert a 1-week break from external beam irradiation and 5-FU. The 5-year actuarial disease-free and overall survival for all 41 patients was 58% and 67%, respectively. For the 19 patients with four or fewer positive nodes, both the 5-year overall survival and the disease-free survival rate were

**TABLE 8-6** Five-Year Actuarial Local Control and Recurrence-free Survival of Adjuvantly Irradiated Patients Based on 5-FU Administration

| | Without 5-FU | | | With 5-FU | | |
|---|---|---|---|---|---|---|
| Stage | Number of Patients | Local Control (%) | Recurrence-free Survival (%) | Number of Patients | Local Control % | Recurrence-free Survival (%) |
| B2 | 16 | 87 | 69 | 7 | 100 | 80 |
| B3 | 37 | 94 | 78 | 16 | 100 | 83 |
| C2 | 41 | 69 | 48 | 14 | 70 | 43 |
| C3 | 24 | 67 | 53 | 15 | 79 | 52 |

61%. For the 20 patients with more than four involved nodes, the 5-year actuarial disease-free and overall survival rates with chemoirradiation were 55% and 74%, respectively. This is higher than the disease-free and overall survival results of 35% and 39% reported in the 5-FU and levamisole intergroup trial. Based on the results, these investigators propose that this regimen be evaluated against 5-FU and levamisole in a phase III trial.

Estes et al.[48] compared patterns of relapse for MAC C2 patients in SWOG 8591 (arms of surgery alone or surgery plus 5-FU/levamisole), SWOG 8572 (whole abdominal irradiation plus tumor bed irradiation and infusion 5-FU), and the surgery-alone arm from the Willett MGH analysis. In SWOG 8591, although lung relapse was decreased from 34% to 21% with the addition of 5-FU/levamisole to surgical resection, the chemotherapy adjuvant had no impact on the rate of local–regional relapse (surgery alone, 20%; 5-FU/levamisole, 27%), which was equivalent to the 32% incidence alone in the MGH analysis. Patients who received chemoirradiation (whole abdominal irradiation and tumor bed irradiation with infusion of 5-FU) in SWOG 8572 had only a 12% tumor bed nodal relapse rate, along with a reduction in liver and peritoneal relapse rates (liver relapse rate of 22% with chemoirradiation vs 54% and 57% in the two arms of SWOG 8591; peritoneal relapse rates of 15% in SWOG 8572 vs. 37% and 40% in SWOG 8591).

## TECHNIQUES OF IRRADIATION OF COLON CANCER

As is true in the treatment of rectal carcinoma, great care must be taken in the postoperative treatment of adenocarcinoma of the colon. Field arrangements will vary to a great degree depending on the exact site of the primary tumor and the areas thought to be at high risk for local recurrence. Although recommendations on specific fields cannot be made, some general suggestions are possible.

One should try to treat the primary tumor site with a 4 to 5 cm margin proximally and distally and a 3 to 4 cm margin medially and laterally, to provide adequate coverage of the local tumor spread. Figure 8-5 shows a standard simulation film of a patient receiving postoperative irradiation of a descending colon cancer. Generally, the lymph nodes in the mesentery beyond the margins of the surgical resection are not treated. At times one may wish to treat lymph nodes draining from adjacent structures that are involved by tumor, such as the para-aortic nodes with deep retroperitoneal involvement. The surgeon can usually obtain good mesenteric nodal margins with standard lymph node dissections. In rare instances, it may be appropriate to treat proximally located lymph nodes in the surgical resection. However, the long-term survival benefit from this type of treatment is likely to be low.

We have often found it helpful to treat patients in the right or left decubitis position. When patients are treated with one side up, often much of the small bowel will fall by gravity away from the radiation field. A special small-bowel series must be obtained in the treatment position and compared to the standard supine position to confirm movement of small bowel and define the exact amount of small bowel in the field. The total radiation dose needs to be adjusted by the amount of small bowel included.

One often finds that part or all of one kidney needs to be irradiated. We have generally accepted the finding that irradiation of a large portion of one kidney results in long-term lack of function in that kidney. We have, however, been willing to treat these patients if their other kidney functions well, and their BUN and creatinine values are within normal limits. An evaluation of the long-term effects of renal irradiation performed at the MGH has shown minimal long-term clinical sequelae from unilateral renal irradiation.[49]

For colon carcinomas, a dose of 45 Gy is delivered through large fields, 1.8 Gy per fraction, as described earlier. At this point, an at-

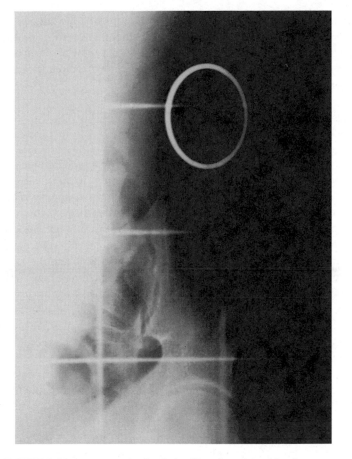

**FIGURE 8-5**   Anteroposterior simulation film of a patient with colon cancer.

tempt is made to design a boost that will exclude as much small bowel as possible from the radiation field. The exact dose delivered to the boost area will vary according to the stage of tumor and the location of normal tissue. For a B3 or C3 tumor, we try to treat with 55 to 60 Gy if this is thought to be safe, given the position of the small intestine. Often two-field reductions are required, one at 45 Gy and one at 50 Gy. The first field reduction may include a small portion of small bowel; beyond 50 Gy, however, small bowel should be completely excluded. Although data are not available at present, the use of intraoperative radiation therapy in certain stage B3 and C3 patients, such as those with uncertain margins, may also be appropriate.

## SUMMARY

Selected subsets of patients with colon cancer have local recurrence risks equivalent to those seen with rectal cancer if surgery alone is used. In view of the positive results seen with combined irradiation and chemotherapy in the adjuvant treatment of rectal cancer, encouraging pilot study results with postoperative irradiation with or without 5-FU for resected high risk colon cancers at MGH and the positive results of 5-FU and levamisole in high risk adjuvant colon cancer, an intergroup randomized trial was conducted comparing 5-FU and levamisole with 5-FU and levamisole and tumor bed irradiaton in patients at high risk for local recurrence following surgical resection (modified Astler–Coller B3,C3 and retroperitoneal C2 lesions; TNM T4b N0 or T4b N1,2; T3,4a N1,2). This protocol did not reach planned accrual objectives, since 6 months of adjuvant 5-FU/leucovorin was shown to be equivalent to 12 months of adjuvant 5-FU/levamisole. A replacement intergroup protocol is being discussed to test the addition of tumor bed with or without nodal irradiation to adjuvant 5-FU leucovorin.

# C. RECTAL CANCER

Carcinoma of the rectum is a heterogeneous disease. At one end of the clinical spectrum, a small number of patients who present with superficially invasive favorable cancers are well served by limited procedures, such as local excision or endocavitary irradiation. The great majority of patients with rectal cancer, however, have mobile but more deeply invasive tumors that require low anterior or abdominoperineal resection. At the other and less favorable end of the clinical spectrum, a subset of patients present with locally advanced tumors that are adherent or fixed to adjoining structures such as the sacrum, pelvic sidewalls, prostate, or bladder. The surgical and oncologic management of these patients varies greatly depending on stage. The following sections review relevant clinical issues in these three presentations: favorable, mobile, and locally advanced rectal cancer.

## FAVORABLE RECTAL CANCER

### Introduction

Approximately 36,000 people will develop carcinoma of the rectum in the United States in 1998.[50] Since the introduction of the abdominoperineal resection by Miles, a surgical approach to removal of this tumor and its adjacent tissues has offered a high probability of local control and survival. Despite its merits, the abdominoperineal resection has profound drawbacks: loss of anorectal function, with a permanent colostomy and a high incidence of sexual and genitourinary dysfunction. To overcome these limitations, an array of surgical procedures has been developed, ranging from simple excision to complex resections with reconstruction. In appropriately staged patients, these operations appear to offer not only comparable rates of local control as the abdominoperineal resection but, importantly, to preserve sphincter integrity. With continued experience, selection criteria and the role of radiation therapy and chemotherapy have become more clearly defined.

One obvious consideration in the selection of patients for sphincter preservation is tumor location within the rectum. Patients with tumors in the upper rectum have long been well managed by a sphincter-preserving anastomosis. With the advent of the end-to-end anastomotic stapling instrument, tumors of the midrectum, even in a narrow pelvis, become amenable to treatment by low anterior resection and preservation of the anal sphincter. Although with the lower anastomoses, there is a real incidence of sexual dysfunction and less than perfect anorectal function, the avoidance of a permanent colostomy is perceived by the patient as an extremely fortunate situation. In contrast to tumors of the upper and middle rectum, management of distal rectal cancer continues to pose a major challenge to the surgeon and oncologist. Clearly, an important consideration in treatment selection of patients with low rectal cancer is the local extent of the primary tumor.

For small tumors in the distal rectum, there has been increasing interest in local excision procedures as an alternative to the abdominoperineal resection. These operations involve an excision of the primary tumor through the anus (per-anal excision), by division of the anal sphincter (transanal, transphincteric, or Park's resection) or using a parasacral approach

(Kraske). The latter two procedures are somewhat more extensive than a simple per-anal excision and have a greater degree of associated morbidity. Clearly, this technique is limited to tumors that can be excised and the excision site closed without significant narrowing of the rectal lumen.

## Clinical and Radiologic Evaluation

The usual criteria for rectal cancers suitable for local excision are as follows: tumor size less than 4 cm, location 8 cm or less from the anal verge, well- or moderately well-differentiated histology, mobile, not ulcerated, and no suspicion of perirectal or presacral nodes.[51] One is attempting to select patients with tumors confined to the rectal wall where there is a low probability of lymph node metastases.

Although impressive advances have been made in the radiologic imaging of rectal cancer, digital examination by an experienced practitioner is one of the most reliable (and inexpensive!) methods of determining the depth of penetration of the primary tumor. The accuracy rate of staging the primary tumor by digital examination has been reported to be approximately 80%.[52] Because lymph node metastases are seen only microscopically in a high percentage of cases, it is not surprising that digital examination is insensitive at identifying metastatic perirectal nodal involvement.

In addition to digital examination, endoscopic ultrasonography (EUS) has been used as a staging tool in assessing local tumor extent as well as lymph node involvement.[53,54] Correlation of ultrasound T stage to pathological T stage ranges from 70% to over 90% in most series.[54] To achieve high accuracy rates ($\geq$ 90%), this examination must be performed by experienced operators. In a study from the University of Minnesota, the accuracy rates rose from 59% during the early phase of the study to 88% in the latter phase of the study.[55] Because ultrasound and other imaging modalities can visualize macroscopic changes only, these techniques are inherently limited in their ability to discriminate lesser degrees of invasion between tumors. In one study, 30% of 24 patients believed on the basis of EUS to have T2 lesions in fact had transmural invasion pathologically.[56] In assessing pararectal nodal involvement, EUS has been less helpful, with reported accuracy rates ranging from 50% to 80%.[15] With these caveats, EUS is generally acknowleged to be complementary to digital examination in staging and more accurate than axial CT and MRI scans.

Although CT and MRI may be inferior to EUS in staging rectal cancer, there are potential advantages of these studies. These imaging modalities offer a larger field of view than EUS, may be less operator and technique dependent, and do allow study of stenotic tumors.[51,53] It is our policy to obtain a CT scan as well as EUS to aid in the selection of patients for local excision. Patients with convincing evidence of transmural penetration or perirectal lymph node involvement are probably best managed by radical surgical resection because of the risk of tumor cut-through and inadequate lymph node removal by local excision procedures.

## Surgery and Pathological Evaluation

The selection of the local excision technique is important. Surgical procedures such as per-anal and trans-sphincteric (York-Mason) excision and excision via midline posterior proctotomy (Kraske) procedure are advocated because these operations permit removal of the tumor and adjoining rectum in one piece without fragmentation of the tumor, and allow assessment of linked margins, histological differentiation, vessel involvement, and depth of penetration through bowel wall. The pathologist should use an ink margin to carefully define the narrowest margin in fresh tissues and on slides. Fulguration or electrocoagulation is not recommended: these procedures are associated with a high likelihood of residual disease after the procedure and inadequate pathological analysis.

A critical limitation of local excision procedures is the inability to sample or resect perirectal and mesenteric lymphatics. The incidence of

**TABLE 8-7   Risk of Perirectal Lymph Nodes by Primary Tumor Histopathology**

Low risk: <10%
  Well-differentiated histology
  Submucosa or inner muscularis propria invasion
Intermediate risk: 10–20%
  Moderately well-differentiated histology
  Muscularis propria invasion
High risk: >30%
  Poorly differentiated histology
  Muscularis propria or perirectal fat invasion
  Lymphatic or venous vessel invasion

perirectal lymph node metastases progressively rises as the tumor penetrates from submucosa through muscularis propria to fat.[57–59] In a collective series, lymph node metastases were observed in 12%, 35%, and 44% of lesions involving the submucosa, muscularis propria, and perirectal fat, respectively.[51] In addition to T stage, histologic grade and vascular involvement are independent predictors of lymph node metastasis. One analysis reported a 29% to 50% risk of perirectal nodal metastasis for patients with T1 and T2 tumors showing poorly differentiated histology or lymphatic/blood vessel involvement.[58] Table 8-7 summarizes the incidence of perirectal nodal metastases by T stage and histologic features of the primary tumor.

Because many patients with pathologically high risk T1 and T2 tumors have perirectal lymph metastases, local excision procedures alone would be inadequate treatment. Studies examining the outcome of patients undergoing local excision show a clear association of local failure rate only to the risk of perirectal nodal metastases as assessed by primary tumor histopathology. In a study from Erlangen, pa-

tients with "low risk" tumors had less than a 10% local failure, whereas patients with "high risk" tumors had greater than 30% local failure.[5] To improve the outcome of these patients, treatment programs of postoperative pelvic irradiation with concurrent 5-FU after local excision of "high risk" tumors are being investigated at many centers in the United States.[60–67] The results of several studies are summarized in Table 8-8.

## Treatment Recommendations and Results

Treatment recommendations should be guided by the surgical and pathological finding of the local excision. For patients with small tumors invading the mucosa and submucosa, local excision alone probably suffices. Studies from several centers have shown that the results of local excision only for patients with T1 lesions with favorable histology is excellent, with local control and recurrence-free survival rates of 90% or greater. Postoperative irradiation is usually not advised for patients with locally excised T1 tumors unless the margins are compromised or the primary tumor exhibits poorly differentiated histology or lymphatic/venous invasion.

In tumors that are somewhat larger or in which there is deeper invasion of the tumor into the rectal wall, more aggressive techniques of combined local excision and radiation therapy and chemotherapy have been employed. Because of the risk of perirectal nodal metastases and reported local failure rates of 20% or greater after local excision only, postoperative pelvic irradiation with 5-FU-based chemotherapy is advised for all patients with T2 lesions.

**TABLE 8-8   Outcome Following Local Excision and Postoperative Irradiation**

| Study | Local Control (%) | Survival (%) |
|---|---|---|
| Princess Margaret Hospital[64] | 76 | 80 (6-year median) |
| Fox Chase Cancer Center[65] | 81 | 75 (5-year disease-free survival) |
| Memorial Sloan-Kettering Cancer Center[66] | 82 | 79 (Overall) |
| CALGB Intergroup[67] | 98 | 96 (2-year) |

Single-institution studies reporting on the results of postoperative irradiation for these patients indicate excellent local control and survival rates. In a report from the M.D. Anderson Hospital, the local control rate of 15 patients with T2 tumors treated by local excision with postoperative irradiation and 5-FU-based chemotherapy was 93%.[62] Similar results were reported by the Massachusetts General Hospital, where all 11 patients with T2 tumors treated by local excision and adjuvant irradiation and 5-FU have maintained local control.[61]

The results from single-institution studies of local excision of T1 and T2 rectal cancer with appropriate selection of postoperative irradiation appear to be supported by preliminary results of the CALGB intergroup phase II study.[67] In this study, 60 patients underwent local excision of T1 tumors without further therapy, whereas 53 patients with T2 tumors received postoperative irradiation with 5-FU after local excision. With a median follow-up of 24 months, 4 of 113 patients were found to have died of their malignant disease, with 2 of 4 patients having distant recurrence only. Only 2 of 113 patients experienced isolated local recurrences: both underwent subsequent resection and remain alive. The investigators of this study conclude that sphincter preservation can be achieved with excellent cancer control without sacrifice of anal function in selected patients with superficial distal rectal cancer.

For patients with tumors invading the perirectal fat (T3), radical surgical resection is recommended (if feasible) because of the risk of tumor cut-through and inadequate lymph node removal by local excision procedures. The experience of local excision with postoperative irradiation and chemotherapy is limited, and the available data suggest higher local failure rates. Three of 15 patients (20%) with T3 tumors from M.D. Anderson experienced local failure following local excision and postoperative irradiation with 5-FU.[62] In a study from Massachusetts General Hospital, three of four patients (75%) with T3 tumors suffered local recurrence after local excision and postoperative irradiation.[61] Unless there is a medical contraindication or patient refusal, we would not advise a treatment program of local excision and postoperative irradiation and chemotherapy for patients with T3 tumors.

## Radiation Therapy Techniques and 5-Fluouracil Administration

At the time of surgery, radiopaque markers are placed at the perimeter of the excision (identifying the high risk region to aid in treatment planning). For patients with disease limited to the submucosa and muscularis propria, pelvic irradiation to 45 Gy in 25 fractions by a four-field technique is given, followed by the first field reduction with lateral fields to 50.4 Gy and a second field reduction (if appropriate) with lateral fields to 54.0 Gy . During the 5.5 to 6 week course of irradiation, our patients receive continuous infusion of 5-fluorouracil (225 mg/m$^2$/24 h), 5 days per week. Chemotherapy alternatives could include bolus 5-FU with leucovorin during the first and last weeks of irradiation.

Patients are treated in the prone position. For the initial fields (45 Gy), the superior border should be 1.5 cm above the level of the sacral promontory and the lower border of the field 4 to 5 cm below the defined tumor bed (Figures 8-6 and 8-7). Laterally, the posteroanterior–anteroposterior (PA-AP) fields extend 1 to 1.5 cm beyond the true bony pelvis. To treat the entire presacral space with adequate margins and full dose, the lateral fields are designed so that the posterior border encompasses the entire sacrum with a 1 cm margin posterior to the sacrum. Anteriorly, the fields are designed to encompass the previous tumor bed, including the posterior wall of the vagina for females and a large portion of the prostate for males. The radiopaque markers placed at surgery are helpful in designing the field reductions (Figure 8-8). After 45 Gy, lateral fields with an approximately 3 cm margin around the "marked" tumor bed are typically used for three fractions to 50.4 Gy. This is followed by a further field reduction with a 2 cm margin around the "marked" tumor bed to 54 Gy. A small-bowel series must be per-

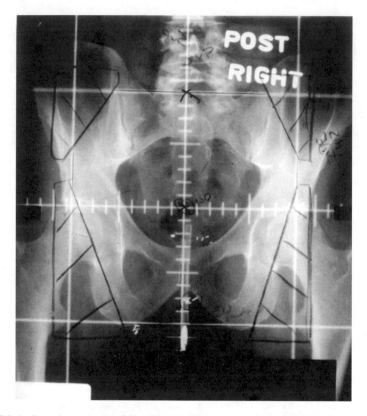

**FIGURE 8-6**    Posterioanterior simulation film of a patient with rectal cancer following local excision.

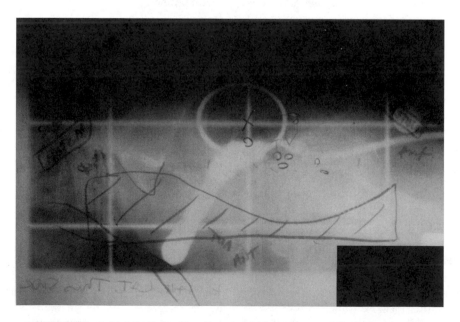

**FIGURE 8-7**    Lateral simulation film of a patient with rectal cancer following local excision.

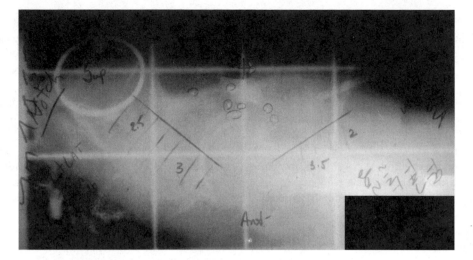

**FIGURE 8-8**   Simulation film showing clip placement to aid in field design.

formed to ensure that no small bowel is within these lateral boost fields. For patients with positive or tight resection margins or poor prognostic features suggesting a higher risk of local recurrence, additional irradiation to 55 to 65 Gy may be appropriate. Specialized techniques, such as interstitial implant, split beams with rectal dilatation, or perineal proton beam irradiation, allow homogeneous irradiation of high risk regions in the rectum and adjacent perirectal fat with sparing of uninvolved rectum, perineum, and pelvic viscera. These techniques may allow a substantial number of patients to obtain local control with good preservation of anorectal function.

## SUMMARY

Local excision and postoperative irradiation and chemotherapy appears to offer not only satisfactory local control and survival but, importantly, sphincter preservation for selected patients with distal rectal cancer. For patients with favorable histology T1 rectal cancer, local excision alone suffices. Postoperative irradiation and chemotherapy should follow local excision procedures for patients with unfavorable histology T1 and all T2 tumors. The data for T3

tumors with this approach is limited; however, results from single-institution studies suggest unacceptably high local failure rates. Radical resection is advised.

## MOBILE RECTAL CANCER

### Adjuvant Therapy

The efficacy of postoperative irradiation and 5-FU-based chemotherapy as adjuvant therapy for resected high risk rectal cancer (stage II or III disease) was established by a series of prospective randomized trials during the 1980s and 1990s.[68-72] These studies examined the role of postoperative irradiation and chemotherapy for rectal carcinoma. The Gastrointestinal Tumor Study Group (GITSG) randomized patients with Duke B2 and C rectal carcinomas to one of four arms: observation; postoperative irradiation only (40 or 48 Gy); chemotherapy only [semustine (methyl-CCNU) and 5-FU]; and postoperative irradiation (40 or 44 Gy) with concurrent 5-FU and maintenance chemotherapy with 5-FU and methyl-CCNU.[68] This study demonstrated improved local control and survival for patients receiving combined irradiation and chemotherapy compared with surgery alone. The National Surgical Adjuvant Breast and Bowel Project (NSABP) randomized patients with Duke B and C rectal cancers to one of three arms: observation only, adjuvant chemotherapy only [methyl-(chloroethyl)cyclohexylnitrogourea (CCNU), vincristine, and 5-FU], or postoperative irradiation only (46–47 Gy).[69] There was a reduction in local recurrence in patients receiving postoperative irradiation but no improvement in survival compared with surgery alone. Male patients receiving chemotherapy had improved survival compared with control patients. The Mayo/North Central Cancer Treatment Group (NCCTG) study compared postoperative irradiation only (50.4 Gy), postoperative irradiation (50.4 Gy) with concurrent 5-FU, and pre- and postirradiation chemotherapy (5-FU and methyl-CCNU).[70] This showed improved local control and survival in patients who received combined modality treatment versus postoperative irradiation only. Most investigators have interpreted these data to indicate that combined pelvic irradiation with concurrent and maintenance 5-FU-based chemotherapy results in both improved pelvic control and longer survival compared with surgery alone for patients with rectal tumors extending through the bowel wall or with nodal involvement.

All these chemotherapy regimens contain methyl-CCNU, a known risk factor for acute nonlymphocytic leukemia. The estimated risk of delayed acute leukemia in patients receiving multiple doses of methyl-CCNU over 12 to 18 months is 2.3 cases per 1000 persons per year (14 cases of leukemia in 2067 patients given methyl-CCNU; 6-year cumulative risk of developing leukemia is 4%). Importantly, two subsequent randomized postoperative trials from the GITSG and the NCCTG have demonstrated that methyl-CCNU does not produce an additive benefit to irradiation plus 5-FU.[71,72] Thus, methyl-CCNU is no longer utilized in the adjuvant chemotherapy regimens in colorectal cancer.

A major issue at present in the adjuvant therapy of rectal cancer is how best to optimize the proven combination of radiation and 5-FU.

If there is a combined modality effect of radiation therapy and 5-FU, it is logical to try to use both modalities optimally. Both the use of 5-FU as a long-term continuous infusion (225 mg/m$^2$/day) and 5-FU combined with leucovorin have been shown to produce higher response rates in patients with metastatic disease than doses of conventional bolus 5-FU. The GI Intergroup has run a study testing the value of continuous infusion 5-FU given with radiation therapy compared with bolus 5-FU during radiation therapy.[72] Both groups of patients also received pre- and postirradiation 5-FU. This study showed a reduction in distant metastases with improved relapse-free and overall survival for patients treated with continuous infusion (Table 8-9). A study has also been recently completed testing the value of pelvic irradiation with combinations of 5-FU, 5-FU and leucovorin, and 5-FU, leucovorin, and levamisole in the adjuvant therapy of rectal cancer.[73] Pre-

**TABLE 8-9  Randomized Postoperative Trials of Rectal Cancer: Radiation Therapy (RT) and/or Chemotherapy (ChT)**

| Study and Treatment | Local Failure (%) | Distant Failure (%) | Overall Survival (%) |
|---|---|---|---|
| GITSG[68] | | | |
| RT + ChT | 11 | 26 | 57 |
| RT | 20 | 30 | 43 |
| ChT | 27 | 27 | 43 |
| Control | 24 | 34 | 28 |
| NSABP[69] | | | |
| RT | 16 | 31 | 50 |
| ChT | 21 | 24 | 58 |
| Control | 25 | 26 | 48 |
| NCCTG/Mayo[70] | | | |
| RT + ChT | 14 | 29 | 53 |
| RT | 25 | 46 | 38 |
| GI Intergroup[72] | | | |
| RT + PVI 5-FU | NS[a] | 31 | 70 |
| RT + Bolus 5-FU | NS[a] | 40 | 60 |

[a]NS, not stated. Although there was a reduction in distant metastases and improved recurrence-free and overall survival in patients receiving peripheral versus infusion (PVI) 5-FU compared to bolus 5-FU, there was no difference in local control rates by 5-FU administration ($p = 0.11$).

liminary analysis indicates that the three-drug regimen is more toxic and no more efficacious than the one- or two-drug regimen. Additional studies will continue to be run to attempt to determine the optimal mode of administration as well as modulation of 5-FU. In a nonstudy setting, we have utilized continuous infusion schedules of 5-FU (225 mg/m$^2$/24 h) throughout the 5 to 6 week course of pelvic irradiation.

## Neoadjuvant Therapy

Because of the success of combined modality treatment in the postoperative setting, there has been intense interest in the neoadjuvant use of this approach. Numerous phase II studies have demonstrated the safety of this program, and preliminary analyses indicate satisfactory local control and survival rates. These studies have also shown higher rates of complete pathological response following chemoirradiation compared with irradiation only. Complete pathological responses occur in only 6% to 12% of patients following moderate to high dose (45–50 Gy) preoperative irradiation (Table 8-10).[74–78]

In some studies, continuous infusion 5-FU programs or various 5-FU-based regimens with irradiation have increased these complete pathological response rates to 20% to 29% (Table 8-8). The significance of increased pathological responses in terms of local control and survival will require further maturation of these and other studies.

Although the techniques and dose of irradiation are similar in these chemoirradiation studies (45–50.4 Gy in 25–28 fractions to the pelvis with a three- or four-field arrangement), there is marked variability in modes of 5-FU administration. Some studies employ a schedule of 5-FU given as a bolus for 3 or 4 consecutive days during the first and last weeks of irradiation, whereas other investigators have utilized a continuous infusion approach throughout irradiation. Additionally, several investigators have incorporated other agents such as leucovorin and cisplatin in combination with 5-FU. Because of the Intergroup trial showing a survival advantage for patients treated with continuous infusion 5-FU throughout irradiation compared with patients treated with bolus 5-FU in the postoperative setting, it would seem appropriate that this approach should be adopted for preoperative irradiation programs in rectal cancer. The value of additional agents such as leucovorin, levamisole, and cisplatin in combination with 5-FU is under active investigation. It is becoming clear from the adjuvant rectal trials that more chemotherapy with irradiation is not necessarily a better situation. As previously discussed, the three-drug combination of 5-FU, levamisole, and leucovorin is more toxic and no more effective than the one- or two-drug regimen. At present, we are using a 5-FU schedule of 225 mg/m$^2$/24 h for 5 days per week throughout the 5.5 week course of preoperative irradiation (45 Gy to

**TABLE 8-10  Correlation of Pathological Response to Preoperative Regimen**

| Study | Number of Patients | Preoperative EBRT Dose (Gy) | Chemotherapy | Complete Pathological Regression Rate (%) |
|---|---|---|---|---|
| University of Florida[74] | 132 | 30–50 | None | 11 |
| Jewish Hospital[75] | 208 | 40–50 | None | 6 |
| M. D. Anderson Hospital[76] | 77 | 45 | 5-FU infusion | 29 |
| Duke University[77] | 43 | 45 | 5-FU and CDDP | 27 |
| Memorial Sloan-Kettering Cancer Center[78] | 20 | 50.4 | 5-FU and leucovorin | 20 |

the pelvis followed by a tumor boost of 5.4 Gy in 28 fractions of 1.8 Gy). In our experience, this 5-FU schedule has been well tolerated.

These is much debate regarding the relative merits and disadvantages of adjuvant versus neoadjuvant combined modality therapy in the treatment of patients with rectal carcinoma. Currently, there is one active randomized trial (NSABP R-03) in the United States assessing the merits of neoadjuvant therapy (5-FU and leucovorin, pelvic irradaition) versus adjuvant therapy (5-FU, leucovorin, pelvic irradiation). In a preliminary analysis of 116 patients, preoperative chemotherapy and irradiation appeared to be as safe and tolerable as postoperative therapy.[79] There appeared to be a trend to tumor downstaging and sphincter preservation in the preoperative arm. Final determination of survival benefit and long-term toxicity awaits completion of this study.

## Technical Aspects of Postoperative or Preoperative Radiation Therapy

In treatment of abdominopelvic tumors, careful attention must be paid to radiation therapy technique. It is generally inappropriate to treat rectal tumors with AP-PA fields alone where the anterior structures, not substantially at risk for local failure, are treated to a high dose. This approach invariably leads to increased toxicity from the treatment, with minimal gain in terms of improved local control. At the Massachusetts General Hospital, patients are generally treated with a four-field box technique, although the use of three fields (right and left lateral fields and a posterior field) is also reasonable. The use of lateral fields allows a portion of the bladder and some anteriorly placed small bowel to be spared.

The AP-PA fields extend from approximately the lower level of the L5 vertebral body to 4 to 5 cm below the anastomosis (or below the tumor when one is treating preoperatively) in patients who had a low anterior resection. For patients with an abdominoperineal resection, the fields always extend to include the

perineum. There are a substantial number of local recurrences in the perineum, and this area needs to be in the high dose volume. Laterally, the fields extend approximately 1.0 to 1.5 cm beyond the bony pelvis so that the lateral pelvic soft tissue receives the full radiation dose. The lateral fields have the same cephalad and caudad extent as the AP-PA fields. Patients are treated prone. The posterior border of the lateral field extends beyond the bony sacrum, ensuring that the full dose is delivered to the presacral space, a common site of local failure. Anteriorly, the fields extends to cover adequately the original tumor with at least a 2 cm margin. Blocks can often be used to spare a portion of the femoral neck on the lateral fields.

Patients are treated with a full bladder, to push some of the small intestine out of the radiation field. When the perineum needs to be treated, a bolus is placed on it so that a full dose will be delivered to the scar in this region. If the reaction becomes marked, the bolus can be removed. Generally, perineal reactions have not produced major symptoms.

Patients are treated at 1.8 Gy, five fractions per week, to a total dose of 45 Gy to these fields. The field size is then reduced and a boost dose is delivered to the tumor bed. Prior to designing the boost field, a special small-bowel radiographic series is obtained to define the exact location of the small bowel with respect to the boost area. Only by defining the exact bowel position can one design the radiation fields to eliminate excess irradiation of the small intestine. Great effort is made to avoid doses greater than 45 Gy to any small bowel that is fixed in the pelvis. In this regard, it is helpful to have the surgeon (at the time of the initial surgical procedure) try to move small intestine out of the pelvis. This can best be accomplished by reperitonealizing the pelvic floor. When this is not possible, it is helpful to have a loop of omentum swung to cover the pelvic floor or to have the uterus retroverted to accomplish the same purpose. Some centers have considered the use of prostheses or artificial mesh, but these are still being investigated. This is most important in treating patients after an abdominoperineal resection, since after a low anterior resection, the remaining rectum and colon prevent some small bowel from being immobilized deep in the pelvis. Examples of a standard field arrangement in the treatment of rectal cancer are shown in Figures 8-9 and 8-10.

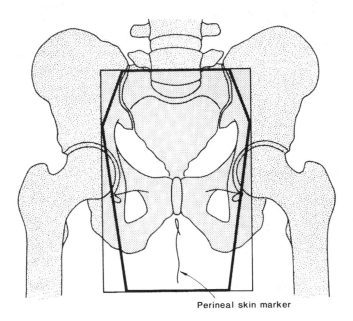

Perineal skin marker

**FIGURE 8-9**  Example of a standard radiation field for patients with rectal cancer.

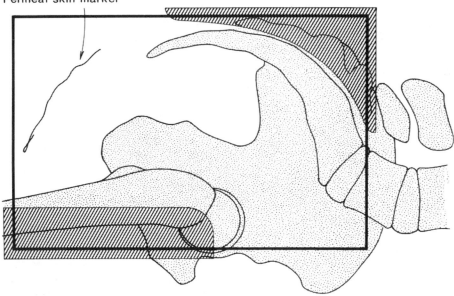

Perineal skin marker

**FIGURE 8-10**  Second example of a standard radiation field for patients with rectal cancer.

## LOCALLY ADVANCED RECTAL CANCER

### Introduction

Within the group of patients categorized as having "locally advanced" rectal cancer, there is also variability in disease extent with no uniform definition of resectability. Depending on the series, a locally advanced lesion can range from a tethered or marginally resectable tumor to a fixed cancer with direct invasion of adjacent organs or structures. The definition will also depend on whether the assessment of resectability is made clinically or at the time of surgery. In some cases, tumors thought to be unresectable at the time of clinical or radiographic examination may be more mobile when the patient is examined under anesthesia. With these caveats, a good working definition of a locally advanced tumor is "a tumor that cannot be resected without leaving microscopic or gross residual disease in the local site because of tumor adherence or fixation to that site." Since these patients do poorly with surgery alone, treatment programs of irradiation, chemotherapy, and surgery have evolved to improve their outcome.

### External Beam Irradiation

In the past, the management of locally advanced rectal cancer has been variable. Some patients have had incomplete surgical resections alone, while others have had radiation alone or surgery combined with post- or preoperative irradiation. The results of high dose external beam irradiation as a primary curative treatment have been unsatisfactory, with local failure rates of at least 90% or greater and 5-year survivals of less than 10%. Wang and Schulz reported that of 58 patients with recurrent, inoperable, or residual rectosigmoid carcinoma treated with 35 to 50 Gy in 4 to 5 weeks, six patients survived 5 years disease free.[80] O'Connell et al. noted that 37 of 44 patients with locally unresectable or recurrent rectal carcinoma treated with 50 Gy in a split-

course fashion over 7 weeks with and without adjuvant immunotherapy had progression of disease.[81] Of 31 patients assessable for sites of initial tumor progression, 17 had local progression only, 11 had concurrent local progression and distant metastases only, and 3 developed only distant metastases. Brierley, Cummings, et al. reported that of 77 patients with clinically fixed tumors who were treated with 50 Gy in 20 fractions over 4 years, local control was 3% and survival was 4%.[82] Unless the patient is not a candidate for surgery, external beam irradiation has no role as definitive treatment.

### External Beam Irradiation and Surgery

Combinations of external beam irradiation and surgical resection have been used to improve local control and survival. Radiation therapy after subtotal resection gives better local control and survival in patients treated for residual microscopic disease than to patients treated with gross residual disease. Allee et al. reported the results of 31 patients with residual microscopic cancer treated with 45 Gy followed by additional radiation therapy to as much as 60 to 70 Gy if small bowel could be moved from the radiation field.[83] Local control rate and 5-year disease-free survival rates were 70% and 45%, respectively. In contrast, these figures were 43% and 11% for 25 patients treated for gross residual disease. A possible dose–response correlation was seen in patients with microscopic residual disease; the risk of local failure was 11% (1 of 9) with doses of 60 Gy or greater versus 40% (8 of 20) if the boost dose was less than 60 Gy. There was no clear dose–response relationship in patients with gross disease. Of 17 patients receiving external beam irradiation after subtotal resection, Schild et al. observed that local control was achieved in 3 of 10 patients (30%) with microscopic residual cancer and one of seven patients (14%) with gross remaining cancer.[84] Four of the 17 patients (24%) have remained disease free for more than 5 years. Ghossein et al. treated patients to 46 Gy in 1.8 Gy fractions followed by a field reduction to the area of persistent disease which received 60 Gy.[85] For patients treated with microscopic disease the incidence of local failure and survival was 16% and 84%, whereas for patients with gross disease, these figures were 50% and 39%, respectively.

For patients presenting with locally advanced disease (unresectable for cure because of tumor fixation), high dose preoperative irradiation (45–50 Gy) has been used to reduce tumor size and facilitate resection. Emami et al. reported that the rate of resectability of 28 patients after full-dose preoperative irradiation was 50%.[86] Dosoretz et al. reported 25 (57%) patients with unresectable tumors in the rectum or rectosigmoid treated with 40 to 52 Gy preoperative radiation therapy.[87] Sixteen of the 25 patients underwent potentially curative resection, and the 6-year survival was 26% (with 3 postoperative deaths). Total pelvic failure after curative resection was 39% (5 of 13 patients). Mendenhall et al. reviewed 23 patients with locally advanced carcinoma who received 35 to 60 Gy of preoperative irradiation.[88] Eleven patients were able to undergo complete resection with a 5-year absolute survival of 18% and a local failure of 55%. As reported by Stevens and Fletcher, 28 of 72 patients (39%) with locally advanced carcinoma of the rectum or rectosigmoid received 50 to 72 Gy preoperatively and were resectable.[89] However, tumor recurred locally in 9 of 28 (32%) of these patients, and the 5-year survival was 10%. Of 20 patients with unresectable rectal cancer undergoing 43 to 55.8 Gy preoperative irradiation reported by Whiting et al., 13 patients (65%) underwent resection with curative intent.[90] Three of 13 (23%) subsequently developed a local failure. The 5-year survival was 40%.

There has been one randomized prospective study examining the merits of preoperative irradiation in patients with locally advanced rectal cancer. Under the auspices of the Northwest Rectal Cancer Group (Manchester, United Kingdom), 284 patients with tethered or fixed rectal cancer were entered into a prospective randomized trial between 1982 and 1986 to assess the effects of preoperative irradiation given one week before surgery.[91] One hundred forty-one patients were allocated to undergo surgical treatment alone, and 143 were allocated to receive 20 Gy in four fractions. This study showed a highly significant reduction in local recurrences in the irradiated group (12.8%) versus the surgery-alone group (36.5%). Although there was no significant difference in either overall survival or cancer-related mortality between the two treatment groups, subset analysis of the patients who underwent curative surgery alone reveals an overall mortality of 53.3% for patients allocated to surgery alone and 44.9% for patients allocated to preoperative radiotherapy. This is a significant reduction in mortality.

In summary, following full-dose preoperative irradiation, most series report that half to two-thirds of patients will be converted to a resectable status. However, despite a complete resection and negative margins, the local failure rate depending on the degree of tumor fixation varies from 23% to 55%.

## Preoperative External Beam Irradiaton with Chemotherapy and Surgery

Because of the efficacy of postoperative irradiation and 5-FU in the adjuvant treatment of rectal cancer, there has been interest in examining this approach preoperatively. These investigations have studied combinations of moderate to full-dose preoperative irradiation (45–50.4 Gy) with 5-FU-based chemotherapy for patients with clinical T3 and T4 rectal cancer. Comments in this section are limited to analyses of patients with clinical T4 tumors. The end points of these studies have included not only resectability, local control, and survival but pathological downstaging and sphincter preservation rates. One such report came in 1995 from the M. D. Anderson Hospital.[92] Patients with locally advanced rectal cancer who received 45 Gy of preoperative irradiation with continuous infusion chemotherapy of 5-FU and/or cisplatin and surgery had a 3-year survival and local recurrence rate of 82% and 3%, respectively. These results contrasted to a 3-year survival and local recurrence rate of 62%

and 33% for 36 similarly staged patients undergoing preoperative irradiation without chemotherapy. Although there was a higher rate of sphincter-preserving procedures in patients receiving chemoirradiation (35%) versus patients undergoing irradiation only (7%), there were no differences in rates of resectability or pathological downstaging between these groups of patients receiving chemotherapy versus no chemotherapy. Other investigations, however, have reported higher resectability and pathological downstaging rates with the use of preoperative chemoirradiation schedules. In an analysis of 36 patients (30 primary and 6 recurrent) with locally advanced/unresectable disease who were treated with 50.4 Gy of pelvic irradiation and concurrent 5-FU and leucovorin at Memorial Sloan-Kettering Cancer Center, the resectability rate with negative margins was 97% and the total complete response rate was 25%.[93] Similarly, a Swedish study reported an enhanced resectability rate in patients with unresectable rectal cancer who received preoperative irradiation, 5-FU, methotrexate, and leucovorin rescue compared with 38 patients who received radiation alone (71% vs. 34%).[94] Investigators from Tom Baker Cancer Centre reported an 89% complete resection rate in 46 patients with tethered and fixed rectal cancer treated with 40 Gy and 5-FU infusion and mi-

tomycin C.[95] Of 31 patients receiving continuous 5-FU infusion throughout irradiation at Thomas Jefferson University, 29 patients (94%) underwent complete resection with negative margins.[96] Enhanced resectability is an important end point, since patients with initially unresectable rectal cancer who have microscopic or gross residual disease have higher local failure and lower survival rates than patients who undergo a complete resection.

Analyses of local control and survival following treatment programs of preoperative chemoirradiation and surgery for locally advanced rectal cancer are limited by small patient numbers and short follow-up. Nevertheless, preliminary results suggest improved outcomes in patients receiving chemoirradiation compared with prior studies evaluating patients undergoing irradiation only (Table 8-11).[92–97] Based on the data, combinations of moderate to high dose preoperative irradiation with concurrent 5-FU-based chemotherapy can be said to result in improved rates of resectability and possibly local control and survival.

Although the dose and techniques of irradiation are similar in these studies (45–50.4 Gy in 25–28 fractions to the pelvis via a three- or four-field arrangement), there is marked variability in 5-FU administration. Some studies

TABLE 8-11 Preoperative Chemotherapy, Radiation Therapy, and Resection of Locally Advanced Rectal Cancer

| Study | Number of Patients | Drug | EBRT Dose (Gy) | Complete Resection Rate (%) | Local Failure (%) | Survival (%) |
|---|---|---|---|---|---|---|
| M. D. Anderson[92] | 38 | 5-FU infusion ± cisplatin | 45 | 84 | 3 (crude) | 82 (3 years) |
| Memorial Sloan-Kettering Cancer Center[93] | 36 | 5-FU/ leucovorin | 50.4 | 97 | 30 (4-year actuarial) | 67 (4 years) |
| Tom Baker Cancer Centre[95] | 46 | 5-FU/Mit-C | 40 | 89 | 16 (2-year actuarial) | 31 (3 years) |
| Thomas Jefferson[96] | 31 | 5-FU, continuous infusion | 55.8 | 94 | 16 (crude) | 68 (3 years) |
| Emory[97] | 20 | 5-FU bolus | 50 | NS | 10 (crude) | 82 (3 years) |

employ a schedule of 5-FU administered as a bolus for 3 consecutive days during weeks 1 and 5 of irradiation, whereas other investigators have utilized a continuous infusion approach throughout irradiation. Additionally, several investigators have used other agents such as leucovorin, cisplatin, and mitomycin-C in combination with 5-FU. Because of the Intergroup trial showing a survival advantage for patients treated with continuous infusion 5-FU throughout irradiation over patients treated with bolus 5-FU in the postoperative setting,[98] it would seem appropriate to adopt the former approach for preoperative irradiation programs in rectal cancer. The value of additional agents such as leucovorin, levamisole, cisplatin, and mitomycin C in combination with 5-FU is under investigation. It is becoming clear from the adjuvant rectal trials that more chemotherapy with irradiation is not necessarily a better situation. In the adjuvant postoperative chemo-irradiation rectal trials, it appears that the three-drug combination of 5-FU, levamisole, and leucovorin is more toxic and no more efficacious than 5-FU only or the two-drug regimen of 5-FU and leucovorin.[99] At present, we are using a 5-FU schedule of 225 mg/m$^2$/24 h for 5 days per week throughout the 5.5 week course of preoperative irradiation (45 Gy to the pelvis followed by a tumor boost of 5.4 Gy in 28 fractions of 1.8 Gy). In our experience, this 5-FU schedule with pelvic irradiation has been well tolerated.

## Intraoperative Electron Beam Irradiation

Despite full-dose preoperative irradiation and complete resection of locally advanced rectal cancer, local failure occurs in at least one-third of patients. These local failure rates are even higher in patients undergoing subtotal resection. At Massachusetts General Hospital, Mayo Clinic, and other centers in the United States, Europe, and Asia, intraoperative electron beam radiation therapy (IOERT) has been used in combination with preoperative irradiation (with and without 5-FU) and surgical resection

when there is gross residual cancer, positive resection margins, or simply tumor adherence.

At MGH, all patients with locally advanced rectal cancer receive full-dose preoperative irradiation with infusional 5-FU (225 mg/m2/day, 5 days per week, throughout irradiation). Surgical exploration is undertaken 4 to 6 weeks later. At surgery, the abdomen is carefully evaluated for liver and peritoneal metastases. If metastases are found, intraoperative irradiation is not performed and treatment ends with surgical resection or external beam radiation therapy alone. If no metastases are found, the patients undergo abdominoperineal resection, low anterior resection, or pelvic exenteration depending on the extent and location of the tumor. Attempts are made to resect as much disease as possible, even if some gross residual disease remains. The surgical specimen and the tumor bed are examined pathologically to define areas of possible residual disease, microscopic positive margins, or gross residual tumor. It is critical to define all high risk areas accurately, to determine the optimal position for the IOERT field. If no tumor adherence and adequate soft tissue radial margins are present (> 1cm), IOERT is usually not used. Patients with residual cancer or with positive or minimal (< 5 mm) radial soft tissue margins are evaluated for IOERT.

The areas at highest risk for local tumor recurrence are defined by the surgeon and radiation oncologist. To direct the IOERT, cones are used with internal diameters ranging from 4 to 8 cm. Some have beveled ends, enabling good apposition of the cone to sloping surfaces in the pelvis. Cone size is selected to cover fully the high risk area generally on the sacrum or pelvic sidewall. These cones allow the geometry of the cone to fit the specific situation of tumor versus normal tissue. The cone must abut the site being treated, which can be difficult if the high risk area is located in an anatomically confined region such as the pelvis. Further, the angle of the edge of the cone should optimally be placed flat against the body surface to maximize dose homogeneity. It is important that the applicator be placed so that the tumor is fully covered, that no sensitive normal tissues be included in the beam, and that no fluid buildup occur in the treatment area. During treatment, suction tubes are positioned to minimize fluid buildup. If necessary, lead sheets can be cut out to block sensitive normal tissues that cannot be removed from the path of the beam: retraction and packing are often necessary to move normal tissues. Most IOERT treatments in rectal cancer are given through the abdomen, but a perineal port is occasionally used to treat a very low-lying tumor involving the coccyx, distal pelvic sidewall, or portions of the prostate and bladder when an exenteration is not performed.

Typical doses of radiation delivered intraoperatively are in the range of 10 to 20 Gy, with the lower doses being given for minimal residual disease and the higher doses for gross residual disease after resection. For patients undergoing complete resection with negative margins, the IOERT dose is usually 10 to 12.5 Gy, whereas for patients undergoing subtotal resection with microscopic residual the dose is 12.5 to 15 Gy. For patients with macroscopic tumor after resection, the dose is 17.5 to 20 Gy. Typical electron energies used are 9 to 15 MeV, depending on the thickness of residual tumor. The dose is quoted at the 90% isodose.

The IOERT program at MGH was started in 1978. Sixty-four patients with locally advanced rectal cancer have undergone full-dose preoperative irradiation and resection with IOERT. The 5-year actuarial local control and disease-specific survival for 40 patients undergoing complete resection with IOERT was 91% and 63%, respectively. For patients undergoing partial resection, local control and disease-specific survival correlated with the extent of residual cancer: 65% and 47%, respectively, for microscopic residual disease, and 57% and 14%, respectively, for gross residual disease.

The 5-year actuarial risk of complications of the 64 patients receiving IOERT was 16%. Two patients developed osteoradionecrosis of the sacrum requiring surgical intervention.

No deaths were seen as a consequence of these complications.

At the Mayo Clinic, the treatment approach of primary locally advanced rectal carcinoma has been similar to that of MGH, combining external beam irradiation with surgery and IOERT to high risk regions.[100] From April 1981 through August 1995, 61 patients with primary locally advanced colorectal cancer received an IOERT dose of 10 to 20 Gy, usually combined with 45 to 55 Gy of fractionated EBRT. The amount of residual disease remaining at IOERT after exploration and maximal resection in the 56 patients was gross in 16, microscopic or less in 39, and unresected in 1. The 5-year survival for the entire group of patients was 46%. Patients with microscopic or less residual disease fared better than those with gross residual, with a 5-year actuarial overall survival of 59% (vs. 21%). Failures within an irradiation field have occurred in 4 of 16 patients (25%) who presented with gross residual after partial resection versus 2 of 39 (5%) with microscopic or less residual after gross total resection. An in-depth analysis of neuropathy following IOERT was also performed. Symptomatic or objective neuropathy was documented in 18 of 56 patients (32%). Ten of 18 (56%) had only grade 1 toxicity, usually manifesting as mild or intermittent paresthesis and/or pain not requiring narcotics. Of the seven patients with presumed treatment-related grade 2 or 3 nerve toxicity, the data suggested a relationship between IOERT dose and the incidence of grade 2 or 3 neuropathy [<12.5 Gy, 1 of 29 (3%); >15 Gy, 6 of 26 (23%), $p = 0.03$]. Because of the high rates of distant metastases in these patients, more routine use of systemic chemotherapy was advised.

In the M. D. Anderson study, 11 of 38 patients (29%) with primary locally advanced rectal cancer received IOERT to high risk regions in the pelvis because of persistent tumor adherence or residual tumor following preoperative irradiation and infusional chemotherapy.[92] No local failures were seen in these patients, although 7 of 11 patients developed distant metastases. One patient developed a sensory neuropathy following 20 Gy of IOERT.

In Europe, the Pamploma group has been investigating IOERT in a variety of disease sites, including rectal cancer.[101] From March 1986 to October 1993, 59 patients with primary locally rectal cancer received IOERT as a treatment component in multimodal strategies including surgery and postoperative external beam radiotherapy (13 patients, group 1) or preoperative chemoirradiation followed by planned surgery (46 patients, group II). Pelvic recurrence has been identified in one patient (simultaneously with lung and liver metastasis) and distant dissemination, as the only site of progression, in nine (42% in group 1 and 9% in group II). Cause-specific survival projected over 80 months was 52% and 77% in group I and II, respectively. Toxicity attributable to IOERT consisted of pelvic pain (delayed neuropathy) observed in four patients (9%) and ureteral stenosis in five patients (11%).

The New England Deaconess Hospital has recently analyzed IORT experience for locally advanced rectal cancer.[102] Between 1982 and 1993, 33 patients with locally advanced rectal cancer (primary, 22 patients; recurrent, 11 patients) received preoperative irradiation with 5-FU-based chemotherapy and curative resection. Intraoperative irradiaton through a 300 $kV_p$ orthovoltage unit was given to 26 patients. The median dose of IORT was 12.5 Gy (range 8–20 Gy). The 5-year actuarial overall survival and local control rates for patients undergoing gross complete resection and IORT were 64% and 75%, respectively. The crude local control rate for patients following complete resection with negative margins was 92% for patients treated with IORT. IORT was ineffective for gross residual disease, with all four patients progressing locally despite therapy. Seventeen patients (65%) developed pelvic soft tissue complications and were treated successfully by posterior thigh myocutaneous flap. The incidence of complications was similar in the patients with primary or recurrent disease.

## SUMMARY

The treatment of locally advanced or clinical stage T4 rectal cancer has evolved over the past 20 years. In the 1980s, treatment programs of moderate to high dose irradiation followed by surgery were carried out at several centers in the United States. These studies showed that a complete resection was possible in half to two-thirds of patients with locally advanced rectal cancer after full-dose preoperative irradiation. Despite irradiation and complete resection, local failure occurred in at least one-third of these patients. Recent efforts to improve local control have included the administration of concurrent chemotherapy with preoperative irradiation and the use of IOERT at resection.

Because of the efficacy of postoperative irradiation and 5-FU in the adjuvant treatment of rectal cancer, there has been interest in investigating this approach neoadjuvantly. These investigations have studied combinations of moderate to full-dose preoperative irradiation (45–50.4 Gy) with 5-FU-based chemotherapy. Although limited by small patient numbers and short follow-up, the data from these studies show improved rates of resectability and possibly local control and survival. Concurrent 5-FU-based chemotherapy should be utilized with moderate to high dose preoperative irradiation programs.

To further improve local control in patients with locally advanced rectal cancer, investigators from the United States and Europe have studied IOERT in combination with treatment programs of external beam irradiation, surgery, and more recently chemotherapy. The data from these studies offer compelling evidence that local control is improved in patients receiving IOERT over patients not receiving this therapy. The result is most beneficial in patients undergoing complete resection versus patients undergoing partial resection. The treatment-related morbidity of IOERT in patients with primary locally advanced rectal cancer has been minimal. In this disease site, IOERT has been integrated successfully into treatment programs utilizing external beam irradiation, chemotherapy, and surgery.

# D. ANAL CANAL

Epidermoid malignancies of the anal region comprise only 1% to 3% of all carcinomas of the lower rectum. Nevertheless, these neoplasms have increased dramatically in importance during the past 15 years as models have developed for effectively employing concomitant radiation therapy and chemotherapy in lieu of radical surgery.[103] For patients with localized carcinoma of the anal canal, sphincter-preserving therapy utilizing a combination of radiation therapy and chemotherapy has become standard treatment. Radical surgery such as abdominoperineal resection is generally reserved for salvage in cases of local tumor recurrence.

Most centers have emphasized the approach of external beam irradiation to the pelvis combined with mitomycin C and 5-FU infusion, pioneered by Nigro[104] at Wayne State University. In the original Wayne State studies, patients received 1000 mg/m$^2$/day of 5-FU as a continuous infusion for the first 4 days of irradiation and mitomycin C as a bolus (15 mg/m$^2$) on day 1 of radiation therapy. Patients received irradiation to the pelvis at a dose of 30 Gy at 2 Gy per fraction. Of the 19 patients treated in this manner, 15 (79%) had no gross evidence of residual disease. Similar protocols at the Princess Margaret Hospital and other centers have shown excellent tumor regression and long-term local control and survival.[105,106] With 50 Gy of external beam irradiation given in 2 Gy fractions, the Princess Margaret Hospital group reported a complete clinical regression rate of 93% and a 5-year cause-specific survival of 75%. In a multi-institutional study, the Radiation Therapy Oncology Group (RTOG), utilizing a treatment regimen of 40.8 Gy of pelvic irradiation and concurrent 5-FU and mitomycin C, reported a 3-year local control rate of 71% and survival of 73%.[107] In this study, patients with tumors less than 3 cm in size had an improved 3-year local control rate (88%) and survival (85%) compared with patients with tumors 3 cm or larger, who had a local control of 62% and survival of 68%. It appears that combinations of chemotherapy and external beam irradiation

obviate abdominoperineal resection in a large percentage of patients.

Despite the wide acceptance of this multimodality approach, the optimal chemotherapy and radiation regimen has not been fully established. Because of its toxicity, investigators have attempted to eliminate mitomycin C from the chemotherapy regimen. A single-institution analysis from Princess Margaret Hospital demonstrated that irradiation with 5-FU and mitomycin C yields the best primary tumor control when compared with irradiation with 5-FU only (85% vs. 60%).[106] This superiority was demonstrated in all tumor stages except for those 2 cm or less in size. These results were confirmed in an RTOG/Eastern Cooperative Oncology Group (ECOG) study.[108] In this study, 310 patients were randomly assigned to receive pelvic irradiation (45 Gy) with 5-fluorouracil alone or pelvic irradiation (45 Gy) with 5-FU and mitomycin C chemotherapy. Patients with negative biopsy results (taken between days 45 and 60) received no other treatment. Patients with positive biopsy results received an additional 9 Gy of irradiation and 5-FU and cisplatin chemotherapy. Posttreatment biopsy results were positive in 15% of the patients in the 5-FU arm versus 7.7% in the 5-FU and mitomycin arm. At 4 years, colostomy rates were lower (95% vs. 23%, $p = 0.002$), colostomy-free survival was higher (71% vs. 59%, $p = 0.014$), and disease-free survival was higher (73% vs. 51%, $p = 0.003$) in the 5-FU and mitomycin C arm. A significant difference in overall survival has not been observed at 4 years. Toxicity was greater in the mitomycin C arm (23% vs. 7% grade 4 and 5 toxicity, $p < 0.001$). Thus despite its toxicity, mitomycin C is necessary for effective treatment. As an alternative to the standard 4-day regimen of 5-FU infusion and mitomycin C, investigators from the M. D. Anderson Cancer Center have studied combinations of 5-FU and cisplatin chemotherapy given 5 days a week continuously throughout irradiation.[109] With this approach, the 2-year local control rate was 85%, suggesting that this combination may be another effective regimen. Similarly, an ECOG phase II protocol utilizing high dose irradiation (59.4 Gy) and a 4-day infusion of 5-FU and cisplatin demonstrated a high overall response rate of 94%.[110] Further evaluation of this regimen is being pursued in a phase III study.

A wide range of radiation doses and schedules have been reported in the literature. Recent data suggest that there is a dose–response relationship in anal cancer. In an analysis of patients treated with radiation and concurrent 5-FU infusional chemotherapy, Rich et al. reported local control rates of 50% in patients who received less than 46 Gy, 73% in those who received 50 to 55 Gy, and 88% in those who received 60 to 66 Gy (by external beam irradiation and interstitial implant boost).[109] In a group of patients treated with pelvic irradiation and 5-fluorouracil and mitomycin C chemotherapy from the Massachusetts General Hospital and Boston University Hospital, radiation doses exceeding 54 Gy were associated with significantly improved survival and local control in anal canal patients.[111] This issue of total dose is an area of active investigation. The RTOG is presently investigating the feasibility and efficacy of a regimen consisting of 60 Gy of irradiation with 5-FU and mitomycin C.

## RADIATION THERAPY TECHNIQUE

The initial radiation field encompasses the pelvis from the S1-S2 level, the inguinal lymph nodes, and the anus with AP-PA portals. Typically 0.5 cm of bolus is placed over the inguinal regions when high energy photons (6–10 MV) are used. After 30 to 36 Gy, the treatment volume is reduced to the low pelvis with the superior border at the inferior margin of the S-I joints. Three-field technique combined with PA (6–10 MV) and lateral (10–24 MV) photon fields is used to carry this low pelvic volume to 45 Gy. The lateral inguinal nodes are excluded at this point unless clinically involved, in which case boost treatment with electrons is employed. Additional therapy

to the primary site is usually given by perineal electrons (9–18 MeV) or high energy opposed laterals or three-field technique. Total dose to the primary tumor is 54 to 56 Gy.

## SUMMARY

For patients with carcinoma of the anal canal, external beam irradiation with 5-fluorouracil and mitomycin C chemotherapy has replaced surgery as primary therapy. Current studies are optimizing chemotherapeutic and radiotherapeutic regimens.

## REFERENCES

1. Willett CG, Rustgi AL, Rossi RL, et al: Cancer of the pancreas and biliary tract, in *Cancer Manual,* 9th ed. Framingham, American Cancer Society, Massachusetts Division, 1996, pp 376–386.

2. Gunderson LL, Willett CG: Pancreas and hepatobiliary cancer, in CA Perez, and LW Brady (eds): *Principles and Practice of Radiation Oncology,* 3rd ed. Philadelphia, Lippincott, 1998.

3. Tepper JE, Nardi GL, Suit HD: Carcinoma of the pancreas—Review of MGH experience from 1963 to 1973: Analysis of surgical failure and implications for radiation therapy. *Cancer* 1976;37:1519.

4. Willett CG, Lewandrowski K, Warshaw AL, Efird J, Compton CC: Resection margins in carcinoma of the head of the pancreas: Implications for radiation therapy. *Ann Surg* 1993; 217:144–148.

5. Kalser MH, Ellenberg SS, for Gastrointestinal Tumor Study Group: Pancreatic cancer—Adjuvant combined radiation and chemotherapy following curative resection. *Arch Surg* 1985; 120:899.

6. Gastrointestinal Tumor Study Group: Further evidence of effective adjuvant combined radiation and chemotherapy following curative resection of pancreatic cancer. *Cancer* 1987; 59:2006.

7. Whittington R, Bryer MP, Haller DG, et al: Adjuvant therapy of resected adenocarcinoma

of the pancreas. *Int J Radiat Oncol Biol Phys* 1991;21:1137.

8. Bossett JF, Pavey JJ, Gillet M, et al: Conventional external irradiation alone as adjuvant treatment in resectable pancreatic cancer: Results of a prospective study. Short communication. *Radiother Oncol* 1992;24:191.

9. Foo ML, Gunderson LL, Nagorney DM, et al: Patterns of failure in grossly resected pancreatic ductal adenocarcinoma treated with adjuvant irradiaton + 5 fluorouracil. *Int J Radiat Oncol Biol Phys* 1993;26:483.

10. Yeo CJ, Cameron JL, Lillemoe KD, et al: Pancreaticoduodenectomy for cancer of the head of the pancreas: 201 patients. *Ann Surg* 1995; 221:721.

11. Hoffman JP, Weese JL, Solin LJ, et al: A pilot study of preoperative chemoradiation for patients with localized adenocarcinoma of the pancreas. *Am J Surg* 1995;169:71.

12. Staley CA, Lee JE, Cleary KR, et al: Preoperative chemoirradiation, pancreaticoduodenectomy, and intraoperative radiation for adenocarcinoma of the pancreatic head: Patient survival and patterns of treatment failure. *Am J Surg* 1996;171:118–125.

13. Ishikawa O, Ohigashi H, Imaoka S, et al: Is the long-term survival rate improved by preoperative irradiation prior to Whipple's procedure for adenocarcinoma of the pancreatic head? *Arch Surg* 1994;129:1075.

14. Sindelar WF, Kinsella TJ: Randomized trial of intraoperative radiotherapy in resected carcinoma of the pancreas. *Int J Radiat Oncol Biol Phys*. 1986;12(5):148.

15. Klaassen DJ, MacIntyre JM, Catton GE, Engstrom PF, Moertel CG: Treatment of locally unresectable cancer of the stomach and pancreas: A randomized comparison of 5-fluorouracil alone with radiation plus concurrent and maintenance 5-fluorouracil—An Eastern Cooperative Oncology Group study. *J Clin Oncol* 1985;3:373–378.

16. Moertel CT, Childs DS Jr, Reitemeir RJ, et al: Combined 5-fluorouracil and supervoltage radiation therapy of locally unresectable gastrointestinal cancer. *Lancet* 1969;2:865.

17. Gastrointestinal Tumor Study Group: Comparative therapeutic trial of radiation with or without chemotherapy in pancreatic carcinoma. *Int J Radiat Oncol Biol Phys* 1979;5: 1643.

18. Gastrointestinal Tumor Study Group: Therapy of locally unresectable pancreatic carcinoma: A randomized comparison of high dose (6000 rads) radiation alone, moderate dose radiation (4000 rads + 5-fluorouracil), and high dose radiation + 5-fluorouracil. *Cancer* 1981;48:1705.

19. Gastrointestinal Tumor Study Group: Radiation therapy combined with adriamycin or 5-fluorouracil for the treatment of locally unresectable pancreatic carcinoma. *Cancer* 1985;56:2563.

20. Gastrointestinal Tumor Study Group: Treatment of locally unresectable carcinoma of the pancreas: Comparison of combined-modality therapy (chemotherapy plus radiotherapy) to chemotherapy alone. *J Natl Cancer Inst* 1988;80:751.

21. Haslam JB, Cavanaugh PJ, Stroup SL: Radiation therapy in the treatment of unresectable adenocarcinoma of the pancreas. *Cancer* 1973;32:1341.

22. Whittington R, Dobelbower RR, Mohiuddin M, et al: Radiotherapy of unresectable pancreatic carcinoma: A six-year experience with 104 patients. *Int J Radiat Oncol Biol Phys* 1981;7:1639.

23. Whittington R, Solin L, Mohiuddin M, et al: Multimodality therapy of localized unresectable pancreatic adenocarcinoma. *Cancer* 1984;54:1991.

24. Mohiuddin M, Cantor RJ, Biermann W, Weiss SM, Barbot D, Rosato FE: Combined modality treatment of localized unresectable adenocarcinoma of the pancreas. *Int J Radiat Oncol Biol Phys* 1987;14:79.

25. Pilepich MV, Miller HH: Preoperative irradiation in carcinoma of the pancreas. *Cancer* 1980;46:1945.

26. Jessup JM, Steele G, Mayer RJ, et al: Neoadjuvant therapy for unresectable pancreatic adenocarcinoma. *Arch Surg* 1993;128:559.

27. Shipley WU, Nardi GL, Cohen AM: Iodine-125 implant and external beam irradiation in patients with localized pancreatic carcinoma: A comparative study to surgical resection. *Cancer* 1980;45:709.

28. Roldan GE, Gunderson LL, Nagorney DM, Martin JK, Ilstrup DM, Holbrook MA, Kvols

LK, McIlrath DC: External beam versus intraoperative and external beam irradiation for locally advanced pancreatic cancer. *Cancer* 1988;61:1110.

29. Shipley WU, Wood WC, Tepper JE, et al: Intraoperative electron beam irradiation for patients with unresectable pancreatic carcinoma. *Ann Surg* 1984;200:289.

30. Tepper JE, Shipley WU, Warshaw AL, Nardi GL, Wood WC, Orlow EL: The role of misonidazole combined with intraoperative radiation therapy in the treatment of pancreatic carcinoma. *J Clin Oncol* 1987;5:579.

31. Gunderson LL, Martin JK, Earle JB, et al: Intraoperative and external beam irradiation + resection: Mayo pilot experience. *Mayo Clin Proc* 1984;59:691.

32. Gunderson LL, Martin JK, Kvols LK, Nagorney DM, Fieck JM, Wieand HS, Martinez A, O'Connell MJ, Earle JD, McIlrath D: Intraoperative and external beam irradiation + 5-FU for locally advanced pancreatic cancer. *Int J Radiat Oncol Biol Phys* 1986;13:319.

33. Gunderson LL, Shipley WU, Suit HD, et al: Intraoperative irradiation: A pilot study combining external beam photons with "boost" dose intraoperative electrons. *Cancer* 1981;49:2259.

34. Gunderson LL, Tepper JE, Biggs PJ, et al: Intraoperative + external beam irradiation. *Curr Probl Cancer* 1983;7:1.

35. Wood W, Shipley WU, Gunderson LL, et al: Intraoperative irradation for unresectable pancreatic carcinoma. *Cancer* 1982;49:1272.

36. Moertel CG, Fleming TR, Macdonald JS, et al: Levamisole and fluorouracil for adjuvant therapy of resected colon carcinoma. *New Engl J Med* 1990;322:352–358.

37. International Multicentre Pooled Analysis of Colon Cancer Trials (IMPACT) Investigators: Efficacy of adjuvant fluorouracil and folinic acid in colon cancer. *Lancet* 1995;345:939–944.

38. O'Connell MJ, Mailliard JA, Kahn MJ, et al: Controlled trial of 5-FU and low-dose leucovorin given for 6 months as postoperative adjuvant therapy for colon cancer. *J Clin Oncol* 1997;15:246, 250.

39. Willett CG, Tepper JE, Cohen AM, et al: Failure patterns following curative resection of colonic carcinoma. *Ann Surg* 1984;200:685–690.

40. Gunderson LL, Sosin H, Levitt S: Extrapelvic colon—Areas of failure in a reoperation series: Implications for adjuvant therapy. *Int J Radiat Oncol Biol. Phys* 1985;11:731–741.

41. Willett CG, Fung CY, Kaufman DS, et al: Postoperative radiation therapy for high-risk colon cancer. *J Clin Oncol* 1993;11:1112–1117.

42. Schild SE, Gunderson LL, Haddock MW, Nelson H: The treatment of locally advanced colon cancer. *Int J Radiat Oncol Biol Phys* 1997;37:97.

43. Amos EH, Mendenhall WM, McCarty PJ, et al: Postoperative radiotherapy for locally advanced colon cancer. *Ann Surg Oncol* 1996;3:431–436.

44. Gastrointestinal Tumor Study Group: Adjuvant therapy with hepatic irradiation plus 5-FU in colon carcinoma. *Int J Radiat Oncol Biol Phys* 1991;21:1151–1156.

45. Wang CS, Harwood AR, Cummings BJ, et al: Total abdominal irradiation for cancer of the colon. *Radiother Oncol* 1984;2:209–214.

46. Brenner HJ, Bibe C, Chaitchik S: Adjuvant therapy for Duke's C adenocarcinoma of the colon. *Int J Radiat Oncol Biol Phys* 1983;9:1789–1792.

47. Fabian C, Giri S, Estes N, et al: Adjuvant continuous infusion 5-FU, whole abdominal radiation and tumor bed boost in high-risk stage III colon carcinoma: A Southwest Oncology Group pilot study. *Int J Radiat Oncol Biol Phys* 1995;32:457–464.

48. Estes NC, Giri S, Fabian C: Patterns of recurrence for advanced colon cancer modified by whole abdominal radiaton and chemotherapy. *Am Surg* 1996;62:546–550.

49. Willett CG, Tepper JE, Orlow E, et al: Renal complications secondary to radiation treatment of upper abdominal malignancies. *Int J Radiat Oncol Biol Phys* 1986;12:1601–1604.

50. Landis S, Murray T, Bolden S, et al: Cancer statistics, 1998. *CA A Cancer J Clin* 1998;47:5–27.

51. Billingham RP: Conservative treatment of rectal cancer: Extending the indication. *Cancer* 1992;70:1355–1363.

52. Nichos RJ, York-Mason AM, Morson BC, et al: The clinical staging of rectal cancer. *Br J Surg* 1982;69:404–407.

53. Ng A, Recht A, Busse PM: Sphincter preservation therapy for distal rectal cancer—A review. *Cancer* 1997;79:671–683.

54. Alexander AA: The effect of endorectal ultrasound scanning on the preoperative staging of rectal cancer. *Surg Oncol Clin North Am* 1992;1:39–56, 1992.

55. Orrom WJ, Wong WD, Rothenberger DA, et al: Endorectal ultrasound in the preoperative staging of rectal tumors: A learning experience. *Dis Colon Rectum* 1990;33:654–659.

56. Hulsmans FJH, Tio TL, Fockens P, et al: Assessment of tumor infiltration depth in rectal cancer with transrectal sonography: Caution is necessary. *Radiology* 1994;190:715–720.

57. Minsky BD, Rich T, Recht A, Harvey W, Mies C: Selection criteria for local excision with or without adjuvant radiation therapy for rectal cancer. *Cancer* 1989;63:1421–1429.

58. Brodsky JT, Richard GK, Cohen AM, Minsky BD: Variables correlated with the risk of lymph node metastasis in early rectal cancer. *Cancer* 1991;69:322–326.

59. Gall FP, Hermanek P: Update of the German experience with local excision of rectal cancer. *Surg Oncol Clin North Am* 1992;1:99–109.

60. Willett CG, Tepper JE, Donnelly S, et al: Patterns of failure following local excision and local excision and postoperative radiation therapy for invasive rectal cancer. *J Clin Oncol* 1989;7:1003–1008.

61. Wood WC, Willett CG: Update of the Massachusetts General Hospital experience of combined local excision and radiotherapy for rectal cancer. *Surg Oncol Clin North Am* 1992;1:131–136.

62. Ota DM, Skibber J, Rich TA: MD Anderson Cancer Center experience with local excision and multimodality therapy for rectal cancer. *Surg Oncol Clin North Am* 1992;1:147–152.

63. Jessup JM, Bothe A, Stone MD, Gray C, Bleday R, Busse PM, et al: Preservation of sphincter function in rectal carcinoma by a multimodality treatment approach. *Surg Oncol Clin North Am* 1992;1:137–145.

64. Wong CS, Stern H, Cummings BJ: Local excision and postoperative radiation therapy for retal carcinoma. *Int J Radiat Oncol Biol Phys* 1993;25(4):669–675.

65. Fortunato L, Ahmad NR, Yeung RS, et al: Long-term followup of local excision and radiation therapy for invasive rectal cancer. *Dis Colon Rectum* 1995;38:1193–1199.

66. Minsky BD, Enker WE, Cohen AM, et al: Local excision and postoperative radiation therapy for rectal cancer. *Am J Clin Oncol* 1994;17:411–416.

67. Steele GD, Herndon JE, Burgess AM, et al: Sphincter sparing treatment for distal rectal adenocarcinoma: A phase II intergroup study. *Proc ASCO* 1997;16:256a.

68. Gastrointestinal Tumor Study Group: Prolongation of the disease-free interval in surgically treated rectal carcinoma. *New Engl J Med* 1985;312:1465–1472.

69. Fisher B, Wolmark N, Rockette H, et al: Postoperative adjuvant chemotherapy or radiation therapy for rectal cancer: Results from NSABP Protocol R-01. *J Natl Cancer Inst* 1988;80:21–29.

70. Krook JE, Moertel CG, Gunderson LL, et al: Effective surgical adjuvant therapy for high-risk rectal cancer. *New Engl J Med* 1991;324:709.

71. Gastrointestinal Tumor Study Group: Radiation therapy and 5-FU with or without semustine for the treatment of patients with surgical adjuvant adenocarcinoma of the rectum. *J Clin Oncol* 1992;10:549–557.

72. O'Connell MJ, Martenson JA, Wieand HS, et al: Improving adjuvant therapy for rectal cancer by combining protracted-infusion 5-FU with radiation therapy after curative surgery. *New Engl J Med* 1995;331:502–507.

73. Tepper JE, O'Connell M, Petroni G, et al: Toxicity in the adjuvant therapy of rectal cancer. *Proc ASCO* 1996;15:210.

74. Mendenhall WM, Bland KI, Copeland EM, et al: Does preoperative radiation therapy enhance the probability of local control and survival in high-risk distal rectal cancer. *Ann Surg* 1992;215:696–706.

75. Myerson RJ, Michalsi JM, King ML, et al: Adjuvant radiation therapy for rectal carcinoma: Predictors of outcome. *Int J Radiat Oncol Biol Phys* 1995;32:41–50.

76. Rich TA, Skipper JM, Ajani JA, et al: Preoperative infusional chemoirradiation for stage T3

rectal cancer. *Int J Radiat Oncol Biol Phys* 1995;32:1025–1029.

77. Chan RS, Tyler DS, Anscher MS, et al: Preoperative radiation and chemotherapy in the treatment of adenocarcinoma of the rectum. *Ann Surg* 1995;221:779–787.

78. Minsky BD, Cohen AM, Kemeny N, et al: Enhancement of radiation-induced downstaging of rectal cancer by 5-FU and high-dose leucovorin chemotherapy. *J Clin Oncol* 1992;10: 79–84.

79. Hyams DM, Mamounas EP, Petrelli N, et al: A clinical trial to evaluate the worth of preoperative multimodality therapy in patients with operable carcinoma of the rectum: A progress report of NSABP R-03. *Dis Colon Rectum* 1997;40:131–139.

80. Wang CC, Schulz MD: The role of radiation therapy in the management of carcinoma of the sigmoid, rectosigmoid, and rectum. *Radiol Soc North Am* 1962;79:1–5.

81. O'Connell MJ, Childs DS, Moertel CG, et al: A prospective controlled evaluation of combined pelvic radiotherapy and methanol extraction residue of BCG (MER) for locally unresectable or recurrent rectal carcinoma. *Int J Radiat Oncol Biol Phys* 1982;8:1115–1119.

82. Brierley JD, Cummings BJ, Wong CS, Keane TJ, O'Sullivan B, Catton CN, Goodman P: Adenocarcinoma of the rectum treated by radical external radiation therapy. *Int J Radiat Oncol Biol Phys* 1995;31:255–259.

83. Allee PE, Tepper JE, Gunderson LL, et al: Postoperative radiation therapy for incompletely resected colorectal carcinoma. *Int J Radiat Oncol Biol Phys* 1989;17:1171–1176.

84. Schild SE, Martenson JA, Gunderson LL, et al: Long-term survival and patterns of failure after postoperative radiation therapy for subtotally resected rectal adenocarcinoma. *Int J Radiat Oncol Biol Phys* 1988;16:459–463.

85. Ghossein NA, Samala EC, Alpert S, et al: Elective postoperative radiotherapy after incomplete resection of colorectal cancer. *Dis Colon Rectum* 1981;24:252–256.

86. Emami B, Pilepich M, Willett CG, Munzenrider JE, Miller HH: Effect of preoperative irradiation on resectability of colorectal carcinomas. *Int J Radiat Oncol Biol Phys* 1982;8:1295–1299.

87. Dosoretz DE, Gunderson LL, Hedberg S, et al: Preoperative irradiation for unresectable rectal and rectosigmoid carcinomas. *Cancer* 1983;52:814–818.

88. Mendenhall WM, Bland KI, Pfaff WW, et al: Initially unresectable rectal adenocarcinoma treated with preoperative irradiation and surgery. *Ann Surg* 1987;205:41–44.

89. Stevens KR, Fletcher WS: High dose preoperative pelvic irradiation for unresectable adenocarcinoma of the rectum or sigmoid. *Int J Radiat Oncol Biol Phys* 1983;9:148.

90. Whiting JF, Howes A, Osteen RT: Preoperative irradiation for unresectable carcinoma of the rectum. *Surgery (Gynecol Obstet)* 1993;176:203–207.

91. Marsh PJ, James RD, Scholfield PF: Adjuvant preoperative radiotherapy for locally advanced rectal carcinoma. *Dis Colon Rectum* 1994; 37:1205–1214.

92. Weinstein GD, Rich TA, Shumate CR, Skibber JM, Cleary KP, Ajani JA, Ota DM: Preoperative infusional chemoradiation and surgery with or without an electron beam intraoperative boost for advanced primary rectal cancer. *Int J Radiat Oncol Biol Phys* 1995;32: 197–204.

93. Minsky BD, Cohen AM, Enker WE, Saltz L, Guillem J, et al: Preoperative 5-FU, low-dose leucovorin, and radiation therapy for locally advanced and unresectable rectal cancer. *Int J Radiat Oncol Biol Phys* 1997;37:289–295.

94. Prykolm G, Glimelius B, Pahlman L: Preoperative irradiation with and without chemotherapy (MFL) in the treatment of primary non-resectable adenocarcinoma of the rectum. Results from two consecutive studies. *Eur J Cancer Clin Oncol* 1989;25:1535–1541.

95. Chan A, Wong A, Langevin J, Khoo R: Preoperative concurrent 5-fluorouracil infusion, mitomycin C and pelvic radiation therapy in tethered and fixed rectal carcinoma. *Int J Radiat Oncol Biol Phys* 1992;25:791–799.

96. Chen ET, Mohiuddin M, Brodovsky H, Fishbein G, Marks G: Downstaging of advanced rectal cancer following combined preoperative chemotherapy and high dose radiation. *Int J Radiat Oncol Biol Phys* 1994;30:169–175.

97. Landry G, Koretz MJ, Wood WC, Bahri S, Smith RG, Costa M, et al: Preoperative irradi-

ation and fluorouracil chemotherapy for locally advanced rectosigmoid carcinoma: Phase I–II study. *Radiology* 1993;188: 423–426.

98. O'Connell MJ, Martenson JA, Wieand HS, et al: Improving adjuvant therapy for rectal cancer by combining protracted-infusion 5-FU with radiation therapy after curative surgery. *New Engl J Med* 1995;331:502–507.

99. Tepper JE, O'Connell M, Petroni G, et al: Toxicity in the adjuvant therapy of rectal cancer. *Proc ASCO* 1996;15:210.

100. Gunderson LL, Nelson H, Martenson JA, Cha S, Haddock M, Devine R, et al: Locally advanced primary colorectal cancer: Intraoperative electron and external beam irradiation ± 5-FU. *Int J Radiat Oncol Biol Phys* 1997;37: 601–614.

101. Azinovic I, Calvo FA, Aristu JJ, Martinez R, Fernandez-Hidalgo O, et al: Intraoperative radiation therapy as a treatment component in primary rectal cancer: Ten-year experience, Personal Communication.

102. Kim HK, Jessup M, Beard CJ, Bornstein B, Cady B, Stone MD, Bleday, et al: Locally advanced rectal carcinoma: Pelvic control and morbidity following preoperative radiation therapy, resection and intraoperative radiation therapy. *Int J Radiat Oncol Biol Phys* 1997;38: 777–783.

103. Flam NS, John MJ, Mowry P, et al: Definitive combined modality therapy of carcinoma of the anus. *Dis Colon Rectum* 1987;30: 495–502.

104. Nigro ND: An evaluation of combined therapy for squamous cell cancer of the anal canal. *Dis Colon Rectum* 1984;27:763–766.

105. Cumming BJ: Anal cancer. *Int J Radiat Oncol Biol Phys* 1990;19:1309–1315.

106. Epidermoid anal cancer: Treatment by radiation alone or by radiation and 5-fluorouracil and without mitomycin C. *Int J Radiat Oncol Biol Phys* 1991;21:1115–1125.

107. Sischy B, Doggett RLS, Krall JM, Taylor DG, Sause WT, Lipsett JA, Seydel HG: Definitive irradiation and chemotherapy for radiosensitization in management of anal carcinoma: Interim report on Radiation Therapy Oncology Group Study No. 8314. *J Natl Cancer Inst* 1989;81:850–856.

108. Flam MS, John M, Pajak J, et al: Radiation and 5-FU vs. radiation 5-FU, mitomycin in the treatment of anal carcinoma: Results of a phase III randomized RTOG/ECOG. *J Clin Oncol* 1996;14:2527–2539.

109. Rich TA, Ajani JA, Morrison WH, Ota D, Levin B: Chemoradiation therapy for anal cancer: Radiation plus continuous infusion of 5-fluorouracil with or without cisplatin. *Radiother Oncol* 1993;27:209–215.

110. Martensen JA, Lipsitz S, Wagner H, et al: Phase II trial of radiation therapy, 5-FU and cisplatin in patients with anal cancer. *Int J Radiat Oncol Biol Phys* 1995;32:158.

111. Constantinou EC, Daly W, Fung CY. Time–dose considerations in the treatment of anal cancer. *Int J Radiat Oncol Biol Phys* 1997;39: 651–657.

# CHAPTER 9

# GENITOURINARY MALIGNANCIES

WILLIAM U. SHIPLEY and ANTHONY L. ZIETMAN

## A. BLADDER CANCER

### INCIDENCE AND PATHOLOGY

Bladder cancer is the fourth most common cancer among men and the eighth most common cancer among women in the United States, with 54,500 new cases and 7700 bladder cancer deaths expected to occur in 1997. The incidence increases with age: the median age of diagnosis in most series is between 64 and 68 years, with less than 1% of bladder cancer occurring in patients under the age of 40. Males are affected at least three times as frequently as females. Bladder cancer represents a wide spectrum of diseases that can be grouped into three major categories: superficial, invasive (of the muscle of the bladder wall), and metastatic. These tumors differ in their clinical behavior, in their prognosis, and in their primary management. For a superficial tumor the goal is to prevent both superficial recurrences and progression to an incurable stage. For muscle-invading tumors, the issue becomes how to determine which tumors can be cured by means of combined modality therapy without surgical removal of the bladder, which require cystectomy for primary control, and which, by virtue of high metastatic potential, require an integrated systemic chemotherapy approach to enhance the possibility of cure. Tumor heterogeneity is so great in bladder cancer that conventional histopathologic classification is clearly inadequate for predicting the behavior of most bladder cancers today. Dedicated efforts are being made to identify the potential prognostic markers that may better stratify and identify a tumor's true malignant potential as well as its response to specific cytotoxic therapies. For comprehensive reviews of the epidemiology, molecular carcinogenesis, and molecular biology of bladder cancer, the reader may consult recent reviews.[1-3]

Transitional cell carcinomas frequently demonstrate a papillary growth pattern in approximately 80% of cases and a solid pattern in the remaining 20%. Solid tumors, either visibly or microscopically, are more likely to be high grade and to invade into the muscularis propria, whereas most superficial bladder tumors are low grade and papillary. Thus, for superficial bladder cancer, grade is an important predictor for aggressiveness. For muscle-invasive disease, however, almost all tumors are high grade, and thus the pathologic predictor of tumor aggressiveness is the depth of invasion into the muscle layer or beyond. The primary carcinoma in situ (Tis) without a concurrent invasive tumor is a rare presentation, accounting for no more than 2% of newly detected bladder cancers. However carcinoma in situ is noted adjacent to or even involving mucosal sites remote from the primary visible

*Clinical Radiation Oncology: Indications, Techniques, and Results, 2nd ed.* Edited by C.C. Wang.
ISBN: 0-471-23803-1   Copyright © 2000 Wiley-Liss, Inc.

tumor, particularly those invading the muscle, high grade tumors, or multiply recurrent superficial tumors. The lymphatic pathways of spread include the external and internal iliac chains as well as the perivesical nodes. The second-echelon lymph nodes include those of the common iliac, para-aortic, and pericaval regions.[4]

Bladder cancer arises from the transitional cell epithelium that lines the bladder. Thus over 90% percent of the tumors are transitional cell cancers, with the remaining cancers being squamous (in about 8%) and adenocarcinomas (about 2%); the frequency of undifferentiated carcinomas, including small-cell carcinoma, is very low.

## CLINICAL EVALUATION

Intermittent hematuria, either microscopic or macroscopic, is the presenting clinical manifestation in over 80% of patients with bladder cancer. This hematuria, which is present throughout micturition, often is referred to as total gross painless hematuria. The second most common presenting symptom is dysuria or occasionally stranguria (pain with straining to urinate). The workup of a patient with unexplained hematuria or a suspected bladder tumor includes analysis of the voided urine, urinary cytology, excretion urography (via intravenous pyelogram), and cystoscopy. The endoscopic evaluation, which forms the mainstay of diagnosis and staging of bladder cancer, includes a bimanual examination under anesthesia, complete inspection of the urethra and the bladder, and cold cup biopsies of all suspicious areas, followed by a transurethral resection of all visible tumor (if possible). The resection should include muscle underlying the visible tumor for staging purposes to assess depth and extent of invasion by the tumor. A careful search should be made for flat, velvety, reddened areas that may harbor carcinoma in situ. Upon completion of the endoscopic procedure, a diagram should be made showing the location of the positive findings, the location of visibly residual disease, and the results of bimanual examination after transurethral resection of the bladder cancer (TURBT) (Figure 9-1). The workup of a patient with an invasive primary tumor includes a chest x-ray, an abdominal and pelvic CT scan, and possibly a bone scan. Unfortunately neither CT nor magnetic resonance imaging precisely predicts the depth of invasion of the primary bladder tumor, nor are these modes particularly sensitive in detecting lymph nodal metastases. Thus, because of this insensitivity in detecting extravesicular disease, clinical evaluation often results in an underestimate of true disease extent. Therefore reported outcomes following treatment differ significantly by stage category according to whether patients were staged clinically or, if a cystectomy specimen was available, pathologically.

The most commonly used staging system is the TNM system, which since 1997 has divided the muscle infiltrating disease into superficial muscle (T2a), deep muscle (T2b), or extravesical (T3 and T4, see Ref. 5 and Table 9-1). However in clinical practice the correlation between the depth of invasion based on endoscopic evaluation and the depth of the tumor invasion in the final cystectomy specimen is only 50% to 60%.[3] The clinical staging system as proposed by the International Union Against Cancer (UICC) is a more practical one (Table 9-2). In patients with tumors invading the muscle, those without a mass or residual induration after TURBT are staged as T2 and those with palpable residual induration or a mass are staged as T3 (Ref. 6, Table 9-2).

## TREATMENT SELECTION

### Treatment for Patients with Superficial Bladder Cancer

Superficial tumors (clinical stage Ta, T1, or Tis), which comprise 70% to 80% of all patients with newly diagnosed bladder cancer, are usually treated successfully by a variety of conservative (bladder-sparing) techniques. These

## CYSTOSCOPY REPORT FORM

PATIENT NAME _____ UNIT # _____

CYSTOSCOPY DATE ___/___/___  SURGEON _____

---

Specify location/origin of primary (at cysto <u>or</u> TURB) _____

| | | |
|---|---|---|
| Visibly complete TURB? | Yes ____ | No ____ |
| Palpable mass or induration persists after TURB? | Yes ____ | No ____ |

Initial largest tumor (diameter): ≤1 cm ____ 1.1-2.9 cm ____ 3-4.9 cm ____ ≥ 5 cm ____

| | | |
|---|---|---|
| Does tumor invade prostate or vagina? | Yes ____ | No ____ |
| Is tumor fixed to pelvic/abdominal wall? | Yes ____ | No ____ |

---

**PLEASE COMPLETE THE FOLLOWING TWO DIAGRAMS:**

**A. TUMOR LOCATION <u>BEFORE TURB</u>**

**B. <u>POST-TURB</u>: IF MACROSCOPIC TUMOR REMAINS AT END OF PROCEDURE, INDICATE ITS LOCATION. IF NOT, CHECK "NONE."**

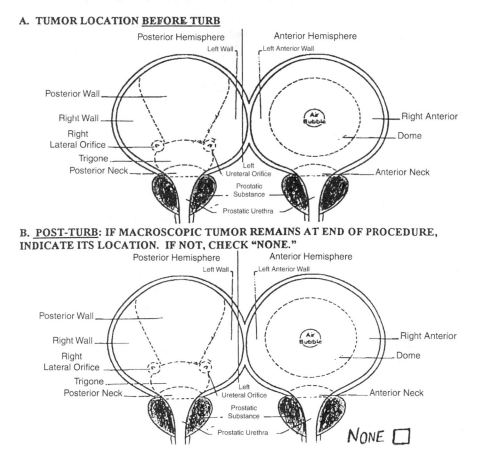

**FIGURE 9-1** Diagram for tumor mapping at the time of the cystoscopy and transurethral resection of the bladder tumor.

include a complete TURBT, and often intravesical therapy is added, based on the risk of tumor progression. Bacillus Calmette–Guérin (BCG) is currently the most effective and most commonly used intravesical agent for treatment. BCG has been shown to be effective in reducing the rates of progression, improving survival, and decreasing recurrence.[1–3] Intravesical chemotherapy with thiotepa, doxorubicin, and mitomycin C has been shown to decrease short-term tumor recurrence rates but not to decrease tumor progression nor to increase patient survival rates, and in several randomized trials such treatment has been shown to be inferior to BCG treatment. Alternative intravesical therapeutic approaches employing interferons or photodynamic therapy are under investigation.[1,2] The role of definitive external beam radiation therapy in the treatment of patients with Ta and T1 tumors is unclear, but in general external radiation therapy is not likely to be beneficial in the majority of patients with superficial disease. Specifically, it is of very questionable benefit in patients presenting af-

ter multiple superficial recurrent tumors when multiple endoscopic resections have failed.[7] Definitive external beam radiation therapy may have a significant impact on the long-term outcome of selected patients with T1 G3 tumors. Recently excellent results with T1 G3 tumors following thorough TURBT and concurrent chemotherapy and radiation therapy have been reported in 53 patients, with overall survival at 5 and 10 years of 77% and 61%, survival with an intact bladder at 5 and 10 years was observed in 55% and 45% of these patients.[8] The reports of the success of external beam radiation therapy in treating carcinoma in situ either primarily or coexistent with invasive tumors are conflicting; some investigators report uniquely poor results[9] and others, using concurrent chemotherapy and radiation following TURBT, report only an increase in the recurrence of superficial tumors.[10] The experience of interstitial radiation therapy in patients with T1 G3 bladder cancer has come mainly from the Netherlands, Belgium, and France. The studies have been limited to single tumors of

**TABLE 9-1   The 1997 AJCC Clinical TNM Staging System for Bladder Cancer**

| *Primary Tumor (T)* | | *Regional Lymph Nodes (N)* | |
|---|---|---|---|
| TX | Primary tumor cannot be assessed | Regional lymph nodes are those within the true pelvis; all others are distant lymph nodes. | |
| T0 | No evidence of primary tumor | | |
| Ta | Noninvasive papillary carcinoma | NX | Regional lymph nodes cannot be assessed |
| Tis | Carcinoma in situ: "flat tumor" | N0 | No regional lymph node metastasis |
| T1 | Tumor invades subepithelial connective tissue | N1 | Metastasis in a single lymph node, 2 cm or less in greatest dimension |
| T2 | Tumor invades muscle | N2 | Metastasis in a single lymph node, more than 2 cm but not more than 5 cm in greatest dimension: or multiple lymph nodes, none more than 5 cm in greatest dimension |
| | T2a  Tumor invades superficial muscle (inner half) | | |
| | T2b  Tumor invades deep muscle (outer half) | N3 | Metastasis in a lymph node more than 5 cm in greatest dimension |
| T3 | Tumor invades perivesical tissue | | |
| | T3a  microscopically | | |
| | T3b  macroscopically (extravesical mass) | | |
| T4 | Tumor invades any of the following: prostate, uterus, vagina, pelvic wall, abdominal wall | *Distant Metastasis (M)* | |
| | T4a  Tumor invades prostate, uterus, vagina | MX | Distant metastasis cannot be assessed |
| | T4b  Tumor invades pelvic wall, abdominal wall | M0 | No distant metastasis |
| | | M1 | Distant metastasis |

*Source:* Ref. 5.

**TABLE 9-2    The 1978 UICC Clinical TNM Staging System for the Primary Tumor**

| Primary Tumor | UICC Clinical TNM |
|---|---|
| Invasion into the lamina propria but not beyond | T1 |
| Muscle invasion (into muscularis propria) and bimanual exam after TURBT do *not* reveal residual induration | T2 |
| Muscle invasion and bimanual exam after TURBT do reveal residual induration | T3a |
| Muscle invasion and bimanual exam after TURBT reveal a residual mobile mass | T3b |
| Tumor invades adjacent organs | T4a |
| Tumor invades pelvic wall or abdominal wall | T4b |

*Source:* Ref. 6.

less than 5 cm and in many cases have been combined with TURBT and of course external beam radiation. Bladder relapse rates vary from 15% to 28%, and actuarial 5-year survival rates of 70% to 80% for this select group of patients[2,11] have been reported.

## Treatment for Patients with Muscle-Invading Tumors

The treatment for patients with muscle-infiltrating disease can be bladder sparing or non–bladder sparing. The most common treatment in this country is surgical removal of the entire organ by radical cystectomy. The standard bladder-sparing treatment has over the last three decades been external beam radiation therapy. In the United States, radiation has been recommended primarily only for patients judged "unfit" for a cystectomy on the basis of age, comorbid conditions, or disease extent. At least in part, because of these negative selection criteria for treatment by radiation, the reported results of retrospective series with radiation alone are inferior to those reported with radical surgery.[11–18] The difference is also due to at least two other factors. First, approximately 15% of patients are excluded from treatment by cystectomy because of identification, at the time of operation, of a previously unrealized, extravesical tumor that is too extensive to be amenable to surgery. Thus in cystectomy series, but not in radiation series, some patients with metastatic tumors are excluded.

Second, the cure rate of the cancer in the bladder with cystectomy is higher than with radiation therapy alone.

## Randomized Comparisons of External Beam Radiation Therapy to Radical Cystectomy

By 1985 four randomized phase III trials had compared cystectomy (with preoperative radiation therapy) with external beam radiation therapy with cystectomy reserved for salvage of patients with persistent or recurrent bladder cancer. In 1977 Miller reported the results of a randomized trial from the M. D. Anderson Hospital for patients with large T3 tumors.[19] Of 35 patients randomized to receive planned cystectomy, 45% survived 5 years, compared with 22% for the 32 patients randomized to external beam radiation. This is the only trial that demonstrated a statistically significant survival advantage to immediate cystectomy. This trial has been criticized because the only patients entered had large T3 tumors (which were relatively unlikely to be cured with radiation therapy alone). The Urologic Cooperative Group from the United Kingdom reported a much larger trial of 189 randomized patients. The recently updated results[20] report 5- and 10- year survival rates for the 98 patients randomized to immediate cystectomy of 39% and 19%, while for the 91 patients randomized to radiation therapy with salvage surgery, the 5- and 10-year survival rates were 28% and 15%. The differences were not statistically significant. Analysis of outcome at 5 years by subgroups within this randomized trial (even though such analysis may not be statistically appropriate) indicated that women had a statistically insignificant trend of a survival benefit if randomized to radiation therapy, and men who were less than 60 years old had a survival advantage if randomized to immediate cystectomy. In 1991 the Danish National Bladder Cancer Group randomized trial also reported no significant difference in overall survival in the two arms (immediate vs. deferred cystectomy).[21] The median follow-up period was 50 months for 183 patients. However, the local/pelvic recurrence rate was significantly lower in the group randomized to receive immediate cystectomy (6.8%) than in the 95 patients randomized to receive external beam radiation therapy alone (35%). Twenty-seven of the patients with persistent or recurrent tumor underwent salvage cystectomy. The incidence of metastatic disease was similar in both groups: 32% and 34% at 5 years. In the randomized trial of 72 patients done by the National Bladder Cancer Group (S. D. Cutler, personal communication, 1983), there was no difference in the 5-year survival rate nor in the rate of distant metastases for patients randomized to immedi-

ate cystectomy (27% and 38%, respectively) versus those having radiation therapy with cystectomy only for recurrence (40% and 31%, respectively). The median follow-up period in that study (Table 9-3) was 66 months. In the two trials that reported the incidence of distant metastases, there was no increased rate of distant metastases in the patients randomized to deferring radical cystectomy for salvage.[22] The Memorial Sloan-Kettering Cancer Center, which used both univariate and multivariate analysis,[23] also reported that deferring cystectomy in patients treated with neoadjuvant M-VAC (methotrexate, vinblastine, Adriamycin, cisplatin) chemotherapy did not alter the overall survival at 5 years.

## Recent Advances with Radical Surgery

Following a radical cystectomy, the urinary flow from the ureters is directed into a conduit (usually an ileal loop) or into a conduit reservoir as a bladder substitute. In the standard ileal loop (Bricker) procedure, the urine drains directly from the ureters into a segment of isolated ileum to the skin surface, where it is collected from the stoma in a external bag. No internal reservoir is created. For continent diversions, bowel segments are created and used

**TABLE 9-3  Randomized Trials of Irradiation That Did or Did Not Defer Radial Cystectomy for Salvage of Recurrence**

| Study and Treatment | Number of Patients | Clinical Stage | 5-Year Survival (%) | 10-Year Survival (%) | Distant Metastases (%) |
|---|---|---|---|---|---|
| M. D. Anderson Hospital[19] | | | | | |
| 50 Gy + cystectomy | 35 | T3 | 46 | | |
| 60 Gy + salvage cystectomy | 32 | T3 | 22 | | |
| U.K. Co-op Group[20] | | | | | |
| 40 Gy + radical cystectomy | 98 | T3 | 39 | 19 | |
| 60 Gy + salvage cystectomy | 91 | T3 | 28 | 15 | |
| National Danish Trial[21] | | | | | |
| 40 Gy + radical cystectomy | 88 | T3 | 29 | | 34 |
| 60 Gy + salvage cystectomy | 95 | T3 | 23 | | 32 |
| National Bladder Cancer Group[a] | | | | | |
| 40 Gy + radical cystectomy | 37 | T2-T4a | 27 | | 38 |
| 60 Gy + salvage cystectomy | 35 | T2-T4a | 40 | | 31 |

[a]S. D. Cutler, personal communication, 1983.

as reservoirs that are either intermittently catheterized by the patient through abdominal wall stoma or are anastomosed to the urethra (the orthotopic neobladders), where the patient can void naturally. The continent urinary diversions have been classified according to the location of the urinary outflow,[14] which include (1) those of the abdominal wall, (2) those anastomosed to the urethra (orthotopic bladder), and (3) those that utilize the rectal sphincter (uncommonly used now). However, although continent reservoirs are becoming increasingly popular, they are not constructed for most patients undergoing radical cystectomy for muscle-invading tumors.[24] The relative contraindications for the continent reservoirs include advanced age, intercurrent disease, impaired renal function, hesitancy to prolong surgery by 1 to 2 hours, dilated ureters, and bowel diseases.[3]

Because patients who have muscle-invading tumors have, at the time of cystectomy, a high rate of occult distant metastases (up to 50%) that manifest themselves clinically usually 1 to 3 years following surgery, chemotherapy following (adjuvant) or preceding (neoadjuvant) surgery has been studied for improvement in overall survival and in a reduction in distant metastases. Three randomized trials have failed to demonstrate any survival benefit from single- or multiple-agent neoadjuvant chemotherapy when added to cystectomy.[17,25,26] Similarly a meta-analysis of several randomized trials showed no benefit from a neoadjuvant chemotherapy approach.[27] By contrast, the phase III Nordic Cooperative Bladder Study 1 has recently been updated and now reports a survival benefit at 5 years of 12% with two cycles of cisplatin and doxorubicin in stage T3 and T4 patients treated by preoperative irradiation and radical cystectomy.[28] None of the randomized trials evaluating postcystectomy single-agent chemotherapy have shown any survival benefit.[13] Three randomized trials of multidrug adjuvant chemotherapy, all from single institutions (and all with some criticisms of trial design), have failed to show a statistically significant survival benefit but have shown a significant increase in recurrence-free survival.[29–31] Many medical oncologists currently recommend systemic chemotherapy for patients with adverse pathologic features following cystectomy; they cite the delay in disease progression as justification for this treatment. Recent assessment of the USC experience with adjuvant multidrug chemotherapy suggests that tumors with p53 alteration as assessed by immunohistochemical staining for p53 accumulation represent a subset that is significantly benefited by adjuvant chemotherapy.[32] This hypothesis is now forming the basis for a national multi-institutional randomized trial.

## Advances in Bladder-Preserving Approaches with Combined Modality Therapy

Multimodality organ-sparing treatment has, over the last decade, become the standard of care in North America and Europe for many common malignancies. Radical mastectomy for breast cancer and limb amputation for soft tissue sarcomas are procedures now primarily used for salvage after failure of first-line management with combined radiation and chemotherapy. Other tumor sites with organ sparing as a standard treatment option include laryngeal cancer, anal cancer, and prostate cancer. When used alone for muscle-invading bladder cancer, transurethral resection alone of the bladder tumor, external beam radiation therapy alone, or chemotherapy alone are all associated with limited local control (Table 9-4[33–40]); combinations of these modalities are considerably more successful (Tables 9-5, 9-6, and 9-7).[8,22,23,36,37,41–61]

In appropriately selected patients, bladder-preserving treatment with transurethral resection, radiation therapy, and concurrent chemotherapy offers a probability of long-term cure and overall survival comparable to cystectomy-based approaches (40% to 63% at 5 years) in patients of similar clinical stage and age. In addition, these selective bladder-preserving approaches allow approximately 80% of the long-term survivors to maintain a

TABLE 9-4   Muscle-Invading Bladder Cancer: Success Rates of Bladder Preservation with Monotherapy

| Treatment | Number of Evaluated Series | Total Number of Patients | With Bladder Preservation, Free of Invasive Recurrence (%) |
|---|---|---|---|
| Transurethral resection alone[33,34,a] | 2 | 331 | 20[b] |
| Radiation therapy alone[35–39,c] | 5 | 949 | 41 |
| Chemotherapy alone (cisplatin + methotrexate)[40,c] | 1 | 27 | 19 |

[a]Used selectively as monotherapy; most patients at these centers had cystectomy.

[b]Intravesical drug therapy often used for noninvasive recurrent tumors.

[c]No transurethral resection of tumor.

TABLE 9-5   Muscle-Invading Bladder Cancer: Complete Response Rates After Monotherapies and Combined Modality Therapies

| Treatment[a] | Number of Evaluated Series | Total Number of Patients | Complete Responses (%) |
|---|---|---|---|
| Radiation therapy alone[36,37,41,42] | 4 | 721 | 45 |
| Chemotherapy alone[43–47] | 6 | 301 | 27 |
| TURBT plus chemotherapy[48–51] | 4 | 225 | 51 |
| TURBT plus chemoradiotherapy[10,52–54] | 4 | 218 | 71 |

[a]TURBT, transurethral resection of tumor.

*Source:* Modified, with permission, from Shipley et al.[22]

normal functioning bladder.[53–57,62,63] The rationale for combining concurrent chemotherapy and radiation is twofold. First, certain cytotoxic agents, in particular cisplatin and 5-fluorouracil (5-FU), are capable of sensitizing tumor tissues to radiation, thus increasing cell kill in a synergistic fashion. Second, about half the patients with muscle-invading transitional cell cancer harbor occult metastases. Thus treatment of the primary tumor with radical surgery alone or with radiation therapy alone provides no treatment for occult systemic disease.

Although a variety of different drugs and radiation dose schedules have been used, it is apparent that the highest clinical complete response (cCR) rates (or a T0 bladder response) are achieved in patients who received concurrent chemotherapy and radiation rather than sequential treatments (Table 9-5, Ref. 3). One of the clearest indicators of the potential

of concurrent radiation therapy and chemotherapy for bladder preservation is reported in a study from the University of Paris.[62,63] In these reports, transurethral resection of the bladder tumor was followed by concurrent cisplatin, 5-FU and accelerated radiation therapy was initially used as a pre-cystectomy regimen. The first 18 patients who demonstrated no residual tumor on cystoscopic reevaluation and re-biopsy all underwent radical cystectomy, as planned. None of these 18 cCR patients had any evidence of malignancy in the cystectomy specimen—a 100% pathologic complete response rate in patients who had been determined cystoscopically to be clinical complete responders. Previous studies employing transurethral surgery and M-VAC chemotherapy found residual tumors in as many as 50% of the patients in the cystectomy specimen of those who had been evaluated cystoscopically and judged to be clinical complete responders.[51] This difference in pathologic Complete Response (pCR) rates for the cCR patients with and without radiation concurrent with chemotherapy (100% vs. 50%) gives a clear indication of the benefit of radiation concurrent with chemotherapy.

In a recent update of the Paris experience[63] of 120 patients with operable tumors, a clinical complete response rate of 77% was reported. The complete responders underwent consolidation chemoradiation, while the incomplete responders underwent immediate radical cystectomy. The overall 5-year survival rate was 63%. At the University of Ehrlangen, 93 patients treated with maximum transurethral resection plus radiation therapy concurrent with cisplatin had a clinical complete response rate of 85%. Five-year overall survival was 61%, with 47% surviving with a functioning bladder at 5 years.[8] We recently updated our experience with 106 patients treated with combined modality therapy using an as maximal transurethral resection of the tumor as was safely possible, then two cycles of neoadjuvant MCV (methotrexate, cisplatin, velban). This was followed by concurrent cisplatin and radiation to a dose of 39.6 Gy.

**TABLE 9-6   Recent Results of TURBT and Chemotherapy with Radiation**

| Series | Treatment[a] | Number of Patients | 5-Year Survival (%) | 5-Year Survival with Bladder Preservation (%) |
|---|---|---|---|---|
| Sauer et al.[8] | TURBT, concurrent cisplatin and XRT | 93 | 61 | 47 |
| Tester et al.[54] | Concurrent cisplatin and XRT | 42 | 52 | 42 |
| Tester et al.[55] | MCV and concurrent cisplatin and XRT | 91 | 62 | 44 |
| Kachnic et al.[56] | TURBT, MCV, concurrent cisplatin and XRT | 106 | 52 | 43 |
| Shipley et al.[57] | TURBT, MCV, concurrent cisplatin and XRT | 123 | 50 | 38 |

[a]TURBT, transurethral resection of tumor; MCV, methotrexate, vinblastine, Adriamycin, cisplatin; XRT, external beam irradiation.

**TABLE 9-7   Recent Results of TURBT and Chemotherapy Without Radiation**

| Series | Treatment[a] | Number of Patients | 5-Year Survival (%) | 5-Year Survival with Bladder Preservation (%) |
|---|---|---|---|---|
| Given et al.[59] | TURBT, MCV, plus, in 49 patients, (53%), concurrent cisplatin and XRT | 93 | 51 | 18 |
| Srougi and Simon[58] | M-VAC and partial cystectomy | 30 | 53 | 20 |
| Sternberg et al.[60] | TURBT + M-VAC, but without cystectomy, in 31 patients | 64 | —[b] | 33[b] |
| Scher et al.[61] and Schultz et al.[23] | M-VAC and conservative surgery | 111 | 48 | 21 |

[a]TURBT, transurethral resection of tumor; MCV, methotrexate, cisplatin, velban; M-VAC, methotrexate, vinblastine, Adriamycin, cisplatin; XRT, external beam irradiation.

[b]Median follow-up 30 months at time of report.

Seventy patients who were clinical complete responders (66%) and 6 who were not but were unsuited for surgery underwent consolidation with concurrent chemotherapy and radiation to a total dose of 64.8 Gy. Nineteen patients underwent radical cystectomy immediately: 13 were less than complete responders and 6 were not able to tolerate the induction chemotherapy plus radiation. The overall survival rate for all 106 entered patients in this prospective study is 52% and the disease-specific survival rate is 60%.[56] The 5-year overall survival with an intact bladder is 43%. The median follow-up period in this series is 4.4 years, with 40 patients being followed for longer than 5 years. No patient has required a cystectomy for a recurrence-related morbidity.

The Radiation Therapy Oncology Group (RTOG) has carried out two separate pilot trials of concurrent cisplatin and radiation for selective bladder preservation, with cystectomy being reserved for patients who were less than clinical complete responders to the induction regimen.[54,55] These two approaches, one with two cycles of neoadjuvant chemotherapy with MCV, resulted in complete response rates of 66% and 75% and 4-year survival rates of 60% and 62%. Most recently, the RTOG has reported results of a randomized trial to assess the long-term efficacy of neoadjuvant MCV chemotherapy in patients with muscle-invading bladder cancer treated by TURBT and concurrent cisplatin and radiation therapy, with consolidation by either cystectomy or cisplatin and radiation based on initial response.[57] With a median follow-up of 60 months, the 5-year overall survival rate was 49%, distributed as follows: 48% in arm 1 (MCV) and 49% in arm 2 (no MCV). Forty percent of the patients have evidence of distant metastases at 5 years (35% in arm 1 and 43% in arm 2). The 5-year survival rate with a functioning bladder is 38% overall (36% in arm 1 and 40% in arm 2). Among the 72 CR patients (61% CR in arm 1 and 55% CR in arm 2), 12% have had an invasive local tumor relapse at 5 years. None of these differences are statistically significant. No patient required a cystectomy for a treatment-related bladder morbidity. The absence of any benefit of two cycles of MCV neoadjuvant chemotherapy and the unexpectedly low (67%) completion rate of the MCV arm due to toxicity has led to trials at several institutions and within the RTOG to assess the feasibility and tolerance of adjuvant chemotherapy rather than neoadjuvant chemotherapy. In both the RTOG randomized trial[57] and the MGH study,[56] superficial disease appeared in the bladders of patients selected for bladder-preserving therapy in over 20% of patients observed for 5 or more years. This superficial recurrence, almost all carcinoma in situ, has responded well to conventional intravesical therapy but emphasizes the need for close cystoscopic follow-up.

Twice-a-day (BID) radiation regimens may be more effective than once-a-day (QD) radiation in their ability to induce and maintain a complete response.[20,64] We recently reported an MGH pilot study to evaluate the use of BID radiation together with cisplatin, and 5-fluorouracil in the treatment of comparable stage T2-T4a bladder cancers for potential bladder preservation.[65] Fifteen of the 18 patients received three cycles of adjuvant chemotherapy consisting of methotrexate, cisplatin, and vinblastine subsequent to definitive local therapy. The clinical complete response rate to induction chemoradiation was 77%. With a median follow-up period of 32 months, the overall survival and the survival with a functioning bladder at 3 years are 83% and 78%. To date, three patients have developed superficial tumors, and these have been managed successfully so far with intravesical BCG. Compared with our previous experience with neoadjuvant MCV,[56] the newer approach using adjuvant MCV is encouraging, with an overall 3-year survival rate of 88% versus 77%. At present we are participating in the RTOG Protocol 97-06 which is a multi-institutional successor protocol based on our pilot study described above. This protocol is for patients with a clinical stage T2-T4a operable bladder cancer with no hydronephrosis in which a maximal transurethral resection is followed by twice-a-day radiation (as 1.6 Gy to the bladder tumor and 1.8 Gy to the bladder and the pelvis) for 12 days (24 fractions) over 2.5 weeks, combined with concurrent outpatient cisplatin (20 mg/m$_2$) on the first 2 days of each of these 3-week sessions. Consolidation chemoradiotherapy is given in complete responding patients following cystoscopic reevaluation in week 6 by BID radiation of pelvis: 1.5 Gy per fraction over 8 days is given with the same cisplatin dose given on the first 2 days of each of these 2 weeks. The total radiation dose will be 45.6 Gy to the pelvis and to the whole bladder and 64.8 Gy to the bladder tumor. Subsequently outpatient adjuvant chemotherapy with methotrexate, cisplatin, and velban will be given every 28 days for three cycles.

## Conclusion

For patients with muscle-invading bladder tumors, bladder-preserving treatment in appropriately selected patients (best based on the response of the tumor to induction therapy) with chemotherapy and radiation therapy offers rates of long-term cure and survival comparable to those with immediate cystectomy-based approaches. The bladder-preserving approach is not suitable for patients with advanced tumors, especially those presenting with a tumor obstructing a ureter. Twenty to 30% of patients cured of their muscle-invading bladder cancer will subsequently develop a new superficial tumor. Such superficial tumors have responded well to the usual intravesical drug therapy. These patients require close urologic surveillance, as do patients with superficial bladder cancer treated conservatively. Bladder-preserving treatment with chemoradiation is not likely to increase the risk of distant metastases if it is used selectively in patients who are complete responders. Bladder-preserving treatment usually results in a normally functioning bladder without incontinence or hematuria. The ideal candidate for bladder preservation would be a patient whose primary tumor is a clinical stage T2; this tumor should have no associated ureteral obstruction, and a visibly complete transurethral resection of the tumor should have been accomplished. Concurrent systemic

chemotherapy and radiation have the potential for systemic morbidity. It is recommended that this treatment be administered by dedicated multimodality teams. This approach exists in many of the over 250 U.S. institutions participating in the RTOG. This treatment should be considered as a reasonable alternative in patients who are deemed medically unfit for cystectomy and for patients who are seeking an alternative to radical cystectomy.

## RADIOTHERAPY TECHNIQUES

Optimizing the treatment of a primary bladder tumor involves including the first-echelon draining regional lymphatics, while sparing as much normal tissue as possible. This requires using linear accelerator beams of high energy photons (10–25 MV). The treatment program includes the combination of a small pelvic field that irradiates the pelvic lymph nodes and the bladder as well as the entire bladder tumor volume and the prostatic urethra tissues to a dose adequate to control microscopic disease (40–50 Gy with conventional fractionation) and a subsequent or concomitant boost to the bladder tumor volume to raise its total dose to at least 64 to 70 Gy via conventional daily fractionation schemes. The volumes are best defined at simulation by information from the CT scan of the pelvis as well as information from the bladder map at cystoscopy and the results of the bimanual exam. Prior to simulation, a 40 to 50 mL of air and contrast cystogram is performed. This program is useful in defining the mucosal service of the bladder. Using cystogram information alone without a planning CT may cause inadequate coverage of the bladder in 60% of the cases, especially in the dorsal caudal dimensions.[66,67] The amount of cystogram contrast material should not be less than the postvoid residual, since this amount of urine will be present in the bladder during treatment. The postvoid residual is determined at the time of catheterization for the contrast introduction. A small rectal tube is inserted prior to simulation, and contrast is administered after completion of the design of the anterior and posterior treatment fields. **The treatment fields are designed to be treated with the patient always voiding immediately prior to the radiation treatment session.**

### The Small Pelvic Field

The target volume includes the bladder, the total bladder tumor volume, the proximal urethra (in the male, the entire prostatic urethra), and the lymph nodes immediately adjacent to the bladder such as the distal hypogastric external iliac and the obturator groups. The planning target volume (PTV) for these small pelvic fields will extend in the cranial–caudal dimension from the lower pole of the obturator foramen to the midsacrum (the anterior aspect of the S2–S3 junction). The PTV width will extend half a centimeter lateral to the bony margin of the pelvis at its widest point. The anterior and posterior fields will extend 1.5 cm outside the planning target volume and will have shaped inferior lateral blocks, which will shield the medial border of the femoral heads (Figure 9-2).

For the lateral fields, the anterior portion of the PTV will be half a centimeter anterior to the most anterior portion of the bladder mucosa seen on the air contrast cystogram. Thus, the field border will be 1.5 cm anterior to that or 2 cm anterior to the mucosal border. Posteriorly, the PTV should extend 1.5 cm posterior to the most posterior portion of the bladder tumor as identifiable on the pelvic CT scan or from information from the bimanual examination. The lateral fields should be shaped inferiorly, with corner blocks to shield tissue outside the symphysis anteriorly and to block the entire anal canal posteriorly. Superiorly, these lateral fields should have anterior blocks to exclude any portion of the bowel that lies anterior to the external iliac lymph nodal group. Wedges (usually 15°) should be considered for lateral fields as compensators if the transverse contour has a significant slope. The AP-PA weighting relative to the paired lateral fields will depend on the technique chosen for the boost treatment to the bladder tumor volume only. This weighting should be chosen to limit the total dose to the femoral heads to no more than 45 Gy and to the posterior rectal wall

**SMALL PELVIC FIELDS**

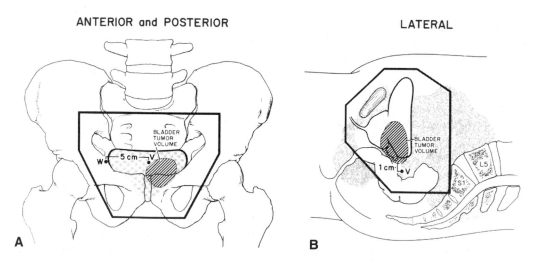

**ANTERIOR and POSTERIOR**          **LATERAL**

**FIGURE 9-2**   Radiation fields for the initial treatment of the bladder tumor and the pelvic lymph nodes: **(A)** anterior/posterior and **(B)** laterals.

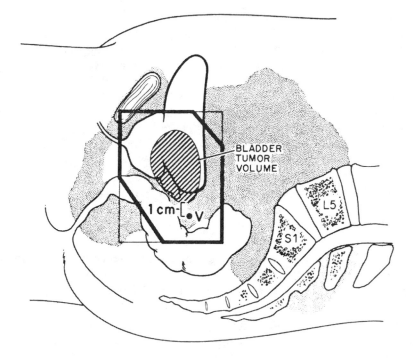

**FIGURE 9-3** Parallel opposed lateral fields for the boost to the tumor volume of a bladder tumor located posteriorly in the bladder (see text).

to no more than 55 Gy. We usually give 30% of the dose to the small pelvic field, using these four isocentric fields by using the paired lateral field and 70% with the anterior and posterior fields. This allows the boost to the bladder tumor volume to be given safely by paired lateral fields without overdosing the femoral heads. There are some unusual anatomic variations in which the PTV will require alterations. For example, in women with vaginal prolapse the bladder may protrude below the lower border of the obturator foramen, while in some male patients, a bladder diverticulum that extends outside the usual target volume may be present.

### The Boost Fields to the Bladder Tumor Volume

Either the entire bladder is treated, including the bladder and the extravesical tumor volume with a 2 cm margin, or the target volume is confined to one portion of the bladder. In the latter in-

stance the boost volume excludes uninvolved areas of the bladder. The information on the extent of the boost target volume is derived from information available from the cystoscopic map, the selective mucosal biopsies, the bimanual exam, and CT imaging data. These fields will be designed during the same simulation with an air contrast cystogram as described above. **The patient must also void prior to each of these treatments.** The boost volume for the clinical tumor volume (CTV) will be equal to the gross tumor volume (GTV). A 0.5 cm margin beyond the GTV will be used as the PTV. The field border should be 1.5 cm outside the PTV. Therefore the light field typically encompasses a 2.0 cm margin beyond the GTV. The majority of the bladder tumors involve the trigone and/or the posterior bladder wall. The optimal field arrangement for the GTV for these tumors utilizes opposed lateral fields with beam energies of 10 MV or higher. A typical lateral boost field is shown in Figure 9-3. To avoid the inward drift of isodose lines at increasing depths, a beam-flattening filter is employed which widens the 95% to 98% isodose lines, making them 6 to 8 mm closer to the light field edge at a depth of 15 to 20 cm.[68] If high energy photons are not available, boost techniques may be delivered by means of lateral arch rotations or via the four-field approach. The usual boost dose given to patients would be 14.4 to 18.0 Gy, given in 1.8 Gy daily fractions, usually concurrent with cisplatin chemotherapy. The dose to the bladder tumor volume in our pilot studies using concurrent chemotherapy with twice-a-day radiation has been 64 to 65 Gy.

## CURRENT RADIATION TREATMENT POLICIES

An algorithm for the evaluation and treatment of patients with nonmetastatic muscle-invading bladder cancer with a selective bladder-preserving approach used present departmental and RTOG protocols as shown in Figure 9-4.

## SPECIAL PRESENTATIONS

**I. Patients presenting with symptomatic pelvic recurrence following radical cystectomy.** Isolated urethral recurrence following radical cystectomy can be approached with hope of cure by radiation therapy. However, we and others have not been successful in curing patients with pelvic wall recurrences following radical cystectomy.[69] We treat patients with proximal urethral recurrences after radical cystectomy and urinary diversion by ileal conduit with external beam irradiation by a four-field external beam approach to doses from 65 to 70 Gy with concurrent cisplatin. With the use of lateral fields for at least half the dose, this can be given without significant risk of injury to the intestine, rectum, or anus. For patients with pelvic sidewall recurrences and pain, we usually begin with a course of concurrent cisplatin and external beam radiation therapy to a dose likely to be tolerated by

the intestine, the ileal loop, and its stoma. This is usually in the 50 to 56 Gy range. This is followed by multidrug systemic chemotherapy. A recent retrospective review from the M. D. Anderson Hospital[70] has documented that pelvic wall recurrence following modern radical cystectomy tends to occur only in patients with clinical stage T3b tumors. These investigators report a 30% to 40% incidence of pelvic recurrence in stage T3b patients treated by radical cystectomy, with or without multidrug chemotherapy before or after surgery. However, when stage T3b patients were treated with preoperative radiation therapy (which this institution used extensively prior to 1980), the pelvic recurrence rate was only 10%. Thus prevention of pelvic recurrence in stage T3b patients by preoperative irradiation seems the best approach presently.

**II. Patients presenting with muscle-invading bladder cancer and hydronephrosis.** For patients with tumor-associated hydronephrosis and clinically modest-sized, operable tumors, we recommend immediate radical cystectomy, with chemotherapy or radiation therapy considered after the pathologic extent of disease has been learned and renal function (if it was originally compromised) has returned. We would offer pelvic radiation therapy only in the face of a positive surgical margin. In this instance, we would treat to a dose of no more than 4000 cGy with concurrent cisplatin, using conventional daily fractionation. This adjuvant combined modality therapy would be combined with several cycles of multidrug adjuvant cisplatin-based systemic chemotherapy. This is because other aspects of the pathology report would likely indicate a very high risk of occult metastatic disease. For patients presenting with hydronephrosis and a locally very advanced tumor of questionable resectability, we would offer (following percutaneous upper tract decompression) a course of concurrent cisplatin and external beam radiation therapy prior to a planned radical cystectomy, provided the patient's medical condition was appropriate and no evidence of metastatic disease had developed.

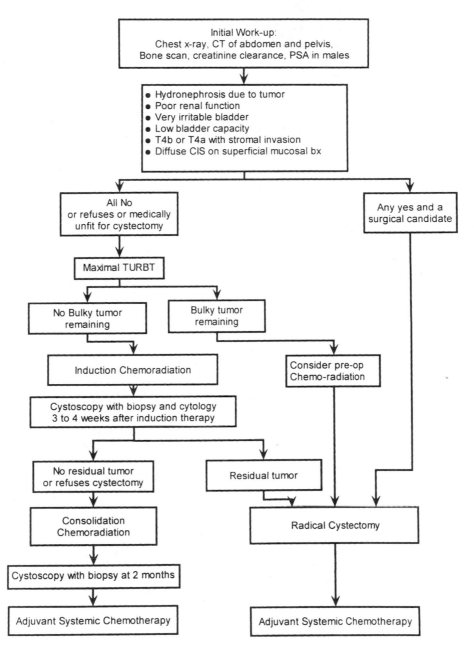

**FIGURE 9-4** Algorithm for evaluation and treatment of nonmetastatic muscle-invading bladder cancer with a selective bladder-preserving approach.

**III. Patients presenting with radiographic imaging evidence of metastatic nodal disease confirmed by percutaneous biopsy.** For these patients we would recommend three or more cycles of systemic multidrug cisplatin-based chemotherapy followed by reevaluation with imaging and cystoscopic evaluation. If the patient has had a good initial response to chemotherapy locally in the bladder and has a reasonable bladder capacity, we would then treat the primary tumor with concurrent cisplatin and external beam radiation therapy to full dose. Target volumes would include the lymph nodes of the pelvis and the entire bladder to 45 to 50 Gy, followed by a total bladder tumor dose of approximately 65 Gy.

**IV. Patients following partial cystectomy for attempted cure found to have a positive surgical margin.** Assuming an adequate bladder capacity and a pT2-T3 tumor, we would restage the patient and offer concurrent cisplatin-based chemotherapy and external beam radiation therapy. If the pelvic lymph nodes were known to be negative, we would treat the whole bladder and the entire abdominal incision to a dose of 45 Gy with a cone-down boost of additional 20 Gy, using conventional fractionation to the section of the bladder judged to be at highest risk of residual microscopic disease.

**V. Palliation of symptomatic metastatic transitional cell carcinoma, usually to bone, lymph nodes, lung, or brain.** If the patient were symptomatic or if the patient had previously undergone maximal systemic chemotherapy, we would initially treat with external beam radiation therapy with cisplatin to doses that are close but not beyond tolerance to the organs or partial organs requiring irradiation. This would usually mean a dose of 50 to 55 Gy or its biologic equivalent. This approach usually yields significant, often long-term, palliative benefit.

**VI. Palliation of bleeding from primary bladder tumor or a metastases to the bladder that cannot be controlled endoscopically.** These patients present to us with three-way catheters for irrigation. We generally offer 30 Gy in 2 weeks either as 10 daily fractions of 3 Gy each or as two BID 1.5 Gy fractions. This usually controls the bleeding and often allows (usually within 2–3 weeks) removal of the catheter. Depending on the expected longevity and the patient's condition, we may then add an additional dose of radiation with 2 Gy daily fractions to a total dose of approximately 56 Gy.

**VII. Patients presenting with a solitary muscle-invading tumor that cannot be completely resected transurethrally and for whom neither radical cystectomy nor systemic chemotherapy is acceptable.** In these instances we have treated with external beam radiation therapy combined with intraoperative boost using electrons, as was initially reported from the National Cancer Center in Tokyo.[71] We have had good success and tolerance in 6 bladder cancer patients using external beam doses with conventional fractionation to 40 to 45 Gy followed by a boost using intraoperative radiation therapy through a cone 6 to 7 cm in diameter, directed at the tumor through an open cystotomy. We have used single intraoperative doses in the range of 15 to 20 Gy with electron energies of 15 to 18 MeV. This regimen has been well tolerated and has given long-term local control. One patient did develop a nearly complete obturator nerve neuropathy.[72]

## INTERSTITIAL RADIOTHERAPY

For brachytherapy of bladder cancer, temporary implants with iridium-192 are now used with success. The use of remote afterloading techniques decreases the radiation hazard to personnel. Interstitial radiation therapy in patients with a solitary bladder cancer of less than 4 to 5 cm in diameter is used in Holland, Belgium, France, and Germany.[73–79] This approach is used exclusively for patients with solitary T1 or T2 or T3a tumors of a diameter 5 cm or less. In almost all instances the interstitial radiation therapy is preceded by external beam radiation therapy. In the majority of series, the patients also undergo a maximum tumor debulking either by a partial cystectomy, if possible, or by transurethral fulguration. For patients with T1 G3 tumors, bladder relapse rates of 15% to 28% are reported with actuarial 5-year survival rates of 70% to 80%. Wijnmaalen and colleagues in Rotterdam recently reported that patients with T3a bladder cancers that were solitary and less than 5 cm had a long-term bladder control rate of over 60%, as well as a 5-

year survival rate of 61%.[77] Thus interstitial radiation therapy in the hands of interested and experienced urologists and radiation oncologists has a high percentage of local control and excellent survival rates. However, in the absence of any prospective randomized trials comparing the results and the toxicities of brachytherapy to those of full-dose external beam radiation therapy with or without concurrent cisplatin chemotherapy, it is not possible to conclude whether the brachytherapy approaches offer any advantage over the more commonly used external beam radiation.

## REFERENCES

1. Vogelzang NJ, Scardino PT, Shipley WU, Coffey DS (eds): *Comprehensive Textbook of Genitourinary Oncology.* Baltimore, Williams & Wilkins, 1996.

2. Petrovich Z, Baert L, Brady LW (eds): *Carcinoma of the Urinary Bladder, Innovations in Management.* Berlin, Heidelberg, Springer-Verlag, 1988.

3. Scher HI, Shipley WU, Herr HW: Cancer of the bladder, in VT DeVita Jr, S Hellman, and SA Rosenberg (eds): *Cancer: Principles and Practice of Oncology,* 5th ed. Philadelphia, Lippincott, 1997, pp 1300–1318.

4. Young RH: The pathology of bladder cancer, in NJ Vogelzang, PT Scardino, WU Shipley, and DS Coffey (eds): *Textbook of Genitourinary Oncology,* Baltimore, Williams & Wilkins, 1996, pp 326–337.

5. American Joint Committee on Cancer: *AJCC Cancer Staging Manual,* 5th ed. Philadelphia, Lippincott-Raven, 1997.

6. Union Internationale Contre le Cancer: *TNM Classification of Malignant Tumors,* 3rd ed. Geneva, UICC, 1978, pp 114–115.

7. Jenkins BJ, Nauth-Misir RR, Martin J, et al: The fate of G3$_p$T1 bladder cancer. *Br J Urol* 1989;64:608–610.

8. Sauer R, Berkenhage S, Kuhn R, et al: Efficacy of radiochemotherapy with platin derivatives compared to radiotherapy alone in organ-sparing treatment of bladder cancer. *Int J Radiat Oncol Biol Phys* 1998;40:121–127.

9. Wolf H, Olsen PR, Hoigaard K: Urothelial dysplasia concomitant with bladder tumors: A determinant for future new occurrences in patients treated by full-course radiotherapy. *Lancet* 1985;8435:1005–1008.

10. Fung CY, Shipley WU, Young RH, Griffin PP, Convery KM, Kaufman DS, Althausen AF, Heney NM, Prout GR Jr: Prognostic factors in invasive bladder carcinoma in a prospective trial of neoadjuvant chemotherapy and radiotherapy. *J Clin Oncol* 1991;9:1533–1542.

11. Gospodarowicz MK, Quilty PM, Scalliet P, Tsujii H, Fossa SD, Horenblas S, Isaka S, Prout GR, Shipley WU, Wijnmaalen AJ, Crawford ED, Jones WG, Kawai T: The place of radiation therapy as definitive treatment of bladder cancer. *Int J Urol* 1995;2(suppl 2):41–48.

12. Zietman AL, Shipley WU, Kaufman DS. The combination of *cis*-platinum based chemotherapy and radiation in the treatment of muscle-invading transitional cell cancer of the bladder. *Int J Radiat Oncol Biol Phys* 1993;27:161–170.

13. Javie M, Raghavan D: Systemic therapy for invasive bladder cancer. *Cancer Control* 1996;3:501–506.

14. McDougal WS: Continent urinary diversion, in JE Osterling and JP Richie (eds): *Urologic Oncology.* Philadelphia, Saunders, 1997, pp 336–340.

15. Jung P, Jaske G: Bladder preservation in invasive locally confined bladder cancer. *Onkologie* 1996;19:296–301.

16. Geven KM, Spera JA, Solin LJ, Morgan T, Hanks GE: Local control after cystectomy alone in bladder carcinoma. *Cancer* 1992;69:2767–2770.

17. Martinez-Pineiro JA, Martin MG, Arocena NF, et al: Neoadjuvant cisplatin chemotherapy before radical cystectomy in invasive transitional cell carcinoma of the bladder: A prospective randomized phase III study. *J Urol* 1995;153:964–973.

18. Pressler LB, Petrylak DP, Olsson CA: Invasive transitional cell carcinoma of the bladder: Prognosis and management, in JE Osterling, and JP Richie (eds): *Urologic Oncology.* Philadelphia, Saunders, 1997, pp 275–291.

19. Miller LS: Bladder cancer: Superiority of preoperative radiation in cystectomy in clinical stage T3. *Cancer* 1977;39:973–980.

20. Horwich A, Pendlebury S, Dearnaley DP: Organ conservation in bladder cancer. *Eur J Cancer* 1995;31(suppl 5):208.

21. Sell A, Jakobsen A, Nerstrom B: Treatment of advanced bladder cancer category T2, T3, T4a. *Scand J Urol Nephrol* 1991;138(suppl):193–201.

22. Shipley WU, Zietman AL, Kaufman DS, Althausen AF, Heney NM: Invasive bladder cancer: Treatment strategies using transurethral surgery, chemotherapy and radiation therapy with selection for bladder conservation. *Int J Radiat Oncol Biol Phys* 1997;39(4):937–943.

23. Schultz TK, Herr HW, Zhang ZF, et al: Neoadjuvant chemotherapy for invasive bladder cancer: Prognostic factors for survival in patients treated with MVAC with 5-year follow-up. *J Clin Oncol* 1994;12:1394–1401.

24. Baert L, Elgamal AA, Van Poppel H: Complications of radical cystectomy, in Z Petrovich, L Baert, and LW Brady (eds): *Carcinoma of the Urinary Bladder, Innovations in Management.* Berlin, Heidelberg, Springer-Verlag, 1998, pp 169–186.

25. Wallace DMA, Raghavan D, Kelley K et al: Neoadjuvant (preemptive) cisplatin therapy in invasive transitional cell carcinoma of the bladder. *Br J Urol* 1991;67:608–612.

26. Hall RR: Neoadjuvant CMV chemotherapy and cystectomy or radiotherapy in muscle invasive bladder cancer: First analysis of MRC/EORTC intercontinental trial. *Proc ASCO* 1996;15:244 (abstr 612).

27. Ghersi D, Stewart LA, Parmar MKB, et al: Does neoadjuvant cisplatin-based chemotherapy improve the survival of patients with locally advanced bladder cancer? A meta-analysis of individual patient data from randomized clinical trials. *Br J Urol* 1995;71:75–206.

28. Malmstrom PU, Rintala E, Wahlquist R, et al: Five-year follow up of a prospective trial of radical cystectomy and neoadjuvant chemotherapy: Nordic Cystectomy Trial 1. *J Urol* 1996;155: 1903–1906.

29. Skinner DG, Daniels JR, Russell CA: The role of adjuvant chemotherapy following cystectomy for invasive bladder cancer: A prospective comparative trial. *J Urol* 1991;145:459–464.

30. Stockle M, Meyenberg W, Wellek S, et al: Advanced bladder cancer (stages pT3b, pT4a, pN1 and pN2): Improved survival after radical cys-

tectomy and 3 adjuvant cycles of chemotherapy. Results of a controlled prospective study. *J Urol* 1992;148:302–308.

31. Freiha F, Reese J, Torti F: A randomized trial of radical cystectomy versus radical cystectomy plus cisplatin, methotrexate and vinblastine chemotherapy for muscle invasive bladder cancer. *J Urol* 1996;155:495–500.

32. Esrig D, Elmajian DA, Groshen S, Freeman J, Stein JP, Chen SC, Nichols P, Skinner DG, Jones PA, Cote RJ: p53 nuclear accumulation and tumor progression in organ confined bladder cancer. *New Engl J Med* 1996;331: 1259–1264.

33. Herr HW: Conservative management of muscle-infiltrating bladder cancer: Prospective experience. *J Urol* 1987;138:1162–1163.

34. Henry K, Miller J, Mort M, Loening S, Fallon B: Comparison of transurethral resection to radical therapies for stage B bladder tumors. *J Urol* 1988;140:964–967.

35. DeNeve W, Lybeert ML, Goor C, et al: Radiotherapy for T2 and T3 carcinoma of the bladder: The influence of overall treatment time. *Radiat Oncol* 1995;36:183–188.

36. Gospodarowicz MK, Hawkins MC, Rawling GA et al: Radical radiotherapy for muscle invasive transitional cell carcinoma of the bladder: Failure analysis. *J Urol* 1989;142:148–154.

37. Jenkins BJ, Blandy JP, Caulfield MJ, et al: Reappraisal of the role of radical radiotherapy and salvage cystectomy in the treatment of invasive bladder cancer. *Br J Urol* 1988;62: 343–346.

38. Mameghan H, Fisher R, Mameghan J, et al: Analysis of failure following definitive radiotherapy for invasive transitional cell carcinoma of the bladder. *Int J Radiat Oncol Biol Phys* 1995;31:247–254.

39. Shearer RJ, Chilvers CE, Bloom HJG, et al: Adjuvant chemotherapy in T3 carcinoma of the bladder. *Br J Urol* 1988;62:558–564.

40. Hall RR: Transurethral resection for transitional cell carcinoma. *Probl Urol* 1992;6:460–470.

41. Quilty P, Duncan W: Primary radical radiotherapy for T3 transitional cell cancer of the bladder: An analysis of survival and control. *Int J Radiat Oncol Biol Phys* 1986;12:853–860.

42. Smaaland R, Akslen LA, Tonder B, et al: Radical radiation treatment of invasive and locally

advanced bladder carcinoma in elderly patients. *Br J Urol* 1991;67:61–69.

43. Farah R, Chodak GW, Vogelzang NI, et al: Curative radiotherapy following chemotherapy for invasive bladder carcinoma (a preliminary report). *Int J Radiat Oncol Biol Phys* 1991;20: 413–417.

44. Hall RR, Roberts JT: Neoadjuvant chemotherapy, a method to conserve the bladder? *ECCO* 1991:6 (abstr 144).

45. (a) Keating J, Zincke H, Morgan WR, et al: Extended experience with neoadjuvant M-VAC chemotherapy for invasive transitional cell carcinoma of the urinary bladder. *J Urol* 1989;141:244a. (b) Kurth KII, Splinter TA, Jacqmin D, et al: Transitional cell carcinoma of the bladder: A phase II study of chemotherapy in T3-4 NO MO of the EORTC GU group, in AR Alderson, RT Oliver, IW Hanham, and HJ Bloom (eds): *Urological Oncology Dilemmas and Developments.* New York, Wiley-Liss, 1991, pp 115–128.

46. Maffezzini M, Torelli T, Villa E, et al: Systemic preoperative chemotherapy with cisplatin, methotrexate, and vinblastine for locally advanced bladder cancer: Local tumor response and early follow-up results. *J Urol* 1991;145: 741–743.

47. Roberts JT, Fossa SP, Richards SB, et al: Results of Medical Research Council phase II study of low dose cisplatin and methotrexate in the primary treatment of locally advanced (T3 and T4) transitional cell carcinoma of the bladder. *Br J Urol* 1991;68:162–168.

48. Hall RR, Newling DWW, Ramsden PD, et al: Treatment of invasive bladder cancer by local resection and high dose methotrexate. *Br J Urol* 1984;56:668–672.

49. Parsons JT, Million RR: Bladder cancer, in CA Perez and LW Brady (eds): *Principles and Practice of Radiation Oncology.* Philadelphia, Lippincott, 1991, pp 1036–1058.

50. Prout GR, Shipley WU, Kaufman D, et al: Preliminary results in invasive bladder cancer with transurethral resection, neoadjuvant chemotherapy and combined pelvic irradiation plus cisplatin chemotherapy. *J Urol* 1990;144: 1128–1134.

51. Scher HI, Herr HW, Sternberg C, et al: Neoadjuvant chemotherapy for invasive bladder cancer. Experience with the MVAC regimen. *Br J Urol* 1989;64:250–256.

52. Cervak J, Cufer T, Marolt F, et al: Combined chemotherapy and radiotherapy in muscle-invasive bladder carcinoma. Complete remission results. *ECCO* 1991:6 (abstr 561).

53. Dunst J, Sauer R, Schrott KM, et al: An organsparing treatment of advanced bladder cancer: A 10-year experience. *Int J Radiat Oncol Biol Phys* 1994;30:261–266.

54. Tester W, Porter A, Asbell S, et al: Combined modality program with possible organ preservation for invasive bladder carcinoma: Results of RTOG protocol 85-12. *Int J Radiat Oncol Biol Phys* 1993;25:783–790.

55. Tester W, Porter A, Heaney J, et al: Neoadjuvant combined modality therapy with possible organ preservation for invasive bladder cancer. *J Clin Oncol* 1996;14:119–126.

56. Kachnic LA, Kaufman DS, Griffin PP, Heney NM, Alfthausen AF, Zietman AL, Shipley WU: Bladder preservation by combined modality therapy for invasive bladder cancer. *J Clin Oncol*, 1997;15:1022–1029.

57. Shipley WU, Winter KA, Lee R, et al: Initial results of RTOG 89-03: A phase III trial of neoadjuvant chemotherapy in patients with invasive bladder cancer treated with selective bladder preservation by combined radiation therapy and chemotherapy. *Proc Am Soc Ther Radiol Oncol* (abstr 41); *Int J Radiat Oncol Biol Phys* 1997 (suppl 2).

58. Srougi M, Simon SD: Primary methotrexate, vinblastine, doxorubicin and cisplatin chemotherapy in bladder preservation in locally invasive bladder cancer: A 5-year follow up. *J Urol* 1994;151:593–597.

59. Given RW, Parsons JT, McCarley D, et al: Bladder-sparing multimodality treatment of muscle-invasive bladder cancer: A 5-year follow up. *Urology* 1995;46:499–505.

60. Sternberg CN, Raghaven D, Ohi Y, et al: Neo-adjuvant and adjuvant chemotherapy in locally advanced disease: What are the effects on survival and prognosis? *Int J Urol* 1995;2(suppl):75–87.

61. Scher H, Herr H, Sternberg C, et al: M-VAC and bladder preservation, in T Splinter and HI Scher (eds): *Neoadjuvant Chemotherapy in Invasive Bladder Cancer.* New York, Wiley-Liss, 1990, pp 179–186.

62. Housset M, Maulard C, Chretien YC, et al: Combined radiation and chemotherapy for invasive transitional-cell carcinoma of the bladder: A prospective study. *J Clin Oncol* 1993;11: 2150–2157.

63. Houssett M, Dufour E, Maulard-Durtux C, et al: Concomitant 5-fluorouracil–cisplatin and bifractionated split course radiation therapy for invasive bladder cancer. *Proc ASCO* 1997;16: 319 (abstr 1139).

64. Cole D, Durrant K, Robert J, et al: A pilot study of accelerated fractionation in the radiotherapy of invasive carcinoma of the bladder. *Br J Radiol* 1992;65:792–798.

65. Zietman AL, Kaufman DS, Shipley WU, et al: A phase I/II trial of transurethral surgery plus cisplatin and radiation therapy followed either by selective bladder preservation or radical cystectomy for patients with muscle-invading bladder cancer but without hydronephrosis. *Proc Am Soc Ther Radiol Oncol* (abstr 42);*Int J Radiat Oncol Biol Phys* 1997(suppl 2).

66. Larsen LE, Engelholm SA: The value of 3-dimensional radiotherapy planning in advanced carcinoma of the urinary bladder based on computed tomography. *Acta Oncol* 1994;33:655–694.

67. Rothwell R, Ash D, Jones W: Radiation treatment planning for bladder cancer: A comparison of cystogram localization with computed tomography. *Clin Radiol* 1983;34:103–111.

68. Biggs PJ, Shipley WU: A beam with improving device for a 25 MV x-ray beam. *Int J Radiat Oncol Biol Phys* 1986;12:131.

69. Fromenti SC: Management of patients with pelvic recurrence following radical cystectomy, in Z Petrovich, L Baert, and LW Brady (eds): *Carcinoma of the Urinary Bladder: Innovations in Management.* Berlin, Heidelberg, Springer-Verlag, 1998, pp 249–258.

70. Cole CJ, Pollack A, Zagars GK, Dinney CP, Swanson DA, von Eschenbach AC: Local control of muscle-invasive bladder cancer. Preoperative radiotherapy and cystectomy versus cystectomy alone. *Int J Radiat Oncol Biol Phys* 1995;32:331–340.

71. Matsumoto L, Kakizoe T, Mikuriya S, et al: Clinical evaluation of intraoperative radiotherapy for carcinoma of the urinary bladder. *Cancer* 1981;47:509–513.

72. Shipley WU: Intraoperative radiation therapy in patients with bladder cancer: A review of techniques allowing improved tumor doses and providing high cure rates without loss of bladder function, in M Abe and JR Dobelbower (eds): *Intraoperative Radiation Therapy.* Boca Raton, FL, CRC Press, 1989, pp 227–236.

73. Batterman JJ, Tierie AH: Results of implantation for T1 and T2 bladder tumors. *Radiother Oncol* 1986;5:85-90.

74. Mazeron J, Crook J, Chopin D, et al: Conservative treatment of bladder carcinoma by partial cystectomy and interstitial iridium-192. *Int J Radiat Oncol Biol Phys* 1988;15:1323–1330.

75. DeNeve W, Lybeert MLM, Goo C et al: T1 and T2 carcinoma of the urinary bladder: Long-term results with external, preoperative or interstitial radiotherapy. *Int J Radiat Oncol Biol Phys* 1992;23:299–304.

76. Rozan R, Albuisson E, Donnarieix D, et al: Interstitial iridium-192 for bladder cancer (a multicentric survey: 205 patients). *Int J Radiat Oncol Biol Phys* 1992;24:469–477.

77. Wijnmaalen A, Helle PA, Koper PCM, et al: Muscle invading bladder cancer treated by transurethral resection followed by external beam radiation and interstitial iridium-192. *Int J Radiat Oncol Biol Phys* 1997;39:1043–1052.

# B.  CARCINOMA OF THE PROSTATE

## INTRODUCTION

Prostate carcinoma is a malignancy of vast national importance. After skin cancer, it is the commonest neoplasm of American men and the second commonest cause of neoplastic death.[1] Early detection programs began in earnest in the late 1980s and have revealed an extraordinary prevalence of the disease in the population. This is manifest as an apparent increase in incidence. Since 1989 the number of new cases per year has at least tripled, reaching

315,000 in 1996. While not all men need radical treatment, the majority elect for it. Radiation therapy is one of the mainstays of treatment, and as a result prostate cancer represents 25% to 30% of the average radiation oncologist's workload.

The apparent "epidemic" of prostate cancer that resulted from early detection campaigns has had several additional consequences. The large caseload has stimulated the analysis and publication of many large, single-institution experiences and allowed the completion of several multi-institution trials. Radiation oncologists and surgeons have learned who may and who may not be treated successfully by conventional treatment and have refined therapy in many ways to improve outcome. A further advantage has been the increased media attention cast on prostate cancer, with a consequent increase in research funding.

## EPIDEMIOLOGY

Prostate cancer is primarily a disease of the western world. In northern Europe and the United States, death rates per 100,000 population are 10 to 20 times those of Japan, China, and the Far East.[2] Though race is an important determinant in the development of prostate cancer, environment plays a role. Japanese men who migrate to the United States demonstrate increased death rates from this disease. African-American men have a higher incidence and higher mortality than white U.S. males. Whether this relates to biology or to a more limited access to health care and early detection remains debatable. The strongest risk factor, however, is age. Many autopsy series have shown that occult prostate cancer may be detectable in the prostates of young men. By 50 years of age approximately 30% of men have occult foci, and by 90 years the figure exceeds 70%. It is interesting that both white and Asian-American men have a similar frequency of histologically detectable cancer within the prostate in autopsy series. What differs is the incidence of progression to clinically significant disease.

Approximately 10% of cases may be familial in nature. First-degree relatives of men with prostate cancer have a threefold higher risk of developing prostate cancer themselves than the general population. Men with three first-degree relatives may have a prostate cancer risk 10 times that of the general population.

Other than age, race, and genetics, issues about which we can do little, there are no clearly demonstrable risk factors for prostate cancer. Unlike many other cancers, there is also no association with alcohol, smoking, or sexually transmitted diseases. Dietary associations have been noticed, however. There appears to be a slightly decreased instance in vegetarians and in those with higher serum levels of retinol, vitamin D, and vitamin E. There is no known association between benign prostatic hyperplasia and prostate carcinoma.

The development of microscopic foci of histologically recognizable prostate cancer appears to be a natural part of the aging process. Most do not progress to clinically overt disease, and much research is now being focused on the determinants of progression at a molecular level. Alterations in the *p53* tumor suppressor gene are seen in 95% of biopsies from metastatic lesions, but in only 38% of early stage, small-volume primary tumors. The loss of *p53* function may therefore be a step that determines a progression to a more aggressive form. Differences in growth factor expression, the expression of oncogenes, and other tumor suppressor genes have also been noted. It is likely that multiple events are involved, and the coming decade will unravel these precise molecular points of activation.

## ANATOMY

The understanding of prostatic anatomy has evolved greatly over the last 15 years, allowing considerable improvements in both surgical and radiotherapy technique. McNeil has described the zonal anatomy of the prostate[3] (Figure 9-5). Three major regions exist within the normal prostate: the peripheral zone, the cen-

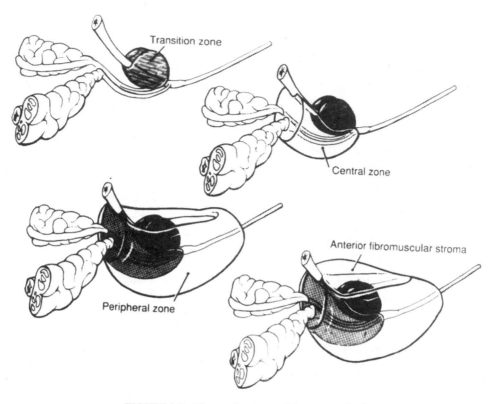

**FIGURE 9-5**   The zonal anatomy of the prostate gland.

tral zone, and the transition zone. The transition zone wraps around the midprostatic urethra and is the origin of benign prostatic hyperplasia (BPH). The position of the transition zone explains the bladder outflow symptoms frequently correlated with BPH. The central zone is situated behind the transition zone. It invests the intraprostatic course of the ejaculatory ducts and extends down to the verumontanum. The largest zone in the normal gland is the peripheral zone. This surrounds the transition and central zones but is incomplete anteriorly. Here the circle is completed by the anterior fibromuscular stroma. The peripheral zone is of importance because the majority of prostatic carcinomas arise within it. The central zone is rarely the site of origin of carcinoma. When involved, it is usually by direct extension from the peripheral zone. Transition zone tumors, owing to their internal location, may

grow very large without breaching the confines of the prostate. These zones are clearly seen by means of transrectal ultrasound.

Knowledge of the anatomy has facilitated the use of directed biopsies. It may also be used by brachytherapists to adjust the distribution of radiation dose across the prostate gland.

## HISTOLOGY

To make a diagnosis of prostate cancer, both architectural and cytologic criteria must be fulfilled. The characteristic adenomatous hyperplasia so common in advanced years may easily be distinguished from cancer, but prostatic intraepithelial neoplasia (PIN) is more difficult. There is good evidence that high grade PIN is a premalignant lesion. The cells are similar cytologically to carcinoma cells but differ in their architectural arrangement in that the normal acini are well preserved. PIN has been broken down into three grades. The third or highest grade is usually restricted to the peripheral zone. The presence of high grade PIN on biopsy greatly raises the likelihood that either a carcinoma will be found on a subsequent biopsy, or, if radical prostatectomy is performed, invasive carcinoma will be seen in an unbiopsied site.

All but 5% of prostatic cancers are adenocarcinomas. The remainder are divided among sarcomatoid, carcinoid, endometrioid, adenocystic, and small-cell histologies. Though rare, these categories are important to recognize because they may not respond to androgen deprivation in the manner typical of adenocarcinomas. Small-cell carcinomas may also be associated with paraneoplastic syndromes due to the secretion of hormones, such as an adrenocorticotropic hormone, or a parathyroid-type hormone. Though transitional cell carcinomas may be detected within the prostate, and may arise from the transitional epithelium within the proximal urethra, it is difficult to distinguish these from transitional cell carcinomas arising in the bladder and spreading in a superficial fashion down into the prostate and its ducts.

The most useful and widely accepted grading system for the common adenocarcinoma of the prostate was described by Gleason in 1977.[4] The primary or dominant pattern of differentiation is graded with a score from 1 to 5, based largely on architecture. The second most commonly encountered pattern also receives a grade, and the two are summed to give a value between 2 and 10. The clinical utility of the system has been demonstrated in many studies of patients managed either expectantly or with radical therapy. There is a stepwise increase in mortality as the Gleason sum increases. The system has been criticized for paying little heed to cytologic characteristics of the tumor and for not taking into account small volumes of high grade tumor. Despite these concerns, it has proved a reproducible system and is currently the standard by which studies are compared. Currently, two-thirds of patients with early stage tumors will have a Gleason sum between 5 and 7. This, however, is not a homogeneous group, since as many fail radical treatment as are cured. Thus pathologists are attempting to further refine this majority group in the interest of tailoring treatment. It is within this group that molecular markers and measurements of DNA content (ploidy) may be useful.

The local spread of carcinoma beyond the prostate most frequently occurs along nerves and lymphatics. These are the lines of least resistance. As a result, extracapsular extension is most commonly found around the neurovascular bundles and at the apex, the sites of entry and exit of neurovascular structures.[5] Direct extension into the seminal vesicles may occur along the ejaculatory ducts. Alternatively, a tumor may embolize or metastasize to the seminal vesicles through blood vessels. It is striking, however, that a primary carcinoma of the seminal vesicles is almost never seen. Why this difference should exist between two adjacent structures, which have similar glandular epithelia, is currently unknown.

## MARKERS OF PROSTATE CANCER

### Prostate-Specific Antigen

Prostate-specific antigen (PSA) is a glycoprotein produced by both benign and malignant prostate cells. It has serine protease activity and appears to be involved in lysis of the seminal coagulum. The normal range for men is between 0 and 4.0 ng/mL (using the Hybritech assay), and elevations may be caused by benign prostatic hyperplasia, and prostatitis, as well as cancer. Approximately one-quarter of men with a serum PSA between 4 and 10 ng/mL will prove to have prostate carcinoma on biopsy. This increases to 44% in men with PSA values exceeding 10 ng/mL. Unfortunately, the probability that the cancer is organ-confined decreases with increasing serum PSA.[6]

Many screening trials have been performed. It is clear that the routine use of annual digital rectal exam (DRE) and PSA screening increases the likelihood of detecting organ-confined cancer. In one study this was 64%, which is higher than the 48% seen in non-screened radical prostatectomy series. It is not however clear that all patients with PSA-detected and organ-confined cancers have clinically significant disease. Many European series have documented a long life expectancy despite palpable disease, certainly for men with lower grade tumors.[7] This may lead to much unnecessary treatment when one considers that many men screened for prostate cancer are 60 and above, with potentially significant comorbid conditions. This debate has not yet been resolved, which is why, despite the recommendations of the American Urologic Association and the American College of Radiology, screening as a national policy has not yet found favor. The Baltimore longitudinal study on aging showed that the lead time bias from PSA elevation to the development of palpable disease is 3 years for poorly differentiated and 7 years for well-differentiated tumors.[8] Whitmore et al. have shown that most patients with palpable T2 tumors will progress locally over the subsequent 15 years, but only a minority of those with lower grade tumors will develop metastases.[9]

Attempts have been made to refine the use of serum PSA in early detection. The PSA density is the ratio of PSA to gland volume and thus takes into account benign hyperplasia. It has not, however, been shown to have clear use either in lowering biopsy rates or in determining prognosis. Age-specific reference ranges for PSA also have been generated in an attempt to reduce unnecessary biopsies on older men with a low probability of cancer. PSA may exist in the blood stream either free or complexed with $\alpha$-antichymotrypsin. The percent of free PSA may help discriminate those with cancer from those with BPH. Cancer is more likely when the free PSA represents less than 20% of the total.

Serum PSA is also useful in the early detection of recurrence after radical treatment. Following a radical prostatectomy, the serum PSA should fall to, and remain at, undetectable levels as the source of all PSA, the cancer and the benign prostatic tissue, has been removed. The situation is less clear following radiation, since the normal prostate remains in place. Radiation undoubtedly depresses the production of PSA just as it affects the production of different proteins in other glandular organs such as the thyroid or pituitary. Men with rectal or bladder cancer receiving incidental irradiation to their prostate have a median serum PSA that is only 50% of aged matched counterparts from the general population (1.1 vs. 0.6 ng/mL).[10] A "normal" PSA level following radiation should probably be less than 1 ng/mL but not undetectable. Experience has shown that unless the PSA declines to these very low levels following radical radiation therapy, cure is unlikely (Figure 9-6). The PSA reaches a nadir approximately 18 months after radiation. The vast majority of those who at this stage have serum PSA values in excess of 1 ng/mL will have a rising PSA by 5 years. Those whose PSA is undetectable at this stage have a less than 10% chance of a rising PSA in 5 years. Since the beginning of the PSA era in the late 1980s, different institutions have reported their results in different ways. Some have declared patients with PSA values below 4 ng/mL to be biochemically disease free; others have used cutoffs of 1.5, 1, or even less than 0.5 ng/mL. In 1996 a consensus committee of the American Society for Therapeutic Radiology and Oncology (ASTRO) met to weigh the evidence. Agreement was reached that a rising serum PSA constitutes evidence for persistent disease and, if sufficient time elapses, will ultimately result in clinical and symptomatic failure.[12] Because there are some inaccuracies in the PSA test and because PSA values may fluctuate, especially in the low range, the definition mandates three *successive* rises above 0.5 ng/mL regardless of the absolute PSA level. Hanks et al. have shown that the rates of PSA rise following radiation therapy predicts subsequent clinical failure: those with a PSA doubling time in excess of 1 year are unlikely to develop symptoms in the next 5 years; those with PSA

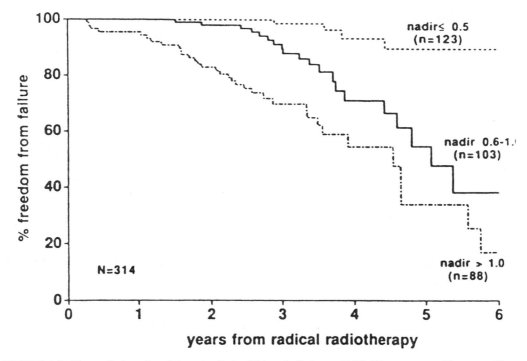

**FIGURE 9-6**  The predictive value of the postradiation PSA nadir. Patients with T1-T2 tumors treated by external beam radiation at the MGH who reached low nadirs (≤ 0.5 ng/mL) were the least likely to have rising PSA profiles 5 years after treatment.

doubling times less than 4 months are extremely likely to develop symptoms or metastatic disease within the next 2 years.[13]

## Acid Phosphatase

Acid phosphatase was the principal serum marker for prostate cancer prior to the discovery of PSA. Both the total acid phosphatase and the prostate-specific fraction are increased in the blood in 70% of patients with disseminated prostate cancer. Though this was previously helpful in identifying patients unsuitable for radical treatment, it is not a very specific test and its utility has been far superseded by PSA.

## PRESENTATION

Up until 10 years ago the commonest presentation for prostate cancer included symptoms of bladder outflow obstruction, such as hesitancy,

frequency, nocturia, and a dwindling urinary stream. These were in part related to prostate cancer and in part to benign prostatic hyperplasia. The latter commonly provoked a transurethral resection of the prostate, the chips revealing carcinoma. At the Massachusetts General Hospital (MGH), two-thirds of patients referred to the Radiation Oncology Department in the late 1980s had palpable disease. The incidence of prostate cancer has appeared to increase almost exponentially over the last decade, primarily as a result of the routine use of serum prostate-specific antigen by internists and urologists. Though no formal screening program is in place, the majority of men between 50 and 70 years who regularly attend a doctor will have a serum PSA performed. When an elevated level is reported, referral is usually made for a transrectal ultrasound examination and biopsy. The majority of patients are, therefore, now detected with impalpable disease, and the presence of obstructive voiding symptoms is far less common.

Symptoms such as hematuria and perineal pain are very worrisome and may signify invasion of the bladder neck or the external sphincter.

Despite a vigorous campaign to promote early detection, a significant proportion of men still present late with the principal symptoms of metastatic disease, bone pain, and tiredness.

## STAGING

The most widely accepted staging system is that of the American Joint Committee on Cancer (Table 9-8). This classification included for the first time in 1992 a new category, the T1c tumor, which now represents the commonest form of prostate cancer seen. In this stage the tumor is impalpable, but is identified on a needle biopsy because of an elevated serum level

**TABLE 9-8   TNM Staging for Prostate Cancer**

| | |
|---|---|
| TX | Primary tumor cannot be assessed |
| T0 | No evidence of primary tumor |
| T1 | Clinically inapparent tumor not palpable nor visible by imaging |
| | T1a   Tumor incidental histologic finding in 5% or less of tissue resected |
| | T1b   Tumor incidental histologic finding in more than 5% of tissue resected |
| | T1c   Tumor identified by needle biopsy (e.g., because of elevated PSA) |
| T2 | Tumor confined within prostate[a] |
| | T2a   Tumor involves one lobe |
| | T2b   Tumor involves both lobes |
| T3 | Tumor extends through the prostate capsule[b] |
| | T3a   Extracapsular extension (unilateral or bilateral) |
| | T3b   Tumor invades seminal vesicle (s) |
| T4 | Tumor is fixed or invades adjacent structures other than seminal vesicles: bladder neck, external sphincter, rectum, levator muscles, and/or pelvic wall |

[a]Tumor found in one or both lobes by needle biopsy, but not palpable or reliably visible by imaging, is classified as T1c.

[b]Invasion into the prostate apex or into (but not beyond) the prostatic capsule is not classified as T3, but as T2.

*Source:* American Joint Committee on Cancer.

of prostate-specific antigen (PSA). Tumors that are palpable are classified in the T2 to T4 categories according to their extent on digital rectal exam. The classification system originally demanded that inpalpable tumors identifiable by radiologic imaging take the T2 stage. This rule has not been consistently applied. Though transrectal ultrasound and endorectal coil MRI may be useful in determining subpalpable extracapsular extension, only a minority of institutions incorporate such studies into staging.

The need for staging investigation beyond an ultrasound and a digital rectal exam is determined by the palpable size of the tumor and the serum PSA. When the serum PSA is less than 10 ng/mL, it is unlikely that imaging of the pelvic lymph nodes by CT or MRI, or surgical sampling will yield useful information. By the same token, bone scan is equally unlikely to detect overt metastases. It has been estimated that only 1 of 180 bone scans performed on patients with a serum PSA below 10 ng/mL will be positive. At the opposite extreme, PSA values in excess of 100 almost invariably indicate metastatic disease. Here it is worth a thorough radiographic staging to exclude patients from fruitless and potentially morbid radical treatment to the prostate. At the MGH the majority of patients with PSA values in excess of 10, or those with high Gleason sum tumors, will undergo a CT scan of the pelvis and a bone scan.

Despite our best efforts to stage prostate cancer with accuracy, many prostatectomy series have shown that 50% or more of clinical T1-T2 patients actually have a pathologic T3 or T4 disease. The likelihood of extraprostatic extension is well predicted by a judicious use of serum PSA, palpation stage, and Gleason sum. Nomograms developed by Partin et al. have proven very useful in this regard.[6]

## MANAGEMENT OF LOCALIZED CARCINOMA

One of the more controversial areas of modern-day clinical medicine is the management of localized carcinoma. The first major issue is to define who actually needs treatment, recognizing the excellent prognosis of untreated small volume, lower grade cancer. The second issue is to determine the most appropriate of several competing therapies in any individual case.

When one is evaluating patients, careful attention must be given to the grade of the tumor and its apparent extent, to the serum PSA level and its rate of rise, and to the age of the patient and his comorbid health conditions. The likelihood that a man with a T1-T2 tumor graded as Gleason 6 or less will develop metastatic disease within the next decade is only 20%. Patients with a life expectancy of 10 years or less may therefore be safely guided away from radical treatment toward close observation. This in itself is an active not a passive strategem, and the patient must be carefully counseled about the importance of regular follow-up to ensure that rapid and unexpected progression is not occurring.

Assuming that treatment is deemed appropriate, prostate cancer may be broken up into four broad groups: early stage disease, locally advanced disease, node-positive disease, and metastatic disease.

### Early Stage Disease (T1-T2b NX M0)

Patients with early stage disease have many radical options available: radiation by external beam or implant, or the radical prostatectomy.

The radical prostatectomy has greatly increased in popularity among urologists over the past 10 years. This is the result of anatomical studies by Walsh and others, who clearly defined the relationship between the neurovascular bundles and the prostate gland.[14] This allowed for the development of the so-called anatomic radical prostatectomy, in which sparing of the neurovascular bundles is possible with potential preservation of erectile potency and urinary continence. Approximately 100,000 radical prostatectomies were performed in the United States in 1996. The radical prostatectomy is often an effective treatment for organ-confined disease. It extirpates not only the tumor but the prostatic ep-

ithelium within which future tumors may develop. Prostatic carcinoma may be multifocal not just in place, but also in time. The prostatectomy also provides prognostic information that may be useful to younger men and may guide adjuvant therapy. Extracapsular extension and positive surgical margins may necessitate postoperative radiation therapy. Seminal vesicle or lymph node invasion likely indicates micrometastatic disease, and consideration can be given to systemic androgen deprivation. Despite its enthusiastic acceptance by surgeons, national studies show the anatomic radical prostatectomy is associated with levels of impotence that may exceed 80% and with a significant degree of stress urinary incontinence.[15] Between 20 and 35% of patients require pads for protection, one or more years beyond their surgery. Most alarming, unless careful selection has taken place, 50% or more of the operated patients prove to have extracapsular disease and thus probably have not been cured by their radical surgery. Though many surgeons feel that the prostatectomy is more likely to be a curative procedure than radical radiation, long-term studies have not borne this out.[16]

Because many patients treated were not destined to die of prostate cancer and because so many prostate cancers remain incurable by surgery, as well as by radiation, any differences between the therapies in terms of mortality will be very difficult to resolve. Long-term studies following patients into the second or even the third decade, such as those published by groups at Stanford University and UCLA, clearly show a continued force of failure, whatever the treatment technique used.[17] It has been argued that in the new era of early detection, late failure will be less common after surgery than after radical radiation therapy. This, however, has yet to be demonstrated.

Radiation oncologists now have a number of radiation techniques from which to choose to treat their early stage patients. While conventional external beam radiation to doses of approximately 68 Gy is the standard, several academic centers have started employing three-dimensional conformal planning techniques, both to reduce the morbidity of treatment and to escalate the radiation dose. Also, increasing in popularity is prostate brachytherapy. Approximately 20,000 regimens of brachytherapy will be prescribed in 1998.

## Locally Advanced Disease (T2b-T4 NX M0)

Patients with locally advanced disease fare rather more poorly than the early stage patients. Strict use of PSA criteria has made it clear that men with bulky primary tumors, men with PSA levels above 15 ng/mL, and men with Gleason scores of 8 and above are infrequently cured by monotherapy, be that radical prostatectomy or conventional external beam radiation (Figure 9-7). Following radiation, both local failure and metastases are common in this group. Approximately 30% to 50% will develop palpable local recurrence over the sub-

sequent 10 years. The majority of the remainder will be found to have histologically persistent disease if rebiopsied. This may well be the source of subsequent metastases. Fuks et al. have demonstrated a second wave of metastases in patients who failed locally following radiation therapy performed in the 1970s.[18] Efforts are thus being made to increase the radiation dose delivered to the primary site by the use of conformal techniques. Such technology is not available to all radiation oncologists, and an alternative strategy is to use the neoadjuvant androgen deprivation to attempt to shrink the tumors prior to radiation. Animal studies using the Shionogi androgen-dependent tumor system have clearly shown that shrinking the tumor volume reduces the radiation dose required for local tumor eradication (Figure 9-8). This measure seems to operate in a synergistic fashion, and mechanisms involving common apoptosis-inducing pathways have been the subject of speculation. Androgen suppression

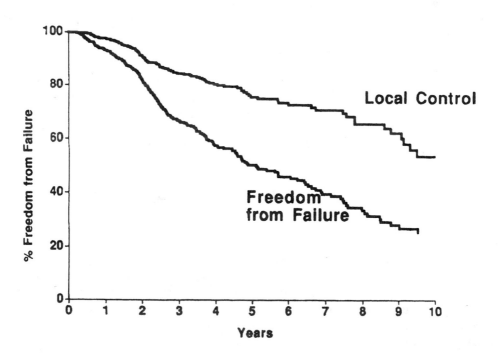

**FIGURE 9-7**   Long-term biochemical and local control rates for men with T3 tumors treated at the MGH with conventional radiation to a median dose of 68 Gy.

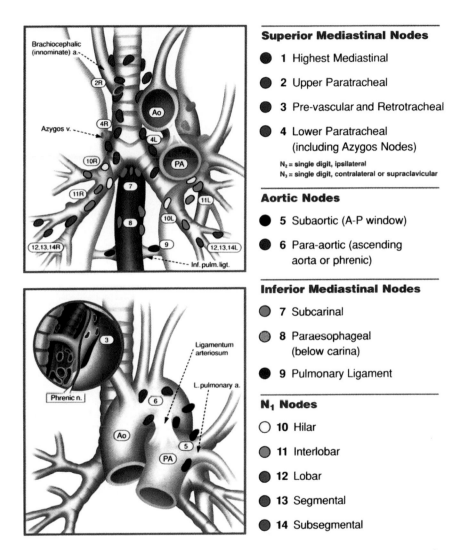

**FIGURE 7-1** Regional nodal stations for lung cancer staging. (From Mountain and Dressler.[8])

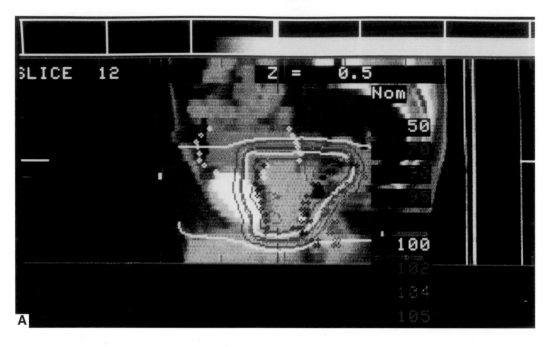

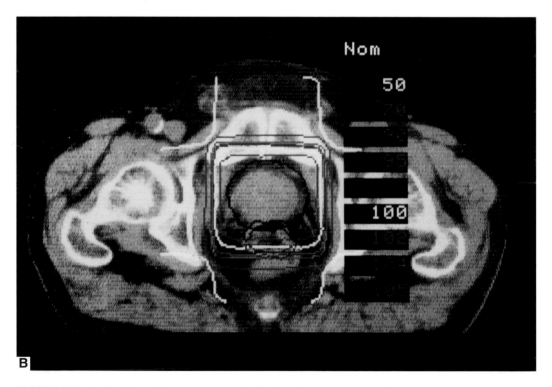

**FIGURE 9-9** **(A)** Sagittal and **(B)** transverse dose distributions for conformal external beam therapy covering the prostate and seminal vesicles. The seminal vesicles are excluded from the boost volume to minimize the rectal volume carried to the full radiation dose.

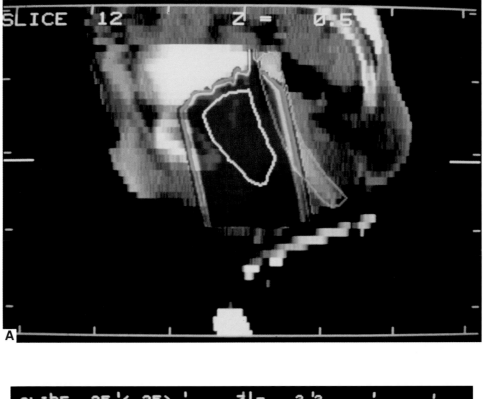

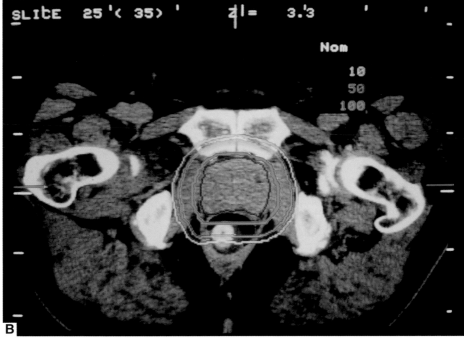

**FIGURE 9-15** **(A)** Sagittal and **(B)** transverse dose distributions for a conformal perineal boost delivered by means of a 160MV proton beam.

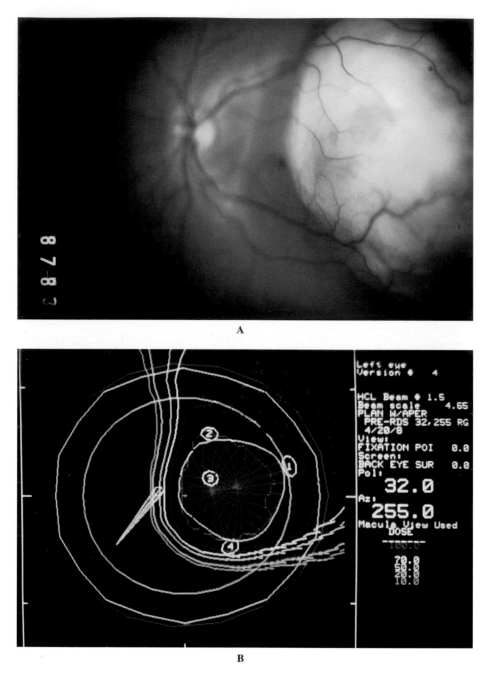

**FIGURE 15-2** **(A)** Narrow-angle fundus photograph showing a large choroidal melanoma. The macula is seen as the dark spot immediately to the left of the midportion of the tumor. The optic disc and retinal vessels are also shown. **(B)** Tumor shown in **(A)**, modeled on the eye treatment planning program.[79] Optic disc shown as cone-shaped structure to the right, with the macula being at the end of the blue line just inside the tumor edge. Clips placed surgically to mark the tumor are shown. Clip 3 was not able to be placed at the posterior tumor edge due to the extreme posterior location of the tumor. Iso-dose curves are shown on the unfolded retina of the patient. Dose is prescribed to the 90% isodose line, which is placed 1.5 mm from the edge of the modeled tumor.[79] Macula (small purple cross) and tumor receive full dose, while the 50% isodose line passes through the center of the disk.

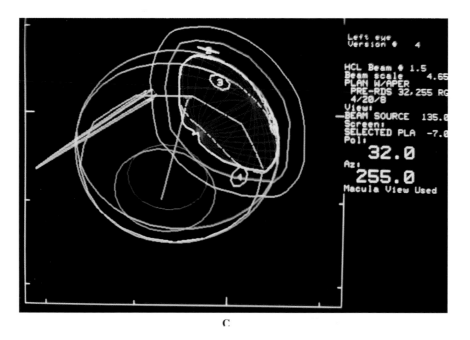

C.

(C) "Beam's eye view" of the proton beam on the anterior eye with patient in treatment position. Eye is voluntarily fixated on an inferior and slightly medial point, as indicated by the projection of the optic axis (blue line) connecting the center of the lens with the macula. The 50% and 90% isodose lines are shown in yellow and red, respectively, as outlined by the aperture. A field light projected through the treatment aperture onto the eye would outline the 50% yellow isodose line and allow verification of patient setup after radiographic alignment had been achieved.

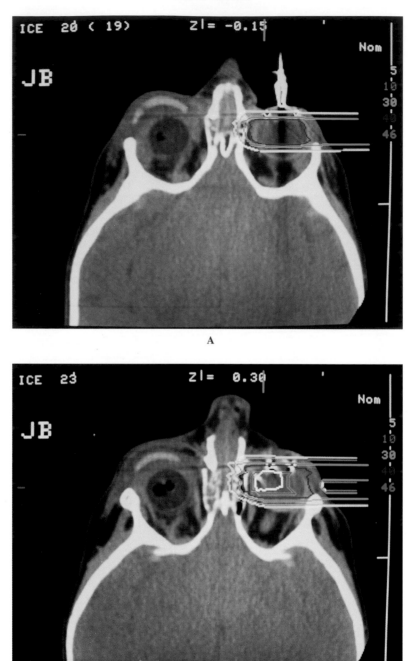

**FIGURE 15-3** **(A)** Dose distribution to a retinoblastoma patient with a single direct lateral proton portal. Scan section is 1.5 mm superior to top of lesion, with dose of 40 CGE delivered at this level. Note stem of suction cup used to fix eye in place for treatment, with artifact in central globe from metallic stem. Radiopaque circles anteriorly are cross sections of a circular wire embedded in the plastic contact lens, which adheres to the cornea by suction during the treatment. The wires in the contact lens define the anterior margin of the eye and are used for radiographic patient setup. Patient has prosthesis with anterior shell in right eye. Prescribed dose (46 CGE, green isodose line) is given to all the tumor defined on this slide. **(B)** Scan 3

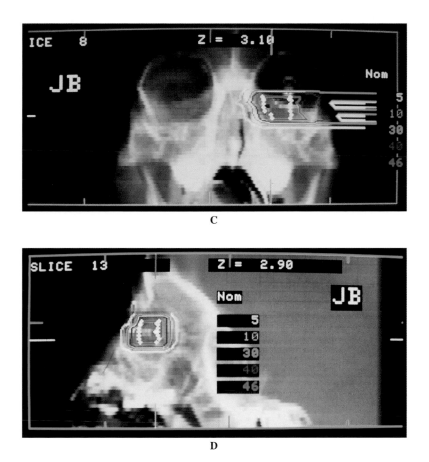

C

D

mm inferior to scan in (A), showing small punctate calcification in tumor medially, and outline of tumor in white. The pre-scribed dose of 46 CGE conforms to virtually all of the defined tumor on this slice. Entrance dose is 40 CGE or less. **(C)** Coronal reconstruction of the planning CT scan. Conformality of prescribed dose (46 CGE) to target is again noted. A small portion of the inferior left lateral orbit is included in the 40 CGE isodose line. **(D)** Sagittal reconstruction of the planning CT scan. Conformality of prescribed dose (46 CGE) to target is again noted, with the dose on this scan appearing to be concentrated solely in the globe. A small portion of the inferior left lateral orbit is included in the 40 CGE isodose line.

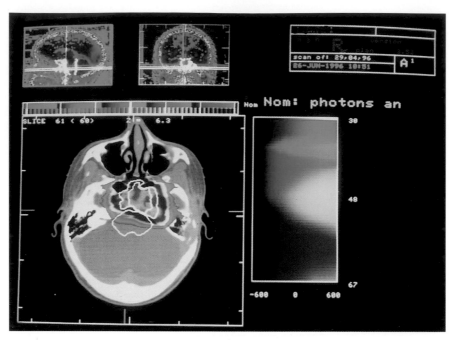

**A**

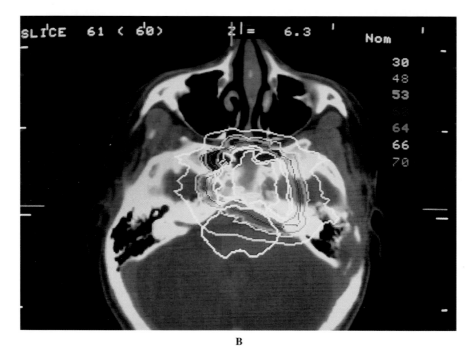

**B**

**FIGURE 15-4** **(A)** Contours shown in white outline the smaller and the larger clinical target volumes (CTVs) defined on this CT image of the planning scan of a 13-year-old girl with a low grade chondrosarcoma of the clivus. The smaller volume is gross residual tumor seen on imaging studies, and the larger contour represents target enlargement to allow for uncertainty in target definition on planning scan, and for microscopic extension. Area shown in magenta received the prescribed dose of 66.6 CGE. Note sparing of the right internal auditory canal, the right cochlea, and the right acoustic nerve, each of which receives less than 30 CGE. **(B)** Same scan as in **(A)**, showing isodose lines instead of color-wash display.

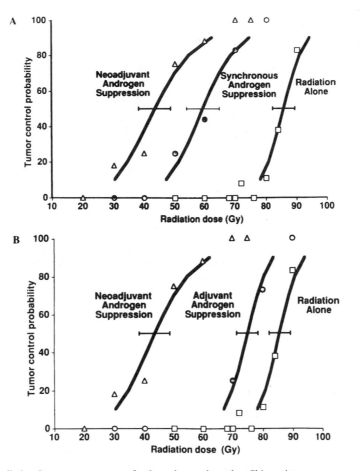

**FIGURE 9-8** Radiation dose–response curves for the androgen-dependent Shionogi tumor grown as allografts in the hind limbs of nude mice. The curve is shifted to the left by androgen deprivation. This effect is most profound when radiation is given at the time of maximal tumor regression after androgen deprivation.

reliably reduces the volume of over 90% of prostate carcinomas. Tumor volume reduction prior to radiation is more attractive than dose escalation to many radiation oncologists because it raises the probability of improved local control without the increased normal tissue damage.

For T2b-T4 disease it has become clear that conventional monotherapy alone, be it radiation or surgery, is insufficient, and patients should be guided toward radical radiation with dose escalation, conventional radiation with neoadjuvant androgen deprivation, or radical prostatectomy with postoperative radiation.

### Node-Positive Disease

There has been no convincing evidence that radical therapy extends the life of patients who are found either radiologically or pathologically to have involved lymph nodes. At least 90% of these patients will ultimately prove to have occult micrometastatic disease. Long-term androgen deprivation either by orchiectomy, monotherapy with an LHRH agonist, or combination total androgen blockade (LHRH agonist plus testosterone receptor blocker) are usually instituted. Sands et al. demonstrated that the first site of androgen independent progression is within the pelvis in 50% of cases.[20] An argument can therefore be made to offer pelvic radiation as a means of impeding the progression, and therefore, extending the symptom-free life of men who cannot be cured. Recent data from the MGH support this contention, with a progression-free advantage at 5 years. The likelihood of patients needing a subsequent intervention for locally uncontrolled tumor is significantly reduced. The RTOG has begun a randomized trial (RTOG-96-08) of adding pelvic irradiation (50 Gy) plus prostate boost (to 65–70 Gy) or not to total androgen for patients with histology-proven metastasis into the pelvic lymph nodes. The data from the Mayo Clinic, in which men with node-positive disease received a radical prostatectomy for local control, together with their orchiectomy, support this concept.[21]

## Metastatic Disease

Androgen deprivation is the mainstay of treatment for metastatic disease. Symptomatic improvement is seen in 90% of the patients, and PSA values usually decline to normal levels, a situation that is maintained for 18 to 24 months on the average. Unfortunately, androgen-independent progression is inevitable, and symptomatic disease will result. Bone pain and fatigue resulting from the anemia of marrow infiltration are common. External beam radiation will reduce pain in two-thirds of irradiated skeletal metastases for the remainder of the patient's life. When metastases are too numerous or pain is very diffuse and poorly controlled by opiates, systemic therapy using radionuclides, such as $^{89}$Sr may be considered. In our experience approximately 25% of men will have complete pain relief with strontium, but the duration is relatively short (7–8 weeks median) and troublesome myelosuppression, in particular thrombocytopenia, may result. Systemic radionucleotides are therefore not suitable for patients who have diffuse marrow involvement and declining blood counts. It is of note that strontium is not suitable for patients who are incontinent: it is concentrated in the urine and may represent a radiation hazard.

External beam radiation may also be used to palliate the consequences of bulky lymphadenopathy. Patients with lower limb edema, as a result of pelvic or para-aortic lymph node enlargement, may respond to doses of 40 to 44 Gy in 2 Gy fractions.

## RADIOTHERAPEUTIC TECHNIQUE

### Radical External Beam Radiation

The modern era of external beam radiation for cancer of the prostate began with the pioneering work of Dr. Bagshaw, at the Stanford University School of Medicine. The techniques developed by his group were widely adopted and were used in most large series currently reporting long-term results. Patients at the MGH are simulated in the supine position and important anatomic structures are identified; 40 mL of air and contrast may be introduced into the bladder by means of a Foley catheter. Barium may be placed within the rectum. The apex may be identified by the use of a urethrogram. It may also be identified by the placement under digital guidance of a fiducial marker, such as an inert gold seed, at the apex, which lies 0.5 to 1.5 cm above the beak of urethrogram. The seed may be introduced with local anesthesia by inserting a needle through the perineum.

The patient may also be CT-scanned in the treatment position to further define the target and the important normal tissue structures. The prostate, the seminal vesicles, and, if indicated, the lower pelvic lymph nodes are treated to 50.4 Gy in 1.8 Gy fractions with four fields The prostate tumor target volume itself is then boosted to a total tumor dose of 68.4 to 72 Gy by means of a combination of opposed lateral fields and 120° lateral arcs (Figure 9-9). Because of this reliance on a lateral field for the boost, the four-field first phase is weighted 20:8 toward the AP-PA. The depth–dose distribution obtained by means of the lateral boost fields may be improved by the use of a small, flattening filter. This device for improving beam width prevents the "waisting" of the beams in the center of the body.[22] At the MGH, beams of 18 to 23

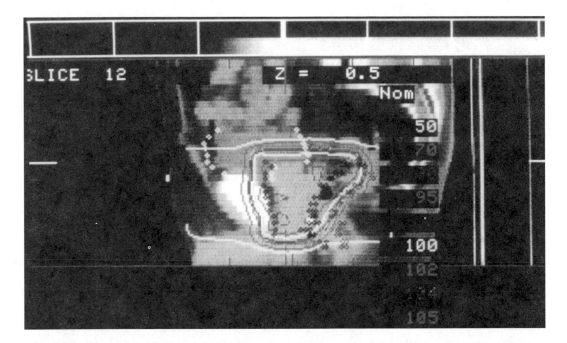

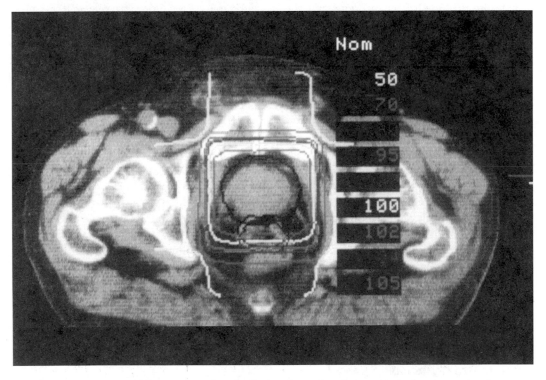

**FIGURE 9-9**   **(a)** Sagittal and **(b)** transverse dose distributions for conformal external beam therapy covering the prostate and seminal vesicles. The seminal vesicles are excluded from the boost volume to minimize the rectal volume carried to the full radiation dose. Figures also appear in Color Figure section.

MV are used for all fields, except the anterior, where the beam is only 6 MV, to reduce the rectal dose.

The dimensions of the fields have long been a source of controversy. Several retrospective studies have suggested that pelvic nodal radiation improves the disease-free survival, but two randomized trials have indicated little or no benefit.[23] Our practice is to utilize low pelvic nodal radiation on the basis of risk of lymph node involvement and on the projected patient tolerance. The previously described Johns Hopkins University nomogram, based on the retrospective analysis of more than 1000 radical prostatectomy specimens, is useful in this regard. We limit the pelvic node radiation to young men with a risk of nodal involvement that exceeds 15% to 20%. We also omit the seminal vesicles from the final boost volume when they are clinically and radiologically uninvolved. Many academic centers now employ sophisticated radiation planning computers for three-dimensional visualization of the prostate and the adjacent normal structures. Radiation fields may be tailored accordingly and dose escalation attempted. There is no current consensus on the direct total dose required to treat the prostate target volume by external beam radiation. Early data from a dose escalation study by Hanks et al. suggest that doses in excess of 72 Gy improve outcome for T1, T2 patients with PSA values exceeding 10 ng/mL, but not for those with values below 10 ng/mL. Patients with the higher PSA values ($>$ 10 ng/mL) may be presumed to have a higher burden of local disease. Other data from the Memorial Sloan-Kettering Cancer Center, using rebiopsy, have suggested that a significant improvement in tumor clearance is not noted until doses of 79 Gy or more are delivered.[25] Many radiation oncologists feel uncomfortable with such high doses of radiation outside a clinical trial. At least two randomized studies of dose escalation are in progress.

## Prostate Brachytherapy

Brachytherapy is an increasingly popular alternative to external beam radiation and radical prostatectomy. Dr. Whitmore, in the 1970s, at the Memorial Sloan-Kettering Cancer Center, first used a retropubic approach to implant $^{125}$I. This required an open procedure with a lymph node dissection and surgical mobilization of the prostate. A free-hand technique was used to implant iodine seeds in an anterior–posterior direction. This technique is not ideal for accurate spacing, however. Further, the distribution of iodine seeds and total activity to be implanted was determined in the operating room on the basis of caliper measurements. This may well have led to a dose delivery substantially lower than would have been achieved had the measurements been made with transrectal ultrasound, a problem that was magnified with larger prostates and prostate tumors. A recent reanalysis with 25-year follow-up identified inadequate radiation dosing as one of the causes of failure in a multivariate analysis.[26] Local control rates consequently were poor and, as external beam techniques improved, the implant fell from favor in the 1980s. By the late 1980s transrectal ultrasonography (TRUS), now in common usage for diagnosis and biopsy, was first used to guide source placement via a transperineal approach. Rigid templates employed for brachytherapy elsewhere in the body began to be used for the prostate, as well as careful preplanning.

At the MGH suitable patients undergo planning TRUS in the lithotomy position in the Radiation Oncology Department. Serial transverse images are recorded at 5 mm intervals from the base of the prostate gland to the apex. Every point within the prostate has a vector location that corresponds in two transverse dimensions to the holes on the template grid, and the third longitudinal dimension matches the 5 mm step position within the prostate gland. The ultrasound images are downloaded onto a planning computer, and an optimal seed distribution to deliver the prescribed radiation dose is determined. The appropriate activity and number of seeds may then be ordered (Figures 9-10 and 9-11). The procedure itself is performed under general anesthesia in the operating room. It is crucial to reposition the patient in the same position used for the planning

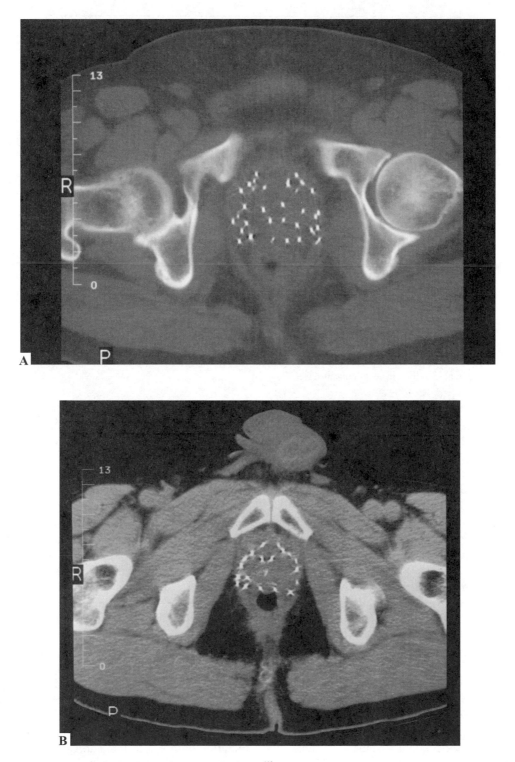

**FIGURE 9-10**   CT scans showing conformal distribution of $^{103}$Pd seeds across the prostate gland: **(A)** homogeneous and **(B)** peripheral arrangements.

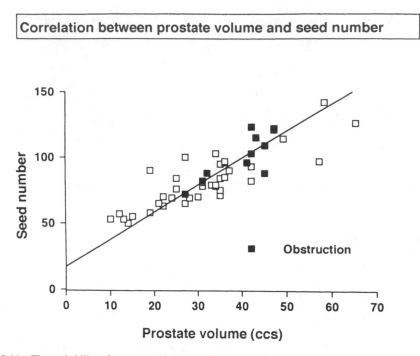

**FIGURE 9-11**   The probability of temporary bladder outflow obstruction (catheter for greater than 2 days) as a function of prostate volume and the number of implanted seeds.

ultrasound. The transrectal probe must be maneuvered into position such that the images obtained correspond with those from the prior planning ultrasound. Then a specially designed immobilization device locks the probe in place. The seeds, which have been preloaded in 18-gauge needles, are then passed through appropriate holes in the template, through the perineum, and into the prostate gland. Seeds may be placed beyond the prostate gland if there is some risk of extracapsular extension. If oncologically appropriate, the periurethral region may be kept cooler to reduce the risk of late morbidity. The seeds in the posterior row are placed 1 to 2 mm within the posterior capsule of the prostate to ensure that the posterior peripheral zone receives full dose, but carefully limiting the dose to the anterior rectal wall.

The most appropriate radiation dose to deliver using the implant, and the ideal choice of radioactive isotope, have not yet been determined. The most popular isotope thus far, [125]I, produces at 28 keV emission but has a low initial dose rate of about 8 cGy/h with a half-life of 60 days. Traditionally, 160 cGy has been prescribed as a matched peripheral dose when this source is used. Because of concerns that the dose rate may be too low, some groups have started using palladium as an alternative; it has a similarly low emission energy but a shorter half-life of 17 days, and a faster dose rate at greater than 20 cGy/h. A matched peripheral dose of 115 cGy is usually prescribed. To date there has been no "head-to-head" comparison between palladium and iodine, and no clear data exist proving the superiority of one over the other. Because of problems with supply of isotopes in 1997 and 1998, the choice at many institutions has been based on availability.

Some institutions combine external beam radiation with a seed implant. Commonly 45 Gy is given prior to a reduced-dose iodine or palladium implant. There are no data yet proving that this combined approach is superior to either conformal external beam radiation or external beam radiation plus neoadjuvant androgen deprivation. The combined approach is certainly more expensive and may well increase the morbidity. At the MGH if we judge the risk of extracapsular disease to be so high that when external beam radiation is required, the entire treatment is delivered in this fashion with neoadjuvant androgen suppression.

Not all patients with early tumors are candidates for prostate brachytherapy. Those who have had a prior transurethral resection of the prostate (TURP) are at significant risk for subsequent superficial urethral necrosis and incontinence. Those with a prostatic volume much in excess of 40 cm$^3$ may be technically difficult to implant. The anterolateral portion of the prostate gland is shielded from a transperineal approach by the pubic arch. In addition, patients with prostate glands over 40 cm$^3$ have a significant risk of bladder outflow obstruction in the first few weeks after the implant. If they are to be implanted at all, these patients need to undergo temporary androgen deprivation to reduce their prostate volume prior to the procedure. Speed and convenience, two potential advantages of prostate brachytherapy, may thus be negated by the need for 3 months of androgen deprivation therapy.

## Postoperative Radiation Therapy

The fate of patients undergoing radical prostatectomy who have unsuspected pathologic T3 disease has been examined in a number of studies. Clinical local failure rates between 25% and 68% have been reported in literature from the pre-PSA era.[27] Modern series now report PSA failure as the primary end point. This occurs in 40% to 75% of those with extensive extracapsular disease, positive margins, or seminal vesicle invasion. For some, the rise in PSA represents the first sign of local failure; for others it is metastatic disease; and for the remainder it is both. Obviously it is only the first group that truly stands to gain from a local therapy, such as tumor bed irradiation. Those with seminal vesicle invasion and Gleason 8–10 tumors are far more likely to have disseminated disease. In addition, those whose serum PSA values do not decline to zero in the first month following radical prostatectomy also are likely have disseminated disease. Upon rebiopsy, these patients are most likely to experience only local recurrence; they also tend to have Gleason 7 or lower tumors, positive surgical margins, negative seminal vesicles and lymph nodes, and undetectable postoperative PSA.

Adjuvant radiation is recommended to those who fulfill the foregoing criteria. We normally wait 6 or more weeks after radical surgery for patients to begin the recovery toward continence before initiating radiation. Not all patients with positive surgical margins or extracapsular disease will experience local recurrence, or even any recurrence at all. If patients wish to be followed expectantly with radiation reserved for salvage when the PSA first rises, this is also a reasonable approach. In our experience, however, once the PSA has risen much beyond 1.5 ng/mL the chance of cure with salvage radiation is low.

The technique used for treating both adjuvant and salvage patients is the same. In the simulator 40 mL of air and contrast are instilled into the bladder by means of a Foley catheter (Figure 9-12). A urethrogram is also performed. The space between the most inferior portion of the bladder and the beak of the urethrogram represents the urethrovesical anastomosis. Ultrasound-guided rebiopsy studies have shown that this is the commonest site for local persistence after prostatectomy.[28] For the lateral fields, barium is introduced into the rectum. Because the prostate is no longer in situ, the rectum has often moved forward into the tumor bed. The target volume may on occasions be limited by the rectal volume within the field. The total tumor dose delivered is 61.2 to 64.8 Gy in 1.8 Gy fractions. A single volume is used throughout.

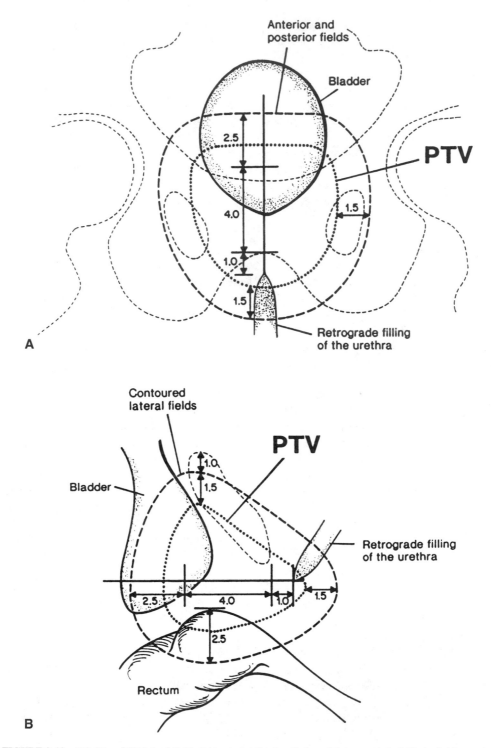

**FIGURE 9-12** **(A)** AP and **(B)** lateral fields for postoperative irradiation of the prostatic bed. These fields are similar for both adjuvant and salvage therapy.

## RESULTS OF RADICAL RADIATION THERAPY

### Early Stage Disease

*External Beam Radiation* External beam radiation has a long and highly documented track record in early stage prostate cancer. When patients are simply observed, 100% of patients will progress locally within 15 years. If the same population is treated with external beam radiation, less than 30% will progress locally within the same time period. Thus a local control advantage is well demonstrated. A survival advantage is more difficult to document. We compared patients treated with external beam radiation with those managed expectantly.[29,30] No advantage was detected in terms of overall survival or survival free from metastases in the first 12 years for the well-differentiated cancers; a small advantage of only about 10% was seen for the moderately differentiated cancers. For the poorly differentiated cancers, though few were ultimately cured, the time to the development of metastasis and the median time to death were considerably extended by radiotherapy.

PSA surrogates are now more commonly used as end points in studies. When these biochemical end points are selected, failure is detected more frequently and earlier over the first 10 years than when clinical end points are used. The likelihood of a rising PSA following external beam radiation is strongly predicted by the pretreatment PSA[31,32] (Figure 9-13). Those with PSA values in excess of 10 ng/mL are infrequently cured by external beam radiation. In selected subgroups (e.g., PSA < 10 ng/mL, Gleason grade $\leq$ 6), over 70% may have lasting biochemical control.[33]

Another important end point is the prostatic rebiopsy. Histologic evidence of cancer within the prostate 3 or more years beyond external beam radiation strongly predicts for subsequent clinical failure. In a prospective series with a minimum follow-up in 4 years, Crook et al. documented 38% of men with T1/T2 tumors treated to a median dose of 66 Gy had locally persistent disease.[34] It therefore seems that conventional doses fit on the steep part of the dose–response curve, suggesting a potential advantage for dose escalation.

Three-dimensional conformal external beam radiation is now being used to more accurately target the prostate and to minimize normal tissue complications. In addition, it allows safer dose escalation. Early data strongly suggest improved biochemical disease-free survival for T1/T2 patients treated with doses in excess of 72 Gy. Rebiopsy data from the Memorial Sloan-Kettering Cancer Center indicate that rebiopsy positive rates of approximately 50% are reduced to below 10% if 80 Gy or more is delivered. At least two randomized

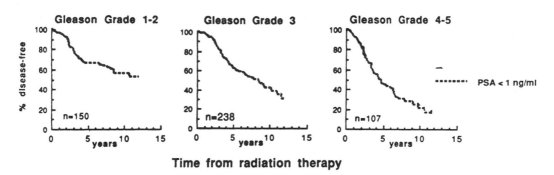

**FIGURE 9-13** Freedom from PSA recurrence for men treated with conventional external beam radiation at the MGH. Patients are stratified by Gleason grade.

trials are in progress to assess the efficacy of dose escalation in patients with probably organ-confined disease.

*Prostate Brachytherapy* The first contemporary prostate brachytherapy series reporting medium-term data is that from Seattle.[35] These authors showed that for selected men with low PSA and low Gleason grade, the probability of remaining free from PSA progression at 7 years is 79%. This subgroup represents a population of patients who might alternatively be considered for either radical prostatectomy or external beam radiation. The 10-year data are not yet available, but bearing in mind that the median PSA for the disease-free survivors in this group is 0.2, the results may well not change a great deal. One must, however, be cautious in making such predictions. Even in the modern Johns Hopkins prostatectomy series, patients with T2a tumors continue to fail well into the second decade.[36] Brachytherapy in selected patients with excellent technique produces good results, comparable to those obtained with surgery or external beam radiation. What is currently not clear is the role of brachytherapy in patients with larger tumors or tumors of higher grade or with higher initial PSA values. Undoubtedly, technique will prove critical.

Quality assurance studies are now being initiated in an attempt to determine whether the high standards of the Seattle group are being reproduced across the nation. An American College of Surgeons study examining nearly 2000 prostatectomies in nearly 400 hospitals reported failure and morbidity rates substantially higher than those of the major centers.[15] A similar study has not yet been performed on patients treated with external radiation in the PSA area, but the Patterns of Care Studies showed no difference in local control and overall survival for men treated by external beam radiation, either in academic or community center.[37] There is evidence therefore that, historically at least, external beam radiation transferred better to the community than radical prostatectomy. How well brachytherapy will transfer remains to be seen.

## Locally Advanced Prostate Cancer

### Neoadjuvant Androgen Deprivation and Radiation

The most compelling data available to date on the use of radiation in combination with neoadjuvant androgen suppression (NAS) come from RTOG Protocol 8610. This study by the Radiation Therapy Oncology Group evaluated the efficacy of the combination of goserelin acetate and flutumide administered prior to external radiation to 471 patients with bulky, locally advanced prostate cancer.[38] Androgen suppression was started 8 weeks prior to radiation and continued throughout for a total of 16 weeks. Patients were randomized, with a median follow-up of 4 years. The estimated cumulative instance of local failure at 5 years was 71% for control patients, but only 54% for the experimental patients. It is of note that local failure rates are higher in the control arm than in many other series reporting results with radiation alone for similar stages of tumor. This most probably reflects the use of more rigorous failure criteria, in particular the rebiopsy of many, but not all, with clinically negative glands. It is also based on the presumption that those with biochemical failure and no clinical evidence of distant metastases had local failure, which well may well result in overestimating the actual incidence. There was also a strong trend toward a reduction in the cumulative incidence of distant metastases at 5 years between the treatment and control group (34% and 41%). The trend had not reached statistical evidence, and it is not clear whether it is the result of improved local control or of the systemic action of androgen suppression on occult micrometastases present at diagnosis.

An interim analysis of a randomized trial from Quebec has also recently been reported.[39] Patients received either radiation alone or 3 months of neoadjuvant androgen suppression

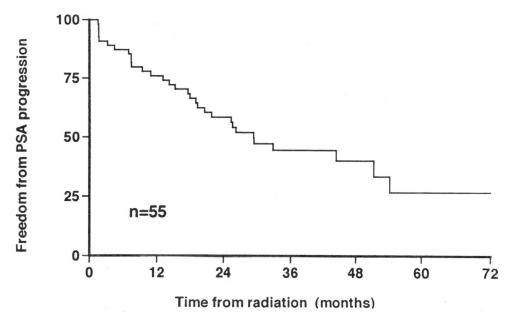

**FIGURE 9-14**    The likelihood of obtaining and maintaining an undetectable PSA for men treated at the MGH with salvage radiation following radical prostatectomy.

and then radiation or 3 months of NAS followed by radiation and a further 6 months of NAS. Thus far 120 patients have reached the 2-year point in the trial and have undergone prostate rebiopsy. The rates of positive rebiopsy were 64%, 28%, and 8%, respectively. A long-term gain from the addition of as little as 3 months of androgen suppression is once again demonstrated.

### Salvage Radiation after Prostatectomy

Radical prostatectomy is not usually performed on patients with clinical T2b-T4 disease because the chance that these patients have organ-confined tumors is low and the procedure is unlikely to represent curative therapy. Nevertheless, many patients with lower clinical stages who undergo radical prostatectomy will turn out to have pathologic T3 disease and therefore, become candidates for adjuvant radiation therapy.

When adjuvant radiation is delivered to patients at high risk of local failure from a radical prostatectomy, 5-year biochemical disease-free survival rates are in the order of 60% to 70%. This is certainly superior to many, but not all, series in which no adjuvant radiation was given. If radiation is reserved as a salvage maneuver, the likelihood that the serum PSA will fall to undetachable levels in well-selected patients is approximately 2 out of 3. Only half of these patients, however, maintain an undetectable PSA at 5 years (Figure 9-14). Either radiotherapy is ineffective in eradicating the local tumor, or, more likely, micrometastases are present and ultimately become apparent.

### MORBIDITY OF RADIATION THERAPY

Side effects during external beam treatment, such as fatigue, urinary frequency, slow urinary stream, dysuria, diarrhea, and occasional rectal bleeding, may occur at varying degrees in over 50% of patients treated. These may be relieved by simple measures, such as anticholinergics to reduce bladder irritability and increase capacity, $\alpha$-adrenoceptor blockers to improve urinary flow, anti-inflammatory agents to relieve prostatic inflammation, and steroid suppositories. The likelihood of late complications from external beam treatment was well documented in an analysis of 331 patients from the MGH, the M. D. Anderson Cancer Center, and the RTOG trial 77-06 with 6.1 years median follow-up.[40] Impotence stood at 63% at 5 years, diarrhea 4%, rectal bleeding 5%, hematuria 5%, and genitourinary strictures 5%. All the post-treatment sequelae described were mild to moderate (grade II and grade III, no grade IV or grade V complications). Only one patient from 331 became incontinent, and he had had three prior transurethral resections. The rate of rectal and bladder neck complications has been related to dose, field size, and the relative volume of organ irradiated. With the newer technique of three-dimensional conformal radiotherapy, the tumor volume can be more accurately localized and the proportion of the adjacent organs irradiated to full tumor dose is lower. These efforts have resulted in a lower proportion of patients with acute reactions. The situation with late effects is less clear, as since smaller volumes of normal tissue are irradiated, they are irradiated to a higher dose. A previous trial from the MGH looking at dose escalation for T3 and T4 tumors using proton beam showed an increase in rectal bleeding at the higher radiation dose despite smaller boost volumes.[41] Over one-quarter (27%) of patients had mild to moderate rectal bleeding after 75.6 Gy, compared with only 8% of patients at 67.2 Gy. Analysis of the data showed, unsurprisingly, that the likelihood of rectal bleeding was greater when larger rectal volumes are irradiated. This was a common event for these bulky tumors. The inclusion of large rectal volumes should not be necessary for T1 or T2 tumors unless significant benign hyperplasia is present.

Radical radiation employing interstitial brachytherapy has its own unique morbidity. In the first week most patients experience dysuria, urinary frequency, hematuria, and a slow urinary stream. This subsides rapidly, but in the second and third weeks a brisk radiation prostatitis occurs in the majority of patients. This, again, is characterized by frequency and dysuria. If there is significant prostatic swelling, urinary outflow obstruction may occur. Postvoid residuals need to be assessed, and when greater than 200 mL a catheter may need to be inserted for an average of 2 weeks until the swelling has subsided. This proves necessary in approximately 20% to 25% of treated patients. The likelihood is substantially higher if the prostate is 35 mL or larger at the time of implantation. Conservative management is the most appropriate as TURP and TUIP (transurethral incision of the prostate) are associated with significant risks of incontinence. The long-term morbidity from brachytherapy is currently unclear, as data are not yet mature. Unless a TURP is required, incontinence is comparably low to external beam. Mild urinary symptoms may persist for 3 to 6 months, but these usually subside completely. Impotence rates, variably reported as between 10% and 25%, are likely to be underestimates, and mature data are awaited.

When external beam radiation follows a radical prostatectomy with doses of 60 to 64 Gy, long-term morbidity is low. There is currently no evidence that incontinence rates are increased with postoperative radiation.[42,43] There is, however, some evidence that the few men who do manage to maintain their potency following a radical prostatectomy may well lose it when adjuvant or salvage radiation is added.

## PARTICLE RADIATION FOR PROSTATE CANCER

### Proton Therapy

Proton beams have been widely used in radiotherapy because of the unique depth–dose characteristics. The dose deposited by a beam of monoenergetic protons increases slowly with depth, but reaches sharp maximum shortly before the end of the particle range, the "Bragg peak." A randomized trial was completed at the MGH to examine the potential for using a high dose proton beam in locally advanced disease (Figure 9-15). All men

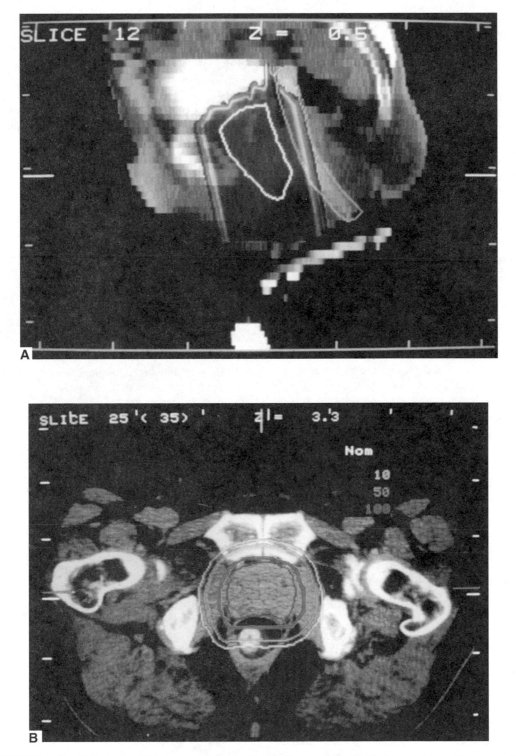

**FIGURE 9-15** **(A)** Sagittal and **(B)** transverse dose distributions for a conformal perineal boost delivered by means of a 160MV proton beam. Figures also appear in Color Figure section.

received 50.4 Gy through a pelvic field from conventional photons. Half the patients received a lateral boost using photons to 67.2 Gy; the other half received a perineal boost with protons to 75.6 Gy. A probe was placed within the rectum and the balloon inflated around it to displace as much rectum from the perineal beam as possible. T3-T4 patients were enrolled from 1982 until 1992, with a median follow-up of 5 years. There was no difference in outcome between the treatment arms with respect to overall survival, recurrence-free survival, or local control. In a subgroup of 58 patients with poorly differentiated tumors, however, the high dose proton arm did result in a significantly higher rate of local control. There was no difference in serum PSA outcome at 7 years. The essentially negative results of this trial are, in retrospect, not surprising. Most patients with T3 and T4 tumors have occult micrometastatic disease, and benefits from improved local control will be difficult to detect. A randomized trial is currently under way for T1, T2 patients who have a lower probability of occult micrometastatic disease. These are the patients who, when they fail following conventional doses, may fail locally alone. In the rebiopsy series of Crook et al., 40% of T1-T2 patients have locally persistent disease three or more years beyond conventional external beam radiation.[29]

## Neutron Beam Therapy

Neutrons have unique radiobiologic properties that make cell killing less dependent on tissue oxygenation. If hypoxia is present in large prostate tumors, this should therefore be a less serious limitation to tumor control if neutrons are used for at least a portion of the treatment. In addition, the injury to DNA from neutrons is less reparable than that caused by photons given a significantly higher radiobiologic effectiveness (RBE). For a worthwhile therapeutic advantage, however, the RBE for tumor control must be higher than that for normal tissue injury. Several trials have examined patients with T3-T4 tumors. Improved rates of

local control were evident, but no improvement in overall or cancer specific survival. The incidence of severe late complications has been consistently higher in patients receiving neutrons as a component of their therapy than in patients receiving photons alone. The neutron delivery techniques are undergoing an evolution, and new data may become available in the future.

## REFERENCES

1. Brawley OW, Kramer BS: Epidemiology of prostate cancer, in NJ Vogelzang, PT Scardino, WU Shipley, and D Coffey (eds): *Comprehensive Textbook of Genitourinary Oncology.* Baltimore, Williams & Wilkins, 1996, pp 565–578.

2. Isaacs WB: Molecular genetics of prostate cancer, in NJ Vogelzang, PT Scardino, WU Shipley, and D Coffey (eds): *Comprehensive Textbook of Genitourinary Oncology.* Baltimore, Williams & Wilkins, 1996, pp 579–592.

3. McNeal JE: Normal histology of the prostate. *Am J Surg Path* 1988;12:619–633.

4. Gleason DF: Histologic grading of prostatic adenocarcinoma: A perspective. *Hum Pathol* 1977;23:273–279.

5. McNeal JE, Redwine EA, Freiha F, Stamey TA: Zonal distribution of prostatic adenocarcinoma: Correlation with histologic pattern and direction of spread. *Am J Surg Path* 1988;12:897–906.

6. Partin AW, Yoo J, Carter HB, Pearson JD, Chan DW, Epstein JI, Walsh PC: Use of prostate-specific antigen, clinical stage, and Gleason score to predict pathological stage in men with localized prostate cancer. *J Urol* 1993;150:110–114.

7. Johansson JE, Adami HO, Andersson JO, Bergstrom R, Krusemo UB: High 10-year survival rate in patients with early, untreated prostate cancer. *JAMA* 1992;267:2191–2196.

8. Carter HB, Pearson JD, Metter EJ: Longitudinal evaluation of prostate-specific antigen levels in men with and without prostatic disease. *JAMA* 1992;267:2215–2220.

9. Whitmore WF, Warner JA, Thompson IM: Expectant management of prostate cancer. *Cancer* 1991;67:1091–1096.

10. Willett CG, Zietman AL, Shipley WU, Coen JJ: The effect of pelvic radiation therapy on the

production of prostatic specific antigen. *J Urol* 1994;151:1579–1581.

11. Zietman AL, Tibbs MK, Dallow KC, Althausen AF, Willett CG, McGovern FG, Shipley WU: The use of PSA nadir to predict subsequent biochemical outcome following external beam radiation therapy for T1-2 adenocarcinoma of the prostate. *Radiother Oncol* 1996;40:159–162.

12. American Society for Therapeutic Radiology and Oncology Consensus Panel: Consensus statement for PSA following radiation therapy. *Int J Radiat Oncol Biol Phys* 1997;37:1035–1041.

13. Hanks GE, D'Amico A, Epstein BE, Schultheiss TE: Prostate-specific antigen doubling times in patients with prostate cancer: A potentially useful reflection of tumor doubling time. *Int J Radiat Oncol Biol Phys* 1993;27:125–127.

14. Reiner WG, Walsh PC: An anatomical approach to the surgical management of the dorsal vein and Santorini's plexus during radical retropubic surgery. *J Urol* 1979;121:198–202.

15. Murphy GP, Mettlin C, Menck H: National patterns of prostate treatment by radical prostatectomy: Results of a survey by the American College of Surgeons Commission on Cancer. *J Urol* 1994;152:1817–1820.

16. Bagshaw MJ, Cox RS, Hancock L: Control of prostate cancer with radiotherapy: Long-term results. *J Urol* 1994;152:1781–1789.

17. Trapasso JG, DeKernion JB, Smith RB, Dorey F: The incidence and significance of detectable levels of serum prostate specific antigen after radical prostatectomy. *J Urol* 1994;152:1821–1825.

18. Fuks Z, Leibel S, Wallner K: The effect of local control on metastatic dissemination in carcinoma of the prostate: Long-term results in patients treated with 125-I implantation. *Int J Radiat Oncol Biol Phys* 1992;21:537.

19. Zietman AL, Prince E, Nakfoor BM, Park JJ: Androgen deprivation and radiation therapy: Sequencing studies using the Shionogi in vivo tumor system. *Int J Radiat Oncol Biol Phys* 1997;38:1067–1070.

20. Sands ME, Pollack A, Zagars GK: Influence of radiotherapy on node-positive prostate cancer treated with androgen deprivation. *Int J Radiat Oncol Biol Phys* 1995;31:13–19.

21. Myers RP, Larson-Keller JJ, Bergstralh EJ: Hormonal treatment at time of radical retropubic prostatectomy for stage D1 prostate cancer: Results of long-term follow-up. *J Urol* 1992;147:910–915.

22. Biggs PA, Shipley WU: A beam width improving device for a 25 MV x-ray beam. *Int J Radiat Oncol Biol Phys* 1986;12:131–135.

23. Asbell SO, Krall JM, Pilepich MV: Elective pelvic irradiation in stage A2, B carcinoma of the prostate: Analysis of RTOG 77-06. *Int J Radiat Oncol Biol Phys* 1986;12:345–351.

24. Hanks GE, Lee WR, Hanlon AL: Conformal technique dose escalation for prostate cancer: Biochemical evidence of improved cancer control with higher doses in patients with pretreatment PSA > 10ng/mL. *Int J Radiat Oncol Biol Phys* 1996;35:862–868.

25. Zelefsky MJ, Leibel SA, Kutcher GJ, Fuks Z: Three-dimensional conformal radiotherapy and dose escalation: Where do we stand? *Semin Radiat Oncol* 1998;8:107–114.

26. Zelefsky MJ, Whitmore WF: Long-term results of retropubic permanent iodine-125 implantation of the prostate for clinically localized prostatic cancer. *J Urol* 1997;158:23–30.

27. Zietman AL, Shipley WU, Willett CG: Residual disease following radical surgery or radiation therapy for prostate cancer: Clinical significance and therapeutic implications. *Cancer* 1993;71:959–969.

28. Connolly JA, Shinohara K, Presti JC, Carroll PR: Local recurrence after radical prostatectomy: Characteristics in size, location, and relationship to prostate-specific antigen and surgical margins. *Urology* 1996;47:225–231.

29. Crook JM, Bahadur YA, Robertson SJ, Perry GA, Esche BA: Evaluation of radiation effect, tumor differentiation, and prostate biopsies after external beam radiotherapy for patients with prostate carcinoma. *Cancer* 1997;79:81–89.

30. Zietman AL, Coen JJ, Dallow KA, Shipley WU: The treatment of prostate cancer by conventional radiation therapy: An analysis of long term outcome. *Int J Radiat Oncol Biol Phys* 1995;32:287–292.

31. Chodak GW, Thirsted RA, Gerber GS, Johansson J-E, Adolfsson J, Jones GW, Chisholm GD, Moskovitz B, Livne PM, Warner J: Results of conservative management of clinically localized prostate cancer. *New Engl J Med* 1994;330:242–248.

32. Zietman AL, Coen JJ, Shipley WU, Efird J: Radical radiation therapy in the management of prostatic adenocarcinoma: The initial PSA value as a predictor of treatment outcome. *J Urol* 1994;151:640–645.

33. Zagars GK, Pollack A, von Eschenbach AC: Prognostic factors for clinically localized prostate cancer. *Cancer* 1997;79:1370–1380.

34. Keyser D, Kupelian PA, Zippe CD, Levin HS, Klein EA: Stage T1-2 prostate cancer with pretreatment prostate-specific antigen level ≤ 10 ng/mL: Radiation therapy or surgery? *Int J Radiat Oncol Biol Phys* 1997;38:723–729.

35. Blasko JC, Wallner K, Grimm PD: Prostate-specific antigen based disease control following ultrasound-guided 125-iodine implantation for stage T1/T2 prostatic carcinoma. *J Urol* 1995; 154:1096–1099.

36. Pound CR, Partin AW, Epstein JI, Walsh PC: Prostate-specific antigen after anatomic radical prostatectomy. *Urol Clin North Am* 1997;24: 395–406.

37. Hanks GE, Diamond JJ, Krall JM: A ten-year followup of 682 patients treated for prostate cancer with radiation therapy in the United States. *Int J Radiat Oncol Biol Phys* 1987;13: 499–505.

38. Pilepich MV, Krall JM, Al-Sarraf M, Scotte-Doggett RL, Sause WT, Lawton CA, Abrams RA, Rotman M, Rubin P, Shipley WU, Grignon D, Caplan R, Cox JD: Androgen deprivation with radiation therapy alone for locally advanced prostatic carcinoma: A randomized comparative trial of the Radiation Therapy Oncology Group. *Urology* 1995;45:616–623.

39. Laverdiere J, Gomez JL, Cusan L, Suburu ER, Diamond P, Lemay M, Candas B, Labrie F: Beneficial effect of combination therapy administered prior to and following external beam radiation in localized prostate cancer. *Int J Radiat Oncol Biol Phys* 1997.

40. Shipley WU, Zietman AL, Hanks GE, Coen JJ, Caplan RJ, Won W, Zagars GK, Asbell SO: Treatment-related sequelae following external beam radiation for prostate cancer: A review with an update in patients with stage T1 and T2 tumors. *J Urol* 1994;152:1799–1805.

41. Benk VA, Adams JA, Shipley WU, Urie MM, McManus PL, Efird JT, Willett CG: Late rectal bleeding following combined x-ray and proton high dose irradiation for patients with stages T3-T4 prostate carcinoma. *Int J Radiat Oncol Biol Phys* 1993;26:551–557.

42. Morris M, Dallow KC, Zietman AL, Park JJ, Heney NM, Shipley WU: Adjuvant and salvage radiation following radical prostatectomy. *Int J Radiat Oncol Biol Phys* 1997;38:731–736.

43. Van Cangh PJ, Richard F, Lorge F, Castille Y, Moxhon A, Opsomer R: Adjuvant radiation therapy does not cause urinary incontinence after radical prostatectomy: Results of a prospective randomized study. *J Urol* 1998;159: 164–166.

44. Shipley WU, Verhey LJ, Munzenrider JE, Suit HD, Urie MM, McManus PL, Young RH, Shipley JW, Zietman AL, Biggs PJ, Heney NM, Goitein M: Advanced prostate cancer: The results of a randomized comparative trial of high dose irradiation boosting with conformal protons compared with conventional dose irradiation using photons alone. *Int J Radiat Oncol Biol Phys* 1995;32:3–12.

# C. CARCINOMA OF THE UPPER URINARY TRACT

## ADULT RENAL CELL CARCINOMA

### Results

The management of patients with localized renal cell carcinoma is primarily surgical. The cure rates for patients selected for treatment by radical nephrectomy are only fair and have not improved much, if at all, over the last three decades. For instance, Skinner et al. reported a 57% 5-year survival and a 44% 10-year survival in such patients.[1] This had improved only slightly, judged by an update from the Massachusetts General Hospital (MGH) nearly 15 years later.[2] Survival following nephrectomy for renal cell carcinoma is significantly influenced by pathologic stage. In the Skinner report, the 5- and 10-year survival for patients with tumors invading into perinephric fat or beyond was 47% and 20%, respectively.[1] For patients with regional lymph node involvement but no other evidence of metastatic disease, the 5- and 10-year survivals were 33% and 17%. There were no long-term survivors when the tumor extended directly into contiguous retroperitoneal visceral structures. No adjuvant radiation therapy was given to these patients.

Patients with renal cell carcinoma can have a variable and protracted natural history. This makes any benefit in survival from radical nephrectomy plus any additional therapy difficult to evaluate. For instance, there are no clear data that radical nephrectomy plus lymphadenectomy provides an enhanced cure rate over that achieved by radical nephrectomy alone.[3] Approximately 20% to 30% of patients have regional lymphadenopathy detected on node dissection, and this value rises to over 45% when there is renal vein involvement. Over half of these patients also have occult distant metastases. Thus the potential survival advantage from any policy of regional treatment is only 10% to 15%, assuming the treatment is fully effective. Many surgeons omit a lymphadenectomy, feeling that the gains do not offset the risks of bowel damage, chylous ascites, and bleeding. Early data from a large European randomized trial of over 600 patients show no survival gain from the addition of a regional node dissection.[4]

Studies looking at the possible benefit of adjuvant irradiation combined with radical nephrectomy are few, dated, and inconclusive. These are outlined in Table 9-9.[5–9] The report by Peeling et al. shows no apparent benefit, but this trial was not controlled either for extended disease or for the addition of radiation therapy postoperatively.[5] Further, the radiation dose was not clearly stated but very likely was less than we can now give safely. The randomized report from England by Finney showed no benefit from 40 Gy postoperatively.[6] However, while the report does not specify the radiation dose and technique, any possible benefit from the radiation therapy was likely compromised by the technique. Four fatal liver complications occurred following the treatment. The one positive report for postoperative radiation therapy was a nonrandomized retrospective analysis in which 96 patients were treated by nephrectomy alone and 36 (37%) patients had a 5-year survival, while 94 patients given postoperative radiation therapy of uncertain dose had a 56%

**TABLE 9-9  Renal Cell Carcinoma: Review of Treatment Results with and Without Adjuvant Radiotherapy (RT)**

| Author | Number of Patients | Local Treatment | 5-Year Survival (%) | Local Recurrence (%) | Comments |
|---|---|---|---|---|---|
| Peeling et al.[5] | 96 | Nephrectomy | 52 | | Not randomized |
| | 68 | Nephrectomy + RT | 25 | | ? RT dose |
| Rafla[7] | 96 | Nephrectomy | 37 | 25 | Not randomized |
| | 94 | Nephrectomy + RT | 56 | 7 | ? RT dose |
| Rafla[7] | 52 | Nephrectomy | 28 | | |
| (pT3 only) | 69 | Nephrectomy + RT | 57 | | |
| Finney[6] | 49 | Nephrectomy | 44 | | Randomized |
| | 51 | Nephrectomy + RT | 36 | | 40 Gy; four fatal liver complications |
| van der Werf-Messing[8] | 85 | Nephrectomy | 50 | | Randomized |
| | 89 | RT + nephrectomy (30 Gy) | 45 | | 37% pT1-2 |
| Juusela et al.[9] | 44 | Nephrectomy | 63 | | Randomized |
| | 38 | RT + nephrectomy (36 Gy) | 47 | | 70% pT1-2 |

(53/94 patients) 5-year survival rate.[7] This survival difference held up for patients with the advanced stage tumors.

Preoperative radiation therapy has been tested in two randomized trials. The first is reported by van der Werf-Messing, in which there was no benefit to a dose of 30 Gy preoperatively followed by nephrectomy.[8] Thirty-seven percent of these patients had small tumors and thus would have been unlikely to benefit from adjuvant therapy. Juusela et al. also reported no benefit from preoperative radiation therapy of 36 Gy with conventional fractionation.[8] However, 70% of the patients in this trial had small tumors (pT1-2) and thus also would have been unlikely to have benefited from any adjuvant treatment. Thus there are no satisfactory retrospective or prospective analyses of the efficacies of modern megavoltage adjuvant postoperative radiation therapy to adequate dose in patients at high risk for local regional failure—those with high pathologic stage tumors.

## Radiation Technique

Appropriately selected patients are treated by daily fractions of 1.8 Gy with 10 or 25 MV beams from linear accelerators to fields that included the renal fossa and the tumor bed as well as the para-aortic and paracaval lymph nodes to a total dose of 45 Gy in 5 weeks. The treatment fields are usually by isocentric and parallel opposed shaped fields. For right-sided tumors, there is often a need for a field reduction at 36 to 40 Gy to include only the tumor bed and the para-aortic and paracaval lymph nodes to a total dose of 45 to 50.4 Gy in 5 to 5.5 weeks, to ensure that not more than 30% of the liver parenchyma is treated to high dose. A postnephrectomy preirradiation therapy abdominal CT scan is done as a baseline for subsequent comparison. The radiation therapy begins usually 3 to 6 weeks following radical nephrectomy. No effort is made to include the surgical incision in patients treated following radical nephrectomy unless there is specific information that significant wound contamination by tumor spill occurred.

## Treatment Policy

The only good candidates for adjuvant postoperative radiation therapy are patients with no known metastatic disease who have histologically confirmed primary unilateral renal cell carcinoma with pathologic evidence of deep invasion of Gerota's fascia, adjacent organs, or regional lymph nodes. Patients with pathologic stage T1 or T2 tumors without lymph node metastases have high cure rates with radical nephrectomy alone—80% or greater for 5- to 10-year survival—and thus are not good candidates for adjunctive therapy.[2,10]

Isolated, and especially late, local recurrences following radical nephrectomy may be managed aggressively by a combination of preoperative external beam radiation to a dose of 45 Gy followed by re-resection and intraoperative radiation. The latter delivers, via 6 to 12 MeV electrons, a single-dose boost of 10 to 15 Gy to microscopic residual tumors and 15 to 20 Gy to gross residual tumors, taking care to avoid spinal cord, small bowel, and duodenum.

## Palliative Radiation Therapy

External beam irradiation can be of significant palliative benefit for painful bony metastases provided adequate radiation doses are administered. Based on recent observations on the duration of palliation, a dose equivalent of at least 50 Gy in 5 to 5.5 weeks is optimal for long-term control of bony metastases. To deliver such high doses, multiple-field (three or more) techniques are often necessary. Where structural integrity of the bone may be compromised and the radiation dose can be administered so as not to exceed spinal cord or other critical normal tissue tolerance, doses in the 60 to 65 Gy range with conventional fractionation are given. If a patient presents with a solitary bony metastasis, he or she is of course very likely to develop multiple bony lesions but also has a 30% to 40% chance of surviving 5 years. Thus, in such settings, it becomes important to assure as durable a palliative response as possible. Reirradiation to adequate dose is not possible. Palliation of large renal bed recurrences by external beam alone has been unsatisfactory. Some relief of pain (usually of short duration) has been achieved in about 50% of the patients.[11]

## CARCINOMA OF THE RENAL PELVIS AND URETER

### Results

Transitional cell carcinoma of the renal pelvis and ureter are relatively uncommon and constitute less than 3% of all genitourinary malignancies. These tumors present usually with hematuria or symptoms of upper urinary tract obstruction, with the preoperative diagnosis now nearly always available from the combination of excretory urography, CT, and ultrasound. The treatment for patients with these tumors is primarily surgical. The results with surgery for those patients with low stage tumors (tumors limited to the submucosa or with no invasion shown pathologically through the ureteral or pelvic muscle layer) is high, with most series reporting less than 20% of patients failing or dying within 5 years following surgical resection.[12,13] For these early tumors, neither the extent of the surgery, nor the presence of carcinoma in situ or other abnormal urothelial findings in the adjacent mucosa, nor the tumor configuration (papillary vs. solid) influences this good overall survival (75–100% at 5 years). Importantly, however, all reports document that between one-third and one-half of all patients with these rare upper tract transitional cell tumors are associated with a previous, concomitant, or subsequent transitional cell tumor at another site in the urinary tract. There seems to be no clear role for adjuvant therapy for these low stage, upper tract transitional cell tumors, although some are exploring the use of percutaneous intraluminal high dose iridium therapy. The results following clinical resection for patients with high stage tumors— those shown pathologically with periureteral, peripelvic, or perirenal extension, or those with regional lymph nodal metastases—are poor,

with less than 30% of patients being cured by surgery alone.[12–14]

Some retrospective reviews suggest that more extensive surgical procedures (radical nephroureterectomy as contrasted to simple nephrectomy) have been associated with improved results in patients with renal pelvis tumors. For patients with ureteral tumors there has been no apparent advantage of nephroureterectomy over segmental resection, although all authors recommend always removing the distal ureteral stump together with a cuff of bladder during the course of a nephroureterectomy to avoid the need of repeated retrograde pyelography at the time of each subsequent cystoscopy. There is relatively limited information on the patterns of failure following surgery alone for patients with the more invasive tumors. Autopsy studies, however, have indicated lymph node involvement in 37% to 82% of patients with renal pelvis tumors[13–16] and from 22% to 41% of patients with ureteral tumors.[16,17] Although very few data exist, the local recurrence rate has been reported higher (43%) following surgery for invasive renal pelvic tumors than for the invasive tumors of the ureter (14%).[12,13]

A retrospective analysis of patients treated for poor risk (high stage and/or grade) transitional cell carcinoma of the renal pelvis and ureter was reported by Brookland and Richter.[14] In patients treated with postoperative radiation therapy (40–50 Gy), lower incidence of local recurrence (11% vs. 46%) and higher 5-year survival (27% vs. 17%) were observed in comparison to patients treated by surgery alone. Forty-five percent of the patients in the poor prognosis group developed distant metastases. More recently, Cozad et al. reviewed 94 patients treated with similar disease.[18] Postoperative irradiation was associated with higher rates of local–regional control in a multivariate analysis and a borderline significant improvement in 5-year survival.

### Treatment Policy

We recommend adjuvant therapy following surgical resection only for patients with locally advanced disease—those with pathologically confirmed periureteral, perirenal, or peripelvic extension of tumor, or those with proven regional lymph node metastases. We recommend, based on the available patterns of failure analysis described above and the overall poor survival, combined upfront chemotherapy and adjuvant radiation therapy to the tumor bed and regional lymph nodes. The chemotherapy recommended in patients with adequate renal function postoperatively is currently the cisplatin-based "MCV" regimen consisting of 30 mg/m$^2$ of methotrexate given on day 1, followed by 70 mg/m$^2$ of cisplatin and 3 mg/m$^2$ of vinblastine on day 2. Methotrexate and vinblastine are then repeated on days 15 and 22. The second cycle is begun on day 29 and completed on day 51. This is followed by external beam radiation to the tumor bed, as well as to the para-aortic and paracaval lymph nodes, to a dose of 40 Gy in 1.8 Gy daily fractions over 4.5 weeks, usually by isocentric parallel opposed anterior and posterior fields. If possible, a boost to the tumor bed is given to 45 Gy, provided this can be done safely without irradiating a significant amount of either liver parenchyma or small intestine. The radiation is accompanied by concurrent single-agent cisplatin chemotherapy for radiation sensitization. If no chemotherapy is given, the dose of radiation therapy administered is higher at 45 Gy in 1.8 Gy fractions over 5 weeks to the tumor bed and the regional lymph nodes, with a boost to the tumor bed, if possible, to 50.4 Gy.

The chemotherapy used in ureteric carcinoma will likely change in the coming few years, tracking, as it does, that used in the more common transitional carcinoma of the bladder.

### Palliation of Ureteral Obstruction by Metastatic Tumor

Patients presenting with ureteral obstruction or periureteral metastases, often from breast cancer, can be palliated by conventional external beam radiation therapy in the majority of cases. For instance, we have maintained a complete response rate with radiation therapy in over 50% of patients treated with metastases from breast

cancer.[19] To protect renal function in the obstructed kidney, a percutaneous nephrostomy is usually done. Following confirmation of the diagnosis by either open surgical exploration or a percutaneous needle biopsy by CT guidance, a dose of 45 to 50 Gy of radiation in conventional 1.8 Gy daily fractions is administered.

## REFERENCES

1. Skinner DG, Colvin RB, Vermillion CD, et al: Diagnosis and management of renal carcinoma, a clinical and pathologic study of 309 cases. *Cancer* 1971;28:1165–1177.

2. Basil B, Dosoretz DE, Prout GR Jr: Validation of the tumor, nodes and metastasis classification of renal cell carcinoma. *J Urol* 1985;134: 450–454.

3. Giuliani L, Giberti C, Martorana G, Rovida S: Radical extensive surgery for renal cell carcinoma: Long-term results and prognostic factors. *J Urol* 1990;143:468–474.

4. Blom JHM: The role of lymphadenectomy in association with radical nephrectomy. *Curr Opin Urol* 1993;3:359–362.

5. Peeling WB, Mantell BS, Shepheard BGF: Postoperative irradiation in the treatment of renal cell carcinoma. *Br J Urol* 1969;41:23–31.

6. Finney R: Radiotherapy in the treatment of hypernephroma—A clinical trial. *Br J Urol* 1973; 45:258–269.

7. Rafla S: Renal cell carcinoma. *Cancer* 1970;25:26–40.

8. van der Werf-Messing B: Carcinoma of the kidney. *Cancer* 1973;32:1056–1062.

9. Juusela H, Maimio K, Alfthan D, et al: Preoperative irradiation in the treatment of renal adenocarcinoma. *Scand J Urol Nephrol* 1977;2: 277–281.

10. Siminovitch JM, Montie JE, Straffon RA: Prognostic indicators in renal adenocarcinoma. *J Urol* 1983;130:20–23.

11. Halperin EC, Harisiadis L: The role of radiation therapy in the management of metastatic renal cell carcinoma. *Cancer* 1983;51:614–617.

12. Heney NM, Nocks BN, Daly JJ, et al: Prognostic factors in carcinoma of the ureter. *J Urol* 1981;125:632–636.

13. Seaman EK, Slawin KM, Benson MC: Treatment options for upper tract transitional cell carcinoma. *Urol Clin North Am* 1993;20: 97–105.

14. Brookland RK, Richter MP: Postoperative irradiation of transitional cell carcinoma of the renal pelvis and ureter. *J Urol* 1985;133:952–955.

15. Johannson S, Walhqvist L: A prognostic study of urothelial renal pelvic tumors. *Cancer* 1979;43:2525–2531.

16. Saitoh H, Hida N, Nakamura K, et al: Distant metastases of urethelial tumors of the renal pelvis and ureter. *Tokai J Exp Clin Med* 1982;7:355–361.

17. Batata MA, Whitmore WF Jr, Hilaris BS, et al: Primary carcinoma of the ureter: A prognostic study. *Cancer* 1985;35:1626–1630.

18. Cozad et al: Transitional cell carcinoma of the renal pelvis or ureter. *J Urol* 1995;216: 796–800.

19. Kopelson G, Munzenrider JE, Kelly RM, et al: Radiation therapy for ureteral metastasis from breast carcinoma. *Cancer* 1981;47:110–124.

# D. TESTIS CANCER

## CLINICAL EVALUATION

The incidence of testicular cancer has an age peak in the third decade. Nonseminomatous germ cell tumors occur mainly between the ages of 18 and 30 years, and seminomatous germ cell tumors occur above the age of 20, and with a much longer tail on the incidence–age curve. This pattern extends beyond the seventh decade. Primary lymphoma of the testis accounts for only 2% of testicular tumors in men under 50 years of age and 25% of those older.

The treatment of germ cell tumors of the testis is one of the most gratifying endeavors in oncologic clinical practice. With the advent of effective multidrug chemotherapy of men, the overall cure rate has increased from 60% to 70% to well over 90% regardless of stage or histologic type. Since patients are young, and cure rates so high, either with primary or salvage therapy, our task now is to develop criteria for safely omitting some therapy in patients with particularly favorable subtypes of testis cancer, to avoid, if possible, the risk of developing late treatment sequelae such as infertility or a second malignancy.

Radical inguinal orchiectomy is the appropriate procedure for the diagnosis and treatment of the primary tumor in the patient presenting with a testicular mass.[1] Previously there was often delay before surgery because the scrotal mass was erroneously diagnosed as a unilateral epididymitis or orchitis and treated conservatively. Now scrotal ultrasound allows reliable discrimination between a definite intratesticular mass surrounded by normal testis tissue and epididymitis, and prompt radical orchiectomy is performed when indicated. All the slides of the tumor specimen should be reviewed by an experienced pathologist to be as certain as possible that the discrimination between a pure seminoma and a nonseminomatous, or mixed, malignant cancer is correct and to determine whether vascular, epididymal, or spermatic cord invasion is present.

Evaluation for possible extragonadal metastatic disease should always include quantitative postorchiectomy serum radioimmunoassays of human chorionic gonadotrophin ($\beta$-hCG) and $\alpha$-fetoprotein (AFP), chest x-ray, retroperitoneal CT scan and, for patients with seminoma, bipedal lymphangiogram. The latter is controversial, but a skilled radiologist may detect a tumor within retroperitoneal nodes of normal size on CT. The "true negative" status of the retroperitoneal lymph nodes can now be ascertained with an 85% accuracy without surgery in the nonseminomatous testis tumors if the radiologic studies (CT and lymphangiogram) and serum markers ($\beta$-hCG and AFP) are negative. Because the serum AFP is never elevated in the presence of seminoma and the serum hCG rarely is, these contribute little to staging in patients with seminoma following orchiectomy. Present best estimates are that in the presence of a normal CT and lymphangiogram, the retroperitoneal lymph nodes are truly negative in approximately 80% of patients with seminoma. Histopathologic absence of both vascular invasion and invasion of the spermatic cord have been recognized as independent and probably significant predictors of a true negative status of the retroperitoneal lymph nodes in nonseminomatous germ cell tumors[2,3]

Following all treatment regimens patients should be followed very closely for 5 years to detect possible metastatic disease. The patients must be specifically counseled in self-examination to detect a second testis tumor, because one can occur for up to at least 20 years with a reported frequency as high as 3%.[4] Seminoma relapses late more often than nonseminoma, and thus vigilance is required for longer.

## SEMINOMA

Testicular seminoma is the most common tumor of the testis, making up about 60% of all germ cell tumors in the adult male. By comparison, the extragonadal seminomatous tumors are very rare primary neoplasms occurring in the mediastinum, retroperitoneum, and brain. Both types of seminoma (as well as dysgerminomas in the female) are exquisitely sensitive to radiation therapy. Radical inguinal orchiectomy followed by external beam radiation therapy to the involved, or potentially involved, regional lymph nodes is the accepted treatment of choice

in early testicular seminoma, that is, stages I and IIA (Tables 9-10 and 9-11[5-9]). While in the past many patients with large masses of metastatic seminoma in the retroperitoneum (stage IIB) or with even more widespread disease (stage III) were cured by radiation therapy, a large minority were not. Now, with the availability of effective chemotherapy, the majority of these patients, as well as those with relapse of metastatic seminoma subsequent to initial treatment, can be cured.

## Radiotherapeutic Techniques

In patients with clinical stages I or IIA testicular seminoma, the radiotherapeutic fields include the para-aortic, paracaval, ipsilateral renal hilar, and the ipsilateral ileoinguinal lymph nodes. The exact definition of the fields depends on the unique characteristics of a given patient and the type of megavoltage equipment available. Lymphangiographic visualization of the retroperitoneal lymph nodes is helpful for

TABLE 9-10    Staging of Pure Seminoma

| | |
|---|---|
| Stage I | Tumor confined to the testis |
| Stage II | Tumor with nodal metastases limited to the infradiaphragmatic lymphatics<br>A. Minimal retroperitoneal disease<br>B. Bulky tumor metastases |
| Stage III | Tumor involving lymphatics above the diaphragm |
| Stage IV | Tumor with extranodal metastases |

TABLE 9-11    Stage I Seminoma Testis: Review of Outcome and Patterns of Failure After Orchiectomy and Adjuvant Radiation

| Study | Radiation Dose (Gy) | Number of Patients | Total Relapses | Abdominal Relapses | CSS |
|---|---|---|---|---|---|
| Fossa et al.[5] | 50 | 249 | 13 | 1 | 99 |
| Hamilton et al.[6] | 30 | 232 | 5 | 0 | 100 |
| Thomas et al.[7] | 25 | 150 | 2 | 0 | 99 |
| Schultz et al.[8] | 34 | 162 | 8 | 1 | 99 |
| Zagars and Babaian[9] | 25 | 162 | 6 | 1 | 97 |
| MGH | 30 | 158 | 2 | 0 | 100 |

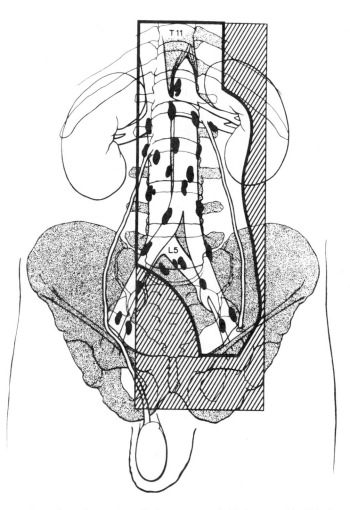

**FIGURE 9-16**   Contoured anterior and posterior radiation treatment fields for men with clinical stages I or IIA left testicular cancer; diagonally shaded area is an individually made, 8-cm thick Cerrobend block.

the careful design at simulation of these treatment fields. An excretory urogram or contrast enhanced CT scan must be carefully evaluated prior to, or at the time of, simulation with the patient immobilized to ensure exact localization of the kidneys with respect to the radiation treatment fields. When such care is taken to localize the kidneys properly, the risk of radiation-induced damage is essentially eliminated.

Figure 9-16 illustrates characteristic paired anterior and posterior fields that are contoured with individually cut Cerrobend blocking and treated with the 10 MV linear accelerator beams. The boundaries of the fields usually are

as follows: superiorly, to include the origin of the thoracic duct or the entire anterior surface of the T11 vertebral body; inferiorly, to include the internal ring (but not necessarily the inguinal incision); laterally, to include the ipsilateral renal hilum, usually more generous with left- than with right-sided tumors; and the contralateral para-aortic or paracaval and common iliac groups. Traditionally these fields have been expanded to include additional areas in the following two, not uncommon, situations:

1. In patients who have a history of prior inguinal herniorhaphy or orchiopexy,

which may predispose atypical lymphatic drainage, the inferior portion of the field has been extended to include the contralateral inguinal region.

2. In patients with histologic evidence of epididymal invasion by the tumor, the field has been enlarged to include the ipsilateral hypogastric lymph nodes as a potential site of metastatic drainage.

With salvage chemotherapy now so successful and concerns about the late effects of large volume irradiation growing, these field extensions are no longer regarded as mandatory. Recent studies have shown that a radiation field that covers only the first-echelon para-aortic lymph nodes is sufficient for most patients.[10,11] Pelvic relapse occurs in less than 4% and may be effectively salvaged with either radiation or

chemotherapy. Randomized trials are awaited, but it is likely that the regimen just described will become standard adjuvant treatment for stage I disease.

When ipsilateral pelvic irradiation is used, the contralateral testis must be adequately shielded to minimize any further risk to fertility. At the MGH we use three additional shields outside the primary beam: a lead shield 10 cm thick immediately above the contralateral testicle, an extension of the Cerrobend block for an additional 5 cm below the inferior border of the field, and a more comprehensive gonadal shield preventing the majority of internally scattered photons from hitting the remaining testicle (Figure 9-17). This combination has lowered the dose received to the contralateral testicle to approximately 0.1% of the treatment dose.[12]

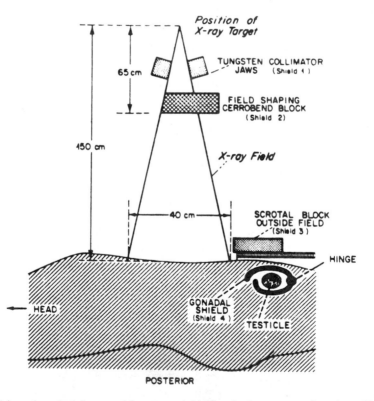

**FIGURE 9-17**   Schematic sagittal diagram of the setup and shielding for the treatment of a patient with testicular seminoma following radical orchiectomy. Patient is supine and the contralateral testis is shown diagramatically. Field size is 40 cm in the longitudinal direction and the treatment distance from source to skin is 150 cm. Four shielding devices are illustrated: 1, the collimator jaws of the linear accelerator; 2, Cerrobend field-shaping blocks; 3, a lead scrotal block; and 4, a gonadal shield whose front or cephalad wall separates the testicle from the horizontal internal scatter.

## Relapse-Free Survival
## Stage I and IIa vs. Stage IIb

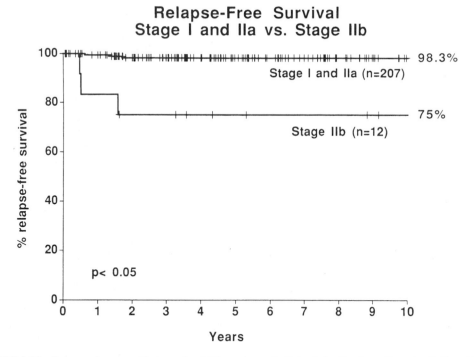

**FIGURE 9-18**    Outcome for men with stages I and IIA seminoma testis treated with retroperitoneal radiation at the MGH. Median follow-up is 6 years.

The retroperitoneal fields are usually treated to a total dose of 25 to 30 Gy in 1.5 Gy fractions, delivered via a 10 MV linear accelerator beam. Both the anterior and posterior fields are treated each day. If the patient has had a massive primary tumor invading into part of the scrotum but not requiring a hemiscrotectomy, or if the patient's tumor has been removed through a scrotal incision (strongly discouraged and generally no longer done), the ipsilateral hemiscrotum is treated by means of a 12 to 15 MV electron beam field that is matched to the lower border of the photon field. A soft clamp (such as an "intestinal clamp" surgical instrument) is used to hold the ipsilateral hemiscrotum to the involved side, while the patient places and holds his remaining testicle high in his (contralateral) inguinal canal and under a 2 cm thick lead cup. In this way, the contralateral testicle can usually be more than 5 cm distance from the electron beam edge and thus usually receive only 3% of the given electron dose by scatter.

### Treatment Results

When no futher treatment follows orchiectomy in stage I, between 15% and 20% of patients will relapse, the majority of relapses occurring in the retroperitoneum.[13] Though salvage is excellent, the likelihood that chemotherapy will need to be used is higher than it would have been if radiation had been delivered at the outset. In addition, follow-up surveillance must be thorough, with CT scans every three to four months for the first 3 years and twice a year for the subsequent 2 years to avoid detecting recurrence only when it is large and late. Surveillance may be costly, may generate anxiety in patients, and is not suitable for either noncompliant individuals or those with a geographically unsettled lifestyle. The majority of patients at the MGH and throughout the United States are thus encouraged to receive adjuvant radiation, which remains the standard of care. When this treatment is given, there is less than a 3% chance of recurrence (Figure 9-18).

**TABLE 9-12  Stage II Seminoma Testis Treated with External Beam Irradiation Following Radical Orchiectomy: Patients Are Divided According to Volume of Para-aortic Lymphadenopathy**

| Study | Lymphadenopathy | |
|---|---|---|
| | <5 cm | >5 cm |
| Lai et al.[14] | 31/33 | |
| Hunter and Peschel[15] | 15/15 | |
| Vallis et al.[16] | 45/48 | |
| Tombolini et al.[17] | 20/20 | |
| Bayens et al.[18] | 22/29 | 7/9 |
| Thomas et al.[7] | 37/40 | 22/46 |
| Mason et al.[19] | 24/25 | 18/24 |
| Evensen et al.[20] | 23/24 | 38/48 |
| Sagerman et al.[21] | 19/21 | 10/11 |
| Ball et al.[22] | 28/33 | 14/23 |
| Zagars and Babaian[9] | | 7/10 |
| Ellerbroek et al.[23] | | 8/15 |
| Jackson et al.[24] | | 13/16 |
| MGH | 48/49 | 9/12 |
| | 312/337 | 146/212 |
| | (93%) | (69%) |

Stage IIA disease is cured over 90% of the time by radiation alone (Figure 9-18, Table 9-12).[14–24] Chemotherapy is reserved for salvage. More bulky stage IIB patients may also be treated with radiation after orchiectomy, but cure rates are lower (at 60%–70%) because of the probability of distant metastases (Table 9-12).

Less than 5% of the total cases of seminoma present at an advanced stage with hematogenous metastases or lymph nodal metastases above the diaphragm. In the era before effective multidrug chemotherapy, the composite experience suggests that about half these patients who were treated with radiation therapy alone following orchiectomy were cured. Now, with effective multidrug chemotherapy, treatment of disseminated seminoma has sharply improved these results to 90% or better survival in patients with this rare type of testis seminoma presentation.

## Current Radiation Treatment Policy

Favorable categories of seminoma treated with radiation therapy alone after orchiectomy are as follows:

1. Stage I testicular seminoma receives adjuvant radiation.
2. Stage IIA testis seminoma receives radical radiation.
3. Extragonadal seminoma of the mediastinum, retroperitoneum, or pineal region.

Patients with stage I seminoma have the retroperitoneal lymph nodes treated as shown in Figure 9-16. No elective mediastinal or supraclavicular irradiation is given. Patients with stage IIA disease are treated with similar fields, also to a dose of 30 Gy, but this is followed by an additional boost of 6 Gy to the areas of disease defined by CT or lymphangiography. No mediastinal or left supraclavicular irradiation is given because of the risk of late cardiac complications and because such extended fields can limit marrow reserve, making the administration of future chemotherapy difficult.

The early published experience with patients with testicular seminoma suggested that patients with an anaplastic histology did uniquely poorly.[25,26] Several large institutions have not borne out this assumption for patients with stage I and IIA disease treated with conventional radiation therapy. Stage I and IIA patients with an elevated hCG are as likely to be cured following conventional treatment with radiation therapy as those who do not have the elevation.[27–29] Indeed, such high hCG levels provide a useful marker for follow-up. Immunoperoxidase staining of the primary seminoma has identified the source of the hCG secretion, which occasionally (in 5% of patients) is seen in pure seminoma to be the associated benign cytotrophoblastic giant cells.

## Categories of Advanced Testicular Seminoma Potentially Requiring Both Chemotherapy and Radiation

1. Stages IIB and III.
2. Relapse with metastatic seminoma subsequent to initial treatment.
3. Massive primary tumor invading the scrotum or beyond.

Patients with advanced seminoma in category 1 or 2 are now treated initially with cis-platin-based multidrug chemotherapy. This may be followed by involved-field radiation therapy to residual masses in excess of 3 cm using daily fractions of 1.5 to 1.8 Gy to a total dose of 30 to 36 Gy. The clinical considerations in favor of treating patients in these categories with subsequent irradiation are as follows:

1. Though residual masses are frequently sterile, the chance that tumor persists increases once the residuum is bulkier than 3 cm. The use of involved-field radiation therapy subsequent to systemic chemotherapy will allay concerns that may exist from radiographic studies that chemotherapy response is neither complete nor permanent. As mentioned, seminoma is exquisitely sensitive to radiation therapy; therefore doses in the range of 30 to 36 Gy will assure local control and thus prevent the need for surgical evaluation, which can often be associated with very severe morbidity or operative mortality.

2. The detection of a relapse is more difficult in seminoma than with nonseminomatous testis tumors. The serum marker hCG is elevated in only 5% of patients with pure seminoma, and the AFP is never elevated. Thus, should disseminated seminoma develop, it may become relatively advanced prior to its detection, perhaps compromising the chance for cure wth second-line therapy.

A strong argument against the use of combined chemotherapy and radiation therapy has recently been becoming considerably more audible. Contemporary analyses are beginning to suggest a small but detectable risk of second malignancy following treatment with conventional radiation for seminoma. These tumors are usually solid malignancies with a far more more fatal potential than a relapsed seminoma. The long-term experience with Hodgkin survivors suggests that this risk is greatly increased when multidrug chemotherapy and radiation are combined. In the Hodgkin series alkylating agents were usually used along with higher radiation doses, but even with these

caveats the concern remains. A recent meta-analysis has not shown any survival advantage to combined modality therapy over chemotherapy alone, even with residual masses, and it is likely that the combined approach will increasingly be reserved for individual cases.

In patients with no detectable metastatic disease who present with a massive testis tumor that cannot be satisfactorily resected by radical orchiectomy or hemiscrotectomy, treatment may be with radiation therapy alone, but the fields will cover the entire hemiscrotum and the immediately adjacent areas thought to be at risk (36 Gy), and fields also will cover the para-aortic and usually the ipsilateral pelvic lymph nodal regions (30 Gy). When the skin of the scrotum is involved by tumor, the femoral nodes are at risk and should also be included. This is done by matching electron beam fields, usually of energies ranging from 10 to 15 MV with 10 MV x-ray treatment fields to the retroperitoneum (see Figure 9-16).

## NONSEMINOMATOUS TUMORS

### Treatment Results

Over the last two decades the treatment of patients with nonseminomatous testicular germ cell tumors with multidrug chemotherapy has evolved dramatically.[30] Now over 85% of men with advanced disease are cured with first-line chemotherapy, compared with historical rates of only 50% to 60% using surgery, radiation therapy, and single-agent chemotherapy. The most effective agents are cisplatin, etoposide, and bleomycin. Current studies are aimed at reducing the overall number of cycles to the minimum necessary and, if possible, eliminating bleomycin, with its risk of pulmonary toxicity and Raynaud phenomenon.[31]

The high success rate with multidrug chemotherapy in advanced disease includes complete response rates of approximately 70% in advanced or bulky retroperitoneal disease. Retroperitoneal lymphadenectomy is selectively used in patients who do not achieve a complete radiographic response.

Lymphadenectomy has been associated with a very low disease recurrence rate in the retroperitoneum (< 5%). The recurrences in this setting are usually in patients in whom residual mature teratoma has been found histologically and, because of massive invasion from microscopic deposits in the region of the great vessels or the diaphragmatic crura, resection has not been done. Nevertheless, the use of preoperative multidrug chemotherapy has been as good or better at preventing retroperitoneal recurrence than the use of preoperative radiation therapy in patients with clinical stage II disease. Thus, although nonseminomatous germ cell testis cancer is relatively radiosensitive, radiation is given in only a limited number of clinical situations. These include patients presenting with very bulky nodal disease with extranodal extension into the regions of the upper abdomen and mediastinum. Here encirclement of or invasion into the great vessels may preclude adequate surgical resection following initial chemotherapy. Such patients may be candidates for radiation.

Historical data clearly documents the sensitivity to radiation of nonseminomatous germ cell tumors. Traditionally, higher doses were given than for seminoma: 45 Gy external beam irradiation with conventional fractionation to the para-aortic and paracaval as well as to the ipsilateral ileoinguinal lymph nodes with a boost dose to bulk disease to 50 Gy was the standard at the MGH before the chemotherapy era. These tumors were treated from the mid-1960s through the early 1970s, and were staged on the basis of lymphangiograms without the additional benefit of CT scanning. A quarter of those whose lymphangiograms were interpreted as normal (stage I) were found to have occult metastases by retroperitoneal node dissection. The true positive rate of the stage II patients with the abnormal lymphangiograms but without the additional information from CT scanning is 90%. Table 9-13 summarizes an 86% 3-year disease-free survival following radiation therapy alone for 140 patients who had received lymph nodal irradiation for clinical stage I tumors.[32–36]

**TABLE 9-13   Radiation Therapy in Nonseminomatous Germ Cell Tumor[a]**

| Institution | Number of Patients | Retroperitoneal Recurrence (%) | 3-Year Disease-Free Survival |
|---|---|---|---|
| *Clinical Stage I* | | | |
| Royal Marsden[34,35] | 84 | 2 | 72 (86%) |
|   Teratocarcinoma | 44 | 2 | 41 (94%) |
|   Embryonal | 40 | 2 | 30 (74%) |
| Walter Reed[36] | 29 | | 25 (86%) |
| Stanford[37] | 14 | | 11 (79%) |
| Rush-Presbyterian[38] | 13 | | 13 (100%) |
| | 140 | | 192; average 87% |
| *Clinical Stage II* | | | |
| Royal Marsden[34,35] | 27 | 37 | 16 (58%) |
| Retroperitoneal metastasis | | | |
|   < 2 cm | 14 | 7 | |
|   > 2 cm | 13 | 69 | |
| Walter Reed[36] | 11 | | 9 (82%) |
| Stanford[37] | 17 | | 10 (58%) |
| | 55 | | 35; average 66% |

[a]Three-year disease-free survival approximates very closely with cure in this disease.

The Royal Marsden Hospital series reports that only two of 84 patients developed a retroperitoneal recurrence—one each in 44 patients with a primary teratocarcinoma and in 40 patients with a primary embryonal carcinoma.[32,33] This shows that subclinical or microscopic disease is very sensitive to doses of radiation therapy in the range of 45 Gy. Approximately 20 of these 84 patients would have had occult metastasis to their lymph nodes, which were controlled in 90% of these patients. Table 9-13 also lists results of 55 patients with clinical stage II disease treated by nodal irradiation who reported a 64% 3-year disease-free survival rate. With the exception of 13 patients in the Royal Marsden Hospital series, essentially all these patients were in the clinical stage IIA category. Retroperitoneal lymph node metastases that were 2 cm or less were sterilized by doses of radiation therapy in 93% of cases. However, the results were significantly worse in patients with bulkier tumors. Only 31% of these were sterilized by radiation therapy. This latter result is greatly inferior to that which can be achieved with multidrug chemotherapy, from which at least three-quarters of the complete responders will have complete sterilization without subsequent recurrence.

### Current Radiation Treatment Policy

For patients with clinical stage I nonseminomatous germ cell testis tumors, patients in the favorable subgroups (no vascular invasion or spermatic cord involvement in the primary tumor and no AFP or hCG elevation following orchiectomy) are either followed on a surveillance protocol or managed with an elective retroperitoneal lymph node dissection. Unlike seminoma, a higher proportion of the relapses will be at sites other than the retroperitoneum. Of this subgroup, 85% will be cured by orchiectomy alone, and radiation has no contemporary role.[37]

In more advanced disease we use "surgical boosts"—retroperitoneal lymph node dissection rather than radiation therapy—as an adjunct after multidrug chemotherapy. Radiation is reserved for patients with particularly large and radiologically unresponsive metastases that, because of their proximity to great blood vessels, are not completely resectable. In this setting, we use doses of 36 Gy at 1.8 Gy fractions following chemotherapy, before or after attempt at surgical resection. Care must be taken if the kidneys must be irradiated following cisplatin-based chemotherapy, which has a potential for nephrotoxicity. The dose to at least two-thirds of the renal parenchyma is kept below 18 Gy. For patients with hematogenous metastases to the CNS or the bones, we recommend following a full course of multidrug chemotherapy with boost doses of radiation to 36 Gy in 4 weeks, inasmuch as these sites often are not amenable to resection without considerable functional loss. Radiation may also be needed in the case of the CNS, since the blood–brain barrier can prevent adequate drug doses from reaching the tumor. As complete response rates to novel aggressive forms of chemotherapy continue to climb, however, these grim scenarios have become increasingly rare.

### LYMPHOMA OF THE TESTIS

Primary lymphoma of the testis is a relatively rare entity but one that must always be considered in the differential diagnosis of an older man with a testicular mass. Such masses are usually of intermediate to high grade B cell histology and have a prognosis comparable to stage IA$_E$ non-Hodgkin lymphoma arising elsewhere in the body. Orchiectomy is the standard initial management but, because of the rarity of this tumor, there are few studies in the literature adequate to guide recommendations about subsequent management.[38-40] Over the last three decades, 26 patients with stage I testicular lymphoma were treated at the MGH. The actuarial 5- and 10-year relapse-free survival for the entire group was 79% and 63%, respectively.[38] In patients receiving adjuvant combination chemotherapy the rate was improved at

5 years (75% vs. 50%), but this advantage was lost by 10 years. No advantage was seen for patients receiving adjuvant radiation to the retroperitoneum. No isolated retroperitoneal relapse was seen in any of the men who did not receive radiation. Older studies from the era before effective chemotherapy have shown an improvement in relapse-free survival when radiation was given. Currently we would not recommend adjuvant radiation unless a patient were unfit for chemotherapy. We treat such a patient as for stage I seminoma but taking the total dose to 36 to 40 Gy. Some have felt that CNS relapse is a common event in this disease and have recommended elective cranial irradiation.[39] This was not seen in any of the 26 MGH patients with median follow-up of 5 years and is, thus, not part of our management.

## REFERENCES

1. Whitmore WF Jr: Surgical treatment of adult germinal testis tumors. *Semin Oncol* 1979;6:85–102.

2. Moriyama N, Daly JJ, Prout GR Jr, et al: Vascular invasion as a prognosticator of metastatic disease in non-seminomatous germ cell tumors of the testis. *Cancer* 1985;56:2492–2498.

3. Herr HW, Whitmore WF Jr., Sogani PC, et al: Selection of testicular tumor patients for omission of retroperitoneal lymph node dissection. *J Urol* 1986;135:500–503.

4. Peckham MJ, McElwain TJ, Hendry FW: Testis and epididymis, in KE Hallman, JL Boak, D Crowther, et al (eds): *The Treatment of Cancer.* New York, Chapman & Hall, 1982, pp 501–528.

5. Fossa SD, Aass N, Kaalhus O: Radiotherapy for testicular seminoma stage I: Treatment results and long range morbidity in 365 patients. *Int J Radiat Oncol Biol Phys* 1989;16:383–388.

6. Hamilton C, Horwich A, Easton D: Radiotherapy for stage I seminoma testis: Results of treatment and complications. *Radiother Oncol* 1986;6:115–120.

7. Thomas GM, Rider WD, Dembo AJ, Cummings BJ, Gospodarowicz MK, Hawkins NV, et al: Seminoma of the testis: Results of treatment and patterns of failure after radiation therapy. *Int J Radiat Oncol Biol Phys* 1982;8:165–174.

8. Schultz HP, von der Maase H, Rorth M, Pedersen M, Nielsen ES, Walbom-Jorgenses S, DATECA Study Group: Testicular seminoma in Denmark 1976–1980: Results of treatment. *Acta Radiol Oncol* 1984;23:263–270.

9. Zagars GK, Babaian RJ: Stage I testicular seminoma: Rationale for post-orchiectomy radiation therapy. *Int J Radiat Oncol Biol Phys* 1987;13:155–162.

10. Kiricuta IC, Sauer J, Bohndorf W: Omission of the pelvic irradiation in stage I testicular seminoma: A study of postorchiectomy paraaortic radiotherapy. *Int J Radiat Oncol Biol Phys* 1996;35:293–301.

11. Fossa SD, Horwich A, Russell JM, Roberts JP, Jakes R, Stenning S, on behalf of MRC Testicular Working Party: Optimal field size in adjuvant radiotherapy (XRT) of stage I seminoma—A randomised trial. *Proc ASCO* 1996; 15:595 (abstr).

12. Kubo HD, Shipley WU: Reduction of the scatter, dose to the testicle outside the radiation treatment fields. *Int J Radiat Oncol Biol Phys* 1982;8:1741–1745.

13. Warde PR, Gospodarowicz MK, Goodman PJ, Sturgeon JF, Jewett MA, Catton CN, et al: Results of a policy of surveillance in stage I testicular seminoma. *Int J Radiat Oncol Biol Phys* 1993;27:11–15.

14. Lai PP, Bernstein MJ, Kim H, Perez CA, Wasserman TH, Kucik NA: Radiation therapy of stage I and IIA testicular seminoma. *Int J Radiat Oncol Biol Phys* 1994;28:373–379.

15. Hunter M, Peschel RE. Testicular seminoma. *Cancer* 1989;64:1608–1611.

16. Vallis KA, Howard GCW, Duncan W, Cornbleet MA, Kerr GR: Radiotherapy for stages I and II testicular seminoma: Results and morbidity in 238 patients. *Br J Radiol* 1995;68:400–405.

17. Tombolini V, Grapulin L, Maurizi Enrici R: Ruolo della radioterapia nel trattamento del seminoma del testicolo. *Radiol Med* 1991;82:334–338.

18. Bayens YC, Helle PA, Van Putten WL: Orchidectomy followed by radiotherapy in 176 stage I and II testicular seminoma patients: Benefits of a 10-year follow-up study. *Radiother Oncol* 1992;25:97–102.

19. Mason BR, Kearsley JH: Radiotherapy for stage 2 testicular seminoma: The prognostic in-

fluence of tumor bulk. *J Clin Oncol* 1988;6: 1856–1862.

20. Evensen JF, Fossa SD, Kjellevold K: Testicular seminoma: Analysis of treatment and failure for stage II disease. *Radiother Oncol* 1985; 4:55–61.

21. Sagerman RH, Kotlove DJ, Regine WF: Stage II seminoma results of post-orchiectomy radiation. *Radiology* 1989;172:565–568.

22. Ball D, Barrett A, Peckham MJ: The management of metastatic seminoma testis. *Cancer* 1982;50:2289–2294.

23. Ellerbroek NA, Tran LM, Selch MT: Testicular seminoma. *Am J Clin Oncol* 1988;11:93–99.

24. Jackson SM, Olivotto I, McLoughlin MG: Radiation therapy for seminoma of the testis: Results in British Columbia. *Can Med Assoc J* 1980;123:507–512.

25. Percarpio B, Clements JC, McLeod DG, et al: Anaplastic seminoma: An analysis of 77 patients. *Cancer* 1979;43:2510–2513.

26. Cockburn AG, Vugrin D, Batata M, et al: Poorly differentiated (anaplastic) seminoma of the testis. *Cancer* 1984;53:1991–1994.

27. Javadpour N, MacIntyre KR, Waidmann TA, et al: Ròle of AFP and hCG in seminoma. *J Urol* 1978;120:687–690.

28. Mauch P, Weichselbaum R, Botnick L: The significance of positive chorionic gonadotropins in apparently pure seminoma of the testis. *Int J Radiat Oncol Biol Phys* 1979;5:887–889.

29. Mirimanof RO, Shiply WU, Dosoretz DE, et al: Pure seminoma of the testis: The results of radiation therapy in patients with elevated human chorionic gonadotropin titers. *J Urol* 1985;134: 1124–1126.

30. Williams SD, Birch R, Einhorn LH, Loehrer PJ: Treatment of disseminated germ-cell tumors with cisplatin, bleomycin, and either vinblastine or etoposide. *New Engl J Med* 1987;316: 1435–1440.

31. Horwich A, Dearnaley D, Nicholls J: Effectiveness of carboplatin, etoposide, and bleomycin combination chemotherapy in good prognosis metastatic testicular non-seminomatous germ cell tumors. *J Clin Oncol* 1991;9:62–69, 1991.

32. Peckham MJ, McElwain TJ: Radiotherapy of testicular tumors. *Proc R Coll Med* 1974;67: 300–307.

33. Tyrrell CJ, Peckham MJ: The response of lymph node metastases of testicular teratoma to radiation therapy. *Br J Urol* 1976;48:363–370.

34. Maier JG, Sulak MH: Radiation therapy in malignant testis tumors. *Cancer* 1973;48:2184–2190.

35. Earle JD, Bagshaw MA, Kaplan HS: Supervoltage radiotherapy of testicular tumors. *Am J Roentgenol* 1973;117:653–661.

36. Lee MS, Hendrickson FR: Analysis of pattern of occurrence in non-seminomatous testicular tumor. *Radiology* 1978;127:775–777.

37. Peckham MJ, Darrett A, Husband JE, et al: Orchiectomy alone in testicular cancer. 1. Non-seminomatous germ cell tumours. *Lancet* 1982;1:678–681.

39. Zietman AL, Coen JJ, Ferry JA, Scully RE, Kaufman DS, McGovern FG: The management and outcome of stage IAE non-Hodgkins lymphoma of the testis. *J Urol* 1996;155:943–946.

39. Crellin AM, Hudson BV, Bennett MH, Harland S, Hudson GV:Non-Hodgkin's lymphoma of the testis. *Radiother Oncol* 1993;27: 99–104.

40. Duncan PR, Checa F, Gowing NF, McElwain TJ, Peckham MJ: Extra-nodal non-Hodgkin's lymphoma presenting in the testicle. A clinical and pathologic study of 24 cases. *Cancer* 1980;45:1578–1585.

# E. PENIS

Because of the prevalence of childhood circumsion, squamous cell carcinoma of the penis is an uncommon tumor in the United States. When it occurs, treatment has traditionally been surgical, with either partial or total penec-tomy. The attendant psychological distress may be considerable, and several larger series document suicide among the causes of death. Radiation can be used effectively for small tumors of the glans and coronal sulcus with high rates

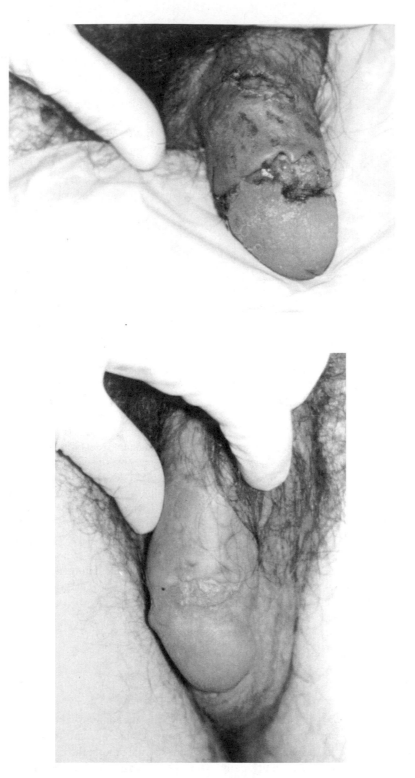

**FIGURE 9-19**   Small squamous cell carcinoma of the penis treated with local electrons to a dose of 52 Gy in 13 fractions.

of local control.[1-6] Surgery may still be used for salvage, and survival rates are comparable to primary penectomy series. Case selection is important. Ideal tumors are distal, less than 4 cm in maximal diameter, with minimal invasion, and well to moderately differentiated.

## TREATMENT TECHNIQUE

Squamous cell carcinoma of the penis is simply a carcinoma of the skin with a high propensity for regional lymph node metastasis. Radiotherapeutic management reflects these two characteristics.

All patients require circumcision to prevent the development of a paraphimosis during radiation as the glans swells. The groins must be carefully palpated. Palpable nodes cannot be assumed to be malignant and are often inflammatory, the result of an ulcerated primary. These men may be treated with a course of antibiotics to see if regression occurs, or fine needle aspiration may be performed. Positive lymph nodes are a grave prognostic sign.

Small, lower grade primary tumors (Figure 9-19) are usually treated by means of an electron beam of appropriate energy with a 2 cm margin. The penis is immobolized between two Lucite plates 5 mm thick that act as bolus and through which the tumor can be clearly seen. A plate of lead protects the testes from radiation. The tumors are treated either with doses of 60 to 66 Gy using 2 Gy fractions or are boosted after 40 Gy with a single- or double-plane interstitial implant, using iridium to deliver a further 25 Gy over 2 days. The latter treatment is not employed if the tumor is greater than 4 cm in diameter or if three planes are required, since the risk of soft tissue necrosis is too high. Very small tumors may be treated with shorter courses of radiation, such as 52 Gy in 13 fractions.

The management of larger or high grade tumors must also address both groins. Patients are treated supine with the penis folded up and taped to the lower anterior abdominal wall. The penis, groins, and low pelvic nodes are encompassed in parallel opposed AP-PA fields and treated with beams of 6 to 10 MV. A bolus of appropriate thickness is applied to the primary tumor. This field is treated to 45 Gy in 1.8 Gy fractions. The penis is then boosted to a total dose in excess of 65 Gy. The final dose is determined by the skin reaction. Moist desquamation is required for a cure.

## RESULTS

Local failure rates in the literature range from 15 to 43% (Table 9-14). Salvage is usually possible with penectomy, and uncontrolled primary tumors as a result of this organ-sparing approach are very unusual. Complications of therapy occur with an incidence that relates to tumor size and treatment technique. Urethral or meatal strictures occur in 14% to 41%, and soft tissue necrosis requiring penectomy in 3% to 15%. The higher figures almost invariably come from series that have employed an

TABLE 9-14   Recent Larger Series (> 50 Patients) Reporting Outcome of the Use of Radiation Therapy for Squamous Cell Carcinoma of the Penis

| Author | Number of Patients | Treatment | Local Failure (%) | Urethral Stricture (%) | Penectomy for Necrosis (%) |
|---|---|---|---|---|---|
| Delannes et al.[1] | 51 | [192]Ir implant | 18 | 41 | 16 |
| Rozan et al.[2] | 259 | [192]Ir implant ± EBRT | 15 | 30 | 7 |
| Ravi et al.[3] | 156 | EBRT or implant | 35 | 24 | 6 |
| Sarin et al.[4] | 69 | EBRT or implant | 43 | 14 | 3 |

implant as sole therapy. Some degree of soft tissue necrosis, which may or may not heal with time and conservative management, is very common when lesions over 4 cm diameter are implanted. When regional lymph nodes are involved, cure is unlikely even if groin dissections are employed because of the high risk of pelvic nodal and distant spread.

Acute reactions usually force patients to abstain from sexual activity during and for a few months after therapy, but afterward they can resume. One small study documented that sexual potency was preserved or only slightly diminished in 10 of 12 radiation-treated patients. It is also our experience that erectile potency is well preserved.[7]

The results clearly show that any man with an early stage penile cancer who wishes to preserve intact both his penis and his sexual function can do so without risk to his life.

## REFERENCES

1. Delannes M, Malavaud B, Douchez J: Iridium-192 interstitial therapy for squamous cell carcinoma of the penis. *Int J Radiat Oncol Biol Phys* 1992;24:479–483.

2. Rozan R, Albuisson E, Giraud B, Donnarieix D, Delannes M: Interstitial brachytherapy for penile carcinoma: A multicentric survey (259 patients). *Radiother Oncol* 1995;36:83–93.

3. Ravi R, Chaturvedi HK, Sastry D: Role of radiation therapy in treatment of carcinoma of the penis. *Br J Urol* 1994;74:646–651.

4. Sarin R, Norman AR, Steel GG, Horwich A: Treatment results and prognostic factors in 101 men treated for squamous cell carcinoma of the penis. *Int J Radiat Oncol Biol Phys* 1997; 38:713–722.

5. Duncan W, Jackson SM: The treatment of early cancer of the penis with megavoltage x-rays. *Clin Radiol* 1972;23:246–258.

6. Salaverria JC, Hope-Stone HF, Paris AM: Conservative treatment of carcinoma of the penis. *Br J Urol* 1979;51:21–37.

7. Opjordsmoen S, Wachre H, Aass N, Fossa SD: Sexuality in patients treated for penile cancer. Patients' experience and doctor's judgement. *Br J Urol* 1994;73:554–560.

# CHAPTER 10

# GYNECOLOGIC CANCER

## A.  Carcinoma of the Endometrium - PATRICIA J. EIFEL

### INTRODUCTION

The uterine fundus is the most common site of gynecologic malignancy in United States women, with about 35,000 cases diagnosed per year.[1] However, because symptoms of endometrial carcinoma, most commonly post-menopausal bleeding, characteristically present at an early stage, most cases are curable, and only about 5000 women die of the disease per year. More than 75% of cases occur in postmenopausal women, and fewer than 5% in women under the age of 40. Factors associated with an increased incidence of the disease include the use of unopposed exogenous estrogens and conditions that result in chronic increased or prolonged endogenous estrogen exposure (estrogen-secreting tumors, low parity, early menarche, late menopause, and morbid obesity).[2,3] Increased risk also has been associated with long-term tamoxifen use,[1] hypertension, and diabetes mellitus. Obesity and comorbid illnesses often complicate treatment.

Endometrial carcinomas usually originate in the endometrial epithelium but may then invade locally to involve the myometrium, gaining access to its rich lymphatic network. Cancers also may spread to involve the uterine cervix or metastasize locally to the ovaries, parametrium, or vagina. Invasive cancers can progress regionally to involve the external or common iliac nodes or can spread directly to the para-aortic nodes via the tubo-ovarian lymphatic vessels. In this respect, uterine cancers differ from primary cervical cancers, which rarely, if ever, involve the para-aortic nodes without pelvic node metastases. The most common sites of distant metastasis are the lung and upper abdomen. Intra-abdominal spread is most commonly seen in patients with high grade papillary serous carcinomas of the endometrium.

Before 1988, a clinical staging system (Table 10-1) was used to classify corpus cancers, which were often treated with radiation before hysterectomy. As treatment preferences shifted to the use of hysterectomy as the initial treatment or immediately (2–3 days) following preoperative intracavitary treatment, interest in developing a "surgical staging system" resulted in the 1998 revisions of the staging system of the International Federation of Gynecology and Obstetrics (FIGO)[4] (Table 10-2).

The 1988 staging system includes important prognostic information about the depth of myometrial infiltration and resolves problems found in the earlier FIGO grading system, providing more detailed descriptions of tumor grades, and for the first time emphasizing the prognostic importance of cytologic grade, particularly for patients with papillary serous

**TABLE 10-1   Clinical Staging in Carcinoma of the Corpus Uteri**

| Stage | Description |
|-------|-------------|
| 0 | Atypical endometrial hyperplasia, carcinoma in situ. Histological findings are suspicious of malignancy. Cases of stage 0 should not be included in any therapeutic statistics. |
| I | The carcinoma is confined to the corpus. |
| IA | The uterine cavity is 8 cm or less in length. |
| IB | The uterine cavity is longer than 8 cm. |
| II | The carcinoma has involved the corpus and the cervix, but has not extended outside the uterus. |
| III | The carcinoma has extended outside the uterus, but not outside the true pelvis. |
| IV | The carcinoma has extended outside the true pelvis or has obviously involved the mucosa of the bladder or rectum. A bullous edema as such does not permit a case to be allotted to stage IV. |
| IVA | Spread of the growth to adjacent organs as urinary bladder. |
| IVB | Spread to distant organs. |

*Source:* International Federation of Gynecology and Obstetrics (FIGO) 1988 correlation with the nomenclature of the International Union Against Cancer (UICC) and the American Joint Cancer Committee on Cancer Staging (AJCC).

adenocarcinomas. However, the surgical staging system presents several other problems.

1. Subgroups of clinical stages I and II are shifted to the surgical stage III category, making it impossible to translate from the surgical to the clinical staging system; consequently, current results cannot be related to those of any studies that include patients treated before 1988.

2. The pre-1988 clinical staging system must still be used to categorize patients who are treated with radiation alone or with preoperative external beam radiation therapy (EBRT).

3. Although surgical staging is mandated, FIGO does not define the extent of the procedure, which varies widely.

4. Positive peritoneal cytology places patients in stage III, although patients for whom this is the sole site of extrauterine disease have an excellent prognosis.

**TABLE 10-2   Surgical Staging in Carcinoma of the Corpus Uteri**

| Stage | Description |
|-------|-------------|
| IA | Tumor is limited to the endometrium. |
| IB | Tumor invades less than half of the myometrial thickness. |
| IC | Tumor invades more than half of the myometrial thickness. |
| IIA | Endocervical glandular involvement only. |
| IIB | Tumor invades the cervical stroma. |
| IIIA | Tumor invades the uterine serosa, adnexa, or positive peritoneal cytology. |
| IIIB | Vaginal metastases are present. |
| IIIC | Tumor has spread to pelvic or para-aortic lymph nodes. |
| IVA | Tumor invades the mucosa of the bladder or rectosigmoid. |
| IVB | Distant metastases are present. |

Tumor grade (G 1, 2, 3) should always be specified in staging (e.g., stage IA G1). Carcinomas should be grouped with regard to the degree of differentiation of the adenocarcinoma as follows:

G1   $\leq$5% of a nonsquamous or nonmorular solid growth pattern

G2   6–50% of a nonsquamous or nonmorular solid growth pattern

G3   >50% of a nonsquamous or nonmorular solid growth pattern

Notes to grading:

1. Notable nuclear atypia, inappropriate for the architectural grade, raises the grade of a G1 or G2 tumor by 1.

2. In serous adenocarcinomas, clear cell adenocarcinomas, and squamous cell carcinomas, nuclear grading takes precedence.

3. Adenocarcinomas with squamous differentiation are graded according to the nuclear grade of the glandular component.

*Source:* FIGO 1988.

## PRETREATMENT INVESTIGATION

The initial diagnosis of endometrial carcinoma is usually made from an endometrial biopsy or curettage. Historically, fractional curettage has been recommended to evaluate the cervix for possible involvement, but the accuracy of this procedure is poor.[5] When cervical involvement is suspected, a cervical biopsy should be performed. In addition to a dilatation and curettage, the pretreatment evaluation should include a careful history and physical examination, laboratory studies, and a chest x-ray. Further studies are probably warranted only in patients with an abnormal pelvic examination. Intravenous pyelogram is rarely helpful and probably should not be part of the routine preoperative workup. Occasionally, magnetic resonance imaging can clarify the primary site in patients with extensive cervical involvement. Some clinicians suggest obtaining a preoperative computed tomographic scan and carbohydrate antigen 125 (CA-125) in women with uterine papillary serous carcinoma (UPSC). For inoperable patients and those who require initial pelvic radiation therapy (RT), clinical stage is determined using the pre-1988 categories. For all other patients, stage is determined after hysterectomy and abdominal exploration using surgical staging schema.

## SURGICAL TREATMENT AND STAGING

A type I, simple extrafascial abdominal hysterectomy with bilateral salpingoopherectomy (TAH-BSO) is the hysterectomy of choice for most patients with endometrial carcinoma. The ovaries are usually removed because most women are post- or perimenopausal at diagnosis and because women with endometrial carcinoma are at significant risk for ovarian metastasis or independent primary ovarian cancer. Some surgeons are now performing laparoscopic-assisted vaginal hysterectomy and lymph node dissection in selected patients. The morbidity of a radical hysterectomy is rarely justified unless a primary surgical approach is being used for a patient with gross cervical involvement.

The current surgical staging system requires surgical evaluation of the abdomen and regional lymph nodes, but FIGO has never specified the operative procedure that should be performed. In practice, intraoperative lymph node evaluations range from none at all or palpation of nodal areas with biopsy of enlarged nodes to extensive pelvic and para-aortic lymphadenectomy. Surgeons may dissect or sample only the pelvic nodes, only the para-aortic nodes, or both.

Most clinicians feel uncomfortable subjecting a patient with a minimally invasive grade 1 tumor (and a negligible risk of regional metastasis) to the morbidity of a full abdominal staging, arguing for intraoperative assessment of the hysterectomy specimen followed by selective lymphadenectomy only for patients with deeply invasive or high grade disease. The spirit of the staging system clearly suggests that both the pelvic and aortic nodes should be evaluated, although many surgeons limit the procedure to a pelvic or para-aortic lymphadenectomy, depending on their treatment philosophy.

## PROGNOSTIC FACTORS

In the absence of sound prospective randomized studies, decisions about the need for adjuvant treatment must be based on a thorough understanding of the natural history of the disease and risk factors for recurrence. In particular, the histologic grade and subtype of the carcinoma, the extent of disease in the uterus, and the presence and distribution of extrauterine disease can be used to predict the risk of tumor recurrence in the vagina, pelvis, abdomen, and in distant sites. This information is used to counsel the patient about the potential value of adjuvant treatment.

### Histologic Subtype and Grade

The four major histologic patterns of Müllerian neoplasia listed in Table 10-3 arise, with varying frequency, in any of the organs that comprise the

**TABLE 10-3   Müllerian Neoplasms**

| Histology | Features | Differentiated Features Similar to | Most Often Seen in Carcinoma of | Clinical Stage I Uterine Cases (%) | Comments |
|---|---|---|---|---|---|
| Endometrioid | Stratified epithelium<br>Cribriform ("back-to-back") glandular pattern<br>Increasingly disorganized glandular formation and solid sheets of cells as grade increases | Hyperplastic endometrium | Endometrium | 75–80 | Squamous elements should not be included in grading |
| Mucinous | Architecture similar to endometrioid neoplasms<br>Abundant intracytoplasmic mucin | Endocervical glandular epithelium | Cervix, Ovary | 5–10 | |
| Papillary serous (UPSC) | Papillary growth pattern often on coarse fibrous stalks<br>Pleomorphic cytology (nuclear anaplasia, macronucleoli)<br>Psammoma bodies in 25–30% | Fallopian tube epithelium | Ovary, fallopian tube | 10–15 (pure or mixed) | Should not be confused with other papillary subtypes (e.g., villoglandular) |
| Clear cell | Glandular, sheetlike, or papillary growth<br>Prominent cytoplasmic clearing<br>Nuclear pleomorphism ("extruded" nuclei in "hob-nail" cells)<br>Often merges with areas of UPSC | Arias–Stella reaction seen in hyperprogestational states | Ovary (cervix or vagina after *in utero* exposure to diethylstilbestrol) | 5–10 | Should not be confused with secretory carcinoma (usually low grade) |

*Two or more types of differentiation are often seen in one tumor. Prognosis is dominated by UPSC if any is present.

so-called extended Müllerian system (ovary, fallopian tube, endometrium, cervix, upper vagina, and pelvic peritoneum).[6] The site of origin of a cancer may be difficult or impossible to determine with certainty from histopathologic examination alone and is often based on the distribution of disease. In some cases (e.g., some adenocarcinomas of the uterine isthmus), the assignment cannot be made with certainty; specification of the primary site in these cases is often based on the probability of a histologic type arising in a given site.

Most endometrial carcinomas are of the endometrioid type and are graded primarily on the basis of their architectural pattern (the proportion of tumor that is solid vs. glandular). Cytologic grade usually parallels architectural grade for endometrioid and mucinous carcinomas. Areas of squamous differentiation may be benign-appearing or frankly malignant. Tumors with benign squamous elements are sometimes called "adenoacanthomas," and those with malignant squamous elements are called "adenosquamous carcinomas." Some authors have reported a relatively poor prognosis for adeno-

squamous cancers, probably because malignant squamous elements are usually associated with high grade adenocarcinomas.[7]

Atypical endometrial hyperplasias and well-differentiated carcinomas represent points on a morphologic continuum. In the absence of discrete criteria for differentiating "benign" from "malignant," pathologists' thresholds have evolved over time and still vary somewhat today. This complicates comparisons among institutions or even with historical controls—a less restrictive threshold for labeling a lesion as cancer will artificially inflate the apparent survival rate of a group of patients with endometrial carcinoma. This is only one of several reasons for viewing with skepticism studies that lack contemporary review of histologic material. The clinical importance of primary UPSC was first recognized in the early 1980s (Figure 10-1).[8] Numerous studies have since confirmed that this form of endometrial cancer, morphologically identical to high grade serous carcinoma of the ovary, behaves very aggressively, with frequent deep myometrial invasion, lymph–vascular space invasion, a

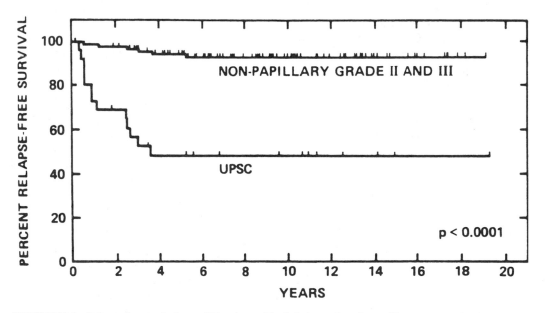

**FIGURE 10-1** Relapse-free survival rate of 26 patients with clinical stage I uterine papillary serous carcinoma compared with that of patients with grade 2-3 tumors of other histologic types. (Patients with evidence of extrauterine disease at hysterectomy were excluded.) (From Ref. 8.)

marked tendency to disseminate intraperitoneally, and a poor survival rate compared with other subtypes. The strictly architectural grading system recommended by FIGO before 1988 was inappropriate for UPSC because the highly ordered papillary architecture of many of these lesions belies their anaplastic cytologic appearance and aggressive behavior. Papillary serous cancers should be distinguished from other papillary lesions (e.g., villoglandular adenocarcinomas) that are not serous, have low grade cytologic features, and enjoy a relatively good prognosis. Clear cell carcinoma is a rare subtype that, when present, is frequently associated with UPSC. When any serous carcinoma is present, the prognosis for patients with clear cell carcinoma is poor; however, there is some evidence that the prognosis of pure clear cell carcinomas is less ominous.[9] Grade 1 carcinomas with secretory vacuolization ("secretory carcinomas") are sometimes erroneously called clear cell carcinoma but have an excellent prognosis.

### Myometrial, Cervical Invasion

The depth of myometrial infiltration is one of the most important predictors of lymph node involvement and prognosis.[10–12] Tumors that have not invaded the myometrium rarely involve lymph nodes and are usually curable with hysterectomy alone (although high grade tumors will occasionally recur in the vaginal apex). UPSC may be an exception, because these tumors have been reported to behave aggressively in the absence of demonstrable myometrial invasion.[13]

Tumors that involve the cervix are classified by FIGO as stage II. Tumors that involve only endocervical glands (FIGO stage IIA) have a relatively good prognosis, probably similar to that of patients with tumors of comparable grade and depth that are confined to the fundus. Tumors that involve the endocervical stroma have a poorer prognosis, with a higher likelihood of extrauterine involvement and disease recurrence. Presumably, the involvement of cervical stroma gives the tumor access to cervical regional routes of spread, placing pelvic nodes at relatively greater risk. Because many clinicians still prescribe preoperative pelvic irradiation for patients with definite clinical evidence of cervical stromal invasion, there is as yet limited data reliably documenting the survival rate of FIGO (1988) stage IIB disease. In a small series of surgically staged patients, Fanning et al. reported recurrences in five of eight with stage IIB disease and no recurrences among 12 patients with stage IIA disease.[14]

### Tumor Size

Schink and colleagues[15] reported a relationship between the size of an endometrial primary tumor and the rates of lymph node metastasis and survival. The predictive value of tumor size appeared to be independent of the grade or depth of invasion of the endometrial cancer. This is one factor that may influence the decision to treat when the indications for adjuvant treatment are in a "gray zone."

### Lymph Node Involvement

With the advent of "routine" surgical staging, more detailed information is becoming available about the incidence and prognostic importance of various patterns of extrauterine spread. However, the results of surgical staging studies still must be viewed with caution. Because node dissections and washings were not routinely performed before 1988, many of the patients in retrospective studies of "pathologic staging" were not surgically staged by FIGO criteria. So far, the only large prospective study of surgical staging (albeit in clinically staged patients) is from the Gynecologic Oncology Group (GOG).[12,16] Though this study is valuable, its significance is compromised somewhat by large numbers of ineligible and inevaluable patients and by inconsistencies in the numbers of patients excluded in different reports of the study. The small number of cases said to have been excluded because of UPSC or clear cell histology suggests that some cases may not have been identified. If so, the incidences of positive cytology, abdominal relapse, and death from disease might be misleading.

Nevertheless, these reports provide some of the best data available about the relationships among hysterectomy findings, regional involvement, and outcome. Overall, lymph node metastases were reported in 70 of 621 (11%) evaluable patients.[16] Approximately half of those with documented nodal involvement had positive para-aortic nodes, 32% of those with pelvic node metastases also had positive para-aortic nodes, and 12 of 70 patients with regional metastases had only para-aortic node involvement. There is a strong correlation between lymph node involvement, particularly aortic involvement, and prognosis (Figure 10-2). However, regional node involvement does appear to be curable in many cases. The Gynecologic Oncology Group reported a 70% survival rate among patients with histologically documented pelvic node involvement and negative aortic node involvement. Although treatment

details were not given, it was stated that most patients had pelvic RT. The survival rate for patients with positive para-aortic nodes in that study was 40%, which is comparable with other reports of patients treated with extended field (EFRT).[17-20]

## Peritoneal Cytology

Although involvement of peritoneal cytology influences the current FIGO staging of patients with uterine cancer, its significance is still uncertain. Some authors have reported a poorer prognosis for patients with abnormal cytology, but these studies have not consistently identified patients with papillary serous cancers.[12,21] Other investigators have concluded that cytology is not an independent risk factor for recurrence.[22,23] In the past, reactive mesothelial cells sometimes were confused with malignant cells. However, even a clear finding of malignant cells in peritoneal washings may be of questionable value. Morrow

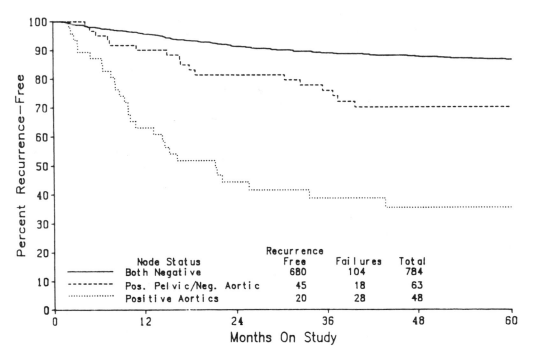

**FIGURE 10-2** Recurrence-free interval in 784 patients with negative pelvic and para-aortic node dissections, 63 patients with positive pelvic but negative para-aortic nodes, or 48 patients with positive para-aortic nodes. (From Ref. 12.)

and colleagues[12] concluded that the data "seem to indicate that positive cytology is associated with not only an increased risk for abdominal recurrence but regional/distant recurrence in general." However, in a multivariate analysis, washings did not add significantly to the predictive value of other extrauterine metastasis. In patients without nodes, adnexal spread, or gross laparotomy findings, positive cytology appeared to have some predictive value for recurrence (RR = 2.4; $p$ = 0.02); however, cytology was a much less powerful predictor than grade or myometrial invasion, and only 2 of 32 evaluable patients who had positive cytology without other extrauterine disease had recurrences in the abdomen. Peritoneal cytology alone is rarely, if ever, an indication that very aggressive adjuvant treatment is needed. Certainly, in a patient with G1-2 non-UPSC histology, minimal myometrial invasion, and no other evidence of extrauterine spread, peritoneal washings should not be considered an indication for whole abdominal RT (WART) or systemic chemotherapy.

### Adnexal Metastases and Simultaneous Ovarian Primary Tumors

Although endometrial carcinomas may metastasize to the ovaries, some patients who present with simultaneous disease in the endometrium and ovary actually have multiple primary tumors. In particular, patients who have low grade endometrioid neoplasms with minimal myometrial invasion and early ovarian disease tend to have an excellent prognosis, with survival rates of 80% to 100%, suggesting that these lesions do not represent either metastatic ovarian or endometrial cancer.[24,25] Women with simultaneous endometrial and ovarian tumors tend to present with disease at a younger age than most patients with cancer of the endometrium or ovary alone (median 40–50 years), adding to the evidence that their tumors represent some kind of field defect. In some cases, it may be impossible to determine the site(s) of origin. Erratic assignment of these patients to one diagnosis or the other may influence the apparent survival rates

of patients with stage IIIa disease, but in most cases these patients are best served by therapy that would be considered appropriate for each disease site. For example, if there is G1 noninvasive disease in the endometrium and a small G1 endometrioid tumor in the ovary, surgery alone is probably sufficient. If the extent of the ovarian or endometrial disease would generally be considered sufficient to warrant adjuvant treatment (e.g., deep myometrial invasion or invasion of adjacent tissues by the ovarian tumor), then appropriate treatment for those conditions is warranted.

## ADJUVANT TREATMENT

Despite decades of study, the role of adjuvant (pre- or postsurgical) treatment has been difficult to define. Several factors have contributed to this.

1. Because treatment failure is expected in only about 15% of patients after surgery alone, the margin for improvement is small and many patients or highly selected populations are needed to demonstrate the effects of adjuvant treatments.

2. Few randomized trials have been completed.

3. Retrospective studies have been compromised by biases in the selection of patients for adjuvant treatment, ambiguities and changes in pathologic and staging classifications, and the widespread use of preoperative RT before the mid-1980s. In this context, treatment decisions often must be based on our understanding of the natural history of the disease, our interpretation of data, which are frequently flawed, reporting the influence of RT on recurrence patterns, and an estimate of the risk of complications in an individual case.

Intracavitary radium was first used to treat uterine cancers shortly after the discovery of radium in 1895. Early investigators described complete tumor responses in subsequent hysterectomy specimens and advocated the use of combined preoperative radium and hysterectomy on theoretical grounds.[26] Preoperative irradiation decreased the vaginal recurrence rates for patients with clinical stage I disease, but was never clearly demonstrated to improve overall survival. As high energy megavoltage linear accelerators became available, the use of EBRT increased, and postoperative intracavitary RT (ICRT) was used increasingly to secure local control of possible microscopic disease in the vaginal cuff. Although there are still some advocates of preoperative ICRT for patients with high grade clinical stage I and IIA disease, most clinicians now prefer to operate first and tailor any adjuvant treatment to the surgical findings.

Preoperative RT may be useful for patients who have gross tumor involvement of the cervix. In these cases, deep cervical stromal invasion probably increases the risk of spread to the paracervical tissues. Preoperative ICRT delivers a higher dose to these regions than postoperative brachytherapy and reduces the risk of having positive margins after a type I simple hysterectomy. Preoperative pelvic irradiation also may be used to shrink cervical tumor but should generally be avoided in patients with UPSC, because these patients are at very high risk for extrapelvic disease. Alternatively, some surgeons might recommend a radical hysterectomy for patients with bulky stage II disease, but the morbidity associated with the more radical surgery is greater, and postoperative RT may still be necessary.

## Postoperative Pelvic Irradiation

Postoperative pelvic irradiation clearly reduces the risk for pelvic recurrence, but no study has yet determined whether it improves the survival rates of patients with high risk features. Only one prospective randomized study, which was conducted at the Norwegian Radium Hospital,[10] has evaluated the benefit of postoperative pelvic irradiation. Patients with clinical stage I disease all had TAH-BSO and postoperative vaginal radium treatment (60 Gy vaginal surface dose). Comprehensive surgical staging was not done, but patients with "proven metas-

tases at surgery" were excluded. The results demonstrated a lower overall rate of pelvic recurrence in patients who had pelvic irradiation, but overall survival was not significantly better. Patients with deeply invasive grade 3 disease appeared to have a somewhat better survival rate, but the number in this subset was small, and the result was not statistically significant. The authors hypothesized that improved pelvic control with pelvic irradiation did not result in a higher survival rate, because patients recurred instead at distant sites. However, subset analysis showed that local control was most improved in patients with deeply invasive tumors, whereas distant metastases appeared to be more frequent in those with superficial or no muscle invasion (Figure 10-3). Unfortunately, even this relatively large prospective study included too few patients with high risk tumors and disease-related deaths to demonstrate or rule out clinically significant differences in survival.

Several authors have argued that excellent (80–90%) survival rates achieved after adjuvant pelvic irradiation in patients with high risk (e.g., high grade or deeply invasive) cancers provide indirect evidence of the treatment's efficacy.[27–30] In particular, Carey and colleagues[27] reported an 81% 5-year, relapse-free survival rate in 157 patients with high risk (G3, deep invasion, or cervical involvement) clinical stage I tumors. The local recurrence rate was 4%, compared with 29% in a separate group of 28 patients who refused adjuvant treatment. In another relatively large study, Kucera and colleagues[28] reported an 88% survival rate in 229 patients with G2-3 tumors that invaded the myometrium by more than one-third or G1 tumors that were invading the outer third, not significantly different from the 91% survival rate of patients with more favorable tumors treated with hysterectomy and vaginal irradiation alone. The 70% projected 5-year survival rate reported by the Gynecologic Oncology Group in 63 patients with positive pelvic nodes (and negative para-aortic nodes) also may provide indirect evidence of the benefit of pelvic RT in high risk patients.[12]

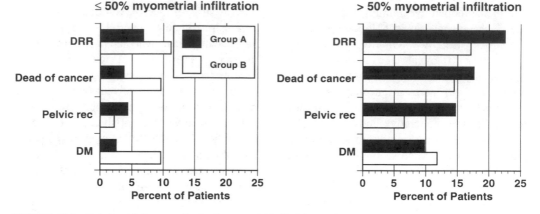

**FIGURE 10-3**  Relationship between depth of myometrial infiltration and recurrence for patients treated with (group B) or without (group A) postoperative pelvic radiotherapy: DRR, death and recurrence rate; DM, distant metastasis. (Adapted from Ref. 10.)

Pelvic RT may be delivered by means of a four-field technique or anterior and posterior opposed fields with 15 to 20 MV photons. Four fields are usually preferred for patients who have had an extensive lymphadenectomy or who have wound problems. The lateral fields should usually receive less weighting than the anterior and posterior fields (e.g., 50:50:40:40, AP:PA:RL:LL) to reduce the lateral applied dose (a computer plan should be done). However, patients are frequently very obese, and wide lateral separations may compromise the day-to-day reproducibility of lateral fields. Anterior fields may be treated by means of a compression device attached to the blocking tray that raises the pannus and reduces the anterior–posterior separation by up to 10 cm. Typical pelvic treatment fields extend from L4-5 to the mid or lower pubic ramus (verifying that there is at least a 4–5 cm margin on the vaginal cuff identified with a radiopaque marker).

The total treatment dose is usually 40 to 50 Gy at 1.8 to 2.0 Gy per fraction. Extracapsular nodal extension or close margins on cervical disease may warrant an external beam boost. Serious complications are observed in about 5% of patients who received standard doses of EBRT but are probably increased in patients who have had a lymphadenectomy.[31] Possible indications for vaginal vault irradiation are discussed below.

## INDICATIONS FOR EFRT OR WART

EFRT is indicated for patients with nonserous endometrial cancers with evidence of extrapelvic disease in the para-aortic nodes only. Expected survival rates are 30% to 50%.[17–20,32,33] There is as yet no evidence that chemotherapy is as effective in this setting as EFRT.

In most cases, the upper border of the field should be T11-12 to cover perirenal nodes that are at risk for direct spread via the tubo-ovarian vessels. Whenever possible, treatment should be with photons of at least 15 MV. Four fields may be used, but care must be taken to monitor the renal dose. CT planning should be obtained to verify the dose to para-aortic nodes as well as to spinal cord and kidney, particularly if four fields are used. Small boost fields may be used to increase the dose to residual gross disease or sites of extracapsular spread to 55 to 60 Gy (depending on the volume). However, the entire extended field probably cannot be taken beyond 45 to 50.4 Gy at 1.8 Gy per fraction without a significant risk of major complications.

A number of investigators have explored the use of WART in the treatment of patients with tumors considered to be at high risk for intra-abdominal recurrence. In particular, patients with UPSC and patients with biopsy-proven evidence of peritoneal involvement who have minimal or no microscopic residual disease after hysterectomy may be good candidates for WART. For the reasons discussed above, involvement of peritoneal washings or lymph nodes alone probably is not sufficient indication for WART in patients with nonserous tumors, although several groups, including the Gynecologic Oncology Group, have included such patients in studies of WART.

Justification for the use of WART in patients with papillary serous tumors arises from the high rate of recurrence in the upper abdomen in patients treated to the pelvis alone[34-36] and the relatively poor results achieved thus far with chemotherapy.[37] Unfortunately, published reports of WART for UPSC are still largely anecdotal, probably because this is a rare disease that has been well recognized for only 10 to 15 years and because it tends to affect elderly women who may not be ideal candidates for aggressive treatment. Reports of unexpected, long-term survivors among patients treated after documentation of upper abdominal involvement suggest that this approach may be effective,[38-41] but larger prospective studies are needed to fully define the role and indications for WART.

Some authors have recommended WART for patients with FIGO stage III nonserous tumors, but studies have been retrospective and have included few patients. In 1992 the GOG completed a large phase II study of WART in 137 patients with stage I–IV UPSC or clear cell carcinoma and 77 patients with stage III–IV endometrial carcinoma of other histologic types. This study is still being analyzed, and the GOG is currently randomizing similar patients between WART and doxorubicin/cisplatin chemotherapy. Scrutiny of the patterns of failure among patients whose pathology has been carefully reviewed suggests that intra-abdominal spread is rare in tumors that have no papillary serous component, suggesting that WART probably is not warranted in most cases, even when the washings are positive.

WART is usually given using AP-PA fields. The photon energy should be based on the thickness of the patient's subcutaneous tissue. The use of beams exceeding 15 MV in very thin women can place peritoneal surfaces in the buildup region. The upper border of the field should be determined under fluoroscopy to give a 1 cm margin on the upper excursion of the diaphragm under quiet respiration. Computed tomography assists in treatment planning and is used to verify the position of the kidneys and the borders of the peritoneal cavity. Use of standard anatomic landmarks can result in underdosage to portions of the peritoneum. Computed tomography studies have shown that the pelvic peritoneum sometimes extends lateral to the anterior iliac crest. A number of treatment schedules have been used for WART. Doses of 25 to 30 Gy at 1.5 Gy per fraction are usually tolerated if the patient is well covered with antiemetics and blood counts are followed closely. The kidneys are usually shielded with posterior 2-5 half-value-layer blocks to restrict the dose to less than 18 Gy and liver blocks to shield the right lobe of the liver after about 25 Gy. Most investigators recommend a boost to the pelvis, bringing the total dose to 45 to 50 Gy. Some investigators also boost the para-aortic nodes and medial diaphragms to approximately 42 Gy.

## POSTOPERATIVE VAGINAL IRRADIATION

Vaginal ICRT may be prescribed in selected cases to prevent vaginal recurrence. Experience suggests that postoperative and preoperative ICRT have the same effect in preventing relapse, although they have never been compared in a prospective study. The magnitude of the benefit of adjuvant ICRT is, however, difficult to define, because clinicians differ in their criteria for adding external pelvic irradiation and because reported vaginal recurrence rates after hysterectomy alone range from 2% to 20%.

The most common site of vaginal recurrence is in the region of the hysterectomy scar in the apical vagina. Recurrences also may occur suburethrally in the distal anterior vagina or uncommonly in other sites. The mechanism of vaginal recurrence is not well understood, but there are at least two possible routes of spread: implantation into disturbed sites, principally in the vaginal apex, and lymph–vascular. The first mechanism is probably most consistent with the relatively high cure rates after aggressive treatment of isolated vaginal recurrences and might explain the wide variation in vaginal recurrence rates reported in different institutions. A number of case reports of episiotomy scar recurrences in women with cervical cancers (adenocarcinoma or squamous) who delivered babies vaginally suggests that implantation is a potential mechanism of gynecologic tumor recurrences.

Vaginal ICRT alone is usually used to treat patients at intermediate risk for recurrence. A possible approach to selecting external beam or intracavitary treatment for patients in various risk groups is illustrated in Figure 10-4. This schema assumes that patients with deeply invasive cancer are a highest risk for regional spread, and the risk increases in parallel with tumor grade. Patients at intermediate risk, particularly those with noninvasive or minimally

invasive high grade lesions, may be at risk for isolated vaginal recurrence and are probably the best candidates for vaginal ICRT alone.

Variations in clinicians' choice of dose and dose rate, and their determination about target volume (vaginal length), and indications for vaginal ICRT probably reflect uncertainties about the degree of risk and mechanisms of recurrence. Some investigators advocate treatment of the entire vaginal length; however this approach increases vaginal morbidity. Because the greatest risk is to the vaginal apex and because the suburethral distal vagina is difficult to cover adequately without undue morbidity, most clinicians treat only the upper one third to one half of the vagina.

The vaginal cuff can be treated with low dose rate (LDR) or fractionated high dose rate (HDR) irradiation. If EBRT is not given, the typical dose delivered with LDR ICRT is 60 to 70 Gy to the vaginal surface in about 72 hours. A variety of applicators have been used, including Delclos or Henschke ovoids; a variety of preloaded or afterloaded Lucite vaginal cylinders exists, as well. The Delclos vaginal cylin-

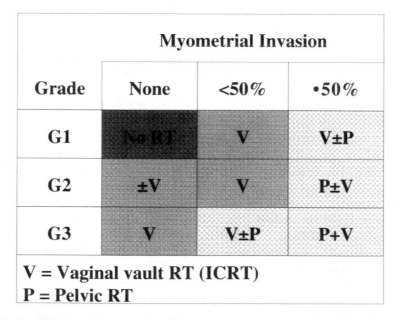

| Grade | Myometrial Invasion | | |
|---|---|---|---|
| | **None** | **<50%** | **•50%** |
| **G1** | No RT | V | V±P |
| **G2** | ±V | V | P±V |
| **G3** | V | V±P | P+V |
| **V = Vaginal vault RT (ICRT)** | | | |
| **P = Pelvic RT** | | | |

**FIGURE 10-4** Possible schema for postoperative treatment based on grade and depth of invasion. However, other prognostic factors, including tumor size and lymph node status, and risk factors for major complications should also be considered in selecting treatment.

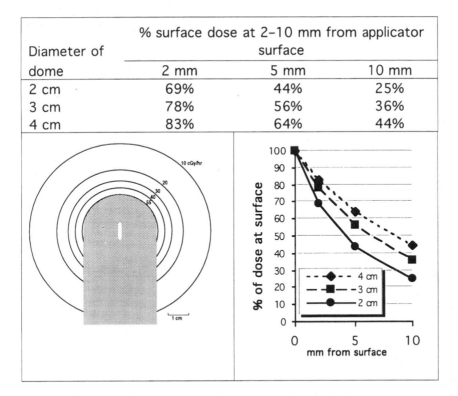

| Diameter of dome | % surface dose at 2–10 mm from applicator surface | | |
|---|---|---|---|
| | 2 mm | 5 mm | 10 mm |
| 2 cm | 69% | 44% | 25% |
| 3 cm | 78% | 56% | 36% |
| 4 cm | 83% | 64% | 44% |

**FIGURE 10-5** Decline in dose from the surface of a Delclos dome cylinder loaded with a single point source of $^{137}$Cs.

der is loaded with a point source of $^{137}$Cs and delivers a homogeneous dose to the surface of the apical vagina (Figure 10-5). Some clinicians give additional ICRT to the vaginal cuff after pelvic RT, although the benefit of this treatment is uncertain. Bliss and Cowie[42] reported a lower vaginal recurrence rate (10% vs. 0%) in patients who had ICRT added to pelvic RT, but gastrointestinal toxicity was also increased. In a similar retrospective review, Randall and colleagues[43] reported no improvement in local control when the vaginal cuff received an ICRT boost. A typical dose prophylactic ICRT of the cuff after pelvic irradiation is 30 Gy in 48 hours (LDR) or 15 to 18 Gy in three fractions (HDR) prescribed to the vaginal surface.

HDR ICRT has some obvious advantages over LDR for prophylactic cuff RT. Placement of the applicator is simple, requires no sedation, and is an outpatient procedure. The standard geometry of the applicators permits rapid cal-

culation of source dwell times. In this setting, the theoretical radiobiological disadvantages of HDR versus LDR are of less concern than in the treatment of primary tumors, because the modest dose required for prophylactic treatment usually does not approach normal tissue tolerance. However, it should be remembered that the dose and fraction size at .5 cm from the vaginal surface is approximately equivalent to the maximum rectal dose for most applicator designs. Dose specification (for LDR or HDR) should always include a calculation of the maximum (i.e., vaginal surface) dose. It is important to remember that the dose falls off very steeply with depth (Figure 10-5). A number of HDR treatment schemes have been used (Table 10-4).[28,44–49] Those that deliver a high dose in large fractions may carry an unacceptably high risk of complications. In a prospective study comparing four fractionation schemes, Sorbe and Smeds[48] reported rectal complications in

**TABLE 10-4   Protocols Used to Treat the Vaginal Cuff Prophylactically with Vaginal Cylinders and HDR Intracavitary Treatment**

| | Treatment (Gy/number of fractions) | | |
| | After 40–45 Gy EBRT | ICRT Alone | |
| Study | | | Prescription Point |
|---|---|---|---|
| Kucera et al.[28] | 32/1 | 32/1 | Surface |
| Lybeert et al.[44] | 5/4 | 5/7 | 5 mm |
| Nori et al.[45] | 7/3 | 7/3 | 5 mm |
| Noyes et al.[46] | | 16/2 | Surface |
| Peschel et al.[47] | | 5/3 | 5 mm |
| | | 7/3 | |
| Sorbe and Smeds[48,a] | | 9/4 | 10 mm |
| | | 6/5 | |
| | | 5/6 | |
| | | 4.5/6 | |
| Thomas et al.[49] | 6/3 | 6/6 | Surface |
| | 5/3 | | |

[a]Rectal complications reported in more than 80% of patients treated with 9 Gy fractions and high rates of severe vaginal shortening with all schedules reported in this study.

more than 80% of patients treated with four fractions of 9 Gy prescribed at 10 mm. Using colpometry measurements, these authors found a strong correlation between vaginal shortening and dose per fraction. The lowest risk, after 4.5 Gy per fraction (at 10 mm), was still 31% at 5 years. More conservative regimens [5–6 Gy in three fractions after pelvic RT or 6 GY in six fractions with ICRT alone (dose prescribed at the vaginal surface)] should be sufficient to control microscopic disease and would be expected to carry less risk of late toxicity.

## RADIATION ALONE FOR MEDICALLY OR SURGICALLY INOPERABLE PATIENTS

Although hysterectomy with or without adjuvant RT is the standard treatment for clinical stage I–II endometrial carcinoma, patients who are at very high risk for major complications from surgery can be effectively treated with RT alone. Reported disease-specific survival rates of 75% to 85% and uterine control rates of 80% to 90% are typical (Table 10-5).[50–59] Prognosis tends to be correlated with clinical stage and tu-

mor grade, but intercurrent disease is the most common cause of death in these patients. Authors disagree somewhat about the relative roles of pelvic RT and ICRT; however, ICRT alone is probably sufficient for most patients with G1 disease. Large uterine size and high grade are generally considered indications for pelvic irradiation to reduce the uterine size before ICRT and to treat regional nodes. Risk factors for radiation morbidity should be considered in determining whether EBRT is indicated.

In general, if the risks of major morbidity and mortality from surgery are greater than 5% to 10%, RT alone should be strongly considered as a treatment option. If there is a post-RT uterine recurrence, the risk–benefit ratio for surgery should be reconsidered, because isolated intrauterine recurrences can sometimes be salvaged.

Adequate treatment of fundal tumors requires a broader radiation dose distribution in the region of the fundus than is typically required in cervical cancer treatment. In a small uterus, this can be accomplished with differential loading of the tip of an intrauterine tandem. For patients with a larger uterine cavity, Heyman packings (rarely available today) or Simon capsules (afterloaded with $^{137}$Cs) can be packed in the uterus to achieve a better distribution to the fundus. Alternatively, a nice dose distribution can sometimes be obtained by inserting two tandems curving away from one another into the cornua of the uterus.

A variety of different methods for prescribing dose in these cases have been described; none of these methods, however, is entirely satisfactory. The target volume is rarely well known, because the size of the uterus and thickness of the uterine wall cannot be accurately determined clinically. When available, magnetic resonance imaging may be helpful[60] but is often impossible to obtain because of the massive obesity of many of these patients. With LDR irradiation, uterine applicators are commonly loaded with 45 to 50 mg Raequiv and are left in place for two 72-hour or three 48-hour treatments (or for two 48-hour treatments after 40–45 Gy to the whole pelvis). With this approach, reported control rates have been high and complication rates low.[53] Alternatively, some investigators prescribe a dose at 1 cm from the sources. The vagina does not re-quire as high a dose as with cervical cancers unless there is cervical stromal involvement. For a clinical stage I tumor, source loadings that yield a vaginal surface dose of 60 to 80 Gy should be sufficient to prevent vaginal recurrence in most patients.

## TREATMENT OF RECURRENT DISEASE

Cure rates for isolated apical vaginal recurrences are 30% to 50% with RT[61–67] (Table 10-6), with the better survival rates reported for patients whose initial treatment was surgery alone. Survival is correlated with the size, extent, location, and grade of the tumor. Some authors have found a correlation between the time to recurrence and outcome. Sears and colleagues[68] reported survival rates of 74% and 30% for patients with tumors 2 cm or less and larger than 2 cm, respectively, emphasizing the probable importance of early detection. Distal vaginal recurrences also may be cured if there is no evidence of other disease.

**TABLE 10-5    Endometrial Carcinoma Treated with Radiation Alone: Local–Regional Control, Disease-Specific Survival, and Major Complication Rates**

| Study | Clinical Stage | Patients | Local–Regional Recurrence (%) | Disease-Specific Survival (%) | Major Complications (%) |
|---|---|---|---|---|---|
| Abayomi et al.[50] | I-II | 50 | 26 | 78 | 15 |
|  | III-IV | 16 |  | 10 |  |
| Grisby et al.[51] | I | 69 | 9 | 88 | 16 |
| Jones and Stout[52] | I-II | 146 | 22 | 61 | 4 |
|  | III | 14 | 79 | 14 |  |
| Kupelian et al.[53] | I-II | 137 | 14 | 85 | 3 |
|  | III-IV | 15 | 32 | 49 |  |
| Landgren et al.[54] | I-II | 124 | 22 | 68 | 7 |
|  | III-IV | 26 | 42 | 22 |  |
| Lehoczky et al.[55] | I | 171 | 20 | 75 | 0 |
| Patanaphan et al.[56] | I-II | 42 | 14 | 64 | 2 |
|  | III-IV | 10 | 60 | 20 |  |
| Taghian et al.[57] | I-II | 94 | 6 | 70 | 17 |
|  | III-IV | 10 | 10 | 27 |  |
| Varia et al.[58] | I-II | 73 | 21 | 43 | 10 |
| Wang et al.[59] | I-II | 41 | 22 | 76 | 5 |

*Source:* Ref. 53.

TABLE 10-6   Survival Rates of Patients with Clinically Isolated Vaginal Recurrences of Endometrial Carcinoma

| Study | Patients (site) | Survived (%) |
|---|---|---|
| Aalders et al.[61] | 42 (apex) | 26 |
| | 42 (Distal) | 14 |
| Badib et al.[62] | 63 (upper vagina) | 38 |
| | 11 (lower vagina) | 27 |
| Curran et al.[63] | 30 (apex) | 39 |
| | 16 (suburethra) | 25 |
| Greven and Olds[64] | 18 | 33 |
| Ingersol[65] | 25 (apex) | 64 |
| | 9 (anterior wall) | 11 |
| Kuten et al.[66] | 17 | 40 |
| Mandell et al.[67] | 11 | 82 |

A combination of EBRT and brachytherapy is usually indicated; brachytherapy should be tailored to the size, extent, and initial response of the lesion. As with primary vaginal cancers, ICRT should not be used to treat tumors 5 mm thick or thicker. A variety of interstitial techniques may be indicated in various situations. For apical lesions, laparotomy or laparoscopy guidance may be necessary. Combined EBRT and interstitial RT is usually indicated for distal (usually suburethral) recurrences. If the target volume cannot be adequately encompassed with brachytherapy, shrinking fields of EBRT can be curative in some cases.

The prognosis is poorer for pelvic wall recurrences, but 10% to 15% of patients may be cured with local–regional treatment if there is no other evidence of disease. Isolated inguinal node recurrences are uncommon, but cures have been reported, presumably because the inguinal nodes are a rare, primary echelon site of spread via the round ligament.

## REFERENCES

1. Wingo PA, Ton T, Bolden S: Cancer statistics, 1995. *CA Cancer J Clin* 1995;45:8–30.
2. Antunes CM, Stolley PD, Rosenshein NB, et al: Endometrial cancer and estrogen use: Report of a large case-control study. *New Engl J Med* 1979;300:9–13.
3. Parazzini F, LaVecchia C, Bocciolone L, et al: Review: The epidemiology of endometrial cancer. *Gynecol Oncol* 1991;41:1–16.
4. International Federation of Gynecology and Obstetrics: Corpus cancer staging. *Int J Gynaecol Obstet* 1989;28:190.
5. Mannel RS, Berman ML, Walker JL, et al: Management of endometrial cancer with suspected cervical involvement. *Obstet Gynecol* 1990;75:1016–1022.
6. Lauchlan SC: Conceptual unity of the Müllerian tumor group. A histologic study. *Cancer* 1968;22:601–610.
7. Zaino RJ, Kurman R, Herbold D, et al: The significance of squamous differentiation in endometrial carcinoma. A Gynecologic Oncology Group study. *Cancer* 1991;68:2293–2302.
8. Hendrickson M, Ross M, Eifel P, et al: Uterine papillary serous carcinoma. A highly malignant form of endometrial adenocarcinoma. *Am J Surg Pathol* 1982;6:93–108.
9. Carcangiu ML, Chambers JT: Early pathologic stage clear cell carcinoma and uterine papillary serous carcinoma of the endometrium: Comparison of clinicopathologic features and survival. *Int J Gynecol Pathol* 1995;14:30–38.
10. Aalders J, Abeler V, Kolstad P, et al: Postoperative external irradiation and prognostic parameters in stage I endometrial carcinoma. *Obstet Gynecol* 1980;56:419–427.
11. Grisby PW, Perez CA, Kuten A, et al: Clinical stage I endometrial cancer: Prognostic factors for local control and distant metastasis and implica-

tions of the new FIGO surgical staging system. *Int J Radiat Oncol Biol Phys* 1992;22:905–911.

12. Morrow C, Bundy B, Kurman R, et al: Relationship between surgical–pathological risk factors and outcome in clinical stage I and II carcinoma of the endometrium: A Gynecologic Oncology Group study. *Gynecol Oncol* 1991; 40:55–65.

13. Silva EG, Jenkins R: Serous carcinoma in endometrial polyps. *Modern Pathol* 1990;3: 120–128.

14. Fanning J, Alvarez PM, Tsukada Y, et al: Prognostic significance of the extent of cervical involvement by endometrial cancer. *Gynecol Oncol* 1991;40:46–47.

15. Schink JC, Rademaker AW, Miller DS, et al: Tumor size in endometrial cancer. *Cancer* 1991;67:2791–2794.

16. Creasman W, Morrow C, Bundy B, et al: Surgical pathologic spread patterns of endometrial cancer. A Gynecologic Oncology Group study. *Cancer* 1987;60:2035–2041.

17. Corn B, Lanciano R, Greven K, et al: Endometrial cancer with para-aortic adenopathy: Patterns of failure and opportunities for cure. *Int J Radiat Oncol Biol Phys* 1992;24:223–227.

18. Feuer G, Calanog A: Endometrial carcinoma. Treatment of positive paraaortic nodes. *Gynecol Oncol* 1987;27:104–109.

19. Potish R: Radiation therapy of periaortic node metastases in cancer of the uterine cervix and endometrium. *Radiology* 1987;165:567–570.

20. Rose P, Cha S, Tak W, et al: Radiation therapy for surgically proven para-aortic node metastasis in endometrial carcinoma. *Int J Radiat Oncol Biol Phys* 1992;24:229–233.

21. Turner DA, Gershenson DM, Atkinson N, et al: The prognostic significance of peritoneal cytology for stage I endometrial cancer. *Obstet Gynecol* 1989;74:775–780.

22. Grimshaw RN, Tupper C, Fraser RC, et al: Prognostic value of peritoneal cytology in endometrial carcinoma. *Gynecol Oncol* 1990; 36:97–100.

23. Milsevic MF, Dembo AJ, Thomas GM: The clinical significance of malignant peritoneal cytology in stage I endometrial carcinoma. *Int J Gynecol Cancer* 1992;2:225–235.

24. Eifel P, Hendrickson M, Ross J, et al: Simultaneous presentation of carcinoma involving the ovary and the uterine corpus. *Cancer* 1982;50: 163–170.

25. Pearl ML, Johnston CM, Frank TS, et al: Synchronous dual primary ovarian and endometrial carcinomas. *Int J Gynaecol Obstet* 1993;43: 305–312.

26. Jones HW: Treatment of adenocarcinoma of the endometrium. *Obstet Gynecol Surv* 1975;30: 147–169.

27. Carey MS, O'Connell GJ, Johanson CR, et al: Good outcome associated with a standardized treatment protocol using selective postoperative radiation in patients with clinical stage I adenocarcinoma of the endometrium. *Gynecol Oncol* 1995;57:138–144.

28. Kucera H, Vavra N, Weghaupt K: Benefit of external irradiation in pathologic stage I endometrial carcinoma: A prospective clinical trial of 605 patients who received postoperative vaginal irradiation and additional pelvic irradiation in the presence of unfavorable prognostic factors. *Gynecol Oncol* 1990;38:99–104.

29. Marchetti DL, Caglar H, Driscoll DL, et al: Pelvic radiation in stage I endometrial adenocarcinoma with high-risk attributes. *Gynecol Oncol* 1990;37:51–54.

30. Piver MS, Hempling RE: A prospective trial of postoperative vaginal radium/cesium for grade 1-2 less than 50% myometrial invasion and pelvic radiation therapy for grade 3 or deep myometrial invasion in surgical stage I endometrial adenocarcinoma. *Cancer* 1990;66:1133–1138.

31. Greven KM, Lanciano RM, Herbert SH, et al: Analysis of complications in patients with endometrial carcinoma receiving adjuvant irradiation. *Int J Radiat Oncol Biol Phys* 1991;21: 919–923.

32. Hicks ML, Piver MS, Puretz JL, et al: Survival in patients with paraaortic lymph node metastases from endometrial adenocarcinoma clinically limited to the uterus. *Int J Radiat Oncol Biol Phys* 1993;26:607–611.

33. Komaki R, Mattingly RF, Hoffman RG, et al: Irradiation of para-aortic lymph node metastases from carcinoma of the cervix or endometrium: Preliminary results. *Radiology* 1983;147: 245–248.

34. Carcangiu ML, Chambers JT: Uterine papillary serous carcinoma: A study on 108 cases with emphasis on the prognostic significance of

associated endometrioid carcinoma, absence of invasion, and concomitant ovarian carcinoma. *Gynecol Oncol* 1992;47:298–305.

35. Greven KM, Lanciano RM, Corn B, et al: Pathologic stage III endometrial carcinoma. Prognostic factors and patterns of recurrence. *Cancer* 1993;71:3697–3702.

36. O'Hanlan K, Levine P, Harbatkin D, et al: Virulence of papillary endometrial carcinoma. *Gynecol Oncol* 1990;37:112–119.

37. Levenback C, Eifel PJ, Burke TW, et al: Hemorrhagic cystitis following radiotherapy for stage Ib cancer of the cervix. *Gynecol Oncol* 1994;55:206–210.

38. Gibbons S, Martinez A, Schray M, et al: Adjuvant whole abdominal irradiation for high risk endometrial carcinoma. *Int J Radiat Oncol Biol Phys* 1991;21:1019.

39. Greer BE, Hamberger A: Treatment of intraperitoneal metastatic adenocarcinoma of the endometrium by the whole-abdomen moving-strip technique and pelvic boost irradiation. *Gynecol Oncol* 1983;16:365–373.

40. Malipeddi P, Kapp DS, Teng NNH: Long-term survival with adjuvant whole abdominopelvic irradiation for uterine papillary serous carcinoma. *Cancer* 1993;71:2076–3081.

41. Potish RA: Abdominal radiotherapy for cancer of the uterine cervix and endometrium. *Int J Radiat Oncol Biol Phys* 1989;16:1453–1458.

42. Bliss P, Cowie VJ: Endometrial carcinoma: Does the addition of intracavitary vault caesium to external beam therapy postoperatively result in improved control or increased morbidity? *Clin Oncol* 1992;4:373–376.

43. Randall ME, Wilder J, Greven K, et al: Role of intracavitary cuff boost after adjuvant external irradiation in early endometrial carcinoma. *Int J Radiat Oncol Biol Phys* 1990;19:49–54.

44. Lybeert MLM, vanPutten WLJ, Ribot JG, et al: Endometrial carcinoma: High dose-rate brachytherapy in combination with external irradiation; a multivariate analysis of relapses. *Radiother Oncol* 1989;16:243–252.

45. Nori D, Merimsky O, Batata M, et al: Postoperative high dose-rate intravaginal brachytherapy combined with external irradiation for early stage endometrial cancer: A long-term follow-up. *Int J Radiat Oncol Biol Phys* 1994;30:831–837.

46. Noyes WR, Bastin K, Edwards SA, et al: Postoperative vaginal cuff irradiation using high dose rate remote afterloading: A phase II clinical protocol. *Int J Radiat Oncol Biol Phys* 1995;32:1439–1443.

47. Peschel RE, Healey GA, Smith RJ, et al: High dose rate remote afterloading for endometrial cancer. *Endocuriether Hypertherm Oncol* 1989;5:209–214.

48. Sorbe BG, Smeds AC: Postoperative vaginal irradiation with high dose rate after loading technique in endometrial carcinoma stage I. *Int J Radiat Oncol Biol Phys* 1990;18:305–314.

49. Thomas H, Pickerine GL, Dunn P, et al: Treating the vaginal vault in carcinoma of the endometrium using the Buchler afterloading system. *Br J Radiol* 1991;64:1044–1048.

50. Abayomi O, Tak W, Emami B, et al: Treatment of endometrial carcinoma with radiation therapy alone. *Cancer* 1982;49:2466–2469.

51. Grigsby P, Kuske R, Perez C, et al: Medically inoperable stage I adenocarcinoma of the endometrium treated with radiotherapy alone. *Int J Radiat Oncol Biol Phys* 1987;13:483–488.

52. Jones D, Stout R: Results of intracavitary radium treatment for adenocarcinoma of the body of the uterus. *Clin Radiol* 1986;37:169–171.

53. Kupelian PA, Eifel PJ, Tornos C, et al: Treatment of endometrial carcinoma with radiation therapy alone. *Int J Radiat Oncol Biol Phys* 1993;27:817–824.

54. Landgren R, Fletcher G, Delclos L, et al: Irradiation of endometrial cancer in patients with medical contraindication to surgery or with unresectable lesions. *Am J Roentgenol Radiat Ther Nucl Med* 1976;126:148–154.

55. Lehoczky O, Bosze P, Ungar L, et al: Stage I endometrial carcinoma: Treatment of nonoperable patients with intracavitary radiation therapy alone. *Gynecol Oncol* 1991;43:211–216.

56. Patanaphan V, Salazar O, Chougule P: What can be expected when radiation therapy becomes the only curative alternative for endometrial cancer? *Cancer* 1985;55:1462–1467.

57. Taghian A, Pernot M, Hoffstetter S, et al: Radiation therapy alone for medically inoperable patients with adenocarcinoma of the endometrium. *Int J Radiat Oncol Biol Phys* 1988;15:1135–1140.

58. Varia M, Rosenman J, Halle J, et al: Primary radiation therapy for medically inoperable patients with endometrial carcinoma—Stages I-II. *Int J Radiat Oncol Biol Phys* 1987;13:11–15.

59. Wang M, Hussey D, Vigliotti A, et al: Inoperable adenocarcinoma of endometrium: Radiation therapy. *Radiology* 1987;165:561–565.

60. Sironi S, Taccagni G, Garancini P, et al: Myometrial invasion by endometrial carcinoma by MR imaging. *Am J Roentgenol* 1992;158:565–569.

61. Aalders JG, Abeler V, Kolstad P: Recurrent adenocarcinoma of the endometrium: A clinical and histopathological study of 379 patients. *Gynecol Oncol* 1984;17:85–103.

62. Badib AO, Kurohara SS, Beitia AA, et al: Recurrent cancer of the corpus uteri: Techniques and results of treatment. *Am J Roentgenol* 1969;105:596–602.

63. Curran WJ, Whittington R, Peters AJ, et al: Vaginal recurrences of endometrial carcinoma: The prognostic value of staging by a primary

vaginal carcinoma system. *Int J Radiat Oncol Biol Phys* 1988;15:803–808.

64. Greven K, Olds W: Isolated vaginal recurrences of endometrial adenocarcinoma and their management. *Cancer* 1987;60:419–421.

65. Ingersol FM: Vaginal recurrences of carcinoma of the corpus—Management and prevention. *Am J Surg* 1971;121:472–477.

66. Kuten A, Grigsby PW, Perez CA, et al: Results of radiotherapy in recurrent endometrial carcinoma: A retrospective analysis of 51 patients. *Int J Radiat Oncol Biol Phys* 1989;17:29–34.

67. Mandell LR, Nori D, Hilaris B: Recurrent stage I endometrial carcinoma: Results of treatment and prognostic factors. *Int J Radiat Oncol Biol Phys* 1985;11:1103–1109.

68. Sears JD, Greven KM, Hoen HM, et al: Prognostic factors and treatment outcome for patients with locally recurrent endometrial cancer. *Cancer* 1994;74:1303–1308.

# B. Vulva - ANTHONY H. RUSSELL

## INTRODUCTION

Starting in the 1930s, en bloc radical vulvectomy in continuity with bilateral inguinofemoral and selective pelvic lymphadenectomy emerged as the standard of operative therapy for primary cancer of the vulva. Consideration of failure sites following local excision, knowledge of the lymphatic drainage of the vulva, and the desire to be surgically rigorous in attacking all potential sites of local and regional spread resulted in this comprehensive approach, which succeeded in more than doubling the cure rates previously obtained by more limited surgery.[1–4] Subsequent technical refinements, including primary closure of the perineal wound, shortened the duration of hospitalization and recovery. Improvements in anesthesia and monitoring, transfusion of blood components, antibiotic therapy, deep venous thrombosis prophylaxis, and increasingly sophisticated postoperative metabolic and nutritional support, resulted in a steady decline in

perioperative mortality. Initially reported at a rate of 6% to 19% by the pioneers of radical vulvar surgery,[3,5] total operative and postoperative deaths had declined to a rate less than 4% by the 1970s.[6,7] Selected patients with locally extensive disease could be treated by anterior, posterior, or total pelvic exenteration with cure rates exceeding 50% when regional nodes were found to be free of metastatic involvement.[8]

Frail patients were relegated to treatment by radiation, along with those patients whose disease extended beyond the boundaries of surgical feasibility.[9] Largely restricted to the palliative treatment of patients who were assessed to be technically unresectable or medically inoperable, radiotherapy was administered (in hindsight) using naive dose and fractionation schedules as well as techniques of limited sophistication.[10–12] Often, eradication of the cancer would exchange the burden of malignancy for the debilitating, chronic sequelae of high dose radiation applied to the vulva and skin of the perineum.[12]

However, the past two decades have witnessed a series of remarkable transformations in the management of this disease. The extent of vulvar cancers at diagnosis has been steadily decreasing in recent years. Among patients undergoing radical groin dissections, the frequency of lymph node metastasis has fallen from approximately 50% to 60% in the 1940s and 1950s,[2,4] to approximately 30% in surgical literature from the 1980s.[13–17] Younger, sexually active patients are being diagnosed with preinvasive disease or focal invasive disease of minimal volume, often with regional nodes both clinically and microscopically free of metastatic contamination.[18] During the past two decades, modifications in the surgical approach to cancer of the vulva have been stimulated by concerns about the chronic morbidities associated with successful extirpative surgery for patients presenting with limited disease. Management of patients with cancer of the vulva has evolved in parallel with successful efforts to preserve structure, function, and cosmesis in the treatment of patients with primary cancers of the head and neck, breast, rectum, and sarcomas of the extremities.

Following radical groin and pelvic node dissection, leg lymphedema may be temporary, lasting a year or longer until collateral lymphatic channels develop, or it may be permanent, massive, and disabling.[6,19] Pelvic relaxation, organ prolapse, and urinary incontinence can develop in some patients, particularly when removal of the distal urethra or a portion of the lower vagina is required. Significant stenosis of the vaginal introitus can occur. Absence of the vulva and venereal fat can have the functional consequence of shortening the effective vaginal depth and removing a protective cushion from the pubic arch, contributing to dyspareunia. Major alterations in body image, decreased capacity for sexual arousal, and reduced frequency of coital activity consequent to dyspareunia, may combine to precipitate feelings of guilt, worthlessness, depression, and anxiety.[20,21]

For selected individuals, conservative excision of a small primary cancer coupled with limited groin dissection can achieve equivalent cancer control to more extensive surgery, with less functional loss and mutilation.[22–24] Adjuvant, postoperative radiation has reduced regional relapse, improved survival, and decreased the indications for pelvic lymphadenectomy in patients with groin node metastases.[25,26] In the United States, approximately half of surgically treated patients with groin node metastases will undergo postoperative radiotherapy.[27] Planned in coordination with conservative surgery, preoperative or postoperative radiation (alone or with concurrent chemotherapy) has permitted salvage of patients who might otherwise have required exenteration for cure and has made possible clitoral preservation in others.[28–44] Extrapolating from the success achieved in the conservative therapy of carcinoma of the anal canal, synchronous chemotherapy coupled with radiation in reduced dose have allowed curative, nonsurgical management of some patients with massive, unresectable disease.[41,42,45–50] Coordinated chemoradiation may accomplish better tumor control with less chronic radiation morbidity than described in previous reports of high dose radiation alone.[12] The array of sensible, effective treatment options now available permits management responsibly tailored to the initial extent of disease, defined clinical and histopathologic prognostic factors, and the hierarchy of concerns of the individual patient.

## ANATOMY

The vulva is composed of the mons veneris, the labia majora, labia minora, clitoris, and the vulvar vestibule, which harbors the urethral meatus and is bounded by the vaginal introitus (Figure 10-6). The labia, limited laterally by the labiocrural folds, are the female analog of the male scrotum and are pigmented and covered by hair lateral to the crests of the labia majora. Medially, the skin of the labia majora is smooth and hairless, with underlying sebaceous glands. Between the labia majora lie the hairless labia minora, whose

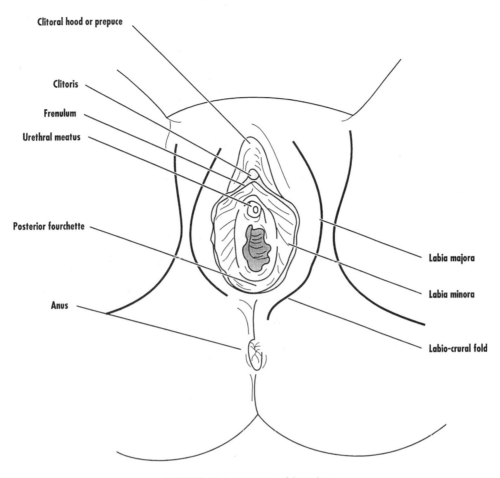

Clitoral hood or prepuce

Clitoris

Frenulum

Urethral meatus

Posterior fourchette

Anus

Labia majora

Labia minora

Labio-crural fold

**FIGURE 10-6**    Anatomy of the vulva.

medial skin also contains multiple sebaceous glands. Coursing posteromedially, the labia minora taper and join in a fold called the posterior fourchette. Anteriorly, the labia minora taper then split to envelop the clitoris, fusing in front of the clitoris to form the prepuce, and behind the clitoris to form the frenulum. The clitoris, an erectile organ analogous to the penis in the male, is composed of the glans, and a body consisting of two corpora cavernosa, which diverge into the two crura that lie attached to the undersurface of the pubic rami. The paired, mucus-secreting Bartholin glands lie deep to the posterior labia majora, and drain by a simple duct to the vulvar vestibule between the hymenal membrane and

the medial borders of the labia minora. The arterial supply of the vulva is from branches of the pudendal arteries, which originate from the hypogastric arteries. The innervation is from branches of the third and fourth sacral nerves via the pudendal nerve.

Metastatic contamination of lymph nodes by epidermoid carcinoma of the vulva proceeds in a sequential, incremental fashion, the somewhat predictable consequence of the lymphatic anatomy of the normal vulva[52–53] (Figures 10-7 and 10-8). The lymphatics of the vulva comprise a network of fine vessels that cover the entire labia minora, fourchette, prepuce, and distal vagina below the hymenal membrane. These coalesce anteriorly, forming

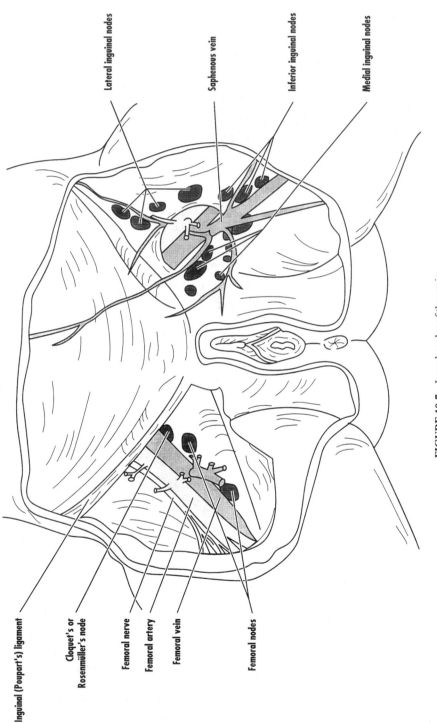

Lateral inguinal nodes

Saphenous vein

Inferior inguinal nodes

Medial inguinal nodes

Inguinal (Poupart's) ligament

Cloquet's or
Rosenmüller's node

Femoral nerve

Femoral artery

Femoral vein

Femoral nodes

**FIGURE 10-7**　Lymph nodes of the groin.

larger trunks that run lateral to the clitoris to the mons veneris, acquiring tributaries from the lymphatics of the labia majora, which run in a parallel fashion anteriorly from the perineal body. The vulvar lymphatics run through the vulva and do not cross the labiocrural fold. The lymphatics of the perineum course lateral to the labiocrural fold through the superficial tissues of the upper medial thigh. In the radiation treatment of patients with cancer extending beyond the vulva to the perineal skin, these more lateral channels must be addressed. Similarly, extension of an advanced vulvovaginal cancer along the vaginal barrel proximal to the hymenal ring requires attention to the direct pelvic lymphatic flow of the middle and upper

vagina. At the mons the vulvar lymphatic trunks deviate laterally to the primary regional nodes, the ipsilateral or contralateral inguinal nodes. Study of the localization of radiolabeled tracer in regional lymph nodes after focal injection of discrete sites in the vulva and on the perineum reveals that the lymphatic drainage of the perineum, clitoris, and anterior labia minora is bilateral, whereas the lymph flow from well-lateralized sites in the vulva is, predominantly, to the ipsilateral groin.[53] Discrete ($\leq$ 2 cm diameter), well-lateralized primary cancers limited to the vulva and not approaching midline structures will rarely manifest spread to contralateral groin nodes in the absence of spread to ipsilateral

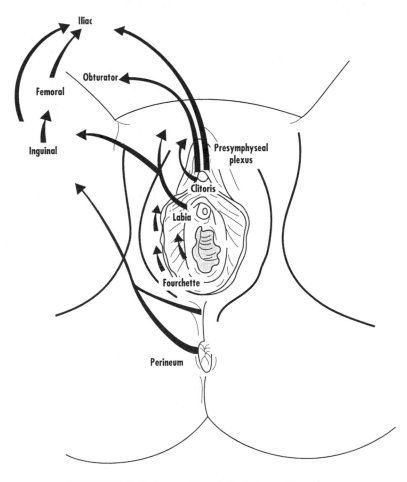

**FIGURE 10-8**  Pathways of lymphatic drainage of the vulva.

nodes.[23,24,54–57] From the inguinal nodes, secondary lymphatic drainage is through the cribriform fascia to the femoral nodes, with subsequent tertiary flow under the inguinal ligaments to the external iliac nodes. Although direct lymphatic channels from the clitoris to the deep pelvic nodes have been described, three surgical series of patients with clitoral involvement by primary cancers of the vulva have failed to find evidence of pelvic node metastasis in the absence of groin metastasis.[13,58,59] Similarly, direct lymphatic channels from the clitoris and anterior vulva to the femoral nodes exist, and though occasional patients with metastatic spread to the deep femoral nodes without inguinal nodal metastasis have been reported,[55,60–62] this is a rare event when the inguinal nodes have been fully dissected and histologically examined. Metastatic spread to pelvic nodes will be found in approximately 15% to 25% of patients with groin node metastasis, but very rarely without prior contamination of the inguinal or femoral nodes.[6,7,14,25,63–68] Based on study of bipedal lymphangiograms, inguinal nodes are located within the femoral triangle, do not lie lateral to the medial 80% of the inguinal ligament, and do not lie medial to the pubic tubercle.[69] Based on cadaveric dissection, the femoral nodes are usually one to four in number and located at the fossa ovalis medial to the femoral vein.[70] Medial and lateral borders of radiation ports intended to treat these nodes can be established accordingly, with additional volume to assure adequate coverage despite minor daily variations in patient setup and to avoid cold spots near the beam edge. Depending on patient size, the depth of the inguinal nodes can be quite variable and impossible to accurately estimate by palpation.[71–73] The depth in tissue of the deep femoral nodes should be measured radiographically by CT, with radiation dose prescribed to the depth of the femoral artery as it passes beneath the inguinal ligament. Failure to measure the depth accurately can result in possible underdosage of the deep nodes, with disastrous sequelae.[74,75]

## EPIDEMIOLOGY

Cancer of the vulva constitutes less than 5% of female genital tract cancer malignancies, and only 1% to 2% of cancer in women. Malignant melanoma,[76–83] adult and embryonal sarcomas of varied histologies,[84–86] Merkel cell tumors,[87,88] histiocytosis-X,[89] Kaposi sarcoma,[90] epidemic (AIDS-associated) Kaposi sarcoma,[91] hemangiopericytoma,[92,93] eccrine carcinoma,[94] primary breast cancers,[95] basal cell carcinomas,[96] adenocarcinomas and adenoid cystic carcinomas (usually arising within Bartholin glands),[97–102] and neuroendocrine small-cell carcinoma,[103] as well as other histologic tumor types, have all been reported as primary malignancies arising from the vulva.[104] However, more than 85% of invasive vulvar malignancies are epidermoid carcinomas,[51,105] leading to the common practice of using the terms "squamous carcinoma of the vulva" and "vulvar carcinoma" synonymously. Because of distinctive histopathology and characteristic clinical behaviors, it is important to recognize verrucous carcinoma[106–109] and so-called spray pattern carcinomas[110,111] as variants of squamous carcinoma representing polar extremes in the spectrum of biologic virulence and potential for metastatic spread.

Cancer of the vulva is most commonly observed in the seventh and eighth decades of life, but the age-specific incidence rates in the United States rise steeply at age 70 and continue to rise beyond age 80.[112] The coincidence of vulvar intraepithelial neoplasia (VIN) or invasive squamous carcinoma of the vulva with in situ or invasive epidermoid carcinoma of the cervix has long been noted, and synchronous or sequential (usually antecedent) cervical lesions may be present in as many as 20% of women with primary vulvar lesions, suggesting a common etiology in at least some patients.[113–119] Appearance of cancer at separate sites within the conserved vulva after local excision of small primary cancers probably represents metachronous appearance of independent primaries rather than true recurrence. Multifocal cancers of the vulva lend further support to the so-called field change model of oncogenesis.[120] Additional risk factors for the development of invasive vulvar cancer include a history of condylomata, VIN, smoking, and chronic vulvar dystrophies.[121-124] Radiation exposure consequent to treatment of a prior cervical malignancy is discounted as an independent risk factor for vulvar neoplasia by comparing prevalence of cancer of the vulva among patients treated with or without radiation for primary cervical cancer.[125]

A rising incidence of VIN and reports of invasive vulvar cancer in young patients may reflect changing sexual mores and transmission of the human papilloma virus (HPV), which has been detected in most younger patients with VIN, and a smaller proportion of patients with invasive lesions. Detection of HPV in VIN or invasive disease is most common in young patients and less frequent as a function of advancing age.[126,127] Invasive cancer of the vulva has been reported in young patients with both naturally occurring and iatrogenic immune compromise.[48,128 130] Detection of the human immunodeficiency virus (HIV) in 4 of 18 young (age < 50) vulvar cancer patients from an inner city population raises concerns that rising rates of vulvar as well as cervical cancer may become apparent as the AIDS epidemic unfolds.[131] Experience with a limited number of HIV-1 infected patients with vulvar intraepithelial neoplasia suggests that VIN will be more likely to persist or recur following standard therapies, and when invasive cancer of the vulva develops in the context of HIV infection, it may prove refractory to conventional treatments.[132,133]

Cancer of the vulva frequently coexists with vulvar dystrophy, particularly in older women,[134-136] however it is unknown whether lesions such as lichen sclerosus et atrophicus, and typical or atypical hyperplastic dystrophy, are true precursor lesions. The vast majority of patients with chronic, irritative vulvar inflammations do not have coexistent vulvar cancer,

and only a small minority will develop vulvar cancer during surveillance follow-up.[137] Cancers in these older patients will much less commonly be associated with HPV infection, leading to the hypothesis that patients with vulvar cancer may be segregated into two broad groups: an older population with cancer arising in association with vulvar dystrophy and unassociated with HPV, and a younger population with HPV-associated tumors frequently adjacent to areas of VIN.[126,138]

## SURGERY

For more than 30 years, en bloc radical vulvectomy and bilateral regional lymphadenectomy (inguinofemoral ± pelvic) has been the standard of care in the United States for patients with operable carcinoma of the vulva. Understanding the results of primary surgical therapy is the foundation for understanding the treatment innovations of the past 20 years. Most of the classic surgical literature analyzes results utilizing the 1969 staging system of the International Federation of Gynecology and Obstetrics (FIGO), which employed clinical evaluation of both the primary tumor and groin nodes (Table 10-7). In 1988 FIGO adopted modifications to this staging system resulting in a hybrid, clinicopathologic staging system (Table 10-8) that incorporated the results of histologic assessment of regional nodes. This explicitly acknowledged the pivotal importance of nodal status in determining prognosis and therapy and implicitly recognized the inaccuracies of assessment of the regional lymph nodes by palpation.

Approximately 20% of patients with clinically uninvolved groin nodes (1969 FIGO N0-1) will have histologic evidence of groin metastasis if the nodes are radically dissected.[3,7,14,63,65,139] Conversely, enlarged, palpably suspicious nodes, including matted nodes tethered to overlying skin, may be the consequence of injury or infection in the lower extremities, prior venereal infection, or a reaction to necrosis or infection of the primary cancer. Approximately 22% of patients with clinically suspicious groin nodes (1969 FIGO N2,3) will show no histologic evidence of nodal spread if the groin nodes are dissected and studied pathologically[3,7,63,65,139] (Table 10-9). If a treat-

**TABLE 10-7   AJCC TNM Classification and 1969 FIGO Stage Grouping**

T: PRIMARY TUMOR

| | |
|---|---|
| Tis | Preinvasive carcinoma (carcinoma in situ) |
| T1 | Tumor confined to the vulva, 2 cm or less in greatest dimension |
| T2 | Tumor confined to the vulva, more than 2 cm in greatest dimension |
| T3 | Tumor of any size with adjacent spread to the urethra and/or vagina and/or perineum and/or anus |
| T4 | Tumor of any size invading any of the following: the upper urethral mucosa, the bladder mucosa, the rectal mucosa, or tumor fixed to the bone |

N: REGIONAL LYMPH NODES

| | |
|---|---|
| N0 | No nodes palpable |
| N1 | Nodes palpable in either groin, not enlarged, mobile (not clinically suspicious of neoplasm) |
| N2 | Nodes palpable in one or both groins, enlarged, firm, and mobile (clinically suspicious of neoplasm) |
| N3 | Fixed or ulcerated nodes |

M: DISTANT METASTASES

| | |
|---|---|
| M0 | No clinical metastases |
| M1a | Palpable pelvic lymph nodes |
| M1b | Other distant metastases |

FIGO STAGE[a]

| | |
|---|---|
| 0 | Tis |
| I | T1N0,1M0 |
| | T2N0,1M0 |
| III | T1,2N2M0 |
| | T3N0,1,2M0 |
| IV | TxN3M0 |
| | T4N0,1,2M0 |
| | TxNxM1a |
| | TxNxM1b |

[a]x denotes any T or N category.

**TABLE 10-8   1992 AJCC TNM Classification and 1988 FIGO Stage Grouping**

T: PRIMARY TUMOR

| | |
|---|---|
| Tis | Carcinoma in situ (preinvasive carcinoma) |
| T1 | Tumor confined to the vulva and perineum[a] 2 cm or less in greatest dimension |
| T2 | Tumor confined to the vulva and perineum[a] more than 2 cm in greatest dimension |
| T3 | Tumor of any size with adjacent spread to the lower urethra and/or vagina and/or anus |
| T4 | Tumor of any size invading any of the following: the upper urethral mucosa, the bladder mucosa, the rectal mucosa, or tumor fixed to the bone |

N: REGIONAL LYMPH NODES[b]

| | |
|---|---|
| N0 | No nodal metastases |
| N1 | Unilateral regional lymph node metastasis |
| N2 | Bilateral regional lymph node metastasis |

M: DISTANT METASTASIS

| | |
|---|---|
| M0 | No evidence of distant metastasis |
| M1 | Any distant metastasis including pelvic lymph nodes |

FIGO STAGE[c]

| | |
|---|---|
| 0 | Tis |
| I | T1N0M0 |
| II | T2N0M0 |
| III | T3N0M0 |
| | T1,2,3N1M0 |
| IVA | T1,2,3N2M0 |
| | T4NxM0 |
| IVB | TxNxM1 |

[a]Lesions extending onto the perineum were formerly classified as T3.

[b]Assessment of inguinofemoral nodes is now histologic.

[c]x denotes any T or N category.

ment decision is contingent upon the histopathologic status of the groin nodes, fine needle aspiration or excisional biopsy prior to treatment is sensible.

The prognosis of surgically treated cancer of the vulva is directly related to the presence or absence of regional node metastasis, the extent of lymph node infestation, and the anatomic level of nodal involvement. Five-year disease-free survival probability is approximately 95% for patients with T1-2 N0 tumors treated surgically,[7,140] decreasing to approximately 70% for stage T3 N0.[7] Metastasis to a single node is less ominous than involvement of multiple nodes.[13,15] Patients with unilateral node metastasis fare better than those with bilateral spread.[140] Five-year disease-free survival drops to approximately 40% with the finding of multiple involved nodes. The size, number, and extent of metastatic deposits in groin nodes correlates with prognosis. Intracapsular metastases less than 5 mm in diameter are prognostically favorable, as opposed to metastases 15 mm or larger, or metastases with extracapsular spread.[141] The combination of metastasis to three or more nodes, extension of metastatic disease beyond the node capsule, and 50% or greater lymph node replacement by cancer is strongly predictive of recurrence with almost half of such patients manifesting distant dissemination.[142] Metastatic involvement of pelvic (iliac) nodes is grave, but approximately 20% of patients with pelvic node metastasis can be cured by local–regional therapies (surgery, radiation, or combined therapy).[6,7,13,63,64,67,143]

The probability of lymph node spread has been correlated with primary tumor size, depth of invasion, invasion of endothelial-lined space (lymph–vascular space invasion), pattern of tumor growth and invasion, and histologic grade, although there is no consensus concerning the relative independent importance of each of these parameters in multivariance analysis.[61,68,110,140,144] Surgical specimens from patients with primary tumors 2 cm or less in diameter (T1) show escalating risk of node metastasis with progressive depth of invasion[24,55,56,62,111,145] as measured from the most superficial dermal papilla adjacent to the tumor or from the basement membrane. Tumors with 3 mm or less invasion will have groin node metastasis in less than 10% of cases, with the risk rising to approximately 25% with depth of invasion 3.1 to 5 mm, and escalating to greater than 35% for invasion greater than 5 mm. The probability of finding node metastasis is less than 10% for tumors 2 cm or less in diameter, approximately 25% for tumors 2.1 to 4 cm in diameter, and approximately 35% for tumors greater than 4 cm in size.[146,147] An infiltrative pattern of growth increases the risk of nodal spread,[61,110] and the presence of vascular or lymphatic space invasion substantially escalates the probability of finding metatases in dissected nodes.[144] Metastatic spread to contralateral groin nodes in the absence of disease in ipsilateral nodes will occur in 15% or less of all patients with metastases to groin nodes,[66] generally in patients with larger lesions. Although contralateral nodal spread has been described in two patients with lateralized T1 lesions,[56] the risk of this condition in the absence of ipsilateral metastasis is less than 1%.[23,24,54,55,57,62] When metastatic disease is present in multiple groin nodes, pelvic lymphadenectomy will detect disease in 15% to

**TABLE 10-9  Assessment of Inguinofemoral Nodes**

| FIGO 1969 Stage | Number of Patients | Number (%) Receiving Each Histological Assessment | |
|---|---|---|---|
| | | Negative | Positive |
| Clinically negative, N0,1 | 451 | 363  (80.5%) | 88  (19.5%) |
| Clinically positive, N2,3 | 243 | 53  (21.8%) | 190  (78.2%) |

*Source:* Pooled data from six institutions.[3,7,14,63,65,139]

25% of patients,[6,7,14,25,63–68] but rarely when only one groin node is microscopically contaminated.[13,15] Appraisal of the risk and anatomic level of lymph node spread is an essential part of determining target volume, dose, and technique for any course of radiation therapy, definitive or adjuvant.

Integration of radiation and surgery for optimal outcomes requires an understanding of the strengths and limitations of primary surgical treatment, and the extent of operative therapy to be performed. Contemporary surgical management of cancer of the vulva is highly individualized. Surgical strategy is predicated on primary tumor parameters, clinical assessment of the groin nodes, the status of adjacent tissues, medical comorbidities, and patient preference. Based on identifying patients with minimal risk of nodal spread, wide local excision omitting node dissection has been reported to be a sensible surgical option in selected circumstances. Discrete tumors, 2 cm or less in diameter, with 1 mm or less of invasion, and without an infiltrating or "spray" pattern of growth, locally excised with at least 1 cm clinical margin, will recur locally in only 5% of cases.[22,24,55,57] Success with this approach is dependent on the diligence of the pathologist, as the risk of groin metastasis escalates with progressive depth of tumor invasion and correlates with pattern of invasion. The consequence of recurrence in an undissected groin will usually be death from cancer,[17,24,56,62,53,148] regardless of the salvage therapy employed. Wide local excision may be appropriate for patients with larger or more deeply invasive primary tumors but should be accompanied by at least ipsilateral groin dissection. For patients with well-lateralized T1 primary tumors, contralateral groin dissection is unwarranted absent spread to more than one node in the ipsilateral groin, as the risk of contralateral spread is otherwise minimal.[23–25,54–57,149] Unless conservation of the clitoris is of importance to the patient, radical vulvectomy will generally be the most appropriate surgical management of the primary tumor for patients with multifocal invasive vulvar cancer, extensive VIN, or

vulvar dystrophy that has been unresponsive to topical steroids.

The most reliable factor predictive of local control is the adequacy of the surgical margin.[150] An 8 mm margin in fixed tissue, corresponding to a clinical margin of approximately 1 cm, is a useful guide in planning conservative surgery for patients with primary tumors that encroach upon functionally important structures such as the anus, urethra, distal vagina, and clitoris. The distal urethra can be removed with preservation of urinary continence in most patients, though removal of only a portion of the anal sphincter may compromise fecal continence.[151] The competing risks of local recurrence and functional loss of normal structures must be assessed in comparison with alternative strategies employing preoperative radiation or chemoradiation coupled with surgery of lesser magnitude, or treatment by chemoradiation alone. Surgical exenteration, even for massive primary disease, should seldom be chosen as initial therapy unless the cancer has already destroyed the functions of the critical normal tissues that might otherwise be preserved, and is rarely appropriate when regional node metastases are present.[8]

The postoperative complication frequently responsible for prolonged hospitalization and delayed recovery is breakdown of the surgical wound in the groins. Associated with the so-called butterfly incision and en bloc resection of the primary and groin nodes with overlying skin, this complication can be reduced in frequency and severity by performance of the vulvectomy and the groin dissections through separate incisions, reducing tension on the skin flaps and preserving vascular supply.[152,153] This refinement in technique comes at the price of the rare, but disheartening, recurrence in the preserved bridge of tissue between the separate incisions, an unlikely event unless groin nodes are contaminated.[153]

Although cancer of the vulva may occasionally disseminate hematogenously, this is uncommon and is rarely seen as the solitary manifestation of failure. Approximately 80% of patients who fail surgical therapy will first

TABLE 10-10    Pattern of Recurrence[a] in 267 Patients Who Failed Regional Therapy[b] for Carcinoma of the Vulva

| Vulva/Perineum | Groin | Pelvis | Distant |
|---|---|---|---|
| 162  (60.7%) | 62  (23.2%) | 42  (15.7%) | 51  (19.1%) |

[a]Total recurrences exceed 267 and total of the percentages exceeds 100 percent because some patients manifested recurrence at more than one site.

[b]The majority of patients underwent radical surgery. Adjunctive radiation was administered in some, and a small number were treated with radiation alone.

*Source:* Pooled data from seven series.[24,154–159]

experience recurrence in residual vulva, on the perineum, at the vaginal margin, in the groins or upper thighs, or in the pelvis, and less than 20% will experience distant recurrence[24,154–159] (Table 10-10). Parameters predictive of local–regional recurrence include a surgical margin less than 8 mm,[150] the presence of groin node metastasis, vascular or lymphatic space invasion, and an infiltrative pattern of growth. The presence of one or more of these factors should prompt consideration of adjuvant radiation.

## RADIATION THERAPY

Radiotherapy is increasingly employed in the curative management of cancer of the vulva,[26-34] often in conjunction with synchronous administration of radiation potentiating cytotoxic chemotherapy (chemoradiation).[35–50] Radiation will salvage some patients with local–regional recurrence after radical vulvectomy and regional node dissection.[160] Adjuvant postoperative radiation directed to the groins and pelvic nodes will improve disease-free survival in patients with metastatic spread to two or more inguinofemoral nodes[25] and may further improve local–regional control and survival if residual vulva and perineum are included within the irradiated volume.[26,161] Preoperative radiation, alone or coordinated with synchronous chemotherapy, has reduced the indications for exenterative surgery and may permit a substantial decrease in the volume of normal tissue that needs to be removed in patients with tumors invading or intimately approximating the anus, clitoris, urethra, and distal vagina.[28–31,33,35–44,162] Radical chemoradiation provides sensible alternative therapy for patients who are technically unresectable or medically inoperable.[46–50]

## SALVAGE THERAPY

Following surgery, central, limited volume local recurrence in residual vulva, at the vaginal introitus, or on the perineum can be successfully salvaged with secondary surgery, radiation, or combined modality therapy.[148,154,158–160,163] A disease-free interval of 2 or more years and lack of involvement of regional nodes initially portend a favorable outcome with salvage therapy,[158] although 2-year actuarial survival after local relapse may be as little as 25%.[26] When the anticipated surgical margin will be less than that of the original surgery, when recurrence approaches or involves critical structures, or when the pattern of recurrence is multifocal, it is prudent to plan for delivery of radiation as at least a component of the salvage strategy. Regional relapse in the groin or in pelvic nodes is much less likely to be cured, regardless of the combination of modalities employed.[148,154,158–160] Radiation alone, in doses ranging from 63 to 72 Gy employing progressive volume reductions or partial treatment with brachytherapy, will often be successful in controlling small-volume recurrence. Preoperative radiation ranging in dose from 45 to 54 Gy followed by local excision may be less damaging in terms of delayed normal tissue effects than a large perineal volume carried to a high radiation dose in the absence of surgery. The majority of patients with cancer of the vulva who develop clinical recurrence will do so within 2 years of initial therapy,[158] and recurrent disease may grow rapidly despite the reputation of the primary cancer for slow, even indolent growth. When a combined approach employing surgery and radiation is planned, it is usually best to commence with radiation. Residual occult cancer after initial salvage surgery may proliferate as rapidly as the wounds heal, with the disheartening appearance of cancer regrowth within granulation tissue inadequately healed to permit initiation of postoperative radiation.

## ADJUVANT POSTOPERATIVE RADIOTHERAPY

In 1977 the Gynecologic Oncology Group (GOG) commenced a randomized trial comparing pelvic lymphadenectomy to radiotherapy directed to the bilateral groins and pelvic nodes (but not including the tumor bed or perineum) for patients found to have groin node metastasis. Because of significant survival differences between the treatment arms at 2 years, the study was closed to accrual of patients in 1984, 2 years ahead of the originally projected date. A total of 114 eligible patients were randomized, of whom 40 had only one groin node positive. Fifteen of 53 patients undergoing pelvic lymphadenectomy had spread to pelvic nodes (28.3%), and 9 of these women (60%) had died of cancer within one year of study entry. The survival advantage for radiation at 2 years (68% survival for radiation, 54% for pelvic node dissection) was statistically limited to patients with metastases in two or more groin nodes (63% survival for radiation, 37% for pelvic node dissection). The benefit of radiation was attributable to a decrease in groin recurrence among the irradiated patients (5.1%) versus patients treated by surgery alone (23.6%). Lymphedema was observed among 19% of patients irradiated and 11% of patients treated with surgery alone. Of the 44 patients who failed, only 11 patients relapsed with a component of "distant" disease (including 3 patients with failure in the thigh,

para-aortic nodes, and abdominal skin), whereas 75% of patients failed with local–regional disease alone (vulvar area, perineum, groins, or pelvis). Eleven patients recurred in the unirradiated vulvar area (25%), of whom 10 had no other apparent sites of failure. Consequent to this study, pelvic lymphadenectomy is less likely to be performed, and regional adjuvant radiation has become the standard of additional care for patients with metastasis to two or more regional nodes.[25] Many patients whose cancer has spread to regional nodes have adverse prognostic factors predictive of local relapse. Inclusion of the primary tumor bed and perineum in the treatment volume should be given serious consideration when postoperative radiation is administered, as this may further improve relapse-free survival and prevent the unsalvageable local recurrence.[26,161]

## PREOPERATIVE RADIATION THERAPY

Whenever the clinical extent of either the primary disease or regional node involvement would indicate postoperative radiation, it is reasonable to consider preoperative radiation if this measure has the potential to reduce the scope of surgery and to conserve normal tissue structure and function.[162] Preoperative radiotherapy may convert the unresectable cancer to an operable status.[28–33,162] An anticipated clinical margin of 1 cm or less from structures that will not be removed surgically is a useful guide for selecting patients for preoperative radiation. Tumors that encroach upon the anal sphincter, abut the pubic arch, or involve more than the distal urethra should be considered for preoperative therapy. Patients with tumors that approach the clitoris or extend more than minimally past the vaginal introitus should be considered for preoperative therapy if conservation of sexual function is desired. Moderate dose (36–54 Gy) preoperative radiation has been given followed by excision of residual palpable abnormalities that have revealed no evidence of persistent cancer in 50% of cases[30–32] (Table 10-11). External beam has been the radi-

**TABLE 10-11  Histologic Tumor Clearance by Preoperative Radiation Employing External Beam Therapy**

| Study | Number of Patients[a] | Dose (Gy) | Number of Negative Specimens | Percent[b] |
|---|---|---|---|---|
| Hacker et al.[30] | 8[c] | 44–54 | 4 | 50 |
| Acosta et al.[31] | 14 | 36–55 | 5 | 36 |
| Jafari et al.[32] | 4 | 30–42 | 4 | 100 |
| | 16 | | 13 | 50 |

[a]Minimum and maximum dose (range) in Gy.

[b]Percent with operative specimens showing no residual cancer.

[c]Includes one patient who received an additional 24 Gy by intravaginal mold.

ation modality most commonly employed. Interstitial or intracavitary brachytherapy may be used to apply a higher dose to a limited volume where an inadequate surgical margin is anticipated.[29] The probability of local tumor control has been excellent when this approach has been used, with conservation of normal tissue integrity in many patients who would otherwise have required exenteration to achieve surgical tumor clearance with secure margins. The observation of complete histologic clearance of malignancy following moderate dose preoperative radiation serves to encourage efforts to control cancer of the vulva with radiation-based therapy. When surgery is technically unfeasible, medically contraindicated, or likely to imply more severe chronic morbidity, radiation-based therapy is an appropriate alternative.

## RADICAL RADIOTHERAPY AND CHEMORADIATION

Definitive radiation has been historically employed to treat medically inoperable or technically unresectable patients, often in circumstances that combine advanced, neglected cancer with major comorbid illnesses. Overall, results have been poor, both in terms of tumor control and normal tissue sequelae, although the tumor control probability for patients with disease of limited volume has approached that of surgery.[12,34,164] With the benefit of hindsight, it is easy to appreciate that historical results were frequently compromised by treatment of inadequate volume, using inadequate technique, employing naive dose–fractionation schemes with primitive dosimetry and equipment. Contemporary experience using high dose radiation alone with sensible technique, equipment, and fractionation is sparse.[34] The favorable clinical experience employing chemotherapy and reduced dose radiation in the treatment of cancers of the anal canal has prompted extrapolation of this approach in the treatment of advanced vulvar cancer. Most published experiences have employed 5-fluorouracil, with or without cisplatin or mitomycin C.[35–50] Experience with bleomycin has been unfavorable.[165]

The small numbers of heterogeneous patients undergoing individualized management with chemoradiation necessarily render conclusions preliminary. Unquestionably, the administration of concurrent chemotherapy augments the acute reaction in normal tissues. Moist desquamation of the vulva will necessitate treatment interruption in many patients. Hybrid dose–fractionation regimens have been developed to preserve dose intensity and to maximize potential synergistic effects. Twice daily fractionation has become a popular strategy to exploit the radiation drug interaction while minimizing the theoretic disadvantages of split course radiation often made necessary by the enhanced acute effects in normal tissues.[46,48,49,162] Frequently, the additional patient and physician effort necessitated by combined modality therapy will be rewarded by dramatic, rapid tumor regression. Protection from late

**TABLE 10-12**   **Results of Radical Chemoradiation for Locally–Regionally Advanced or Recurrent Cancers of the Vulva**

| Study | Stages (number of patients) | Drugs[a] | Radiation Dose (Gy) | Complete Response | Subsequent Failure[b] | No Evidence of Disease at Follow-up (months)[c] |
|---|---|---|---|---|---|---|
| | | *Previously Untreated Patients* | | | | |
| Thomas et al.[46] | "Advanced" | F,M | 40–64 | 6 (67%) | 3 (50%) | N/A |
| Berek et al.[47] | 12 | | | | | |
| | III (8) | F,P | 44–54 | 8 (67%) | 0 | 7–60 |
| | IV (4) | | | | | |
| Russell et al.[48] | 18[d] | | | | | |
| | II (1) | F,P | 46.8–56 | 16 (89%) | 2 (13%) | 2–52 |
| | III (10) | M | | | | |
| | IV (6) | | | | | |
| Koh et al.[49] | 14[d] | | | | | |
| | III (4) | F,P | 34–63.1 | 8 (57%)[e] | 1 (17%) | 5–75 |
| | IV (10) | M | | | | |
| Cunningham et al.[50] | 14 | | | | | |
| | III (9) | F,P | 50–65 | 9 (64%) | 1 (11%) | 7–81 |
| | IV (5) | | | | | |
| Eifel et al.[42] | 12 | | | | | |
| | II (1) | F,P | 40–50 | 6 (50%)[e] | 1 (16%) | 17–37 |
| | III,IV (11) | | | | | |
| Total | 79 | | | 53 (67%) | 8 (15%) | |
| | | *Patients with Recurrent Disease* | | | | |
| Thomas et al.[46] | 15 | F,M | 40–64 | 8 (53%) | 0 | N/A |
| Russell et al.[48] | 7 | F,P | 54–72 | 4 (57%) | 1 (25%) | 2–35 |
| Total | 22 | | | 12 (55%) | 1 (13%) | |

[a]F, 5-fluorouracil; P, cisplatin; M, mitomycin.

[b]Recurrence within the irradiated volume.

[c]Length of follow-up in patients continuously cancer free.

[d]Includes one patient in each series dying of treatment-related complications (neutropenia and sepsis).

[e] Includes patients who undergo surgery following completion of chemoradiation because of clinically suspected residual disease. Surgical specimens without residual cancer.

effects in normal tissue has been achieved by reducing dose per fraction, as well as total dose. Fraction size should never exceed 1.8 Gy. Fraction size as low as 1.6 Gy has been recommended to reduce late sequelae.[166] Potential enhancement of late normal tissue effects, as well as the virtual impossibility of exploiting the skin-sparing effects of megavoltage radiation when treating what is fundamentally a skin cancer, renders it advisable that total dose not exceed approximately 54 Gy in 30 fractions, 59.5 Gy in 35 fractions, or 64 Gy in 40 fractions to gross disease when chemoradiation is employed, and that the volume carried to full dose be as small as possible consistent with inclusion of all areas of initial measurable clinical involvement. Results of 5-fluorouracil-based radical chemoradiation for locally advanced or recurrent cancer of the vulva are compiled in Table 10-12.

## ELECTIVE GROIN RADIATION

A major contributing factor to perioperative complications and chronic morbidity is the dissection of the inguinofemoral nodes. Postoperative wound breakdown is frequent, and chronic lymphedema is a common consequence of radical surgical treatment of the groins.[16,19] For patients with very small, minimally invasive primary cancers, omission of the node dissection may be prudent. In others, limiting the groin dissection to nodes superficial to the cribriform fascia (if histopathologically negative) may be an effective strategy to reduce acute and chronic surgical morbidity. Dissection of the groin nodes through a separate incision from that used to remove the vulvar primary will substantially reduce the probability of acute wound dehiscence, but will not significantly diminish the risk of lymphedema. Elective irradiation of clinically negative groins is an alternative strategy that has the theoretical advantage of treating all the regional nodes rather than leaving all, or some portion, untreated. This approach may also be applicable to patients with locally advanced primary tumors, in whom less than radical bilateral groin dissection would be inadequate surgical therapy. Several series[29,34,167–170] have reported favorable results with elective or pro-

phylactic groin irradiation (Table 10-13) but frequently in settings that would lead one to expect groin nodes to be histologically uninvolved if treated surgically (T1,2 primary tumors of limited extent).[170] The Gynecologic Oncology Group embarked on a prospective randomized trial comparing groin irradiation to groin surgery in selected patients with vulvar cancer.[74] The study was terminated early because an unacceptable rate of groin node failures (5 of 27 patients, 18.5%) was observed in the group assigned to radiation. Technical inadequacies in radiation administration may have inadvertently caused substantial underdosage of inguinofemoral nodes,[75] resulting in the observed failures and serving to emphasize the importance of technique, treatment planning, and proper dosimetry in contriving a treatment strategy based all, or in part, on radiation.[71,72] Chemoradiation may be a mechanism to improve the results of elective groin irradiation, but the simplest expedient is to deliver treatment with adequate dose distribution to the tissues at risk. At the Radiation Oncology Centers of Northern California, 23 previously untreated patients with locally advanced primary squamous cancers of the vulva [stages T2 (2), T3 (19), $T_4$ (2)] and clinically negative groin nodes have undergone chemoradiation to a volume electively including the inguinofemoral nodes.

**TABLE 10-13    Results of Elective Groin Radiation in Patients with Vulvar Cancer and Clinically Negative Inguinofemoral Lymph Nodes**[a]

| Study | Number of Patients | Groin Failure | |
|---|---|---|---|
| | | Number | Percent[b] |
| Frankendal et al.[167] | 12 | 0 | 0 |
| Simonsen et al.[168] | 65 | 11 | 16.9 |
| Boronow et al.[29] | 13 | 0 | 0 |
| Perez et al.[34] | 39 | 2 | 5.1 |
| Lee et al.[169] | 16 | 3 | 18.8 |
| Petereit et al.[170] | 23 | 2 | 8.7 |
| Stehman et al.[74] | 27 | 5 | 18.5 |
| | 195 | 23 | |

[a]Patients with FIGO 1969 N0,1 clinically evaluated groin nodes.

[b]Percent of total number of patients (195) who relapsed in the groin.

No patient underwent prior or subsequent surgical therapy to the groins. With follow-up of 6 to 98 months (mean 45, median 42), no patient has relapsed in an irradiated groin.[73] Similarly favorable results have been reported elsewhere.[41] Elective groin irradiation is likely to remain a controversial issue in the therapy of patients with limited-volume operable primaries and clinically negative nodes, in whom radiation may be entirely avoided if the histopathologic results of radical surgery are favorable. For patients who are already undergoing preoperative or definitive radiation-based therapy because of the extent of the primary tumor, extension of the treatment volume to encompass the regional nodes is a sensible alternative to groin dissection.

## RADIATION THERAPY TECHNICAL FACTORS

There is no standard target volume, technique, or dose–fractionation schedule in the radiation treatment of cancer of the vulva. The clinical context, including whether radiation is to be done postoperatively (with pathology report in hand), preoperatively (based on clinical assessment of the extent of disease), or as definitive treatment, will influence the designation of target volume, fractionation, and dose. Clinical and histopathologic characteristics of the primary and regional nodes will independently impact on the selection of technique and dose, which will be further dependent upon the scope of any coordinated surgery and chemotherapy.

### Target Volume

In the assessment of any one patient, particularly an aged individual, the radiation oncologist must first appraise that patient's general health for the presence of coincidental illnesses that may compromise the optimal use of radiation. This will necessitate considering the health of all normal tissues (small and large bowel, blood vessels, nerves, bones, urinary bladder, and skin of the vulva and perineum)

that might be included in the treatment volume. Comorbidities may require alterations in treatment volume and technique analogous to tailoring a suit of clothes to accommodate the physiognomy of the person intended to wear it.

### Volume for Postoperative Radiation

The target volume in patients undergoing treatment for groin node involvement detected at the time of radical vulvectomy should, in general, include both groin areas and the pelvic nodes. If there has been no surgical assessment of the pelvic nodes, a CT scan or equivalent imaging modality should be used to define whether pelvic nodes are grossly enlarged, and a percutaneous fine needle aspiration (FNA) performed if suspicious nodes are detected. In the absence of clinical pelvic node involvement, the superior border of the treatment volume should encompass the caudal external iliac nodes and should not extend higher than the middle of the sacroiliac joints. A 2 cm margin lateral to the medial bony margin of the pelvis will assure adequate coverage of lymph nodes that may lie lateral to the external iliac vessels. If there has been invasion of overlying skin, inclusion of at least an additional 5 cm of the skin flaps is prudent to encompass potential contamination of dermal lymphatics. In the groins, the lateral border of the treatment volume should extend close to the anterior iliac crest. If there has been extensive nodal involvement (more than microscopic, subcapsular embolization) the caudal border of the treatment volume should encompass the vertical chain of femoral lymph nodes in the upper medial thigh because of the possibility of contamination of these nodes by retrograde lymphatic spread. Under circumstances dictating irradiation of the groin and pelvic nodes, it is wise to consider including the primary tumor bed and adjacent perineal skin. Frequently patients with multiple groin node metastases have unfavorable prognostic factors associated with the primary tumor. Substantial risk of recurrence in tissues shielded by a midline block has been reported when such shielding has been employed during postoperative radiotherapy directed to the groins and pelvic nodes.[25,161] When an infiltrating or "spray" pattern of tumor growth is detected in the primary, wider margins of clinically normal tissue should be included around the tumor bed and perineum. If the primary tumor has grown across the labiocrural fold, treatment volume should include the lymphatics that run through the upper medial thighs. Some patients with histologically negative groin nodes will have indications for local tumor bed irradiation only. A microscopic margin less than 8 mm constitutes an example.[150] In this circumstance, the treatment volume should not be extended to encompass the groins or pelvic nodes because this measure will only increase the risk of subsequent lymphedema.

## Volume for Preoperative Radiation

Utilization of radiation prior to surgery should be considered either when surgical margins are anticipated to be inadequate ($\leq$ 1 cm of clinically normal tissue) or when the scope of initial surgery would compromise the functional integrity of important normal tissues (anus, urethra, clitoris, bladder). Usually such patients will have T3,4 primary tumors, but occasional patients, particularly thin individuals, will have predictably inadequate margins with T2 primary tumors. Fixed or matted groin nodes, or nodes invading or ulcerating through overlying skin, are additional indications for preoperative radiation. If preoperative radiation is to be employed, the histopathologic status of groin and pelvic nodes should be assessed prior to treatment by fine needle aspiration of palpable groin nodes exceeding 1 cm in size, or by excisional biopsy if they are superficial, accessible, and FNA has been inconclusive. CT through the pelvis and inguinal areas should be used both diagnostically and for treatment planning, with FNA assessment of abnormal findings.

At the Radiation Oncology Centers of Northern California, it has become standard practice to include groin and external iliac nodes in the initial target volume for most patients undergoing preoperative chemoradiation, even if these nodes are clinically uninvolved.

Generally, the extent of the primary lesion will suggest a substantial probability of microscopic nodal contamination. Moderate dose radiation (36–45 Gy) is applied with the intention of sterilizing occult micrometastases, and the groins are not dissected when the primary is removed. If groin nodes are histologically confirmed to be involved, preoperative chemoradiation is administered and limited dissection of residual palpable nodes is carried out at the same time as removal of the primary. Alternatively, removal of all nodes 1 cm or larger may be accomplished prior to chemoradiation. The anatomic extent of the target volume is determined in a fashion similar to that used to define the target volume for postoperative radiation. However, a full pelvic node volume is treated if the primary extends to involve middle or upper vagina, proximal urethra, bladder, or rectum, or if groin nodes are extensively involved (multiple, matted, or ulcerated).

## Volume for Radical Radiation

Treatment with radiation alone, or with concurrent chemotherapy, should be reserved for patients who have advanced local–regional disease that cannot be converted to resectable status with preoperative therapy. Although chemoradiation may eventually supplant surgery for many patients in analogy to the evolution of treatment of cancers of the anal canal, vulvectomy remains the standard of care at present. Rarely are resectable patients medically inoperable on the basis of severe comorbidities. Patients who are resectable only by exenteration may chose radiation-based therapy as an alternative, as well as sexually active patients among the approximately 15% of patients with cancer of the vulva whose primary tumor involves the clitoris. Treatment volume considerations will be similar to those for patients undergoing preoperative radiation with the exception that patients who are unresectable because of extensive skin involvement with dermal lymphatic invasion (peau d'orange) will require inclusion of larger areas of clinically uninvolved skin to achieve secure lateral margins.

## TECHNIQUE

Selection of technique will depend on the availability of equipment and the sophistication of medical dosimetry support. In addition to the care needed to select appropriate target volumes for gross and microscopic cancer, attention must be directed to the composition and volumes of normal tissue unavoidably included. Vulnerable normal tissues include the femoral necks (which lie posterior to lateral inguinal nodes), small bowel, bladder, urethra, clitoris, and anus. For patients who may be undergoing definitive radiation-based therapy, an essential step is meticulous, written recording of the anatomic extent of initial disease involvement. Clinical photographs documenting initial tumor extent will permit accurate volume reductions and sensible selection of limited, high dose volumes when the original anatomy has been obscured by rapid

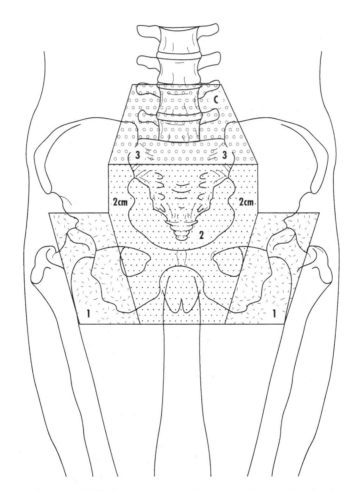

**FIGURE 10-9** Target volumes for irradiation of the vulva, pelvis, and inguinofemoral nodes. Areas labeled 1 denote volumes encompassing lateral inguinal nodes; these may be treated with anterior photons of energies 4 to 6 MV to deliver prescribed inguinofemoral node dose to a depth defined by the depths of the femoral arteries passing beneath the inguinal ligament, or with mixed photon and electron energies (12–18 MeV). Area labeled 2 indicates the volume encompassing the vulva and portions of the perineum in continuity with the true pelvic nodes; it will be treated with parallel opposed photon beams. This area may be encompassed by a partial transmission block if a large anterior photon field is used exclusively to treat the inguinal nodes.[170] Volume labeled 3 may be added to the pelvic volume if that lymph node metastasis is verified in the caudal pelvic nodes.

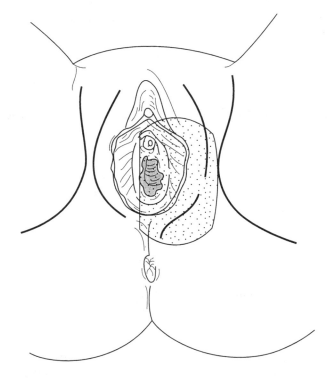

**FIGURE 10-10**  Shaped perineal port for electron beam or orthovoltage boost to vulvar primary.

tumor shrinkage. Reasonable techniques include the use of a large anterior photon field designed to encompass the entire target volume, a smaller posterior photon field designed to encompass the perineum and pelvic nodes while excluding the femurs, and supplemental anterior electron fields to bring up the dose to the groin areas that overlie the femoral necks (Figure 10-9).[34,48] Alternatively, a large anterior photon field can be used to encompass the entire target volume and to deliver the full dose to the groin areas, employing a partial transmission block centrally to attenuate dose to the midplane of the low pelvis (central axis) to 50% of the daily dose, the remaining 50% being administered through a smaller posterior pelvic photon port that excludes the femoral necks.[171] When available, use of lower energy photons (4–6 MV) anteriorly and higher energy photons (10–20 MV) posteriorly will further reduce dose to the femurs. Because of the contour of the perineum in the sagittal plane, the dose to the vulva and perineum may be as much as 20% greater than the central axis midplane dose, depending on the patient's size and the beam energy employed. Thermoluminescent dosimetry (TLD) may be helpful to clarify the magnitude of this effect, and use of a compensator may be advisable to minimize dose heterogeneity.

Successful use of these techniques mandates that dose to the groin area be applied at an appropriate depth in tissue.[71,72] This depth is conventionally defined as the depth of the femoral artery as it passes beneath the inguinal ligament. This may best be measured by CT, and will depend markedly on patient size and whether nodes have been dissected or are enlarged. Arbitrarily specifying a depth of 3 cm will adequately treat 18% of patients. Femoral nodes will be more than 5 cm deep to the skin in more than half of adult women.[71] Treatment to a reduced volume encompassing the primary disease can be accomplished by small opposed anterior and posterior photon fields, but more normal tissue can be excluded using an en face perineal electron or orthovoltage port (Figure 10-10). When disease has extended up the vagina for several centimeters, interstitial or intracavitary brachytherapy may be useful in lieu of a perineal teletherapy port.

## FRACTIONATION AND DOSE

Definitive radiation-based therapy for cancer of the vulva is difficult because of the requirement to administer a high dose to tissue that is frequently moist from perspiration and lack of ventilation and subject to continual friction. Acute radiation dermatitis with moist desquamation and pain is the frequent consequence of a course of continuous, conventionally fractionated radiation. Topical application of Silvadene cream will be soothing to many patients. Gentle debridement with sitz baths, followed by air exposure, will reduce the risk of infection and promote reepithelialization. Occlusive dressings, such as are used for thermal burn patients, may be helpful to patients with severe moist desquamation. Interruption of therapy, either mandated by skin reaction or planned to avoid severe acute effects, is common and may prolong the elapsed time required to complete a course of radiation by 2 or more weeks. Compensatory increase in the total dose may not be the best tactic to address this difficulty. While 63 to 72 Gy can often control gross cancer in the vulva, the predictable late sequelae induced by non-skin-sparing treatment, even when administered in fractions of 1.8 Gy, render such an approach inadvisable. Thin, atrophic skin with prominent telangiectasis may result. This tissue is vulnerable to interruption of epithelial integrity with formation of "greasy ulcers" with chronic weeping of serum and infection. Over years, progressive subcutaneous fibrosis and contracture can be the sequelae of high dose radiation in this area, resulting in significant disability if a large volume has been treated to high dose. Topical application of testosterone-containing cream to the vulva may thicken and toughen vulvar skin rendered atrophic by radiation in a

fashion analagous to the use of topical estrogen for radiation vaginitis. Pentoxifylline (Trental) has been used to treat fibrosis and contracture, but its efficacy is not established.

For more than a decade, chemoradiation has been used in an effort to obtain improved cancer control with lesser late sequelae (improved therapeutic ratio), in a fashion extrapolated from its successful use to treat primary cancers of the anal canal. Synchronous administration of chemotherapy complicates the treatment program by substantially potentiating acute radiation effects on all cycling cell systems (cancer and normal epithelia), as well as subjecting the patient to the hazards of systemic treatment. However, the total radiation dose employed is 15% to 20% less than might be employed if radiation alone were used, and effects on the infrequently cycling cell populations responsible for late radiation injury do not appear to be as pronounced as effects on cycling cell populations responsible for acute effects. Enhanced acute effects appear to be the price for reduced late sequelae, and treatment interruption is the common consequence. Acute skin reactions, enhanced acute gastrointestinal toxicity, and hematopoietic suppression may all contribute to treatment delay.

In an effort to preserve dose intensity by keeping elapsed treatment time as short as possible while minimizing vulnerability to tumor cell repopulation, hybrid fractionation regimens have evolved. Twice-daily fractionation (for all or some portion of the treatment) has been coupled with short, planned treatment interruptions to avoid excessive acute skin toxicity while allowing hematologic recovery.[46,48,49] Multiple daily fractions during chemotherapy infusion will, theoretically, maximize radiation–drug synergism. The chemotherapy agent most commonly employed has been 5-fluorouracil (5-FU) in doses from 750 to 1000 mg/m$^2$/24 h for 72 to 120 continuous hours. Success has also been reported with low dose continuous infusion 5-FU at 250 mg/m$^2$/24 h with 96-hour cycles weekly during 4 weeks of radiotherapy. Cisplatin at 50 to 100 mg/m$^2$ has been used as a second agent (renal function permitting), as well as mitomycin C at 6 to 12.5 mg/m². Continuous infusion cisplatin at 4 mg/m²/24 h has been coordinated with continuous infusion 5-FU.[42] Reported results of such therapy are compiled in Table 10-12. The preoperative fractionation scheme recently employed by the Gynecologic Oncology Group[162] (Table 10-14) is a rational approach to preserving dose intensity, maximizing radiation–drug synergy, minimizing treatment interruption, and minimizing late effects in normal tissue through the use of reduced dose per fraction twice-daily radiation. Guidelines for radiation dose, alone or in combination with concurrent chemotherapy, are summarized in Table 10-15 and are compartmentalized for volume of disease (microscopic vs. gross) and treatment intent (preoperative, adjuvant postoperative, or radical).

## BARTHOLIN GLAND CARCINOMA

Malignancy arising from a Bartholin gland constitutes approximately 4% to 7% of malignancies of the vulva. The criteria established by the Armed Forces Institute of Pathology for the diagnosis of Bartholin gland carcinoma enjoy the broadest contemporary acceptance.[98] A primary Bartholin gland cancer should show areas of apparent transition from normal elements to neoplastic ones on histologic study, should be histologically compatible with origin from Bartholin gland, and should exist without evidence of primary cancer elsewhere. The Bartholin complex comprises a duct lined by squamous epithelium as it enters the distal vagina. The more proximal portions of the ductal system are lined by transitional epithelium and may be lined by columnar epithelium

**TABLE 10-14    Time–Dose–Fractionation Schedule for GOG Protocol 101: A Phase II Evaluation of Preoperative[a] Chemoradiation for Advanced Vulvar Cancer**

| Treatment[b] | M | T | W | Th | F | Sa | Su | M | T | W | Th | F |
|---|---|---|---|---|---|---|---|---|---|---|---|---|
| | | | | | *Cycle 1* | | | | | | | |
| Radiation: 1.7 Gy/fraction | R | R | R | R | R | 0 | 0 | R | R | R | R | R |
| 5-FU: 1000 | R | R | R | R | | | | | | | | |
| mg/m²/24 h | F | F | F | F | | | | | | | | |
| Cisplatin: 50 mg/m² | | P | | | | | | | | | | |
| | | | | 1.5–2.5 weeks planned rest | | | | | | | | |
| | | | | | *Cycle 2* | | | | | | | |
| Radiation: 1.7 Gy/fraction | R | R | R | R | R | 0 | 0 | R | | R | | |
| R | | R | R | | | | | | | | | |
| 5-FU: 1000 | R | R | R | R | | | | | | | | |
| mg/m²/24 h | F | F | F | F | | | | | | | | |
| Cisplatin: 50 mg/m² | | P | | | | | | | | | | |
| | | | | 1.5–2.5 weeks planned rest | | | | | | | | |

[a]Patients who are judged to be unresectable following completion of 47.6 Gy preoperative chemoradiation receive additional 20 Gy in fractions of 1.7 to 2.0 Gy with reduced treatment volume encompassing gross residual disease; or they may receive additional radiation dose via brachytherapy. A third cycle of chemotherapy is recommended if teletherapy is employed. The author would suggest restricting the cumulative dose to 59.5 Gy in 35 fractions in the interest of avoiding severe late skin effects.

[b]R denotes a fraction of external radiation. A 4-hour minimum intertreatment interval is mandatory, but 6 or more hours is suggested when practically feasible; F signifies 5-fluorouracil by continuous intravenous infusion; P indicates bolus administration of cisplatin.

**TABLE 10-15   Dose Guidelines[a] for Microscopic and Gross Volumes**

| | Dose Guidelines (Gy) | | | |
| | Radiation Alone | | Chemoradiation | |
| Intent | Microscopic | Gross | Microscopic | Gross |
| --- | --- | --- | --- | --- |
| Preoperative | 45–56 | 45–56 | 36–48 | 36–48 |
| Postoperative | 45–56 | 54–64 | 36–48 | 45–56 |
| | | (+ margin) | | (+ margin) |
| Radical | 45–56 | 63–72 | 36–48 | 45–64 |

[a]Dose guidelines assume that treatment will be administered in fractions of 1.6 to 1.8 Gy and that multiple daily fractions may be employed for all or a part of the treatment. Higher total doses imply fraction size of 1.6 Gy, and lower total doses imply fraction size of 1.8 Gy. Dose guidelines should be interpreted in the contexts of tumor bulk, health of normal tissues unavoidably included within the treatment volume, tolerance, and response to treatment. Use of doses in the lower end of the range for gross disease is predicated on a biopsy at the completion of treatment to confirm histologic clearance. Doses for gross disease should be applied with progressively shrinking volumes that confine high dose to not more, and possibly less, than the original volume of measurable disease.

before arborization into secretory glandular elements. A variety of histologic tumor types may arise. Squamous carcinoma constitutes approximately 35% to 50% of cases, with adenocarcinoma only slightly less common.[97–100,102] Adenosquamous carcinomas and transitional cell carcinomas are a small minority of cases. Adenoid cystic carcinoma (cylindroma) represents a distinct subset[101] thought to be less likely to spread to regional nodes, and associated with a long natural history and late recurrences that may be either local or hematogenous. Bartholin gland carcinomas have been reported in younger women and in association with pregnancy,[97,98] although an etiological relationship is not apparent. A small minority of patients will have a history of recurrent bouts of bartholinitis, but the irritative effects of multiple infections cannot be etiologically implicated in most patients. Often presenting with a mass deep in the labia with intact overlying skin, a patient with Bartholin gland carcinoma, particularly if she is young, may experience delay in correct diagnosis owing to misdiagnosis as a Bartholin cyst or abcess. There is no persuasive evidence that squamous carcinomas of Bartholin gland behave differently or should be managed differently from squamous cancers arising from other structures in the vulva. Patients with

other histologic types are so rare that it is not credible to assert standard treatment policies. Rather it is probably wiser to manage such patients according to generally accepted oncologic principles, and without doctrinal rigidity. A role for radiotherapy has not been specifically established for patients with Bartholin gland carcinoma, but the majority of patients who fail primary surgical therapy will have at least a component of local–regional recurrence.[100,102] A retrospective review of 36 nonrandomized patients at M. D. Anderson Hospital and Tumor Institute revealed that 6 of 22 patients (27%) treated with surgery alone developed local recurrence, whereas only 1 of 14 higher risk patients (7%) selected to receive adjuvant radiation manifested local failure.[102]

## VERRUCOUS CARCINOMA

Verrucous carcinoma is a variant of squamous cancer characterized by minimal nuclear anaplasia, infrequent mitotic figures, exuberant hyperkeratosis and parakeratosis, and reactive inflammation consisting of plasma cells, mononuclear cells, and polymorphonuclear leukocytes. Often this cancer is associated with condyloma acuminata.[109] Generally large, pearly gray to white, and with gross morphology similar to a cauliflower, these cancers characteristically invade with a sharply circumscribed pushing margin. While locally destructive, this cancer will rarely metastasize to regional lymph nodes or distantly[107–109] but will often recur at the margin of surgical resection. Radiation therapy has generally been considered ineffective, and possibly dangerous. Transformation of verrucous lesions to more anaplastic histology following unsuccessful radiation treatment has been attributed to radiation mutagenesis or accelerated repopulation, although the evidence for this is anecdotal. However, reports of any favorable outcomes after radiation are infrequent.[108] It would seem prudent to limit the use of radiation and other innovative therapies to circumstances in which potentially curative surgery cannot be performed.

## MELANOMA

Cases of vulvar melanoma-76–83 represent a small minority of female patients with mucocutaneous melanoma (approximately 2%) as well as a minority of patients with primary malignancies of the vulva ($\leq$ 10%). Memorial Sloan-Kettering Cancer Center recorded 44 patients between 1934 and 1973[79] and the Mayo Clinic reported 48 patients between 1950 and 1980.[80] Because of the rarity of this clinical problem, even in tertiary referral centers, no single institution or physician is likely to accumulate a significant number of patients with uniform initial assessment or standardized treatment. Retrospective reviews have revealed several clear clinical parameters that distinguish this disease from squamous cancer. Patients are more likely to have nodal and hematogenous metastases at the time of diagnosis. Patients with nodal spread are rarely cured.[79] Although an overall 5-year survival rate as high as 50% has been reported,[78] most series record 5-year survival between 15% and 30%. As with melanoma arising at other sites, the spectrum of biologic virulence is broad. Recurrences and metastases 10 years or longer

after initial treatment are not uncommon.[77,79–81] The reported patterns of recurrence reveal a high frequency of relapse locally, in the groins, and in pelvic soft tissues, which often antedates the clinical appearence of hematogenous metastases.[77–81] Prognosis can be correlated with the level of invasion using Clark's methodology[172] or the depth of invasion using Breslow's classification,[173] which may be useful tools in selecting prognostically unfavorable node-negative patients for potential adjuvant therapies, as well as in discriminating between patients who warrant therapeutic node dissection from those who do not.

Controversy surrounds the issue of the extent of surgical intervention in vulvar melanoma. Some advocate local excision without groin dissection reserving groin dissection, for patients with clinical groin metastases at presentation and those relapsing in the groin after initial management.[82] Others argue that aggressive surgery (radical vulvectomy and inguinal lymphadenectomy) remains the standard of care from which one deviates cautiously.[83] The rarity of this condition, coupled with a long natural history of the disease in some patients and a lack of effective systemic therapy, renders it implausible that this divergence of views will be reconciled soon. A role for radiation therapy has not been established. Anecdotal information suggests that melanoma arising in this location may be more radiocurable than melanoma from other cutaneous sites.[76] Given the high local–regional recurrence rate following what is often extensive and sometimes mutilating surgery, prospective investigation of adjuvant regional radiotherapy, alone or in combination with chemotherapy, would appear warranted.

## CONCLUSION

The management of carcinoma of the vulva is in rapid transition. Indeed, the very biology and anatomic extent of the disease to be treated may be changing as a result of changes in sexual mores and improved access to health care. The past two decades have seen major modifications in treatment techniques, reflecting alterations in the goals of therapy. No longer is cancer eradication at any cost the sole objective. Preservation of normal tissue integrity and function has become equally important as results of therapy have improved. As clinical experience with newer combinations of treatment modalities accumulates and matures, guidelines for patient selection, treatment volume, technique, dose, fractionation, and use of adjunctive therapies are anticipated to become increasingly refined. During this period of rapid evolution, it is unwise to become rigid or doctrinaire in the application of existing treatment modalities and techniques. They are quite likely to change.

At the pinnacle of his distinguished career, Stanley Way, the English surgeon perhaps most deserving of credit for the acceptance of radical vulvectomy and inguinofemoral lymphadenectomy as the standard of surgical therapy for cancer of the vulva, addressed the annual meeting of the American Association of Obstetricians and Gynecologists in Hot Springs, Virginia.[3] In concluding his remarks he stated: "This operation is, I think, but a passing phase in cancer therapy, and it is my hope that one day it will become obsolete."

# REFERENCES

1. Taussig FJ: Cancer of the vulva: An analysis of 155 cases. *Am J Obstet Gynecol* 1940;40: 764–779.

2. Way S: The anatomy of the lymphatic drainage of the vulva and its furtherance on the radical operation for carcinoma. *Ann R Coll Surg Engl* 1948;3:187–209.

3. Way S: Carcinoma of the vulva. *Am J Obstet Gynecol* 1960;79:692–697.

4. Green TH Jr, Ulfelder H, Meigs JV: Epidermoid carcinoma of the vulva: An analysis of 238 cases. Parts I and II. *Am J Obstet Gynecol* 1958;73:834–847.

5. Collins CG, Collins JH, Barclay DL, et al: Cancer involving the vulva. A report on 109 consecutive cases. *Am J Obstet Gynecol* 1963; 87:762–769.

6. Green TH Jr: Carcinoma of the vulva: A reassessment. *Obstet Gynecol* 1978;52:462–469.

7. Morley GW: Infiltrative carcinoma of the vulva. Results of surgical treatment. *Am J Obstet Gynecol* 1976;124:874–888.

8. Cavanagh D, Shepherd JH: The place of pelvic exenteration in the primary management of advanced carcinoma of the vulva. *Gynecol Oncol* 1982;13:318–322.

9. Lifshitz S, Savage JE, Yates SJ, Buchsbaum HJ: Primary epidermoid carcinoma of the vulva. *Surg Gynecol Obstet* 1982;155:59–61.

10. Helgason NM, Hass AC, Latourette HB: Radiation therapy in carcinoma of the vulva: A review of 53 patients. *Cancer* 1972;30:997–1000.

11. Kuipers T: Carcinoma of the vulva. *Radiol Clin (Basel)* 2975;44:475–483.

12. Frischbier HJ, Thomsen K: Treatment of cancer of the vulva with high energy electrons. *Am J Obstet Gynecol* 1971;111:431–435.

13. Curry SL, Wharton JT, Rutledge F: Positive lymph nodes in vulvar squamous carcinoma. *Gynecol Oncol* 1980;9:63–66.

14. Iversen T, Aalders JG, Christensen A, Kolstad P: Squamous cell carcinoma of the vulva: A review of 424 patients, 1956–1974. *Gynecol Oncol* 1980;9:271–279.

15. Hacker NF, Berek JS, Lagasse LD, Leuchter RS, Moore JG: Management of regional lymph nodes and their prognostic influence in vulvar cancer. *Obstet Gynecol* 1983;61:408–412.

16. Podratz KC, Symmonds RE, Taylor WF, Williams TJ: Carcinoma of the vulva: Analysis of treatment and survival. *Obstet Gynecol* 1983;61:63–74.

17. Monaghan JM, Hammond IG: Pelvic node dissection in the treatment of vulval carcinoma—Is it necessary? *Br J Obstet Gynaecol* 1984;91:270–274.

18. Woodruff JD, Julian C, Puray T, Mermut S, Katayama P: The contemporary challenge of carcinoma in situ of the vulva. *Am J Obstet Gynecol* 1973;115:677–686.

19. McKelvey JL, Adcock LL: Cancer of the vulva. *Obstet Gynecol* 1965;26:455–466.

20. Andersen BL, Hacker NF: Psychosexual adjustment after vulvar surgery. *Obstet Gynecol* 1983;62:457–462.

21. Stellman RE, Goodwin JM, Robinson J, Dansak D, Hilgers RD: Psychological effects

of vulvectomy. *Psychosomatics* 1984;25: 779–783.

22. DiSaia PJ, Creasman WT, Rich WM: An alternative approach to early cancer of the vulva. *Am J Obstet Gynecol* 1979;133:825–832.

23. Iversen T, Abeler V, Aalders J: Individualized treatment of stage I carcinoma of the vulva. *Obstet Gynecol* 1981;57:85–91.

24. Hacker NF, Berek JS, Lagasse LD, Nieberg RK, Leuchter RS: Individualization of treatment for stage I squamous cell vulvar carcinoma. *Obstet Gynecol* 1984;63:155–162.

25. Homesley HD, Bundy BN, Sedlis A, Adcock L: Radiation therapy versus pelvic node resection for carcinoma of the vulva with positive groin nodes. *Obstet Gynecol* 1986;68:733–740.

26. Faul CM, Mirmow D, Huang Q, Gerszten K, Day R, Jones MW: Adjuvant radiation for vulvar carcinoma: Improved local control. *Int J Radiat Oncol Biol Phys* 1997;38:381–389.

27. Creasman WT, Phillips JL, Menck HR: The National Cancer Data Base report on early stage invasive vulvar carcinoma. The American College of Surgeons Commission on Cancer and the American Cancer Society. *Cancer* 1997;80:505–513.

28. Boronow RC: Therapeutic alternative to primary exenteration for advanced vulvo-vaginal cancer. *Gynecol Oncol* 1973;1:233–255.

29. Boronow RC, Hickman BT, Reagan MT, Smith RA, Steadham RE. Combined therapy as an alternative to exenteration for locally advanced vulvovaginal cancer. *Am J Clin Oncol* 1987;10:171–181.

30. Hacker NF, Berek JS, Juillard GJ, Lagasse LD: Preoperative radiation therapy for locally advanced vulvar cancer. *Cancer* 1984;54: 2056–2061.

31. Acosta AA, Given FT, Frazier AB, Cordoba RB, Luminari A: Preoperative radiation therapy in the management of squamous cell carcinoma of the vulva: Preliminary report. *Am J Obstet Gynecol* 1978;132:198–206.

32. Jafari K, Magalotti F, Magalotti M: Radiation therapy in carcinoma of the vulva. *Cancer* 1981;47:686–691.

33. Fairey RN, MacKay PA, Benedet JL, Boyes DA, Turko M: Radiation treatment of carcinoma of the vulva, 1950–1980. *Am J Obstet Gynecol* 1985;151:591–597.

34. Perez CA, Grigsby PW, Galakatos A, Swanson R, Camel HM, Kao MS, Lockett MA: Radiation therapy in management of carcinoma of the vulva with emphasis on conservation therapy. *Cancer* 1993;71:3707–3716.

35. Kalra JK, Grossman AM, Krumholz BA, Chen S, Tinker MA, Flores GT, Molho L, Cortes EP: Preoperative chemoradiotherapy for carcinoma of the vulva. *Gynecol Oncol* 1981;12:256–260.

36. Levin W, Goldberg G, Altaras M, Bloch B, Shelto MG: The use of concomitant chemotherapy and radiotherapy prior to surgery in advanced stage carcinoma of the vulva. *Gynecol Oncol* 1986;25:20–25.

37. Whitaker SJ, Kirkbride P, Arnott SJ, Hudson CN, Shepherd JH: A pilot study of chemoradiotherapy in advanced carcinoma of the vulva. *Br J Obstet Gynaecol* 1990;97: 436–442.

38. Evans LS, Kersh CR, Constable WC, Taylor PT: Concomitant 5-fluorouracil, mitomycin-C, and radiotherapy for advanced gynecologic malignancies. *Int J Radiat Oncol Biol Phys* 1988;15:901–906.

39. Carson LF, Twiggs LB, Adcock LL, Prem KA, Potish RA: Multimodality therapy for advanced and recurrent vulvar squamous cell carcinoma. A pilot project. *J Reprod Med* 1990;35:1029–1032.

40. Rotmensch J, Rubin SJ, Sutton HG, Javaheri G, Halpern HJ, Schwartz JL, Stewart M, Weichselbaum RR, Herbst AL: Preoperative radiotherapy followed by radical vulvectomy with inguinal lymphadenectomy for advanced vulvar carcinomas. *Gynecol Oncol* 1990; 36:181–184.

41. Wahlen SA, Slater JD, Wagner RJ, Wang WA, Keeney ED, Hocko JM, King A, Slater JM: Concurrent radiation therapy and chemotherapy in the treatment of primary squamous cell carcinoma of the vulva. *Cancer* 1995;75: 2289–2294.

42. Eifel PJ, Morris M, Burke TW, Levenback C, Gershenson DM: Prolonged continuous infusion cisplatin and 5-fluorouracil with radiation for locally advanced cancer of the vulva. *Gynecol Oncol* 1995;59:51–56.

43. Lupi G, Raspagliesi F, Zucali R, Fontanelli R, Paladini D, Kenda R, di Re F: Combined preoperative chemoradiotherapy followed by radical

surgery in locally advanced vulvar carcinoma. A pilot study. *Cancer* 1996;77:1472–1478.

44. Landoni F, Maneo A, Zanetta G, Colombo A, Nava S, Placa F, Tancini G, Mangioni C: Concurrent preoperative chemotherapy with 5-flourouracil and mitomycin C and radiotherapy (FUMIR) followed by limited surgery in locally advanced and recurrent vulvar carcinoma. *Gynecol Oncol* 1996;61: 321–327.

45. Roberts WS, Hoffman MS, Kavanagh JJ, Fiorica JV, Greenberg H, Finan MA, Cavanagh D: Further experience with radiation therapy and concomitant intravenous chemotherapy in advanced carcinoma of the lower female genital tract. *Gynecol Oncol* 1991;43:233–236.

46. Thomas G, Dembo A, DePetrillo A, Pringle J, Ackerman I, Bryson P, Balogh J, Osborne R, Rosen B, Fyles A: Concurrent radiation and chemotherapy in vulvar carcinoma. *Gynecol Oncol* 1989;34:263–267.

47. Berek JS, Heaps JM, Fu YS, Juillard GJ, Hacker NF: Concurrent cisplatin and 5-fluorouracil chemotherapy and radiation therapy for advanced-stage squamous carcinoma of the vulva. *Gynecol Oncol* 1991;42:197–201.

48. Russell AH, Mesic JB, Scudder SA, Rosenberg PJ, Smith LH, Kinney WK, Townsend DE, Trelford JD, Taylor MH, Zukowski CL, McMahon KG: Synchronous radiation and cytotoxic chemotherapy for locally advanced or recurrent squamous cancer of the vulva. *Gynecol Oncol* 1992;47:14–20.

49. Koh WJ, Wallace JH III, Greer BE, Cain J, Stelzer KJ, Russell KJ, Tamimi HK, Figge DC, Russell AH, Griffin TW. Combined radiotherapy and chemotherapy in the management of local–regionally advanced vulvar cancer. *Int J Radiat Oncol Biol Phys* 1993;26:809–816.

50. Cunningham MJ, Goyer RP, Gibbons SK, Kredentser DC, Malfetano JH, Keys H: Primary radiation, cisplatin, and 5-fluorouracil for advanced squamous carcinoma of the vulva. *Gynecol Oncol* 1997;66:258–261.

51. Plentl AA, Friedman EA: *Lymphatic System of the Female Genitalia.* Philadelphia, Saunders, 1971.

52. Parry-Jones E: The management of premalignant and malignant conditions of the vulva. *Clin Obstet Gynaecol* 1976;3:217–228.

53. Iversen T, Aas M: Lymph drainage from the vulva. *Gynecol Oncol* 1983;16:179–189.

54. Wharton JT, Gallagher S, Rutledge FN: Microinvasive carcinoma of the vulva. *Obstet Gynecol* 1974;118:159–162.

55. Parker RT, Duncan I, Rampone J, Creasman W: Operative management of early invasive epidermoid carcinoma of the vulva. *Am J Obstet Gynecol* 1975;123:349–355.

56. Magrina JF, Webb MJ, Gaffey TA, Symmonds RE: Stage I squamous cell cancer of the vulva. *Am J Obstet Gynecol* 19979;134:453–459.

57. Buscema J, Stern JL, Woodruff JD: Early invasive carcinoma of the vulva. *Am J Obstet Gynecol* 1981;140:563–569, 1981.

58. Way S: *Aspects and Treatment of Vulvar Cancer.* Basel, Karger, 1972, p 18.

59. Piver MS, Xynos FP: Pelvic lymphadenectomy in women with carcinoma of the clitoris. *Obstet Gynecol* 1977;49:592–595.

60. Chu J, Tamimi HK, Figge DC: Femoral node metastases with negative superficial inguinal nodes in early vulvar cancer. *Am J Obstet Gynecol* 1981;140:337–339.

61. Hacker NF, Nieberg RK, Berek JS, Leuchter RS, Lucas WE, Tamimi HK, Nolan JF, Moore JG, Lagasse LD: Superficially invasive vulvar cancer with nodal metastases. *Gynecol Oncol* 1983;15:65–77.

62. Hoffman JS, Kumar NB, Morley GW: Microinvasive squamous carcinoma of the vulva: Search for a definition. *Obstet Gynecol* 1983; 61:615–618.

63. Rutledge F, Smith JP, Franklin EW: Carcinoma of the vulva. *Am J Obstet Gynecol* 1970; 106:1117–1130.

64. Dean RE, Taylor ES, Weisbrod DM, Martin JW: The treatment of premalignant and malignant lesions of the vulva. *Am J Obstet Gynecol* 1974;119:59–68.

65. Morris JM: A formula for selective lymphadenectomy: Its application to cancer of the vulva. *Obstet Gynecol* 1977;50:152–158.

66. Krupp PJ, Bohm JW: Lymph gland metastases in invasive squamous cell carcinoma of the vulva. *Am J Obstet Gynecol* 1978; 130: 943–952.

67. Benedet JL, Turko M, Fairey RN, Boyers DA: Squamous carcinoma of the vulva: Results of

treatment, 1938–1976. *Am J Obstet Gynecol* 1979;134:201–207.

68. Boyce J, Fruchter RG, Kasambilides E, Nicastri AD, Sedlis A, Remy JC: Prognostic factors in carcinoma of the vulva. *Gynecol Oncol* 1985;20:364–377.

69. Nicklin JL, Hacker NF, Heintze SW, van Eikeren M, Durham NJ: An anatomical study of inguinal lymph node topography and clinical implications for the surgical management of vulvar cancer. *Int J Gynecol Cancer* 1995; 5:128–133.

70. Borgno G, Micheletti L, Barbero M, Cavanna L, Preti M, Valentino MC, Ghiringhello B, Bocci A: Topographic distribution of groin lymph nodes. A study of 50 female cadavers. *J Reprod Med* 1990;35:1127–1129.

71. McCall AR, Olson MC, Potkul RK: The variation in inguinal lymph node depth in adult women and its importance in planning elective irradiation for vulvar cancer. *Cancer* 1995;75: 2286–2288.

72. Kalidas H: Influence of inguinal node anatomy on radiation therapy techniques. *Med Dosim* 1995;20:295–300.

73. Leiserowitz G, Russell AH, Kinney WH, Smith LH, Taylor MH, Scudder SA: Prophylactic chemoradiation of inguinofemoral lymph nodes in patients with locally extensive vulvar cancer. *Gynecol Oncol* 1997:66: 509–514.

74. Stehman FB, Bundy BN, Thomas G, Varia M, Okagaki T, Roberts J, Bell J, Heller PB: Groin dissection versus groin radiation in carcinoma of the vulva: A Gynecologic Oncology Group study. *Int J Radiat Oncol Biol Phys* 1992; 24:389–396.

75. Koh WJ, Chiu M, Stelzer KJ, Greer BE, Mastras D, Comsia N, Russell KJ, Griffin TW: Femoral vessel depth and the implications for groin node radiation. *Int J Radiat Oncol Biol Phys* 1993;27:969–974.

76. Cascinelli N, Di Re F, Lupi G, Balzarini GP: Malignant melanoma of the vulva. *Tumori* 1970;56:345–352.

77. Fenn ME, Abell MR: Melanomas of vulva and vagina. *Obstet Gynecol* 1973;41:902–911.

78. Morrow CP, Rutledge FN: Melanoma of the vulva. *Obstet Gynecol* 1972;39:745–752.

79. Chung AF, Woodruff JM, Lewis JL Jr: Malignant melanoma of the vulva: A report of 44 cases. *Obstet Gynecol* 1975;45:638–646.

80. Podratz KC, Gaffey TA, Symmonds RE, Johansen KL, O'Brien PC: Melanoma of the vulva: An update. *Gynecol Oncol* 1983;16: 153–168.

81. Brand E, Fu YS, Lagasse LD, Berek JS: Vulvovaginal melanoma. Report of seven cases and literature review. *Gynecol Oncol* 1989;33: 54–60.

82. Tasseron EW, van der Esch EP, Hart AA, Brutel de la Riviere G, Aartsen EJ: A clinicopathologic study of 30 melanomas of the vulva. *Gynecol Oncol* 1992;46:170–175.

83. Piura B, Egan M, Lopes A, Monaghan JM: Malignant melanoma of the vulva: A clinicopathologic study of 18 cases. *J Surg Oncol* 1992;50:234–240.

84. DiSaia PJ, Rutledge F, Smith JP: Sarcoma of the vulva: Report of 12 patients. *Obstet Gynecol* 1971;38:180–184.

85. Davos I, Abell MR: Soft tissue sarcomas of vulva. *Gynecol Oncol* 1976;4:70–86.

86. LiVolsi VA, Brooks JJ: Soft tissue tumors of the vulva, in EJ Wilkinson (ed): *Pathology of the Vulva and Vagina.* New York and Edinburgh, Churchill Livingstone, 1987, pp 209–238.

87. Copeland LJ, Cleary K, Sneige N, Edwards CL: Neuroendocrine (Merkel cell) carcinoma of the vulva: A case report and review of the literature. *Gynecol Oncol* 1985;22;367–378.

88. Husseinzadeh N, Wesseler T, Newman N, Shbaro I, Ho P: Neuroendocrine (Merkel cell) carcinoma of the vulva. *Gynecol Oncol* 1988; 29:105–112.

89. Rose PG, Johnston GC, O'Toole RV: Pure cutaneous histiocytosis-x of the vulva. *Obstet Gynecol* 1984;64:587–590.

90. Hall DJ, Burns JC, Goplerud DR: Kaposi's sarcoma of the vulva: A case report and brief review. *Obstet Gynecol* 1979;54:478–483.

91. Macasaet MA, Duerr A, Thelmo W, Vernon SD, Unger ER: Kaposi's sarcoma presenting as a vulvar mass. *Obstet Gynecol* 1995;86: 695–697.

92. Reymond RD, Hazra TA, Edlow DW, Bawab MS: Haemangiopericytoma of the vulva with

metastasis to bone 14 years later. *Br J Radiol* 1972;45:765–768.

93. Ambrosini A, Becagli L, De Bastiani BM: Hemangiopericytoma of the vulva: A study of two cases. *Eur J Gynaecol Oncol* 1980;1: 198–200.

94. Wilner RB, Greenwald M, Wendelken H: Eccrine carcinoma of the vulva: Report of a case. *J Am Osteopath Assoc* 1976;76:282–285.

95. Cho D, Buscema J, Rosenshein NB, Woodruff JD: Primary breast cancer of the vulva. *Obstet Gynecol* 1985;66(suppl):79S–81S.

96. Breen JL, Neubecker RD, Greenwald E, Gregor CA: Basal cell carcinoma of the vulva. *Obstet Gynecol* 1975;46:122–129.

97. Barclay DL, Collins CG, Macey HB: Cancer of the Bartholin gland: A review and report of 8 cases. *Obstet Gynecol* 1964;24:329–336.

98. Chamlian DK, Taylor HB: Primary carcinoma of Bartholin's gland: A report of 24 patients. *Obstet Gynecol* 1972;39:489–494.

99. Leuchter RS, Hacker NF, Voet RL, Berek JS, Townsend DE, Lagasse LD: Primary carcinoma of the Bartholin gland: A report of 14 cases and review of the literature. *Obstet Gynecol* 1982;60:361–368.

100. Wheelock JB, Goplerud DR, Dunn LJ, Oates JF III: Primary carcinoma of the Bartholin gland: A report of ten cases. *Obstet Gynecol* 1984;63:820–824.

101. Copeland LJ, Sneige N, Gershenson DM, Saul PB, Stringer CA, Seski JC: Adenoid cystic carcinoma of Bartholin gland. *Obstet Gynecol* 1986;67:115–120.

102. Copeland LJ, Sneige N, Gershenson DM, McGuffee VB, Abdul-Karim F, Rutledge FN: Bartholin gland carcinoma. *Obstet Gynecol* 1986;67:794–801.

103. Cliby W, Soisson AP, Berchuck A, Clarke-Pearson DL: Stage I small cell carcinoma of the vulva treated with vulvectomy, lymphadenectomy, and adjuvant chemotherapy. *Cancer* 1991;67:2415–2417.

104. Figge DC. Rare vulvar malignancies, in BE Greer and JS Berek (eds): *Gynecologic Oncology: Treatment Rationale and Techniques.* New York, Elsevier, 1991, pp 239–257.

105. Hunter DJ: Carcinoma of the vulva: A review of 361 patients. *Gynecol Oncol* 1975;3: 117–123.

106. Foye G, Marsh MR, Minkowitz S: Verrucous carcinoma of the vulva. *Obstet Gynecol* 1969; 34:484–488.

107. Gallousis S: Verrucous carcinoma: Report of three vulvar cases and review of the literature. *Obstet Gynecol* 1972;40:502–507.

108. Lucas WE, Benirschke K, Lebherz TB: Verrucous carcinoma of the female genital tract. *Am J Obstet Gynecol* 1974;119:435–440.

109. Japaze H, Van Dinh T, Woodruff JD: Verrucous carcinoma of the vulva: A study of 24 cases. *Obstet Gynecol* 1982;60:462–466.

110. Crissman JD, Azoury: Microinvasive carcinoma of the vulva. *Diagn Gynecol Obstet* 1981;3:75–80.

111. Wilkinson EJ, Rico MJ, Pierson KK: Microinvasive carcinoma of the vulva. *Int J Gynecol Pathol* 1982;1:29–39.

112. Henson D, Tarone R: An epidemiologic study of cancer of the cervix, vagina, and vulva based on the Third National Cancer Survey in the United States. *Am J Obstet Gynecol* 1977;129:525–532.

113. Marcus SL: Multiple squamous cell carcinomas involving the cervix, vagina, and vulva: The theory of multicentric origin. *Am J Obstet Gynecol* 1960;80:802–812.

114. Stern BD, Kaplan L: Multicentric foci of carcinomas arising in structures of cloacal origin. *Am J Obstet Gynecol* 1969;104:255–266.

115. Jimerson GK, Merrill JA: Multicentric squamous malignancy involving both the cervix and vulva. *Cancer* 1970;26:150–153.

116. Franklin EW III, Rutledge FN: Epidemiology of epidermoid carcinoma of the vulva. *Obstet Gynecol* 1972;39:165–172.

117. Figge DC, Gaudenz R: Invasive carcinoma of the vulva. *Am J Obstet Gynecol* 1974;119: 382–395.

118. Choo YC, Morley GW: Double primary epidermoid carcinoma of the vulva and cervix. *Gynecol Oncol* 1980;9:324–333.

119. Sherman KJ, Daling JR, Chu J, McKnight B, Weiss NS: Multiple primary tumours in women with vulvar neoplasms: A case-control study. *Br J Cancer* 1988;57:423–427.

120. Microinvasive cancer of the vulva: Report of the ISSVD Task Force. *J Reprod Med* 1984; 29:454.

121. Daling JR, Chu J, Weiss NS, Emel L, Tamimi HK: The association of condylomata acuminata and squamous carcinoma of the vulva. *Br J Cancer* 1984;50:533–535.

122. Newcomb PA, Weiss NS, Daling JR: Incidence of vulvar carcinoma in relation to menstrual, reproductive, and medical factors. *J Natl Cancer Inst* 1984;73:391–396.

123. Mabuchi K, Bross DS, Kessler II: Epidemiology of cancer of the vulva: A case-control study. *Cancer* 1985;55:1843–1848.

124. Brinton LA, Nasca PC, Mallin K, Baptiste MS, Wilbanks GD, Richart RM: Case-control study of cancer of the vulva. *Obstet Gynecol* 1990;75:859–866.

125. Boice JD, Day NE, Andersen A, Brinton LA, et al: Second cancers following radiation treatment for cervical cancer: An international collaboration among cancer registries. *J Natl Cancer Inst* 1985;74:955–975.

126. Crum CP: Carcinoma of the vulva: Epidemiology and pathogenesis. *Obstet Gynecol* 1992;79:448–454.

127. Ansink AC, Heintz APM: Epidemiology and etiology of squamous cell carcinoma of the vulva. *Eur J Obstet Gynecol Reprod Biol* 1993;48:111.

128. Porreco R, Penn I, Droegemueller W, Greer B, Makowski E: Gynecologic malignancies in immunosuppressed organ homograft recipients. *Obstet Gynecol* 1975;45:359–364.

129. Caterson RJ, Furber J, Murray J, McCarthy W, Mahoney JF, Sheil AG: Carcinoma of the vulva in two young renal allograft patients. *Transplant Proc* 1984;16:559–561.

130. Halpert R, Fruchter RG, Sedlis A, Butt K, Boyce JG, Sillman FH: Human papillomavirus and lower genital neoplasia in renal transplant patients.*Obstet Gynecol* 1986;68: 251–258.

131. Levine P, Maiman M, Zavalas E, et al: Invasive vulvar cancer and HIV infection. *Proceedings of the Society of Gynecologic Oncologists,* 1994 (abstr).

132. Korn AP, Abercrombie PD, Foster A: Vulvar intraepithelial neoplasia in women infected with human immunodeficiency virus-1. *Gynecol Oncol* 1996;61:384–386.

133. Wright TC, Koulos JP, Liu P, Sun XW: Invasive vulvar carcinoma in two women infected with human immunodeficiency virus. *Gynecol Oncol* 1996;60:500–503.

134. Bucsema J, Stern J, Woodruff JD. The significance of the histologic alterations adjacent to invasive vulvar carcinoma. *Am J Obstet Gynecol* 1980;137:902–909.

135. Zaino RJ, Husseinzadeh N, Nahhas W, Mortel R. Epithelial alterations in proximity to invasive squamous carcinoma of the vulva. *Int J Gynecol Pathol* 1982;1:73–84.

136. Borgno G, Micheletti L, Barbero M, Preti M, Cavanna L, Ghiringhello B: Epithelial alterations adjacent to 111 vulvar carcinomas. *J Reprod Med* 1988;33:500–502.

137. Jeffcoate TNA: Chronic vulvar dystrophies. *Am J Obstet Gynecol* 1966;95:61–74.

138. Leibowitch M, Neill S, Pelisse M, Moyal-Baracco M: The epithelial changes associated with squamous cell carcinoma of the vulva: A review of the clinical, histological and viral findings in 78 women. *Br J Obstet Gynaecol* 1990;97:1135–1139.

139. Goplerud DR, Keettel WC: Carcinoma of the vulva: A review of 156 cases from the University of Iowa Hospitals. *Am J Obstet Gynecol* 1968;100:550–553.

140. Rutledge FN, Mitchell MF, Munsell MF, Atkinson EN, Bass S, McGuffee V, Silva E: Prognostic indicators for invasive carcinoma of the vulva. *Gynecol Oncol* 1991;42:239–244.

141. Origoni M, Sideri M, Garsia S, Carinelli SG, Ferrari AG: Prognostic value of pathologic patterns of lymph node positivity in squamous cell carcinoma of the vulva stage III and IVA FIGO. *Gynecol Oncol* 1992;45:313–316.

142. van der Velden J, van Lindert AC, Lammes FB, ten Kate FJ, Sie-Go DM, Oosting H, Heintz AP: Extracapsular growth of lymph node metastases in squamous cell carcinoma of the vulva. *Cancer* 1995;75:2885–2890.

143. Boutselis JG: Radical vulvectomy for squamous cell carcinoma of the vulva. *Obstet Gynecol* 1972;39:827–836.

144. Binder SW, Huang I, Fu YS, Hacker NF, Berek JS: Risk factors for the development of lymph node metastasis in vulvar squamous cell carcinoma. *Gynecol Oncol* 1990;37:9–16.

145. Kneale B, Elliott P, Fortune D: Microinvasive carcinoma of the vulva. *Proceedings of the*

*International Society for the Study of Vulvar Disease,* Sixth World Congress, Cambridge, England, 1981.

146. Franklin EW III, Rutledge FN: Prognostic factors in epidermoid carcinoma of the vulva. *Obstet Gynecol* 1971;37:892–901.

147. Krupp PJ, Lee FY, Bohm JW, Batson HW, Diem JE, Lemire JE: Prognostic parameters and clinical staging criteria in epidermoid carcinoma of the vulva. *Obstet Gynecol* 1975; 46:84–88.

148. Jeppesen JT, Sell A, Skjoldborg H: Treatment of cancer of the vulva. *Acta Obstet Gynec Scand* 1972;51:101–107.

149. Dvoretsky PM, Bonfiglio TA, Helmkamp BF, Ramsey G, Chuang C, Beecham JB: The pathology of superficially invasive thin vulvar squamous cell carcinoma. *Int J Gynecol Pathol* 1984;3:331–342.

150. Heaps JM, Fu YS, Montz FJ, Hacker NF, Berek JS: Surgical–pathologic variables predictive of local recurrence in squamous cell carcinoma of the vulva. *Gynecol Oncol* 1990; 38:309–314.

151. Hoffman MS, Roberts WS, LaPolla JP, Fiorica JV, Cavanagh D: Carcinoma of the vulva involving the perianal or anal skin. *Gynecol Oncol* 1989;35:215–218.

152. Byron RL, Mishell DR, Yonemoto RH: The surgical treatment of invasive carcinoma of the vulva. *Surg Gynecol Obstet* 1965;121:1243.

153. Hacker NF, Leuchter RS, Berek JS, Castaldo TW, Lagasse LD: Radical vulvectomy and bilateral inguinal lymphadenectomy through separate groin incisions. *Obstet Gynecol* 1981;58:574–579.

154. Podratz KC, Symmonds RE, Taylor WF: Carcinoma of the vulva: Analysis of treatment failures. *Am J Obstet Gynecol* 1982;143: 340–351.

155. Malfetano J, Piver MS, Tsukada Y: Stage III and IV squamous cell carcinoma of the vulva. *Gynecol Oncol* 1986;23:192–198.

156. Cavanagh D, Fiorica JV, Hoffman MS, Roberts WS, Bryson SC, LaPolla JP, Barton DP: Invasive carcinoma of the vulva: Changing trends in surgical management. *Am J Obstet Gynecol* 1990;163:1007–1015.

157. Bryson SCP, Dembo AJ, Colgan TJ, et al: Invasive squamous cell carcinoma of the vulva: Defining low and high risk groups for recurrence. *Int J Gynecol Cancer* 1991;1:25.

158. Tilmans AS, Sutton GP, Look KY, Stehman FB, Ehrlich CE, Hornback NB: Recurrent squamous carcinoma of the vulva. *Am J Obstet Gynecol* 1992;167:1383–1389.

159. Piura B, Masotina A, Murdoch J, Lopes A, Morgan P, Monaghan J: Recurrent squamous cell carcinoma of the vulva: A study of 73 cases. *Gynecol Oncol* 1993;48:189–195.

160. Prempree T, Amornmarn R: Radiation treatment of recurrent carcinoma of the vulva. *Cancer* 1984;54:1943–1949.

161. Dusenbery KE, Carlson JW, LaPorte RM, Goswitz JJ, Roback DM, Adcock LL, Potish RA: Radical vulvectomy with postoperative nodal radiotherapy: A reappraisal of the vulvar central block. *Int J Radiat Oncol Biol Phys* 1993;27(suppl 1):199.

162. Moore DH, Thomas GM, Montana GS, Saxer A, Gallup DG, Olt G: Preoperative chemoradiation for advanced vulvar cancer: A phase II study of the Gynecologic Oncology Group. *Int J Radiat Oncol Biol Phys* 1998;42:79–85.

163. Buchler DA, Kline JC, Tunca JC, Carr WF: Treatment of recurrent carcinoma of the vulva. *Gynecol Oncol* 1979;8:180–184.

164. Pirtoli L, Rottoli ML: Results of radiation therapy for vulvar carcinoma. *Acta Radiol Oncol* 1982;21:45–48.

165. Iversen T: Irradiation and bleomycin in the treatment of inoperable vulval carcinoma. *Acta Obstet Gynecol Scand* 1982;61:195–197.

166. Thomas GM, Dembo AJ, Bryson SC, Osborne R, DePetrillo AD: Changing concepts in the management of vulvar cancer. *Gynecol Oncol* 1991;42:9–21.

167. Frankendal B, Larsson LG, Westling P: Carcinoma of the vulva: Results of an individualized treatment schedule. *Acta Radiol Ther Phys Biol* 1973;12:165–174.

168. Simonsen E, Nordberg UB, Johnsson JE, Lamm IL, Trope C: Radiation therapy and surgery in the treatment of regional lymph nodes in squamous cell carcinoma of the vulva. *Acta Radiol Oncol* 1984;23:433–442.

169. Lee WR, McCollough WM, Mendenhall WM, Marcus RB, Parsons JT, Million RR: Elective inguinal lymph node irradiation for pelvic carcinomas. *Cancer* 1993;72:2058–2065.

170. Petereit DG, Mehta MP, Buchler DA, Kinsella TJ: Inguinofemoral radiation of N0,N1 vulvar cancer may be equivalent to lymphadenectomy if proper radiation technique is used. *Int J Radiat Oncol Biol Phys* 1993;27:963–967.

171. Kalend AM, Park TL, Wu A, Kalnicki S, Meek AG, Bloomer WD, Solowsky EL: Clinical use of a wing field transmission block for the treatment of the pelvis including the inguinal node. *Int J Radiat Oncol Biol Phys* 1990;19:153–158.

172. Clark WH Jr, From L, Bernardino EA, Mihm MC: The histogenesis and biologic behavior of primary human malignant melanomas of the skin. *Cancer Res* 1969;29:705–727.

173. Breslow A: Thickness, cross-sectional areas, and depth of invasion in the prognosis of cutaneous melanoma. *Ann Surg* 1970;172:902–908.

# C. Ovary - ANTHONY H. RUSSELL

## INTRODUCTION

Epithelial ovarian cancer is the most frequently lethal of the common forms of gynecologic cancer. The American Cancer Society estimated 26,800 new cases in the United States in 1997, with 14,200 fatalities from the disease. While the age-specific incidence rises with age, 52% of patients are younger than 65 years at the time of diagnosis, and the peak incidence is between 65 and 69.[1]

## EPIDEMIOLOGY

Environmental, dietary, viral, reproductive, endocrine, and genetic factors have been implicated in the epidemiology of ovarian cancer. These variables may not be independent, but a unifying hypothesis for the pathogenesis of epithelial ovarian cancer has remained elusive.

Parity is inversely related to risk of ovarian cancer, with relative risk declining with increasing numbers of pregnancies.[2] Breast feeding has been reported to reduce the risk of ovarian cancer,[2] and several studies have confirmed that women with a history of oral contraceptive use have a lower risk of ovarian cancer than women without this history.[3–6] Use of ovulation-inducing fertility drugs has been associated with an increased risk of ovarian cancer.[7,8] These observations have led to the hypothesis that ovarian cancer is the result of an error in the reparative processes of the ovarian surface epithelium, which is ruptured and repaired with each ovulatory cycle.[9,10] Factors that reduce the number of ovulatory cycles (pregnancy, multiparity, breast feeding, oral contraceptives) may be protective, while factors that increase the lifetime number of ovulations (ovulatory infertility, ovulation-inducing drugs) may increase risk.

Hereditary or familial ovarian cancer is seen in the context of the Lynch type II cancer family syndrome (hereditary nonpolyposis colorectal cancer associated with excessive risk of endometrial and other cancers) accounting for approximately 5% of the total number of cancers in families with this syndrome.[11] Hereditary breast–ovarian cancer syndromes are associated with mutations in the *BRCA1* and *BRCA2* susceptibility loci.[12,13] *BRCA1* is believed to be a tumor suppressor gene producing a protein that is a negative regulator of tumor growth. Inheritance of the mutant allele predisposes a person to the development of cancer when the wild-type allele is damaged or inactivated. Inheritance mimics that of an autosomal dominant trait of incomplete penetration, with 50% of children of both genders at risk for carrying the mutant allele. A second mutation in the normal allele is thought to be required for "phenotypic" expression. Women with familial ovarian cancer are frequently diagnosed in their forties, in contrast to women with sporadic ovarian cancer, which has its peak 15 to 20 years later. Once thought to be extremely rare, familial ovarian cancer may be more common than originally appreciated. Consequent to increased awareness by both the medical profession and the lay public, more accurate recording and reporting may lead to more accurate appraisal of the genetic contribution to ovarian cancer risk. Families of Ashkenazi (European) Jewish descent have a higher prevalence of carriers of *BRCA1* and *BRCA2* mutations than the general public. Approximately 10% of ovarian cancers and 7% of breast cancers have been attributed to inherited mutations at the *BRCA1* and *BRCA2* genes.[14]

Ovarian cancer is usually diagnosed in an advanced stage, and the majority of afflicted women will die of the disease despite treatment. Efforts to prevent the disease include the use of oral contraceptives. Five years of oral contraceptive use may reduce the risk in nulliparous women to a level comparable to parous women who have not used oral contraceptives. Ten years of oral contraceptive use by women with a family history of ovarian cancer may reduce the risk below that of women without a family history who have not used oral contraceptives.[15] Prophylactic oophorectomy has been advocated for women with a strong, verified family history of ovarian cancer (two or more first-degree relatives affected). However, prophylactic oophorectomy with removal of histologically normal ovaries will not eliminate the risk of subsequent abdominal carcinomatosis, which can be histopathologically identical with and clinically indistinguishable from ovarian cancer.[16–19] This phenomenon has been attributed to malignant transformation of the peritoneal mesothelium, which shares embryologic origin with the ovaries.

The serum carbohydrate antigen 125 (CA-125) assay is a marker for epithelial ovarian cancer, although elevations in CA-125 can occur in nonmalignant disease such as endometriosis, uterine fibroids, pelvic inflammatory disease, and other conditions that produce irritation of the peritoneal surfaces, as well as pregnancy. In postmenopausal women, elevation of the CA-125 to levels greater than 65 U/mL has a sensitivity of 97% for ovarian cancer, with a specificity of 78%, but this measure is less reliable in premenopausal women.[20] The use of CA-125, along with detection procedures such as pelvic examinations and transvaginal ultrasound, has been advocated as a screening strategy for women at high risk for ovarian cancer. The efficiency of these screening interventions and their cost effectiveness will depend markedly on the level of risk in the population targeted for screening. There is no national consensus concerning the usefulness of screening in the general population, nor has consensus been achieved concerning the frequency and nature of screening for high risk patients. CA-125 has been found useful to monitor therapy in women with ovarian cancer. CA-125 elevation is an early warning alarm for women relapsing after complete clinical response to treatment for ovarian cancer, and may antedate clinical symptoms of relapse by several months. Because of the extremely low curative potential for salvage therapies in epithelial ovarian cancer, there is controversy over whether a rising CA-125 level should be an indication for treatment in an otherwise asymptomatic woman manifesting relapse following first-line therapy.

## HISTOLOGY

The histologic classification of ovarian tumors is complex. Tumors are categorized as serous, mucinous, endometrioid, clear cell, and transitional cell. Further categories include mixed tumors, and undifferentiated carcinomas. Within each category except the undifferentiated carcinomas, tumors may be benign or malignant. Histologic grade in malignant tumors is from I to III, corresponding to progressive loss of differentiation. Mixed epithelial and sarcomatous tumors exist, as well as homologous and heterologous mesodermal (Müllerian) mixed tumors, stromal sarcomas, and tumors of germ cell and sex-cord-stromal origin. This chapter focuses primarily on the common epithelial tumors.

It is essential to appreciate that within the serous, mucinous, clear cell, and endometrioid variants exist tumors categorized as "borderline," or tumors of low malignant potential.

This can be a subtle distinction, requiring the evaluation of an experienced gynecologic pathologist able to integrate operative and histopathologic findings. Because of the characterisitically indolent behavior of these tumors and the lack of persuasive evidence that therapy other than surgery alters the prognosis of patients with borderline "LMP" tumors, identifying these tumors is critical both in defining prognosis and prescribing therapy. Death from progressive tumor is very unusual among patients with stages I and II borderline tumors, regardless of whether adjuvant therapy is administered, and regardless of the adjuvant therapy chosen.[21,22] Among patients presenting with stage III or IV borderline tumors, it is more difficult to make this diagnosis as well as to refrain from intervention. Survival at 5 years is not indicative of cure, as relapses after 5 years are common and disease-related mortality can be 25% to 35%.[21] Cellular DNA content may be a useful tool to identify patients with aggressive borderline tumors who might benefit from therapy in addition to surgery. In a retrospective study, patients over age 60 with advanced diploid borderline tumors had a 15-year survival of 75% compared to a 20% survival among patients with aneuploid tumors.[23]

Endometrioid carcinomas of the ovary represent a special set of problems. Up to 25% of patients will have synchronous endometrial cancers of the endometrium, which may represent independent primary tumors and multifocal malignant transformation of the Müllerian tract, or may represent metastasis from the endometrium (stage IIIA).[24-30] Some endometrioid "ovarian" cancers arise in association with benign endometriosis,[31] with a transition apparent histologically. These may be seen in the context of unopposed estrogen replacement therapy in postmenopausal women, sometimes in the context of prior hysterectomy. Under these circumstances, dissemination through the peritoneal cavity is less common. For clinically localized disease (stages I and II) local–regional therapies (surgery and radiation) may be critically important components of therapy. Historically, patients with endometrioid can-

cers of the ovary were considered to be more radiocurable, often with radiation target volumes that would now be considered suboptimal for the more common serous and mucinous cancers. This may reflect the fact that some of these patients had "endometrial" cancer arising in ectopic endometrium, with a clinical behavior more reminiscent of primary uterine cancer than typical serous or mucinous ovarian tumors.

## SURGERY

Staging of ovarian cancer is primarily operative. Except for patients presenting with extra-abdominal disease such as cytologically confirmed, malignant pleural effusion, assignment of stage is based on operative findings (Table 10-16). Exploration should be carried out through an incision permitting access to the entire peritoneal cavity and allowing sampling of all sites at risk for dissemination; maximal removal of all apparent sites of tumor should be attempted. Ascites, if present, should be aspirated for cytological evaluation. Peritoneal wash should be obtained from the pelvis, paracolic gutters, and undersurfaces of the leaves of the diaphragm. Clinically encapsulated ovarian masses should be removed without rupture if technically feasible. With intraoperative confirmation of malignancy, vigorous surgical efforts should be made to define disease extent and remove all accessible sites of disease. In the absence of clinically apparent dissemination, a rigorous abdominal exploration should be undertaken with evaluation of all peritoneal surfaces. Random biopsy samples of clinically normal areas should be obtained, as well as sames from sites of apparent benign adhesions. Omentectomy, sampling of para-aortic and pelvic nodes, and biopsies of the cul-de-sac, paracolic gutters, and undersurface of the diaphragm should be routinely performed. With rare exceptions, total hysterectomy and bilateral salpingoophorectomy should be carried out. When such extensive sampling is performed, 31% of patients who are clinically

**TABLE 10-16   AJCC/FIGO Staging of Ovarian Cancer**

| TNM Categories | FIGO Stages | Description |
|---|---|---|
| TX | | Primary tumor cannot be assessed. |
| T0 | | No evidence of primary tumor. |
| T1 | I | Tumor limited to ovaries (one or both). |
| T1a | IA | Tumor limited to one ovary; capsule intact, no tumor on ovarian surface. No malignant cells in ascites or peritoneal washings.[a] |
| T1b | IB | Tumor limited to both ovaries; capsules intact, no tumor on ovarian surface. No malignant cells in ascites or peritoneal washings.[a] |
| T1c | IC | Tumor limited to one or both ovaries with any of the following: capsule ruptured, tumor on ovarian surface, malignant cells in ascites, or peritoneal washings. |
| T2 | II | Tumor involves one or both ovaries with pelvic extension. |
| T2a | IIA | Extension and/or implants on uterus and/or tube(s). No malignant cells in ascites or peritoneal washings.[a] |
| T2b | IIB | Extension to other pelvic tissues. No malignant cells in ascites or peritoneal washings.[a] |
| T2c | IIC | Pelvic extension (2a or 2b) with malignant cells in ascites or peritoneal washings. |
| T3 and/or N1 | III | Tumor involves one or both ovaries with microscopically confirmed peritoneal metastasis outside the pelvis and/or regional lymph node metastasis. |
| T3a | IIIA | Microscopic peritoneal metastasis beyond the pelvis. |
| T3b | IIIB | Macroscopic peritoneal metastasis beyond pelvis 2 cm or less in greatest diameter. |
| T3c and/or N1 | IIIC | Peritoneal metastasis beyond pelvis more than 2 cm in greatest dimension and/or regional lymph node metastasis. |
| M1 | IV | Distant metastasis[b] (excludes peritoneal metastasis). |

[a]The presence of ascites does not affect assignment of stage unless malignant cells are present.

[b]Liver capsule metastases are stage AJCC T3 and FIGO stage III. Parenchymal liver metastasis is categorized AJCC M1 and FIGO stage IV. Malignant cells must be present in pleural effusion for assignment to AJCC M1 and FIGO stage IV.

stage I or II will be upstaged,[32] commonly to stage III.

Increasingly, performance of rigorous operative staging has resulted in so-called stage migration. A smaller proportion of patients will be diagnosed with stage I and II disease who, however, may enjoy a better prognosis than historic stage I and II disease with unrecognized disease dissemination at the time of initial surgery. Similarly, the correspondingly larger proportion of patients with stage III disease in the era of aggressive staging will include patients with only subclinical evidence of microscopic dissemination who may have a somewhat better prognosis than individuals with grossly apparent dissemination at diagno-

sis. This phenomenon necessarily has the effect of limiting conclusions that can be drawn from clinical trials that antedated aggressive surgical staging, particularly trials employing local–regional radiation targeted to volumes that may have been inadequate in the light of current knowledge.

In the context of clinically apparent stage IIIC disease, effort should be expended to remove all visible and palpable disease down to microscopic volumes. Multiple retrospective series[33–49] correlate extent of residual disease after surgery with duration of survival, usually in the context of treatment with subsequent chemotherapy. Clearly patients with smaller volumes of residual disease have longer survival. It is not fully clear, however, that the surgical debulking has contributed to this outcome. Patients who can be surgically cytoreduced to volumes of less than 1 cm residual masses may well have had less extensive disease to begin with, or may have patterns of dissemination subtly different from those of patients whose disease extent and distribution are not amenable to optimal cytoreduction. In the absence of a prospective randomized trial validating aggressive cytoreduction, this approach has generally been adopted by gynecologic oncologists. The rationale for surgical debulking includes removal of potential tumor sanctuary sites in bulky tumors consisting of poorly vascularized foci of cancer not adequately exposed to chemotherapeutic agents. Bulky tumors may harbor foci of relatively resistant cells that possibly are less vulnerable to chemotherapeutic agents because they are not proliferating or progressing through the cell cycle.

When debulking surgery is not initially feasible, it may be performed following initial cytoreduction with chemotherapy, with similar results obtained. A prospective randomized trial for patients with suboptimal residual disease after initial laparotomy (residual disease > 1 cm diameter) compared three cycles of chemotherapy followed by interval cytoreductive surgery with a treatment strategy based exclusively on chemotherapy. Preliminary results show an improvement in progression-free interval and median survival for patients undergoing interval debulking.[50]

Second-look surgery was popularized as a means to identify patients without identifiable residual tumor for whom discontinuation of chemotherapy might be feasible. In addition to acute toxicities, late induction of leukemia has been linked to the prolonged use of alkylating chemotherapeutic drugs.[51,52] Despite refinements in body imaging, the most reliable method for assessing whether morphologically persistent cancer is present after chemotherapy remains second surgery. Even when the CA-125 level in marker-positive patients has fallen to within normal limits, persistent cancer can be identified in up to 62% of patients.[53,54] Second surgery, as a research tool, will provide the most accurate measure of complete response rates when new drugs or innovative treatment strategies are investigated.

While second surgery may be a useful tool in identifying patients in whom complete response permits cessation of therapy, systematic use of second surgery has not resulted in improvement in ultimate survival statistics. Despite negative findings at second surgery, as many as 50% of patients with negative second-look procedures after platinum-containing chemotherapy will relapse,[55] with probability of relapse correlating with higher initial stage, higher histologic grade, and extent of residual disease after initial surgery.[56] Second-look surgery may be used to select patients for consolidative therapy (intraperitoneal chemotherapy, immunotherapy, radiophosphorus) after complete response to first-line chemotherapy. However, at present, there is no generally accepted technique for consolidative therapy, nor is there persuasive evidence that such therapy alters survival or relapse rates.

Patients who relapse after negative second surgery, particularly if the interval to relapse is 12 months or longer, will have a significant likelihood of response to second-line chemotherapy and may remain sensitive to the agents that induced the initial complete response. However, curative management is rarely, if ever, achieved.

Patients with persistent disease detected at second laparotomy may be candidates for additional systemic therapy, possibly including high dose chemotherapy with stem cell rescue. Selected patients may be appropriate for treatment with whole-abdomen radiation. There is no national standard of care for these patients at present.

## CHEMOTHERAPY

In the United States, the majority of patients receiving postsurgical therapy will be treated with systemic agents. Patients with grade I or

II, stages IA or IB ovarian cancer based on rigorous surgical staging can be kept under observation with no further therapy, as relapse-free survival exceeds 90% in this group of patients.[57] Patients with grade III cancer or higher operative stage will usually be treated with polyagent chemotherapy.

Chemotherapy has evolved through several generations. Initially, melphalan (L-phenylalanine mustard) was the drug most frequently employed, usually as a single-agent. A prospective randomized trial of polyagent chemotherapy versus single agent therapy demonstrated a higher probability of complete response among patients treated with multiple drugs.[58] With the introduction of cisplatin in the early 1980s, platinum-based chemotherapy regimens became the standard of care in advanced ovarian cancer after prospective comparison with non-platinum-containing chemotherapy.[59] Paclitaxel, first found to be active in advanced ovarian cancer in the late 1980s, was rapidly integrated into first-line chemotherapy consequent to a randomized trial of the Gynecologic Oncology Group (GOG) that compared cisplatin and paclitaxel to cisplatin and cyclophosphamide and found the paclitaxel regimen to be superior.[60] Carboplatin, a cisplatin analog less likely to cause emesis, neurotoxicity, and renal toxicity, has been established as equivalent to cisplatin in antitumor effect.[61] Because carboplatin is more myelosuppressive (thrombocytopenia being dose limiting), platinum-based chemotherapy may employ both cisplatin and carboplatin in an effort to promote platinum dose intensity by alternating the platinum drugs and exploiting their somewhat different toxicity spectra. The current national standard of care for first-line chemotherapy is paclitaxel and one or both platinum agents.

## RADIOTHERAPY

The use of radiation to treat patients with ovarian cancer has a long and storied history. Radiation has been used as primary therapy following surgical diagnosis with or without surgical cy-toreduction. Radiation has been used in an effort to consolidate complete response to surgery and chemotherapy, and radiation has been used in an effort to salvage patients with persistent disease at the time of second laparotomy. Radiation treatment has targeted the pelvis or other partial abdominal volumes, or the whole abdominal contents by external beam. Intraperitoneal isotope administration has been used with the intent to treat the entire peritoneal surfaces. Clearly radiation is an active agent in ovarian cancer, but the goal of identifying clinical circumstances when radiation can be applied with predictable benefit has remained elusive.

## Radiophophorus

Intraperitoneal installation of colloidal suspensions of radioactive isotopes of gold and phosphorus ($^{198}$Au and $^{32}$P) represents a theoretically attractive treatment strategy for ovarian cancer patients. Ovarian cancer can be expected to manifest diffuse dissemination to multiple foci scattered throughout the peritoneal surfaces without demonstrating extra-abdominal spread until late in the clinical course of the disease. Intraperitoneal isotope administration has minimal acute toxicity and will theoretically result in the treatment of all peritoneal surfaces without the acute and chronic gastrointestinal toxicities, acute hematopoietic suppression and destruction of marrow stem cells, and time commitment associated with whole-abdomen radiation by external beam. Because of the partial $\gamma$ emission of $^{198}$Au and concerns about radiation exposure to individuals other than the patient, $^{32}$P, a pure $\beta$ emitter, has become the isotope of choice. Radiophosphorus has been used as postsurgical therapy for patients with completely resected stage I and II disease with adverse prognostic factors (ruptured capsule, tumor on the external surface of the ovary, ascites or positive peritoneal cytology, or high grade histology). A randomized trial in the Gynecologic Oncology Group comparing $^{32}$P and melphalan in this group of patients showed no survival difference at 5 years.[57] While associated with favorable survival, treatment with adjuvant $^{32}$P carries a higher risk of bowel sequelae than treatment with systemic chemotherapy.[62]

A prospective randomized trial in Norway compared radiophosphorus to six courses of cisplatin as a single agent in patients with completely resected stages I, II, and III ovarian cancer after thorough surgical staging. There was no statistically significant difference in actuarial relapse-free survival,[63] but there was a 5% rate of bowel obstruction requiring surgical intervention among the group treated with $^{32}$P. The GOG conducted a prospective randomized trial comparing $^{32}$P with three cycles of cisplatin and cyclophosphamide (GOG 95) for patients with selected unfavorable IA and IB ovarian cancers, and patients with IC and stage II A,B,C disease. Preliminary, unpublished analysis shows no significant survival difference, but a lower relapse rate among patients receiving chemotherapy. A prospective study in Italy for patients with stage IC disease randomizing between six courses of cisplatin or $^{32}$P showed no survival difference, but disease-free survival was longer in the chemotherapy-treated patients.[64]

Methodological concerns hamper interpretation of each of the foregoing studies with respect to adequacy of surgical staging in some patients, dose of $^{32}$P employed, technical aspects of $^{32}$P administration, and statistical methods. Despite these caveats, the use of $^{32}$P has largely been abandoned in the setting of low stage or completely debulked ovarian cancer. This isotope emits β particles with average energy of 0.7 MeV, which will potentially treat 3 mm deep to the peritoneal surface. Predictably, $^{32}$P will be inefficacious for patients with disease diameter larger than 5 mm, or for patients with metastasis to retroperitoneal nodes. Because inflammatory adhesions begin to form within hours after surgery, radiocolloid distribution will be problematic unless all adhesions are fully lysed at the time of laparotomy and free flow of peritoneal fluid is documented with a tracer isotope prior to installation of a therapeutic dose of isotope. Treatment should be accomplished within

hours of surgery. Catheter placement should be accomplished at the time of surgery to prevent inadvertent bowel injury, which can occur when blind catheter placement is delayed to the postoperative period. A carefully choreographed sequence of patient position changes is necessary to assure the most uniform possible distribution of radioisotope in the peritoneal cavity.[65,66] Failure to observe all these precautions may result in areas of underdosage and treatment failure, or loculation of radioisotope with focal soft tissue injury, usually manifesting as bowel obstruction.

The radioisotope $^{32}$P has been used in an effort to consolidate chemotherapeutic complete response at the time of second laparotomy,[67-69] or to treat small-volume persistent disease.[70,71] Results in phase II trials have been conflicting, and no standard role for this intervention is established at this time. When $^{32}$P is combined with pelvic external beam radiotherapy, complication rates have been unacceptably high, and this particular combination of radiation modalities should be avoided.[72]

## External Radiation

External radiation administered to a portion of the abdomen, or to the whole abdomen, has been used as first-line therapy following maximal surgical resection for patients with stages I, II, and III ovarian cancer.[73] Currently, most such patients are treated with systemic chemotherapy. Chemotherapy is perceived as less likely to cause late sequelae such as bowel injury or obstruction, and sequential chemotherapy regimens will often prolong survival for patients not cured of their cancer who can, however, live for periods of time in reasonable symbiosis with their disease. Systemic chemotherapy is difficult, if not impossible, to administer following failure of wide field radiotherapy. Thus chemotherapy has assumed primacy in the postoperative therapy of adult epithelial ovarian cancer, and the use of radiotherapy has been virtually abandoned.

Adjuvant pelvic radiotherapy was historically employed, alone or sometimes in combination with $^{32}$P, for patients with completely resected stage I and II disease in the era antedating the adoption of aggressive surgical staging. While pelvic radiotherapy was successful in reducing pelvic relapse, the high frequency of extrapelvic, upper abdominal relapse in patients with occult stage III disease limited the value of these efforts, resulting in modest, if any, survival benefit. Analysis of treatment failures, and the findings from rigorous surgical staging, made it apparent that the appropriate target volume for the first-line radiotherapeutic management of ovarian cancer is the whole abdomen.[73]

Since only limited daily doses (1.0–1.5 Gy) of radiation can be symptomatically tolerated when the entire abdomen is being irradiated, radiation is likely to be less effective in the treatment of tumors that may be proliferating rapidly. Results of abdominopelvic radiation tend to be better for patients with tumors of lower grade. Because of the limited total radiation dose that can be absorbed by sensitive structures such as the kidneys, liver, and small bowel, radiation will predictably fail when bulky disease must be eradicated. Results are better for patients with no residual disease following surgery than for patients with residual disease less than 2 cm in diameter.

The most extensive and best-analyzed data on whole-abdomen radiation as first-line therapy after surgery come from Canada[73] and Australia.[74] Patients with residual pelvic disease 2 cm or larger should not be managed in this fashion, nor should patients with residual macroscopic disease in the upper abdomen. Results are best for patients with grade I or II disease and low stage. Patients with stage III disease should be managed in this fashion only if tumor is grade I. Following these guidelines, long-term results with abdominal radiation delivered in the modern era[74] may be equivalent to those reported for polyagent chemotherapy.

Whole-abdomen radiation has been administered by means of either a "moving-strip" technique or open fields that encompass the entire abdomen from the domes of the diaphragm to the pelvic floor. The strip technique originated in an era when therapy machines could not generate fields large enough to encompass the whole abdomen in continuity. Treatment of strips in higher than conventional dose per fraction (2.25 Gy) theoretically might decrease treatment time and improve local effectiveness of radiation, provided the tumor "targets" for treatment would not move between treatments. The cancer control outcomes associated with these two techniques are equivalent, but the late effects in normal tissues have been consistently more damaging with strip technique than with open fields, leading to the abandonment of the former technique.[75,76] Sample portals for abdominal radiation using open fields are depicted in Figure 10-11. Dose and fractionation guidelines are presented in Table 10-17.

It has not been possible to prospectively compare the long-term results of abdominal radiation and contemporary chemotherapy as first-line treatments following maximal surgical effort. Attempts to conduct prospective clinical trials have been unsuccessful, probably because the treatments are so different that patient and investigator bias precluded patient participation in adequate numbers to complete a trial. There is a misconception that late radiation sequelae attributed to abdominal radiation in modest dose are more frequent than, in fact, they are. Bowel obstruction is a complication of abdominopelvic radiotherapy, but is also a common event in the natural history of recurrent ovarian cancer. Bowel obstruction after abdominopelvic radiation, in the absence of tumor recurrence, is actually an uncommon event. Analyses of complications among more than 600 patients treated with abdominopelvic radiation as first-line therapy after surgery reveal that between 2.7% and 6.4% required operative intervention for bowel complications.[74,75]

Retrospective comparisons are hampered by the bulk of the radiation data antedating the era of aggressive surgical staging that resulted in "stage migration." The impact of surgical debulking on outcome is an additional variable. Patients with similar volumes of residual disease after laparotomy and biopsy without

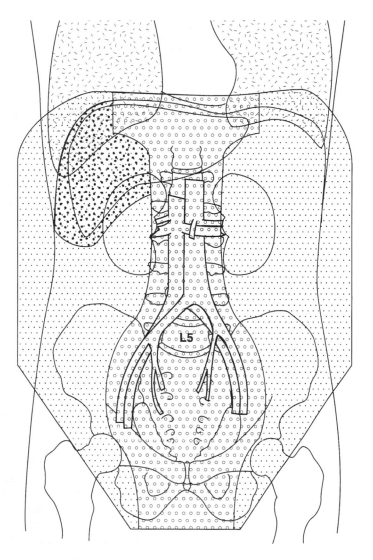

**FIGURE 10-11**   Lightly stippled large volume is intended to encompass the entire peritoneal cavity as well as the pelvic floor and vagina. Shaped secondary collimation should be designed with the assistance of fluoroscopy at the time of simulation to assure full coverage of both leaves of the diaphragm despite respiratory motion. Lateral "shine-off" is preferable to inadequate coverage of the peritoneal cavity, as the skin dose will be modest and unlikely to result in late sequelae. The more heavily stippled T-shaped volume is intended to encompass the pelvis and retroperitoneal pelvic, para-aortic, and aortocaval nodes, broadening to encompass the coalescence of the peritoneal lymphatics in the medial right leaf of the diaphragm and the diaphragmatic crus. The most heavily stippled volume corresponds to the right lobe of the liver, which should be shielded to limit dose to 24.0 to 27.0 Gy if abdominal radiation is administered at 1.5 Gy per fraction. The kidney silhouettes should be shielded from the posterior beam with 5 half-value layers or equivalent to restrict the dose to the renal parenchyma to 22.0 Gy or less, including scatter radiation as well as transmitted dose.

debulking as opposed to laparotomy with maximal effort at surgical cytoreduction may fall into prognostically different groups. The relative merits of radiation and chemotherapy as first-line postsurgical therapy for a subset of optimal patients are likely to continue to be debated. What is clear from the historic results of radiation therapy is that radiation is an agent

TABLE 10-17  Dose Guidelines for Whole-Abdomen Radiotherapy: Open Field Technique

| Structure | Dose Range (Gy) | Fraction Size (Gy)[a] |
|---|---|---|
| Whole abdomen | 22.5–30.0 | 1.0–1.5 |
| Kidneys | 22[b] | 1.2 Gy or less per fraction (5 HVL[b] posterior shielding) |
| Liver | 22.5–30.0 | 1.0–1.5: Shield right lobe[c] for a portion of treatment depending on fraction size |
| Pelvis | 45.0–51.0 | 1.5–1.8 total[d] |
| Spinal cord[e] | 45.0–48.6 | 1.5–1.8 total[e] |
| Lung bases[f] | 22.5–48.6 | 1.5–1.8[g] |

[a] Assumes treatment comprising 5 fractions weekly.

[b] Five half-value layers of posterior shielding of renal parenchyma based on IVP or CT at simulation. Total dose includes scatter contribution.

[c] Entire liver will tolerate 30 Gy delivered at 1.0 Gy per fraction.[76] If fractions of 1.5 Gy are used to treat the whole abdomen, it is appropriate to shield the right lobe of the liver after 24 to 27.0 Gy to reduce the risk of radiation hepatitis (hepatic veno-occlusive disease), which can be fatal.

[d] May be treated as field-within-field concurrent boost during whole-abdomen radiation, or as sequential boost following completion of treatment to the larger volume. Total daily dose should not exceed 1.8 Gy per fraction.

[e] May be included as part of treatment of para-aortic and aortocaval lymph nodes, either as field-within-field concurrent boost during whole-abdomen treatment, or as part of sequential boost after completion of treatment to the larger volume. Total daily dose should not exceed 1.8 Gy per fraction.

[f] Dependent portions of both the right and left lower lobes will be necessarily irradiated to assure adequate inclusion of the undersurfaces of the diaphragms and the coalescence of the peritoneal lymphatics under the right leaf of the diaphragm. Shaped lung blocks should be designed at simulation to include approximately 1.0 to 1.5 cm of lung over each diaphragm with gentle respiration.

[g] Does not account for decreased beam attenuation by lung. Pneumonitis may be symptomatic in some patients at this dose.

with a significant response rate in ovarian cancer, with substantial curative potential in selected patients. Useful integration of this partially effective modality remains elusive and controversial.

## Radiation Following Chemotherapy

In a phase II study in Toronto, a selected population of prognostically unfavorable patients (based on expected outcome with radiation as first-line therapy) with stage II or III disease, optimally cytoreduced, was treated with six courses of cisplatin-based chemotherapy. Subsequently abdominopelvic radiation was administered, and results were compared with results from matched control patients treated with radiation alone. Median survival was extended to 5.7 years versus 2.4 years in the control population; relapse-free survival in the study population was 42.6% at 5 years and

21.6% in the historical controls.[77] This study suggested that radiation may be a feasible modality to consolidate response to chemotherapy in patients at high risk of relapse based on initial extent or grade of disease. How such patients might be selected is controversial; possibilities include assessments such as operative or nonoperative findings, histologic grade, volume of residual tumor after cytoreductive surgery, and location of suspected residual. A role for routine consolidative abdominopelvic radiotherapy has not been established, nor should such treatment be administered outside the sanctions of a clinical trial.

A phase II trial from Israel could show no benefit from consolidative abdominopelvic radiation in 25 women with complete pathologic response ($n = 14$), or surgically accomplished complete response ($n = 11$) after 3 to 14 cycles of platinum-based chemotherapy.[78] In a Swiss report, consolidative whole-abdomine radiation was administered to 24 of 45 patients with pathologic complete response to cisplatin-containing chemotherapy. While the 3-year time to progression percentage was 83% for those irradiated and 49% for those not irradiated, it is discouraging that five patients had relapsed despite consolidative whole-abdomen irradiation.[79]

When whole-abdomen radiation is administered to consolidate chemotherapy response, hematologic toxicity can be expected to significantly delay completion of the planned course of radiation in up to a third of patients[80,81] and to preclude completion of treatment in 10% to 33%. Early and aggressive use of colony-stimulating factors (G-CSF, GM-CSF) to maintain circulating granulocyte counts could favorably impact on the ability to administer consolidative therapy. Depression of the circulating platelet count is the most common hematologic cause of treatment interruption and failure to complete planned radiation. Use of a recently approved cytokine (recombinant interleukin 11, Oprelvekin, NEUMEGA) may sustain circulating platelet counts at levels sufficient to press on to complete treatment,[82] although the use of this agent in this context is speculative and of unproven efficacy. The major side effect associated with this agent is fluid retention.

Partial abdominal radiation, directed to limited volumes of known persistent disease after initial surgery, may be given to consolidate response to chemotherapy. This makes sense if only one or two discrete target volumes can be treated, thus limiting both acute side effects and the potential for late sequelae, as well as increasing the likelihood that radiation will be delivered in an uninterrupted fashion, and to a higher dose. While this approach is intuitively reasonable, there are no validating data validating.

## Radiation as Salvage

An extensive literature[81,83–99] reports the results of radiation therapy employed to salvage patients identified with persistent disease at second or third laparotomy after one or more regimens of cytotoxic chemotherapy. Overall results are mediocre, but selected patients may derive substantial benefit. Clearly, patients who would have been poor candidates for initial radiation therapy should not be considered for radiation as salvage therapy. Patients with macroscopic disease at laparotomy, even if cytoreduced to microscopic disease, fare substantially less well than patients with only microscopically persistent disease.[92] Patients with limited prior chemotherapy are more likely to be able to complete salvage abdominopelvic radiation therapy than are patients who have been more heavily treated. Hematopoietic suppression, particularly thrombocytopenia, may interrupt and delay or preclude completion of radiation. Thus, if radiation is to be employed as a salvage strategy, it would seem to be sensible to confine this effort to patients with surgically defined persistent microscopic disease after optimal first-line platinum and paclitaxel-based chemotherapy. Though such patients may have prolonged survival with second-line chemotherapy, cure is rarely, if ever, accomplished with conventional therapies.

A recent report and review of the literature review[99] suggests that approximately one-third of patients with microscopic recurrent or persistent cancer after platinum-based chemotherapy will have prolonged cancer survival after abdominopelvic radiation administered as salvage therapy. Patients with macroscopic disease generally fare poorly, with only 6.8% long-term survival. This survival experience needs to be compared with the survival experience of prognostically similar patients given no further therapy until symptomatic progression, treated with second-line chemotherapy, or subjected to high dose chemotherapy with stem cell support.

## Technique for Whole-Abdomen Radiation

Irradiation of the entire abdominal contents is best planned with a fluoroscopic simulator to assure adequate coverage of the diaphragm throughout the respiratory cycle. Care must be taken to encompass the entire peritoneal surface. The use of extensive secondary collimation (blocking) in an effort to shield noncritical normal tissues can risk marginal miss, particularly when patients are treated at extended distance in both the prone and supine positions.[100] Because there are no critical tissues lateral to the peritoneal cavity, and the fraction size and total doses are modest, there is no major contraindication to treating with lateral "shine-off" or "fall-off" to assure full coverage of peritoneal surfaces in these circumstances. Posterior kidney shielding (5 half-value layers) is used to restrict the cumulative dose to the renal parenchyma to 22 Gy if the dose to the abdomen will be higher. Kidney shields may be planned based on intravenous pyelography at the time of simulation, or with the assistance of CT simulation. Depending on total dose prescribed, a portion of the liver may be shielded to restrict the dose to 24 to 27 Gy if fractions of 1.5 Gy are employed. Liver shielding will not be necessary if the abdomen is treated to 22.5 to 25 Gy in fractions of 1.0 to 1.25 Gy. Generally, the entire abdomen is treated to 22.5 to 30 Gy in fractions of 1.0 to 1.5 Gy. Limited volumes may be carried to higher dose including the medial leaves of the diaphragm where lymphatics coalesce, aortocaval nodes in patients with confirmed nodal metastasis either at the time of the initial diagnostic laparotomy or at the time of second surgery, and the pelvis. Cumulative dose to limited boost volumes may be as high as 51 Gy, with boost fractions administered in fractions of 1.5 to 1.8 Gy.

Acute and chronic toxicities associated with whole-abdomen irradiation are substantial. Hematopoietic suppression will delay treatment in approximately 27% of chemotherapy-naïve patients[101] but will more frequently interrupt therapy in patients heavily pretreated with chemotherapy. The radiation oncologist using whole-abdomen radiation as second-line or salvage therapy should be prepared to continue to treat patients with absolute neutrophile counts as low as 1000/mm$^3$ and platelet counts as low as 35,000/mm$^3$ if prolonged treatment interruption is to be avoided.

Sequelae of abdominopelvic radiation can include scarring at the lung bases (with the rare patient experiencing clinical symptoms of radiation pneumonitis), bowel obstruction, radiation hepatitis (hepatic veno-occlusive disease), which can be fatal or result in chronic portal hypertension and transudative ascites, and chylous ascites.[102] With appropriate shielding, renal damage is highly unlikely.[103] Many patients will manifest asymptomatic elevation of hepatic enzymes,[75] which may persist for months, or a year, or longer. Risks can be anticipated to be higher for patients undergoing salvage whole-abdomen radiation for persistent or recurrent disease in the setting of prior chemotherapy and second-look laparotomy.[104,105] Myelosuppression will be more severe and is more likely to interrupt therapy as well as to preclude completion of the planned course of treatment in 20% of patients. Bowel obstruction requiring surgery, in the absence of recurrent neoplasm, will affect approximately 9% to 14% of patients.[104,105]

## Future Directions with Radiation

Chemotherapy has largely supplanted radiation as first-line therapy following surgery for epithelial ovarian cancer. However, the majority of patients have stage III and IV disease at diagnosis, and most such patients will ultimately die from progressive disease despite high initial response rates to contemporary polyagent chemotherapy. Results might be improved by integrating radiation earlier into the management of selected prognostically unfavorable patients who have experienced partial or complete clinical response to chemotherapy. Radiation should be considered as potential salvage therapy for patients with microscopically persistent disease at second laparotomy, particularly if persistent disease is grade I or II. This approach merits prospective evaluation in the context of clinical trials. Interpretation of historical results has been hampered by lack of uniform reporting. Disease volume and distribution at presentation, histologic tumor grade, quantitation of residual disease following surgical cytoreduction, dose intensity of chemotherapy with first-line agents, and extent and distribution of persistent disease (if any) before and after secondary surgical cytoreduction, are all variables that could be expected to influence outcome.

Efforts to improve the effectiveness of whole-abdomen radiation might include the use of multiple daily fractions with accelerated dose delivery, use of radioprotective compounds that selectively protect normal tissues, and synchronous administration of radiation with chemotherapeutic agents known to be active in the treatment of ovarian cancer (cisplatin, paclitaxel).

The novel mechanism of action of paclitaxel could potentially be exploited in combination with synchronous radiation. Paclitaxel binds to and stabilizes intracellular microtubules, which ordinarily assemble and disassemble in a choreographed fashion as part of progression of cells through the cell cycle and mitosis. Paclitaxel prolongs cells in the $G_2$/M phases of the cell cycle in which they are more vulnerable to radiation. Cisplatin has been found to be a radiation sensitizer in vitro, and it has profitably been administered with radiation in the treatment of other tumor types.

Clearly a strategy employing either paclitaxel or cisplatin or both these agents synchronously with abdominal radiation would be potentially quite toxic. Modifications in dose and schedule of both drugs and radiation, coupled with aggressive supportive therapies such as marrow stimulants and antiemetics, might allow exploitation of potential therapeutic synergism without exceeding the acute tolerance of normal tissues.

## Radiation for Rare Ovarian Neoplasms

Dysgerminoma is a germ cell line neoplasm analogous to testicular seminoma in the male. In contrast to seminoma, dysgerminoma will be bilateral in up to 20% of cases. Because this tumor is exquisitely radiosensitive, radiation therapy has been historically employed in the adjuvant therapy of patients with bulky stage I disease as well as patients with more advanced disease. When dysgerminoma metastases were found in aortocaval nodes, prophylactic radiation was administered to the mediastinum and supraclavicular nodes in addition to partial or total abdominal volumes.[106–111] While of historical interest, the use of radiation has been appropriately abandoned since the advent of highly effective platinum-based BEP chemotherapy (**b**leomycin, **e**toposide, **c**isplatin). Platinum-based chemotherapy will salvage approximately 90% of patients presenting with stage II, III, and IV incompletely resected disease as well as patients relapsing after surgery for stage I disease.[112–114] Dysgerminoma is commonly diagnosed in women in their twenties. Use of chemotherapy, in contrast to wide field radiation, will permit conservation of fertility in some patients with advanced disease. Because of high salvage rates with chemotherapy, a policy of postsurgical observation in resected stage I disease will spare many patients the need to undergo adjuvant therapy of any sort.

Dermoid cysts are mature cystic teratomas composed largely of epidermis and skin appendages. While mature tissue elements derived from all three embryonic germ cell layers may be present and undergo malignant transformation, squamous cancers comprise the most common malignancy found within dermoids. These rare cancers tend to behave like squamous cancers arising in other sites, with the predominant pattern of early spread being local extension and metastasis to regional nodes. Radiation may be useful in the curative treatment of patients with limited stage II and III disease (local extension and/or regional node metastasis without diffuse peritoneal dissemination), although the heterogeneity of these uncommon patients precludes any generalization concerning target volumes, dose, or fractionation. Other tumors arising within dermoids include malignant neural tumors, malignant thyroid tumors (malignant struma ovarii), melanoma, sarcomas, carcinoids, basal cell carcinomas, and tumors of the skin appendages.

Granulosa cell tumors are malignant stromal tumors that can occur in infants and children but are found much more commonly in adults. The adult form of the disease is histologically different from the rare juvenile tumor and is most commonly diagnosed in women in their early fifties, comprising about 5% of malignant ovarian tumors. Adult granulosa cell tumors are frequently hormonally active, producing circulating estrogens, which may be the precipitating factor leading to diagnosis, since many of these patients seek medical attention because of menstrual irregularities (e.g., menometrorrhagia, postmenopausal bleeding). Progesterone production can be seen from these tumors, as well as androgen production with hirsutism, virilization, and oligomenorrhea in premenopausal patients.

Granulosa cell tumors will be associated with endometrial pathology in more than half of patients, with endometrial hyperplasia or endometrial cancer (in situ or invasive) arising in response to prolonged unopposed estrogenic stimulation of the endometrium.[115,116] Most granulosa cell tumors will be stage I at diagnosis. Reflecting an indolent rate of growth, granulosa cell tumors may recur or metastasize many years after surgery.[115,117,118] Hormonally active tumors may have endocrine effects, such as breast tenderness, which may antedate clinical tumor recurrence by many months. Recurrences may be focal and confined to the pelvis or retroperitoneal nodes.

As patients with resected stage I disease have 5-year survival in excess of 90%,[115,119] it is doubtful that any adjuvant intervention is indicated. Recurrence is much more common among patients with fully resected stage II or III disease.[115] Radiotherapy has been employed in an adjuvant fashion, with equivocal results.[115,120,121] Some granulosa cell tumors have hormone receptors,[122] and response to medroxyprogesterone acetate and luprolide acetate has been reported.[123-126] Radiation may be very effective in the palliative treatment of local–regional disease recurrence, but its curative salvage potential is unknown.

## REFERENCES

1. Yancik R, Ries LG, Yates JW: Ovarian cancer in the elderly: An analysis of Surveillance, Epidemiology, and End Results program data. *Am J Obstet Gynecol* 1986;154:639–647.

2. Greene MH, Clark JW, Blayney DW: The epidemiology of ovarian cancer. *Semin Oncol* 1984;11:209–226.

3. The Cancer and Steroid Hormone Study of the Centers for Disease Control and the National Institute for Child Health and Human Development: The reduction in risk of ovarian cancer associated with oral-contraceptive use. *New Engl J Med* 1987;316:650–655.

4. Rosenblatt KA, Thomas DB, Noonan EA: High-dose and low-dose combined oral contraceptives: Protection against epithelial ovarian cancer and the length of the protective effect. The WHO Collaborative Study of Neoplasia and Steroid Contraceptives. *Eur J Cancer* 1992;28A:1872–1876.

5. Cramer DW, Hutchison GB, Welch WR, Scully RE, Knapp RC: Factors affecting the association of oral contraceptives and ovarian cancer. *New Engl J Med* 1982;307:1047–1051.

6. Hartge P, Schiffman MH, Hoover R, McGowan L, Lesher L, Norris HJ: A case-control study of epithelial ovarian cancer. *Am J Obstet Gynecol* 1989;161:10–16.

7. Rossing MA, Daling JR, Weiss NS, Moore DE, Self SG: Ovarian tumors in a cohort of infertile women. *New Engl J Med* 1994;331:771–776.

8. Whittemore AS: The risk of ovarian cancer after treatment for infertility. *New Engl J Med* 1994;331:805–806.

9. Casagrande JT, Pike MC, Russ RK, Louie EW, Roy S, Henderson BE: Incessant ovulation and ovarian cancer. *Lancet* 1979;2:170–173.

10. Fathalla MF: Incessant ovulation—A factor in ovarian neoplasia? *Lancet* 1971;2:163.

11. Watson P, Lynch HT: Extracolonic cancer in hereditary nonpolyposis colorectal cancer. *Cancer* 1993;71:677–685.

12. Ford D, Easton DF, Bishop DT, Narod SA, Goldgar DE, and the Breast Cancer Linkage Consortium: Risks of cancer in *BRCA1*-mutation carriers. *Lancet* 1994;343:692–695.

13. Wooster R, Neuhausen SL, Mangion J, Quirk Y, Ford D, Collins N, Nguyen K, Seal S, et al: Localization of a breast cancer susceptibility gene, *BRCA2,* to chromosome 13q12-13. *Science* 1994;265:2088–2090.

14. Claus EB, Schildkraut JM, Thompson WD, Risch NJ: The genetic attributable risk of breast and ovarian cancer. *Cancer* 1996;77: 2318–2324.

15. Gross TP, Schlesselman JJ: The estimated effect of oral contraceptive use on the cumulative risk of epithelial ovarian cancer. *Obstet Gynecol* 1994;83:419–424.

16. Struewing JP, Watson P, Easton DF, Ponder BA, Lynch HT, Tucker MA: Prophylactic oophorectomy in inherited breast/ovarian cancer families. *J Natl Cancer Inst Monogr* 1995;17:33–35.

17. Tobacman JK, Tucker MA, Kase R, Greene MH, Costa J, Fraumeni JF: Intra-abdominal carcinomatosis after prophylactic oophorectomy in ovarian-cancer-prone families. *Lancet* 1982;2:795–797.

18. Dalrymple JC, Bannatyne P, Russell P, Solomon HJ, Tattersall MH, Atkinson K, Carter J, Duval P, Elliot P, Friedlander M, et al: Extra-ovarian peritoneal serous papillary carcinoma—A clinicopathologic study of 31 cases. *Cancer* 1989;64:110–115.

19. Piver MS, Jishi M, Tsukada Y, Nava G: Primary peritoneal carcinoma after prophylactic oophorectomy in women with a family history of ovarian cancer. *Cancer* 1993;71:2751–2755.

20. Malkasian GD Jr, Knapp RC, Lavin PT, Zurawski YR Jr, Podratz KC, Stanhope CR, Mortel R, Berek JS, Bast RC Jr, Ritts RE: Preoperative evaluation of serum CA-125 levels in premenopausal and postmenopausal patients with pelvic masses: Discrimination of benign from malignant disease. *Am J Obstet Gynecol* 1988;159:341–346.

21. Chambers JT: Borderline ovarian tumors: A review of treatment. *Yale J Biol Med* 1989; 62:351–365.

22. Creasman WT, Park R, Norris H, DiSaia PJ, Morrow CP, Hreshchyshyn MM: Stage I borderline ovarian tumors. *Obstet Gynecol* 1982; 59:93–96.

23. Kaern J, Trope C, Kjorstad KE, Abeler V, Pettersen EO: Cellular DNA content as a new prognostic tool in patients with borderline tumors of the ovary. *Gynecol Oncol* 1990;38: 452–457.

24. Eisner RF, Nieberg RK, Berek JS: Synchronous primary neoplasms of the female reproductive tract. *Gynecol Oncol* 1989;33: 335–339.

25. Ayhan A, Yalcin OT, Tuncer ZS, Gurgan T, Kucukali T: Synchronous primary malignancies of the female genital tract. *Eur J Obstet Gynecol Reprod Biol* 1992;45:63–66.

26. Tidy J, Mason WP: Endometrioid carcinoma of the ovary: A retrospective study. *Br J Obstet Gynaecol* 1988;95:1165–1169.

27. Czernobilsky B, Silverman BB, Mikuta JJ: Endometrioid carcinoma of the ovary. A clinicopathologic study of 75 cases. *Cancer* 1970;26:1141–1152.

28. Kline RC, Wharton JT, Atkinson EN, Burke TW, Gershenson DM, Edwards CL: Endometrioid carcinoma of the ovary: Retrospective review of 145 cases. *Gynecol Oncol* 1990;39:337–346.

29. Falkenberry SS, Steinhoff MM, Gordinier M, Rappoport S, Gajewski W, Granai CO. Synchronous endometrioid tumors of the ovary and endometrium. A clinicopathologic study of 22 cases. *J Reprod Med* 1996;41:713–718.

30. Pearl ML, Johnston CM, Frank TS, Roberts JA: Synchronous dual primary ovarian and endometrial carcinomas. *Int J Gynaecol Obstet* 1993;43:305–312.

31. Heaps JM, Neiberg RK, Berek JS: Malignant neoplasms arising in endometriosis. *Obstet Gynecol* 1990;75:1023–1028.

32. Young RC, Decker DG, Wharton JT, Piver MS, Sindelar WF, Edwards BK, Smith JP: Staging laparotomy in early ovarian cancer. *JAMA* 1983;250:3072–3076.

33. Griffiths CT: Surgical resection of tumor bulk in the primary treatment of ovarian carcinoma. *Monogr Natl Cancer Inst* 1975;42:101–104.

34. Hacker NF, Berek JS, Lagasse LD, Neiberg RK, Elashoff RM: Primary cytoreductive surgery for epithelial ovarian cancer. *Obstet Gynecol* 1983;61:413–420.

35. Vogl SE, Pagano M, Kaplan BH, Greenwald E, Arseneau J, Bennett B: Cisplatin bases combination chemotherapy for advanced ovar-

ian cancer: High overall response rate with curative potential only in women with small tumor burdens. *Cancer* 1983;51:2024–2030.

36. Piver MS, Lele SB, Marchetti DL, Baker TR, Tsukada Y, Emrich LJ: The impact of aggressive debulking surgery and cisplatin-based chemotherapy on progression-free survival in stage III and IV ovarian carcinoma. *J Clin Oncol* 1988;6:983–989.

37. Hainsworth JD, Grosh WW, Burnett LS, Jones HW III, Wolff SN, Greco FA: Advanced ovarian cancer: Long term results of treatment with intensive cisplatin based chemotherapy of brief duration. *Ann Intern Med* 1988;108: 165–170.

38. Delgado G, Oram DH, Petrilli ES: Stage III epithelial ovarian cancer: The role of maximal surgical reduction. *Gynecol Oncol* 1984;18: 293–298.

39. Neijt JP, ten Bokkel Huinink WW, van der Burg ME, van Oosterom AT, Willemse PH, Heintz AP, van Lent M, Trimbos JB, Bouma J, Vermarken JB, et al: Randomized trial comparing two combination chemotherapy regimens (CHAP-5 vs. CP) in advanced ovarian carcinoma. *J Clin Oncol* 1987;5:1157–1168.

40. Pohl R, Dallenbach-Hellweg G, Plugge T, Czernobilsky B: Prognostic parameters in patients with advanced ovarian malignant tumors. *Eur J Gynaecol Oncol* 1984;5:160–169.

41. Redman JR, Petrini GR, Saigo PE, Geller NL, Hakes TB: Prognostic factors in advanced ovarian carcinoma. *J Clin Oncol* 1986;4: 515–523.

42. Conte PF, Sertoli MR, Bruzzone M, Rubagotti A, Rosso R, Bentivoglia G, Conio A, Pescetto G: Cisplatin, methotrexate and 5-fluorouracil combination chemotherapy for advanced ovarian cancer. *Gynecol Oncol* 1985;20:290–297.

43. Louie K, Ozols R, Myers E, Ostchega Y, Jenkins J, Howser D, Young RC: Long term results of cisplatin-containing combination chemotherapy regimen for the treatment of advanced ovarian carcinoma. *J Clin Oncol* 1986;4: 1579–1585.

44. Posada JG Jr, Marantz AB, Yeung KY, Smith FP, Delgado G, Edwards BK, Schein PS: The cyclophosphamide, hexamethylmelamine, 5-fluorouracil regimen in the treatment of advanced and recurrent ovarian cancer. *Gynecol Oncol* 1985;20:23–31.

45. Sutton GP, Stehman FB, Einhorn LH, Roth LM, Blessing JA, Ehrlich CE: Ten-year follow-up of patients receiving cisplatin, doxorubicin, and cyclophosphamide chemotherapy for advanced epithelial ovarian carcinoma. *J Clin Oncol* 1989;7:223–229.

46. Hoskins WJ, Bundy BN, Thigpen JT, Omura GA: The influence of cytoreductive surgery on recurrence-free interval and survival in small-volume stage III epithelial ovarian cancer: A Gynecologic Oncology Group study. *Gynecol Oncol* 1992;47:159–166.

47. Hoskins WJ: Surgical staging and cytoreductive surgery of epithelial ovarian cancer. *Cancer* 1993;71:1534–1540.

48. Hoskins WJ, McGuire WP, Brady MF, Homesley HD, Creasman WT, Berman M, Ball H, Berek JS: The effect of diameter of largest residual disease on survival after primary cytoreductive surgery in patients with suboptimal residual epithelial ovarian carcinoma. *Am J Obstet Gynecol* 1994;170:974–979.

49. Del Campo JM, Felip E, Rubio D, Vidal R, Bermejo B, Colomer R, Zanon V: Long-term survival in advanced ovarian cancer after cytoreduction and chemotherapy treatment. *Gynecol Oncol* 1994;53:27–32.

50. Van der Burg ME, van Lent M, Buyse M, Kobierska A, Colombo N., Favalli G, Lacave AJ, Nardi M, Renard J, Pecarelli S: The effect of debulking surgery after induction chemotherapy on the prognosis in advanced epithelial ovarian cancer. *New Engl J Med* 1995;332:629–634.

51. Reimer RR, Hoover R, Fraumeni JF Jr, Young RC: Acute leukemia after alkylating agent therapy for ovarian cancer. *New Engl J Med* 1977;297:177–181.

52. Kaldor JM, Day NE, Pettersson F, Clarke EA, Pederson D, Mehnert W, Bell J, Host H, Prior P, Karjalainen S, et al: Leukemia following chemotherapy for ovarian cancer. *New Engl J Med* 1990;322:1–6.

53. Rubin SC, Hoskins WJ, Hakes TB, Markman M, Reichman BS, Chapman D, Lewis JL Jr, et al: Serum CA-125 levels and surgical findings in patients undergoing secondary operations for epithelial ovarian cancer. *Am J Obstet Gynecol* 1989;160:667–671.

54. Berek JS, Knapp RC, Malkasian GD, Lavin PT, Whitney C, Niloff JM, Bast AC Jr: CA-125 serum levels correlated with second-look operations among ovarian cancer patients. *Obstet Gynecol* 1986;67:685–689.

55. Rubin SC, Hoskins WJ, Hakes TB, Markman M, Cain JM, Lewis JL Jr: Recurrence after negative second-look laparotomy for ovarian cancer: Analysis of risk factors. *Am J Obstet Gynecol* 1988;159:1094–1098.

56. Advanced Ovarian Cancer Trialists Group: Chemotherapy in advanced ovarian cancer: An overview of randomised clinical trials. *Br Med J* 1991;303:884–893.

57. Young RC, Walton LA, Ellenberg SS, Homesley HD, Wilbanks GD, Decker DG, Miller A, Park R, Major F Jr: Adjuvant therapy in stage I and II epithelial ovarian cancer. Results of two prospective randomized trials. *New Engl J Med* 1990;322:1021–1027.

58. Young RC, Chabner BA, Hubbard SP, Fisher RI, Bender RA, Anderson T, Simon RM, Canellos GP, DeVita VT Jr: Advanced ovarian adenocarcinoma: A prospective clinical trial of melphalan (L-PAM) versus combination chemotherapy. *New Engl J Med* 1978;299: 1261–1266.

59. Omura G, Blessing JA, Ehrlich CE, Miller A, Yordan E, Creasman WT, Homesley HD: A randomized trial of cyclophosphamide and doxorubicin with or without cisplatin in advanced ovarian carcinoma. *Cancer* 1987;57: 1725–1730.

60. McGuire WP, Hoskins WJ, Brady MF, Kucera PR, Partridge EE, Look KY, Clarke-Pearson DL, Davidson M: Cyclophosphamide and cisplatin versus paclitaxel and cisplatin: A phase III randomized trial in patients with suboptimal stage III/IV ovarian cancer (from the Gynecologic Oncology Group). *Semin Oncol* 1996;23:40–47.

61. Mangioni C, Bolis G, Pecorelli S, Bragman K, Epis A, Favalli G, Gambino A, Landoni F, Presti M, Torri W, et al: Randomized trial in advanced ovarian cancer comparing cisplatin and carboplatin. *J Natl Cancer Inst* 1989;81: 1464–1471.

62. Condra KS, Mendenhall WM, Morgan LS, Marcus RB Jr: Adjuvant $^{32}$P in the treatment of ovarian carcinoma. *Radiat Oncol Invest* 1997; 5:300–304.

63. Vergote IB, Vergote-DeVos LN, Abeler VM, Aas M, Lindegaard MW, Kjorstad KE, Trope CG: Randomized trial comparing cisplatin with radioactive phosphorus or whole abdominal irradiation as adjuvant treatment of ovarian cancer. *Cancer* 1992;69:741–749.

64. Bolis G, Colombo N, Pecorelli S, Torri V, Marsoni S, Bonazzi C, Chiari S, Favalli G, Mangili G, Presti M, et al: Adjuvant treatment for early epithelial ovarian cancer: Results of two randomised clinical trials comparing cisplatin to no further treatment or chromic phosphate ($^{32}$P). Gruppo Interregionale Collaborativo in Ginecologia Oncologica. *Ann Oncol* 1995;6: 887–893.

65. Spanos WJ Jr, Day T, Abner A, Jose B, Paris K, Pursell S: Complications in the use of intra-abdominal $^{32}$P for ovarian carcinoma. *Gynecol Oncol* 1992;45:243–247.

66. Walton LA, Yadusky A, Rubinstein L: Intraperitoneal radioactive phosphate in early ovarian carcinoma: An analysis of complications. *Int J Radiat Oncol Biol Phys* 1991;20: 939–944.

67. Peters WA III, Smith MR, Cain JM, Lee RB, Yon JL Jr: Intraperitoneal P-32 is not an effective consolidation therapy after a negative second-look laparotomy for epithelial carcinoma of the ovary. *Gynecol Oncol* 1992;47:146–149.

68. Spencer TR Jr, Marks RD Jr, Fenn JO, Jenrette JM III, Lutz MH: Intraperitoneal P-32 after negative second-look laparotomy in ovarian carcinoma. *Cancer* 1989;63:2434–2437.

69. Varia M, Rosenman J, Venkatraman S, Askin F, Fowler W, Walton L, Halle J, Currie J: Intraperitoneal chromic phosphate therapy after second-look laparotomy for ovarian cancer. *Cancer* 1988;61:919–927.

70. Reddy S, Sutton GP, Stehman FB, Hornback, Ehrlich CE: Ovarian carcinoma: Adjuvant treatment with P-32. *Radiology* 1987;165: 275–278.

71. Soper JT, Wilkinson RH Jr, Bandy LC, Clarke-Pearson DL, Creasman WT: Intraperitoneal chromic phosphate P-32 as salvage therapy for persistent carcinoma of the ovary after surgical restaging. *Am J Obstet Gynecol* 1987;156:1153–1158.

72. Klaassen D, Starreveld A, Shelly W, Miller A, Boyes D, Gerulath A, Levitt M: External beam

pelvic radiotherapy plus intraperitoneal radioactive chromic phosphate in early stage ovarian cancer: A toxic combination. A National Cancer Institute of Canada Clinical Trials Group Report. *Int J Radiat Oncol Biol Phys* 1985;11:1801–1804.

73. Dembo AJ: Epithelial ovarian cancer. The role of radiotherapy. *Int J Radiat Oncol Biol Phys* 1992;22:835–845.

74. Hruby G, Bull CA, Langlands AO, Gebski V: WART revisited: The treatment of epithelial ovarian cancer by whole abdominal radiotherapy. *Australas Radiol* 1997;41:276–280.

75. Fyles AW, Dembo AJ, Bush RS, Levin W, Manchul LA, Pringle JF, Rawlings GA, Sturgeon JF, Thomas GM, Simm J: Analysis of complications in patients treated with abdomino-pelvic radiation therapy for ovarian carcinoma. *Int J Radiat Oncol Biol Phys* 1992;22:847–851.

76. Fazekas JT, Maier JG: Irradiation of ovarian carcinomas. A prospective comparison of the open-field and moving-strip techniques. *Am J Roentgenol* 1974;120:118–123.

77. Ledermann JA, Dembo AJ, Sturgeon JF, Fine S, Bush RS, Fyles AW, Pringle JF, Rawlings GA, Thomas GM, Simm J: Outcome of patients with unfavorable optimally cytoreduced ovarian cancer treated with chemotherapy and whole abdominal radiation. *Gynecol Oncol* 1991;41:30–35.

78. Fuks Z, Rizel S, Biran S: Chemotherapeutic and surgical induction of pathological complete remission and whole abdominal irradiation for consolidation does not enhance the cure of stage III ovarian carcinoma. *J Clin Oncol* 1988;6:509–516.

79. Goldhirsch A, Greiner R, Dreher E, Sessa C, Krauer F, Forni M, Jung FW, Brunner KW, Veraguth P, Engeler V, et al: Treatment of advanced ovarian cancer with surgery, chemotherapy, and consolidation of response by whole-abdominal radiotherapy. *Cancer* 1988;62:40–47.

80. Buser K, Bacchi M, Goldhirsch A, Greiner R, Diener P, Sessa C, Jungi WF, Forni M, Leyvraz S, Engeler V: Treatment of ovarian cancer with surgery, short-course chemotherapy and whole abdominal radiation. *Ann Oncol* 1996;7:65–70.

81. Arian-Schad KS, Kapp DS, Hackl A, Juettner FM, Leitner H, Porsch G, Lahousen M, Pickel H: Radiation therapy in stage III ovarian cancer following surgery and chemotherapy: Prognostic factors, patterns of relapse, and toxicity: A preliminary report. *Gynecol Oncol* 1990;39:47–55.

82. Tepler I, Elias L, Smith JW II, Hussein M, Rosen G, Chang AY, Moore JO, Gordon MS, Kuca B, Beach KJ, Loewy JW, Garnick MB, Kaye JA: A randomized placebo-controlled trial of recombinant human interleukin-11 in cancer patients with severe thrombocytopenia due to chemotherapy. *Blood* 1996;87:3607–3614.

83. Hacker NF, Berek JS, Burnison CM, Heintz PM, Juillard GJ, Lagasse LD: Whole abdominal radiation as salvage therapy for epithelial ovarian cancer. *Obstet Gynecol* 1985;65:60–66.

84. Peters WA III, Blasko JC, Bagley CM Jr, Rudolph RH, Smith MR, Rivkin SE: Salvage therapy with whole-abdominal irradiation in patients with advanced carcinoma of the ovary previously treated by combination chemotherapy. *Cancer* 1986;58:880–882.

85. Piver MS, Barlow JJ, Lee FJ, Vongtama V: Sequential therapy for advanced ovarian adenocarcinoma: Operation, chemotherapy, second-look laparotomy, and radiation therapy. *Am J Obstet Gynecol* 1975;122:355–357.

86. Cain JM, Russell AH, Greer BE, Tamimi HK, Figge DC: Whole abdomen radiation for minimal residual epithelial ovarian carcinoma after surgical resection and maximal first-line chemotherapy. *Gynecol Oncol* 1988;29:168–175.

87. Hainsworth JD, Malcolm A, Johnson DH, Burnett LS, Jones HW III, Greco FA: Advanced minimal residual ovarian carcinoma: Abdominopelvic irradiation following combination chemotherapy. *Obstet Gynecol* 1983;61:619–623.

88. Hoskins WJ, Lichter AS, Whittington R, Artman LE, Bibro MC, Park RC: Whole abdominal and pelvic irradiation in patients with minimal disease at second-look surgical reassessment for ovarian carcinoma. *Gynecol Oncol* 1985;20:271–280.

89. Kucera PR, Berman ML, Treadwell P, Sheets EE, Micha JP, Rettenmaier MA, Colman M,

DiSaia PJ: Whole abdominal radiotherapy for patients with minimal residual epithelial ovarian carcinoma. *Gynecol Oncol* 1990;36:338–342.

90. Rosen EM, Goldberg ID, Rose C, Come S, Goldstein M, Simon L, Botnick LE: Sequential multi-agent chemotherapy and whole abdominal irradiation for stage III ovarian carcinoma. *Radiother Oncol* 1986;7:223–231.

91. Rizel S, Biran S, Anteby SO, Brufman G, Sulkes A, Milwidsky A, Weshler Z, Fuks Z: Combined modality treatment for stage III ovarian carcinoma. *Radiother Oncol* 1985;3:237–244.

92. Schray MF, Martinez A, Howes AE, Podratz KC, Ballon SC, Malkasian GD Jr, Sikic BI: Advanced epithelial ovarian cancer: Salvage whole abdominal irradiation for patients with recurrent or persistent disease after combination chemotherapy. *J Clin Oncol* 1988;6:1433–1439.

93. Steiner M, Rubinov R, Borovik R, Cohen Y, Robinson E: Multimodal approach (surgery, chemotherapy, and radiotherapy) in the treatment of advanced ovarian carcinoma. *Cancer* 1985;55:2748–2752.

94. Reddy S, Lee MS, Yordan E, Graham J, Sarin P, Hendrickson FR: Salvage whole abdomen radiation therapy: Its role in ovarian carcinoma. *Int J Radiat Oncol Biol Phys* 1993;27:879–884.

95. Bolis G, Zanaboni F, Vanoli P, Russo A, Franchi M, Scarfone G, Pecorelli S: The impact of whole-abdomen radiotherapy on survival in advanced ovarian cancer patients with minimal residual disease after chemotherapy. *Gynecol Oncol* 1990;39:150–154.

96. Chiara S, Orsatti M, Franzone P, Scarpati D, Bruzzone M, Repetto L, Vitale V, Conte PF, Rosso R: *Clin Oncol (R Coll Radiol)* 1991;3:340–344.

97. Haie C, Pejovic-Lenfant MH, George M, Michel G, Gerbaulet A, Prade M, Chassagne D: Whole abdominal irradiation following chemotherapy in patients with minimal residual disease after second look surgery in ovarian carcinoma. *Int J Radiat Oncol Biol Phys* 1989;17:15–19.

98. Cmelak AJ, Kapp DS: Long-term survival with whole abdominopelvic irradiation in platinum-refractory persistent or recurrent ovarian cancer. *Gynecol Oncol* 1997;65:453–460.

99. Sedlacek TV, Spyropoulus P, Cifaldi R, Glassburn J, Fisher S: Whole-abdomen radiation therapy as salvage treatment for epithelial ovarian carcinoma. *Cancer J Sci Am* 1997;3:358–363.

100. LaRoure J, Perez-Tamayo C, Fraass B, Tesser R, Lichter AS, Roberts J, Hopkins M: Optimal coverage of peritoneal surface in whole abdominal radiation for ovarian neoplasms. *Int J Radiat Oncol Biol Phys* 1989;17:607–613.

101. Schray MF, Martinez A, Howes AE: Toxicity of open-field whole abdominal irradiation as primary postoperative treatment in gynecologic malignancy. *Int J Radiat Oncol Biol Phys* 1989;16:397–403.

102. Lentz SS, Schray MF, Wilson TO: Chylous ascites after whole-abdomen irradiation for gynecologic malignancy. *Int J Radiat Oncol Biol Phys* 1990;19:435–438.

103. Irwin C, Fyles A, Wong CS, Cheung CM, Zhu Y: Late renal function following whole abdominal irradiation. *Radiother Oncol* 1996;38:257–261.

104. Schray MF, Martinez A, Howes AE, Ballon SC, Podratz KC, Sikic BI, Malkasian GD: Advanced epithelial ovarian cancer: Toxicity of whole abdominal irradiation after operation, combination chemotherapy, and reoperation. *Gynecol Oncol* 1986;24:68–80.

105. Whclan JT, Dembo AJ, Bush RS, Sturgeon JF, Fine S, Pringle JF, Rawlings GA, Thomas GM, Simm J: Complications of whole abdominal and pelvic radiotherapy following chemotherapy for advanced ovarian cancer. *Int J Radiat Oncol Biol Phys* 1992;22:853–858.

106. DePalo G, Lattuada A, Kenda R, Musumeci R, Zanini M, Pilotti S, Bellani FF, Di Re F, Baufi A: Germ cell tumors of the ovary: The experience of the National Cancer Institute of Milan: I. Dysgerminoma. *Int J Radiat Oncol Biol Phys* 1987;13:853–860.

107. Freed JH, Cassir JF, Pierce VK, Woodruff J, Lewis JL Jr, et al: Dysgerminoma of the ovary. *Cancer* 1979;43:798–805.

108. Krepart G, Smith JP, Rutledge F, Delclos L: The treatment for dysgerminoma of the ovary. *Cancer* 1978;41:986–990.

109. Lawson AP, Adler GF: Radiotherapy in the treatment of ovarian dysgerminomas. *Int J Radiat Oncol Biol Phys* 1988;14:431–434.

110. Marks RD, Underwood PB, Othersen HB: Dysgerminoma—100% control with combined therapy in six consecutive patients with advanced disease. *Int J Radiat Oncol Biol Phys* 1978;4:453–456.

111. Slayton RE: Management of germ cell and stromal tumors of the ovary. *Semin Oncol* 1984;11:299–313.

112. Williams SD, Blessing JA, Hatch KD, Homesley HD: Chemotherapy of advanced dysgerminoma: Trials of the Gynecologic Oncology Group. *J Clin Oncol* 1991;9:1950–1955.

113. Gershenson DM, Morris M, Cangir A, Kavanagh JJ, Stringer CA, Edwards CL, Silva EG, Wharton JT: Treatment of malignant germ cell tumors of the ovary with bleomycin, etoposide, and cisplatin. *J Clin Oncol* 1990;8: 715–720.

114. Williams SD, Blessing JA, DiSaia PJ, Major FJ, Ball HG, Liao S: Second-look laparotomy in ovarian germ cell tumors: the Gynecologic Oncology Group experience. *Gynecol Oncol* 1994;52:287–291.

115. Evans AT, Gaffey TA, Malkasian GD Jr, Annegers JF: Clinicopathologic review of 118 granulosa and 82 theca cell tumors. *Obstet Gynecol* 1980;55:231–238.

116. Gusberg SB, Kardon P: Proliferative endometrial response to theca-granulosa-cell tumors. *Am J Obstet Gynecol* 1971;111:633–643.

117. Bjorkholm E, Silfversward C: Prognostic factors in granulosa-cell tumors. *Gynecol Oncol* 1981;11:261–274.

118. Stenwig JT, Hazekamp JT, Beecham JB: Granulosa-cell tumors of the ovary. A clinicopathological study of 118 cases with long-term follow-up. *Gynecol Oncol* 1979;7: 136–152.

119. Malmstrom H, Hogberg T, Risberg B, Simonsen E: Granulosa-cell tumors of the ovary: Prognostic factors and outcome. *Gynecol Oncol* 1994;52:50–55.

120. Smith JP, Day TG: Review of ovarian cancer at the University of Texas Systems Cancer Center. *Am J Obstet Gynecol* 1979;135:984–993.

121. Ohel G, Kaneti H, Schenker JG: Granulosa-cell tumors in Israel: A study of 172 cases. *Gynecol Oncol* 1983;15:278–286.

122. Chadha S, Rao BR, Slotman BJ, van Vroonhoven CCJ, van der Kwast TH: An immunohistochemical evaluation of androgen and progesterone receptors in ovarian tumors. *Hum Pathol* 1993;24:90–95.

123. Fishman A, Kudelka A, Tcesukosol D, Edwards CL, Freedman RS, Kaplan AL, Girtanner RE, Kavanagh JJ: Leuprolide acetate for treating refractory or persistent ovarian granulosa-cell tumor. *J Reprod Med* 1996;41: 393–396.

124. Martikainen H, Penttinen J, Huhtaniemi I, Kauppila A: Gonadotropin-releasing hormone agonist analog therapy effective in ovarian granulosa-cell malignancy. *Gynecol Oncol* 1989;35:406–408.

125. Isaacs R, Forgeson G, Allan S: Progestagens for granulosa-cell tumours of the ovary. *Br J Cancer* 1992;65:140.

126. Malik ST, Slevin ML: Medroxyprogesterone acetate (MPA) in advanced granulosa-cell tumours of the ovary—A new therapeutic approach? *Br J Cancer* 1991;63:410–411.

# D. Vagina - ANTHONY H. RUSSELL

## INTRODUCTION

Cancer of the vagina is a rare disease. The American Cancer Society estimates that fewer than 2300 cases were diagnosed in 1997, representing less than 0.4% of the 596,000 new cancers diagnosed in American women.[1] According to the staging conventions of the AJCC and FIGO (Table 10-18) a cancer that extends to the portio vaginalis and reaches the external os of the cervix must be classified as a cervical primary. Similarly, a cancer that extends to involve any portion of the vulva is classified as a primary cancer of the vulva. These formalisms will inevitably lead to classifying some cancers whose bulk is in the proximal vagina as stage II

**TABLE 10-18   AJCC TNM Staging Classification for Carcinoma of the Vagina with FIGO Stages**

| TNM | FIGO Stage | Description |
|---|---|---|
| PRIMARY TUMOR (T)[a] | | |
| TX | | Primary tumor cannot be assessed. |
| T0 | | No evidence of primary tumor. |
| Tis | 0 | Carcinoma in situ. |
| T1 | I | Tumor confined to the vagina. |
| T2 | II | Tumor invades paravaginal tissues but not to pelvic wall. |
| T3 | III | Tumor extends to pelvic wall. |
| T4 | IVA | Tumor invades mucosa of the bladder or rectum and/or extends beyond the true pelvis. Bullous edema is not sufficient evidence to classify a tumor as T4. |
| M1 | IVB | Distant metastases. |
| REGIONAL LYMPH NODES (N) | | |
| NX | | Regional lymph nodes cannot be assessed. |
| N0 | | No regional lymph node metastasis. |
| N1 | | Pelvic or inguinal lymph node metastasis. |
| DISTANT METASTASIS (M) | | |
| MX | | Distant metastasis cannot be assessed. |
| M0 | | No distant metastasis. |
| M1 | | Distant metastasis. |

*PTNM Pathologic Classification*

The pT, pN, and pM categories correspond to the T, N, and M categories.

| FIGO Stage | AJCC Grouping[b] |
|---|---|
| 0 | Tis N0 M0 |
| I | T1 N0 M0 |
| II | T2 N0 M0 |
| III | T3 N0 M0 |
| | T1,2,3 N1 M0 |
| IVA | T4 Nx M0 |
| IVB | Tx Nx M1 |

[a]The classification applies to primary carcinoma only. A tumor that has extended to the portio and reached the external os should be classified as carcinoma of the cervix. A tumor involving the vulva should be classified as carcinoma of the vulva.

[b]x denotes any T or N.

or higher stage cervical cancer. Other cancers whose center and probable origin is in the distal vagina will be scored as T3 primary cancers of the vulva or termed "vulvovaginal cancer." The rare stage IIIA cervical cancer may reflect the idiosyncrasies of the staging nomenclature rather than an entity meaningfully distinct from vaginal cancer.

## HISTOLOGY AND EPIDEMIOLOGY

Most cancers of the vagina (80–85% in clinical series) are squamous cancers. Patients with vaginal intraepithelial neoplasia (VAIN) or invasive squamous cancer of the cervix will often have concurrent or prior cervical intraepithelial neoplasia (CIN) or invasive cervical cancer.[2–11] In a 30-year review of 100 cases from a single institution, 47 patients had a total hysterectomy prior to the diagnosis of vaginal cancer. Hysterectomy was carried out because of in situ cervical cancer in 10 patients, and invasive cervical cancer in 5 additional patients.[12]

Human papillomavirus appears to be implicated in the pathogenesis of VAIN as well as CIN,[13] and patients with multifocal transformation of the epithelium of the anogenital tract[7] presumably suffer from a "field change" effect initiated by the virus. It may not be possible to clinically distinguish between synchronous but separate squamous cancers of the vagina and cervix, which by convention would be scored as cervical cancer of higher stage. Similarly, metachronous appearance of vaginal cancer after treatment for cervical cancer would be conventionally counted as recurrence or metastasis unless 5 or more years have elapsed between the two events. The higher incidence of CIN and invasive cervical cancer than VAIN and vaginal cancer appear to relate to the vulnerability of the cervical transformation zone to viral mediated carcinogenesis.

The absence of glandular tissue in the normal stratified squamous vaginal epithelium may account for the relative rarity of true adenocarcinoma of the vagina. Adenocarcinoma accounts for approximately 10% to 20% of vaginal cancers.[14,15] Some patients treated for primary adenocarcinoma of the vagina may bear metastasis from another primary site. Cancers of the endometrium, ovary, large bowel, kidney, and breast are sources for this pattern of metastatic spread, and primary adenocarcinoma of the vagina should be considered a diagnosis of exclusion. Historically, the adverse prognosis associated with adenocarcinoma of the vagina and the higher rates of distant dissemination associated with this diagnosis may be consequent to failure to recognize some lesions as metastatic from an occult primary site. With modern diagnostic tools and a diligent search, this should be a rare event. Adenocarcinoma of the vagina may occur as a consequence of malignant degeneration of vaginal endometriosis, and endometrial stromal sarcoma has been reported in this context as well.[16]

Because of the rarity of primary adenocarcinomas of the vagina, which occur predominantly in postmenopausal women, the clustered appearance of clear cell adenocarcinomas in women in their late teenage years and early twenties elicited immediate attention. Careful medical detective work led to the linkage of these otherwise extremely rare cancers to in utero exposure to diethylstilbestrol (DES).[17,18,19] DES-associated clear cell carcinoma of the vagina is almost invariably seen accompanied by vaginal adenosis, which may microscopically consist of endocervical, endometrial, or tubal Müllerian epithelium. Prognosis for patients with stages I clear cell adenocarcinoma of the vagina is excellent when the disease is managed by radiation alone,[20] vaginectomy alone, or local excision alone, or with radiation.[21] Both 5- and 10-year survival rates should be in the vicinity of 90%. Survival is approximately 80% at 5 years and 65% at 10 years in patients with stage II disease managed by surgery including vaginectomy, radical hysterectomy with vaginectomy, partial or total exenteration, radiation alone, or combinations of these therapies.[22]

Malignant melanomas account for approximately 3% to 5% of primary vaginal malignancies. The prognosis for these patients is grim. There are no consensus treatment guidelines for these patients, for whom management usually reflects physician and patient bias rather than evidence-based therapy.

Rare tumors of the vagina include primary lymphoma, small-cell neuroendocrine cancers, and sarcomas usually derived from smooth or striated muscle. Sarcoma botryoides, a form of embryonal rhabdomyosarcoma, is the most common vaginal tumor in children. Most will be diagnosed in infants and children under the age of 5 years. Treatment is based on polyagent cytoreductive chemotherapy prior to conservative surgery, with selective use of radiotherapy for patients not amenable to surgery or for incomplete removal. Occasional patients will have complete tumor clearance after chemotherapy alone. With this approach, excellent local–regional control has been achieved, as well as long-term disease-free survival in over 80% of patients.[23]

## TREATMENT

Generalizations concerning treatment of adults with vaginal cancer are largely limited to management of the most common form of vaginal cancer, squamous cancer and its precursor lesion, vaginal intraepithelial neoplasia (VAIN). Treatment of primary adenocarcinoma of the vagina parallels treatment of the statistically more frequent squamous cancers, but may have worse outcome.[14] Patients with clear cell adenocarcinoma of the vagina in the context of in utero DES exposure are, on average, 40 years younger than typical patients with other histologies of vaginal cancer. Surgical therapy is often selected for these patients in an effort to avoid the perceived late morbidities (endocrine and reproductive ablation, vaginal stenosis) associated with primary radiation therapy. Management of melanoma primary in the vagina is highly individualized, and is based heavily on physician and patient bias rather than consensus or widely accepted standards.

Treatment of VAIN, which is often multifocal, must first include careful examination and directed biopsies to exclude invasive disease. In the interests of conserving vaginal function, surgical excision is generally avoided. Initial management usually consists of topical 5-fluorouracil cream,[24] which may be useful to treat VAIN developing in patients previously irradiated for cervical cancer.[25–29] Alternatively, laser vaporization to a controlled depth (2–3 mm) to the level of the lamina propria will focally destroy the vaginal mucosa with minimal deleterious effect on vaginal caliber and elasticity. Owing to the multifocal nature of the problem, repeat treatments may be required.[11,30,31] Laser should be employed only when the full extent of the lesion can be visualized, and will probably not be effective therapy when VAIN is buried in the vaginal cuff repair after hysterectomy.

Intravaginal radiation[32,33] employing mucosal doses from 65 to 80 Gy, and doses from 15 to 45 Gy employing high dose rate technique,[34,35] will control VAIN in a substantial majority of patients but will result in ablation of ovarian function in premenopausal women and may cause significant vaginal stenosis and inelasticity, leading to dyspareunia.[32,33] Vaginal brachytherapy should not be used unless more conservative interventions have failed. Total vaginectomy with split-thickness skin grafting has been employed as a surgical solution for patients with multifocal disease and recurrent disease, but this approach has been associated with dyspareunia as well as the anecdotal occurrence of in situ cancer in the grafted skin.[36] Surgery is generally reserved for failures of less morbid interventions, and circumstances in which minimal invasive disease is suspected.

Management of invasive disease will depend on the tumor stage, size, and gross morphology. The patient's age, reproductive history (parity), vaginal size, desires regarding sexual capacity and reproductive integrity, and medical comorbidities will all potentially impact on the selection and implementation of therapies. Numerous series reporting management of patients with squamous cancers of the vagina detail an astonishing array of radiotherapeutic and surgical treatment techniques[14,15,37–40] that might superficially seem lacking in constancy. In all likelihood, these diverse therapeutic strategies reflect the heterogeneity of the patient population treated and are consistent with the individualization of care that is the foundation of excellence in clinical medicine.

Stage I disease may be managed either by surgery or radiation. Small cancers, generally less than 2 cm in diameter, may be managed by transmural local excision with good results, depending on location in the vagina. Posterior lesions overlying the rectovaginal septum may not permit achievement of a deep surgical margin. Surgical management of anterior lesions will be similarly constrained by the bladder outlet and urethra. Lesions of the fornix may be managed by radical hysterectomy with upper vaginectomy and pelvic lymphadenectomy. Lesions located on the lateral walls will be most amenable to successful surgical treatment by wide local excision without major compromise of vaginal function, but care must be used in employing surgery to address distal lesions that encroach upon the vaginal introitus. Skin grafting may be required rather than primary surgical closure to avoid narrowing of the vagina and dyspareunia. Because of the young age at diagnosis in many patients with DES-associated clear cell cancer of the vagina, concerns about preserving endocrine and reproductive functions as well as sexual capacity may lead to a choice of surgical management of most such patients with stage I disease. Postmenopausal patients with squamous lesions of similar extent may well be treated with radiation. Extensive surgical procedures are likely to adversely impact vaginal function to a greater degree than carefully planned and administered radiotherapy, which will be associated with cancer control probability of 75% to 80% in experienced hands.[37,38,41]

For very small primaries with limited thickness, radiation may be accomplished by brachytherapy alone or transvaginal cone radiation. For patients with more extensive disease, teletherapy should generally precede brachytherapy because of better long-term outcomes.[14] Techniques of endovaginal (endocavitary) brachytherapy such as colpostats, cylinders, and molds will effectively irradiate tumors with a thickness up to 5 mm, and may represent a good technical solution for flat, sessile tumors of limited diameter. The largest possible endocavitary apparatus that can be comfortably tolerated should be employed to minimize the dose inhomogeneity within the target volume. The larger the distance between the brachytherapy sources and the vaginal mucosa, the lower the mucosal dose will be required to deliver a therapeutic dose at the depth where the tumor is thickest.

At the Radiation Oncology Centers of Northern California in Sacramento, endocavitary technique is the brachytherapy technique employed if the dose achievable at depth is 75% or greater of the calculated surface (mucosal) dose. This guideline is employed whether the brachytherapy is the only treatment, or is used to supplement a course of fractionated teletherapy. If this ratio cannot be attained, brachytherapy is accomplished with a combination of interstitial and endocavitary technique, usually employing a transperineal technique with a template to stabilize needle placement in a geometric array. For stage I disease, needles are placed a single row parallel to the vaginal wall and parallel to a vaginal obturator (cylinder) with a central linear source. Needles are placed 5 to 10 mm deep in tissue. Needles should not be placed directly on the vaginal mucosa, as the focally intense dose thus delivered could result in vaginal ulceration and possible fistula formation.

Virtually all patients with stage II disease should have radiation therapy initiated by external beam. Based on surgical evaluation, the risk of lymph node involvement escalates from 6% in stage I (1 of 17 patients) to 26% with stage II (8 of 31).[42] The target volume for teletherapy will depend on the location of the primary within the vagina and whether pretreatment assessments have clinically or histopathologically documented node metastasis. The lymphatic drainage of the proximal third of the vagina is through the parametria to the pelvic nodes. The distal vagina has dual lymphatic drainage consisting of pathways caudally to the inguinofemoral nodes, and drainage cephalad to the lymphatics of the proximal vagina, cervix, and parametria.

Diagnostic evaluations of regional nodes may include abdominopelvic computed axial tomography (CT), lymphangiography, or magnetic resonance imaging, in addition to careful palpation of the groins. Examination by CT or ultrasound will be necessary to measure the depth of the deep inguinofemoral nodes, whose assessment is notoriously inaccurate by clinical palpation. Groin nodes that are clinically suspicious (or > 1 cm as measured by palpation or CT) should be assessed by fine needle aspiration (FNA) or excisional biopsy. Pelvic or extrapelvic nodes that are enlarged on CT or suspicious by lymphography, should be aspirated under CT guidance. For tumors which, in their entirety, are confined to the upper third of the vagina, the teletherapy ports may target only the pelvic nodes caudal to the bifurcations of the common iliac arteries (approximately the L5–S1 interspace).

If pelvic node metastasis can be histologically confirmed, the target volume should be extended cephalad to encompass the para-aortic nodes. When vaginal cancer involves the middle or caudal third of the vagina, the inguinofemoral nodes are encompassed in addition to pelvic nodes. The inguinofemoral nodes are encompassed electively by means of the same techniques used when these nodes are addressed in the treatment of cancer of the vulva.[43–46] External beam is employed to administer 45 to 50.4 Gy in fractions of 1.8 Gy to nodal groups receiving elective or prophylactic treatment because of potential contamination by clinically occult micrometastases. Up to 70.2 Gy in fractions of 1.8 Gy may be administered via shrinking volumes to bulky, unresected regional nodes histologically confirmed. Interstitial brachytherapy or a combination of interstitial and intracavitary radiation is used to carry the primary disease and regional extensions to a cumulative dose of 65 to 75 Gy, with the upper limit of dose being defined by the dose unavoidably administered to adjacent normal tissues (Figure 10-12).

When brachytherapy is used as a boost technique for stage II, more extensive interstitial technique may be required with several rows of needles. Transrectal ultrasound[47] or endorectal coil magnetic resonance imaging[48] as well as fluoroscopy may be useful technical adjuncts to needle placement. If placement of needles into the parametria or cephalad to the vaginal vault is required for adequate tumor coverage, control of needle placement with concurrent laparotomy or laparoscopy is desirable to assure placement of needles within disease without perforation of adjacent tissues.

Patients with advanced disease (stages III and IV) should have disease extent verified by cystoscopy and/or proctosigmoidoscopy prior

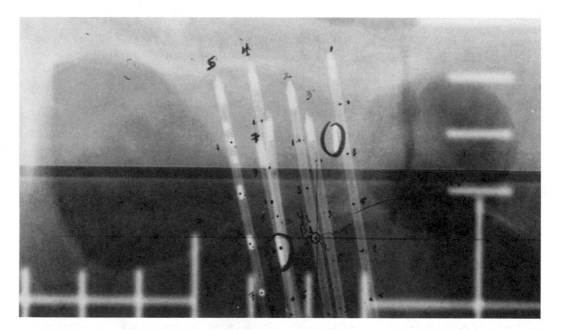

**FIGURE 10-12** Anteroposterior radiograph of volume interstitial implant of a patient with stage II carcinoma of the right lateral wall of the midvagina. Film obtained for confirmation of position and dosimetric calculations. Numbers used to identify catheters (7) and dwell positions for treatment by high dose rate afterloading technology. Dummy sources are 1 cm apart. Circled clips represent marker seeds embedded deep to the proximal and distal mucosal edges of the residual tumor volume after teletherapy.

to treatment. The target volume for external radiation should be determined in the same fashion as for stage II, but will almost invariably include both pelvic and inguinofemoral nodes. Additionally, the pretreatment volume and distribution should be documented with body imaging, preferably with MRI. Treatment should commence with teletherapy in all patients, as cure accomplished by brachytherapy alone is extraordinarily unlikely.[49] Extensive interstitial implantation may be used to supplement teletherapy in an attempt to treat gross disease to a radical therapeutic dose of radiation. This may require placement of needles at the time of laparotomy to assure optimal placement of needles in relation to disease, as well as to avoid perforation of bowel and urinary bladder. Risk of bowel perforation will be greatest for patients with antecedent hysterectomy, and, at a minimum, laparoscopic surveillance of needle placement should be considered in such patients.[48] Alternatively, treating progressively smaller volumes with shrinking teletherapy ports will permit prescription of dose to approximately 70 Gy without exceeding generally acknowledged limits of normal tissue tolerance. Repeat body imaging after 45 to 50.4 Gy will assist in the delineation of reduced target volumes and selection of technique. Treating with aggressive radiation will salvage approximately one third of patients with stage III disease.[14,37,49] Cures with stage IV disease are anecdotal. Fewer than 20% of stage IV patients will be disease-free at 5 years.

At the Radiation Oncology Centers of Northern California in Sacramento, it has been the practice, for almost a decade, to treat patients with bulky stage II cancers or stage III or IV disease with a combination of 5-fluorouracil based chemotherapy and concurrent teletherapy. Techniques, radiation and chemotherapy doses, and schedules of administration have been adapted from programs used to advantage in the treatment of patients with epidermoid cancers of the anus and vulva. Not surprisingly, squamous cancer of the vagina appears to respond favorably to this strategy, and the following preliminary clinical impressions are offered anticipating the outcomes from a formal analysis now ongoing.

Patients treated with external radiation and concurrent chemotherapy will generally manifest rapid tumor shrinkage. This, in turn, permits substantial reductions in target volume for "boost" doses. Brachytherapy, when employed, can often be accomplished by intracavitary technique, and interstitial therapy is less likely to be required to generate isodose lines that encompass residual disease. Bulky tumors flatten rapidly. Cancers have been controlled using cumulative radiation doses that, if given alone, would be considered subtherapeutic. Total radiation doses have been approximately 10% to 15% lower than might be utilized were radiation the sole modality of therapy. While acute normal tissue reactions and side effects have been enhanced, late effects in normal tissues have not been noticeably different from what would be anticipated from radiation alone. In particular, vaginal effects have been quite mild, and some patients with initially bulky cancers remain sexually active without discomfort. It seems plausible that this approach will gain broader acceptance over time as more patients are treated in this fashion. The unsatisfactory results historically obtained in stage III and stage IV patients justify innovative treatment strategies. Simply escalating radiation dose is unlikely to achieve more than modest gains in local control at the hazard of increased complications.

Melanoma of the vagina is associated with a very high mortality ($\geq 90\%$) regardless of therapeutic intervention employed, with local–regional and distant failures almost equally common.[50] Aggressive attempts to accomplish surgical cure have been justified by the clinical resistance of melanoma to conventional total radiation dose administered in conventional fraction size with conventional technique. The poor prognosis of vaginal melanoma may relate to delay in diagnosis compared to cutaneous melanoma. Prognosis appears to correlate with depth of invasion.[51] The high mortality from this disease, despite aggressive surgical interventions including partial or total vaginectomy with anterior, posterior, or total pelvic exenteration, should prompt a diligent search for tumor dissemination before embarking on what may be a mutilating undertaking. Documentation of spread of melanoma should temper surgical enthusiasm for procedures that may markedly diminish quality of life without a realistic prospect for cure or prolonged disease-free survival. Conversely, the overall poor results should not be grounds for therapeutic nihilism justifying undertreatment of the few women for whom surgical cure can be attained. Metabolic imaging with [18F]fluorodeoxyglucose (positron emission tomography, or PET) has been reported to be both highly sensitive and specific for detection of metastatic melanoma when correlated with subsequent clinical course and histopathology.[52,53] This imaging modality might prove useful in the pretreatment evaluation of melanomas of the vagina and vulva, assisting in the selection of patients for aggressive surgical therapy, as well as in establishing the scope of surgical therapy predicated on the presence or absence of demonstrable metastases in regional nodes.

## Brachytherapy with High Dose Rate

High dose rate remote-afterloading technology offers several potential technical advantages for patients with limited vaginal cancers who will receive all, or a portion, of their treatment with brachytherapy. Long-term vaginal function will depend intimately on the volume of vagina that is carried to high dose. The total length of the vagina will usually be treated to an intermediate dose of radiation (45–50.4 Gy) to address multifocality and the possibility of clinically occult disease in the lymphatics of the vaginal mucosa. However, it is not necessary to carry the full length of the vagina to the full therapeutic dose that need be directed only to gross disease with a narrow margin. Since varying dwell times of a miniaturized source permits flexibility in designing dose distributions, isodose distributions that closely parallel disease distribution can be created. Equivalent dose distributions cannot be attained by treatment using low dose rate sources of larger size with a limited range of source activities.

Because of the short treatment times (minutes), patients can be effectively immobilized, permitting treatment of more tightly tailored volumes. Despite the best efforts of both physicians and patients, some potential for movement of the treatment apparatus (interstitial or endocavitary) must be taken into account when one is designing dose distributions for treatments that will last for days rather than for minutes. A patient may be able to tolerate a tighter fit from an intravaginal cylinder if that cylinder is in place for minutes rather than hours. A tighter insertion will compress and flatten a tumor and improve dose distribution at depth. A larger cylinder or colpostats will decrease the mucosal dose relative to tumor dose at depth. By inserting a cylinder to the vaginal vault under modest tension, and securing it rigidly in place by fixation to a locking baseplate, discrete portions of the vagina can be reproducibly treated under remote computer control by varying dwell times of the miniaturized high intensity gamma source. Limited segments of the long axis of the vaginal barrel can be targeted for full therapeutic dose, while restricting dose to adjacent segments. Additionally, partially shielded cylinders are commercially available that allow sparing up to 75% of the circumference of the vagina in the treatment of well-circumscribed lesions. This will inevitably result in decreased fibrosis, inelasticity, and mucosal atrophy, with consequently lesser physical barriers to sexual enjoyment. Conservation of structure and function represent major goals for radical radiation. Often these goals constitute the rationale for treatment by radiotherapy rather than ablative radical surgery. Meticulous technique must be employed to confine areas of high radiation dose to structures that require them.

## Follow-Up

Following completion of a course of radiation, patients should be encouraged to use a vaginal dilator daily. Topical estrogen cream will aid in the healing of the vagina and may be necessary on a chronic basis to mitigate against symptomatic vaginal mucosal atrophy.[54,55] For most patients to remain sexually active, exogenous vaginal lubrication will be required. For many women treated for vaginal cancer, remaining sexually active is both a desirable and an achievable goal.

Treatment failures may be local, regional, or distant. In most clinical series of vaginal cancer, local–regional recurrences are substantially more common than distant failures,[14,38,56] and are a component of the pattern of failure in approximately 75% of cases. This fact is grounds for some optimism that efforts focused on improvements in radiotherapeutic technique and dose delivery may ultimately yield improvements in survival. Improved brachytherapy techniques with better tumor coverage are clearly one avenue to improved results.[57] Retrospective series consistently demonstrate better outcomes in patients receiving brachytherapy versus patients treated by teletherapy alone, and better outcomes with more sophisticated (interstitial) brachytherapy techniques,[58] than with intracavitary techniques.

Changes in the radiotherapeutic management of squamous cancers of the cervix and vulva have been the consequence of improvements in diagnostic imaging and target volume definition, and integration of radiopotentiating chemotherapy in the management of patients with locally–regionally advanced disease. Since squamous cancers of the vagina comprise a rare and heterogeneous condition, it should not be a surprise that reports of extrapolating the foregoing interventions to vaginal patients have lagged. Neither should it come as a surprise when such reports inevitably appear. The clinical paradigms for anogenital squamous cancer and the principles for management are probably more powerful and general than the factors that distinguish the behavior and treatment of squamous cancer at different anatomic sites within the lower female reproductive tract. Similarly, the prognosis and management of patients with melanoma of the vagina and vulva are probably most sensibly correlated with the paradigms for cutaneous melanoma, and to a lesser extent governed by paradigms for management of cancer at a particular anatomical locale.

Radiation therapy has a dual agenda: permanent eradication of cancer within an appropriate target volume intended to cure the patient, and conservation of both structure and function of normal tissues unavoidably included within that target volume. The vagina, itself a functionally important structure, is in intimate association with other functionally important structures including the urinary bladder, urethra, rectum, and vulva. Perhaps more than any other primary site in the female pelvis, the vagina requires unremitting attention to technique and technical detail if treatment of primary tumors is to achieve results serving both goals. Pay attention. Measure twice, cut once.

## REFERENCES

1. American Cancer Society: *Cancer Facts and Figures—1997.* Atlanta, ACS.

2. Rubin SC, Young J, Mikuta JJ: Squamous carcinoma of the vagina: Treatment, complications, and long-term follow-up. *Gynecol Oncol* 1985; 20:346–353.

3. Benedet JL, Murphy KJ, Fairey RN, Boyes DA: Primary invasive carcinoma of the vagina. *Obstet Gynecol* 1983;62:715–719.

4. Peters WA III, Kumar NB, Morley GW: Carcinoma of the vagina: Factors influencing treatment outcome. *Cancer* 1985;55:892–897.

5. Kolstad P, Klem V: Long-term follow-up of 1121 cases of carcinoma in situ. *Obstet Gynecol* 1976;48:125–129.

6. Choo YC, Anderson DG: Neoplasms of the vagina following cervical carcinoma. *Gynecol Oncol* 1982;14:125–132.

7. Choo YC, Morley GW: Multiple primary neoplasms of the anogenital region. *Obstet Gynecol* 1980;56:365–369.

8. Eddy GL, Singh KP, Gansler TS: Superficially invasive carcinoma of the vagina following treatment for cervical cancer: A report of six cases. *Gynecol Oncol* 1990;36:376–379.

9. Kanbour AI, Klionsky B, Murphy AI: Carcinoma of the vagina following cervical cancer. *Cancer* 1974;34:1838–1841.

10. Lee RA, Symmonds RE: Recurrent carinoma in situ of the vagina in patients previously treated for in situ carcinoma of the cervix. *Obstet Gynecol* 1976;48:61–64.

11. Lenehan PM, Meffe F, Lickrish GM: Vaginal intraepithelial neoplasia: Biologic aspects and management. *Obstet Gynecol* 1986;68:333–337.

12. Stock RG, Chen ASJ, Seski J: A 30-year experience in the management of primary carcinoma of the vagina: Analysis of prognostic factors and treatment modalities. *Gynecol Oncol* 1995; 56:45–52.

13. Wright VC, Chapman W: Intraepithelial neoplasia of the lower female genital tract: Etiology, investigation, and management. *Semin Surg Oncol* 1992;8:180–190.

14. Chyle V, Zagars GK, Wheeler JA, Wharton JT, Delclos L: Definitive radiotherapy for carcinoma of the vagina: Outcome and prognostic factors. *Int J Radiat Oncol Biol Phys* 1996;35: 891–905.

15. Fine BA, Piver MS, McAuley M, Driscoll D: The curative potential of radiation therapy in the treatment of primary vaginal carcinoma. *Am J Clin Oncol* 1996;19:39–44.

16. Granai CO, Walters MD, Safaii H, et al: Malignant transformation of vaginal endometriosis. *Obstet Gynecol* 1984;64:592–595.

17. Herbst AL, Ulfelder H, Poskanzer DC: Adenocarcinoma of the vagina: Association of maternal stilbestrol therapy with tumor appearance in young women. *New Engl J Med* 1971;284: 878–881.

18. Greenwald P, Barlow JJ, Nasca PC, Burnett WS: Vaginal cancer after maternal treatment with synthetic hormones. *New Engl J Med* 1974;285:390–392.

19. Herbst AL, Anderson S, Hubby MM, Haenszel WM, Kaufman RH, Noller KL: Risk factors for the development of diethylstilbestrol-associated clear cell adenocarcinoma: A case control study. *Am J Obstet Gynecol* 1986;154:814–822.

20. Fletcher GH: Tumors of the vagina and female urethra, in GH Fletcher (ed): *Textbook of Radiotherapy,* 3rd ed. Philadelphia, Lea & Febiger, 1980, pp 821–824.

21. Senekjian EK, Frey KW, Anderson D, Herbst AL: Local therapy in stage I clear cell adenocarcinoma of the vagina. *Cancer* 1987;60: 1319–1324.

22. Senekjian EK, Frey KW, Stone C, Herbst AL: An evaluation of stage II vaginal clear cell adenocarcinoma according to substages. *Gynecol Oncol* 1988;31:56–64.

23. Andrassy RJ, Hays DM, Raney RB, Wiener ES, Lawrence W, Lobe TE, Corpron CA, Smith M, Maurer HM: Conservative surgical management of vaginal and vulvar pediatric rhabdomyosarcoma: A report from the Intergroup Rhabdomyosarcoma Study III. *J Pediatr Surg* 1995;30:1034–1036.

24. Woodruff JD, Parmley TH, Julian CG: Topical 5-fluorouracil in the treatment of vaginal carcinoma in situ. *Gynecol Oncol* 1975;3:124–132.

25. Piver MS, Barlow JJ, Tsukada Y, Gamarra M, Saudecki A: Postirradiation squamous cell carcinoma of the vagina: Treatment by topical 20% 5-fluorouracil cream. *Am J Obstet Gynecol* 1979;135:377–380.

26. Audet-LaPointe P, Body G, Vauclair R, Drouin P, Ayoub J: Vaginal intraepithelial neoplasia. *Gynecol Oncol* 1990;36:232–239.

27. Ballon SC, Roberts JA, Lagasse LD: Topical 5-fluorouracil in the treatment of intraepithelial neoplasia of the vagina. *Obstet Gynecol* 1979; 54:163–166.

28. Daly JW, Ellis GF: Treatment of vaginal dysplasia and carcinoma in situ with topical 5-fluorouracil. *Obstet Gynecol* 1980;55:350–352.

29. Sillman FH, Sedlis AH, Boyce JG: A review of lower genital intraepithelial neoplasia and the use of topical 5-fluorouracil. *Obstet Gynecol Surv* 1985;40:190–220.

30. Capen CV, Masterson BJ, Magrina JF, Calkins JWL: Laser therapy of vaginal intraepithelial neoplasia. *Am J Obstet Gynecol* 1982;142: 973–976.

31. Townsend DE, Levine RU, Crum CP, Richart RM: Treatment of vaginal carcinoma in situ with the carbon dioxide laser. *Am J Obstet Gynecol* 1982;143:565–568.

32. Perez CA, Camel HM: Long-term follow-up in radiation therapy of carcinoma of the vagina. *Cancer* 1982;49:1308–1315.

33. Rutledge F: Cancer of the vagina. *Am J Obstet Gynecol* 1967;97:635–655.

34. Ogino I, Kitamura T, Okajima H, Matsubara S: High-dose-rate intracavitary brachytherapy in the management of cervical and vaginal intraepithelial neoplasia. *Int J Radiat Oncol Biol Phys* 1998;40:881–887.

35. MacLeod C, Fowler A, Dalrymple C, Atkinson K, Elliott P, Carter J: High-dose-rate brachytherapy in the management of high-grade intraepithelial neoplasia of the vagina. *Gynecol Oncol* 1997;65:74–77.

36. Imrie JE, Kennedy JH, Holmes JD, McGrouther DA: Intraepithelial neoplasia arising in an artificial vagina. *Br J Obstet Gynaecol* 1986;93:886–888.

37. Perez CA, Camel HM, Galaktos AE, Grigsby PW, Kuske RR, Buchsbaum G, Hederman MA: Definitive irradiation in carcinoma of the vagina: Long-term evaluation of results. *Int J Radiat Oncol Biol Phys* 1988;15:1283–1290.

38. Reddy S, Saxena VS, Reddy S, Lee MS, Yordan EL, Graham JE, Phillips R, Hendrickson FR: Results of radiotherapeutic management of primary carcinoma of the vagina. *Int J Radiat Oncol Biol Phys* 1991;21:1041–1044.

39. Boronow RC, Hickman BT, Reagan MT, Smith RA, Steadham RE: Combined therapy as an alternative to exenteration for locally advanced vulvovaginal cancer. II. Results, complications, and dosimetric and surgical considerations. *Am J Clin Oncol* 1987;10:171–181.

40. Lindeque BG: The role of surgery in the management of carcinoma of the vagina. *Baillieres Clin Obstet Gynaecol* 1987;1:319–329.

41. Brown GR, Fletcher GH, Rutledge FN: Irradiation of "in situ" and invasive squamous cell carcinomas of the vagina. *Cancer* 1971;28:1278–1283.

42. Davis KP, Stanhope CR, Garton GR, Arkinson EJ, O'Brien PC: Invasive vaginal carcinoma: Analysis of early-stage disease. *Gynecol Oncol* 1991;42:131–136.

43. Russell AH, Mesic JB, Scudder SA, Rosenberg PJ, Smith LH, Kinney WK, Townsend DE, Trelford JD, Taylor MH, Zukowski CL, McMahon KG: Synchronous radiation and cytotoxic chemotherapy for locally advanced or recurrent squamous cancer of the vulva. *Gynecol Oncol* 1992;47:14–20.

44. Petereit DG, Mehta MP, Buchler DA, Kinsella TJ: Inguinofemoral radiation of N0,N1 vulvar cancer may be equivalent to lymphadenectomy if proper radiation technique is used. *Int J Radiat Oncol Biol Phys* 1993;27:963–967.

45. Kalend AM, Park TL, Wu A, Kalnicki S, Meek AG, Bloomer WD, Solowsky EL: Clinical use of a wing field transmission block for the treatment of the pelvis including the inguinal node. *Int J Radiat Oncol Biol Phys* 1990;19:153–158.

46. Leiserowitz G, Russell AH, Kinney WH, Smith LH, Taylor MH, Scudder SA: Prophylactic chemoradiation of inguinofemoral lymph nodes in patients with locally extensive vulvar cancer. *Gynecol Oncol* 1997;66:509–514.

47. Stock RG, Chan K, Terk M, Dewyngaert JK, Stone NN, Dottino P: A new technique for performing the Syed–Neblett template interstitial implants for gynecologic malignancies using transrectal–ultrasound guidance. *Int J Radiat Oncol Biol Phys* 1997;37:819–825.

48. Corn BW, Lanciano RM, Rosenblum N, Schnall M, King S, Epperson R: Improved treatment planning for the Syed–Neblett template using endorectal-coil magnetic resonance and intraoperative (laparotomy/laparoscopy) guidance: A new integrated technique for hysterectomized women with vaginal tumors. *Gynecol Oncol* 1995;56:255–261.

49. Kucera H, Vavra N: Radiation management of primary carcinoma of the vagina: Clinical and histopathological variables associated with survival. *Gynecol Oncol* 1991;40:12–16.

50. Reid GC, Schmidt RW, Roberts JA, Hopkins MP, Barrett RJ, Morley GW: Primary melanoma of the vagina: A clinicopathologic analysis. *Obstet Gynecol* 1989;74:190–199.

51. Bonner JA, Perez-Tamayo C, Reid GC, Roberts JA, Morley GW: The management of vaginal melanoma. *Cancer* 1988;62:2066–2072.

52. Damian DL, Fulham MJ, Thompson E, Thompson JF: Positron emission tomography in the detection and management of metastatic melanoma. *Melanoma Res* 1996;6:325–329.

53. Steinert HC, Boni RAH, Buck A, Boni R, Berthold T, Marincek B, Burg G, von Schulthess GK: Malignant melanoma: Staging with whole-body positron emission tomography and 2-[F-18]-fluoro-2-deoxy-D-glucose. *Radiology* 1995;195:705–709.

54. Pitkin RM, Bradbury JR: The effect of topical estrogen on irradiated vaginal epithelium. *Am J Obstet Gynecol* 1965;92:175–182.

55. Pitkin RM, van Voorhis LW: Postirradiation vaginitis. An evaluation of prophylaxis with topical estrogen. *Radiology* 1971;99:417–421.

56. Urbanski K, Kojs Z, Reinfuss M, Fabisiak W: Primary invasive vaginal carcinoma treated with radiotherapy: Analysis of prognostic factors. *Gynecol Oncol* 1996;60:16–21.

57. Erickson B, Gillin MT: Interstitial implantation of gynecologic malignancies. *J Surg Oncol* 1997;66:285–295.

58. Stock RG, Mychalczak B, Armstrong JG, Curtin JP, Harrison LB: The importance of brachytherapy technique in the management of primary carcinoma of the vagina. *Int J Radiat Oncol Biol Phys* 1992;24:747–753.

# E. Cervix - ANTHONY H. RUSSELL

## INCIDENCE AND MORTALITY

Cervical cancer is the second most common malignancy among women worldwide and the most common in the developing world. In 1985 an estimated 437,000 women were diagnosed worldwide representing 12% of cancers in women.[1] The American Cancer Society estimated that 12,800 patients would develop the disease in the United States in 1999, and 4800 women would die of it.[2] While the incidence figures for invasive disease and associated mortality statistics have declined in populations with access to organized screening programs based on the Papanicolaou (Pap) smear,[3,4] cancer of the cervix remains a leading cause of death from malignant disease in developing nations. In the United States, substantial demographic differences exist based on age, ethnicity, and geography which may reflect diverse sexual mores and varying access to health care and screening.[5] Absent effective preventive strategies, the most effective available strategy to reduce mortality from cervical cancer remains early diagnosis of precursor lesions that may be detectable 5 to 20 years before the onset of invasive disease,[6] and lowering the stage at diagnosis of invasive disease. Carcinoma in situ, readily detectable by exfoliative cytology, is generally acknowledged to be a harbinger of ultimate invasive disease. Although spontaneous involutions occur, many patients will ultimately progress to invasive disease.[7] Current reporting of exfoliative cytology is based upon a National Cancer Institute consensus conference held in 1988, with further refinement in 1991.[8] Methods for further clarification of an abnormal smear include colposcopy with directed biopsy, dilatation and curettage, and conization of the cervix with either the cold knife or diathermy (loop electrosurgical excision procedure: LEEP).

## EPIDEMIOLOGY

It has long been recognized that cervical cancer is a disease related to sexual activity, although the precise steps involved in its pathogenesis remain elusive. Early age of first intercourse, multiple sexual partners, male partners with multiple partners, and a history of sexually transmitted infectious disease (STD) correlate with risk. Socioeconomic status, race or ethnicity, number of pregnancies, diet, and smoking may be additional surrogate indexes that reflect vulnerability for exposure to a sexually transmitted agent.[9] Cancer of the cervix is rare in women who are not sexually active.[10] Increasing epidemiologic and laboratory evidence accumulates that infection with the human papillomavirus (HPV) is the initiating event.[11–16] Other sexually transmitted diseases as well as smoking may be active cofactors or promoters.

While HPV infection may be cleared in some individuals or remain latent in others, the immunologic competence of the infected woman is likely to play an integral role in that process. Carcinoma in situ and cervical cancer in women infected with the human immunodeficiency virus (HIV) are associated with poor cancer outcome despite appropriate therapy.[17,18] Identification of HPV as the probable etiologic agent for most cervical cancer creates opportunities for reduced mortality from cervical cancer based on two strategies. Prophylactic vaccination may ultimately prevent development of the disease in populations at risk for HPV infection. Therapeutic vaccines, now in early clinical testing, may benefit cancer patients with antigenic proteins associated with viral transfection.[19,20]

## SYMPTOMS LEADING TO DIAGNOSIS

A thorough history should be obtained from each patient before diagnostic assessments are initiated, since focused questions will often assist in determining the direction and intensity of the subsequent workup. Symptoms leading patients to seek medical attention often include spotting, or bleeding associated with coitus. A sexual history should be obtained from all patients. This may alert the physician to a need to screen for HIV and other sexually transmitted diseases, and will additionally serve to establish a baseline for sexual function and expectations that may be important in the counseling and sexual rehabilitation of patients following completion of treatment. Patients may attribute irregular or excessive bleeding to menstruation, but this probably reflects tumor vascularity rather than cyclical bleeding related to fluctuating hormone levels. A cloudy yellow or gray discharge, often malodorous, accompanies tumors with necrosis and the inevitable saprophytic infection that follows. Pain is unusual when gross cancer is confined to the cervix and vagina, and when present should alert the clinician to possible extensions of disease. The cramping pain of uterine contractions may reflect occlusion of the endocervical canal with the accumulation of blood (hematometra) and uterine decidua in the uterine fundus in a menstruating patient, or occasionally in a post-

menopausal woman with cancer extension to the lower uterine segment or uterine cavity. Fever, chills, and intense pelvic pain may accompany infection in the uterine cavity (pyometra), which should be drained transvaginally by canalizing the cervix followed by treatment with antibiotics before therapy is initiated. Lateralized pain experienced in the groin may accompany parametrial extension with obstruction of a ureter. Pain in the pelvis or gluteal area, or pain radiating to a leg, will usually indicate direct tumor extension to the pelvic sidewall via the uterine suspensory ligaments, or extensive metastatic deposits in regional lymph nodes. Leg lymphedema caused by obstruction will generally be seen in the context of extensive nodal disease on the pelvic sidewall. Compression of the pelvic veins will be responsible for the deep pelvic vein thrombosis and embolic phenomena sometimes manifest in the context of very extensive disease, and superficial or deep thrombophlebitis in a leg should alert the clinician to this hazard. Alterations in urinary frequency, urgency, and urinary flow are most commonly due to mass effects on the bladder and urinary outflow tract and less frequently due to direct invasion of the bladder or urethra, but should indicate the need for cystoscopic evaluation. True hematuria is rare, and spurious hematuria may result from the admixture of urine with vaginal blood. Discomfort with defecation and alteration in bowel habit is sometimes experienced in the context of severe retroflexion of the uterus accentuated by the presence of a bulky cervical tumor and consequent external pressure on the midrectum. Passage of blood per rectum (hematochezia) should mandate endoscopic evaluation prior to treatment. Constitutional symptoms including anorexia, dysgeusia, and weight loss usually reflect advanced disease.

## HISTOLOGY

The most common histology for cervical cancer is squamous carcinoma and its variants, which comprise approximately 80% to 85% of instances. Squamous cancers usually arise at or near the transformation zone, and usually manifest a component visible through the vagina. Historically, most squamous cancers have been triaged into keratinizing and nonkeratinizing large-cell cancers or small-cell nonkeratinizing squamous cancers.[21] The classification of the World Health Organization segregates squamous cell carcinoma into keratinizing, nonkeratinizing, verrucous, papillary transitional, and lymphoepithelioma-like.[22]

Efforts to correlate grade and histologic category with prognosis been neither reproducible nor universally accepted, and with the possible exception of the verrucous variant of squamous cancer, discrimination between these growth patterns does not give grounds for selection of treatment. Verrucous cancers are characteristically strikingly exophytic, well-differentiated squamous cancer associated with exuberant keratinization; although they uncommonly disseminate to lymph nodes, they tend to recur locally after surgical therapy and to persist locally after radiation.[23,24] Verrucous cancers may thus warrant use of hybrid therapeutic strategies.

Lymphoepithelioma-like carcinoma, histologically similar to cancers with the same name in the nasopharynx and associated with marked infiltration of inflammatory cells in the stroma, are thought to carry a more favorable prognosis when stratified by stage.[25]

Adenocarcinoma will comprise about 15% to 20% of invasive cervical cancer in most contemporary series. Adenocarcinomas are subclassified by the World Health Organization into mucinous adenocarcinoma (endocervical type and intestinal type), endometrioid adenocarcinoma, serous adenocarcinoma, mesonephric adenocarcinoma, and clear cell adenocarcinoma.[22] Adenocarcinomas, which arise in the cervical canal without grossly disrupting the mucosa of the exocervix, comprise a disproportionate percentage of patients with bulky, expansile tumors of the endocervix. Adenocarcinoma is reputed to carry a more ominous prognosis than cervical cancer, but this adverse effect on prognosis is seen primarily in patients with bulky stage I tumors 4 cm or larger in diameter, and patients with stage II disease.[26,27] The finding of spread to regional nodes in patients with adenocarcinoma treated by surgery carries a higher risk of recurrence than is found in comparable patients with squamous cancer.[28,29] Stage for stage, the prognosis for patients treated by radiation alone is marginally less than that for patients with squamous cancer, but the differences in prognosis are small.[30] The decrement in prognosis for patients with larger stage I and stage II adenocarcinoma relative to comparable patients with squamous cancer is attributed to a higher rate of distant metastatic failure rather than to major differences in the ability to control pelvic disease.

Clear cell adenocarcinoma of the cervix is a histologic variant of adenocarcinoma of the cervix, found primarily on the exocervix in girls and young women with a history of in utero exposure to exogenous synthetic estrogens such as diethylstilbestrol (DES) who are also susceptible to vaginal clear cell carcinomas.[31] Treatment of these patients will parallel treatment by stage for other cell types, except that the young age at diagnosis will generally result in a recommendation of surgical therapy for patients with stages I and IIA disease.

Adenoma malignum[32] is a rare variant of adenocarcinoma of the cervix whose paradoxical appellation has been "justified by a deceptively bland histologic appearance (adenoma) accompanied by a bad prognosis (malignum)." Minimal deviation adenocarcinoma (MDA) is used as an alternative descriptor for this lesion, which is frequently misdiagnosed as benign and is often an incidental finding in hysterectomy specimens from surgeries carried out for other indications. Delay in diagnosis or inappropriately gentle treatment occasioned by the appearance of low histologic grade may be contributing factors to a high risk of recurrence and mortality after treatment.[33]

Adenosquamous cancers are admixtures of malignant glandular elements and malignant squamous elements that tend to be poorly differentiated in both components. In the WHO classification, adenosquamous cancers are divided into those having mucin production as their only manifestation of glandular differentiation and those having identifiable glandular structure.[22] Glassy cell cancers[34] of the cervix are believed to be an extremely poorly differentiated variant of adenosquamous cancer with a bulky, exophytic growth pattern. Microscopically, these tumors have cells with large nuclei, prominent nucleoli, and a characteristic ground glass appearance to their cytoplasm. Typically, these tumors will exhibit an intense inflammatory infiltrate with abundant plasma cells and eosinophils, and some patients will have elevated eosinophil counts in their peripheral blood. These cancers, which are characterized by explosively rapid growth with a high risk of recurrence even when diagnosed in stage I and treated by appropriately aggressive surgery, are reputed to have a high failure rate when treated by radiation.[35] Because these cancers are most commonly diagnosed in stage I, combined modality therapy with surgery, radiation, and chemotherapy has been advocated when this histology is encountered.[36,37]

Small-cell neuroendocrine cancers may be found in the cervix. The historic use of the term "small-cell cancer"[21] (Reagan and Wentz) to describe some poorly differentiated squamous cancers has been a source of understandable confusion. This term (small-cell cancer) should be used to refer to the rare cervical cancers that are associated with a histologic appearance, natural history, patterns of dissemination, prognosis, and clinical management similar to small-cell neuroendocrine cancers of the lung and other sites ("oat cell" carcinoma).[38–40] Small-cell neuroendocrine cancers of the cervix will usually have neurosecretory granules that can be identified by electron microscopy. Endocrine paraneoplastic syndromes will occasionally accompany small-cell neuroendocrine tumors or the rare carcinoid tumors of the cervix that represent the biologically less aggressive end of the spectrum of small-cell malignancy, which extends from carcinoid tumors through atypical carcinoid tumors to small-cell carcinoma.

## ANATOMY

The cervix, or neck of the uterus, is composed of the portio vaginalis, which consists of the exocervix and transformation zone that protrude into the vaginal vault, and the portio supravaginalis, which contains much of the endocervical canal. The endocervical canal is lined by columnar glandular epithelium that extends through a transformation zone (squamocolumnar junction) to squamous epithelium that covers the exocervix. The cervix is separated from the uterine body by a narrow isthmus that broadens to form the muscular uterine body. The uterus and cervix are retained in the pelvis by a lattice of connective tissue through which course smooth muscle, nerves, and vessels. The paired uterosacral ligaments extend posterolaterally from the caudal portion of the uterus to run along the rectouterine peritoneal folds to insert on the sacrum. The cardinal ligaments or transverse cervical ligaments originate at the upper, lateral portions of the cervix and insert into the fascia that covers the pelvic diaphragm laterally. Regional spread of cervical cancer through these structures can result in the presence of cancer significantly posterior to the cervix. This fact must be taken into consideration when a four-field technique is employed for pelvic teletherapy.[41] The uterine corpus is attached to the lateral pelvic wall by the broad ligament and secured anterolaterally by the round ligaments. The broad ligament consists of a two-layered fold of peritoneum, sandwiching a layer of connective tissue termed the parametria, which extends from the lateral uterus to the pelvic sidewalls, with the fallopian tubes lying along the superior border of this structure. The round ligaments originate anterolaterally on the uterine fundus and course laterally and anteriorly over the pelvic brim to the internal inguinal ring, then pass through the canal to merge with the fascia of the labia majora. The rare cervical cancer metastasis to inguinal nodes in the absence of vaginal extension is believed to represent spread through the lymphatic channels in the round ligaments.

The primary lymphatics of the cervix course through the parametria, which contain small lymphoid aggregates that may harbor secondary cancer deposits as an early manifestation of metastatic spread. Lymphatic drainage proceeds initially to the obturator nodes lying at the superior pole of the obturator foramen, and then to the external iliac and internal iliac nodes, which lie along the course of their associated named vessels. Subsequent lymphatic drainage is to the common iliac nodes and the para-aortic or aortocaval nodes, which lie in parallel with their associated blood vessels. Lymphatics of the uterine body may drain through the parametria to pelvic nodes, but portions of the uterine fundus, including the cornual areas, have draining lymphatics that course through the broad ligament to merge with the ovarian lymphatics running through the infundibulopelvic ligament and parallel to the ovarian vessels.

Thus, metastases in the para-aortic nodes on the right, and metastases in para-aortic nodes or at the hilus of the kidney on the left, may be the first echelon of nodal metastatic spread in patients with cervical cancers with major extension to the upper uterine cavity. However, the upper retroperitoneal nodes will rarely be contaminated by metastatic spread in the absence of concurrent or prior metastasis to pelvic nodes. Para-aortic lymphatics then coalesce in the cysterna chyli lying as high as the level of the twelfth thoracic vertebra, with lymph flow progressing through the thoracic duct to the left subclavian vein. Knowledge of the location of these nodes is of critical importance in the design of radiation fields and will facilitate communication with surgeons and diagnostic radiologists.

In most patients, the aorta will bifurcate into the common iliac arteries at the level of the third lumbar vertebra. The common iliac arteries bifurcate above the lumbosacral promontory in 87% of patients.[41] The internal iliac vessels run posteriorly in the pelvis, and use of a four-field technique for pelvic teletherapy will hazard underdosing the associated nodes if the posterior border on the lateral fields is not placed sufficiently posterior.

The lymphatics of the upper vagina drain through the cervical lymphatics. The rare, apparently discontiguous spread of cervical cancer to the vagina is believed to represent retrograde lymphatic dissemination, and, in general, the teletherapy target volume should include the full length of the vagina when cervical cancer has extended caudally below the vaginal fornix to involve the vaginal wall. As the distal half of the vagina has direct lymphatic drainage to the inguinofemoral nodes, teletherapy treatment volume and technique must be adjusted to encompass those nodes when cervical cancer extends to involve the lower vagina.

The arterial supply of the uterus is from the uterine arteries, branches of the internal iliac arteries. The uterine arteries run through the broad ligament to cross the ureters at points just above and slightly lateral to the vaginal fornix within the medial parametria; shortly thereafter they send off branches to the vagina, the uterine fundus, the fallopian tubes, and smaller branches contributing to the ovarian blood supply. On each side of the cervix, the point at which the uterine artery and ureter cross is designated "point A" and is arbitrarily designated to lie 2 cm lateral to a point 2 cm cephalad to the cervical os measured along the axis of the endocervical canal. These points, right and left, have been historically used as prescription points for intracavitary brachytherapy, and dose to these points is designated as the "medial parametrial dose," or the "paracentral dose." Points 3 cm lateral to points A are called points B and have been arbitrarily designated to represent the right and left lateral parametria.

## STAGING

Staging systems serve multiple purposes. Extent of disease (stage distribution) at diagnosis is an indicator to assess efficacy of public health efforts in education and screening. Correction for clinical stage is important in the assessment of other possible prognostic factors such as tumor

**TABLE 10-19  Staging of Cervical Cancer: AJCC[a] and FIGO[b]**

| TNM Stage | FIGO Stage | Description |
|---|---|---|
| TX | | Primary tumor cannot be assessed. |
| T0 | | No evidence of primary tumor. |
| Tis | | Carcinoma in situ. |
| T1 | I | Cervical carcinoma confined to uterus. Extension to corpus should be disregarded. |
| T1a | IA | Invasive carcinoma diagnosed only by microscopy. All macroscopically visible lesions—even with superficial invasion—are T1b/IB. Stromal invasion with a maximum depth of 5 mm measured from the base of the epithelium and a horizontal spread of 7 mm or less. Vascular or lymphatic space involvement does not affect stage. |
| T1a1 | IA1 | Measured stromal invasion 3 mm or less in depth and 7 mm or less horizontal spread. |
| T1a2 | IA2 | Measured stromal invasion more than 3 mm but not more than 5 mm with a horizontal spread 7 mm or less. |
| T1b | IB | Clinically visible lesion confined to the cervix or microscopic lesion greater than T1a2/IA2. |
| T1b1 | IB1 | Clinically visible lesion 4 cm or less in greatest dimension. |
| T1b2 | IB2 | Clinically visible lesion more than 4 cm in greatest dimension. |
| T2 | II | Cervical carcinoma invades beyond uterus but not to pelvic wall or to the caudal third of the vagina. |
| T2a | IIA | Tumor without parametrial invasion. |
| T2b | IIB | Tumor with parametrial invasion. |
| T3 | III | Tumor extends to the pelvic wall and/or involves the caudal third of the vagina and/or causes hydronephrosis or nonfunctioning kidney. |
| T3a | IIIA | Tumor involves the caudal third of the vagina. No extension to pelvic wall. |
| T3b | IIIB | Tumor extends to pelvic wall and/or causes hydronephrosis or nonfunctioning kidney. |
| T4 | IVA | Tumor invades mucosa of the bladder or rectum and/or extends beyond true pelvis. (Bullous edema is not sufficient to classify tumor as T4/IVA.) |
| M1 | IVB | Distant metastasis. |

[a]AJCC T categories correspond to FIGO stages.

[b]The FIGO staging system is a mixed clinical and pathological staging system. Permitted clinical assessments include pelvic examination (inspection and palpation) under anesthesia, colposcopy, endocervical curretage, hysteroscopy, cervical conization, cystoscopy, proctoscopy, excretory urography (IVP), and plain radiography of the chest and skeletal system. Performance of additional assessments such as computed tomography (CT), lymphangiography, ultrasound, magnetic resonance imaging (MRI), positron emission tomography (PET), arteriography, venography, laparoscopy, and fine needle aspiration biopsy of nodes may assist in planning treatment. However, the results of these assessments do not alter or impact the assignment of clinical stage. For patients who are treated surgically, the clinical findings at surgery do not alter assigned clinical stage. Histopathologic findings from surgery (hysterectomy and/or lymphadenectomy) do not alter stage, although they may be reported as pathologic stage (pTNM) in the AJCC classification.

histology, histopathologic indices such as DNA content or S-phase fraction,[42] and in vitro radiosensitivity,[43] as well as potentially important patient "host" factors such as immune competence. Assignment of preintervention clinical stage permits comparison of treatment outcomes (cancer control and treatment morbidity) achieved by means of alternative therapeutic strategies, and aids in the assessment of experimental or innovative therapies.

The earliest international staging system was that promulgated by the League of Nations in 1929. Currently, the most widely employed formalism is that of the International Federation of Gynecology and Obstetrics, most recently revised in 1995. The FIGO staging system (Table 10-19) permits grouping of patients based on local tumor extent prior to major therapeutic intervention. It is a staging system that should be applicable worldwide, and appropriately must acknowledge that invasive cervical cancer is most prevalent in geographic areas associated with poverty, limited access to modern medical imaging technology, and economically constrained medical resources. A staging system must inevitably reflect its constituency, and should be useful and practical in settings that may have limited access to expensive, high technology assessments. It cannot be overemphasized that assignment of FIGO stage is not sufficient information upon which to predicate a course of treatment based all, or in part, on radiotherapy.

## RADICAL RADIOTHERAPY: SELECTION OF TARGET VOLUME

The FIGO staging system for cervical cancer recognizes the potential contributions of diagnostic imaging by allowing the results of chest radiography, skeletal radiography, excretory urography (IVP), and barium enema to be considered in the assignment of clinical stage. With the exception of the IVP, these assessments are most useful in defining disease extent for patients with very advanced cancer that is often beyond realistic hope of cure with available therapeutic modalities. While tumor size and the presence and level of lymph node metastases are generally acknowledged to be of prognostic importance,[44–47] the FIGO staging system largely ignores these factors.

Except for the use of linear dimensions for stratification within stages IA and IB to serve as surrogates for primary tumor size, volume is not considered in the FIGO system. Assessment of regional lymph node status is also largely irrelevant in the FIGO staging classification. However, these parameters may be of pivotal importance in making treatment decisions for patients whose treatment will be radiation based. The ability of sophisticated contemporary imaging modalities (computed tomography, magnetic resonance imaging, lymphography) to demonstrate cytologically verifiable regional and remote cancer spread substantially exceeds that of the imaging modalities permitted in the FIGO staging formalism. Information from such studies, when available, should be intelligently integrated into rational clinical decision making, but it will not alter assignment of clinical stage.

The American College of Surgeons Commission on Cancer conducted a patient care evaluation survey for U.S. patients with cervical cancer that attempted to quantify the use of various pretreatment diagnostic assessments employed during the study years 1984 and 1990.[48] Based on a total of 9338 patients of known clinical stage (approximately 30% of the estimated total national cases for the two study years) this study revealed a rapidly widening gulf between the assessments actually obtained in clinical practice in the United States and those allowed under FIGO staging rules. Use of body imaging studies increased dramatically between the two survey years, although the use of lymphography remained rare. Qualitatively similar observations have been reported by the American College of Radiology[49] in studying patients treated primarily by radiation.

The FIGO clinical stage, though important to specify and record, does not, alone, provide sufficient information upon which to base treatment decisions (target volume, fractionation, dose, brachytherapy dose distribution) for patients whose management will be radiation based. Failure to include the entire cancer and its regional extensions within the treatment volume is usually fatal. This dictates assessment of all sites of possible gross cancer involvement by direct extension (bladder, rectum, parametria and uterine suspensory ligaments, uterine fundus) as well as investigation of potential clinically apparent (macroscopic) metastases to retroperitoneal lymph nodes. In addition to delineating sites of gross cancer extension and metastasis, the physician must make an intelligent estimation of the statistical risk of subclinical involvement by micrometastatic deposits in anatomic levels of retroperitoneal lymph nodes historically not targeted in pelvic radiation portals.

Accumulating evidence testifies to the curative capability of extended volume radiation for a significant percentage of patients with histologically confirmed metastasis to the para-aortic nodes.[50–56] The statistical risk of extrapelvic nodal metastasis must be carefully weighed against the relative hazard of extending treatment volume, which increases the risk of acute radiation morbidity (which can compromise the timely completion of treatment) as well as chronic radiation injury to the expanded volume of normal tissues exposed. Defining the target volume will be of increasing importance in an era when concurrent use of radiation and cytotoxic chemotherapy is

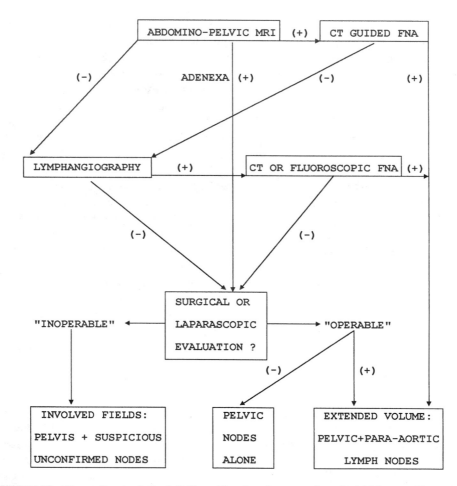

**FIGURE 10-13**  Diagnostic cascade for definition of lymph node target volume for initial external beam radiotherapy FIGO clinical stages IB–IVA cervical cancer. (+), imaging result suspicious for retroperitoneal node metastasis or cytologic confirmation of metastasis by biopsy; (−), normal lymph node exam, or absence of malignant cells on biopsy; ADENEXA (+), abnormal imaging findings in the tubes or ovaries, either potentially neoplastic or inflammatory; FNA, fine needle aspiration biopsy.

rapidly emerging as the national standard of care in the United States.[57,58] A recent prospective randomized study has provided persuasive evidence that synchronous administration of radiopotentiating cytotoxic agents enhances both pelvic control and survival compared with state-of-the-art radiation alone.[59] Concurrent chemotherapy clearly adds to acute gastrointestinal and hematologic toxicity. Appropriate selection of radiation target volume becomes even more critical when combined modality therapy is planned. It seems profligate with normal tissue tolerance to routinely extend the volume of treatment to the para-aortic nodes in all patients with bulky FIGO IB and more advanced stages of disease, as the majority of patients with FIGO stages IB through IIIB will have uninvolved para-aortic nodes if assessed surgically. The majority of patients with FIGO IB, IIA, and IIB will have negative pelvic nodes as well.[60,61] Conversely, it may be unwise to confine radiation to a pelvic target volume when there is histologically confirmed evidence of nodal metastasis in pelvic nodes and treatment of the next echelon of nodes in an extended volume would be entirely consistent with radiotherapeutic custom and convention for primary cancers at other anatomic sites. The schema outlined in Figure 10-13 represents a cascade of diagnostic maneuvers that may be sequentially employed to define the extent of the nodal target volume.[62]

## SURGICAL ASSESSMENT OF LYMPH NODES PRIOR TO RADIATION THERAPY

Definition of nodal target volume may be most accurately accomplished by surgical assessment of the retroperitoneal nodes. Some data support this maneuver as being of therapeutic as well as diagnostic value. Surgical cytoreduction may increase the probability of control of regional lymph node disease otherwise compromised by the limited teletherapy dose that can be prudently directed at grossly contaminated nodes.[56,63–65] Operative definition of disease extent may also allow access for radiation by interstitial implantation or electron beam to be directed to bulky nodes that cannot be removed surgically. Balancing these theoretic advantages are the disadvantages of delay in treatment initiation, cost, and the potential for increased complications.

Whenever feasible, surgical assessment of the nodes should be conducted through an extraperitoneal approach to reduce the subsequent hazard of bowel obstruction occasioned by adhesions and aggressive teletherapy. Late sequelae of treatment can be minimized by effective communication between the treating radiation oncologist and the operating surgeon. With the exception of removal of clinically enlarged, grossly contaminated nodes, the operative invention should be understood as primarily a diagnostic exercise. Complete therapeutic node dissection with stripping of all named node groups from the adventitia of the major vessels with which they are associated will only increase the risk of acute complications (e.g., bleeding, infection, lymphocoele, deep vein thrombosis) without a clear therapeutic benefit. Complete node dissection followed by teletherapy will inevitably yield some unhappy patients who, while cured of their cancer, will be encumbered by what may be a lifetime of leg lymphedema. Removal of one contaminated para-aortic node histologically verified by intraoperative frozen section will suffice to define the need for extended volume radiation. Further dissection of clinically normal nodes to be included within the target volume is probably superfluous and is likely to increase the risk of deleterious sequelae without a compensatory increase in probability of treatment success. Surgical assessment of upper retroperitoneal lymph nodes will detect metastatic disease in approximately 25% to 33% of patients with stage IIB and IIIB disease.

Frequently, the target volume for external beam radiation can be defined nonoperatively with contemporary imaging modalities. Detection of lymph node metastases by lymphography, third-generation CT scanners, or MRI can often be cytologically confirmed by fine needle aspiration under fluoroscopic or CT guidance. Under such circumstances, surgical intervention can be justified only for purposes of therapeutic cytoreduction[64,65] or for preradiation identification and treatment of comorbidities that may complicate radiotherapy (e.g., adenexal pathology such as chronic tubo-ovarian abcesses that may flare up or rupture under the influence of external radiation).

## TECHNIQUES

### Teletherapy

Design of radiation treatment portals is most effectively accomplished by integrating an understanding of normal anatomy with information concerning cancer extent in a particular patient. Morbid anatomy, distorted by mass effects of tumor, reactive inflammation and scarring, intrauterine hemorrhage or infection, and adenexal pathology, may differ substantially from the normal anatomy illustrated in reference texts.[66,67] Radiation technique must be predicated on knowing where things are as opposed to where they ought to be. Guidelines in reference texts should be understood to be only guidelines, not rigid formulations, and not a substitute for intimate knowledge of disease distribution in an individual patient. It is impossible to overstate the concept that there exist no such entities as "standard" radiation treatment volumes, "standard" portal design, or "standard" field sizes. To assert otherwise is the intellectual equivalent of arguing that one size and style of shoe should fit all feet. Intelligent individualization of treatment is the essence of excellence in medical care.

Commonly, radiation therapy for cervical cancer is carried out with a four-field technique employing anterior, posterior, and opposed lateral ports. Careful sculpting of rectangular fields with secondary collimation will reduce radiation dose and the risk of collateral damage to normal tissues. This technique will allow sparing bowel anteriorly, but

comes at the price of irradiating more pelvic bone (iliac wings), skin, and subcutaneous tissue than would be included in treatment accomplished by parallel opposed anterior and posterior fields utilizing high energy photons. A four-field pelvic technique is generally of no advantage for very slender patients, but it will permit reduction of maximal bowel dose for patients with a protuberant abdomen, and for most patients requiring treatment to an extended volume.

Tailored four-field techniques allow delivery to reduced volumes of gross cancer of higher doses than can be achieved under the limitations imposed by anterior and posterior fields. However, the use of this technique will increase the hazard of failing to adequately irradiate disease at the margins of lateral fields[66-68] and will be accomplished with greatest security with the assistance of diagnostic imaging to verify the location of cancer and potentially contaminated normal structures. Portals designed to shield the posterior rectal wall and portions of the sacrum and coccyx will hazard marginal recurrences in internal iliac nodes, presacral nodes, and uterosacral ligaments[66,67] (Figure 10-14). Anterior shielding may cause underdosage of external iliac nodes.[68] Treating slightly expanded pelvic volumes to assure adequate geographic coverage does not appear to augment late normal tissue sequelae compared to the treatment of traditional fields.[69] Sample anterior and lateral portals for the treatment of an extended volume are illustrated in Figures 10-15 and 10-16.

The inferior border of the treatment volume will, in general, be determined by the extent of vaginal wall invasion. The bottom of the obturator space is a commonly employed landmark. With extension confined to the proximal third of the vagina, a 2 cm margin of normal vagina caudal to the tumor will ordinarily suffice. When cancer extends to the midvagina, it is prudent to cover the full length of the vaginal canal and to electively treat the inguinal lymph nodes if the distal half of the vagina is involved. The infrequent patient will have one or more foci of discontiguous vaginal contamina-

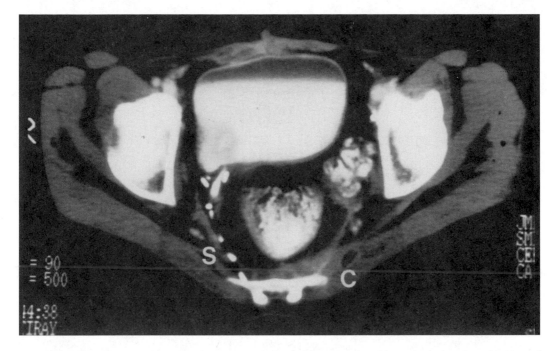

**FIGURE 10-14**   Transverse CT image of the pelvis at the level of the acetabulae with contrast in the urinary bladder and the rectum. This patient underwent radical hysterectomy for stage IB cervical cancer. Hemostatic surgical clips on the patient's right side (S) were placed during dissection of the internal iliac nodes. Note the posterior extent of this dissection. The patient received adjuvant postoperative radiation administered with a four-field technique. The posterior border of the lateral fields "split" the rectum by transecting the S2–S3 interspace. The patient developed biopsy-confirmed recurrent disease in residual uterosacral ligament on the patient's left side (C) adjacent to the sacrum and at the margin of the lateral fields.

tion representing retrograde spread through the lymphatics of the vaginal wall. Under these circumstances, the full length of the vagina should be treated. Some patients will have an exuberantly exophytic primary tumor, which will extend far down the vaginal canal without invading the vaginal walls. Insertion of a radiopaque marker at the time of treatment planning will aid in assuring an adequate inferior margin, a technique also useful for patients with pelvic relaxation and uterine prolapse.

The anterior and posterior fields will have lateral borders most accurately defined by reviewing the vascular and late filling images of the lymphangiogram, through the location of hemostatic clips placed at the time of operative assessment of the retroperitoneal lymph nodes, or with body imaging. In the absence of these aids, the field borders should be drawn to traverse the tips of the transverse processes

of T12–L3. In the pelvis, the beam edge should be placed 2 cm lateral to the inner edge of the bony pelvis at its maximal aperture (approximately 16–17 cm width). Lines connecting the points of greatest width in the pelvis to the tips of the transverse processes of L3 will include the common iliac and external iliac nodes with adequate margin in most patients. Low in the pelvis, the field margins should be constructed to shield most of the femoral heads and necks while including the obturator lymph nodes (which may not be opacified by lymphography) that lie at the superior and lateral corners of the obturator foraminae. It is not feasible to fully shield the femoral heads, since to do so would entail skimping on the margins of these nodes. When involvement of the distal vagina indicates treatment of the inguinal nodes, this can be accomplished by expanding the anterior field to include the

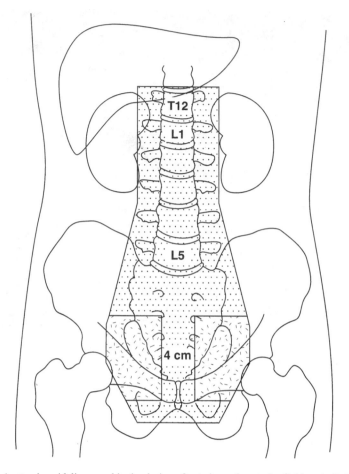

**FIGURE 10-15** Anatomic guidelines used in the design of anterior and posterior fields to include the pelvis and para-aortic lymph nodes: in the absence of radiographic markers, the superior border of the fields may be placed at L2–L3 if coverage of only common iliac nodes is to be assured. The superior border may be lowered to L4–L5 if only nodes below the bifurcation of the common iliac arteries are to be included. The superior border of the treatment volume should be at the T11–T12 interspace to encompass the cisterna chyli. Cervical cancer will occasionally spread to retrocrural lymph nodes at the T10–T11 level, but routine inclusion of this additional volume is probably not warranted in the absence of gross involvement of upper para-aortic nodes.

inguinal areas but employing a posterior field that does not. Compensatory dose to the inguinal nodes may be delivered through small anterior photon or high energy electron fields in order to limit dose to the femoral necks.

The reduced volumes to the right and left of a 4 cm wide midline bar correspond to the parametrial tissues, which may receive additional external beam therapy to supplement the dose absorbed through brachytherapy, while limiting dose to the rectum and bladder outlet.

These reduced portals may be designed with the assistance of coronal plane MRI and findings from physical examination.

The anterior border of the lateral fields will most accurately be determined by the combination of sagittal MRI or CT and lymphography. It will be defined by the need to encompass lymph nodes in the para-aortic and external iliac chains as well as the body of the uterus. For patients with gross invasion of the posterior wall of the urinary bladder, the bladder dome should be included. In the absence of gross nodal involvement visualized by MRI or CT, the lymphangiogram will provide the most effective information to define this border. When a lymphangiogram is unavailable, the para-aortic area from the top of T12 to the bottom of L3 can be encompassed by a curvilinear line parallel to the anterior border of the spine and separated by 3.5 to 4 cm. The course of the external iliac lymph nodes can be approximated by a line connecting the anterior caudal border of L4 to the apex of the pubic arch. A line parallel to this and displaced 2 cm anterior will achieve sufficient coverage of external iliac nodes allowing for beam divergence. Information from the sagittal MRI or CT is used to assure adequate coverage of the uterine fundus if there is any possibility of cancer extension up the endocervical canal to involve the lower uterine segment or the endometrial cavity.

The posterior border of the lateral fields is constructed to encompass the para-aortic nodes while including, at most, the anterior half of the kidneys. It is best defined by information yielded by the MRI or CT, and lymphography. In the absence of such information, the border can be defined by constructing a curved line that traverses the midpoints of vertebral bodies T12–L3. Caudally, the posterior border of the lateral fields should course behind most of the vertebral bodies of L4 and L5, as the common iliac nodes may lie directly lateral to these structures. Below L5, the posterior border of the lateral fields should be drawn to include the sacral silhouette to assure inclusion of internal iliac and presacral lymph nodes as well as the posterolateral extent of the uterosacral and cardinal ligaments. Efforts to spare posterior rectal wall can be hazardous and should be undertaken (if ever) only when the uterine suspensory ligaments are free of involvement both by imaging and by examination under anesthesia. At the caudal end of the lateral fields, a portion of the rectum, the buttocks, the anal canal, and the intergluteal fold can be shielded.

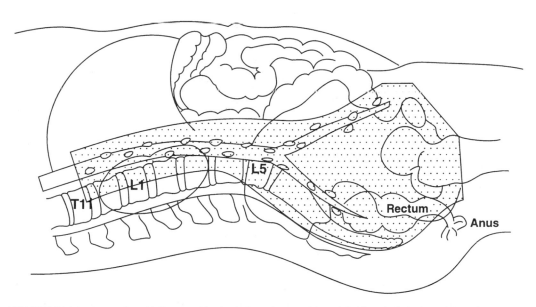

**FIGURE 10-16** Anatomic guidelines used in the design of opposed lateral fields to include the pelvis and para-aortic lymph nodes: in the absence of radiographic markers, the superior border of the fields may be placed at L2–L3 if coverage of the common iliac nodes is to be assured. The superior border may be lowered to L4–L5 if only nodes below the bifurcation of the common iliac arteries are to be included. The cephalad and caudal borders of the lateral portals will correspond to the superior and inferior borders of the anterior and posterior fields.

This can be accomplished using radiopaque markers or contrast material at the time of treatment simulation.

## Brachytherapy

The relative tolerance of the cervix, uterine body, distal ureters, and upper vagina to high dose radiation makes brachytherapy ideal for the treatment of cervical cancer. Endocavitary brachytherapy permits delivery of differentially higher dose to the cancer than the surrounding normal tissues. The history of endocavitary treatment of cervical cancer is long and rich, and well beyond the scope of this chapter to consider in detail. But a cursory consideration of medical history[70] provides valuable perspective on new technologies and their place in the evolution of endocavitary therapies.

Roentgen discovered x-rays in 1895, and investigators looking into this new imaging modality soon appreciated the acute biologic impact on skin consequent to prolonged fluoroscopic exposures. The Curies discovered the radioactivity of radium in 1898. Some of the biologic consequences of brachytherapy employing radioisotopes were appreciated by Becquerel, a colleague of the Curies, who received a skin burn from carrying a radium sample in his waistcoat pocket. As a result of equipment limitations, inability to administer exposure at significant depth, and problems in quantitating absorbed dose, transvaginal administration of roentgen rays became a logical technique for the administration of radiation to the cervix and was first used circa 1901. Radium was first used to treat cervical cancer in 1902, and brachytherapy became the foundation of effective radiotherapy until the advent of megavoltage teletherapy.

Interstitial implantation of radioisotopes was suggested by Alexander Graham Bell in 1903. Radium needle parametrial implantation was popularized in the 1940s to improve dose distribution for patients with bulky parametrial extension. Hyperthermia was utilized to treat cervical cancer early in this century, with an instrument resembling a soldering iron. The tissue thermometer was the surgeon's hand applied to the uterus. When the surgeon's hand became uncomfortably hot, the rheostat would be turned down.[70]

Since these early efforts, technology has become increasingly refined, permitting elegant radiation dose distributions, based on diagnostic imaging, to define treatment volume and the proximity of sensitive normal tissues. Computerized calculations rooted in sophisticated dosimetric algorithms allow accurate specification of absorbed dose at particular points within a target volume treated by brachytherapy, as well as within surrounding normal tissues. Precision afterloading applicators, miniaturized sources utilizing new isotopes, and computer control of source position and dwell times now permit accurate placement of treatment apparatus and optimization of dose distribution within the patient while incurring minimal, if any, radiation exposure to the medical team. It may be a relatively short time until commercially available CT- and MRI-compatible applicators are in routine clinical use, permitting brachytherapy dose distributions to be optimized and treatment prescribed based on three-dimensional reconstruction of cancer and normal tissue volumes with the brachytherapy apparatus in situ. A working knowledge of the techniques and outcomes of conventional low dose rate brachytherapy employing $^{226}$Ra and $^{137}$Cs with stereotypical dose distributions and dose expressed as exposure in milligram-hours (the mathematical product of the total number of milligrams of radium or radium-equivalent cesium and the duration of the implant in hours), or absorbed dose to idealized anatomic points such as point A, provides a reference standard against which new techniques should be compared for cancer control and late normal tissue sequelae.[71] However, the empiric prescriptions of the past, developed in an era without sophisticated soft tissue imaging and without refined computational techniques, should be understood as reference guidelines rather than immutable rules or orthodoxy. The fundamental purpose of brachytherapy is the exploitation of radioisotopes to selectively administer higher radiation dose to cancer than to adjacent normal tissues. The object is to create isodose lines that parallel the actual distribution of disease and encompass target volumes potentially contaminated. The patients in Figures 10-17 and 10-18 clearly should be treated with very different intracavitary dose distributions despite having similar stage (FIGO IIB) disease. Figures 10-19 and 10-20 are AP and lateral radiographs of a tandem and shielded ovoids insertion illustrating a patient with favorable anatomy.

## TREATMENT BY STAGE

In the United States, the majority of patients with in situ or stages IA and IB disease are currently managed by surgery.[72] Surgical cure rates will approach 100% for patients with

stage IA disease, and controversy is confined to the extent of the procedure required to reliably effect cure while minimizing functional surgical sequelae. Patients with stage IA1 disease are unlikely to harbor occult nodal metastases, and extrafascial hysterectomy is highly likely to effect cure with minimal probability of complications. Selected patients desiring conservation of reproductive integrity may be managed by cervical conization alone. For patients with more extensive disease, some form of extended hysterectomy is generally advised.

Patients with in situ cancer and stage IA cancer can be treated with radiation alone with cure probability approaching 100%.[73–77] Treatment may be successfully carried out with brachytherapy alone for patients with in situ or IA1 disease. Patients with more extensive disease will have a small, but not negligible risk of parametrial spread or nodal

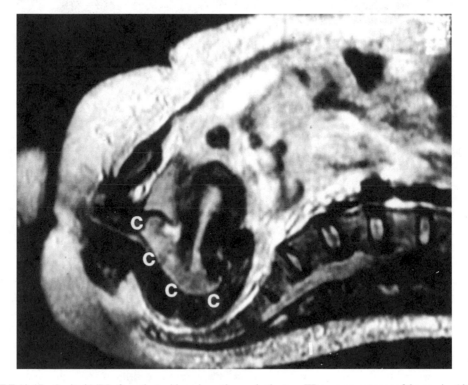

**FIGURE 10-17** Sagittal MRI of a patient with exuberantly exophytic stage IIB squamous cancer of the cervix. Although quite large in transverse diameter, the tumor extended minimally up the endocervical canal, and the uterine cavity was not grossly contaminated. A uterine tandem would be loaded in such a fashion sufficient to provide lateral dose to the medial parametria, but the full length would not be loaded to avoid unnecessary irradiation of the posterior bladder wall.

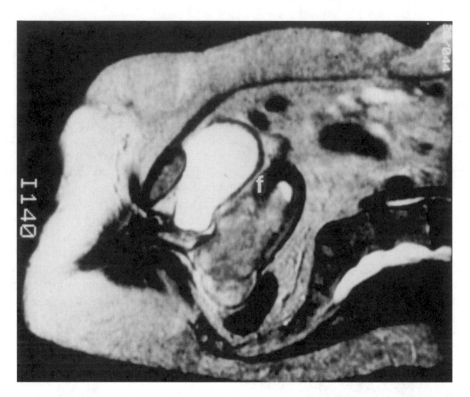

**FIGURE 10-18**   Sagittal MRI of a patient with stage IIB squamous cancer of the cervix with gross extension to the uterine fundus (f) and destruction of the uterine wall anteriorly with extension of neoplasm to the vesicouterine pouch. A uterine tandem would need to be loaded to the tip with heavy weighting to address this pattern of extension.

involvement.[77] Patients with such limited volume disease will usually be referred for radiotherapy only when comorbidities render them medically inoperable. The approximate 3% risk of occult nodal involvement in patients with IA2 and small IB tumors up to 1 cm in diameter needs to weighed against the toxicities of external beam therapy for such compromised patients.

Patients with stage IB and IIA may be managed with either radical radiation or radical surgery. Vigorous controversy surrounds selection of treatment modality and interpretation of outcomes. Alleged superior survival results for surgery will sometimes reflect case selection in that patients with smaller cancers may be selected for surgical therapy, while patients with larger cancers may be relegated to treatment with radiation. Patients surgically explored and found to have gross metastatic adenopathy may have radical surgery aborted and may be dropped from analyses of surgical outcome. Inclusion of such patients in outcome analyses for radiation will further obscure interpretation of results.

A large prospective randomized trial[78] from Milan compared 5-year survival and disease-free survival outcomes for 337 eligible and analyzable patients with IB/IIA cervical cancer randomized to radiation (167 patients) or surgery with selective adjuvant postoperative radiotherapy (170 patients). Analysis was based on initial treatment intent, and overall and relapse-free survivals were identical in the two groups at 83% and 74%, respectively. To interpret the results of this trial, one must appreciate that postoperative radiotherapy was recommended to women with surgical stage greater than pT2a, less than 3 mm of uninvolved cervical stroma, cut-through, or lymph node metastasis. Importantly, the use of these criteria resulted in 62 of 114 patients with tumors 4 cm or less in diameter receiving postoperative radiation (54.4%), and 46 of 55 patients with tumors larger than 4 cm in diameter receiving combined modality therapy (83.6%). Serious late sequelae were reported in 28% of the surgery group and 12% of the radiotherapy group, with the highest risk of late sequelae observed among patients undergoing combined modality therapy.

The advantages of surgery include the conservation of ovarian function in some younger patients, the avoidance of potential late carcinogenic effects of radiation, and better conservation of vaginal function. Conservation of ovaries carries a small risk of preserving occult ovarian metastases, a risk that may be slightly

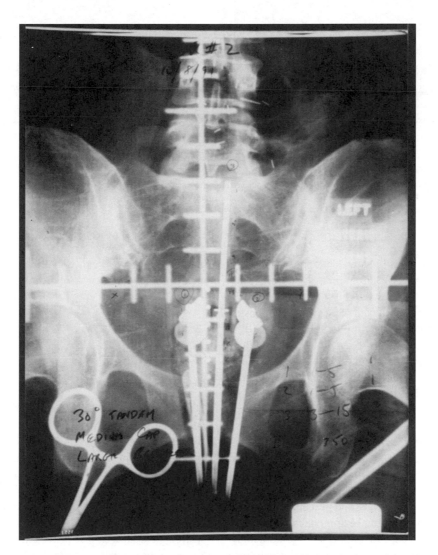

**FIGURE 10-19** AP dosimetry radiograph of a tandem and partially shielded ovoids insertion in a patient with stage IIB disease treated with high dose rate afterloading apparatus. Note that the tandem bisects the space between the ovoids, which are placed in the lateral fornices. Indelible ink markings are for dosimetry purposes and form part of the patient's permanent record.

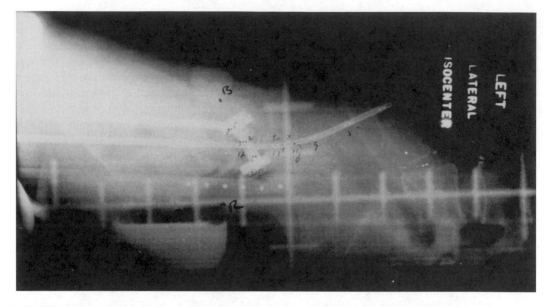

**FIGURE 10-20**   Lateral dosimetry radiograph of a tandem and partially shielded ovoids insertion in a patient with stage IIB disease treated with high dose rate afterloading apparatus. Note contrast in the Foley catheter balloon used to calculate dose to the mucosa of the bladder outlet. Contrast and air in the rectum are used to estimate dose to the anterior rectal wall. BBs lie in a Lucite tongue blade (rectal retractor) placed behind the ovoids and used to displace the anterior rectal wall posteriorly. The tandem bisects the ovoids in the AP dimension. Indelible ink markings are for dosimetry purposes and form part of the patient's permanent record.

higher among patients with adenocarcinoma or adenosquamous carcinoma.[79–85] Generally, ovarian metastases will be seen in the context of one or more other major adverse prognostic factors, and this finding is associated with a high probability of recurrence and death.[85] Anatomic preservation of the ovaries does not assure their endocrine viability in the context of extended hysterectomy. Many women with retained ovaries will experience premature menopause as well as developing ovarian cysts, torsion, and other pathologies.[84,86] Sexual dysfunction after treatment for cervical cancer is multifactorial, with physical, social, and psychological components. It is not clear that with appropriate counseling and precautions (use of vaginal dilator, vaginal estrogen, exogenous lubrication) sexual functioning after radiotherapy for stages IB/IIA need be less satisfactory than after radical surgery.

Regardless of the merits of the argument, the use of surgery has increased for patients with lower stage cervical cancer coincident with the increasing involvement of gynecologic oncologists in the management of these patients.[58,72]

## POSTHYSTERECTOMY RADIATION

### After Simple Hysterectomy

The radiation oncologist will occasionally be requested to evaluate a patient for consideration of radiation following inadvertent simple hysterectomy in the setting of invasive carcinoma.[87–89] This circumstance may occur when invasive cervical cancer is a surprise finding in an individual operated for benign pathology, such as uterine myomata. Patients appropriately evaluated for potentially invasive disease will occasionally have the true pathological extent of disease underestimated by cervical conization performed by means of either the cold knife technique or the loop electrocautery excision procedure (LEEP). Reasons for inappropriate simple hysterectomy include failure to obtain cervical cytology and failure to fully evaluate an abnormal smear or cervical biopsy sample. Misinterpretation of pathology results, and failure to recognize or evaluate positive conization margins or to perform an indicated conization, are common, avoidable causes. Some patients will have abnormal bleeding that either was not investigated prior to hysterectomy or was attributed to other causes.

When careful study of the operative specimen reveals cancer invasion of 3 mm or less, with less than 7 mm horizontal spread and no evidence of endothelial lined space invasion (lymphovascular invasion), the vast majority of such patients will have been adequately treated and can be followed without additional intervention. When more than microinvasive disease is encountered, additional therapy is mandated because of a significant risk of residual disease detectable by reoperation and an approximate 40% risk of recurrence in stage IB disease treated by simple hysterectomy. Sensible treatment options include external pelvic radiation supplemented by vaginal vault brachytherapy,[90–92] or reoperation.[93–95]

Historical results of radiotherapy in this setting have been generally favorable. Long-term results are approximately equivalent to those obtained for patients treated initially by appropriate extended hysterectomy or radical radiotherapy, and radiation will remain the treatment of choice when the patient's body habitus, age, or comorbidities contraindicate reoperation, or when the requisite surgical expertise is not available. Prior to radiation, the pelvis should be imaged to identify possible macroscopic disease requiring more aggressive radiation dose. External radiation in a dose of 45 Gy to 50.4 Gy over 5 to 5.5 weeks will generally suffice, supplemented by a 20 Gy vaginal vault mucosal dose boost by conventional low dose rate brachytherapy or three fractions of 5 Gy using high dose rate brachytherapy.

Controversy exists concerning the prognostic significance of positive margins and palpable residual disease. The bulk of evidence available suggests that patients with gross residual disease have substantially greater risk of both local recurrence and death. For patients who have had gross tumor transection ("cut-through") with macroscopic residual disease, the prognosis is ominous. Generally this will occur in the setting of failure to recognize clinical stage IIB or IIIB disease. Because of lateral and posterior retraction of the parametrial tissues and uterine suspensory ligaments following simple hysterectomy, residual disease in the central portions of these structures is likely to be beyond the effective range of endocavitary brachytherapy. The consequence is outcomes inferior to those expected from treating comparable stages of patients with radiation on intact uterus. Interstitial brachytherapy techniques with placement under operative visualization may allow these patients to reap the benefits of brachytherapy. Treatment with higher radiation dose employing progressively shrinking volumes will salvage some patients. Use of concurrent radiopotentiating chemotherapy to maximize the efficacy of the subtherapeutic doses of teletherapy is not unreasonable.

In patients without obvious tumor transection, reoperation consists of the technically challenging task of completing the surgical removal of the same volume of tissue that should have been removed by radical hysterectomy, absent having the uterine body to provide traction on the parametria and uterine suspensory ligaments. This surgery may be a reasonable approach in selected patients for whom initial treatment by radical hysterectomy would have been appropriate, had the diagnosis of invasive cancer been apparent prior to hysterectomy. When radical parametrectomy and lymphadenectomy are carried out with no residual disease detected, risk of recurrence is minimal.[94] Morbidity of this procedure, in skilled hands, should not exceed that of planned radical hysterectomy.[93] Should residual disease be encountered in the parametria or regional lymphatics, additional adjuvant therapy may be useful. This approach, employing selective radiation for patients with detectable disease revealed by second surgery, results in overall survival results approximately equivalent to patients uniformly given radiation, while avoiding the need for radiation therapy in 73% to 84% of patients.[93-95]

### Adjuvant Radiation Supplementing Radical or Modified Radical Hysterectomy in Patients with Adverse Prognostic Factors

Although survival results after radiotherapy or surgery are equivalent, in the United States surgery has become the most common form of treatment for patients with FIGO stages IB and IIA disease.[72] Retrospective analyses of surgical outcome have identified categories of patients who are at increased risk of pelvic recurrence and distant metastases based on histopathologic study of the operative specimen.[96] Primary tumor size, depth of cervical stromal invasion, and presence of capillary-like space involvement are predictive of lymph node metastasis but may also represent indepedent increments of risk in the absence of nodal spread.[97] Metastasis in regional lymph nodes is universally acknowledged to be the single most important risk factor, with a decrement in prognosis related to the most cephalad location of the nodal metastases[96] (pelvic, common iliac, para-aortic). Decrements in prognosis are observed when the burden of nodal contamination is grossly apparent rather than occult (microscopic)[98] and when multiple nodes are involved compared to cases of single-node contamination.[99,100] Involvement of multiple node groups is more ominous than spread to only one anatomic cluster of nodes, and bilateral metastasis is prognostically worse than unilateral. With metastasis to only one pelvic node, risk of failure is 25% to 27%.[99,101] With multiple nodes involved, the risk of failure rises to 35% to 55%. Although treatment failure may be manifest as hematogenous dissemination or spread to extrapelvic lymph nodes, the majority ($\geq$ 70%) of patients failing surgical therapy will manifest clinically apparent pelvic recurrence as a component of the composite pattern of failure.[102-108]

Because pelvic relapse is uncommonly salvaged, particularly when lymph nodes were originally involved,[109-112] adjuvant postoperative radiation has been historically employed in an effort to prevent pelvic relapse. This strategy is supported by the observation that postoperative radiation will control known residual pelvic cancer in some patients.[113] Although such treatment will reduce the expected rate of pelvic recurrence, failure within the irradiated volume remains a frequent component of the pattern of failure,[100,102-105,114,115] and the theoretical potential survival benefit has not been apparent in case-controlled or matched-pair retrospective series.[102,103] Pelvic radiation consisting of 45 Gy to 50.4 Gy, often supplemented by limited vault brachytherapy (20 Gy by low dose rate or three fractions of 5 Gy by high dose rate), is commonly employed. Recurrence in para-aortic nodes can be expected in 15% or more of patients relapsing after hysterectomy and postoperative pelvic radiotherapy for node-positive cervical cancer,[116] but accompanied by distant disease in half such patients. Favorable survival statistics were reported from Japan when the treatment volume was extended to electively include the para-aortic nodes,[117] and this would seem reasonable when multiple pelvic nodes are contaminated ($\geq$ 4 nodes). However, treating an extended volume has not shown consistent benefit and has resulted in some increased morbidity, including insufficiency fractures of the lumbar vertebrae.[118]

In an effort to enhance pelvic control as well as to reduce distant metastases, the Southwest Oncology Group (SWOG), the Gynecologic Oncology Group (GOG), and the Radiation Therapy Oncology Group (RTOG) initiated a prospective randomized investigation (Intergroup Protocol 0107) in 1991. This study compared adjuvant postoperative pelvic teletherapy alone to pelvic teletherapy plus two cycles of concurrent 5-fluorouracil (5-FU) and cisplatin followed by two additional cycles of sequential 5-FU and cisplatin after completion of radiotherapy. Eligible patients had parametrial extension (pT2B) and/or metastasis to pelvic nodes, and/or a positive surgical margin. Preliminary analysis reveals that synchronous chemotherapy improves cancer control within the irradiated volume and improves progression-free survival from 63% at 4 years with radiation alone to 81% with chemoradiation.[119]

A cooperative effort between Memorial Sloan-Kettering Cancer Center, the Mayo Clinic, the Uniformed Services Health University, and the University of Miami prospectively compared adjuvant systemic chemotherapy alone versus systemic chemotherapy followed by adjuvant pelvic radiotherapy. This study concluded that adjuvant pelvic radiotherapy did not favorably impact on either survival or pelvic control.[120] Because of the delay in initiating radiotherapy after hysterectomy, the somewhat low dose of external radiotherapy employed in that study, and the omission of vaginal vault brachytherapy, it is possible that the benefit of optimal adjuvant pelvic radiotherapy was obscured by the study design. Accelerated repopulation of clinically occult residual clonogens may have occurred during the prolonged interval between surgery and initiation of adjuvant radiation. If adjuvant pelvic radiation is to be employed, it should be initiated within 6 weeks from the date of hysterectomy, and preferably sooner. An additional possible cause of treatment failure in adjuvantly irradiated patients is failure to encompass the entire volume at risk when a four-field pelvic "box" technique is employed. When the uterine suspensory ligaments are surgically divided, residual soft tissues retract laterally and posteriorly. Lateral fields that attempt to spare the posterior half of the rectum may result in substantial underdosage of residual posterior tissues at risk. The patient whose CT scan is illustrated in Figure 10-14 was treated with adjuvant postoperative teletherapy employing a four-field technique, splitting the rectum on the lateral fields. This resulted in an underdosage and recurrence in residual uterosacral ligament. To avoid such an outcome, lateral fields should encompass the entire silhouette of the sacrum and coccyx, sparing only the gluteal muscles, skin, and the anal canal, while sparing small and large bowel anteriorly.

Approximately half of patients failing radical hysterectomy will be patients without lymph node metastasis.[121] Among node-negative patients, primary tumor size, depth of cervical stromal invasion, parametrial extension, presence of vascular or lymphatic space invasion, and histology are parameters that may identify patients at increased risk for recurrence. As with node-positive patients, the largest component of the pattern of failure is local–regional recurrence. Under the aegis of the Gynecologic Oncology Group, a prospective investigation (GOG Protocol 92, RTOG Protocol 87-06) randomized node-negative, parametria-negative, "intermediate risk" patients to observation versus adjuvant pelvic teletherapy following radical hysterectomy. Patient eligibility was based on tumor size, depth of cervical stromal invasion, and presence of lymphatic space invasion. In this study, 277 patients were randomized to pelvic radiation versus no further treatment. Among patients randomized to radiotherapy, 15% experienced recurrence, comparing favorably to the 28% rate among patients randomized to no further treatment. The majority of recurrences in both groups were vaginal and/or pelvic. A modest improvement in relapse-free survival (88% vs. 79% at 2 years) appears to be the benefit of treatment, which is associated with a small risk of increased complications (6% vs. 2%).[122]

Adjuvant postoperative radiation will reduce pelvic failure 39% to 45% compared to surgery alone in intermediate and high risk patients, but pelvic recurrence remains the largest component of the pattern of failure despite adjuvant radiation.[100,102,103,105,114,115,122] This reduction in pelvic recurrences may not be a sufficiently large effect to result in marked improvement in overall or relapse-free survival. Further improvement is likely to come from the synchronous administration of concurrent, radiopotentiating chemotherapy, and it is probable that this strategy will continue to be investigated by the GOG.

Since 1990, 38 intermediate to high risk node-negative patients in northern California have been treated in a multi-institutional effort using a pelvic radiation regimen of 45 Gy in 5 weeks with limited vault brachytherapy. Two cycles of 5-FU (1000 mg/m$^2$/24 h × 96 h) and cisplatin (100 mg/m$^2$) have been administered during the first and fifth weeks of teletherapy. With median follow-up of 42 months for patients without recurrence, five patients have failed. All failures have been distant, with no recurrences in the irradiated volume. In a separate study at the Radiation Oncology Centers of Northern California beginning in 1988, 59 patients with metastasis to one or more pelvic nodes have been treated with the identical adjuvant regimen. With median follow-up in excess of 5 years, 8 patients have relapsed, with only 2 manifesting recurrence within the irradiated volume. Among 32 patients available for 5-year minimum follow-up, actuarial freedom from relapse is 84.3%. This experience suggests that synchronous administration of chemotherapy with radiation can reduce the rate of pelvic recurrence below that expected following adjuvant radiation alone.

Adjuvant chemotherapy has been used to treat high risk patients, primarily patients with metastasis to regional nodes.[123–125] However, prospective randomized study of adjuvant postoperative systemic chemotherapy has failed to show benefit.[125,126]

Late sequelae of adjuvant radiation include injury to the small bowel with obstruction requiring surgery, rare injuries to pelvic bones (insufficiency fractures), greater likelihood of bladder dysfunction, and leg lymphedema. Delayed injury to the bladder mucosa and rectum are unusual with adjuvant dose schedules. Following surgical amputation of the proximal 25% to 33% of the vagina, irradiation of a portion of the residual vagina may significantly increase the risk of dyspareunia even if appropriate precautions are observed, including regular use of a vaginal dilator, vaginal estrogen, and exogenous lubrication prior to intercourse. In contrast to patients treated with radiation without surgery for cervical cancer on intact uterus, patients undergoing pelvic radiation following therapeutic lymphadenectomy will develop some degree of lower extremity lymphedema in approximately 20% of cases. This may vary from intermittent and minimally symptomatic swelling around the ankles to disabling, massive edema extending from the toes to the pelvis and requiring medical therapy including diuretics, massage therapy, and external compression devices.

### Bulky IB2 or Barrel-Shaped Cervical Cancer Stages IB/IIA

The prognosis of stage IB and IIA cervical cancer, treated either by surgery or radiation, declines with increasing tumor size.[44,45,78,127,128] Cancer control should approach 100% for tumors less than 1 cm in diameter, dropping to approximately 65% to 75% for tumors 4 cm or larger. Following completion of radiation therapy, some patients will undergo supplementary extrafascial hysterectomy to clear suspected persistent central disease. Controversy exists regarding whether such treatment should be considered for patients with tumors larger than 4 cm in size (IB2), or whether it should be reserved for patients with "barrel-shaped" tumors. Large, expansile lesions of the endocervical canal and lower uterine segment are sometimes referred to as "barrel-shaped" cancers because of the resemblance the resulting primary mass bears to a wooden barrel or keg. Large primary tumor size alone should not confer this appellation, particularly when a tumor is exuberantly exophytic. Rather, the term should be reserved for tumors arising in the endocervical canal and concentrically expanding the cervix to 6 cm or larger in transverse diameter. Such tumors are associated with a high risk of positive margins or of finding extracervical spread to parametria or nodes when treated by initial surgery. Conversely, such patients have a substantial risk of initial central failure when treated with radiation alone.

Contributing to radiation failures may be suboptimal brachytherapy dose distribution when intracavitary brachtherapy is used to treat these patients.[129] These observations and outcomes resulted in the historical development of a hybrid treatment strategy combining conventional external beam radiotherapy with a slightly reduced dose of brachytherapy supplemented by extrafascial hysterectomy. Five-year survival is approximately 55% to 65% whether patients are treated by radiation alone or by combined modality therapy.[130-132] A modest benefit in central tumor control with a combined modality approach has not translated into consistently improved survival because such patients are at higher risk of distant dissemination than patients with smaller or exophytic tumors. The GOG and RTOG carried out a randomized prospective study for patients with "bulky" IB cancers of the cervix ($\geq$ 4 cm in diameter) comparing radiotherapy alone and preoperative radiation and extrafascial hysterectomy (GOG Protocol 71, RTOG Protocol 84-22). Final results have not been published, but differences, if any, in long-term survival outcome are expected to be minimal. Among patients undergoing combined modality therapy, persistence of tumor in the hysterectomy specimen is associated with a higher probability of relapse.[133,134]

The GOG-RTOG trial has been the object of criticism. Inadequately aggressive radiation therapy may have been used in the radiation-alone arm (80 Gy cumulative to point A via external and intracavitary combined), and patients with exophytic tumors were included who could be expected to fare well with radiotherapy alone. Based on preliminary analysis that suggested prolongation of the relapse-free interval in the patients undergoing adjuvant hysterectomy, the preoperative regimen (75 Gy to point A, 55 Gy to point B from the summation of external beam therapy and intracavitary brachytherapy) became the control arm in the successor GOG study.

In the successor study patients were randomized to receive the same preoperative radiotherapy with or without weekly cisplatin at 40 mg/m$^2$. This trial (GOG Protocol 123) was recently reported[135] to show 57% of hysterectomy specimens with residual cancer after radiation alone, and 47% with residual cancer when weekly cisplatin was added to the preoperative radiotherapy. Both survival (89% vs. 79%) and recurrence-free interval (81% vs. 69%) at 2 years were statistically better in the patients treated by preoperative radiation plus cisplatin than in the patients randomized to preoperative radiotherapy alone.

Management of patients with IB2 or classic "barrel-shaped" cancer IB/IIA has become a source of conflict and contention between radiation oncologists and gynecologic oncologists, possibly owing to doctrinal rigidity where none need be present. When a patient is diagnosed with bulky, or "barrel-shaped" FIGO IB/IIA cancer, determination of the final treatment strategy can be delayed pending an evaluation of tumor response and the adequacy of brachytherapy dose distribution. It is probably not helpful to surgically remove a cervix and uterus in which there has been complete histologic clearance of cancer by radiation. Neither is it sensible to leave, in situ, a cervix suspicious for persistent cancer because the routine use of adjunctive hysterectomy has not had a measurable impact on the survival statistics for the aggregate population of patients with these volumes of disease.

If there has been substantial, objective tumor shrinkage in response to teletherapy, and if favorable geometry obtains at the time of initial intracavitary insertion, it would seem reasonable to complete treatment by radical radiation. Brachytherapy should be administered sufficient to complete an aggressive cumulative dose comprising 85 Gy to 95 Gy to point A. Conversely, if minimal tumor shrinkage is achieved by teletherapy and/or unsatisfactory geometry is encountered at the time of initial intracavitary insertion (rendering the eventualities of tumor persistence and late radiation complications somewhat more predictable), it would seem prudent to truncate the brachytherapy dose and to proceed with extrafascial hysterectomy. This strategy should limit the hazards of combined modality therapy to selected higher risk patients who are most likely to benefit, and for whom potentially more complex therapy can be justified.

### Management of Stages IIB, III, and IVA
Management of patients diagnosed with locally advanced cervical cancer will be radiation

based. The role of surgery is limited. Extraperitoneal surgical assessment of regional nodes may assist in planning radiotherapy, and surgical cytoreduction[64,65] of enlarged metastatic nodes may contribute to radiocurability. However, neither of these interventions has been proven to favorably impact on survival in the context of a prospective randomized trial. The rare patient with stage IVA disease presenting with a vesicovaginal or rectovaginal fistula may be appropriately treated by primary exenterative surgery, usually coordinated with preoperative or postoperative teletherapy. However, the vast majority of patients in these stages of disease will be managed with radiation-based therapy without diagnostic or therapeutic surgery.[72] Increasingly, chemotherapy will be administered concurrently with radiation therapy because of randomized clinical trials yielding results supporting its use.[58,59]

The critical first step in radiotherapeutic management is determination of initial teletherapy target volume based on assessment of regional tumor extent and risk of lymph node metastases. Because of the curative potential of extended field radiation[50–56] and because 25% or more of patients with these stages of disease will have extrapelvic lymph node involvement if the para-aortic nodes are assessed surgically, routine use of extended volume teletherapy has been advocated. Prospective evaluations of extended volume teletherapy versus pelvic teletherapy conducted by the RTOG[136] and the EORTC[137] suggest at most minimal benefit from routine use of extended volumes. When appropriate technique is employed,[52] extending treatment volume to the L1–L2 interspace (encompassing the renal vessels) adds minimally to acute and chronic morbidity if radiation alone is administered and patients have not had pretreatment transperitoneal surgical evaluation of nodes or prior laparotomy. The toxicity implications of extended volume treatment are more important if synchronous chemotherapy will be administered.

At the Radiation Oncology Centers of Northern California, treatment policy is to irradiate an extended volume to the top of T12 in all patients with cervical cancer treated on intact uterus who have documented lymph node metastasis. Patients without node metastasis based on diagnostic imaging and/or operative assessment of the retroperitoneum will customarily have only a pelvic volume irradiated. Patients with major contraindications to extended volume radiation, such as a history of inflammatory bowel disease, may have teletherapy limited to the pelvis even if pelvic node metastasis is documented. The diagnostic cascade in Figure 10-13 has been the historic basis for determining target volume. Recently, because of a lack of experienced lymphangiographers, increasing reliance has been placed on MRI and CT assessment of nodes. Positron emission tomography (PET) may eventually play a role in the noninvasive assessment of cancer extent by exploiting differences in the metabolic activity of cancer deposits compared to normal tissue. Surgical sampling of nodes has been done less frequently because of increasing confidence in the sensitivity of modern body scanners. Greater experience and sophistication in anticipating and managing the acute toxicities of extended volume radiation, even when given synchronously with cytotoxic chemotherapy, have allowed more latitude in the treatment of extended volumes.

Treatment is generally administered at 1.8 Gy per fraction and 9.0 Gy weekly. Areas at risk for occult, microscopic contamination are treated to 45 Gy in 25 fractions. Areas of gross nodal involvement receive 54 Gy to 63 Gy by external beam therapy, usually employing multiple fixed fields of limited size based on body imaging. Higher doses are restricted to small volumes encompassing gross disease with 1.5 to 2.0 cm margin. A midline block 4 cm wide is used to shield the bladder outlet and the distal rectum in anticipation of brachytherapy. This will be placed to restrict the direct teletherapy dose to these structures to 45 Gy, although this shielding may be placed as early as 36 Gy in selected patients in whom brachytherapy geometry is anticipated to be favorable. Gross parametrial disease will be boosted with limited volume teletherapy treatment for an additional 9 Gy to 14.4 Gy. These limited volumes should be designed based on information obtained from body imaging with MRI or CT integrated with physical findings from bimanual examination.

Teletherapy is coordinated with one or two low dose rate tandem and ovoid insertions. Dose from brachytherapy is recorded at points A and points B. However, brachytherapy dose distributions are designed based on an understanding of gross tumor distribution derived from pretreatment MRI and physical examination. Brachytherapy dose is prescribed based on the principle that one cannot overdose cancer, but normal tissues are vulnerable to excess radiation dose. Cumulative dose (external plus brachytherapy) to the bladder outlet reference point is not allowed to exceed 75 Gy in unfavorable geometry circumstances, and is generally restricted to 70 Gy when favorable geometry obtains. Cumulative dose to the anterior rectal wall is limited to 70 Gy. Dose to the anterior rectal wall may be estimated at more than one point using orthogonal dosimetry films. The ratio of average point A dose to the higher of the two (bladder or rectum) dose limiting normal tissues is calculated. (Half the arithmetic sum of the dose rates at points A on the right and left then is divided by the higher of dose rates at the bladder and rectal points.) Favorable geometry is considered to be a ratio of 1.6 or higher. This will allow prescription of 40 Gy or more to points A by brachytherapy while limiting dose to the rectum and bladder to 25 Gy. When added to 45 Gy administered by external beam, cumulative dose to points A should be 85 Gy or more. Under circumstances with extremely favorable anatomy (wide, capacious upper vagina permitting effective intravaginal packing displacing the bladder outlet and anterior rectal wall from the implant hardware, coupled with well-preserved, deep vaginal fornices) a ratio exceeding 2.0 may occasionally be achieved. By placement of a midline block earlier in the course of teletherapy, a cumulative dose to points A as high as 95 Gy may be attained without exceeding 70 Gy to the bladder outlet and anterior rectal wall.

Standard or orthodox weightings of brachytherapy sources are not employed in deference to a policy of individualization of dose distribution based on physical examination and tumor imaging by MRI. When cancer extends to the uterine cavity, the full length of the uterine tandem is loaded to treat the entire uterine cavity, and the highest source in the tandem will be of higher activity. If a cervical cancer is exophytic, does not extend far up the cervical canal, and minimally involves the medial parametria, the upper portion of the tandem will not be loaded, a measure that will avoid unnecessary exposure to small bowel, sigmoid colon, and posterior wall of the bladder. Generally 6 cm of tandem will be loaded with 2 cm $^{137}$Cs sources to assure adequate lateral dose distribution in these circumstances, but a shorter active length may be utilized when high dose rate equipment is used.

Since May 1991, the majority of patients at the Radiation Oncology Medical Centers of Northern California have been treated with high dose rate remote-afterloading technology using a high intensity $^{192}$Ir source. Almost all patients have been treated with five tandem and ovoid insertions. Placement of the intrauterine tandem is often facilitated by the use of ultrasound guidance, which is particularly helpful when the cervical canal is obstructed by tumor and anatomic landmarks are obliterated. The first brachytherapy fraction is generally administered during the third week of external radiation, and the final insertion is timed to coincide with the end of external beam treatment. A maximum of two insertions is performed in a week. External beam therapy is not administered on days when brachytherapy is applied. To minimize total elapsed treatment time (targeted at 7 to 8 weeks), no treatment interruptions are planned. Relative to brachytherapy administered by low dose rate $^{137}$Cs, a 25% reduction in total brachytherapy dose to the rectum and bladder has been adopted to account for increased late effects in normal tissues associated with the higher dose rate. In a manner analogous to the fashion in which low dose rate brachytherapy dose has been prescribed, doses are recorded at points A and points B, but dose distribution is individualized based on pretreatment magnetic resonance imaging of tumor and findings from physical examination. Dose with each brachytherapy fraction and cumulative brachytherapy dose is prescribed based on dose absorbed by adjacent normal tissues. Up to 7.5 Gy may be given to point A with a single fraction when favorable geometry is achieved. Doses to the bladder and rectal points are not allowed to exceed 4 Gy per treatment, and generally no more than two fractions of 4 Gy are given to either structure during a series of five insertions. Customarily, total brachytherapy dose to the bladder and rectum does not exceed 18.75 Gy if 45 Gy is planned for teletherapy to the whole pelvis. Average dose to points A has been between 26 Gy and 35 Gy, but will usually fall in a narrower range, between 30 and 33 Gy. With this formulation, late radiation sequelae have not been appreciably different from those experienced with conventional low dose rate brachytherapy. Because of the flexibility to tailor dose distributions made possible by the use of a high intensity, miniaturized source with multiple dwell positions 5 mm apart, more favorable ratios of dose prescribed to points A to dose-limiting normal structures may be attained, and a ratio of 1.75 is considered favorable. Figures 10-19 and 10-20 are radiographs of a typical tandem and ovoids insertion in which ovoids are used with partial anterior and posterior shielding to diminish dose to the bladder outlet and the anterior rectal wall.

Controversy continues to surround the issue of whether high dose rate brachytherapy is isoeffective with conventional low dose rate brachytherapy. When appropriate radiobiological corrections are applied[138] and care taken to exploit the ability to optimize dose distribution, late sequelae from HDR do not appear to be appreciably different from those seen following LDR.[139,140] Improved dose distributions appear to compensate for the inherent hazards to normal tissues posed by the increased dose rate. The Gynecologic Oncology Group allows the use of HDR brachytherapy in their cur-

rently active protocol for locally advanced cervical cancer (GOG Protocol 165: A Randomized Comparison of Radiation vs. Radiation Plus Weekly Cisplatin vs. Radiation Plus Protracted Venous Infusion of 5-FU in Patients with Stage IIB, IIIB, and IVA Carcinoma of the Cervix). In that study, 40 Gy to points A by LDR in one or two insertions is assumed to be approximately isoeffective for cancer control and complications with five fractions of 6 Gy (30 Gy) to points A by HDR. The RTOG will also permit HDR in developing protocols for advanced cervical cancer, although the fractionation schedule is anticipated to be more flexible.

Final teletherapy dose should be adjusted depending on the brachytherapy dose delivered. When low dose rate brachytherapy is used, dose to the lateral parametria and pelvic sidewall will be administered at 15 to 20 cGy/h. When high dose rate brachytherapy is used, 1.5 to 1.8 Gy may be given over 10 minutes to these structures in the context of administering 6.0 Gy to points A. This could result in significant differences in biologic impact both in cancer and normal tissues. At the Radiation Oncology Centers of Northern California, involved lateral parametria (FIGO stage IIIB) are carried to 66 to 68 Gy summing dose contributions from external beam and LDR intracavitary therapy. Comparable patients treated with high dose rate brachytherapy will have cumulative dose of 63 to 65 Gy.

Interstitial brachytherapy may be used to treat patients with gross parametrial involvement and bulky lateral disease not well encompassed by dose distribution achieved by intracavitary technique. Free-hand insertions of active $^{226}$Ra needles have been supplanted by afterloading techniques using $^{192}$Ir. Insertions are generally accomplished under regional or general anesthesia employing hollow guide needles, which are inserted into the parametria through a perineal template. Often this is accomplished with guidance from laparoscopy or open laparotomy to assure placement of the guide needles in the parametria while avoiding perforation of the bladder, rectosigmoid, and small intestine. When carried out by experienced practitioners, this technique should permit delivery of differentially higher dose to tumor than could historically be accomplished via teletherapy. For a multiplicity of possible reasons, this approach has not gained widespread acceptance, and less than 5% of patients with advanced cervical cancer treated with brachytherapy will receive interstitial brachytherapy. The vast majority will be treated with intracavitary technique.[57] Despite encouraging preliminary reports, late results with this approach have been disappointing and late sequelae substantial.[141] Comparison of outcomes of patients with bulky stage II, III, and IVA cancers treated with interstitial versus intracavitary technique suggested improved local control and disease-free survival in stage II disease with intracavitary technique, and no difference in stage III or IVA disease.[142] Complication rates were comparable.

When radiotherapy is used alone, 5-year relapse-free survival for patients with stage IIB cancer should be 65% to 75%. Patients with IIIB disease will have a 5-year cure rate approaching 40% to 50%. Patients with IVA disease can be salvaged in approximately 20% of cases.[46,142–145]

## Extended Volume Radiation: Pelvic and Para-Aortic Radiation for Cervical Cancer on Intact Uterus

Based on operative assessment of para-aortic nodes, approximately 30% of patients with FIGO IIB/III carcinoma of the cervix will have metastases outside the volume traditionally included in pelvic radiotherapy ports.[60] Some of these patients will be cured with extended volume radiation. Elective irradiation of the para-aortic nodes has been investigated in an effort to determine whether routine inclusion of this volume will improve survival by decreasing the rate of distant failure, including relapse in the upper retroperitoneum. Two randomized prospective phase III trials have examined this issue.[136,137] The RTOG randomized

367 patients with bulky IB/IIA tumors greater than 4 cm in diameter and stage IIB patients to receive pelvic radiation or extended volume radiation with identical brachytherapy in both treatment arms.[136] Although there was no significant difference in disease-free survival, overall survival was statistically significantly better at 5 years (67% vs. 55%) and at 10 years (55% vs. 44%) in the group that was treated to an extended volume. Although the local failure rate at 10 years was not significantly different in the two arms (35% pelvic, 31% extended volume), a significantly higher percentage of patients with local failures after initial complete response were salvaged on the extended volume arm (28% vs. 8%). There was also a trend for reduction in first distant failures in the extended volume group. Major complications were 11% in the extended volume group of patients and only 2% in the pelvic group, including 6% fatal complications in the extended volume group. It is difficult to justify routine use of extended fields in this group of patients if careful assessment of retroperitoneal nodes, either by contemporary diagnostic imaging (CT, MRI, lymphography) or retroperitoneal surgical sampling, fails to reveal evidence of at least pelvic node metastasis.

The EORTC randomized 441 patients with stages IB and IIB with evidence of pelvic node metastasis defined by surgery or lymphography, or extensive stage IIB or stage III disease independent of pelvic node status.[137] Four-year relapse-free survival was not statistically different in the two groups (49.8% pelvic vs. 53.3% extended volume). More para-aortic recurrences were seen in the pelvic radiotherapy arm, and the rate of distant metastases was higher in this group of patients achieving local control. Bowel complications were again higher in the group treated to an extended volume.

Patients most likely to benefit from extended volume radiation would seem to be the subset of patients who have evidence of pelvic or para-aortic metastasis without evidence of hematogenous dissemination, and pelvic disease that can be locally controlled by radiation alone or in combination with other modalities. Identification of this subset of patients may not be straightforward.

## Pelvic Failure and Efforts to Improve Results

Approximately 65% of patients who fail primary treatment by radiation will have a component of pelvic persistence or recurrence.[146] The majority of patients who fail radiation-based therapy will die of their disease, often of the consequences of uncontrolled pelvic cancer. Local persistence of cancer in patients with bulky disease has been attributed to the presence of tissue hypoxia with resulting radioresistant cells that remain clonogenic and repopulate after eradication of more sensitive cell populations. Clinical investigations attempting to deal with this theoretic basis for local failure have included the use of hyperbaric oxygen, neutron teletherapy and brachytherapy, and the hypoxic cell sensitizer misonidazole.

Results from prospective evaluation of adjuvant hyperbaric oxygen in the setting of locally advanced disease have shown no advantage over conventionally fractionated photon radiation.[147,148] Higher complication rates can be anticipated when higher than conventional dose per fraction radiation is used to minimize the inconvenience and hazards of multiple hyperbaric dives. A nonrandomized comparison of patients treated with mixed beam photon/neutron versus photon teletherapy for stage IIIB cervical cancer in Chiba, Japan, revealed identical 49% 5-year survival rates.[149] A prospective randomized RTOG evaluation of mixed beam photon/neutron teletherapy versus photon teletherapy in patients with stages IIB-IVA cervical cancer has shown a statistically nonsignificant trend to worse survival and higher complications for patients receiving a portion of their treatment with neutrons.[150] Intracavitary brachytherapy with neutron emitting $^{252}$Cf has been compared to historical results with brachytherapy using $^{137}$Cs and has shown no survival advantage for patients with stage IIIB cervical cancer.[151] The pharmacologic attack

on hypoxia has involved the prospective evaluation of 746 patients with locally advanced cervical cancer in three studies comparing radiation alone with radiation plus misonidazole,[152,153] and radiation with hydroxyurea versus radiation plus misonidazole.[154] There has been no suggestion of benefit either in pelvic control or survival. The cumulative effect of these clinical trials has been a waning clinical research interest in the issue of hypoxia, and a growing conviction by some that hypoxia is not a clinically significant cause of local failure for patients treated by fractionated radiation.

The most compelling evidence for the clinical significance of hypoxia is provided by retrospective observations and limited prospective data that link hemoglobin levels during radiotherapy with cancer control outcome and suggest a survival benefit consequent to red cell transfusion.[155,156]

The broadest effort to improve outcomes has been directed at the use of chemotherapy administered in a coordinated fashion with radiation either as neoadjuvant therapy prior to radiation, or concurrently with radiation.

The rationale for sequential neoadjuvant chemotherapy followed by radiation includes the potential to cytoreduce pelvic cancer, thus improving anatomy for brachytherapy and decreasing the number of clonogens requiring sterilization by radiation. Neoadjuvant chemotherapy is less likely to complicate or delay completion of radiation once it has started, and neoadjuvant chemotherapy theoretically will address the problem of occult micrometastases without delay and without dilution of the chemotherapy attack. Most regimens have been cisplatin based, since this agent appears to be the most active as a single drug in the setting of disseminated disease. Despite a substantial number of phase II studies reporting favorable experience, the prospective randomized phase III testing has proven uniformly disappointing,[157-161] and in several clinical trials patients undergoing neoadjuvant chemotherapy have done less well than patients treated by radiation alone. A small percentage of patients have died from chemotherapy toxicity, and a small number developed progressive disease while receiving chemotherapy. There has been no compensatory improvement in pelvic control, and this line of investigation has been largely abandoned. Potential explanations for the observed failure of this strategy to impact on local–regional control include the possible emergence of tumor clonogens with cross-resistance to cisplatin and radiation, as well as possible accelerated repopulation.

Despite the failure of this strategy prior to radiation, a similar approach has been utilized in the treament of patients with potentially operable cervical cancers. Neoadjuvant chemotherapy prior to surgery, with or without postoperative pelvic radiotherapy, has been the subject of numerous phase I/II investigations.[162] A randomized prospective trial in Argentina[163] studied neoadjuvant chemotherapy with *cis*-platinum, vincristine, and bleomycin given for three cycles (each of 3 days duration) at 10-day intervals prior to surgery. Two hundred and five patients were randomly allocated to immediate surgery versus neoadjuvant chemotherapy followed by surgery. Unresectable patients were treated by radiotherapy. All patients received 50 Gy adjuvant pelvic radiotherapy following hysterectomy. No apparent advantage to neoadjuvant chemotherapy was seen for patients with cancers 2 to 4 cm in diameter, but for patients with tumors 4 cm or larger there was a survival and disease-free survival advantage to neoadjuvant chemotherapy (80% survival with neoadjuvant chemotherapy vs. 61% in the control group). Pathological downstaging occurred in the group receiving neoadjuvant chemotherapy, with statistically significant reductions in the rate of vascular space invasion, parametrial extension, and lymph node metastasis compared with the patients undergoing immediate hysterectomy.[163] A similar regimen, without bleomycin, has undergone favorable phase I testing[164] in the GOG, and this combination is now undergoing prospective phase III evaluation (GOG Protocol 141: Treatment of Patients with Suboptimal "Bulky" Stage IB Carcinoma of the Cervix: A Randomized Comparison of Radical Hysterec-

tomy and Pelvic and Para-aortic Lymphadenectomy with or Without Neoadjuvant Vincristine and Cisplatin Chemotherapy).

Treatment of patients with advanced disease with concurrent cytotoxic chemotherapy and radiation continues to be an actively pursued avenue of clinical investigation attempting to improve results over those obtained from radiation alone. This approach avoids delay in initiation of radiation as well as theoretical concerns about selection of cross-resistant clonogens refractory to both chemotherapy and radiation. Based on preclinical and radiobiological data,[165–169] hydroxyurea was believed to be directly toxic to S-phase cells,[165] while acting to arrest cells in the more radiation-sensitive $G_1$–S portion of the cell cycle[167] and inhibiting DNA repair.[168] In vitro synergism was demonstrated with radiation,[166] and no increased effects were seen in normal tissues when radiation and hydroxyurea were given together.[169] The foregoing observations led to a series of controversial clinical trials[170–173] that suggest modest benefit from the use of hydroxyurea with radiation in advanced cervical cancer. Apparent improved outcomes with hydroxyurea have been attributed to suboptimal radiation and outcomes in the radiation control arms. Studies have been plagued by eligibility problems and patients lost to follow-up. However long-term results[173] suggest a marginal advantage conferred by hydroxyurea in progression-free interval and a nonstatistically significant trend to improved survival in comparison to radiation with misonidazole (in effect, compared with radiation alone).

The GOG and SWOG conducted a phase III trial randomizing 368 eligible patients to radiation with oral hydroxyurea versus radiation potentiated with cisplatin and 5-FU (GOG Protocol 85) for FIGO stages IIB, III, and IVA cervical cancer.[174] This study reported a survival benefit and progression-free survival benefit conferred by the use of cisplatin and 5-FU compared to hydroxyurea.

A recently reported GOG trial comparing radiation with hydroxyurea to radiation plus weekly cisplatin or radiation plus cisplatin,

hydroxyurea, and 5-FU for patients with locally advanced cervical cancer reveals longer
progression-free intervals in both groups of patients treated with cisplatin-containing regimens compared to the patients treated with
hydroxyurea alone.[175]

Weekly cisplatin administered in conjunction with preoperative external and intracavitary radiation for patients with IB2 cancer of
the cervix has been reported to improve survival and reduce relapses in a trial conducted
by the GOG. Hysterectomy specimens revealed
residual cancer in 57% of patients treated with
radiation, and in only 47% of patients treated
with radiation and weekly cisplatin.[176]

Support for the use of 5-FU concurrently
with radiation in the treatment of cervical cancer is partly derived from a prospective trial
conducted in Toronto, Canada, which revealed
a trend for better survival for patients randomized to receive 5-FU during the first 4 and last
4 days of teletherapy compared to those treated
with radiation alone.[177]

The RTOG recently completed a trial
(RTOG 90-01) in which patients with FIGO
stages IIB-IVA or bulky IB were randomized
to extended volume (pelvic and para-aortic)
radiation alone versus pelvic radiation with
concurrent 5-FU and cisplatin. That study reported 75% 3-year survival for patients get-
ting chemoradiation compared to 63% for
patients treated by extended volume radiation
alone.[59]

Based on the accumulating evidence that
synchronous administration of chemotherapy
with radiation improves survival for patients
with locally advanced cervical cancer, the National Cancer Institute issued a clinical announcement in February 1999 releasing
summary results of several studies prior to
their publication.[58,59,174–176] The radiation-only
control arm of an ongoing GOG study (GOG
Protocol 165) was closed for patient accrual
shortly thereafter, reflecting the growing national consensus that radiation with synchronous chemotherapy should be the standard of
care for patients with locally advanced cervical
cancer.

## Time to Complete Therapy

Prolonged courses of therapy are the rule in the
treatment of locally advanced cervical cancer.
The necessity to integrate brachytherapy insertions, and treatment interruptions, either elective or due to toxicity, may prolong the elapsed
time to complete treatment to 10 weeks or
longer. Numerous retrospective studies have
examined the issue of time to complete treatment and its impact on tumor control.[178–184]
Without exception, these studies have revealed
deleterious effects of prolongation of treatment
that cannot be simply explained on the basis of
tumor stage or volume. Shorter overall treatment schemes do not appear to increase the
likelihood of symptomatic late sequelae in normal tissues. The simplest expedient to assure
the best possible outcomes with conventionally
fractionated therapy is to deliver treatment in
an uninterrupted fashion. At the Radiation Oncology Centers of Northern California, treatment for stage IIB-IVA disease is designed to
be completed in 8 weeks, including reduced
volume boost fields, brachytherapy, and synchronous chemotherapy.

## Salvage Therapy

Some patients who fail in the pelvis after radical hysterectomy or after radical radiation
will be amenable to salvage with local therapies. In general, a crossover treatment strategy
should be followed.[185] The best chance for
surgical cure is with the initial hysterectomy.
Recurrences should be treated with radiation.
Similarly, prior treatment with radiation,
either as primary or adjuvant therapy, will
usually preclude radical retreatment with
radiation. Patients should have a diligent
search for distant metastases, and if local recurrence is solitary, aggressive salvage therapies should be pursued.

Radiation salvage may include brachytherapy or intraoperative radiotherapy,[186–188] depending on the size and location of the
recurrence. Approximately 30% of patients
will be long-term disease-free survivors after

aggressive salvage radiotherapy.[189–192] Results might be improved by the synchronous administration of cytotoxic chemotherapy.[193]

Patients failing primary radiation may be amenable to surgical salvage by partial or total exenteration. Central recurrence is more readily salvaged, but disease on the pelvic sidewall may be resected in conjunction with brachytherapy or intraoperative radiation. In the modern era, low colorectal or coloanal anastamosis may preserve fecal continence in some patients. New surgical techniques allow creation of continent urinary pouches. Construction of a neovagina may be feasible in some patients with use of myocutaneous flaps. Five-year survival can be expected in approximately one-third of patients treatable by exenteration,[194] with approximately one quarter salvageable despite limited lymph node metastasis.[195]

## SPECIAL CIRCUMSTANCES

### Bleeding, Anemia, and the Need for Urgent Radiation

In an effort to secure hemostasis, the occasional patient presenting with massive hemorrhage may propel the radiation oncologist to initiate radiotherapy in a precipitous fashion to an arbitrarily selected volume. The error of selecting an improper target volume can be further compounded by the use of high dose per fraction teletherapy, potentially compromising the eventual completion of a course of carefully fractionated treatment. Once absorbed, radiation cannot be extracted. When the bleeding slows, it is natural to credit this change to radiation. However, most cervical tumors bleed in a sporadic and unpredictable fashion, with the most reliable stimulants being pelvic examinations and biopsies. It is the exceptional patient with untreated cervical cancer in whom bleeding cannot be slowed to a non-life-threatening pace through the judicious use of simple interventions such as superficial cauterization, vaginal packing with Monsel's solution, and bed rest. Topical application of acetone will usually cause prompt cessation of bleeding from the exocervix. If the cervix can be adequately visualized for placement of a transvaginal cone or brachytherapy appliance, emergency radiotherapy is probably not required, since bleeding is not so severe that the patient could not be supported by transfusion until such time as appropriate radiotherapy can be planned. Under the rare circumstance that bleeding remains refractory to all other maneuvers, urgent teletherapy may be initiated through parallel opposed anterior and posterior pelvic fields with little likelihood that gross tumor will be transected by the beam edge. The risk of late normal tissue sequelae occasioned by the use of high dose per hemostatic fraction can be obviated by the simple expedient of treating with two or three fractions per day. In this manner, up to 10.8 Gy can be administered within 36 hours of starting therapy using three daily fractions of 1.8 Gy separated by 6 or more hours.

### Cancer of the Cervical Stump

Cancer of the cervical stump following remote supracervical hysterectomy has become less frequent as that operation has declined in popularity, having been supplanted by more sophisticated techniques of vaginal repair and bladder suspension. Cancer of the cervical stump can be treated surgically by radical trachelectomy and lymphadenectomy when disease is clinically confined to the cervix and proximal vagina, but this may be technically more difficult than radical hysterectomy. Currently, most women with this clinical condition will be elderly, and the potential advantages of surgical therapy in younger patients are largely irrelevant. With more extensive disease, radiation is frequently curative but will require modifications in technique because of lesser ability to achieve satisfactory lateral dose distribution to residual parametria and suspensory ligaments because of the short length of the tandem. A decrease in brachytherapy dose with a corresponding increase in teletherapy dose to limited parametrial volumes will sometimes provide a solution to this technical problem.

Treatment by external beam alone, targeting progressively shrinking volumes with concurrent chemotherapy, will sometimes be effective when brachytherapy is not feasible. Trachelectomy following preoperative radiation may be a solution for patients with bulky central disease and poor brachytherapy anatomy. Following supracervical hysterectomy, small and large bowel may fall into the pelvis in the space formerly occupied by the uterine body, and may become adherent to the residual cervix. Bowel complications, not surprisingly, are somewhat more common in such patients attributable to unfavorable brachytherapy geometry in comparison to patients with intact uterus.[196] Stage by stage, the prognosis for these uncommon patients is approximately equivalent to patients treated for cervical cancer on intact uterus.[197,198]

## Gross Metastatic Adenopathy at the Time of Hysterectomy

Controversy surrounds the issue of whether hysterectomy and therapeutic lymphadenectomy should be completed in patients explored for radical hysterectomy who are found, intraoperatively, to have clinically apparent metastases to pelvic nodes. One option is completion of the planned surgery (usually by modified radical hysterectomy) followed by adjuvant radiotherapy; another is to abort the planned procedure and complete treatment by radiation with the cervix in situ. On occasion, the radiation oncologist will be asked to participate in this decision while the patient is in the operating theater. In a matched-pair analysis, Potter and colleagues[199] could discern no advantage to completion of the hysterectomy, noting a trend for improved local control in the patients treated by radiotherapy. However, removal of grossly contaminated nodes was accomplished in these patients prior to termination of the operative procedure. Kinney and colleagues[200] have argued persuasively that surgical results are equivalent or better than radiotherapy results leaving gross adenopathy on the pelvic sidewall; these investigators could discern no survival advantage to administering adjuvant

radiotherapy. Adjuvant radiation in that report was more commonly given to patients with more ominous histopathologic findings.

There is no resolution to this debate, and the policy adopted reflects the biases of the treating physicians. In Sacramento, California, such patients will usually have modified radical hysterectomy completed, followed by routine postoperative radiation with concurrent 5-FU and cisplatin. Cure probability approaches 75%.

## Cervical Cancer During Pregnancy

Approximately 1% to 1.5% of patients with invasive cervical cancer are pregnant when the diagnosis is established. Management will be contingent, in part, on the clinical stage of disease at diagnosis, gestational age, and whether continuation of the pregnancy is desired. Evaluation of disease extent may need to be reduced in intensity to avoid potentially injurious radiation exposure to the fetus. In the modern era, the former practice of employing transvaginal radiation to diminish bleeding from cervical cancer late in pregnancy has been abandoned, to avoid fetal exposure that may be leukemogenic. In many instances, treatment may be delayed[201] until fetal maturity (assessed biochemically and by ultrasound), with only rare instances[202] of tumor progression under observation. A cervix extensively replaced by cancer will not dilate appropriately, and delivery will generally be accomplished by cesarian section rather than vaginally to avoid the possibility of obstructed labor and the rare complication of wound implantation in an episiotomy site.[203] Delivery by hysterotomy will avoid these concerns and can be accompanied by radical hysterectomy with ovarian conservation for patients with limited disease, or with surgical definition of disease extent for patients subsequently to be treated by radiation.

Adjusted for stage at diagnosis, the prognosis for pregnant patients does not appear to differ from the prognosis for nongravid patients.[203–206] Most pregnant patients in the United States will be diagnosed with cancer in stages IA and IB[207] and will be potentially treatable surgically. The estimated cure rate for patients with stage I disease managed surgically exceeds 90%.[208] For patients with more advanced stages of disease at diagnosis, irradiation in the context of first-trimester pregnancy will inevitably result in fetal death and abortion with spontaneous expulsion of the products of conception, although this may prove emotionally trying for both the patient and the oncologist. Pretreatment surgical evacuation is preferred by some. Cervical cancer detected during the third trimester may indicate a desired pregnancy, and treatment can be delayed, with observation and monitoring of potential tumor progression by means of ultrasound or MRI, pending fetal maturation.

Accurate quantitation of the hazards of delay in cancer treatment is difficult. Such information as exists suggests that delay of treatment does not incur major incremental risk and is appropriate in the context of a desired pregnancy or when the patient's ethical or religious principles preclude termination of pregnancy. Management of the pregnant cervical cancer patient may require exceptional patience and sensitivity, and individualization of care is appropriately the rule.

## AFTERTREATMENT

Following completion of a course of radiation therapy, the radiation oncologist should play a role in the recognition and management of normal tissue sequelae, as well as cancer surveillance.[209] At the Radiation Oncology Centers of Northern California, follow-up is recommended every 3 months for the first 2 years, every 4 months for the third year, every 6 months for the fourth and fifth years, and annually thereafter. Follow-up consists of obtaining an interval history, assessment of bowel, bladder, and sexual function, a general physical examination including patient weight, and a pelvic examination. Scans are not obtained in asymptomatic patients, and Pap smears are not obtained for the first 2 years, since detection and misinterpretation of radiation-induced

atypia will be more likely to cause confusion than to promote early detection of recurrent disease.

Bowel obstruction will generally, but not invariably, require operative intervention. The risk of small-bowel obstruction will be highest for patients undergoing pretreatment laparotomy (actuarial risk 14.5% at 10 years) as opposed to nonoperative assessment of tumor extent (actuarial risk 3.7% at 10 years).[210] The risk of small-bowel injury will be greater in patients undergoing extended volume radiation[136,137] than for patients treated to a pelvic volume alone, but the increased risk should be minimized by good technique.[52] The rare patient with a rectovaginal or vesicovaginal fistula consequent to radiation treatment will require surgical intervention. Not all such patients will require permanent urinary or bowel diversion if managed by surgeons experienced in operating on heavily irradiated tissue. However, most symptomatic late radiation sequelae will not require operative intervention, and the radiation oncologist should take an active role in recognition of late effects of treatment and their symptomatic management.

Most rectal complications of radiation are seen in the first 2 years of follow-up. Chronic radiation proctitis or sigmoiditis will be the source of sporadic bleeding in some patients. Focal laser ablation of bleeding rectal vessels may control this symptom, but should be employed only to treat limited volumes refractory to topical steroid enema therapy. Symptoms of urgency and pain with defecation require pharmacologic and dietary management.

Urinary tract complications may continue to become manifest many years after treatment.[210] Chronic radiation cystitis[211] will mimic recurrent urinary tract infections, with urgency and bladder spasms, accompanied by microscopic or gross hematuria. Misdiagnosis may result in the needless and ineffective prescription of antibiotics. The diagnosis should be verified by cystoscopy. The urothelium contains a class of polysaccharides called glyosaminoglycans, which protect the bladder wall from toxic substances excreted in the urine leaking past the transitional epithelium. When mucosal injury permits leakage, inflammation and hemorrhage may result. Pentosan polysulfate sodium (Elmiron), a macromolecular carbohydrate that chemically resembles naturally occurring glyosaminoglycans, is used to replenish depleted epithelial polysaccharides and is effective in the treatment of chronic interstitial cystitis in an oral dose of 100 mg three times a day. Anecdotal experience has been favorable in the treatment of chronic cystitis associated with radiation injury.[211,212]

Pentoxyifylline (Trental), a drug used to treat arterial insufficiency (peripheral vascular disease), decreases blood viscosity by altering the deformability characteristics of the erythrocyte membrane with consequent improvement in tissue oxygenation. It has been used in the treatment of radiation-induced soft tissue injury, including fibrosis and necrosis, but its value is not established. Hyperbaric oxygen may also promote healing of soft tissue necroses, but such treatment is logistically complex and should be reserved for failure of simpler therapies.

Microfractures in the pelvic girdle are complications of pelvic radiation that are difficult to diagnose and may cause pain and findings on isotope bone scans that mimic cancer recurrence. Many fractures are asymptomatic, and the incidence of this complication is proportional to the diligence of the search to discern them.[213] The best imaging modalities are bone window CT or MRI. Commonly such fractures are multiple, and they may occur in a symmetrical distribution. The finding on a bone scan of one or more areas of increased isotope uptake on a bone scan that are confined to the irradiated volume should be the clue that the abnormalities represent insufficiency fractures rather than cancer. Irradiation of an extended volume may cause insufficiency fractures in the lumbar spine, sometimes of sufficient severity to produce vertebral collapse.[118]

Radiation damage to the vagina should be expected following pelvic radiotherapy, with the most severe injury observed in women undergoing endovaginal brachytherapy. Radiation vaginitis will cause gross abnormalities that can vary from a pale, atrophic vaginal mucosa to severe inflammation with tissue necrosis.[214] Pressure injury associated with aggressive packing with low dose rate conventional brachytherapy will further predispose patients to the formation of vaginal adhesions and the obliteration of the upper vagina. Functional sequelae of radiation vaginitis are better prevented than treated. Daily use of a vaginal dilator immediately following completion of treatment will prevent adhesions and obliteration of the vaginal canal. Regular use of the dilator will minimize narrowing and shortening of the vaginal canal in women who are not regularly sexually active, and should be encouraged among patients who are only sporadically sexually active. Following radiation, the normal stratified squamous epithelium of the vagina will not fully regenerate, and months may elapse before a basal layer of cells is reconstituted in areas in proximity to brachytherapy sources. Systemic administration of estrogen will not reliably promote reepithelialization or maturation of stratified squamous epithelium, and direct vaginal administration of estrogen has proven the most effective method to promote healing. Continued topical estrogen stimulation will be required in many women following radiation, to prevent relapse of mucosal atrophy.[215,216] Therapy is initiated at 1 g vaginally daily for 3 to 6 weeks, and then may often be reduced to two or three treatments weekly as maintenance. Systemic absorption may be sufficient to produce effects such as breast tenderness in postmenopausal women.

Systemic hormone replacement therapy should be considered in all premenopausal women who have not had surgical displacement of at least one ovary from the irradiated volume. Oophoropexy will not always result in viable endocrine function and is associated with an accelerated rate of premature ovarian failure when ovaries are transposed out of the pelvis.[217–220] Scatter dose to ovaries transposed outside the direct radiation beam may be sufficient to accelerate ovarian failure in 29% to 83% depending on volume treated, technique, and energy.[218,221,222] Development of cysts, torsion, or tumor recurrence in ovaries transposed to the paracolic gutters may be the source of otherwise unexplained flank pain.[222]

In women treated for cervical cancer on intact uterus, hormonally sensitive endometrium may persist in portions of the uterine fundus despite brachytherapy.[223,224] Unopposed estrogen administration may cause intrauterine bleeding. Obliteration of the cervical canal by radiation will result in hematometra with cramping pelvic pain and symptoms of uterine enlargement that may require hysterectomy to relieve. This complication can be avoided by initiating hormone replacement with progesterone for at least 3 weeks prior to commencement of combined estrogen/progesterone replacement therapy. Estrogen alone may be used in patients who have undergone hysterectomy, but combined hormone replacement therapy should be used in individuals with a history of endometriosis.

Sexual dysfunction following radiotherapy for gynecologic malignancies is common and may be the result of complex psychosocial and physical factors.[225] Decrease in vaginal depth and diameter as well as loss of spontaneous lubrication will result in dyspareunia in many patients. The anticipation of physical pain with intercourse will lead to a learned, but involuntary response of contraction of the muscles of the pelvic floor, further aggravating discomfort with penetration. Alterations in sexual positioning may reduce or eliminate discomfort associated with vaginal intercourse. Female astride position will serve to limit the depth of vaginal penetration and allow the patient greater control over the vigor of the sexual encounter. Intercourse with thighs adducted following penetration will serve to simulate greater vaginal depth, allowing the male partner to experience the sensation of full penetration necessary for male gratification while avoiding the female discomfort associated with full penetration in the context of a shortened vaginal vault.

The diagnosis of cancer and anxieties concerning the future may precipitate depression and a loss of libido. After treatment, each surveillance follow-up examination will entail pelvic examination that may be associated with significant anticipatory anxiety, as well as suspense concerning the outcome of diagnostic tests.

Loss of procreative capacity may have unpredictable consequences for sexual function. While freedom from contraceptive concerns may be liberating for some, enhancing the spontaneity of sexual encounters, others may experience a debilitating loss of self-worth. In some cultures, the perceived worth of a woman is inextricably linked to her procreative capacity. General cultural background as well as religious convictions will be important in this regard. Loss of sexual self-confidence may be precipitated by temporary physical change consequent to treatment (weight loss, epilation in patients treated with cytotoxic chemotherapy). Endocrine ablation and menopausal symptoms (vasomotor instability) may convince some women that they have lost their sexual attractiveness. Some patients are aware that cervical cancer is related to a virus that is usually transmitted through sexual contact. Concerns regarding transmission of disease to sexual partners will diminish sexual enjoyment in some patients. Concern of sexual partners regarding infliction of pain or damage, as well concerns regarding cancer transmission, may restrict the opportunities for sexual enjoyment. Frank conversations including the patient and her sexual partner (together or separately), both before and after treatment, will provide the best opportunity for helping a patient to remain enjoyably sexually active.

## REFERENCES

1. Parkin DM, Pisani P, Ferlay J: Estimates of the worldwide incidence of eighteen major cancers in 1985. *Int J Cancer* 1993;54:594–606.

2. American Cancer Society: *Cancer Facts and Figures—1999*. Atlanta, ACS.

3. Papanicolaou, G: *Atlas of Exfoliative Cytology*. Boston, Massachusetts Commonwealth Fund; University Press, 1954.

4. Guzick DS: Efficacy of screening for cervical cancer: A review. *Am J Public Health* 1978; 68:125–134.

5. Reis LAG, Miller BA, Hanker BF, Kosary CL, Harras A, Edwards BK (eds): *SEER Cancer Statistics Review, 1973–1991: Tables and Graphs,* NIH Pub 94-2789. Bethesda, MD: National Cancer Institute, 1994.

6. Kashigarian M, Dunn JE: The duration of intraepithelial and preclinical squamous cell carcinoma of the cervix. *Am J Epidemiol* 1970; 92:211–222.

7. Kolstad P, Klem V: Long term follow up of 1121 cases of carcinoma in situ. *Obstet Gynecol* 1976;48:125–129.

8. Kurman RJ, Solomon D: *The Bethesda System for Reporting Cervical/Vaginal Cytologic Diagnoses: Definitions, Criteria and Explanatory Notes for Terminology and Specimen Adequacy.* New York, Springer-Verlag, 1994.

9. Brinton LA: Epidemiology of cervical cancer—Overview. *IARC Sci Publ* 1992;119: 3–23.

10. Taylor RS, Carroll BE, Lloyd JW: Mortality among women in three Catholic religious orders with special references to cancer. *Cancer* 1959;12:1207–1225.

11. Reid R, Crum CP, Herschman BR, Fu YS, Braun L, Shah KV, Agronow SJ, Stanhope CR, et al: Genital warts and cervical cancer. III. Subclinical papillomaviral infection and cervical neoplasia are linked by a spectrum of continuous morphologic and biologic change. *Cancer* 1984;53:943–953.

12. Reeves WC, Brinton LA, Garcia M, Brenes MM, Herrero R, Gaitan E, Tenorio F, deBritton RC, Rawls WE: Human papillomavirus infection and cervical cancer in Latin America. *N Engl J Med* 1989;320:1437–1441.

13. McCance DJ, Kopan R, Fuchs E, Laimins LA: Human papillomavirus type 16 alters human epithelial cell differentiation in vitro. *Proc Natl Acad Sci USA* 1988;85:7169–7173.

14. Munoz N, Bosch FX, de Sanjose S, Tafur L, Izarzugaza I, Gili M, Viladiu P, Navarro C, Martos C, Ascunce N, Gonzalez LC, Kaldor JM, Guerreo E, Lorincz A, Santamari M, Alonso de Ruiz P, Aristizabal N, Shah K: The causal link between human papillomavirus and invasive cervical cancer. A population-based case control study in Colombia and Spain. *Int J Cancer* 1992;52: 743–749.

15. Bosch FX, Manos MM, Munoz N, Sherman M, Jansen AM, Peto J, Schiffman MH, Moreno V, Kurman R, Shah KV: International Biological Study on Cervical Cancer (IBSCC) Study Group. Prevalence of human papillomavirus in cervical cancer: A worldwide perspective. *J Natl Cancer Inst* 1995;87:796–802.

16. Schiffman MH, Brinton LA: The epidemiology of cervical carcinogenesis. *Cancer* 1995;76(10 suppl):1888–1901.

17. Fruchter RG, Maiman M, Sedlis A, Bartley L, Camilien L, Arrastia CD: Multiple recurrences of cervical intraepithelial neoplasia in women with the human immunodeficiency virus. *Obstet Gynecol* 1996;87:338–344.

18. Maiman M, Fruchter RG, Clark M, Arrastia CD, Matthews R, Gates EJ;Cervical cancer as an AIDS-defining illness. *Obstet Gynecol* 1997;89:76–80.

19. Steller MA, Schiller JT: Human papillomavirus immunology and vaccine prospects. *J Natl Cancer Inst Monogr* 1996;21:145–148.

20. Tindle RW: Immunomanipulative strategies for the control of human papillomavirus associated cervical disease. *Immunol Res* 1997;16: 387–400.

21. Wentz WB, Reagan JW: Survival in cervical cancer with respect to cell type. *Cancer* 1959; 12:384–388.

22. Kurman RJ, Norris HJ, Wilkinson EJ: Tumors of the cervix, vagina, and vulva, in *Atlas of Tumor Pathology,* 3rd series, fasc 4. Washington, DC: Armed Forces Institute of Pathology, 1992, pp 29–36.

23. Kraus FT, Perez-Mesa C: Verrucous carcinoma: Clinical and pathological study of 105 cases involving oral cavity, larynx and genitalia. *Cancer* 1966;19:26–38.

24. Lucas WE, Benirschke K, Lebherz TB: Verrucous carcinoma of the female genital tract. *Am J Obstet Gynecol* 1974;119:435–440.

25. Hasumi K, Sugano H, Sakamoto G, Masubuchi K, Kubo H: Circumscribed carcinoma of the uterine cervix with marked lymphocytic infiltration. *Cancer* 1977;39:2503–2507.

26. Eifel PJ, Burke TW, Morris M, Smith TL: Adenocarcinoma as an independent risk factor for disease recurrence in patients with stage

IB cervical carcinoma. *Gynecol Oncol* 1995; 59:38–44.

27. Eifel PJ, Morris M, Oswald MJ, Wharton JT, Delclos L: Adenocarcinoma of the uterine cervix. Prognosis and patterns of failure in 367 cases. *Cancer* 1990;65:2507–2514.

28. Shingleton HM, Bell MC, Fremgen A, Chmiel JS, Russell AH, Jones WB, Winchester DP, Clive RE: Is there really a difference in survival of women with squamous cell carcinoma, adenocarcinoma, and adenosquamous cell carcinoma of the cervix? *Cancer* 1995;76(10 suppl):1948–1955.

29. Samlal RA, van der Velden J, Schilthuis MS, Gonzalez Gonzalez D, Ten Kate FJ, Hart AA, Lammes FB: Identification of high risk groups among node-positive patients with stage IB and IIA cervical carcinoma. *Gynecol Oncol* 1997;64:463–467.

30. Grigsby PW, Perez CA, Kuske RR, Camel HM, Kao MS, Galakatos AE, Hederman MA: Adenocarcinoma of the uterine cervix: Lack of evidence for a poor prognosis. *Radiother Oncol* 1988;12:289–296.

31. Herbst AL, Robboy SJ, Scully RE, Poskanzer DC: Clear-cell adenocarcinoma of the vagina and cervix in girls: Analysis of 170 Registry cases. *Am J Obstet Gynecol* 1974;119: 713–724.

32. Mulvaney, NJ, Monostori, SJ: Adenoma malignum of the cervix: A reappraisal. *Pathology* 1997;29:17–20.

33. Gilks CB, Young RH, Aguirre P, DeLellis RA, Scully RE: Adenoma malignum (minimal deviation adenocarcinoma) of the uterine cervix. A clinicopathological and immunohistochemical analysis of 26 cases. *Am J Surg Pathol* 1989;13:717–729.

34. Glucksman A, Cherry C: Incidence, histology and response to radiation of mixed carcinoma (adenoacanthoma) of the uterine cervix. *Cancer* 1956;9:971–979.

35. Littman P, Clement PB, Henriksen B, Wang CC, Robboy SJ, Taft PD, Ulfelder H, Scully RE: Glassy cell carcinoma of the cervix. *Cancer* 1976;37:2238–2246.

36. Tamimi HK, Ek M, Hesla J, Cain JM, Figge DC, Greer BE: Glassy cell Carcinoma of the cervix redefined. *Obstet Gynecol* 1988;71: 837–841.

37. Lotocki RJ, Krepart GV, Paraskevas M, Vadas G, Heywood M, Fung Kee Fung M: Glassy cell carcinoma of the cervix: A bimodal treatment strategy. *Gynecol Oncol* 1992;44:254–259.

38. Gersell DJ, Mazoujian G, Mutch DG, Rudloff MA: Small-cell undifferentiated carcinoma of the cervix: A clinicopathologic, ultrastructural, and immunocytochemical study of 15 cases. *Am J Surg Pathol* 1988;12:684–698.

39. Walker AN, Mills SE, Taylor PT: Cervical neuroendocrine carcinoma: A clinical and light microscopic study of 14 cases. *Int J Gynaecol Pathol* 1988;71:64–74.

40. O'Hanlan, KA, Goldberg GL, Jones JG, Runowicz CD, Ehrlich L, Rodriguez-Rodriguez L: Adjuvant therapy for neuroendocrine small cell carcinoma of the cervix: Review of the literature. *Gynecol Oncol* 1991;43:167–172.

41. Greer BE, Koh W-J, Figge DC, Russell AH, Cain J, Tamimi HK: Gynecologic radiotherapy fields defined by intraoperative measurements. *Gynecol Oncol* 1990;38:421–424.

42. Kristensen GB, Kaern J, Abeler VM, Hagmar B, Trope CG, Petterson EO: No prognostic impact of flow-cytometric measured DNA ploidy and S-phase fraction in cancer of the uterine cervix: A prospective study of 465 patients. *Gynecol Oncol* 1995;57:79–85.

43. West CM, Davidson SE, Roberts SA, Hunter RD: The independence of intrinsic radiosensitivity as a prognostic factor for patient response to radiotherapy of carcinoma of the cervix. *Br J Cancer* 1997;76:1184–1190.

44. Piver MS, Chung WS: Prognostic significance of cervical lesion size and pelvic node metastases in cervical cancer. *Obstet Gynecol* 1975;45, 507–510.

45. Homesley HD, Raben M, Blake DD, Feree CR, Bullock MS, Linton EB Greiss FC, Rhyne AL: Relationship of lesion size to survival in patients with stage IB squamous cell carcinoma of the cervix uteri treated by radiation therapy. *Surg Gynecol Obstet* 1980;150: 529–531.

46. Perez CA, Grigsby PW, Nene SM, Camel HM, Galakatos A, Kao MS, Lockett MA: Effect of tumor size on the prognosis of carcinoma of the uterine cervix treated with irradiation alone. *Cancer* 1992;69:2796–2806.

47. Stehman FB, Bundy BN, DiSaia PJ, Keys HM, Larson JE, Fowler WC: Carcinoma of the cervix treated with irradiation therapy. I. A multi-variate analysis of prognostic variables in the Gynecologic Oncology Group. *Cancer* 1991;67:2776–2785.

48. Russell AH, Shingleton HM, Jones WB, Fremgen A, Winchester DP, Clive R, Chmiel JS: Diagnostic assessments in patients with invasive cancer of the cervix: A National Patterns of Care Study of the American College of Surgeons. *Gynecol Oncol* 1996;63: 159–165.

49. Montana GS, Hanlon AL, Brickner TJ, Owen JB, Hanks GE, Ling CC, Komaki R, Marcial VA, Thomas GM, Lanciano R: Carcinoma of the cervix: Patterns of Care studies: Review of 1978, 1983, and 1988–1989 surveys. *Int J Radiat Oncol Biol Phys* 1995;32:1481–1486.

50. Berman ML, Keys HM, Creasman WT, DiSaia PJ, Blessing J, Bundy B: Survival and patterns of recurrence in cervical cancer metastatic to periaortic lymph nodes. *Gynecol Oncol* 1984;19:8–16.

51. Potish RA: Radiation therapy of periaortic node metastases in cancer of the uterine cervix and endometrium. *Radiology* 1987;165:567–570.

52. Russell AH, Jones DC, Russell KJ,Gerdes AJ, Figge DC, Greer BE, Tamimi HK, Cain JM: High dose para-aortic lymph node irradiation for gynecologic cancer: Technique, toxicity, and results. *Int J Radiat Oncol Biol Phys* 1987;13:267–271.

53. Lovecchio JL, Averette HE, Donato D, Bell J: 5-year survival of patients with periaortic nodal metastases in clinical stage IB and IIA cervical carcinoma. *Gynecol Oncol* 1989;34: 43–45.

54. Podczaski E, Stryker JA, Kaminski P, Ndubisi B, Larson J, DeGeest K, Sorosky J, Mortel R: Extended-field radiation therapy for carcinoma of the cervix. *Cancer* 1990;66:251–258.

55. Nori D, Valentine E, Hilaris BS: The role of para-aortic node irradiation in the treatment of cancer of the cervix. *Int J Radiat Oncol Biol Phys* 1985;11:1469–1473.

56. Vigliotti AP, Wen BC, Hussey DH, Doornbos JF, Staples JJ, Jani SK, Turner DA, Anderson B: Extended field irradiation for carcinoma of the uterine cervix with positive periaortic nodes. *Int J Radiat Oncol Biol Phys* 1992;23: 501–509.

57. Russell AH, Shingleton HM, Jones WB, Fremgen A, Ocweija K, Winchester DP, Clive R, Chmiel JS: Trends in the use of radiation and chemotherapy in the initial management of patients with carcinoma of the uterine cervix: A study of the American College of Surgeons Commission on Cancer. *Int J Radiat Oncol Biol Phys* 1998;40:605–613.

58. National Cancer Institute: Clinical Announcement: Concurrent chemoradiation for cervical cancer. National Institutes of Health, Bethesda, MD, February 1, 1999.

59. Morris M, Eifel PJ, Lu J, Grigsby PW, Levenback C, Stevens RE, Rotman M, Gershenson DM, Mutch DG: Pelvic radiation with concurrent chemotherapy compared with pelvic and para-aortic radiation for high-risk cervical cancer. *N Engl J Med* 1999;340:1137–1143.

60. Lagasse LD, Creasman WT, Shingleton HM, Ford JH, Blessing JA: Results and complications of operative staging in cervical cancer: Experience of the Gynecologic Oncology Group. *Gynecol Oncol* 1980;9:90–98.

61. Burghardt E, Pickel H: Local spread and lymph node involvement in cervical cancer. *Obstet Gynecol* 1978;52:138–145.

62. Russell AH: Integration of diagnostic imaging in the management of cervical cancer. *J Nat Cancer Inst Monogr* 1996;21:35–41.

63. Inoue T, Chihara T, Morita K: The prognostic significance of the size of the largest nodes in metastatic carcinoma from the uterine cervix. *Gynecol Oncol* 1984;19:187–193.

64. Potish RA, Downey GO, Adcock LL, Prem KA, Twiggs LB: The role of surgical debulking in cancer of the uterine cervix. *Int J Radiat Oncol Biol Phys* 1989;17:979–984.

65. Hacker NF, Wain GV, Nicklin JL: Resection of bulky positive lymph nodes in patients with cervical carcinoma. *Int J Gynecol Cancer* 1995;5:250–256.

66. Russell AH, Walter JP, Anderson MW, Zukowski CL:. Sagittal magnetic resonance imaging in the design of lateral radiation treatment portals for patients with locally advanced squamous cancer of the cervix. *Int J Radiat Oncol Biol Phys* 1992;23:449–455.

67. Kim RY, McGinnis LS, Spencer SA, Meredith RF, Jenelle RL, Salter MM: Conventional four-field pelvic radiotherapy technique without computed tomography—Treatment planning in cancer of the cervix: Potential geographic miss and its impact on pelvic control. *Int J Radiat Oncol Biol Phys* 1995;31:109–112.

68. Chun M, Timmerman RD, Mayer R, Ling MN, Sheldon J, Fishman EK: Radiation therapy of external iliac lymph nodes with lateral pelvic portals: Identification of patients at risk for inadequate regional coverage. *Radiology* 1994;194:147–150.

69. Greer BE, Koh WJ, Stelzer KJ, Goff BA, Comsia N, Tran A: Expanded pelvic radiotherapy fields for treatment of local-regionally advanced carcinoma of the cervix: Outcome and complications. *Am J Obstet Gynecol* 1996;174:1141–1149.

70. Corscaden JA: *Gynecologic Cancer,* 2nd ed. Baltimore, Williams & Wilkins, 1956, pp 176–118.

71. Fletcher GH (ed): *Textbook of Radiotherapy.* Philadelphia, Lea & Febiger, 1964.

72. Jones WB, Shingleton HM, Russell AH, Chmiel JS, Fremgen A, Clive RE, Zuber-Ocwieja KE, Winchester DP: Patterns of care for invasive cervical cancer: Results of a national survey of 1984 and 1990. *Cancer* 1995;76:1934–1947.

73. Grigsby PW, Perez CA: Radiotherapy alone for medically inoperable carcinoma of the cervix: Stage IA and carcinoma in situ. *Int J Radiat Oncol Biol Phys* 1991;21:375–378.

74. Kolstad P, Klem V: Long-term followup of 1121 cases of carcinoma in situ. *Obstet Gynecol* 1976;48:125–129.

75. Kolstad P: Follow-up study of 232 patients with stage Ia1 and 411 patients with stage Ia2 squamous cell carcinoma of the cervix (microinvasive carcinoma). *Gynecol Oncol* 1989;33:265–272.

76. Hamberger AD, Fletcher GH, Wharton JT: Results of treatment of early stage I carcinoma of the uterine cervix with intracavitary radium alone. *Cancer* 1978;41:980–985.

77. Greer BE, Figge DC, Tamimi HK, Cain JM, Lee RB: Stage IA2 squamous carcinoma of the cervix: Difficult diagnosis and therapeutic dilemma. *Am J Obstet Gynecol* 1990;162:1406–1409.

78. Landoni F, Maneo A, Colombo A, Placa F, Milani R, Perego P, Favini G, Ferri L, Mangioni C: Randomised study of radical surgery versus radiotherapy for stage Ib-IIa cervical cancer. *Lancet* 1997;350:535–540.

79. Toki N, Tsukamoto N, Kaku T, Toh N, Saito T, Kamura T, Matsukuma K, Nakano H: Microscopic ovarian metastasis of the uterine cervical cancer. *Gynecol Oncol* 1991;41:46–51.

80. Brown JV, Fu YS, Berek JS: Ovarian metastases are rare in stage I adenocarcinoma of the cervix. *Obstet Gynecol* 1990;76:623–626.

81. Kjorstad KE, Kolbenstvedt A, Stricker T: The value of complete lymphadenectomy in radical treatment of cancer of the cervix, stage IB. *Cancer* 1984;54:2215–2219.

82. Parente JT, Silberblatt W, Stone M: Infrequency of metastasis to ovaries in stage I carcinoma of the cervix. *Am J Obstet Gynecol* 1964;90:1362.

83. Sutton GP, Bundy BN, Delgado G, Sevin BU, Creasman WT, Major FJ, Zaino R: Ovarian metastases in stage Ib carcinoma of the cervix: A Gynecologic Oncology Group study. *Am J Obstet Gynecol* 1992;166:50–53.

84. Feeney DD, Moore DH, Look KY, Stehman FB, Sutton GP: The fate of the ovaries after radical hysterectomy and ovarian transposition. *Gynecol Oncol* 1995;56:3–7.

85. Wu HS, Yen MS, Lai CR, Ng HT: Ovarian metastasis from cervical carcinoma. *Int J Gynaecol Obstet* 1997;57:173–178.

86. Anderson B: Ovarian function after radical hysterectomy. *Gynecol Oncol* 1995;56:1–2.

87. Roman LD, Morris M, Eifel PJ, Burke TW, Gershenson DM, Wharton JT: Reasons for inappropriate simple hysterectomy in the presence of invasive cancer of the cervix. *Obstet Gynecol* 1992;79:485–489.

88. Heller PB, Barnhill DR, Mayer AR, Fontaine TP, Hoskins WJ, Park RC: Cervical carcinoma found incidentally in a uterus removed for benign disease. *Obstet Gynecol* 1986;67:187–190.

89. Hopkins MP, Peters WA, Anderson W, Morley GW: Invasive cervical cancer treated initially by standard hysterectomy. *Gynecol Oncol* 1990;36:7–12.

90. Andras EJ, Fletcher G, Rutledge F: Radiotherapy for carcinoma of the cervix following simple hysterectomy. *Am J Obstet Gynecol* 1973;115:647–655.

91. Davy M, Bentzen H, Jahren R: Simple hysterectomy in the presence of invasive cervical cancer. *Acta Obstet Gynecol Scand* 1977;56: 105–108.

92. Choi DH, Huh SJ, Nam KH: Radiation therapy results for patients undergoing inappropriate surgery in the presence of invasive cervical carcinoma. *Gynecol Oncol* 1997;65:506–511.

93. Orr JW Jr, Ball GC, Soong S-J, Shingleton HM: Surgical treatment of women found to have invasive cervical cancer at the time of total hysterectomy. *Obstet Gynecol* 1986;68: 353–356.

94. Kinney WK, Egorshin EV, Ballard DJ, Podratz KC: Long-term survival and sequelae after surgical management of invasive cervical carcinoma diagnosed at the time of simple hysterectomy. *Gynecol Oncol* 1992;44:24–27.

95. Chapman JA, Mannel RS, DiSaia PJ, Walker JL, Berman ML: Surgical treatment of unexpected invasive cervical cancer found at total hysterectomy. *Obstet Gynecol* 1992;80:931–934.

96. van Bommel PFJ, van Lindert ACM, Kock HCLV, Leers WH, Neijt JP: A review of prognostic factors in early-stage carcinoma of the cervix (FIGO IB and IIA) and implications for treatment strategy. *Eur J Obstet Gynecol Reprod Biol* 1987;26:69–84.

97. Zaino RJ, Ward S, Delgado G, Bundy B, Gore H, Fetter G, Ganjei P, Frauenhoffer E: Histopathologic predictors of the behavior of surgically treated stage IB squamous cell carcinoma of the cervix. A Gynecologic Oncology Group study. *Cancer* 1992;69:1750–1758.

98. Burghardt E, Pickel H, Haas J, Lahousen M: Prognostic factors and operative treatment of stages IB and IIB cervical cancer. *Am J Obstet Gynecol* 1987;156:988–996.

99. Piver MS, Chung WS: Prognostic significance of cervical lesion size and pelvic node metastases in cervical carcinoma. *Obstet Gynecol* 1975;46:507–510.

100. Fuller AF Jr, Elliott N, Kosloff C, Lewis JL Jr: Lymph node metastases from carcinoma of the cervix, stages IB and IIA: Implications for prognosis and treatment. *Gynecol Oncol* 1982; 13:165–174.

101. Delgado D, Bundy B, Zaino R, Sevin BU, Creasman WT, Major FJ: Prospective surgical-pathological study of disease-free interval in patients with stage IB squamous cell carcinoma of the cervix: A Gynecologic Oncology Group study. *Gynecol Oncol* 1990;38:352–357.

102. Morrow CP: Panel Report. Is pelvic radiation beneficial in the postoperative management of stage IB squamous cell carcinoma of the cervix with pelvic node metastasis treated by radical hysterectomy and pelvic lymphadenectomy? *Gynecol Oncol* 1980;10:105–110.

103. Kinney WK, Alvarez RD, Reid GC, Schray MF, Soong S, Morley GW, Podratz KC, Shingleton HM: Value of adjuvant whole-pelvis irradiation after Wertheim hysterectomy for early-stage squamous carcinoma of the cervix with pelvic nodal metastasis: A matched-control study. *Gynecol Oncol* 1989;34:258–262.

104. Soisson AP, Soper JT, Clarke-Pearson DL, Berchuk A, Montana G, Creasman WT: Adjuvant radiotherapy following radical hysterectomy for patients with stage IB and IIA cervical cancer. *Gynecol Oncol* 1990;37: 390–395.

105. Hogan MW, Littman P, Griner L Miller CL, Mikuta JJ: Results of radiation therapy given after radical hysterectomy. *Cancer* 1982;49: 1278–1285.

106. Larson DM, Stringer CA, Copeland LJ, Gershenson DM, Malone JM Jr, Rutledge FN: Stage IB cervical carcinoma treated with radical hysterectomy and pelvic lymphadenectomy: Role of adjuvant radiotherapy. *Obstet Gynecol* 1987;69:378–381.

107. Chung CK, Nahhas WA, Stryker JA, Curry SL, Abt AB, Mortel R: Analysis of factors contributing to treatment failures in stage IB and IIA carcinoma of the cervix. *Am J Obstet Gynecol* 1980;138:550–556.

108. Nahhas WA, Sharkey FE, Whitney CW, Husseinzadeh N, Chung CK, Mortel R: The prognostic significance of vascular channel involvement and deep stromal penetration in early cervical carcinoma. *Am J Clin Oncol* 1983;6:259–264.

109. Deutsch M, Parsons JA: Radiotherapy for carcinoma of the cervix recurrent after surgery. *Cancer* 1974;34:2051–2055.

110. Potter ME, Alvarez RD, Gay FL, Shingleton HM, Soong SJ, Hatch KD: Optimal therapy for pelvic recurrence after radical hysterectomy for early-stage cervical cancer. *Gynecol Oncol* 1990;37:74–77.

111. Larson DM, Copeland LJ, Stringer CA, Gershenson DM, Malone JM, Edwards CL: Recurrent cervical carcinoma after radical hysterectomy. *Gynecol Oncol* 1988;30:381–387.

112. Fuller AF, Elliott N, Kosloff C, Hoskins WJ, Lewis JL Jr: Determinations of increased risk for recurrence in patients undergoing radical hysterectomy for stage IB and IIA carcinoma of the cervix. *Gynecol Oncol* 1989;33:34–39.

113. Guttmann R: Significance of post-operative irradiation in carcinoma of the cervix: A ten year survey. *Am J Roentgenol* 1970;108:102–108.

114. Russell AH, Tong DY, Figge DC, Tamimi HK, Greer BE, Elder SJ: Adjuvant postoperative pelvic radiation for carcinoma of the uterine cervix: Pattern of cancer recurrence in patients undergoing elective radiation following radical hysterectomy and pelvic lymphadenectomy. *Int J Radiat Oncol Biol Phys* 1984;10:211–214.

115. Jobson VW, Girtanner RE, Averette HE: Therapy and survival of early invasive carcinoma of the cervix uteri with metastases to the pelvic nodes. *Surg Obstet Gynecol* 1980;151:27–29.

116. Takahashi M, Mitsuhashi N, Sakurai H, Hayakawa K, Niibe H: Para-aortic lymph node recurrence in patients with cervical cancer treated with postoperative irradiation to the pelvis. *Anticancer Res* 1997;17:2265–2268.

117. Inoue T, Morita K: Long-term observation of patients treated by postoperative extended-field irradiation for nodal metastases from cervical carcinoma stages IB, IIA, and IIB. *Gynecol Oncol* 1995;58:4–10.

118. Chatani M, Matayoshi Y, Masaki N, Narumi Y, Teshima T, Inoue T: Prophylactic irradiation of para-aortic lymph nodes in carcinoma of the uterine cervix. A prospective randomized study. *Strahlenther Onkol* 1995;171:655–660.

119. Peters WA III, Liu PY, Barrett R, Gordon W Jr, Stock R, Berek JF, DiSaia PJ, Souhami L, Grigsby P, Alberts DS: Cisplatin, 5-fluorouracil plus radiation therapy are superior to radiation therapy as adjunctive therapy in high-risk, early stage carcinoma of the cervix after radical hysterectomy and pelvic lymphadenectomy: Report of a phase III inter-group study. *Proceedings of the 30th Annual Meeting of the Society of Gynecologic Oncologists,* San Francisco, March 22, 1999 (abstr 1).

120. Curtin JP, Hoskins WJ, Venkatraman ES, Almadrones L, Podratz KC, Long H, Teneriello M, Averette HA, Sevin BU: Adjuvant chemotherapy versus chemotherapy plus pelvic irradiation for high-risk cervical cancer patients after radical hysterectomy and pelvic lymphadenectomy (RH-PLND): A randomized phase III trial. *Gynecol Oncol* 1996;61.

121. Thomas GM, Stehman FB: Early invasive disease: Risk assessment and management. *Semin Oncol* 1994;21:17–24.

122. Sedlis A, Bundy BN, Rotman MZ, Lentz SS, Muderspach LI, Zaino RJ: A randomized trial of pelvic radiation therapy versus no further therapy in selected patients with stage IB carcinoma of the cervix after radical hysterectomy and pelvic lymphadenectomy: A Gynecologic Oncology Group study. *Gynecol Oncol* 1999;73:177–183.

123. Wertheim MS, Hakes TB, Daghestani AN, Nori D, Smith DH, Lewis JL: A pilot study of adjuvant therapy in patients with cervical cancer at high risk of recurrence after radical hysterectomy and pelvic lymphadenectomy. *J Clin Oncol* 1985;3:912–916.

124. Killackey MA, Boardman L, Carroll DS: Adjuvant chemotherapy and radiation in patients with poor prognostic stage IB/IIA cervical cancer. *Gynecol Oncol* 1993;49:377–379.

125. Lai C, Lin T, Soong Y, Phil M, Chen H: Adjuvant chemotherapy after radical hysterectomy for cervical carcinoma. *Gynecol Oncol* 1989;35:193–198.

126. Tattershall MHN, Ramirez C, Coppleson M: A randomized trial of adjuvant chemotherapy after radical hysterectomy in stage IB-IIA cervical cancer patients with pelvic lymph node metastases. *Gynecol Oncol* 1992;46:176–181.

127. Perez CA, Grigsby PW, Nene SM, Camel HM, Galaktos A, Kao MS, et al: Effect of tumor size on the prognosis of carcinoma of the uterine cervix treated with irradiation alone. *Cancer* 1992;69:2796–2806.

128. Eifel PJ, Morris M, Wharton JT, Oswald MJ: The influence of tumor size and morphology on the outcome of patients with FIGO stage IB squamous cell carcinoma of the uterine cervix. *Int J Radiat Oncol Biol Phys* 1994;29:9–16.

129. Eifel PJ, Thoms WW Jr, Smith TL, Morris M, Oswald MJ: The relationship between brachytherapy dose and outcome in patients with bulky endocervical tumors treated with radiation alone. *Int J Radiat Oncol Biol Phys* 1994;28:113–118.

130. Mendenhall WM, McCarty PJ, Morgan LS, Chafe WE, Million RR: Stage IB or IIA-B carcinoma of the intact uterine cervix greater than or equal to 6 cm in diameter: Is adjuvant extrafascial hysterectomy beneficial? *Int J Radiat Oncol Biol Phys* 1991;21:899–904.

131. Thoms WW Jr, Eifel PJ, Smith TL, Morris M, Delclos L, Wharton JT, et al: Bulky endocervical carcinomas: A 23-year experience. *Int J Radiat Oncol Biol Phys* 1992;23:491–499.

132. Perez CA, Grigsby PW, Camel HM, Galaktos AE, Mutch D, Lockett MA: Irradiation alone or combined with surgery in stage IB, IIA, and IIB carcinoma of the uterine cervix: Update of a non-randomized comparison. *Int J Radiat Oncol Biol Phys* 1995;31:703–716.

133. Russell AH, Burt AR, Ek M, Russell KJ, Cain JM, Tamimi HK, Greer BE, Figge DC: Adjunctive hysterectomy following radiation for bulky carcinoma of the uterine cervix: Prognostic implications of tumor persistence. *Gynecol Oncol* 1987;28:220–224.

134. Maruyama Y, van Nagell JR, Yoneda J, Donaldson E, Gallion HH, Higgins R, Powell D, Kryscio R, Berner B: Dose–response and failure pattern for bulky or barrel-shaped stage IB cervical cancer treated by combined photon irradiation and extrafascial hysterectomy. *Cancer* 1989;63:70–76.

135. Keys HM, Bundy BN, Stehman FB, Muderspach LI, Chafe WE, Suggs CL III, Walker JL, Gersell D: Cisplatin, radiation, and adjuvant hysterectomy compared with radiation and adjuvant hysterectomy for bulky stage IB cervical carcinoma. *N Engl J Med* 1999;340:1154–1161.

136. Rotman M, Pajak TF, Choi K, Clery M, Marcial V, Grigsby PW, Cooper J: Prophylactic extended-field irradiation of para-aortic lymph nodes in stages IIB and bulky IB and IIA cervical carcinomas. Ten-year results of RTOG 79–20. *JAMA* 1995;274:387–393.

137. Haie C, Pejovic MH, Gerbaulet A, Horiot J, Pourquier H, Delouche J, Heinz JF, Brune D, Fenton J, Pizzi G, et al: Is prophylactic para-aortic irradiation worthwhile in the treatment of advanced cervical carcinoma? Results of a controlled clinical trial of the EORTC radiotherapy group. *Radiother Oncol* 1988;11:101–112.

138. Stitt JA, Fowler JF, Thomadsen BR, Buchler DA, Paliwal BP, Kinsella TJ: High dose rate intracavitary brachytherapy for carcinoma of the cervix: The Madison system: I. Clinical and radiobiological considerations. *Int J Radiat Oncol Biol Phys* 1992;24:335–348.

139. Kapp KS, Stuecklschweiger GF, Kapp DS, Poschauko J, Pickel H, Hackl A: Carcinoma of the cervix: Analysis of complications after primary external beam radiation and Ir-192 HDR brachytherapy. *Radiother Oncol* 1997;42:143–153.

140. Han I, Malviya V, Chuba P, Orton C, Devi S, Deppe G, Malone J Sr, Christensen C, Ahmad K, Kim Y, Porter A: Multifractionated high-dose-rate brachytherapy with concomitant daily teletherapy for cervical cancer. *Gynecol Oncol* 1996;63:71–77.

141. Hughes-Davies L, Silver B, Kapp D: Parametrial interstitial brachytherapy for advanced or recurrent pelvic malignancy: The Harvard/Stanford experience. *Gynecol Oncol* 1995;58:24–27.

142. Monk BJ, Tewari K, Burger RA, Johnson MT, Montz FJ, Berman ML: A comparison of intracavitary versus interstitial irradiation in the treatment of cervical cancer. *Gynecol Oncol* 1997;67:241–247.

143. Lowrey GC, Mendenhall WC, Million RR: Stage IB or IIA-B carcinoma of the intact uterine cervix treated with irradiation: A multivariate analysis. *Int J Radiat Oncol Biol Phys* 1992;24:205–210.

144. Horiot JC, Pigneaux J, Pourquier H, et al: Radiotherapy alone in carcinoma of the intact cervix according to G. H. Fletcher guidelines: A French cooperative study of 1383 cases. *Int J Radiat Oncol Biol Phys* 1988;14:605–611.

145. Lanciano RM, Won M, Coia L, Hanks GE: Pretreatment and treatment factors associated

with improved outcome in squamous cell carcinoma of the uterine cervix: A final report of the 1973 and 1978 Patterns of Care studies. *Int J Radiat Oncol Biol Phys* 1991;20:667–676.

146. Jampolis S, Andras J, Fletcher GH: Analysis of sites and causes of failure of irradiation in invasive squamous cell carcinoma of the intact uterine cervix. *Radiology* 1975;115:681–685.

147. Fletcher GH, Lindberg RD, Caderao JB, Wharton JT: Hyperbaric oxygen as a radiotherapeutic adjuvant in advanced cancer of the uterine cervix: Preliminary results of a randomized trial. *Cancer* 1977;39:617–623.

148. Brady LW, Plenk HP, Hanley JA, Glassburn JR, Kramer S, Parker RG: Hyperbaric oxygen therapy for carcinoma of the cervix stages IIB, IIIA, IIIB and IVA: Results of a randomized study by the Radiation Therapy Oncology Group. *Int J Radiat Oncol Biol Phys* 1981; 7:991–998.

149. Morita S, Arai T, Nakano T, Ishikawa T, Tsunemoto H, Fukuhisa K, Kasamatsu T: Clinical experience of fast neutron therapy for carcinoma of the uterine cervix. *Int J Radiat Oncol Biol Phys* 1985;11:1439–1445.

150. Maor MH, Gillespie BW, Peters LJ, Wambersic A, Griffin TW, Thomas FJ, Cohen L, Connor N, Gardner P: Neutron therapy in cervical cancer: Results of a phase III RTOG study. *Int J Radiat Oncol Biol Phys* 1988;14:885–891.

151. Gallion HH, Maruyama Y, van Nagell JR Jr, Donaldson ES, Rowley KC, Yoneda J, Beach JL, Powell DE, Kryscio RJ: Treatment of stage IIIB cervical cancer with californium-252 fast-neutron brachytherapy and external photon therapy. *Cancer* 1987;59:1709–1712.

152. Leibel S, Bauer M, Wasserman T, Marcial V, Rotman M, Hornback N, Cooper J, Gillespie B, Pakuris E, Conner N, et al: Radiotherapy with or without misonidazole for patients with stage IIIB or stage IVA squamous cell carcinoma of the uterine cervix: Preliminary report of a Radiation Therapy Oncology Group randomized trial. *Int J Radiat Oncol Biol Phys* 1987;13:541–549.

153. Overgaard J, Bentzen SM, Kolstad P, Kjoerstad K, Davy M, Bertelsen K, Mantyla M, Frankendal B, Skryten A, Loftquist I, et al: Misonidazole combined with radiotherapy in the treatment of carcinoma of the uterine cervix. *Int J Radiat Oncol Biol Phys* 1989;16: 1069–1072.

154. Stehman FB, Bundy BN, Keys H, Currie JL, Mortel R, Creasman WT: A randomized trial of hydroxyurea versus misonidazole adjunct to radiation therapy in carcinoma of the cervix. A preliminary report of a Gynecologic Oncology Group study. *Am J Obstet Gynecol* 1988;159: 87–94.

155. Bush RS, Jenkin RD, Allt WE, Beale FA, Bean H, Dembo AJ, Pringle JF: Definitive evidence for hypoxic cells influencing cure in cancer therapy. *Br J Cancer* 1978;37(suppl):302–306.

156. Grogan M, Thomas GM, Melamed I, Wong FL, Pearcey RG, Joseph PK, Portelance L, Crook JM, Jones KD: The importance of maintaining high hemoglobin levels during radiation treatment of carcinoma of the cervix. *Proceedings of the 30th Annual Meeting of the Society of Gynecologic Oncologists,* San Francisco, March 24, 1999 (abstr 43).

157. Souhami L, Gil RA, Allen SE, Canary PC, Araujo CM, Pinto LH, Silveira TR: A randomized trial of chemotherapy followed by pelvic radiation therapy in stage IIIB carcinoma of the cervix. *J Clin Oncol* 1991;9:970–977.

158. Chauvergne J, Lhomme C, Rohart J, Heron JF, Ayme Y, Goupil A, Fargeot P, David M: [Neoadjuvant chemotherapy for uterine cervix cancer stages IIB and III: Long-term results of a multicenter randomized trial in 151 patients.] A cooperative study of the French Oncology Centres. *Bull Cancer* 1993;80:1069–1079.

159. Kumar L, Kaushal R, Nandy, M, Biswal BM, Kumar S, Kriplani A, Singh R, Rath GH: Chemotherapy followed by radiotherapy versus radiotherapy alone in locally advanced cervical cancer. A randomized study. *Gynecol Oncol* 1994;54:307–315.

160. Tattersall MHN, Lorvidhaya V, Vootiprux V, Cheirsilpa A, Wong F, Azhart T, Lee HP, Kang SB, Manalo A, Yen M-S, Kampono N, Aziz F, for the Cervical Cancer Study Group of the Asian Oceanian Clinical Oncology Association: Randomized trial of epirubicin and cisplatin chemotherapy followed by pelvic radiation in locally advanced cervical cancer. *J Clin Oncol* 1995;13:444–451.

161. Sundfor K, Trope CG, Hogberg T, Onsrud M, Koern J, Simonsen E, Bertelsen K, Westberg R: Radiotherapy and neoadjuvant chemotherapy for cervical carcinoma. A randomized multicenter study of sequential cisplatin and 5-fluorouracil and radiotherapy in advanced cervical carcinoma stage 3B and 4A. *Cancer* 1996;77:2371–2378.

162. Eddy GL Sr: Neoadjuvant chemotherapy before surgery in cervical cancer. *J Natl Cancer Inst Monogr* 1996;21:93–99.

163. Sardi JE, Giaroli A, Sananes C, Ferreira M, Soderini A, Bermudez A, Snaidas L, Vighi S, Gomez Rueda N, di Paola G: Long-term follow-up of the first randomized trial using neoadjuvant chemotherapy in stage Ib squamous carcinoma of the cervix: The final results. *Gynecol Oncol* 1997;67:61–69.

164. Eddy GL, Manetta A, Alvarez RD, Williams L, Creasman WT: Neoadjuvant chemotherapy with vincristine and cisplatin followed by radical hysterectomy and pelvic lymphadenectomy for FIGO stage IB bulky cervical cancer: A Gynecologic Oncology Group pilot study. *Gynecol Oncol* 1995;57:412–416.

165. Sinclair WK: The combined effect of hydroxyurea and x-rays on Chinese hamster cells in vitro. *Cancer Res* 1968;28:198–201.

166. Piver MS, Howes AE, Suit HD, Marshall N: Effect of hydroxyurea on the radiation response of C3H mouse mammary tumors. *Cancer* 1972;29:407–412.

167. Fu KK: Biological basis for the interaction of chemotherapeutic agents and radiation therapy. *Cancer* 1985;55:2123–2130.

168. Phillips RA, Tolmach LJ: Repair of potentially lethal damage in x-irradiated HeLa cells. *Radiat Res* 1966;29:413–432.

169. Phillips TL, Wharam MD, Margolis LW: Modification of radiation injury to normal tissues by chemotherapeutic agents. *Cancer* 1975;35:1678–1684.

170. Piver MS, Barlow JJ, Vongtama V, et al: Hydroxyurea: A radiation potentiator in carcinoma of the uterine cervix: A randomized double-blind study. *Am J Obstet Gynecol* 1983;147:803–808.

171. Piver MS, Vongtama V, Emrich LJ: Hydroxyurea plus pelvic radiation versus placebo plus pelvic radiation in surgically staged stage IIIB cervical cancer. *J Surg Oncol* 1987;35:129–134.

172. Hreshchyshyn MM, Aron BS, Boronow RC, Franklin EW III, Shingleton HM, Blessing JA: Hydroxyurea or placebo combined with radiation to treat stages IIIB and IV cervical cancer confined to the pelvis. *Int J Radiat Oncol Biol Phys* 1979;5:317–322.

173. Stehman FB, Bundy BN, Thomas G, Keys HM, d'Ablaing G III, Fowler WC Jr, Mortel R, Creasman WT: Hydroxyurea versus misonidazole with radiation in cervical carcinoma: Long-term follow-up of a Gynecologic Oncology Group trial. *J Clin Oncol* 1993;11:1523–1528.

174. Whitney CW, Sause W, Bundy BN, Malfetano JH, Hannigan EV, Fowler WC Jr, Clarke-Pearson DL, Liao SY: Randomized comparison of fluorouracil plus cisplatin versus hydroxyurea as an adjunct to radiation therapy in stage IIB-IVA carcinoma of the cervix with negative para-aortic lymph nodes: A Gynecologic Oncology Group and Southwest Oncology Group study. *J Clin Oncol* 1999;17:1339–1348.

175. Rose PG, Bundy BN, Watkins EB, Thigpen JT, Deppe G, Maiman MA, Clarke-Pearson DL, Insalaco S: Concurrent cisplatin-based radiotherapy and chemotherapy for locally advanced cervical cancer. *N Engl J Med* 1999;340:1144–1153.

176. Keys HM, Bundy BN, Stehman FB, Muderspach L, Chafe WE, Suggs CL III, Walker JL, Gerself D: Cisplatin, radiation, and adjuvant hysterectomy compared with radiation and adjuvant hysterectomy for bulky stage IB cervical carcinoma. *N Engl J Med* 1999;340:1154–1161.

177. Thomas G, Dembo A, Ackerman I, Franssen E, Balogh J, Fyles A, Levin W: A randomized trial of standard versus partially hyperfractionated radiation with or without concurrent 5-fluorouracil in locally advanced cervical cancer. *Gynecol Oncol* 1998;69:137–145.

178. Lanciano RM, Pajak TF, Martz K, Hanks GE: The influence of treatment time on outcome for squamous cell cancer of the uterine cervix treated with radiation: A Patterns of Care study. *Int J Radiat Oncol Biol Phys* 1993;25:391–397.

179. Perez CA, Grigsby PW, Castro-Vita H, Lockett MA: Carcinoma of the uterine cervix.

I. Impact of prolongation of overall treatment time and timing of brachytherapy on outcome of radiation therapy. *Int J Radiat Oncol Biol Phys* 1995;32:1275–1288.

180. Petereit DG, Sarkaria JN, Chappell R, Fowler JF, Hartmann TJ, Kinsella TJ, Stitt JA, Thomadsen BR, Buchler DA: The adverse effect of treatment prolongation in cervical carcinoma. *Int J Radiat Oncol Biol Phys* 1995; 32:1301–1307.

181. Fyles AW, Pintilie M, Kirkbride P, Levin W, Manchul LA, Rawlings GA: Prognostic factors in patients with cervix cancer treated by radiation therapy. *Radiother Oncol* 1995;35: 107–117.

182. Delaloye JF, Coucke PA, Pampallona S, De Grandi P: Effect of total treatment time on event-free survival in carcinoma of the cervix. *Gynecol Oncol* 1996;60:42–48.

183. Girinsky T, Rey A, Roche B, Haie C, Gerbaulet A, Randrianarivello H, Chassagne D: Overall treatment time in advanced cervical carcinomas: A critical parameter in treatment outcome. *Int J Radiat Oncol Biol Phys* 1993; 27:1051–1056.

184. Chatani M, Matayoshi Y, Masaki N, Inoue T: High-dose rate intracavitary irradiation of the uterine cervix. The adverse effect of treatment prolongation. *Strahlenther Onkol* 1997;173: 379–384.

185. Lanciano R: Radiotherapy for the treatment of locally recurrent cervical cancer. *J Natl Cancer Inst Monogr* 1996;21:113–115.

186. Larson DM, Copeland LJ, Stringer CA, Gershenson DM, Malone JM Jr, Edwards CL: Recurrent cervical carcinoma after radical hysterectomy. *Gynecol Oncol* 1988;30:381–387.

187. Krebs HB, Helmkamp BF, Sevin BU, Poliakoff SR, Nadji M, Averette HE: Recurrent cancer of the cervix following radical hysterectomy and pelvic node dissection. *Obstet Gynecol* 1982;59:422–427.

188. Jobsen JJ, Leer JW, Cleton FJ, Hermans J: Treatment of locoregional recurrence of carcinoma of the cervix by radiotherapy after primary surgery. *Gynecol Oncol* 1989;33: 368–371.

189. Potter ME, Alvarez RD, Gay FL, Shingleton HM, Soong SJ, Hatch KD: Optimal therapy for pelvic recurrence after radical hysterectomy for early-stage cervical cancer. *Gynecol Oncol* 1990;37:74–77.

190. Garton GR, Gunderson LL, Webb MJ, Wilson TO, Martenson JA Jr, Cha SS, et al: Intraoperative radiation therapy in gynecologic cancer: The Mayo Clinic experience. *Gynecol Oncol* 1993;48:328–332.

191. Stelzer KJ, Koh WJ, Greer BE, Cain JM, Tamimi HK, Figge DC, et al: The use of intraoperative radiation therapy in radical salvage for recurrent cervical cancer: Outcome and toxicity. *Am J Obstet Gynecol* 1995;172: 1881–1888.

192. Mahe MA, Gerard JP, Dubois JB, Roussel A, Bussieres E, Delannes M, et al: Intraoperative radiation therapy in recurrent carcinoma of the uterine cervix: Report of the French Intraoperative Group on 70 patients. *Int J Radiat Oncol Biol Phys* 1996;34:21–26.

193. Thomas GM, Dembo AJ, Myhr T, Black B, Pringle JF, Rawling G: Long-term results of concurrent radiation and chemotherapy for carcinoma of the cervix recurrent after surgery. *Int J Gynecol Cancer* 1993;3:193–198.

194. Rutledge FN, Smith JP, Wharton JT, O'Quinn AG: Pelvic exenteration: Analysis of 296 patients. *Am J Obstet Gynecol* 1977;129: 881–892.

195. Rutledge FN, McGuffee VB: Pelvic exenteration: Prognostic significance of regional lymph node metastasis. *Gynecol Oncol* 1987; 26:374–380.

196. Wimbush PR, Fletcher GH: Radiation therapy of carcinoma of the cervical stump. *Radiology* 1969;93:655–658.

197. Kovalic JJ, Grigsby PW, Perez CA, Lockett MA: Cervical stump carcinoma. *Int J Radiat Oncol Biol Phys* 1991;20:933–938.

198. Wolff JP, Lacour J, Chassagne D, Berend M: Cancer of the cervical stump: A study of 173 patients. *Obstet Gynecol* 1972;39:10–16.

199. Potter ME, Alvarez RD, Shingleton HM, Soong SJ, Hatch KD: Early invasive cervical cancer with pelvic lymph node involvement: To complete or not to complete radical hysterectomy? *Gynecol Oncol* 1990;37:78–81.

200. Kinney WK, Hodge DO, Egorshin EV, Ballard DJ, Podratz KC: Surgical treatment of patients with stages IB and IIA carcinoma of the

cervix and palpably positive lymph nodes. *Gynecol Oncol* 1995;57:145–149.

201. Greer BE, Easterling TR, McLennan DA, Benedetti TJ, Cain JM, Figge DC, Tamimi HK, Jackson JC: Fetal and maternal considerations in the management of stage I-B cervical cancer during pregnancy. *Gynecol Oncol* 1989;34:61–65.

202. Dudan RC, Yon JL Jr, Ford JH Jr, Averette HE: Carcinoma of the cervix and pregnancy. *Gynecol Oncol* 1973;1:283–289.

203. Hopkins MP, Morley GW: The prognosis and management of cervical cancer associated with pregnancy. *Obstet Gynecol* 1992;80:9–13.

204. Creasman WT, Rutledge FN, Fletcher GH: Carcinoma of the cervix associated with pregnancy. *Obstet Gynecol* 1970;36:495–501.

205. Sall S, Rini S, Pineda A: Surgical management of invasive carcinoma of the cervix in pregnancy. *Am J Obstet Gynecol* 1974;118:1–5.

206. Sivanesaratnam V, Jayalakshmi P, Loo C: Surgical management of early invasive cancer of the cervix associated with pregnancy. *Gynecol Oncol* 1993;48:68–75.

207. Jones WB, Shingleton HM, Russell AH, Fremgen AM, Clive RE, Winchester DP, Chmiel JS: Cervical carcinoma and pregnancy. A national patterns of care study of the American College of Surgeons. *Cancer* 1996;77:1479–1488.

208. Magrina JF: Primary surgery for stage IB-IIA cervical cancer, including short-term and long-term morbidity and treatment in pregnancy. *J Natl Cancer Inst Monogr* 1996;21:53–59.

209. Grigsby PW, Russell A, Bruner D, Eifel P, Koh WJ, Spanos W, Stetz J, Stitt JA, Sullivan J: Late injury of cancer therapy on the female reproductive tract. *Int J Radiat Oncol Biol Phys* 1995;31:1281–1299.

210. Eifel PJ, Levenback C, Wharton JT, Oswald MJ: Time course and incidence of late complications in patients treated with radiation therapy for FIGO stage IB carcinoma of the uterine cervix. *Int J Radiat Oncol Biol Phys* 1995;32:1289–1300.

211. Parsons CL: Successful management of radiation cystitis with sodium pentosanpolysulfate. *J Urol* 1986;136:813–814.

212. Hampson SJ, Woodhouse CRJ: Sodium pentosanpolysulphate in the management of hemorrhagic cystitis: Experience with 14 patients. *Eur Urol* 1994;25:40–42.

213. Blomlie V, Rofstad EK, Talle K, Sundfor K, Winderen M, Lien HH: Incidence of radiation-induced insufficiency fractures of the female pelvis: Evaluation with MR imaging. *Am J Roentgenol* 1996;167:1205–1210.

214. Abitol MM, Davenport JH: The irradiated vagina. *Obstet Gynecol* 1974;44:249–256.

215. Pitkin RM, Bradbury JR: The effect of topical estrogen on irradiated vaginal epithelium. *Am J Obstet Gynecol* 1965;92:175–182.

216. Pitkin RM, Van Voorhis LW: Postirradiation vaginitis. An evaluation of prophylaxis with topical estrogen: *Radiology* 1971;99:417–421.

217. Anderson B: Ovarian function after radical hysterectomy. *Gynecol Oncol* 1995;56:1–2.

218. Anderson B, LaPolla J, Turner D, Chapman G, Buller R: Ovarian transposition in cervical cancer. *Gynecol Oncol* 1993;49:206–214.

219. Chambers SK, Chambers JT, Holm C, Peschel RE, Schwartz PE: Sequelae of lateral ovarian transposition in unirradiated cervical cancer patients. *Gynecol Oncol* 1990;39:155–159.

220. Chambers SK, Chambers JT, Kier R, Peschel RE: Sequelae of lateral ovarian transposition in irradiated cervical cancer patients. *Int J Radiat Oncol Biol Phys* 1991;20:1305–1308.

221. Owens S, Roberts WS, Fiorica JV, Hoffman MS, LaPolla JP, Cavanaugh D: Ovarian management at the time of radical hysterectomy for cancer of the cervix. *Gynecol Oncol* 1989;35:349–351.

222. Feeney DD, Moore DH, Look KY, Stehman FB, Sutton GP: The fate of the ovaries after radical hysterectomy and ovarian transposition. *Gynecol Oncol* 1995;56:3–7.

223. Barnhill D, Heller P, Dames J, Hoskins W, Gallup D, Park R: Persistence of endometrial activity after radiation therapy for cervical carcinoma. *Obstet Gynecol* 1985;66:805–808.

224. McKay MJ, Bull CA, Houghton CR, Langlands AO: Persisting cyclical uterine bleeding in patients treated with radical radiation therapy and hormonal replacement for carcinoma of the cervix. *Int J Radiat Oncol Biol Phys* 1990;18:921–925.

225. Andersen BL: Stress and quality of life following cervical cancer. *J Natl Cancer Inst Monogr* 1996;21:65–70.

# CHAPTER 11

# SOFT TISSUE SARCOMAS

IRA J. SPIRO and HERMAN D. SUIT

## INTRODUCTION

Soft tissue sarcomas are rare mesenchymal tumors, comprising approximately 0.66% of newly diagnosed malignant tumors in the U.S. population.[1] That is, there are approximately 9100 such tumors per year. Of these, 6600 arise in soft tissue and 2500 in bone. The relative rarity of soft tissue sarcoma is better appreciated when compared with 178,000, 181,000, and 334,500 newly diagnosed annual cancers of the lung, breast, and prostate, respectively. The yearly incidence of soft tissue sarcoma has remained stable.[2] The male-to-female ratio is approximately 1.2:1. It is estimated that there are approximately 100 benign for each malignant tumor of soft tissue.[3] These tumors can occur at any site within the body, including parenchymal organs. The most common sites are the lower and upper extremities (Table 11-1). Within the lower extremity, the proximal thigh and buttock comprise the majority of the lesions. These lesions can occur at all body sites, which makes their treatment challenging and requires the individualization of patient treatment.

Most soft tissue sarcomas occur sporadically, although in rare cases there is an association with familial disease syndromes.[4–7] Examples include desmoid tumors among patients with familial polyposis,[8] sarcomas of soft tissue and bone in patients with hereditary or bilateral retinoblastoma, neurofibromatosis type 1, in which benign neurofibromas and malignant neurofibrosarcomas are seen,[9–11] and bone and soft tissue sarcomas in patients with Li–Fraumeni syndrome.[4,12] Also, malignant schwannoma may complicate the multiple endocrine neoplasia syndrome.[13]

In addition to genetic causes, soft tissue sarcomas are associated, though rarely, with exposure to carcinogens. For example, radiation therapy has been linked to the development of bone and soft tissue lesions, although cohort studies of this phenomenon are rare.[14] The frequency of radiation-induced sarcoma is higher following treatment of children, particularly those with Ewing sarcoma and retinoblastoma.[15–18] In addition to radiation, exposure to several classes of industrial chemicals is related to the development of sarcomas.[19–22] Soft tissue sarcomas (usually lymphangiosarcomas) may be observed in the setting of chronic and massive edema.[23]

## NATURAL HISTORY

Sarcomas tend to grow by local extension, infiltrating adjacent tissues and extending along tissue planes, but rarely do they traverse major fascial planes or bone, except in locally advanced disease. Sarcomas infrequently spread to regional lymph nodes, except for

*Clinical Radiation Oncology: Indications, Techniques, and Results, 2nd ed.* Edited by C.C. Wang.
ISBN: 0-471-23803-1 Copyright © 2000 Wiley-Liss, Inc.

**TABLE 11-1** Anatomic Distribution of Sarcoma of Soft Tissues in 788 Patients at the Massachusetts General Hospital

| Region | Proportion (%) |
| --- | --- |
| Lower extremity | 44 |
| Upper extremity | 21 |
| Head and neck | 12 |
| Torso | 10 |
| Retroperitoneum | 6 |
| Other | 7 |

rhabdomyosarcoma, epithelioid sarcoma, and high grade synovial sarcoma. Clear cell sarcoma and alveolar soft parts sarcoma may also rarely show lymph node metastases. The rate of metastasis to the regional lymph nodes by soft tissue sarcomas at diagnosis or as the first metastasis is approximately 4% and increases as a function of grade: grade I, 0/63; grade II, 2/118; and grade III, 17/142.[24]

At diagnosis, over 90% of sarcoma patients will have localized disease.[25] Eventual tumor spread to distant sites is a common development, especially for the large and high grade sarcomas. Among patients with distant failure, 70% to 82% develop disease in the lung as the first metastatic site.[26,27] Patients with liposarcoma are the exception to the observation above, with 59% showing isolated extrapulmonary disease as the site of first metastasis.[28]

## BIOLOGY

An interesting feature of soft tissue sarcomas is that a number of these tumors display stable chromosomal translocations, which serve as diagnostic criteria. Many of these chromosomal abnormalities have been characterized at the molecular level, and the chimeric genes that are associated with these cytogenetic changes have been cloned. These developments have provided clues to the molecular

alterations that are fundamental for the development of soft tissue sarcomas. Myxoid liposarcomas display a t(12;16)(q13;p11) translocation.[29-32] The fusion gene, known as *TLS-CHOP,* fails to induce $G_1/S$ arrest, while the nononcogenic form of *CHOP* induces a normal $G_1/S$ arrest.[32] Synovial cell sarcomas are characterized by the translocation t(x;18) (p11.2;q11.2), which has been cloned and has led to the identification of two novel genes, *SYT* and *SSX.*[33] Alveolar rhabdomyosarcomas show a translocation at t(2;13) (q35;q14). This chimeric gene has also been cloned and has been termed *PAX3-FKHR.*[34]

Molecular determination of minimal residual disease in alveolar rhabdomyosarcoma is possible, but the clinical significance of this finding is uncertain.[35] Clear cell sarcomas often exhibit a t(12;22)(q13;q13) translocation. This entity is sometimes referred to as malignant melanoma of soft parts, although the clear cell sarcoma translocation is not seen in cutaneous malignant melanoma.[36] Molecular characterizations of these chromosome abnormalities now serve as diagnostic criteria for soft tissue sarcomas with the expectation that diagnoses will increasingly be made on the basis of standard histochemistry, immunohistochemistry, cytogenetics, and molecular biology.[37]

Alterations of *Rb,* the retinoblastoma gene, are commonly found in the sporadic development of soft tissue sarcomas. Loss of *Rb* immunoreactivity[38] and *Rb* loss of heterozygosity[39] have each been correlated with a poorer outcome. Somatic alterations of the *p53* gene are also common in soft tissue sarcomas.[40-47] It is now well recognized that the high cancer incidence in patients with the Li–Fraumeni syndrome, in which soft tissue and bone sarcomas are prominent, is the consequence of germ line mutations on the *p53* gene.[48-51] Recently, the *MDM2* gene, located at 12q13-14, was observed to be frequently amplified in soft tissue sarcomas,[52-58] and a gene designated *SAS,* also located at 12q13-14, was amplified in soft tissue sarcomas.[59,60]

## CLINICAL FEATURES

Patients with a soft tissue sarcoma commonly present with a painless mass of a few months' duration. Occasionally, patients present with pain secondary to pressure effects or direct invasion of neural structures by the tumor. Frequently, patients will recall a history of a traumatic incident, predating the awareness of the mass, suggesting that the trauma merely brought the patient's attention to the presence of the mass.

The preferred management of sarcoma patients is by a multidisciplinary and multispecialty sarcoma team, comprising individuals who have a primary clinical and research interest in connective tissue oncology. Team members should include bone and soft tissue diagnostic radiologists, sarcoma pathologists, orthopedic and general oncologic surgeons, medical and pediatric oncologists, radiation oncologists, nurses, physiotherapists, and data managers. In this manner, diagnostic evaluation, treatment, and follow-up are performed by the team, at a major cancer center, where these patients are seen in substantial numbers.

The diagnostic evaluation includes a complete history and physical examination that defines the involved anatomic part and defines evidence of involvement of skin, major vessels, nerves or bone, and regional lymph nodes. Plain radiographs are useful for indicating primary bone tumors with soft tissue masses, bone involvement by soft tissue tumors, and calcification within the soft tissue mass (e.g., synovial sarcoma), as well as for ruling out benign tumors such as myositis ossificans. MRI is the most useful method of imaging the primary site. If plain films indicate either a periosteal reaction or other bone involvement, a CT scan of the primary site with bone windows should be performed. A chest CT is used for assessment of lung metastases in patients with grade II and III lesions. For patients with retroperitoneal sarcoma, evaluation of the liver is recommended, as this is often a first site of metastatic involvement. Patients with large, high grade extremity liposarcomas should undergo abdominal CT scans, since these tumors can metastasize to the retroperitoneum and liver.

Biopsy may be either by CT-guided core needle or incisional. CT-guided core needle biopsies are rapid and less costly and may be better suited for deeply situated pelvic or retroperitoneal lesions. The needle biopsy should be performed by an experienced radiologist, and the sample should lie within tissue planes to be encompassed in the primary resection. The incisional biopsy should be performed by the surgeon who will perform the definitive surgery. It placed along the long axis of the limb, short in length, with meticulous attention paid to hemostasis. Inappropriate biopsy with large areas of potential contamination may preclude limb salvage techniques.[61]

The diagnosis and grading of sarcomas is facilitated by cytohistochemistry, immunohistochemistry, electron microscopy, flow cytometry, cytogenetics, and molecular genetics. Accurate assignment of histopathologic grade is important for the accurate staging of patients. Also the histopathologic subtype should be determined, since certain entities such as epithelioid sarcoma and liposarcoma can have unique patterns of spread. Soft tissue sarcomas are subtyped according to the normal cell or tissue type they resemble. For example, the cells of a liposarcoma resemble fat cells, leiomyosarcomas resemble smooth muscle cells, and fibrosarcomas resemble fibroblasts. For other sarcomas, the designation reflects the histological pattern the tumor mimics, such as alveolar sarcoma, which resembles lung parenchyma. The two most common histopathologic subtypes are the malignant fibrous histiocytoma and liposarcoma. Recently, there has been less use of terms such as spindle cell sarcoma and fibrosarcoma, while the diagnosis of malignant fibrous histiocytoma now accounts for 40% of soft tissue diagnoses (Table 11-2).

The fourth edition of the American Joint Cancer Commission (AJCC) staging of soft tissue sarcoma was based primarily on grade and secondarily on size.[62] The revised fifth edition has made significant changes to the staging system (Table 11-3).[63] Compartmentation is now incorporated based on the finding that superficial tumors have a better prognosis.[64] Also, the three-tiered grading system used in the fourth edition has essentially been replaced by a two-tiered system, although low grades are designated as 1 (well differentiated) or 2 (moderately differentiated), while high grades are designated as 3 (poorly differentiated) or 4 (undifferentiated). Tumors smaller than 5 cm are still designated T1, tumors exceeding 5 cm as T2, superficial tumors as a, and deep tumors as b. The new staging system

was designed to be based on treatment as well as prognosis. Stage I tumors are generally felt to manageable by surgery alone, stage II tumors are managed by surgery and radiation therapy, and treatment for stage III tumors includes chemotherapy. Future retrospective and prospective studies will be needed to validate this system.

## TREATMENT

Surgery is the primary treatment for soft tissue sarcomas. Historically, treatment by marginal surgery was associated with local failure rates of 70% or greater. To reduce local failure rates to less than 20%, the surgical procedure was extended to remove large volumes of grossly normal tissue at the expense of function and cosmesis. For large tumors, compartmental resection or amputation may be required. The randomized trial of surgery versus surgery plus brachytherapy at Memorial Sloan-Kettering Cancer Center demonstrated the results of surgery alone at a modern academic center.[65] In the surgery-alone arm, the local failure rate was 33% despite aggressive surgery by highly experienced oncologic surgeons. Other series of treatment by surgery alone have shown local failure rates of 0% for amputation to 31% for limb-sparing techniques.[66–71] In general, patients who have undergone an unplanned tumor resection or resection by a non-oncologic surgeon will require additional surgery. A number of studies indicate that 37% to 59% of such patients will have residual tumor in the subsequent reresection specimen.[72–75]

To improve the morbidity, functional outcome, and cosmesis of patients who undergo radical surgery, radiation therapy has been combined with more conservative surgical procedures. The expectation is that moderate doses of radiation can inactivate microscopic deposits of tumor in grossly appearing normal tissue beyond the surgical resection margin. The merit of this approach has been shown in a randomized trial at the National Cancer Institute.[76] In addition, a number of clinical studies have shown

**TABLE 11-2    Histopathologic Subtypes at the Massachusetts General Hospital: 1988–1995**

| Subtype | % |
| --- | --- |
| Malignant fibrous histiosarcoma | 40 |
| Liposarcoma | 14 |
| Synovial sarcoma | 13 |
| Neurofibrosarcoma | 12 |
| Leiomyosarcoma | 9 |
| Clear cell sarcoma | 3 |
| Angiosarcoma | 3 |
| Alveolar soft parts sarcoma | 2 |
| Fibrosarcoma | 1 |
| Epithelioid sarcoma | 1 |
| Spindle cell sarcoma | <1 |
| Not specified | <1 |

**TABLE 11-3    AJCC Stage Grouping, 5th Edition, 1997**

| | | TNM Stage | | |
| --- | --- | --- | --- | --- |
| Group | Grade | T[a] | N | M |
| IA | 1–2 | 1a-b | 0 | 0 |
| IB | 1–2 | 2a | 0 | 0 |
| IIA | 1–2 | 2b | 0 | 0 |
| IIB | 3–4 | 1a-b | 0 | 0 |
| IIC | 3–4 | 2a | 0 | 0 |
| III | 3, 4 | 2b | 0 | 0 |
| IV | Any | Any | 1 | Any |
| | Any | Any | Any | 1 |

[a]T1, ≤ 5 cm; T2, > 5 cm; a, superficial; b, deep.
*Source:* Ref. 63.

that local control rates with the combined modality approach are equivalent to those seen with radical surgery alone.[77-89] The success of this approach is reflected by the drop in amputation rate for primary tumors at most major centers to under 5%. A recent study from the National Cancer Institute has also shown a local control benefit to radiation plus conservative surgery versus conservative surgery alone.[90]

Radiation in combination with surgery, may be delivered pre- or postoperatively or intraoperatively. Postoperative radiation will produce fewer delays in wound healing.[91] Also, the entire untreated pathologic specimen can be assessed for grade, histopathologic subtype, and the extent of necrosis in patients receiving preoperative chemotherapy. Preoperative radiation allows treatment volumes to be limited to the radi-

ographically evident disease and tissues judged to be microscopically involved. In contrast, postoperative radiation must include all the tissues handled operatively, including drain sites and scars. A prospective study of portal sizes showed a 62% increase for postoperative treatment versus preoperative.[92] Preoperative radiation is also advantageous for radioresponsive tumors such as liposarcomas, where a significant reduction in tumor volume can be achieved. Another advantage of preoperative radiation is that the risk of tumor autotransplantion is virtually eliminated, as is the establishment of distant metastases from cells exfoliated into vascular spaces during surgery. When surgery precedes radiation, wound complications can delay the start of radiation therapy, permitting residual tumor cells to proliferate. Table 11-4 shows the

**TABLE 11-4  Local Control Results in Patients Treated by Surgery and Radiation**

| Center[a] | Number of Patients | Local Failure (%) | Ref. |
|---|---|---|---|
| POSTOPERATIVE RADIATION | | | |
| MGH | 176 | 14 | 114 |
| MDAII | 300 | 22 | 115 |
| IGR | 89 | 14 | 116 |
| RPMI | 53 | 14 | 117 |
| NCI | 128 | 10 | 71 |
| Toronto | 23 | 9 | 118 |
| St. Louis | 35 | 14 | 119 |
| Amsterdam | 64 | 8 | 120 |
| University of Pennsylvania/Fox Chase | 67 | 13 | 121 |
| University of Chicago | 50 | 24 | 122 |
| PREOPERATIVE RADIATION | | | |
| MGH | 181 | 10 | 114 |
| MDAH | 110 | 10 | 123 |
| Toronto | 39 | 3 | 118 |
| University of Florida | 58 | 9 | 124 |
| BRACHYTHERAPY | | | |
| Memorial | 55 | 18 | 63 |
| Mayo Clinc | 63 | 8 | 125 |
| IA/IV ADRIAMYCIN + RADIATION | | | |
| UCLA | 371 | ~10 | 126 |
| University of Virginia | 55 | 2 | 127 |

[a]MGH, Massachusetts General Hospital; MDAH, M. D. Anderson Hospital; IGR, Institut Gustave-Roussy; RPMI, Roswell Park Memorial Institute; NCI, National Cancer Institute; Memorial, Memorial Sloan-Kettering Cancer Center; UCLA, University of California, Los Angeles.

local control rates for combined surgery and radiation for a number of institutions. Our own results at the Massachusetts General Hospital indicate that there may be a local control advantage for large lesions when preoperative radiation therapy is used (Table 11-5). The National Cancer Institute of Canada is addressing the question of the clinical benefits of pre- versus postoperative radiation in a phase III trial.

In a number of studies, positive surgical margins are a predictor of local failure in soft tissue sarcomas (Table 11-6). Of interest, for patients treated with preoperative radiation, local control was the same for patients with close (e.g., < 1 mm) but negative margins

versus those with no tumor in the resection specimen.[93] Also, this study showed no influence of tumor size on local control for patients with negative margins. Similarly, there was no influence of primary versus recurrent disease when patients were stratified by margin status.

Radiation alone is a treatment option for the small number of patients who are medically inoperable or who refuse an operation. Even for T1 tumors, doses of 75 to 80 Gy are required if tumor control probabilities of 90% are anticipated. For larger tumors, 5-year control rates of 33% have been reported.[94] Other authors have reported similar control rates when they used radiation alone.[95–97]

**TABLE 11-5    5-Year Actuarial Local Control (LC) Results According to Size of Primary Soft Tissue Sarcoma: Massachusetts General Hospital**

| Size (mm) | Postoperative | | Preoperative | |
|---|---|---|---|---|
| | Number of Patients | LC (%) | Number of Patients | LC (%) |
| < 25  20 | 100 | | 11 | 80 |
| 26–49  45 | 95 | | 16 | 100 |
| 50–100 | 64 | 83 | 63 | 93 |
| 101–150 | 12 | 91 | 34 | 100 |
| 151–200 | 6 | 50 | 25 | 79 |
| > 200 | 3 | 67 | 11 | 100 |
| Total: | 150 | | 160 | |
| Average: | | 87 | | 92 |

**TABLE 11-6    Surgical Margins and Local Control**

| Study | Local Control (%) | |
|---|---|---|
| | Negative Margins | Positive Margins |
| Sadoski et al.[93] | 97 | 81 |
| Herbert et al.[128] | 100 | 55 |
| Tanabe et al.[129] | 91 | 62 |
| LeVay et al.[101] | 87 | 76 |
| Pisters et al.[64] | 80 | 60 |

## WOUND HEALING

Wound healing was assessed in 202 consecutive patients treated at the Massachusetts General Hospital (MGH) by preoperative radiation therapy.[98] The overall wound complication rate was 37%. Secondary surgery was necessary in 16.5% of the cases, including 6 patients (3%) who required amputation. Multivariate analyses of the data show that the following factors were significantly associated with wound morbidity: tumor in the lower extremity ($p < 0.001$), increasing age ($p = 0.004$), and postoperative boost with interstitial implant ($p = 0.016$). Wound healing among 180 patients treated with conservative surgery and radiation has been reported.[99] The significant factors associated with increased risk of wound healing delay were size of the specimen, use of preoperative radiation, history of smoking, and vascular disease.

Surgery alone can also result in significant wound healing problems, with rates reported to be as high as 33%.[100] This is comparable to results obtained with preoperative radiation therapy. However, in the surgery-alone series there were no amputations performed for wound-related morbidity and the percentage of patients requiring a secondary procedure was only 3%. Higher wound complication rates are reported for patients treated with radiation preoperatively compared with postoperatively treated patients.

Based on current results and the experience of others as described in the literature, we suggest the following strategies that may lead to reduced wound morbidity:

1. More gentle handling of tissue during surgery.
2. Meticulous attention to achieve hemostasis before wound closure.
3. Avoidance of closure under tension.
4. Elimination of all dead space in the wound. If rotation of a flap is needed to fill the space, it should be used.
5. Drainage of the wound, with the tubes left in place until the drainage is approximately 15 mL/day.
6. In many situations use of a compression dressing is advantageous.
7. Immobilization of the affected part for approximately 7 days.
8. Special attention needs to be directed toward defining the subgroup[s] of patients in whom the postoperative boost dose could be omitted. For example, patients whose specimens have negative histological margins could be one such group for study of this question.

## FUNCTIONAL OUTCOME

Data regarding the functional outcome of patients undergoing limb salvage procedures are limited. In a series of 88 patients treated with either preoperative or postoperative radiation therapy, 68 patients had acceptable functional results and 61 of these patients returned to work.[101] In this series, large tumors, neural sacrifice, proximal thigh tumors, and postoperative complications were associated with a poor outcome. The authors suggested that limiting wound healing complications would impact favorably on functional outcome. In a group of patients with lower limb sarcomas, it was concluded that radiation therapy was associated with reduced muscle power and range of motion, compared with patients treated with surgery alone.[102] Regardless, most patients retained good to excellent limb function and quality of life. These authors also noted that large doses per fraction were associated increased fibrosis and poorer outcome.

Long-term treatment complications were analyzed in sarcoma patients undergoing limb sparing therapy at the National Cancer Institute.[103] All patients received radiation therapy and surgery. Bone fracture was observed in 6%, contracture in 20%, edema greater than 2+ in 19%, moderate to severe decrease in strength in 20%, and induration in 57%. The percentage of patients ambulating without assistive devices with mild or no pain was 84%.

## CHEMOTHERAPY

Distant metastases remain the principal cause of failure in patients with stage IIB and IIIB soft tissue sarcomas treated with surgery and radiation. This knowledge has led to a number of trials of adjuvant chemotherapy. In general, comparisons of disease-free survival and survival with historical controls have often shown a gain for the chemotherapy (Table 11-7). The results of the European Organization for Research and Treatment of Cancer (EORTC) experience with adjuvant cyclophosphamide, vincristine, doxorubicin, and dacarbazine (CYVADIC) chemotherapy has shown that relapse-free survival was 56% in the chemotherapy group versus 43% in control patients.[104] This difference was largely due to a decrease in local failure in the chemotherapy arm (17% vs. 31%), and in fact freedom from distant metastasis was identical in both groups.

A meta-analysis has been performed, combining the results of 15 published randomized trials.[105] These data suggested an improvement in survival at 5 years, although the authors felt the data needed to be viewed with caution. These data are being reanalyzed using individual patient data, and results should be published in the near future. Analysis of the more recent data has shown improvement in disease-free survival but not in overall survival. Recent studies have shown that the addition of ifosfamide to doxorubicin-based chemotherapy produces higher response rates in advanced disease,[106,107] although in a recent EORTC trial, patients receiving doxorubicin alone fared no better than those receiving doxorubicin plus ifosfamide or CYVADIC.[108] Currently, in the United States, many high risk patients are being offered adjuvant multiagent chemotherapy as the "standard of care."

## RADIATION THERAPY TECHNIQUES

The goal in planning radiation therapy for a sarcoma patient is to accurately define a target volume and to estimate the distribution of reproductively intact tumor cells within that target. MRI scanning, and more recently, dynamic MRI have greatly improved and simplified this task. These imaging techniques allow the radiation oncologist to discern the

**TABLE 11-7  Randomized Trials of Multiagent Chemotherapy**

| Study | Treatment[a] | Site | Number of Patients | Survival % Relapse-Free | Overall |
|-------|-----------|------|-------------------|-------------|---------|
| M. D. Anderson[130] | CTX | Limb | 20 | $54_{p=0.04}$ | $65_{p=0.25}$ |
| | Control | | 23 | 35 | 36 |
| Mayo Clinic[131] | CTX | Limb/other | 30 | $90_{p=0.55}$ | |
| | Control | | 31 | 77 | |
| NCI[132–134] | CTX | Limb | 39 | $75_{p=0.04}$ | $82_{p=0.12}$ |
| | Control | | 28 | 54 | 60 |
| Foundation Bergonie[135,136] | CTX | All | 31 | | $87_{p=0.002}$ |
| | Control | | 28 | | 53 |
| EORTC[137–140] | CTX | All | 145 | $56_{p=0.007}$ | $63_{p=0.64}$ |
| | Control | | 172 | 43 | 56 |

[a]CTX, cyclophosphamide.

*Source:* Adpated from EORTC.[104]

extent of tumor spread and edema in the muscle in which the tumor arises and adjacent muscles. Minimizing radiation dose to nontarget tissues is essential for improving cosmetic and functional outcome and to permit an increase of dose to the target.

Preoperative radiation therapy is planned using current MRI or CT imaging information. Biopsy incisions and needle tracks are included within the treatment volume. Generally, 50 Gy is delivered in 25 fractions over 5 to 5.5 weeks, followed by a 3-week rest period before surgery. Occasionally, a daily dose per fraction of 1.8 Gy is employed if the treatment volume is large (linear dimension $\geq$ 30 cm) or encompasses visceral organs, or for patients of advanced age or comorbid disease. We also have treated a small number of patients on a twice-daily schedule to a dose of 46.4 Gy using a daily dose per fraction of 1.6 Gy BID without additional wound healing morbidity. This schedule has been mainly used to accelerate the treatment as a convenience to the patient but has also been used for patients with rapidly growing tumors. For patients with microscopically positive surgical margins,* a postoperative boost of 16 Gy is delivered at 2.5 to 3 weeks after surgery or when the wound is adequately healed. This boost is intended to cover only the tumor bed with a small margin, not the entire surgical bed. For patients with greater than microscopic residual tumor, reoperation to obtain negative margins should be considered. If this is not feasible, a boost of 26 Gy is given to a small volume of tissue where the margins are known to be positive. It is advantageous if the surgeon identifies the tumor bed with single large clips and areas of suspected margin involvement. Brachytherapy and intraoperative techniques can be utilized for the boost if the margin status is known at the time of surgery or if otherwise indicated.

Postoperative radiation therapy starts 3 weeks after surgery to allow for adequate wound healing. Additional time may be needed following the resection of large tumors if a seroma has developed. The initial treatment volume includes all tissues handled at the time of surgery, including drain sites, and is carried to a dose of 50 Gy. For the situation in which all gross disease has been removed, a total dose of 60 to 66 Gy is usually delivered through two subsequent field reductions. If gross residual disease remains and cannot be resected, the dose is carried to 72 to 76 Gy with appropriate field reductions. Planning of postoperative radiation therapy following resection of a large tumor requires an understanding of how normal tissue planes may be altered or shifted in the postoperative state.

If feasible, a sector of uninvolved tissue should be spared from full radiation dose preserve lymphatic drainage. Treatment plans that incorporate more than two fields can minimize normal tissue effects and generally improve homogeneity within the treatment volume. Poorly vascularized skin such as the pretibial, prepatellar, and preolecrenon skin should also be protected, as these areas tend to receive minor but repeated trauma, which may become significant if full radiation dose has been delivered. Also, dose maxima should be avoided in areas where surgical wounds will be placed.

Our historical practice has been to use longitudinal margins of at least 10 cm for grade III lesions. MRI scanning has greatly improved the ability to detect tumor and edema and has aided in the ability to reduce treatment volumes. In general, longitudinal margins extend to cover edema by several centimeters and usually extend beyond the tumor mass by about 8 cm for grade II and III lesions. For grade I lesions, longitudinal margins extend beyond the tumor by about 5 cm. Longitudinal margins need not extend into uninvolved compartments or across joint spaces, beyond the need to ensure adequate buildup and setup error. Similarly, radial portal margins need extend only to uninvolved compartments to ensure sufficient buildup and setup error, such that full dose is achieved within the involved compartment. In general, radiation therapy portals need not

---

*Tumor present at a resection edge. Ink on the intact pseudocapsule of the tumor is not considered a positive margin.

encompass clinically negative lymph nodes. This is true even for tumors arising in the medial proximal thigh. These considerations assume that patients are securely and reproducibly immobilized during treatment. Clinically positive lymph nodes should be biopsied prior to beginning preoperative radiation therapy. Pathologically involved lymph nodes are exceedingly rare in the setting of small low grade tumors except for epithelioid sarcoma.

Brachytherapy involves placement of catheters in the long axis of the extremity. Catheters are spaced at 1 cm intervals in a single plane. The implant volume is intended to cover the tumor bed plus margin and is not intended to cover the entire surgical bed or drain sites. As practiced at Memorial Sloan-Kettering Cancer Center, catheters are loaded on postoperative day 5 and a dose of 45 Gy is prescribed to a distance of 1 cm from the implant plane. Catheters can be safely placed over neurovascular structures and adjacent to pedicle and free flaps. This technique has the advantage that treatment is complete at approximately 10 days after surgery. These investigators recommend that brachytherapy not be used for low grade lesions and that it constitute only a fraction of the treatment for patients with positive surgical margins. The Massachusetts General Hospital experience is to use brachytherapy as a boost modality at doses of 16 to 30 Gy (prescribed at 0.5 cm). We have found the technique well suited for smaller sarcomas. Intraoperative radiation is also generally used as a boost technique and is particularly advantageous for retroperitoneal sarcomas where external beam doses are limited by small bowel and liver. The doses used typically are in the range of 15 Gy.

## BENIGN SOFT TISSUE TUMORS

Desmoid tumors are uncommon locally aggressive but nonmalignant lesions with significant local recurrence rates following surgical extirpation. These tumors can uncommonly recur proximally or distal to the primary site and even more rarely in the contralateral limb. Treatment of primary lesions is surgical if grossly negative margins can be obtained. Patients with microscopically positive margins after primary surgery can be observed, if they will comply with follow-up, inasmuch as roughly 25% to 50% will not recur by 5 years.[109] Patients with primary tumors with grossly positive margins or recurrent tumors with microscopically positive margins are recommended to receive postoperative radiation therapy to dose of 56 to 60 Gy. In addition, external beam radiation therapy can control gross disease in either recurrent or primary disease.[110–112] Dermatofibrosarcoma protuberans are low grade tumors of the dermis, managed by surgery with wide margins (2 cm). Three of three patients managed at the MGH by radiation alone are locally controlled at 9 years or more.[113]

## RADIATION THERAPY FOR THE TREATMENT OF BONE TUMORS

The role of radiation therapy in the treatment of malignant bone tumors is frequently misunderstood by clinicians. There is a commonly held misconception that except for Ewing sarcoma and primitive neuroectodermal tumors, bone tumors are not "sensitive" to radiation. What then is the role of radiation in the treatment of non-Ewing malignant bone tumors? For patients who have had resections of malignant bone tumors and who have microscopic or gross residual disease, postoperative radiation can be combined with surgery and chemotherapy. In addition, radiation can be used for selected patients with inoperable tumors or tumors arising from sites where en bloc resections are difficult or impossible. These sites include, but are not limited to the skull base, vertebral bodies, and proximal sacrum. In these situations, radiation therapy that combines standard external beam treatment with implant techniques or proton irradiation can be considered.

## Radiotherapy in Combination with Surgery

In specialized situations, radiation therapy may be recommended following surgical resection of malignant bone tumors. Radiation in the postoperative setting is usually given for patients with positive margins of resection, tumor spill, or tumor violation at the time of surgery. The decision to give radiation in the postoperative setting is also influenced by whether the patient has received or will receive chemotherapy. Also, the percentage of necrosis in the surgical specimen following chemotherapy will influence the decision to give postoperative radiation. For patients with primary high grade osteosarcoma who have received chemotherapy prior to surgery, we have developed the following algorithm for recommending postoperative radiation therapy.

TUMOR NECROSIS (%)

|  | < 50 | 50–90 | > 90 |
|---|---|---|---|
| Margin ≥ 1 mm | Observe | Observe | Observe |
| Margin < 1 mm | XRT | XRT | Observe |
| Margin positive | XRT* | XRT* | XRT* |

For patients who do not receive chemotherapy, the same guidelines apply except that patients with margins of 1 to 2 mm are more frequently offered radiation therapy. It should be emphasized that treatment recommendations are highly individualized. For example, the tissue material at the margin must be considered when the need for adjuvant radiotherapy is assessed. A 1 mm margin of dense fascial connective tissue or periosteum may be more than adequate, while a similar margin in loose connective tissue, fat, or muscle may not be adequate. Also, postoperative radiation therapy is recommended for high grade chondrosarcoma if there are close margins or tumor spillage.

The general principles of postoperative radiation therapy are similar to those described for soft tissue tumors. For patients with positive margins, doses in the range of 55 to 60 Gy are given using a dose per fraction of 1.6 Gy twice a day. For patients not receiving chemotherapy, with tumor cut-through or multiple positive margins, an attempt is made to cover all surgically handled tissues. On the other hand, for patients receiving chemotherapy, with focally positive margins with good chemotherapy responses, treatment volumes may be limited to the tissues in the vicinity of positive margins.

Occasionally we see patients in whom preoperative radiation is recommended. This situation usually occurs in patients not receiving chemotherapy, who have extensive tumors and in whom close or positive margins are anticipated by the surgeon. Preoperative radiation has the advantage that smaller treatment volumes can be used than in the postoperative setting. Also, there is a theoretical advantage that irradiated tumor cells are less likely to seed the wound or disseminate at the time of surgery. In the preoperative setting, 45 to 50 Gy is delivered followed by a break of 3 weeks before surgery for limb lesions. For patients with extensive pelvic lesions, the break is extended to 3 to 4 weeks. If positive margins are found, a postoperative boost is given after suitable wound healing has occurred, such that the total dose is brought to 60 to 66 Gy. If gross disease remains after surgery, the dose may be brought to 70 to 76 Gy if possible. The boost volume usually need not cover the entire preoperative tumor volume or the surgical bed but can be limited to the tumor bed or the area of positive margins.

## Radiation Alone for Primary Bone Tumors

Primary malignant bone tumors treated by radiation alone requires the judicious use of local high local doses of radiation. Dose for tumor control may range from 66 Gy for low grade chondrosarcoma of the skull base to more than 76 Gy for chordoma. Such high doses require the use of precision immobilization systems,

*Reoperate to achieve a negative margin if feasible.

computer-assisted three-dimensional treatment planning systems, and specialized conformal treatments such as proton radiation therapy. Careful attention must also be directed to critical normal dose-limiting structures adjacent to treatment volumes. Such treatment can be administered only at tertiary treatment centers specializing in this type of treatment.

Currently, proton irradiation is available at only two facilities in the United States: Loma Linda University, in California, and the Massachusetts General Hospital in Boston. This form of heavy charged particle radiotherapy has the advantage that protons exhibit Bragg peak energy dissipation in tissue. Therefore, beams can be designed that travel a specified distance in the body, with no exit dose beyond the treatment volume. Proton radiotherapy results in local control rates in excess of 90% for patients with skull base chondrosarcomas. Substantial numbers of patients with chordomas are controlled, although the results are inferior to those of the chondrosarcomas. These excellent local control rates are generally achieved in patients with gross residual disease remaining following subtotal resection or biopsy and attest to the efficacy of radiation in the treatment of bone tumors.

## REFERENCES

1. American Cancer Society: Cancer Statistics 1997. *CA Cancer J Clin* 1997;47(1):8.
2. Ross JA, Severson RK, Davis S, Brooks JJ: Trends in the incidence of soft tissue sarcomas in the United States from 1973 through 1987. *Cancer* 1993;72:486–490.
3. Enzinger FM, Weiss SW: *Soft Tissue Tumors.* St. Louis, Toronto, and London, CV Mosby, 1983.
4. Li FP: Cancer families: Human models of susceptibility to neoplasia—The Richard and Hinda Rosenthal Foundation award lecture. *Cancer Res* 1988;48:5381–5386.
5. Strong LC: Genetic considerations in pediatric oncology, in WW Sutow et al (eds): *Clinical Pediatric Oncology.* St. Louis, CV Mosby, 1977, pp 16–32.
6. Littlefield JW: Genes, chromosomes and cancer. *J Pediat* 1984;104:489–494.
7. Rowley JD: Human oncogene locations and chromosome observations. *Nature* 1983;301: 290–291.
8. McAdam WAF, Goligher JC: The occurrence of desmoids in patients with familial polyposis coli. *Br J Surg* 1970;57:618–631.
9. Fraumeni JF: Cancer medicine, in JF Holland and EM Frei (eds): *Genetic Factors in the Etiology of Cancer.* Philadelphia, Lea & Febiger, 1973, pp 7–15.
10. Storm FK, Eilber FR, Mirra J, Morton DL: Neurofibrosarcoma. *Cancer* 1980;45:126–129.
11. Heard, G: Malignant disease in von Recklinghausen's neurofibromatosis. *Proc R Soc Med* 1963;56:502.
12. Li FP, Fraumeni JF Jr: Soft-tissue sarcomas, breast cancer, and other neoplasms. *Ann Intern Med* 1969;71:747–749.
13. Pizzo PA, Miser JS, Cassady JR, Filler RM: Solid tumors of childhood, in VT DeVita, S Hellman, and SA Rosenberg (eds): *Cancer: Principles & Practice of Oncology.* Philadelphia, Lippincott 1985, pp 1511–1589.
14. Taghian A, DeVathaire F, Terrier M, Auquier A, Mouriesse H, et al: Long-term risk of sarcoma following radiation treatment for breast cancer. *Int J Radiat Oncol Biol Phys* 1991;21: 361–367.
15. Strong LC, Herson J, Osborne BM: Risk of radiation-related subsequent malignant tumors in survivors of Ewing's sarcoma. *J Natl Cancer Inst* 1979;62:1401–1406.
16. Eng C, Li FP, Abramson DH, Ellsworth RM, Wong FL, Goldman MB, Seddon J, Tarbell N, Boice JD Jr: Mortality from second tumors among long-term survivors of retinoblastoma. *J Natl Cancer Inst* 1993;85:1121–1128.
17. Hawkins MM, Wilson LM, Burton HS, et al: Radiotherapy, alkylating agents, and risk of bone cancer after childhood cancer. *J Natl Cancer Inst* 1996;88:270–278.
18. Tucker MA, D'Angio GJ, Boice JD, Strong LC, et al: Bone sarcomas linked to radiotherapy and chemotherapy in children. *New Engl J Med* 1987;317(10):588–593.
19. Hardell L, Eriksson M: The association between soft tissue sarcoma and exposure to phenoxyacetic acids. *Cancer* 1988;62:652–656.

20. Lander JJ, Stanley RJ, Sumner HW, Boswell DC, Aach RD: Angiosarcoma of the liver associated with Fowler's solution (potassium arsenite). *Gastroenterology* 1975;68(6):1582–1586.

21. Wingren G, Fredrikson M, Brage N, Nordenskjold B, Axelson O: Soft tissue sarcoma and occupational exposures. *Cancer* 1990;66: 806–811.

22. Vineis P, Faggiano F, Tedeschi M, Ciccone G: Incidence rates of lymphomas and soft tissue sarcomas and environmental measurements of phenoxy herbicides. *J Natl Cancer Inst* 1991; 83:362–363.

23. Stewart FW, Treves N: Lymphangiosarcoma in postmastectomy lymphedema: A report of six cases in elephantiasis chirurgica. *Cancer* 1948; 1:64–81.

24. Mazeron JJ, Suit HD: Lymph nodes as sites of metastases from sarcomas of soft tissue. *Cancer* 1987;60:1800–1808.

25. Rydholm A, Berg NO, Gullberg B, Thorngren K-G, Persson BM: Epidemiology of soft-tissue sarcoma in the locomotor system. *Acta Path Microbiol Immunol Scand* 1984;92: 363–374.

26. Rydholm A, Berg NO: Prognosis for soft tissue sarcoma in the locomotor system. *Acta Pathol: Microbiol Immunol Scand* 1984;92: 375–386.

27. Potter DA, Glenn J, Kinsella T, Glatstein E, Lack EE, Restrepo C, White DE, Seipp CA, Wesley R, Rosenberg SA: Patterns of recurrence in patients with high grade soft tissue sarcomas. *J Clin Oncol* 1985;3:353–366.

28. Cheng EY, Springfield DS, Mankin HJ: Frequent incidence of extrapulmonary sites of initial metastasis in patients with liposarcoma. *Cancer* 1995;75:1120–1127.

29. Crozat A, Aman P, Mandahl N, Ron D: Fusion of *CHOP* to a novel RNA-binding protein in human myxoid liposarcoma. *Nature* 1993; 363:640–644.

30. Rabbits TH, Forster A, Larson R, Nathan P: Fusion of the dominanat negative transcription regulator *CHOP* with a novel gene *FUS* by translocation t(12; 16) in malignant liposarcoma. *Nature Genet* 1991;4:175–180.

31. Aman P, Ron D, Mandahl N, Fioretos T, et al: Rearrangement of the transcription factor gene *CHOP* in myxoid liposarcomas with t(12;16)(q13;p11). *Genes Chromosomes Cancer* 1992;5:278–285.

32. Barone MV, Crozat A, Tabaee A, Philipson L, Ron D: *CHOP(GADD153)* and its oncogenic variant, *TLD-CHOP,* have opposing effects on the induction of $G_1/S$ arrest. *Genes Dev* 1994; 8(4):453–464.

33. Clark J, Rocques PJ, Crew AJ, Gill S, et al: Identification of novel genes, *SYT,* and *SSX,* involved in the t(X; 18)(p112; q112) translocation found in human synovial sarcoma. *Nature Genet* 1994;7:502–508.

34. Barr FG, Galli N, Hollick J, et al: Rearrangement of the *PAX3* in the solid tumour alveolar rhadbomyosarcoma. *Nature Genet* 1993;3: 113–117.

35. Kelly KM, Womer RB, Barr FG: Minimal disease detection in patients with alveolar rhabdomyosarcoma using a reverse transcriptase-polymerase chain reaction method. *Cancer* 1996;78:1320–1327.

36. Fletcher JA: Translocation (12;22)(q13-14; q12) is a non-random aberration in soft tissue clear cell sarcoma. *Genes Chromosomes Cancer* 1992;5(2):184.

37. Barr FG, Chatten J, D'Crus CM, et al: Molecular assays for chromosomal translocations in the diagnosis of pediatric soft tissue sarcomas. *JAMA* 1995;273:553–557.

38. Cance WG, Brennan MF, Dudas ME, et al: Altered expression of the retinoblastoma gene product in human sarcomas. *New Engl J Med* 1990;323:1457–1462.

39. Feugeas O, Guriec N, Babin-Boilletot A, et al: Loss of heterozygosity of the *RB* gene is a poor prognostic factor in patients with osteosarcoma. *J Clin Oncol* 1996;14:467–472.

40. Toguchida J, Yamaguchi T, Ritchie B, Beauchamp RL, et al: Mutation spectrum of the *p53* gene in bone and soft tissue sarcomas. *Cancer Res* 1992;53:6194–6199.

41. Wadayama F, Toguchida J, Yamaguchi T, et al: *p53* Expression and its relationship to DNA alterations in bone and soft tissue sarcomas. *Br J Cancer* 1993;68:1134–1139.

42. Stratton MR, Moss S, Warren W, et al: Mutation of the *p53* gene in human soft tissue sarcomas: Association with abnormalities of the *RB1* gene. *Oncogene* 1990;5:1297–1301.

43. Patterson H, Gill S, Fisher C, et al: Abnormalities of the *p53 MDM2* and *DCC* genes in human leiomyosarcomas. *Br J Cancer* 1994; 69:1052–1058.

44. Simms WW, Ordonez NG, Johnston, et al: *p53* Expression in dedifferentiated chondrosarcoma. *Cancer* 1995;76:223–227.

45. Komuro H, Hayashi Y, Kawamura M, et al: Mutations of the *p53* gene are involved in Ewing's sarcomas but not in neuroblastomas. *Cancer Res* 1993;53:5284–5288.

46. Andreassen A, Oyjord T, Hovig E, et al: *p53* Abnormalities in different subtypes of human sarcomas. *Cancer Res* 1993;53:468–471.

47. Mulligan LM, Matlashewski GJ, Scrable HJ, Cavenee WK: Mechanisms of *p53* loss in human sarcomas. *Proc Natl Acad Sci USA* 1990; 87:5863–5867.

48. Malkin D: *p53* and the Li–Fraumeni syndrome. *Cancer Genet Cytogenet* 1993;66(2):83–92.

49. Malkin D, Jolly KW, Barbier N, Look AD, et al: Germline mutations of the *p53* tumor-suppressor gene in children and young adults with second malignant neoplasms. *New Engl J Med* 1992;326(20):1309–1315.

50. Toguchida J, Yamaguchi T, Dayton SH, et al: Prevalence and spectrum of germline mutations of the *p53* gene among patients with sarcoma. *New Engl J Med* 1992;326:1301–1308.

51. McIntyre JF, Smith-Sorensen B, Friend SH, et al: Germline mutations of the *p53* tumor suppressor gene in children with osteosarcoma. *J Clin Oncol* 1994;12:925–930.

52. Oliner JD, Kinzler KW, Meltzer PS, et al: Amplification of a gene encoding a *p53*-associated protein in human sarcomas. *Nature* 1992; 358:80–83.

53. Leach FS, Tokino T, Meltzer P, Burrell M, et al: *p53* Mutation and *MDM*² amplification in human soft tissue sarcomas. *Cancer Res* 1993; 53:2233–2234.

54. Cordon-Cardo C, Latres E, Drobnjak M, Oliva MD, et al: Molecular abnormalities of *mdm*² and *p53* genes in adult soft tissue sarcomas. *Cancer Res* 1994;54:794–799.

55. Florenes VA, Mœlandsmo GM, Forus A, et al: *MDM2* gene amplification and transcript levels in human sarcomas: Relationship to *TP53* gene status. *J Natl Cancer Inst* 1994;86 :1297–1302.

56. Pedeutour F, Suijkerbuijk RF, Forus A, et al: Complex composition and co-amplification of *SAS* and *MDM2* in ring and giant rod marker chromosomes in well-differentiated liposarcoma. *Genes Chromosomes Cancer* 1994; 10:85–94.

57. Khatib ZA, Matsushime H, Valentine M, et al: Coamplification of the *CDK4* gene with *MDM2* and *GLI* in human sarcomas. *Cancer Res* 1993;53:5535–5541.

58. Nilbert M, Rydholm A, Willén, et al: *MDM2* gene amplificant correlates with ring chromosomes in soft tissue tumors. *Genes Chromosomes Cancer* 1994;9:261–265.

59. Smith SH, Weiss SW, Jankowski SA, Coccia MA, Meltzer PS: *SAS* amplification in soft tissue sarcomas. *Cancer Res* 1992;52: 3746–3749.

60. Forus A, Florenes VA, Maelandsmo GM, et al: Mapping of amplification units in the q13-14 region of chromosome 12 in human sarcomas: Some amplification units do not include *MDM2. Cell Growth Differ* 1993;4:1065–1070.

61. Mankin HJ, Lange TA, Spanier SS: The hazards of biopsy in patients with malignant primary bone and soft tissue tumors. *J Bone Joint Surg* 1982;64A:1121–1127.

62. Beahrs OH, et al (eds): *Manual for Staging of Cancer,* ___ ed. Philadelphia, Lippincott, 1992.

63. American Joint Committee on Cancer, American Cancer Society, et al: *Manual for Staging,* Philadelphia, Lippincott, 1997.

64. Pisters PW, Leung DH, Woodruff J, et al: Analysis of prognostic factors in 1041 patients with localized soft tissue sarcomas of the extremities. *J Clin Oncol* 1996;14:1679–1689.

65. Harrison LB, Franzese F, Gaynor JJ, Brennan MF: Long-term results of a prospective randomized trial of adjuvant brachytherapy in the management of completely resected soft tissue sarcomas of the extremity and superficial trunk. *Int J Radiat Oncol Biol Phys* 1993; 27:259–265.

66. Enneking WF, Spanier SS, Malawer MM: The effect of the anatomic setting on the results of surgical procedures for soft parts sarcoma of the thigh. *Cancer* 1981;47:1005–1022.

67. Alvegård TA, Sigurdsson H, Mouridsen H, et al: Adjuvant chemotherapy with doxorubicin in high-grade soft tissue sarcoma: A ran-

domized trial of the Scandinavian Sarcoma Group. *J Clin Oncol* 1989;7:1504–1513.

68. Singer S, Corson JM, Gonin R, Labow B, Eberlein TJ: Prognostic factors predictive of survival and local recurrence for extremity soft tissue sarcoma. *Ann Surg* 1994;219:165–173.

69. Keus RB, Rutgers EJ, Ho GH, Gortzak E, Albus-Lutter CE, Hart AAM: Limb-sparing therapy of extremity soft tissue sarcomas: Treatment outcome and long-term functional results. *Eur J Cancer* 1994;30:1459–1463.

70. Azzarelli A: Surgery in soft tissue sarcomas. *Eur J Cancer* 1993;29A:618–623.

71. Potter DA, Kinsella T, Glatstein E, et al: High-grade soft tissue sarcomas of the extremities. *Cancer* 1986;58:190–205.

72. Eilber FR, Giuliano A, Huth J, Mirra J, Rosen G, Morton D: Neoadjuvant chemotherapy, radiation, and limited surgery for high grade soft tissue sarcoma of the extremity. Recent concepts in sarcoma treatment, in *Proceedings of International Symposium on Sarcomas, Tarpon Springs, Florida, 1987.* Dordrecht, Netherlands: Kluwer Academic Publishers, 1988, p 115.

73. Zornig C, Peiper M, Schroder S: Re-excision of soft tissue sarcoma after inadequate initial operation. *Br J Surg* 1995;82:278–279.

74. Noria S, Davis A, Kandel R, et al: Residual disease following unplanned excision of a soft-tissue saracoma of an extremity. *J Bone Joint Surg (Br)* 1996;78A:650–654.

75. Goodlad JR, Fletcher CDM, Smith MA: Surgical resection of primary soft tissue sarcoma. *J Bone Joint Surg (Br)* 1996;78B:658–661.

76. Rosenberg SA, Tepper J, Glatstein E, et al: The treatment of soft tissue sarcoma of the extremities. *Ann Surg* 1982;196:305–314.

77. Suit HD, Mankin HJ, Wood WC, Proppe KH: Radiation and surgery in the treatment of primary sarcoma of soft tissue: Pre-operative, intra-operative and post-operative. *Cancer* 1985;55:2659–2667.

78. Suit HD, Mankin HJ, Wood WC, Gebhardt MC, Harmon DC, Rosenberg A, Tepper JE, Rosenthal D: Treatment of the patient with stage $M_0$ sarcoma of soft tissue. *J Clin Oncol* 1988;6(5):854–862.

79. Atkinson L, Garvan J, Newton NC: Behavior and management of soft connective tissue sarcomas. *Cancer* 1963;16:1552–1562.

80. Karakousis CP, Emrich LJ, Rao U, Krishnamsetty RM: Feasibility of limb salvage and survival in soft tissue sarcomas. *Cancer* 1986; 56:484–491.

81. Mansson E, Willems J, Aparisi T, Jakobsson P, Nilsonne U, Ringborg U: Preoperative radiation therapy of high malignancy grade soft tissue sarcoma. *Acta Radiol Oncol* 1983; 22:461–464.

82. Barkley HT, Martin RG, Romsdah MM, Lindberg R, Zagard GK: Treatment of soft tissue sarcomas by pre-operative irradiation and conservative surgical resection. *Int J Radiat Oncol Biol Phys* 1988;14:693–699.

83. Bell RS, O'Sullivan B, Liu FF, Powell J, Langer F, Fornasier VL, Cummings B, Miceli PH, Hawkins N, Quirt I, Warr D: The surgical margin in soft tissue sarcoma. *J Bone Joint Surg* 1989;71A:370–375.

84. Abbatucci JS, Bouler N, DeRanier J, Mandarad AM, Tanguy A, Vernhes JC, Lozier JC, Busson AP: Local control and survival in soft tissue sarcomas of the limbs, trunk walls and head and neck: A study of 113 cases. *Int J Radiat Oncol Biol Phys* 1986;12:579–586.

85. Brant TA, Parson JT, Marcus RB, Spanier SS, Heare TC, van der Griend RA, Enneking WF, Million RR: Preoperative irradiation for soft tissue sarcomas of the trunk and extremities in adults. *Int J Radiat Oncol Biol Phys* 1990; 19:899–906.

86. Pao WJ, Pilepick MV: Postoperative radiotherapy in the treatment of extremity soft tissue sarcomas. *Int J Radiat Oncol Biol Phys* 1990; 19:907–911.

87. Schray MF, Gunderson LL, Sim FH, Pritchard DJ, Shives TC, Yeakel PD: Soft tissue sarcoma. Integration of brachytherapy, resection and external irradiation. *Cancer* 1990;66: 451–456.

88. Shiu MH, Hilaris BS, Harrison L, Brennan MF: Brachytherapy and function-saving resection of soft tissue sarcoma arising in the limb. *Int J Radiat Oncol Biol Phys* 1991;21: 1485–1492.

89. Robinson M, Cassoni A, Harmer C, Fisher C, Thomas J, Westbury G: High dose hyperfractionated radiotherapy in the treatment of extremity soft tissue sarcomas. *Radiother Oncol* 1991;22:118–126.

90. Yang JC, Chang AE, Baker AR, et al: Randomized prospective study of the benefit of adjuvant radiation therapy in the treatment of soft tissue sarcomas of the extremity. *J Clin Oncol* 1998;16:197–203.

91. Cheng EY, Dusenbery KE, Winters MR, Thompson RC: Soft tissue sarcoma:Pre-operative versus postoperative radiotherapy. *J Surg Oncol* 1996;61:90–99.

92. Neilson OS, Cummings B, O'Sullivan B, et al: Preoperative and postoperative irradiation of soft tissue sarcomas: Effect on radiation field size. *Int J Radiat Oncol Biol Phys* 1991; 21:1595–1599.

93. Sadoski C, Suit H, Rosenberg A, Mankin H, Convery K: Preoperative radiation, surgical margins and local control of extremity sarcomas of soft tissues. *J Surg Oncol* 1993;52: 223–230.

94. Tepper JE, Suit HD: Radiation therapy alone for sarcoma of soft tissue. *Cancer* 1985;56: 475–479.

95. Cade S: Soft tissue tumors: Their natural history and treatment. *Proc R Soc Med* 1951; 44:19.

96. Windeyer B, Dische S, Mansfield CM: The place of radiotherapy in the management of fibrosarcoma of the soft tissues. *Clin Radiol* 1966;17:32–40.

97. McNeer GP, et al: Effectiveness of radiation therapy in management of sarcoma of soft somatic tissues. *Cancer* 1968;22:391–397.

98. Bujko K, Suit HD, Springfield DS, Convery K: Wound healing after surgery and preoperative radiation for sarcoma of soft tissues. *Surg Gynecol Obstet* 1992;176:124–134.

99. Peat BG, Bell RSQ, Davis A, O'Sullivan B, Mahoney J, Manktelow RT, Bowen V, Catton C, Fornasier VL, Langer F: Wound healing complications after soft tissue sarcoma surgery, presented at the American Academy of Orthopedic Surgeons, Washington, DC, February 1992.

100. Arbeit JM, Hilaris B, Brennan MF: Wound complications in the multimodality treatment of extremity and superficial truncal sarcomas. *J Clin Oncol* 1987;5:480–488.

101. LeVay J, O'Sullivan B, Catton C, Bell R, Fornasier V, Cummings B, Hao Y, Warr D, Quirt I: Outcome and prognostic factors in soft tissue sarcoma in the adult. *Int J Radiat Oncol Biol Phys* 1993;27:1091–1099.

102. Robinson MH, Spruce L, Eeles R, et al: Limb function following conservation treatment of adult soft tissue sarcoma. *Eur J Cancer* 1991; 27:1567–1574.

103. Stinson SF, Delaney TF, Greenberg J, et al: *Int J Radiat Oncol Biol Phys* 1991;21:1493–1499.

104. Bramwell V, Rouesse J, Steward W, Santoro A, Schraffordt-Koops H, Buesa J, Ruka W, Priario J, Wagener T, Burgers M, et al: Adjuvant CYVADIC chemotherapy for adult soft tissue sarcoma-reduced local recurrence but no improvement in survival: A study of the European Organization for Research and Treatment of Cancer Soft Tissue and Bone Sarcoma Group. *J Clin Oncol* 1994;12(6):1137–1149.

105. Tierney JF, Mosseri V, Stewart LA, et al: Adjuvant chemotherapy for soft-tissue sarcoma: review and meta-analysis of the published results of randomised clinical trials. *Br J Cancer* 1995;72:469–475.

106. Edmonson JH, Ryan LM, Blum RH, Brooks JSJ, Shiraki M, Frytak S, Parkinson DR: Randomized comparison of doxorubicin alone versus ifosfamide plus doxorubicin or mitomycin, doxorubicin, and cisplatin against advanced soft tissue sarcomas. *J Clin Oncol* 1993;11:1269–1275.

107. Antman K, Crowley J, Balcerzak P, Rivkin SE, Weiss GR, Elias A, Natale RB, Cooper RM, Barlogie B, Trump DL, Doroshow JH, Aisner J, Pugh RP, Weiss RB, Cooper BA, Clamond GH, Baker LH: An intergroup phase III randomized study of coxorubicin and dacarbazine with or without ifosfamide and mesna in advanced soft tissue and bone sarcomas. *J Clin Oncol* 1993;11:1276–1285.

108. Santoro A, Tursz T, Mouridsen H, et al: Doxorubicin versus CYVADIC versus doxorubicin plus ifosfamide in first-line treatment of advanced soft tissue sarcomas: A randomized study of the European Organization for Research and Treatment of Cancer Soft Tissue and Bone Sarcoma Group. *J Clin Oncol* 1995; 13:1537–1545.

109. Spear MA, Jennings LC, Mankin HJ, Spiro IJ, Springfield DS, Gehardt MC, Rosenberg AE, Efird JE, Suit HD: Individualizing management of aggressive fibromatoses. *Int J Radiat Oncol Biol Phys* 1997.

110. Acker JC, Bossen EH, Halperin EC: The management of desmoid tumors. *Int J Radiat Oncol Biol Phys* 1993;26:851–858.

111. Bataini JP, Belloir C: Desmoid tumors in adults: The role of radiotherapy in their management. *Am J Surg* 1988;155:754–760.

112. McCollough WM, Parsons JT, van der Griend R, Enneking WF, Heare T: Radiation therapy for aggressive fibromatosis: The experience at the University of Florida. *J Bone Joint Surg* 1993;73A(5):717–725.

113. Suit HD, Spiro IJ, Mankin HJ, et al: Radiation in management of patients with dermatofibrosarcoma protuberans. *J Clin Oncol* 1996; 14:2365–2369.

114. Suit HD, Rosenberg AE, Harmon DC, Mankin HJ, Wood WC, Rosenthal D: Soft tissue sarcomas, in K Halnan and K Sikora (eds): *Treatment of Cancer,* 2nd ed. London, Chapman and Hall, 1990, pp 657–677.

115. Lindberg RD, Martin RG, Romsdahl MM, Barkley HT Jr: Conservative surgery and postoperative radiotherapy in 300 adults with soft-tissue sarcomas. *Cancer* 1981;47:2391–2397.

116. Abbatucci JS, Boulier N, de Ranieri J, et al: Local control and survival in soft tissue sarcomas of the limbs, trunk walls and head and neck: A study of 113 cases. *Int J Radiat Oncol Biol Phys* 1986;12:579–586.

117. Karakousis CP, Emrich LJ, Rao U, Krishnamsetty RM: Feasibility of limb salvage and survival in soft tissue sarcomas. *Cancer* 1986; 57:484–491.

118. Wilson AN, Davis A, Bell RS, et al: Local control of soft tissue sarcoma of the extremity: The experience of a multidisciplinary sarcoma group with definitive surgery and radiotherapy. *Eur J Cancer* 1994;30A:746–751.

119. Pao WJ, Pilepich MV: Postoperative radiotherapy in the treatment of extremity soft tissue sarcomas. *Int J Radiat Oncol Biol Phys* 1990; 19:907–911.

120. Keus RB, Bartelink H: The role of radiotherapy in the treatment of desmoid tumours. *Radiother Oncol* 1986;7:1–5.

121. Fein DA, Lee WR, Lanciano RM, et al: Management of extremity soft tissue sarcomas with limb-sparing surgery and postoperative irradiation: Do total dose, overall treatment time, and the surgery-radiotherapy interval impact on local control? *Int J Radiat Oncol Biol Phys* 1995;32:969–976.

122. Mundt AJ, Awan A, Sibley GS, et al: Conservative surgery and adjuvant radiation therapy in the management of adult soft tissue sarcoma of the extremities: Clinical and radiobiological results. *Int J Radiat Oncol Biol Phys* 1995; 32:977–985.

123. Barkley HT, Martin RG, Romsdahl MM, Lindberg R, Zagard GK: Treatment of soft tissue sarcomas by preoperative irradiation and conservative surgical resection. *Int J Radiat Oncol Biol Phys* 1988;14:693–699.

124. Brant TA, Parsons JT, Marcus RB, Spanier SS, Heare TC, van der Griend RA, Enneking WF, Million RR: Preoperative irradiation for soft tissue sarcomas of the trunk and extremities in adults. *Int J Radiat Oncol Biol Phys* 1990; 19:899–906.

125. Schray MF, Gunderson LL, Sim FH, Pritchard DJ, Shives TC, Yeakel PD: Soft tissue sarcomas. Integration of brachytherapy, resection, and external irradiation. *Cancer* 1990;6: 451–456.

126. Eilber FR, Eckardt JJ, Rosen G, Fu YS, Seeger LL, Selch MD: Neoadjuvant chemotherapy and radiotherapy in the multidisciliniary management of soft tissue sarcomas of the extremity. *Surg Oncol Clin North Am* 1993;2(4): 611–620.

127. Wanebo HJ, Temple WJ, Popp MB, et al: Preoperative regional therapy for extremity sarcoma. A tricenter update. *Cancer* 1995; 75:2299–2306.

128. Herbert SH, Corn BW, Solin LJ, Lanciano RM, Schultz DJ, McKenna WG, Coia LR: Limb-preserving treatment for soft tissue sarcomas of the extremities. *Cancer* 1993;72: 1230–1238.

129. Tanabe KK, Pollock RE, Ellis LM, Murphy A, Sherman M, Romsdahl MM: Influence of surgical margins on outcome in patients with preoperatively irradiated extremity soft tissue sarcomas. *Cancer* 1994;73:1652–1659.

130. Benjamin RS, Terjanian TO, Genoglio CJ, et al: The importance of combination chemotherapy for adjuvant treatment of high risk patients with soft tissue sarcomas of the extremities, in SE Salmon (ed): *Adjuvant Therapy of Cancer V.* New York, Grune & Stratton, 1987, pp 735–744.

131. Edmonson JH, Fleming TR, Ivans JS, et al: A randomized study of systemic chemotherapy following complete excision of non-osseous sarcomas. *J Clin Oncol* 1984;2:1390–1396.

132. Chang AE, Kinsella T, Glatstein E, et al: Adjuvant chemotherapy for patients with high grade soft tissue sarcomas of the extremity. *J Clin Oncol* 1988;6:1491–1500.

133. Glenn J, Kinsella T, Glatstein E, et al: A randomized, perspective trial of adjuvant chemotherapy in adults with soft tissue sarcomas of the head and neck, breast and trunk. *Cancer* 1985;55:1206–1214.

134. Rosenberg SA: Prospective randomized trials demonstrating the efficacy of adjuvant chemotherapy in adult patients with soft tissue sarcomas. *Cancer Treat Rep* 1984;68:1067–1078.

135. Bui NB, Maree D, Coindre JM, et al: First results of a prospective randomized study of CYVADIC adjuvant chemotherapy in adults with operable high risk soft tissue sarcoma. *Proc ASCO* 1989;8:318 (abstr).

136. Ravaud A, Bui NB, Coindre JM, et al: Adjuvant chemotherapy with CYVADIC in high risk soft tissue sarcoma: A randomized prospective trial, in SE Salmon (ed): *Adjuvant Therapy of Cancer VI.* Philadelphia, Saunders, 1990, pp 556–566.

137. Bramwell VHC, Rouesse J, Santoro A, et al: European experience of adjuvant chemotherapy for soft tissue sarcoma: A randomized trial comparing CYVADIC with control (preliminary report). *Cancer Treat Symp* 1985;3: 99–107.

138. Bramwell V, Rouesse J, Steward W, et al: European experience of adjuvant chemotherapy for soft tissue sarcoma: Interim report of a randomized trial of CYVADIC versus control, in JR Ryan and LO Baker (eds): *Recent Concepts in Sarcoma Treatment.* Dordrecht, Netherlands: Kluwer Academic Publishers, 1988, pp 157–164.

139. Bramwell V, Rouesse J, Steward W, et al: Reduced rate of local recurrence following CYVADIC chemotherapy in localized soft tissue sarcoma. *Proc ASCO* 1989;8:320 (abstr).

140. Bramwell V, Rouesse J, Steward W, et al: Prognostic index for survival in soft tissue sarcoma, in the setting of a randomized trial of adjuvant chemotherapy. *Proceedings of the Fifth European Conference on Clinical Oncology,* London, September 3–7, 1989 (abstr 0-0437).

# CHAPTER 12

# CENTRAL NERVOUS SYSTEM TUMORS

JAY S. LOEFFLER

## INTRODUCTION

The SEER (Surveillance, Epidemiology, and End Results) registry data of the National Cancer Institute from 1973 to 1987 indicate that the combined incidence of recorded primary intracranial and spinal axis tumors is between 2 and 19 in 100,000 persons per year. There appears to be an early peak between 0 and 4 years (3.1 in 100,000) and then a steady rise after the age of 24 years that reaches a plateau (17.9–18.7 in 100,000) between 65 and 79 years of age. While there have been great improvements in our ability to cope with other malignancies, an analysis of trends in survival over the last 20 years in the United States shows a less attractive situation in tumors of the central nervous system. Survival rates in patients with primary malignant brain tumors were recently updated from the SEER data of 1973–1991.[1] This review gave estimates of survival rates at 2 and 5 years after diagnosis for most histological groups and overall improvements in survival rates of patients across these time periods, adjusting for age at diagnosis. There were improvements in 2- and 5-year survival rates over the three time periods for children and adults with medulloblastoma and for adults with astrocytoma and oligodendroglioma. Improvements in survival rates for pediatric patients with medulloblastoma have leveled off in the most recent time period, and

gender differences in survival rates for patients with this tumor, which were present in the 1970s, have disappeared. Glioblastoma multiforme, the most common primary brain tumor, remains intractable, although 2-year survival rates for these patients have improved twofold. Clinically significant improvements in survival rates were not apparent in patients aged 65 years and older. Changes in diagnostic and treatment procedures since the mid-1970s have resulted in improved survival rates for these selected young patients. These improvements are not explained by a shift in the patient age at diagnosis over time and suggest that we have made therapeutic advances in some brain tumor histologies. However, significant improvement in survival rates do not compare favorably with gains with respect to other malignancies. For instance, in Hodgkin disease comparable survival rates for the same periods have risen, respectively, from 50% to 80%. In addition to primary brain tumors, the problem of metastatic involvement by tumors originating in other organs and spreading hematogenously represents a significant health care problem. Also, certain tumors arise in tissues adjacent to the brain or spinal cord and may extend by direct invasion to cause neurologic sequelae, too. It is estimated that between 30% and 40% of patients who have a malignant diagnosis will at some point experience and suffer the consequences of involvement of the central nervous system.

*Clinical Radiation Oncology: Indications, Techniques, and Results, 2nd ed.* Edited by C.C. Wang.
ISBN: 0-471-23803-1   Copyright © 2000 Wiley-Liss, Inc.

## EPIDEMIOLOGY

Very little is known of the epidemiology of primary tumors of the central nervous system (CNS). Although differences in the age, sex, and ethnic distribution of primary brain tumors by histologic subtypes suggest that some types have distinct causes, few analytic epidemiologic studies have separated these tumors based on subtypes. Clearly, there are some genetic conditions known to carry an increased propensity, as in neurofibromatosis type 1 (NF-1), where both benign and malignant CNS tumors occur more frequently than in a normal population.[2] NF-1 is an autosomal dominant disorder associated with defective production of the protein neurofibromin coded for by a gene on chromosome 17. Approximately 15% of NF-1 patients have low grade optic pathway gliomas, cerebellar astrocytomas, pilocytic astrocytomas of the third ventricle, and high grade gliomas. NF-2, a much less common autosomal dominant disorder, typically manifests as a bilateral eighth nerve schwannoma and ependymomas, meningiomas, and other cranial nerve schwannomas. Li–Fraumeni syndrome is an autosomal dominant aggregation of osteosarcoma and other soft tissue sarcomas, breast cancer and, to a lesser degree, gliomas. Turcot syndrome is an inherited adenomatous polyposis coli associated with astrocytomas and medulloblastoma. Other CNS tumors that can be inherited include retinoblastomas and paragangliomas. In addition to these specific genetic syndromes associated with brain tumors, it has been estimated that 4% of families with an affected child carry a "brain tumor gene." With respect to adults, genetic factors appear to play a strong role in the development of primary brain tumors with up to 30% of patient with glioblastoma multiforme having a first-degree relative with cancer.

Ionizing radiation is a known induction agent, and cases of glioma, meningioma, schwannoma, and sarcoma of the CNS have been recorded in patients who underwent irradiation (1.5 Gy) to the scalp in childhood for tinea capitis.[3] It has been estimated that the risk of second tumor formation following irradiation is between 1% and 3% at 20 years following therapy.[4] Dose and volume of CNS irradiated are important parameters associated with second tumor formation. This must be kept in mind when one is informing children and young adults about their risks; moreover, it represents an added incentive to reduce the irradiated volume by using conformal techniques when possible. Exposure to electromagnetic fields, CNS trauma, the use of cellular phones, and other environmental and occupational factors have not clearly been associated with brain tumor formation.

## CLINICAL PRESENTATION

The clinical presentation of brain tumors is best considered by relating signs and symptoms to anatomy. Intracranial tumors produce symptoms primarily by two mechanisms: mass effect from the tumor and mass effect from vasogenic edema leading to increased intracranial pressure. Headaches and seizures are the most common general signs and symptoms of brain tumors. However, gastrointestinal symptoms such as nausea, loss of appetite, or even vomiting can be seen, particularly with infratentorial tumors of childhood. Sometimes the only presenting symptoms are changes in personality, mood, mental capacity, and concentration. Occasionally a slow deterioration of psychomotor activity is the antecedent symptoms of intracranial tumor. Some patients present with a constellations of signs that are specific for exact tumor location. For instance, patients with tectal or pineal region tumors often have a complete or partial Parinaud syndrome, defined as a lack of convergence, pupillary areflexia, and paralysis of upward gaze. It must be remembered, however, that none of these symptoms are unique to brain tumors and can easily be confused with nonneoplastic disorders. Benign tumors of the skull base can present with cranial nerve abnormalities including hearing loss (vestibular schwannoma), visual disturbances (parasellar tumors), and endocrine abnormalities (pituitary adenomas).

## NEUROIMAGING

The diagnosis of intracranial and spinal tumors requires sophisticated neuroimaging. Today MRI and CT scanning are routine diagnostic procedures for patients suspected of harboring a brain tumor. Angiography is rarely required except in cases of large vascular benign tumors such paragangliomas and meningiomas, where the angiography is used for surgical planning or for preoperative embolization. CT imaging is based on electron density, whereas MRI is based on proton density. Unlike CT, MRI can generate images in all three orthogonal planes and offers high resolution and contrast without associated bone artifacts (an extremely important property when it is necessary to evaluate posterior fossa tumors). MRI is superior to CT in detecting and localizing brain tumors and evaluating edema, hydrocephalus, and hemorrhage. CT is superior to MRI in detecting calcifications in tumors such as oligodendroglioma and craniopharyngioma, as well as in detecting bony abnormalities of the skull. The use of contrast agents with CT and MRI provides tumor visualization and an improved ability to discern tumor type and grade. At our institution, contrast material is included when any patient suspected of having a brain tumor is evaluated, as well as in postradiotherapy follow-up visits. Approximately 50% of patients with low grade and anaplastic astrocytoma present with tumors that do not exhibit contrast enhancement.

Essentially all glioblastoma, meningioma, ependymoma, lymphoma, germinoma, and craniopharyngioma metastasis lesions exhibit brisk, but often irregular enhancement. In the evaluation of intramedullary and extramedullary spinal cord lesions, MRI is the diagnostic study of choice. Indications for myelography are limited, because multiplanar MRI with contrast can visualize almost all intrinsic tumors as well as aiding in the diagnosis of leptomeningeal disease. MRI is also extremely important in radiotherapy treatment planning because of the ability to delineate the extent of edema as well as the ability to use sagittal and coronal images. Techniques of CT and MRI imaging fusion have recently been developed and are routinely employed for our efforts in stereotactic radiation and proton planning. Following high dose radiotherapy, routine MRI or CT often cannot help in the differential of tumor recurrence from radiation injury based on morphological changes. We often use functional MRI, MR spectroscopy, single-photon emission tomography (SPECT), and positron emission tomography (PET) alone, or in combination to aid in this important distinction.[5]

## PATHOLOGY

The goal of this chapter is not to review in detail issues concerning neuropathology. Before treatment recommendations are made, however, a brief review is required. All intracranial tumors, whether histologically well differentiated and relatively "benign" or undifferentiated and malignant, are potentially lethal because of their confinement within the cranium. Neuroglial tumors as a group are referred to as gliomas. They are derived from neuroglia or, more specifically, from astrocytes, oligodendrocytes, and ependymal cells. Astrocytomas represent the most varied spectrum histologically of all other glial tumors. Differentiation, pleomorphism, hyperchromasia, degree of cellularity, mitotic index, necrosis, and vascular proliferation are used to determine whether a given tumor is an astrocytoma low grade, anaplastic, or a glioblastoma multiforme. The modified Ringertz[6] method places predominant emphasis on cellularity and nuclear pleomorphism for the second tier (anaplastic astrocytoma, grade 2/3), with necrosis and pseudopalisading defining glioblastoma (grade 3/3). The Daumas-Duport scheme[7] places equal weight on each of four histologic features: pleomorphism, mitoses, vascular proliferation, and necrosis. Since most well-differentiated astrocytomas have some nuclear pleomorphism they are grade 2/4, while those of higher grade are grade 3/4 or 4/4, depending on the number of negative pathological features.

In our experience at the Massachusetts General Hospital (MGH), we have found that the Daumas-Duport system predicts survival better than the modified Ringertz system.[8] Pilocytic astrocytomas are not classified in either system, since they are clinically and histologically distinct. With the use of MRI, more cases of gliomatosis cerebri are diagnosed, particularly in the elderly population. In this case the gliomas diffusely infiltrate the brain, often without a single mass lesion. Regardless of histology (low grade vs. high grade), these patients respond poorly to radiotherapy and have a projected survival measured in months. In general, well-differentiated oligodendrogliomas have a better prognosis than well-differentiated astrocytomas.

Often "mixed tumors" are seen that appear to have features of both astrocytes and oligodendrogliomas. Anaplastic oligodendrogliomas have a different natural history, and treatment recommendations differ quite distinctly from those of their well-differentiated counterpart. Ependymomas, as the name implies, arise from ependymal lining of the ventricular system. Although they occur at any age, the majority occur near the fourth ventricle of children. Ependymomas and astrocytomas are the most common spinal cord tumors. Transitions in ependymoma to regions of frank anaplasia with hypercellularity, pleomorphism, abundant mitoses, necrosis, and vascular endothelial hyperplasia may occur. We refer to this variant as an anaplastic ependymoma. Myxopapillary ependymoma is often included within the ependymoma family because the prominent cellular constituent is the ependymal cell. However, it is clinically and pathologically different from a classical ependymoma, occurring most often in the filum terminale.

Tumors that contain neoplastic ganglionic and glial elements are called ganglioglioma. These tumors were rarely seen in the CT era, but with the use of MRI the diagnosis is more frequently made. They, in general, are well-circumscribed lesions that rarely require radio-

therapy. Medulloblastoma is the most common tumor of the posterior fossa in children. In some institutions it is referred to as a primitive neuroectodermal tumor (PNET). These lesions differ in their biological character from glial tumors in that almost all medulloblastomas will seed the pathways of the cerebrospinal fluid (CSF) without craniospinal therapy. Extracranial metastases (particularly bone) are seen more frequently in recent years with improved therapies to control CNS disease.

Meningiomas as a group are most prevalent in middle age, even though they can occur throughout life. There is a striking predilection for women, with an occurrence of 2:1 for intracranial lesions and up to 9:1 for intradural spinal lesions. Children rarely develop meningiomas, but when they do the tumors often behave in a more aggressive fashion. Meningiomas are called atypical when they exhibit high cellularity, nuclear pleomorphism, prominent nucleoli, mitotic activity, micronecrosis, and high nuclear–cytoplasmic ratios. When brain invasion and cytological evidence of frank malignancy is found, the term "malignant meningioma" is applied. The most common tumors involving the pineal region, in decreasing order of frequency, are germ cell tumors, pineal parenchymal tumors, glial tumors, and metastatic lesions. The histologic confirmation is required, since the treatments for the various histologies vary greatly.

Primary central nervous system lymphoma (PCNSL) grows in sheets of cells, infiltrating the brain parenchyma between blood vessels in a characteristic vasocentric pattern. In the immunocompetent patients the vast majority of lymphomas within the CNS are of B-lymphocyte origin. According to the Working Formulation definitions, 50% of PCNSLs in immunocompetent patients were large cell, with the next most common histologic type being immunoblastic. AIDS-associated PCNSLs are small and noncleaved in a much higher proportion than in their immunocompetent counterparts.

We sometimes use lumbar puncture for examination of the cerebral spinal fluid in patients without evidence on CT or MRI of mass effect; this practice permits us to evaluate tumor markers or cytology to aid in radiation treatment planning. These studies are particularly helpful in determining the risk of CSF dissemination that would influence the use of limited-field radiotherapy versus craniospinal therapy or pre- or postradiotherapy chemotherapy. In these patients we examine the CSF for malignant cells, protein, glucose, and specific markers such as β-human chorionic gonadotrophic hormone (b-HCG) and α-fetoprotein (AFP).

A schematic presentation of CNS tumors is presented in outline form follows.

### Congenital Tumor of Maldevelopmental Origin

1. Teratoma [e.g., pineal tumor (central), spinal cord cysts (peripheral)]
2. Dermoid and epidermoid
3. Craniopharyngioma

### Dysgenetic Syndrome Associated with Tumor

1. Lindau syndrome (capillary hemangioblastoma)
2. Tuberous sclerosis
3. von Recklinghausen neurofibromatosis
4. Neurocutaneous melanosis–melanoma of the leptomeninges

### Tumors of Glial Origin

1. Astrocytoma
2. Oligodendroglioma
3. Ependymoma
   a. Subependymoma
   b. Choroid plexus papilloma
   c. Colloid cyst

### Tumors of Neuron Origin

1. Medulloblastoma
2. Medulloepithelioma

3. Neuroblastoma
4. Ganglioneuroma and ganglioglioma

## TREATMENT

### Surgery

While this textbook deals mainly with the radiotherapeutic approach to malignancies, it is impossible to discuss neuro-oncology without mentioning some aspects of surgery. No other modality can reduce tumor bulk as quickly as surgery. Surgery is the most important initial therapy of patients with operable brain tumors. Recent advances in image-guided surgery have made operative approaches to tumors in even the most remote areas of the CNS possible and reasonably safe. Functional mapping during surgery, stereotactic navigation systems, and intraoperative MR-guided surgery are recent examples in new technologies applied to brain tumor surgery. The goal of brain tumor surgery is to resect and cure the tumor completely without the requirement of any adjuvant therapy. This is possible for the majority of patients with convexity meningiomas, pituitary microadenomas, vestibular schwannomas, pilocytic astrocytomas, neurocytomas, and gangliogliomas. If surgical cure is not possible (e.g., for malignant gliomas), there must be tumor reduction and decompression of the brain to allow for adjuvant therapies to be initiated. The extent of surgical resection in patients with medulloblastoma, low grade astrocytoma, and ependymoma correlates with survival even though all these patients require postoperative radiotherapy. Patient tolerance of cranial radiotherapy is improved dramatically when surgical debulking has been done. Another benefit of surgical resection is to provide enough tissue for adequate histopathological examination. We rarely recommend radiotherapy to a patient without a histological tissue diagnosis. Exceptions are discussed later, in the radiotherapy section.

## Low Grade Hemispheric Astrocytoma, Oligodendroglioma, and "Mixed Tumors"

Well-differentiated or low grade gliomas constitute a heterogeneous group of intracranial and spinal tumors. Over 2000 cases of low grade gliomas are diagnosed per year in the United States. The vast variability of their behavior has led to uncertainties regarding their prognosis as well as debate about the form and timing of therapy. In our experience at the MGH, approximately 25% are amenable to complete gross resection. Over the past several years, our understanding of the clinical behavior of low grade astrocytomas has increased through studies of tumor proliferation, DNA content, and both cytogenetic and molecular genetic studies. The variety of methods we use at the MGH to measure proliferation include proliferating cell nuclear antigen (PCNA) labeling index, flow cytometry, and Ki-67. Others have used bromodeoxyuridine (BUdR) given 30 minutes before surgery, as well as determining the labeling index of the pathological specimen. Several groups have observed a correlation between labeling index with survival. A labeling index of below 1% is a very good prognostic feature, and in fact in a multivariate analysis is a better predictor of survival than grade.

The mean age at presentation at our hospital is 35 years, with some patients being younger than 10 and some older than 70 years of age. Seizure activity is the most common presenting symptom in our experience. Patients who present with seizures with no other neurological symptoms have a better prognosis than patients who have mental status changes or other neurological signs or symptoms. Age is clearly the most important clinical factor associated with survival. Mean survival from diagnosis in patients less than 40 years of age is approximately 8 years, versus 5 years for the patients over the age of 40 years. MRI (both T2- and T1-weighted images) is clearly the imaging technique of choice, since it can best delineate the extent of tumor. Approximately one-third of the low grade astrocytoma patients at our institution have some mild enhancement on MRI scanning. The T2-weighted image is very important for the radiation oncologist, since the treatment volume should include the T2 extent with a few centimeters of "normal brain" with the full-dose prescription isodose contour.

It should not be standard practice to observe a patient who has had a seizure and is seen, on MRI, to have a hemispheric, nonenhancing lesion. Depending on the age of the patient, up to 25% of younger patients and up to 50% of older patients ($> 40$ years) will actually have a diagnosis of anaplastic astrocytoma at the time of resection or biopsy. Historically, the decision to observe a patient after a histologic diagnosis of low grade astrocytoma has been justified in the literature for several reasons, including lack of proven benefit of any invasive intervention including surgery with or without radiotherapy and the potential morbidity of any treatment. The Mayo Clinic has recently published that institution's experience with patients with supratentorial low grade astrocytomas, oligoastrocytomas, and oligodendrogliomas.[9] The observed survival curve is statistically worse than that of an age- and sex-matched control population, in which the expected survival is greater than 95%. Based on this observation, the argument could be made for having these patients undergo aggressive resection when possible, and postoperative radiotherapy. However, a survival benefit from aggressive surgery and radiotherapy has not been demonstrated in a prospective, randomized clinical trial. The European Organization for the Research and Treatment of Cancer (EORTC) has completed a prospective, randomized trial (EORTC 22845) in patients with low grade hemispheric gliomas of all histologic types (excluding pilocytic astrocytomas) in which patients following surgery were randomized to observation (with radiotherapy reserved at the time of radiographic or clinical regrowth) versus an initial 54 Gy of limited field radiotherapy. The trial has completed the accrual process, and when the results have matured, they will be analyzed and published.

If patients are recommended for postoperative radiotherapy, the decision of total dose has not been established. The EORTC trial 22844 was recently published addressing this issue.[10] This trial randomized 379 patients following surgery or biopsy with cerebral low grade gliomas to receive either 45 Gy in 5 weeks or 59.4 Gy in 6.6 weeks. With a median follow-up period of 74 months, there was no significant difference in survival (58% for low dose arm and 59% for the high dose arm) or the progression-free survival (47% and 50%) between the two dose arms. In a subset analysis, T classification (stage based on size and extent of central invasion), performance status (favoring higher performance status), extent of surgery (more tumor removed better survival), and histologic type (pure astrocytomas faring the worst) were all independent prognostic factors for survival. It is possible that with further follow-up a survival difference will be seen.

At the MGH, the decision to recommend radiotherapy depends on biological indicators of proliferation (labeling) and the consequence of radiotherapy. For instance a patient might have a small tumor, but a labeling index exceeding 3. In this patient we would recommend postoperative radiotherapy. However, a patient with a very large lesion with a low proliferative index might be observed because of our concern of the known late effects of treating such a large volume of the brain in a patient with a projected survival of 5 years or more. If contrast enhancement (possibly representing a higher grade component) is present on CT and/or MRI scanning, we recommend that area be biopsied in helping to determine the need of possible radiotherapy. The appropriate radiation volume should included the MRI T2-weighted extent of the tumor plus a 2 to 3 cm circumferential margin. Conformal radiotherapy techniques are strongly encouraged to reduce normal CNS irradiation. Figure 12-1 demonstrates a dose distribution by means of conformal techniques for a patient with a subtotally resected low grade astrocytoma. We currently prescribe 54 Gy in 30 fractions.

There is no clear role of chemotherapy for patients with low grade gliomas. For young children, preirradiation chemotherapy has been used as a modality to delay radiotherapy until further development in an attempt to reduce radiation late effects to the CNS. An intergroup study of the Radiation Therapy Oncology

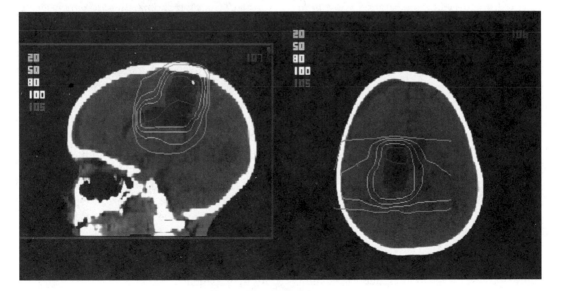

**FIGURE 12-1**    Dose distribution for conformal radiotherapy for a 42-year-old woman being treated for a subtotally resected low grade astrocytoma. Patient received 54 Gy in 30 fractions.

Group (RTOG 94-02), Eastern Cooperative Oncology Group (ECOG R94-02), and the Southwestern Oncology Group (SWOG 94-02) has recently begun for patients with low grade oligodendrogliomas and anaplastic oligodendrogliomas. The study will randomize patients to radiotherapy alone (59.4 Gy in 33 fractions) versus four cycles of procarbazine, vincristine, and CCNU (PCV) followed by the same radiotherapy. This study was initiated after it was found that patients with anaplastic oligodendrogliomas often exhibit dramatic (albeit of short duration) responses to PCV at the time of recurrence following radiotherapy.

The late toxicity of limited-field radiotherapy to doses has recently been studied. Taphoorn et al.[11] studied patients with histologically confirmed low grade gliomas who were followed or irradiated using conformal techniques to doses of between 45 and 63 Gy. The patients were studied prospectively with detailed neuropsychological testing, with an average follow-up period of 3.5 years. There were no differences in performance status and results of neuropsychological testing in the group observed versus the group irradiated. It has been our observation that patients undergo a bimodal pattern of neurocognitive effects following limited-field radiotherapy for low grade gliomas. At about 6 months patients complain of some short-term memory problems, but 6 to 12 months later feel that their memory skills have returned to normal. Clearly, neurocognitive effects of radiotherapy are related to volume irradiated, location of the irradiation, total dose and fractionation employed, technique, and any preexisting neurocognitive damage from the tumor and/or surgery.

## Malignant Gliomas

In this section we will review high grade anaplastic astrocytoma (AA) and glioblastoma multiforme (GBM). These tumors represent the majority of primary CNS tumors of adults. They occur 10 times more frequently in adults than in children. AA and GBM can appear hypodense, isodense, or hyperdense on nonenhanced CT scanning. Following intravenous contrast, essentially all GBM will enhance, and approximately 50% of AA, on CT scanning. MRI has superseded CT scanning for diagnostic and follow-up imaging as well as for surgery and radiation planning. The volume of tumor cell containing edema is usually larger on MRI than on CT. Among the major prognostic variables that have been identified are histology (GBM vs. AA), age, and performance status.[12] These prognostic variables are important to understand when one is evaluating treatment results of clinical trials.

The therapy for these lesions begins with surgery. Maximum surgical resection allows for rapid reduction of mass effect as well as permitting adjuvant therapies to be delivered with reduced acute effects and the need of corticosteroids. Several retrospective studies restricted to GBM of the cerebral hemispheres support the role of maximum resection in extending median survival. If resection cannot be performed because of tumor location or comorbid illness, a biopsy is required before irradiation can be recommend. We have had several cases at the MGH over the last several years where a diagnosis other than high grade astrocytoma was found. These included multiple sclerosis, primary CNS lymphoma, infection, metastatic disease, and atypical meningioma.

For all patients with AA and GBM, radiotherapy is recommended following surgical intervention. Radiotherapy remains the most important adjunct to surgery. The 12-month survival of surgery alone is 3%, versus 24% with surgery and radiotherapy.[13] Radiotherapy should start no earlier than 2 weeks following surgery to allow for wound healing. The treatment volume should include the entire preoperative T2-weighted extent plus a 1 to 2 cm margin for potential setup error. Opposed lateral fields should be avoided if possible to reduce the dose to the cerebral cortex as well as to the scalp. CT- and/or MRI-based three-dimensional treatment planning is recommended for these patients.

Conventional radiotherapy for AA and GBM is delivered to a total dose of 60 Gy in approximately 30 fractions, 1.8 to 2.0 Gy per fraction. Attempts to use higher total doses with routine fractionation have not been successful and have been associated with unacceptable complications. Altered fractionation schemes have been used not only to increase the total dose, but also to reduce treatment time. Hyperfractionation refers to the administration of a larger number of individual treatments, each of smaller fraction size, in the conventional time. Phase I and II trials sponsored by the RTOG found that survival rates were higher for patients receiving 72 Gy (1 Gy BID) than for three alternative fraction schemes.[14] A phase III trial has been proposed to study 72 Gy delivered in a hyperfractionated scheme versus 60 Gy given once daily.

We recently completed an accelerated hyperfractionation phase II study for patients with GBM at the MGH. Accelerated fractionation reduces the overall treatment time, which has shown to be important in certain head and neck tumor trials.[15] We treated 23 patients to a total dose of 90 Gy at 1.8 Gy BID over 4.5 weeks. The median survival of this group was 20 months, but the rate of symptomatic radiation necrosis was quite high.[16]

Other methods to escalate the dose of radiation in a conformal fashion involve stereotactic technology. The two most commonly used techniques are stereotactic brachytherapy and stereotactic radiosurgery. The results for highly selected patients (relatively small tumors in patients with good performance) treated with stereotactic "boost" therapy using temporary high activity $^{125}$I seeds or radiosurgery following 60 Gy of external beam radiotherapy demonstrate the following: (1) median survival rates for GBM patients are 18 to 27 months; (2) 30% to 50% of patients become steroid dependent and require a reoperation for radiation tumor necrosis; (3) brachytherapy and radiosurgery produce equivalent survival and complication rates; and (4) the most common site of tumor progression is immediately outside the boost volume.[17] Since radiosurgery is a single-day outpatient procedure, it has become the more commonly used technique. These sur-

vival results using stereotactic techniques have been criticized because of the potential patient selection biases that are intrinsic to these radiation modalities. The RTOG is currently conducting a phase III trial randomizing patients with GBM lesions less than 4 cm following surgery to radiotherapy and BCNU alone versus radiosurgery and radiotherapy and BCNU.

## Primary CNS Lymphoma (PCNSL)

PCNSL is defined as a non-Hodgkin lymphoma that is confined to the craniospinal axis without systemic involvement. It should not be confused with systemic lymphoma that has spread to the CNS. PCNSL can occur in the immunocompetent and immunocompromised populations. Since the treatment and outcomes for these two groups are different, they are discussed separately in this chapter.

PCNSL is seen in patients with acquired and congenital immunodeficiencies.[18] The largest group of immunocompromised patients seen with PCNSL consists of those infected with the human immunodeficiency virus (HIV). In particular, patients with the diagnosis of acquired immunodeficiency syndrome (AIDS) are at particularly high risk for PCNSL. The median age of an immunocompromised PCNSL patient is 31 years. The lymphoma tends to occur at the end of the disease process when these patients are most immunosuppressed. Since a patient with AIDS who has an enhancing lesion on CT or MRI with mental status changes may not have PCNSL (e.g., toxoplasmosis), we recommend a stereotactic biopsy before radiotherapy is initiated. We recommend that 30 to 40 Gy be given to the whole brain in 3 to 4 weeks. Chemotherapy has no role in these terminally ill patients.

PCNSL in the immunocompetent patient has a median age at diagnosis of 55 years and pathologically is usually a large-cell or immunoblastic lymphoma.[18] Radiographic findings are indicative of single or multiple lesions, usually with some periventricular involvement. The lesions often are hyperdense on CT and can dramatically respond to corticosteroid therapy. Systemic workup for extracranial lymphoma is not required. Radiotherapy alone (40 Gy whole brain with a 20 Gy boost) can produce a 12-month median survival. The use of preradiation chemotherapy of high dose systemic methotrexate (MTX 3.5 g/m$^2$ × 3) followed by whole-brain radiotherapy has produced median survival of nearly 4 years.[19] Other chemotherapy regimens that include intravenous and intraventricular MTX and cytarabine have also produced far better survival than seen in those patients treated with radiotherapy alone. It has been our experience, however, that older patients can develop significant neurocognitive damage from this combined modality approach, and we currently recommend either chemotherapy or radiotherapy alone for patients over the age of 60 years. The vitreous fluid must be carefully evaluated by slit-lamp examination before radiotherapy is initiated, since chemotherapy does not get access to the vitreous fluid. For these patients, the vitreous fluid must be included in the whole brain field. The RTOG is currently completing a trial of combined modality therapy for immunocompetent patients with PCNSL based on the regime developed by investigators from Memorial Sloan-Kettering Cancer Center.

## Meningioma

Meningioma accounts for 14% of intracranial tumors overall and 3% of childhood intracranial tumors. Spinal meningioma is rarer; only 10% to 12% of all meningiomas are in this category. Meningioma occurs most commonly in the middle years and more frequently in women. Hyperostosis is often associated with these lesions, and trauma may well play a role in etiology. Four types of benign tumor—syncytial, transitional, fibroblastic, and angioblastic—are generally recognized. Psammoma bodies are very characteristic of these tumors.

Complete surgical resection is curative in the vast majority of patients with benign meningiomas. Radiotherapy is restricted to patients with incompletely resected or recurrent lesions. Some patients with inoperable progressive le-

sions benefit from radiotherapy. Our review of the recurrence and progression patterns following neurosurgical resection at MGH was published in 1985.[20] Surgery has always been the treatment of choice in this disease and perhaps the only treatment to be considered. There were 225 cases eligible for full review: 168 women and 57 men; 20% were convexity lesions, 17% parasagittal and falx, 16% spheroid ridge, 14% posterior fossa, 12% parasellar, 10% olfactory groove, and 8% spinal lesions. Radiological progression was scored and in patients thought to have complete removal we recognized that at 5, 10, and 15 years there was a probability of second surgery for recurrence of 6%, 15%, and 20%, respectively. Comparable figures for subtotally resected lesions were 37%, 55%, and 91%, respectively. Clearly, the extent of surgery is key, and at certain sites (e.g., the spheroid ridge), where removal is rarely complete, the recurrence rate was highest. The probability of a third resection was 45% at 5 years and 56% at 10 years. Only 10 patients not operated on for a third time were alive and well with no evidence of meningioma, with a mean follow-up time of 4 years at the time of the analysis.

In 1975 Wara et al.[21] reported their data on the role of irradiation following subtotal resection. It appeared that recurrence was less common and substantially delayed when external beam doses of 45 to 55 Gy were used. Goldsmith et al.[22] recently updated the experience from the University of California, San Francisco, showing that in the CT era postoperative radiotherapy can prevent tumor regrowth in more than 90% at 10 years.

Our current recommendations for patients with benign meningiomas are the following: (1) following complete resection observation only; (2) following subtotal resection, 54 Gy of conformal external beam radiotherapy in 30 fractions to the enhancing residual tumor only; (3) observation and radiotherapy at the time of documented tumor growth; and (4) conformal radiotherapy for patients with symptomatic inoperable lesions. Figure 12-2 shows a dose distribution for a patient with an optic nerve sheath meningioma treated with stereotactic ra-

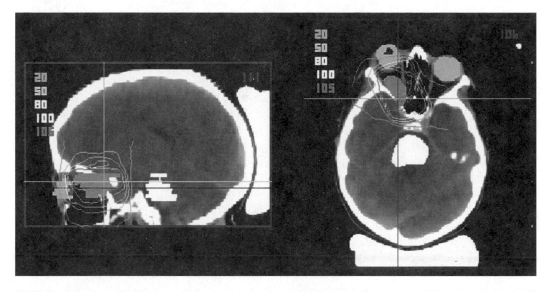

**FIGURE 12-2**   Dose distribution using stereotactic fractionated radiotherapy for a patient with an optic nerve sheath meningioma. Patient's vision improved during the first 3 months following therapy and remains stable 4 years later. He received 54 Gy in 30 fractions using four noncoplanar fields of stereotactically directed radiation. Independent jaws were used for the arc therapy.

diotherapy. We and others have a growing experience with radiosurgery for selected patients with residual or recurrent small meningiomas. Control rates appear to be similar to those seen following fractionated radiotherapy with serious complication rates of less than 5%. Radiosurgery cannot be used if any component of the optic apparatus receives more than 8 Gy.[23]

Recommendations are quite different for patients with atypical or malignant meningiomas and for patients with benign meningiomas. Based on the results of a retrospective review of these patients treated at our institution, we recommend high dose (> 60 Gy) larger volume postoperative therapy even in the absence of postoperative disease. We are currently conducting a phase II trial with these patients in which a combination of photons and protons serves to deliver 68.4 Gy in 38 fractions.

## Pituitary Tumors

Pituitary tumors are almost always benign. The rare malignant form accounts for less than 1% of the total. As a group they come to medical attention in three principal ways: (1) as a mass lesion, sometimes causing raised intracranial pressure; (2) with effects on the optic pathway (classically, chiasmal compression, although eccentric growth patterns may lead to a unilateral field defect in some patients); and (3) by altered endocrine states.

Substantially more is now known about secretory or functioning adenomas, which represent 75% of the group.[24] Some 65% secrete prolactin: when the normal inhibitory mechanism exerted by the hypothalamus fails, serum prolactin rises, leading to amenorrhea and infertility in the female. While many patients simply have microadenoma, studies have shown that serum levels greater than 100 ng/mL commonly indicate tumor, and such patients should be evaluated accordingly.

Fifteen percent of pituitary tumors secrete growth hormone. Fasting levels less than 3 ng/mL exclude this; values greater than 30 ng/mL are diagnostic. It is interesting that there is no meaningful correlation between high serum levels and severity of acromegaly by clinical criteria. It is believed currently that levels of somatomedin C or insulin-like growth factor 1 (IGF-1) levels are a more accurate correlation of treatment success than growth hormone alone. Interestingly, between 25% and 40% of acromegalic patients also show raised prolactin levels related to pituitary "stalk effect." Clearly both situations need regular monitoring for optimum patient care. It is also worth noting that occasionally growth hormone may be produced ectopically by other tumors; for example, lung cancer and stomach and breast primaries have all been identified in this setting.

Cushing disease is now a term that should be limited to the overproduction of corticotropin by the pituitary itself. Nelson syndrome, which represents the extreme when a frank pituitary tumor follows bilateral adrenalectomy, is often associated with hyperpigmentation. Other hypersecretion syndromes of pituitary tumor are thyroid-stimulating hormone, which accounts for less than 1% of all functioning tumors, and tumors secreting both follicle-stimulating hormone (FSH) and luteinizing hormone (LH), although the latter two cases are exceedingly rare.

Hardy and Vezina[25] have proposed a staging system for pituitary tumors that would include tumor size, amount and type of bone destruction, and supra- and extrasellar extension. This would allow better comparisons of treatments offered currently. It grades tumors I to IV for sellar size, with 4 degrees of suprasellar extension: types I through IV.

Surgery, irradiation, and medical management are all relevant in the treatment of pituitary tumors. The goal of treatment can be summarized thus: to reduce or eliminate tumor and to prevent recurrence, while restoring or maintaining anterior pituitary function with prolactin levels remaining within the normal range. As our understanding of pituitary function has increased, it has become clear that for many patients a combination of treatment approaches is often better than one treatment alone. Surgery is the primary need in many patients—for example, to deal speedily with the effects of large mass lesions with secondary hydrocephalus. A shunting procedure may also

be required initially. When the visual pathway is compromised, surgery is also strongly indicated. Prior to 1970 craniotomy was required, carrying with it a mortality quoted at between 2% and 35% in different series, and often significant morbidity ensued too.

Transsphenoidal surgery, which has gained great currency since 1970, has now superseded craniotomy and carries with it no more than a 0.9% risk of mortality and an overall morbidity of 14%, which consists of CSF leak, infection, and (rarely) visual pathway damage.[26] It offers decompression and the opportunity to sample sufficient tissue for detailed staining to document the functional nature of each individual tumor. By this approach, the goal of long-term cure can be best served. Many series exist documenting the late recurrence of microadenoma treated by surgery alone. A recent survey of 80 neurosurgeons who use the procedure frequently suggests an 80% control rate of this process by surgery alone, meaning that some 20% of patients develop other lesions.[26]

External beam irradiation as fractionated therapy plays a major role in the management of macroadenomas, whether functioning or nonfunctioning. Primary surgery will commonly be the initial treatment, but the control of suprasellar or extrasellar disease requires the alternative of irradiation. Bromocriptine in a prolactin-secreting tumor is a viable alternative to surgery or radiotherapy, with the later two being reserved for medical failure or toxicity. Ketaconazole has been used as adjunct to surgery and radiotherapy for Cushing disease and Octreotide as an adjunct for patients with acromegaly.

When radiotherapy is indicated, several techniques can be employed. Fractionated stereotactic radiotherapy using multiple noncoplanar arcs produces a very conformal dose distribution, reducing dose to the hypothalamus and temporal lobes.[27] Three-field static technique using high energy photons is another approach. In this approach opposed lateral fields are complemented by a superior anterior oblique field, with the chin being rested against the sternum. Single-dose proton radiosurgery and fractionated protons are also used in our institution in special clinical situations. Since the target is a benign lesion and the patients have a long survival, every effort should be employed to use these conformal techniques when possible. Our current recommendation is to deliver 45 Gy in 25 fractions for hormonally inactive adenomas and between 55.8 and 60 Gy for hormonally active lesions. It must be remembered that normalization of the abnormally produced hormones takes several years, and these patients should stay on medical therapy until that occurs. Secondary pituitary dysfunction requiring hormonal replacement develops in over 50% of patients by 5 years from the completion of pituitary radiotherapy.[28] These patients required careful endocrinological follow-up, particularly younger patients who might need growth hormone replacement as well as follow-up for fertility issues.

***Tumors of the Pineal Region*** Tumors arising in the pineal region, around the region of the third ventricle and in the suprasellar region, represent less than 1% of all intracranial tumors of adults and between 5% and 11% in children. Clinical symptoms and signs at presentation are extremely helpful in reaching a likely diagnosis, even in the absence of a histologic confirmation. The presence of diabetes insipidus in a teenage patient with delayed or absent development of secondary sexual characteristics or other pituitary dysfunction nearly always indicates a pineal region tumor. Other less common findings related to the compression of the dorsal tectum or its projection include nystagmus, hearing loss, and ataxia.[5]

Tumors of the pineal region may be classified into four different histogenic groups:

1. Tumors of germ cell origin (germinoma, teratoma, embryonal carcinoma, choriocarcinoma, and endodermal sinus tumor).
2. Tumors of pineal parenchymal cell origin (pineocytoma and pineoblastoma).
3. Tumors originating from glial or other surrounding tissues (malignant glioma, ganglioneuroma, ganglioglioma, meningioma, hemangiopericytoma, chemodectoma).
4. Nonneoplastic cysts and vascular lesions.
5. Metastatic tumors: in particular, adenocarcinoma of the lung and breast.

Over 50% of pineal region tumors are germ cell tumors. Among the germ cell tumors listed above, only the germinomas and teratomas develop in appreciable numbers. Both biologically and histopathologically, all these tumors resemble the germ cell tumors of the gonads and other specific extragonadal sites. The germ cell tumors originate within the pineal gland or in the surrounding leptomeningeal tissues or in the suprasellar area.

A less common germ cell tumor of the pineal gland is the well-differentiated teratoma. It is usually partially encapsulated, noninvasive, lobulated, multicystic, and solid. The pineal gland itself is often totally replaced, and the quadrigeminal plate may be destroyed. As with germinomas, the obstruction of CSF outflow with symmetrical hydrocephalus is an invariable finding. Calcifications are more common in teratomas than germinomas, but are not found in the majority of cases. Rarely, areas of dedifferentiation are found within the teratoma (teratocarcinoma).

Pineocytomas are benign tumors of adults and account for approximately one-third of the parenchymal cell tumors of the pineal. They appear to be more frequent among women. The majority of pineocytomas are well-circumscribed tumors that are confined to the posterior third ventricle. The more undifferentiated pineocytomas are more invasive into the ventricular system and tissue surrounding the posterior third ventricle.

Pineoblastomas are primitive malignant neoplasms, which account for approximately two-thirds of the pineal parenchymal cell tumors. These tumors usually originate in childhood and are somewhat more common in males. They are usually frankly invasive, gray-white gelatinous tumors that extend into the third ventricle and subarachnoid space and destroy tissues surrounding the posterior third ventricle. Extension of tumor into the posterior fossa, with involvement of the superior surface of the cerebellum and anterior vermis, can be found. Pineoblastomas found in this region have been clinically confused with medulloblastoma because of their location. Necrosis, hemorrhage, and calcifications are not ordinarily observed, while cystic degeneration is observed occasionally. In these instances the tumor is histologically indistinguishable from medulloblastoma and primitive neuroectodermal tumors. Pineoblastomas and bilateral retinoblastoma (so-called trilateral retinoblastoma) have been described in some patients.

Endocrine dysfunction is such a frequent concomitant of tumors of the pineal region that the endocrine status of all patients with these tumors must be assessed thoroughly. Endocrine dysfunction is more common when the hypothalamus is involved with tumor. Although precocious puberty in males is the most widely known endocrine abnormality, it is merely one of several endocrine disturbances that occur in patients with such neoplasms. These tumors are frequently associated with isolated hypogonadism, diabetes insipidus, and anterior pituitary insufficiency. These findings may be less obvious than precocious puberty, but are more threatening to the survival of the patient.

The reported incidence of sexual precocity among patients with pineal region tumors varies markedly in the literature. In one series of 606 patients with these tumors, 46 cases of precocious puberty were found.[29] Pineal region tumors, in contrast, are found in only a small proportion of the children with precocious puberty (15–20%). Precocious puberty associated with tumors of the pineal region was reported in one study to occur mainly in boys. Diabetes insipidus is an important clinical manifestation of these tumors. Its presence may herald the diagnosis, and it is the most common endocrine abnormality associated with these tumors. The exact incidence is not known because of the different criteria used by previous investigators to make this diagnosis. Diabetes insipidus can

be reversed if rapid tumor regression occurs secondary to surgery or irradiation.

The use of serum and CSF fluid to measure tumor markers is very helpful in the diagnosis, quantitative measurement of tumor burden, management, and prognosis in patients with pineal region tumors. As a reflection of tumor burden, serum and CSF fluid may allow evaluation of response to therapy and detection of early tumor recurrence. $\alpha$-Fetoprotein (AFP) is an oncofetal glycoprotein that has been useful in the evaluation of certain diseases. Primary germ cell tumors of the pineal region—specifically endodermal sinus tumors, yolk sac tumors—have been reported to elevate CSF AFP with normal serum levels or to have abnormal CSF-serum gradients. Human chorionic gonadotropin (hCG), a placental glycoprotein, is secreted by the placental trophoblastic epithelium. The immunologically specific $\beta$ subunit (b-hCG) is found normally only in fetal blood and in the serum of pregnant women. Elevated b-hCG levels have been found in patients with pineal region choriocarcinomas, embryonal cell tumors, and teratocarcinomas. Forty to fifty percent of germinomas and embryonal carcinomas of the pineal region are b-hCG producing.

One of the most controversial aspects of the management of pineal region tumors involves the indications for, timing of, and approach used in surgical assault on these lesions. The controversy takes root from the complexity of the surgical procedures, which results from the anatomy of the pineal region itself.

In the past, the high morbidity and mortality rates of surgery for tumors of the pineal region led investigators to explore the use of radiation therapy. Rubin and Kramer[30] reviewed the available literature in 1965 and could find no long term survivors in patients with germinomas treated with surgery alone. In contrast, the authors reported 50% of their patients alive without disease 5 years after radiation therapy. This early report focused attention on the radiocurability of pineal germinomas. It also encouraged the use of radiotherapy without biopsy for tumors in the pineal and suprasellar locations. The approach of using radiotherapy alone was particularly attractive because of the relatively high cure rate with little associated morbidity.

The interpretation of published treatment results with radiation therapy is difficult. Most series suffer from small numbers of patients treated over a prolonged period of time without a consistent treatment policy and the absence of histologic diagnosis. Only recently has information become available to provide guidelines for establishing treatment policies for germ cell and non-germ cell tumors of the pineal region.

We recently reviewed the experience at Children's Hospital in Boston concerning 40 cases of histologically confirmed dysgerminoma.[31] The 10-year disease-free survival was 97% following radiotherapy. Most of these patients received craniospinal radiotherapy. The only patient who failed radiotherapy was a child with abdominal disease, probably related to a ventriculoperitoneal shunt. That patient was salvaged with abdominal radiotherapy and chemotherapy. One patient died several years following radiotherapy with a radiation-associated glioblastoma.

The Children's Cancer Study Group (CCSG) reported on 118 patients treated with radiotherapy from twelve institutions.[32] With follow-up ranging from 2 to 15 years, 65% of patients are alive. A diagnosis was obtained in 57 of 65 (88%) of patients before the initiation of irradiation. Seventy-two percent (26 of 36) of patients with germinoma survived, versus only 22% (3 of 14) of patients with a pineal parenchymal tumor or malignant teratoma. The survival of patients with biopsy-proven germinoma was comparable to that of patients treated without a biopsy. A recent report from the University of California, San Francisco, describes the results of 13 patients with biopsy-proven germinoma treated with primarily cranial irradiation (40–55 Gy).[33] With a median follow-up time for these 13 patients of 5.3 years, no patient had a recurrence or died, resulting in a 5-year actuarial relapse-free survival of 100%. Shibamoto et al.[34] from Kyoto recently reported

their results in 70 patients with histologic proven (42 of 70) or radiographically suspected pineal region germinoma. Radiation volumes ranged from inclusion of only the primary tumor site (34 patients) to craniospinal irradiation. Doses to the primary site ranged from 50 to 55 Gy. The 5- and 10-year survival rates were 86% and 79%, respectively, with only four patients failing intracranially near the primary site.

The use of prophylactic spinal irradiation to treat biopsy-confirmed germinoma patients is controversial. Germinomas may infiltrate locally, spread along the ventricular walls, or seed throughout the leptomeninges. The exact incidence of seeding at presentation is difficult to determine from the present literature, but it is believed, in general, to be less than 15%. Surgery may increase the risk of spinal seeding. Sung et al.[35] reported 14 patients with biopsy-proven germinomas treated without spinal irradiation. Six eventually developed spinal metastases, with an actuarial risk of greater than 40% at 5 years. In the CCSG experience, 9 of 109 (8%) patients with pineal or suprasellar tumors who did not receive spinal irradiation developed metastases in the spine. In a review of nine series (including Sung's) and their own, Linstadt et al.[33] compiled the results of patients treated with and without adjuvant spinal irradiation and analyzed spinal failure rates. Combined, these reports yield a total of 39 patients with biopsy-proven germinomas who were treated without prophylactic spinal irradiation. Nine patients (23%) failed in the spine versus 1 of 13 (8%) of patients receiving spinal radiation. Although the number of patients is small, the data suggest that only 15% of patients actually benefit from adjuvant spinal irradiation. In the absence of a biopsy or surgical exploration, the incidence of spinal seeding appears low, and some authors believe that routine spinal irradiation is not warranted.

The data on spinal recurrence after cranial irradiation alone must be viewed with caution, however. In the CCSG data, the risk of spinal failure of 8% is a crude value of patients followed for a relatively short period of time. It would be helpful to know an actuarial value for the risk of spinal failure at a longer follow-up period. If the spinal axis is not going to be treated, the use of myelography and/or enhanced MR is mandatory, including CSF cytology. Regardless of whether spinal axis irradiation is used, large brain fields should be used initially in patients with germinomas. We recommend the use of opposed lateral cranial fields that encompass the whole brain and the meninges for 25 to 30 Gy, followed by a three-field cone down to the pineal region for a total dose of 45 Gy. The exact dose of radiation needed to control pineal region tumors is dependent on tumor histology. Pure germinomas appear to be similar in their radio-responsiveness to testicular seminomas, while some "germinomas" contain embryonal cell elements that appear to require a higher dose. The intracranial relapse rate in patients receiving 50 Gy is substantially less than that in patients receiving a lower dose.

If the histologic diagnosis is unknown, CSF cytology and myelogram and/or MR of the spine are negative, and serum and CSF markers are absent, many authors have recommended a nonsurgical approach to tumors of the pineal region. They recommend using the radiation response of the tumor by CT/MR as an aid in the diagnosis and a guide to management. CT scanning has documented rapid tumor response in verified germinoma with doses of radiation as low as 10 to 20 Gy. A rapid response to irradiation has been interpreted as diagnostic of germinoma, thereby obviating the need for histologic confirmation for certain selected cases. The slowly responding or nonresponding tumors include choriocarcinoma, embryonal cell carcinoma, endodermal sinus tumor, malignant teratoma, pineocytoma, astrocytic tumor, and benign tumors (teratoma). These investigators generally deliver 20 Gy to the tumor and repeat the CT scan. If substantial tumor regression has occurred (presumed germinoma or pineoblastoma), they initiate cranial–spinal irradiation. If little or no response is noted by CT, the smaller field is continued to a dose of 55 Gy at 180 cGy per fraction. If tumor regrowth is noted after full-dose irradiation, surgical exploration and tumor excision and/or chemotherapy may salvage some patients.

It is noteworthy that nongerminomatous tumors appear also to have a worse prognosis than germinoma following radiation therapy. Historically, survival rates for pineocytomas are approximately half that of germinomas, and while pineoblastomas respond initially to radiotherapy, the vast majority of these lesions will recur within 2 years of diagnosis. In a report[36] from the Children's Hospital of Philadelphia on the use of aggressive multimodality therapy, 15 of 22 (69%) of patients with pineoblastoma (5), pineocytoma (3), embryonal cell carcinoma (5), glioma (8), and ganglioneuroblastoma (1) are alive from 6 months to 13 years after radiation.

There is growing information about the potential role of systemic chemotherapy in the treatment of pineal region tumors. The absence of a blood–brain barrier in the pineal gland suggests that such lesions may have an increased vulnerability to systemic chemotherapy. Germ cell tumors with similar histologies are known to respond in other extragonadal sites, and there is no reason to believe that the same response would not occur in the pineal region. Allen et al.[37] reported their experience with 15 children treated with newly diagnosed germ cell tumors by means of neoadjuvant (preirradiation) chemotherapy. When cyclophosphamide either alone or in combination with vincristine, bleomycin, and cisplatinum was used, 10 of 11 germinoma patients had complete disappearance of all evaluable disease after two cycles of drug therapy. Radiation doses to the primary were reduced from 54 Gy to 30 Gy and to the cranial–spinal axis from 36 Gy to 20 Gy. Ten patients remain in continuous disease-free remission from 20 to 89+ months from diagnosis.

In conclusion, previously untreated germ cell tumors are highly sensitive to chemotherapy, and patients who have achieved a complete radiographic response appear to tolerate a significant radiation dose reduction without compromising long-term survival and perhaps avoiding some of the late effects of irradiation. Chemotherapy for pineal parenchymal tumors cannot be recommended at this time except in very young patients, for whom preradiation chemotherapy may enable the delay of radiation to the developing nervous system.

## Primary Spinal Tumors

The incidence of primary tumors of the spinal cord represents about 10% of all primary tumors of the CNS. Most spinal lesions seen in radiation oncology practice are extradural tumors that are metastatic from systemic cancers. Intradural, extramedullary tumors include meningiomas, neurilemmomas, chordomas, and epidermoids. These lesions (with chordoma being the exception) are usually controlled with surgery alone and rarely require postoperative radiotherapy. Intradural, intramedullary tumors include, in order of frequency, ependymomas, astrocytomas of various histology, oligodendrogliomas, and hemangioblastomas. These tumors are often not cured with surgery alone and require postoperative radiotherapy. As a rule, doses of 45 to 54 Gy are given, to ensure that the risk of spinal cord injury from radiation will be less than from the tumor itself. If higher doses are needed, hyperfractionated schemes are recommended, such as 1 Gy BID. MRI scanning has greatly aided the determination of treatment volume. In general, a 2 cm margin is added below and above the T2-weighted MRI abnormality. A posterior field alone is strongly discouraged because of the inhomogeneity of dose across the spinal cord, as well as the toxicity of the exit dose anteriorly. We generally use three fields with a pair of posterior obliques and a posterior field. In some situation a 180° arc rotation is employed to reduce non–target dose delivery. Radiation has been shown to decrease the rate of local recurrence in patients with subtotally resected cellular and myxopapillary ependymomas and low grade astrocytomas. High grade lesions (anaplastic astrocytoma or glioblastoma) represent a significant problem, with most tumors recurring locally within several months of radiotherapy and the patient succumbing rapidly from local and disseminated disease throughout the spinal axis.

Schwade et al.[38] reviewed the results of treatment in seven patients with astrocytoma treated at University of California in San Francisco between 1950 and 1975. Three patients had subtotal resections and four had biopsies only. Doses ranged from 31 Gy in 50 fractions to 50 Gy in 28 fractions. Four of the seven patients were alive without evidence of disease 4 to 11 years after treatment.

The MGH experience between 1962 and 1979 was reported in 1980. Kopelson et al.[39] reviewed the outcome of treatment in 23 patients with intramedullary spinal cord tumors. Nine patients with astrocytomas received 35 to 43 Gy in 13 to 22 fractions. Seven patients were treated with irradiation alone after a biopsy, and five achieved local control at 6 to 105 months. There was no evidence of a dose–response relationship, although the number of patients was small. In 19 patients irradiated for either an astrocytoma or an ependymoma, there were 45 neurologic deficits present before the irradiation. Of these, 34 deficits became totally normal and eight improved. In a second report from MGH, Kopelson, Linggood et al.[40] reviewed the effect of histologic grade on prognosis. There were no long-term survivors among the five patients with spinal cord glioblastoma. The nine patients with low grade astrocytomas had a 5-year actuarial survival of 89%. This difference suggests that even with modern surgical and irradiation techniques, histologic grade is the most important prognostic factor. Garrett and Simpson[41] reviewed the results of treatment in 41 patients with spinal cord ependymomas. Six were treated after a complete removal. In these six patients it was thought that there was a high chance of local recurrence because of the difficulty of the surgery. The remainder of the patients were treated after a subtotal excision or biopsy. The 5-year survival for these patients was 83%.

## Epidural Compression

Spinal cord compression results from malignant tumor in the epidural space and may cause permanent neurologic damage. Spinal cord compression is a relative emergency, which requires rapid diagnosis and treatment. Most epidural tumors causing spinal cord compression arise from metastatic foci in the vertebral body that invade directly into the spinal extradural space. The bulk of the tumor is often anterior to the spinal cord. The most common primary tumor sites causing cord compression are lung, breast, lymphoma, and unknown primary lesion. Together these account for half of all cord compressions. Spinal cord compression may occur at any level of the spinal cord.

Successful treatment of spinal cord compression depends on early recognition of the problem. Symptoms may occur acutely or insidiously. Four symptoms characterize spinal cord compression: pain, weakness, sensory loss, and autonomic dysfunction. Almost all patients experienced pain as the initial symptom. Many patients have local pain, which was usually located close to the site of the compression. Radicular pain is more common with cervical and lumbosacral locations than thoracic lesions. Thoracic radicular pain was often bilateral. Weakness is rarely the initial symptom but is common by the time the diagnosis is made At the time of diagnosis, approximately half the patients have sensory symptoms consisting of numbness or paresthesias in the extremities or trunk. Metastases to the conus medullaris or cauda equine can cause saddle anesthesia with impaired control of micturation. Bowel and bladder dysfunction are present in approximately half of the patients at diagnosis.

MRI imaging of the spine has superseded the traditional use of myelography to diagnosis epidural compression. MRI of the entire spinal axis is recommended, since 10% to 30% of patients with epidural compression at one site will have secondary sites of disease. Once the diagnosis of spinal cord compression is established, the patient is started on high dose steroids. The choice of surgery or irradiation as the primary treatment modality depends on the primary tumor the level of the block and other clinical factors.[42]

Surgical decompression is almost always accomplished by means of wide laminectomy in the region of the tumor mass. Since many tumors causing cord compression arise ulterior to the spinal cord, this posterior approach rarely results in complete removal of the tumor. For this reason postoperative irradiation is given. Since the treatment of spinal cord compression is palliative, the index of success is neurologic function. If the initial treatment is radiation therapy, treatments should be initiated promptly after diagnosis. The volume of treatment includes the upper and lower extent of the compression plus a margin of one vertebral body above and below. A posterior field and lightly weighted anterior field are often used, although the technique can be altered depending on the anatomical region. Most patients receive 30 to 40 Gy in 2 to 4 weeks, depending on fractionation and histology. Patients with myeloma and lymphoma have a higher recovery rate after treatment than do patients with carcinomas.

Decompressive surgery should be the first intervention when there has already been irradiation in the area of the compression and when the nature of the primary tumor is not known. Rapid progression of neurologic dysfunction has been thought to be an indication for immediate surgery. It would seem reasonable to proceed with surgery initially in patients with rapidly progressive symptoms and tumors less responsive to radiation therapy. The patient's pretreatment neurologic function is the best predictor of a favorable outcome. Most patients who are ambulatory at the time of treatment remain ambulatory following irradiation.

## Brain Metastases

Radiation therapy has been the mainstay of the treatment of patients with brain metastases for nearly 40 years. The role of radiotherapy has been greatly influenced by improved brain imaging techniques such as CT and MRI. Although the major goal of radiotherapy is the palliation of neurological signs and symptoms, there are selected patients for whom radiotherapy also significantly improves overall survival.

There have been many measures of the effectiveness of radiotherapy for patients with brain metastases. Reported end points include symptom relief, steroid requirements, local control, failure patterns both within the CNS and extracranially, as well as overall survival. The most frequently reported end point, the relief of specific symptoms, is often reported as percentage of overall symptom response rate, complete symptom response rate, promptness of response, and duration of response. Quality of life measures reported have been few, but have included "Palliation Index," as used by the RTOG.[43] This index represents the percentage of survival time spent in an improved or stable neurologic function class. Another measure of quality of life has been termed "functional independence" and measures the length of time during which the patient has a Karnofsky score of 70% or higher. Survival is an important end point and is usually reported as median survival, although actuarial survival and actuarial "neurologic" survival including deaths due to neurological causes only are end points more frequently being reported.

The major result of radiation is the improvement of specific neurological symptoms. The overall published response rate is symptom dependent, but ranges from 70% to 90%.[44] Over half the patients with headaches, seizures, or symptoms of increased intracranial pressure have a complete response to whole-brain radiotherapy, although the duration of response continues for one year in only 65% of patients. Cranial nerve deficits will improve in approximately 40% of patients, but the potential for improvement is directly related to the interval from diagnosis to radiotherapy.[44] Patients with known systemic cancer with new cranial nerve(s) deficits should undergo contrast-enhanced MRI within 24 hours if possible. If

metastatic disease is present at the skull base or meninges, radiotherapy and corticosteroids should promptly be administered. The expected improval of neurological function is dependent on the function class at the time of initiation of whole-brain radiotherapy. The majority of patients with significant neurological dysfunction improve with the use of steroids and radiotherapy, while less than 50% of patients with moderate neurological dysfunction will improve following therapy.

Even in 1998, the ultimate role of postoperative whole-brain radiation therapy as adjuvant treatment to surgery has not been clearly defined. Theoretically, postoperative radiotherapy is expected to destroy microscopic residual cancer cells at the site of resection and at other locations in the brain if they exist. This should reduce the recurrence rate, prolonging survival, and sparing the patient the anguish of reoperation. Although most authors recommend postoperative whole-brain radiotherapy, only four retrospective studies have specifically examined this question.[45] Three of these studies have demonstrated that recurrence rate is, indeed, reduced by adjuvant whole-brain radiotherapy.

The most important argument against the routine use of postoperative whole-brain radiotherapy involves the significant risk of radiation-induced cognitive changes and other long-term neurotoxicity, as discussed in the section on complications from radiation therapy. One of the most important benefits of surgical excision of brain metastasis is the significant chance some patients have of becoming long-term survivors. If whole-brain radiotherapy given at the time of craniotomy renders these patients neurocognitively impaired, the value of surgery is greatly diminished. A randomized trial examining the effects of whole-brain radiotherapy has been completed through the Southwestern Oncology Group to define its advantages and toxicity. Until these results have been released, if adjuvant whole-brain radiotherapy is to be given, a dose/fraction schedule should be utilized which specifically minimizes the risk of long-term complications.

Occasionally, patients are reirradiated with whole-brain or partial-brain radiotherapy at the time of brain recurrence. The percentage of patients who undergo reirradiation is quite small, since most patients who recur within the CNS also have progressive extracranial disease and are treated with supportive measures only. A review of three series with a combined experience involving 189 patients was published in 1992.[44] The overall clinical response rate ranged from 42% to 75%, with median survival from the time of reirradiation of between 3.5 and 5 months. Although there is no consensus on reirradiation with conventional techniques, some investigators have argued that reirradiation should be considered for patients who remain in good general condition but experience neurological deterioration 4 or more months after a satisfactory response to the initial course of whole-brain radiotherapy. Brain tolerance is probably exceeded by reirradiation, but since the expected survival is so limited, few clinical data exist documenting the effects of this approach. If reirradiation is being considered, radiosurgery (see below) is probably the best radiotherapeutic approach, since the amount of normal brain reirradiated is significantly reduced with these highly sophisticated radiation delivery systems.

Radiosurgery is a technique of external irradiation that utilizes multiple convergent beams to deliver a high single dose of radiation to a small volume (Figure 12-1). In radiosurgery, multiple, highly collimated beams of radiation are stereotactically directed toward a radiographically discrete treatment site. The hallmark of all stereotactic radiation techniques is the rapid dose falloff at the target edges. The biological and physical characteristics of metastases (radiographically discrete, small, spherical, noninvasive) appear to make them ideal radiosurgery targets. The potential advantages of radiosurgery over surgery are reduced morbidity and reduced health care costs.

Results obtained by treating metastases with radiosurgery indicate that local control is obtained in 73% to 98% of patients, with median follow-up of 5 to 26 months.[46] In a multi-institu-

tional trial involving 116 patients treated with radiosurgery for single brain metastasis using a mean dose of 17.5 Gy, local tumor control was obtained in 99 patients (85%).[47] The 2-year actuarial tumor control rate for the whole group was 67% ± 8% with a plateau in the curve at 18 months. In a multivariate analysis, better local control was obtained in patients who received whole-brain radiotherapy in addition to radiosurgery and in patients with "radioresistant" histologies (melanoma and renal cell carcinoma).

In summary, there is compelling evidence to suggest that aggressive local therapy (surgery and radiotherapy) for patients with a single brain metastasis produces survival and quality of life superior to results obtained from whole-brain radiotherapy alone. However, the current data suggest that aggressive therapy should be restricted to the minority of patients for whom brain metastases represent the life-threatening site of their disease. For an asymptomatic or mildly symptomatic patient with a small lesion, radiosurgery appears to be an excellent alternative to surgery.

Late complications following whole-brain radiotherapy can be severe and debilitating in some patients. Brain atrophy, necrosis, endocrine dysfunction, and leukoencephalopathy with neurocognitive deterioration and frank dementia can occur. The incidence of late complications is related to many factors, including total dose, fraction size, patient age, extent of CNS disease, and preexisting neurological impairment. For the same total dose, the larger the daily fraction size, the greater the risk of late CNS sequelae. Thus for patients with favorable prognostic features (absence of extracranial disease, young age, long interval from primary disease diagnosis to brain metastases) and a projected survival of greater than 6 months, it is recommended that smaller daily fraction sizes be used (< 2.5 Gy/day).

## REFERENCES

1. Davis FG, Freels S, Grutsch J, et al: Survival rates in patients with primary malignant brain

tumors stratified by patient age and tumor histological type: An analysis based in Surveillance, Epidemiology, and End Results (SEER) data, 1973–1991. *J Neurosurg* 1998;88: 1–10.

2. Bohnen NI, Radhakrishman K, O'Neill DP, Kurland LT: Descriptive and analytic epidemiology of brain tumors, in PMcL Black and JS Loeffler (eds): *Tumors of the Nervous System.* Cambridge, Blackwell Science, 1997, pp 3–24.

3. Ron E, Modan B, Joice JD, et al: Tumors of the brain and nervous system after radiotherapy in childhood. *N Engl J Med* 1988;319:1033–1039.

4. Brada M, Ford D, Ashley S, et al: Risk of second brain tumour following conservative surgery and radiotherapy of pituitary adenoma. *Br Med J* 1992;304:1343–1346.

5. Schwartz RB: Functional imaging of brain tumors, in PMcL Black and JS Loeffler JS (eds): *Tumors of the Nervous System.* Cambridge, Blackwell Science, 1997, pp 98–105.

6. Ringertz N: Grading of gliomas. *Acta Pathol Microbiol Scand* 1950;27:51–64.

7. Daumas-Duport C, Scheithauer BW, O'Fallon J, Kelly P: Grading of astrocytomas: A simple and reproducible method. *Cancer* 1988;62: 2152–2165.

8. Kim TS, Halliday AL, Hedley-White ET, Convery K: Correlation of survival and the Daumas-Duport grading system for astrocytomas. *J Neurosurg* 1991;74:27–31.

9. Shaw EG, Scheithauer BW, O'Fallon JR, et al: Oligodendrogliomas: The Mayo Clinic experience. *J Neurosurg* 1992;76:428–434.

10. Karim ABMF, Maat B, Hatlevol R, et al: A randomized trial on dose–response in radiation therapy of low-grade cerebral glioma: European Organization for Research and Treatment of Cancer (EORTC) study 22844. *Int J Radiat Oncol Biol Phys* 1996;36:549–556.

11. Taphoorn MJB, Schiphorst AK, Snoek FJ, et al: Cognitive function and quality of life in patients with low-grade gliomas: The impact of radiotherapy. *Ann Neurol* 1994;36:48–54.

12. Curran WJ, Scott CB, Horton J, et al: Recursive partitioning analysis of prognostic factors in three Radiation Therapy Oncology Group malignant glioma trials. *J Natl Cancer Inst* 1993; 85:704–710.

13. Walker MD, Strike TA, Sheline GE: An analysis of dose–effect relationship in the radiotherapy of malignant gliomas. *Int J Radiat Oncol Biol Phys.* 1979;5:1725–1731.

14. Nicholas MK, Prados MD, Larson DA, Gutin PH: Malignant astrocytomas, in PMcL Black and JS Loeffler (eds): *Tumors of the Nervous System.* Cambridge, Blackwell Science, 1997, pp 464–491.

15. Wang CC, Suit H, Blitzer P: Twice-a-day radiation therapy for supraglottic carcinoma. *Int J Radiat Oncol Biol Phys* 1986;12:3–7.

16. Fitzek M, Thornton A, Rabenow J, et al: Results of 90 Gy proton/photon radiation therapy for glioblastoma multiforme. *Int J Radiat Oncol Biol Phys* 1997;39:139 (abstr).

17. Loeffler JS, Shrieve DC, Wen PY, et al: Radiosurgery for intracranial malignancies. *Semin Radiat Oncol* 1995;5:225–234.

18. Fine HA, Mayer RJ: Primary central nervous system lymphoma. *Ann Intern Med* 1993;119: 1093–2001.

19. Fine HA, Loeffler JS: Primary central nervous system lymphoma, in GP Canellos, TA Lister, and JL Sklar (eds): *The Lymphomas.* Philadelphia, Saunders, 1998, pp 481–494.

20. Mirimanoff RO, Dosoretz DE, Linggood RM, et al: Meningioma: Analysis of recurrence and progression following neurosurgical resection. *J Neurosurg* 1985;62:18–24.

21. Wara WM, Sheline GE, Newman H, et al: Radiation therapy of meningiomas. *Am J Radiol* 1975;123:453–458.

22. Goldsmith BJ, Wara WM, Wilson CB, Larson DA: Postoperative irradiation for subtotally resected meningiomas. *J Neurosurg* 1994;80: 195–201.

23. Tishler RB, Loeffler JS, Lunsford LD, et al: Tolerance of cranial nerves of the cavernous sinus to radiosurgery. *Int J Radiat Oncol Biol Phys* 1993;27:215–221.

24. Wen PY, Loeffler JS: Advances in the diagnosis and management of pituitary tumors. *Curr Opin Oncol* 1995;7:56–62.

25. Hardy J, Vezina J: Transsphenoidal neurosurgery of intracranial neoplasms. *Adv Neurol* 1976;15:261–274.

26. Black PMcL, Zervas NT, Ridgeway ED, et al: *Secretory Tumors of the Pituitary Gland,* Vol 1,

in *Progress in Endocrine Research and Therapy* Series. New York, Raven Press, 1984.

27. Shrieve DC, Tarbell NJ, Kooy HM, Loeffler JS: Fractionated (relocatable) stereotactic radiotherapy, in VT DeVita, S Hellman, and SA Rosenberg (eds): *Cancer: Principles and Practice of Oncology,* 5th ed. Philadelphia, Lippincott-Raven, 1997, pp 3107–3114.

28. Constine LC, Woolf PD, Cann D, et al: Hypothalmic-pituitary dysfunction after radiotherapy for brain tumors. *N Engl J Med* 1993;328:87–94.

29. Kitay JI, Altschule MD: *The Pineal Gland.* Cambridge, MA: Harvard University Press, 1954.

30. Rubin P, Kramer S: Ectopic pineoloma: A radiocurable neuroendocrinologic entity. *Radiology* 1965;85:512–523.

31. Harrigan PH, Golden J, Billet A, et al: Intracranial germinomas: The case for low dose radiation therapy. *Int J Radiat Oncol Biol Phys* 1997; 39:419–426.

32. Wara W, Jenkin DT, Evan A, et al: Tumors of the pineal and suprasellar region: Children's Cancer Study Group treatment results 1960–1975. *Cancer* 1979;43:698–701.

33. Linstadt D, Wara WM, Edwards MJB, et al: Radiotherapy of primary intracranial germinomas: The case against routine craniospinal irradiation. *Int J Radiat Oncol Biol Phys* 1985;15: 291–297.

34. Shibamoto Y, Abe M, Yamashita J, et al: Treatment results of intracranial germinomas as a function of the irradiation volume. *Int J Radiat Oncol Biol Phys* 1988;15:285–290.

35. Sung DI, Harisiadis L, Chang CH: Midline pineal tumors and suprasellar germinomas: Highly radiocurable by irradiation. *Radiology* 1978;128:745–751.

36. Packer RJ, Sutton LN, Rosenstock JG, et al: Pineal region tumors of childhood. *Pediatrics* 1984;74:97–102.

37. Allen JC, Kim JH, Packer RJ: Neoadjuvant chemotherapy for newly diagnosed germ-cell

tumors of the central nervous system. *J Neurosurg* 1987;67:65–70.

38. Schwade JG, Wara WM, Sheline GE, et al: Management of primary spinal cord tumors. *Int J Radiat Oncol Biol Phys* 1978;4:389–393.

39. Kopelson G, Linggood RM, Kleinman GM, et al: Management of intramedullary spinal cord tumors. *Radiology* 1980;135:473–479.

40. Kopelson G, Linggood RM: Intramedullary spinal cord astrocytoma versus glioblastoma: The prognostic importance of histologic grade. *Cancer* 1982;50:732–735.

41. Garrett PG, Simpson WJ: Ependymomas: Results of irradiation treatment. *Int J Radiat Oncol Biol Phys* 1983;9:1121–1124.

42. Lablaw DA, Laperriere NJ: Emergency treatment of malignant extradural spinal compression: An evidence-based guideline. *J Clin Oncol* 1998;16:1613–1624.

43. Borgelt B, Gelber R, Kramer S, et al: The palliation of brain metastases: Final results of the first three studies of the Radiation Therapy Oncology Group. *Int J Radiat Oncol Biol Phys* 1980;6:1–10.

44. Coia LR: The role of radiation therapy in the treatment of brain metastases. *Int J Radiat Oncol Biol Phys* 1992;23:22–32.

45. Loeffler JS, Patchell RA, Sawaya R: Metastatic brain cancer, in VT DeVita, S Hellman, and SA Rosenberg (eds): *Cancer: Principles and Practice of Oncology,* 5th ed. Philadelphia, Lippincott-Raven, 1997, pp 2523–2536.

46. Loeffler JS, Flickinger JC, Shrieve DC, et al. Radiosurgery for the treatment of intracranial lesions, in VT DeVita, S Hellman, and SA Rosenberg (eds): *Important Advances in Oncology.* 5th ed. Philadelphia, Lippincott-Raven, 1997, pp 141–152.

47. Flickinger JC, Konziolka D, Lunsford LD, et al: A multi-institutional experience with stereotactic radiosurgery for solitary brain metastasis. *Int J Radiat Oncol Biol Phys* 1994;28:797–802.

# CHAPTER 13

# THE LYMPHOMAS

ALAN C. AISENBERG and YUHCHYAU CHEN

The malignant lymphomas are the complex group of primary neoplasms of the lymphoid system: they arise in the lymph nodes and spleen, and, less frequently, in extranodal sites. These two dozen or more disorders, with widely varying natural histories, account for about 4% of the total cancer incidence and a similar percentage of cancer deaths in the United States (approximately 61,000 new cases with 26,000 deaths were reported in 1997).[1,2] Lymphoma treatment, both radiotherapy and chemotherapy, has made remarkable strides since the end of World War II when these conditions were considered uniformly fatal. The therapy of Hodgkin disease, which constitutes about one-eighth of malignant lymphomas, is one of the triumphs of modern oncology: it may provide a pattern on which to base our approach to the more common but less tractable epithelial neoplasms and a benchmark against which to judge this other progress. Optimal management of malignant lymphoma requires the closest collaboration between medical and radiation oncologists. The voluminous and disputatious lymphoma literature attests to the many unresolved controversies arising from this collaboration. This chapter presents the approach to lymphoma that has evolved over the past three decades at the Massachusetts General Hospital (MGH). While some alternative views will be presented, our goal is not an encyclopedic presentation.

## HODGKIN DISEASE

### Histological Classification

The diagnosis of Hodgkin disease is based on identification of unequivocal Reed–Sternberg (R-S) cells (multinucleate giant cells with inclusion-like nucleoli) in a mixed inflammatory infiltrate of lymphocytes, histiocytes, eosinophils, and plasma cells. Current opinion favors an unusual B lineage for the R-S cell: immunophenotype HLA-DR+, CD30+ (Ki-1, an activation antigen), CD15+ (a granulocyte/monocyte antigen), and CD45− (leukocyte common antigen). An adequate biopsy sample, optimally fixed and stained, and reviewed by an expert hematopathologist, is essential for diagnosis. Opinions based on frozen material are unreliable.

Table 13-1 presents the REAL (Revised European–American Classification of Lymphoid Neoplasms) classification for Hodgkin disease,[3] which has gained widespread acceptance. As with other referral centers, about 5% of the MGH cases fall into the favorable lymphocyte predominance category and 5% into the unfavorable lymphocyte depletion category. The major fraction (approximately 60%) exhibits the broad bands of connective tissue and lacunar Reed–Sternberg cells that characterize nodular sclerosis, and the remainder (about 30%), the nondescript pattern of mixed cellularity. The phenotype of the Reed–Sternberg

*Clinical Radiation Oncology: Indications, Techniques, and Results, 2nd ed.* Edited by C.C. Wang.
ISBN: 0-471-23803-1  Copyright © 2000 Wiley-Liss, Inc.

**TABLE 13-1  Histological Classification of Hodgkin Disease**

Lymphocyte predominance (paragranuloma)
Nodular sclerosis
Mixed cellularity
Lymphocyte depletion
Lymphocyte-rich classical Hodgkin disease[a]
Anaplastic large-cell lymphoma, Hodgkin-like[a,b]

[a]Provisional subtype.
[b]Subtype of non-Hodgkin lymphoma.
*Source:* Ref. 3.

cells in the lymphocyte predominance (para-granuloma) type and the clinical behavior of this subtype closely resemble those of a very low grade B-cell non-Hodgkin lymphoma. On-cologists treating Hodgkin disease should also be aware of the newly described provisional non-Hodgkin lymphoma subtype termed "anaplastic large-cell lymphoma, Hodgkin-like," because of its poor response to Hodgkin disease treatment programs. In comparison with the non-Hodgkin lymphomas, histological subclassification of Hodgkin disease plays a less crucial role in management.

## Staging Classification

*In Hodgkin disease, the extent of disease at the time of diagnosis provides the most useful guide to treatment, prognosis and curability.* The Ann Arbor Staging Classification,[4] pre-sented in Table 13-2 is commonly employed to describe the disease extent. The designation *pathological stage* (*PS*) is used when patho-logical confirmation has been obtained by staging laparotomy and splenectomy; when this surgery has not been performed, the term *clinical stage* (*CS*) should be employed. The presence of systemic manifestations (fever and/or weight loss) are major negative prog-nostic criteria, and their presence should be sought with care.

This staging classification represents an at-tempt to reduce into simple terms the complex process by which Hodgkin disease spreads and disseminates. In brief, Hodgkin disease evolves

through two principal mechanisms. Dissemina-tion to adjacent lymph nodes via connecting lymphatic channels characterizes the first, or contiguous, mode of spread. While Hodgkin disease, whose spread is restricted to the con-tiguous mode, is not always cured by radiation alone, contiguous spread implies regional (lo-calized) disease. The second route of dissemi-nation is hematogenous: the presence or absence of such hematogenous spread is a crit-ical point to be established by the staging workup. Further, in our clinic, the presence of splenic involvement at staging laparotomy has always been considered to be strong evidence that hematogenous spread has occurred and

**TABLE 13-2  Staging Classification of Hodgkin Disease**

| | |
|---|---|
| Stage I. | Involvement of a single lymph node region |
| Stage II. | Involvement of two or more lymph node regions on the same side of the diaphragm (II), which may be accompanied by localized involvement of an extralymphatic organ or site (II$_E$) |
| Stage III. | Involvement of lymph node regions on both sides of the diaphragm (III), which may also be accompanied by involvement of the spleen (III$_S$) or by localized involvement of an extralymphatic organ or site (III$_E$) |
| Stage IV. | Diffuse or disseminated involvement of one or more extralymphatic organs or tissues, with or without associated lymph node involvement |

*Notes:*

1. The presence or absence of fever and/or unexplained weight loss of 10% or more of body weight in the preceding 6 months are denoted by the suffix letters B and A, respectively.

2. If staging laparotomy/splenectomy has been per-formed, the designation is pathological stage (PS); if not, it is clinical stage (CS).

3. Stage III may be subdivided into III$_1$ to designate in-volvement of only the upper abdominal nodes and/or spleen, and III$_2$ to designate involvement of the para-aortic and/or pelvic nodes as well.

that cure will require combination chemotherapy. In support of this view, we point to the steadily mounting relapse rates seen when radiation alone is employed in pathological stage III disease.[5]

Figure 13-1 summarizes the stage distribution in the first 250 patients subject to staging laparotomy and splenectomy at the MGH (findings are expressed per 100 patients). Of note is the compelling observation that while 90% of patients appear to be localized on initial examination, the number is reduced to 60% after lymphangiogram, and to 40% after staging laparotomy.

## Diagnostic Workup

The diagnostic workup employed in Hodgkin disease is outlined in Table 13-3. Points of particular interest in the history (fever and weight loss) and physical examination (nodes, liver, and spleen) are self-evident. Routine chemical and hematologic (including a sedimentation rate) studies of the blood are done, but by themselves, do not alter stage. Bilateral lymphangiographic study of the lower extremities is still a useful procedure to detect para-aortic and pelvic adenopathy. Because of the low return, needle biopsy of bone is reserved for symptomatic patients, while needle biopsy of the liver is not employed in the initial diagnostic work-up.

In our experience, bone scan and liver/spleen scan are rarely useful in the initial staging workup. Gallium scans can be obtained in patients who present with a large ($\geq$ one-third the chest diameter) mediastinal mass (LMM) or other bulky adenopathy ($\geq$ 10 cm) to provide a baseline for posttreatment study. The mediastinum cannot be adequately assessed

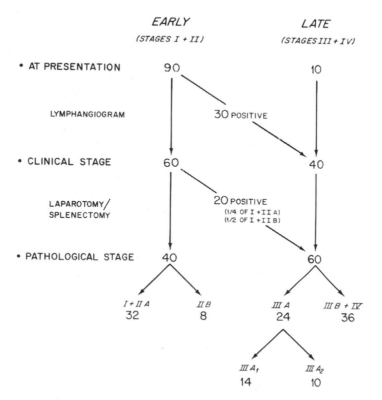

**FIGURE 13-1** Stage distribution in Hodgkin disease expressed per 100 patients: at presentation, after lymphangiogram, and after staging laparotomy.

**TABLE 13-3  Diagnostic Workup in Hodgkin Disease**

1. History: fever, night sweats, weight loss and alcohol-induced pain; physical examination (nodes, spleen, and liver); routine hematological studies and blood chemistries.
2. Chest radiogram and chest CT; MRI as indicated.
3. Abdominal and pelvic CT scan.
4. Bilateral lower extremity lymphangiogram in patients not surgically staged with negative CT scan.
5. Needle biopsy of bone in those with symptoms.
6. Gallium scan for those with large mediastinal mass or other bulky disease.
7. Staging laparotomy only if findings will alter treatment.
   A. Explore:
      i. Some CS IIA patients in neither the very favorable nor the unfavorable categories (see Table 13-4).
      ii. Some CS II patients with equivocal symptoms and IIIA patients with equivocal findings on CT scan and/or lymphangiogram.
   B. Avoid laparotomy in stages IIIB and IV, sick or febrile patients, young children, the elderly, and those with complicating disease or compromised airway.

without a CT examination, and MRI may provide additional information about the extent of involvement of the heart and other mediastinal structures by mediastinal lymphoma.

A positive abdominal CT image avoids the more taxing lymphangiogram and, in patients who are not explored, supplements that study the upper abdomen, where nodes are not opacified by lymphangiographic dye. However, our experience agrees with that of others: lymphangiography is more sensitive in detecting abnormal pelvic and para-aortic lymph nodes. The role of the PET (positron emission tomogram) scan in detecting Hodgkin disease in both the thorax and abdomen is under investigation.

Staging laparotomy with splenectomy, which played a central role in understanding the mode of spread of Hodgkin disease, was widely used in the past at the MGH to guide treatment decisions. However, it has been used with decreasing frequency in the 1990s. We never performed staging laparotomy in sick IIIB patients or those in stage IV (though many patients in stage IIIB and IV are so staged on the basis of laparotomy findings), or the young, the old, or those with major complicating disease. Early on, it became clear that the yield of positive findings was too low (5–10%) to justify the morbidity and potential mortality of the procedure in certain patient groups.[6–8] We successively excluded individuals in CS IA restricted to the mediastinum, CS IA presenting in the groin with negative lymphangiogram, CS IA with lymphocyte predominance histology, and, in women, those in CS IA and some in CS IIA with nodular sclerosis histology (see Table 13-4). At the same time, it became clear that the cure rate with radiotherapy alone was too low (of the order of 50%) in many unfavorable stage I and II presentations: patients with mediastinal masses that equaled or exceeded one-third of the chest diameter were excluded early, with later extension to the other groups listed in Table 13-4.

However, a small fraction of Hodgkin disease patients remain for whom a case can still be made for staging laparotomy. There are usually individuals who present with localized disease that is neither very favorable nor unfavorable (see Table 13-4) or have equivocal symptoms or equivocal findings on lymphangiogram and/or abdominal CT. The morbidity and mortality from staging laparotomy at institutions such as ours (2 operative deaths in the first 500 patients at the MGH) is less than the risk of fatal treatment-induced neoplasms following a single course of irradiation,[9,10] grave cardiac complications following mantle treatment,[11] acute nonlymphocytic leukemia and other neoplasms following MOPP (methotrexate, Oncomycin, procarbazine, and prednisone),[12] or fatal bleomycin lung toxicity following ABVD (Adriamycin, bleomycin, vineristine, and dacarbazine).[13] In our view, a splenectomy has less risk than radiation to the

**TABLE 13-4    Primary Treatment of Hodgkin's Disease**[a]

| Clinical Stage | Primary Treatment |
|---|---|
| I AND II | |
| Very favorable | No laparotomy |
| CS IA LP, | EF; *or* |
| Female; IA NS, IIA NS <2 6 years | Mantle (IF) after negative lap (investigative); *or* |
| Age 11–60 years | Female < 27 years or smokers, ABVD × 6 (investigative) |
| No restrictions listed below | |
| Favorable | Negative laparotomy, EF; *or* |
| ≤ 3 sites | No laparotomy |
| No restrictions listed below | ABVD × 4–6 + mantle (IF); *or* |
| | ABVD × 6 + RT to residual disease*; *or* |
| | Female < 27 years or smokers, ABVD × 6 (investigative) |
| Unfavorable | No laparotomy |
| > 3 sites | ABVD × 6 + mantle (IF); *or* |
| Fever and/or weight loss | ABVD × 4 + mantle (IF); *or* |
| LMM or bulky (≥10 cm) adenopathy | ABVD × 6 + RT to residual disease*; *or* |
| Pericardial or bilateral | MOPP/ABVD × 8 (4 + 4) + mantle (IF) *or* |
| hilar adenopathy | RT to residual disease* |
| Involvement of pericardium, | |
| pleura, or lung | |
| Lymphatic permeation or | |
| obstruction | |
| IIIA | Laparotomy for equivocal CT and LAG only |
| | No laparotomy |
| | ABVD × 6 + RT to bulk *or* residual disease* |
| IIIB AND IV | No laparotomy |
| | MOPP/ABVD × 8 + RT to residual *or* bulk disease; *or* |
| | ABVD × 6 + RT to bulk *or* residual disease* |

[a]Abbreviations and symbols:

> CT, computed tomography; EF, extended field; IF, involved field; LAG, lymphangiogram; LMM, large mediastinal mass (≥ 1/3 chest diameter); LP, lymphocyte predominance histology; NS, nodular sclerosis histology; RT, radiation therapy
>
> MOPP, nitrogen mustard, 6 mg/m$^2$, and vincristine, 1.4 mg/m$^2$ (maximum 2 mg), IV, days 1 and 8, procarbazine, 100 mg/m$^2$, PO days, 1–10; prednisone, 40 mg/m$^2$, PO, days 1–14; 28-day cycles
>
> ABVD, doxorubicin, 25 mg/m$^2$, vinblastine, 6 mg/m$^2$, and bleomycin, 15 units, all IV, and DTIC (immidazole carboxamide), 250 mg/m$^2$, PO; all days 1 and 14 of a 28-day cycle
>
> MOPP/ABVD, alternating cycles of MOPP and ABVD

*Residual radiographic abnormalities without positive gallium or PET scan, or biopsy confirmation are not considered residual disease.

splenic bed. Nonetheless, we assiduously immunize patients with vaccines to the pneumococci and to *H. influenzae* prior to laparotomy/splenectomy,[14] undertaking the surgery only if major treatment decisions depend on the operative findings.

## Treatment

In 2000 the treatment of Hodgkin disease remains in a state of flux. This is not because we lack effective treatments. Indeed, a variety of effective treatment regimens is available. Most of the few individuals who now die of Hodgkin disease itself are old or present with stage IV disease (in 1994 only 1440 individuals died of the disorder in the United States[1]). However, increasingly, treatment-related morbidity and mortality has been demonstrated to compromise the quality of life and longevity of the cured patient. Thus, treatment-related complications (discussed in a later section of this chapter) have become a major consideration in therapy. Available evidence indicates that the risk of treatment-induced solid neoplasms, probably the most grave and intractable complication of Hodgkin disease therapy, continues unabated through three decades.

Another source of contention results from the historical accident that for many years radiation therapy was the only curative modality available for Hodgkin disease. Only recently, appropriate trials have been begun to address the role of radiation therapy in combined modality programs. With the availability of ABVD, a drug regimen without the leukemia or sterility risks of MOPP, there has been a widespread movement away from staging laparotomy, and toward treatment of an increasing fraction of Hodgkin disease patients with ABVD combined with irradiation in lower dosage (36 Gy) to more restricted fields.[15,16] We are reluctant to apply this policy to all (or most) comers without more adequate evidence. Table 13-4 outlines the middle road we recommend, which incorporates incremental changes based on past experience.

Localized Hodgkin disease (CS I and II) is subdivided into three groups.[17] The *very favorable* group (not explored because the likelihood of a positive staging laparotomy is < 10%) includes CS IA disease with lymphocyte predominance histology, and women with nodular sclerosis histology in CS IA and in IIA if age 25 or younger. This group is further restricted to those aged 11 through 60 without large mediastinal or bulky adenopathy, fewer than 3 sites of disease, or with systemic complaints or any of the other adverse clinical features of CS I and II listed in Table 13-4. Standard treatment remains extended field ir-

radiation, but options under investigation include involved field (mantle) irradiation alone, following negative laparotomy,[18] and, because of their high risk of breast cancer, ABVD chemotherapy as alternative to irradiation for women less than 27 years of age.[10]

The *unfavorable* category of CS I and II patients is defined by any of a large number of clinical characteristics; more than 3 sites, bulky mediastinal or other bulky adenopathy, fever and/or weight loss, pericardial or bilateral hilar adenopathy, involvement of pericardium, pleura, or lung, or significant lymphatic permeation or obstruction. Such individuals have a high likelihood of positive findings at laparotomy and/or of recurrence if treated by irradiation alone. This group is also spared exploration, since chemotherapy is indicated without regard to laparotomy findings. Standard treatment has been six cycles of ABVD followed by involved field (mantle) irradiation. Others propose limiting irradiation of these patients to sites of prior bulk disease—or, more restrictively, to residual disease after chemotherapy (positive gallium or PET scan, or biopsy)—or to limit ABVD to four cycles; we occasionally make such modifications based on particular clinical considerations. We may employ alternating MOPP/ABVD followed by mantle irradiation for those age 40 or less with systemic symptoms and prognostically unfavorable large mediastinal masses.

The residual and important fraction of patients in CS I and II, who qualify for neither the *very favorable* or *unfavorable* categories, are defined as *favorable*. At the present time we see no objection to staging laparotomy for this group followed by involved field irradiation for individuals without abdominal disease, as employed in the past. However, if the patient and/or his or her physician are opposed to surgery, there are reasonable alternatives: namely, four to six cycles of ABVD and involved field irradiation, or six cycles of ABVD followed by irradiation of residual disease. ABVD alone is an option in women under age 27 and in smokers who are at high risk for lung cancer following irradiation.

Patients in CS IIIA are explored only if the abdominal and pelvic node studies (abdominal CT scan and lymphangiogram) are equivocal. Treatment is six cycles of ABVD followed by radiation to residual or original bulk disease.

Patients who present in CS IIIB and IV are not explored. We prefer MOPP/ABVD for those age 40 or less with significant fever and/or weight loss, and add irradiation to residual or, less frequently, prior bulk disease. We spare older individuals the leukemia risk following MOPP by restricting their chemotherapy to six cycles of ABVD, and we consider that regimen a reasonable choice also for those in stage IVA. At the present time we do not employ high dose therapy with peripheral stem cell support as part of primary therapy for any subset of Hodgkin disease patients.

## Treatment of Relapse

Patients who relapse after radiation therapy are treated with chemotherapy with survival results that approximate those of an untreated Hodgkin disease population. Most now receive ABVD, though some under age 40 with unfavorable prognostic features (weight loss and/or fever and/or stage IV disease) may receive alternating MOPP/ABVD.

Relapses following primary chemotherapy with or without irradiation present a more difficult problem because such patients are infrequently cured by conventional salvage chemotherapy. We identify those with favorable ($\geq$ 12 months disease-free interval, stage I or IIA disease at relapse) and unfavorable ($<$ 12 months disease-free interval, B symptoms, extranodal disease, or stage III or IV disease at relapse) clinical features.[19-21]

Patients who relapse after chemotherapy, particularly those with favorable prognostic features after a four-drug regimen, can be treated again with the same or another chemotherapy program. Occasional, highly selected individuals, usually with a localized recurrence without systemic complaints, have been irradiated with good disease control.[22,23]

## High Dose Therapy with Autologous Peripheral Stem Cell Support (PST)

Recognizing the poor record of conventional salvage regimens for chemotherapy failures, and the unfavorable results achieved with PST in patients in drug-resistant relapse after multiple drug regimens, we prefer early stem cell transplantation.[24-26] Thus we are inclined to prompt PST in those who fail to achieve an initial complete response (particularly after seven- or eight-drug programs), or who relapse early ($<$ 12 months) or exhibit other negative prognostic features at relapse, PST can be deferred until second relapse for those with favorable prognostic features. We anticipate a 40% to 50% event-free survival at 3 to 5 years from PST in these patients. Allogeneic transplants are under study.

Patients are cytoreduced with conventional or salvage regimens prior to transplantation and frequently receive irradiation to bulk and/or residual disease as tolerated. Individuals who require irradiation to achieve a complete remission following PST are reported to enjoy the same survival advantage as those who achieve complete remission without this radiotherapy.[27] The preparative regimen employed for PST does not include total-body irradiation in patients whose mediastinum has been irradiated.

## Treatment Complications

In some recent reports, the cumulative mortality from treatment complications has surpassed the mortality from Hodgkin disease itself. The first alarming complication noted was the high incidence of treatment-induced acute nonlymphocytic leukemia (ANLL). In the MGH series, 11 cases of ANLL were observed in 220 patients receiving chemotherapy with the MOPP combination (none were observed in an almost equal number receiving radiation alone).[12] Following MOPP treatment, the actuarially calculated leukemia risk was 11% at 13 years. Those over age 40, or who presented in stages IIIB and IV and frequently require repeated courses of leukemogenic drugs for successive relapses, were identified as high risk groups. Fortunately, the incidence of leukemia was low in patients in stages I, II, and IIIA who received MOPP either as part of primary curative treatment or for radiation failure.

Few cases of leukemia have been reported in patients treated with the equally or more[13] effective ABVD regimen, and fertility has been well preserved. For these reasons, ABVD has widely replaced MOPP. However, the bleomycin in this combination can cause severe pulmonary fibrosis, resulting in a 1% to 3% fatality rate following six cycles of ABVD.[13] Advanced age, increased drug dose, and prior mediastinal radiation increase the incidence of grave bleomycin toxicity.

Treatment-induced solid neoplasms are the most frequent serious complications of Hodgkin disease therapy. The magnitude of the problem cannot be accurately assessed yet, since second cancers are still being observed at the end of the third decade following treatment. Approximately 80% of these neoplasms are within or at the edge of the treatment field and can thus be attributed to irradiation therapy, usually to the mantle or para-aortic areas.

We recently assessed the incidence of treatment-induced breast cancer and other neoplasms in 111 women with follow-ups ranging from 10 to 30 years.[10] Thirteen breast cancers were tightly clustered in women irradiated at ages 14 through 25, and detected in years 11 through 25 after treatment. In women under age 20 at the time of irradiation, who were at the highest risk for breast cancer, the incidence was 34% by actuarial calculation after 25 years. We have also observed a markedly increased incidence of sarcomas and unusual epithelial neoplasms, and an increase of lung carcinoma within or at the margins of radiation fields. The latter were restricted to patients with a history of smoking. The few second lymphomas and melanomas followed MOPP chemotherapy rather than irradiation.

Seventeen of the same cohort of women followed 10 to 30 years developed major symptomatic cardiac disease. Cardiac manifestations included coronary and valvular heart disease, as well as pancarditis. In most patients the response to medical and surgical cardiac intervention was encouraging. However, three sudden deaths from myocardial infarction were observed in young men who were the male counterpart of this female cohort.

Finally, less important treatment complications should be noted. MOPP regularly produces sterility in the male and premature menopause in the female, particularly if treatment is given after age 30. In addition, the prednisone in MOPP has been responsible for aseptic necrosis of the femoral head, requiring replacement surgery. Chemical and clinical hypothyroidism frequently follows thyroid irradiation in the setting of prior administration of iodized lymphangiographic dye.

## Prognosis

The most recent national figures available indicate an 80% 5-year survival for Hodgkin disease.[1,2] Figures from the Massachusetts General Hospital for survival and disease-free survival are similar to those from other large treatment centers. Our most recent compilation of 122 patients treated in 1975–1981 indicates an actuarially calculated 5-year survival of 91% in PS IA and IIA, and a disease-free survival of 75%.[28] The respective figures are 93% and 82% for individuals in PS IA, and 85% and 68% for those in IIA. Seventeen of 26 radiation failures were salvaged with chemotherapy, giving an actuarially calculated freedom from second relapse of 55% at 5 years for this subgroup. Of 38 patients in stage IIIA (35 surgically staged), both actuarially calculated 5-year survival and disease-free survival were 83%.[29]

The major function of disease-related (and treatment-related) mortality occurs in patients who present in stages IIIB and IV. For patients treated in the period 1969–1977, the actuarially calculated 5-year survival figure was only 72% and that for disease-free survival 38%.[30]

The major future gains in the longevity of the Hodgkin disease patient must come from treatment regimens that induce fewer second neoplasms and less cardiac disease, rather than from programs that more effectively cure the primary disease. Unfortunately, we still do not have accurate incidence figures for the various grave complications of irradiation and chemotherapy, nor will we know for 20 to 30 years how successful modifications of dose and irradiation technique, now being empirically applied, will be in reducing these catastrophic events. However, it must be kept in mind that this continuing problem reflects an outstanding success of modern cancer treatment.

## RADIATION THERAPY TECHNIQUE

Hodgkin disease predominantly spreads in a pattern that follows contiguous lymphatic chains. This pattern of spread forms the basis for radiotherapy field design. The success of therapy lies in the adequate coverage, by the treatment volume, of the site of lesion and potentially involved lymphatic regions. As discussed earlier, the major gains in the longevity of the Hodgkin disease patient must balance with treatment-induced side effects such as second neoplasm, cardiac disease, and growth defects in children. The criteria of patient selection and the treatment volume definition are in evolution, with the intent of maximizing cures while minimizing therapy-related side effects. The following recommendations represent the current standard with the expectation of fine-tuning patient selection and improved definition of treatment volume in coming years.

The *very favorable* group of localized disease (stage IA and IIA) described earlier in this chapter can be effectively treated with radiotherapy alone. At present the standard radiation treatment portal remains the mantle plus para-aortic irradiation. At the Massachusetts General Hospital a radiation dose of 39.6 to 41.4 Gy is given to all the lymph node areas in the mantle at 1.8 Gy/day at the midplane central axis reference point, and 150 cm skin-to-source distance (SSD). Areas of disease involvement within the mantle volume receive an additional 3.6 to 5.4 Gy boost. After a 10- to 21-day interval, the para-aortic lymph node area is also treated to a total dose of 39 to 41.4 Gy, which is given at either 1.5 Gy/day or 1.8 Gy/day at midplane, depending on patient tolerance. If chemotherapy precedes irradiation, as in patients with *unfavorable category* (B symptoms, bulky mediastinal disease) or patients with IIIA disease, lower radiation doses are given: 36 Gy to the mantle with a boost to a total of approximately 40 Gy to involved sites, and the para-aortic nodes are treated to 36 Gy. In reducing the radiation dose, it is assumed that the chemotherapy makes up for the dose reduction and that the lower radiation dose will reduce the risk of combined modality toxicities.

### The Mantle Field

A mantle field encompasses all the major lymphatic chains above the diaphragm. The field includes lymph node regions of the cervical chains, supraclavicular and infraclavicular regions, the axillae, and the mediastinal nodal regions. In the design of the mantle field, Cerrobend blocks, made individually for each patient, are used to protect the maximum amount of heart and lungs. These blocks are often redesigned during a course of therapy, since as the tumor retracts it may be possible to protect more lung and heart. In addition, blocks are used to protect the humeral heads.

A linear accelerator of 6 MV photon, or 10 MV with a 0.25 in. Lucite sheet called a beam spoiler can be used. A treatment distance of 150 cm is used to both provide a large field size ($\leq 52 \times 52$ cm$^2$), and to homogenize the depth dose distribution. This requires that a removable auxiliary couch be used, since the standard accelerator couch cannot be retracted that far from the source. The dose to superficial lymph nodes in the buildup region is a concern with 10 MV but not the 6 MV, since the maximum dose for 10 MV photons occurs at 2.5 cm with 90% at 0.92 cm and a surface dose of 25%. When 10 MV is to be used, a beam spoiler is positioned 25 cm above the patient's surface to modify the beam, so that 90% falls at 0.48 cm and the surface dose is increased to 52%. In general, patients with a chest separation under 25 cm are best treated with 6 MV, while those with greater separation are well treated with 10 MV. The skin reaction is moderately greater with the 10 MV because of the beam spoiler, while the dose inhomogeneity becomes troublesome with 6 MV and robust patients. The blocks are bolted onto Lucite blocking trays, which are positioned in an accessory tray holder 64 cm from the target. At 20 Gy, Cerrobend blocks to protect the cervical spinal cord posteriorly and the larynx anteriorly are added, provided the initial nodal distribution permits this without compromising tumor control. After the blocks have been fab-

ricated, their alignment is checked in the simulator, and field shape and separation for key lymph node groups are determined, so that each nodal site can be monitored as dose accumulates at different rates in this complex volume. We use a Clarkson computer calculation in this assessment, though in the future, comprehensive three-dimensional calculations will be used. Figures 13-2 and 13-3 show our treatment attitudes schematically.

Field junctions for multiple radiation treatment fields required to treat Hodgkin disease can be complex. When large complex fields abut, there is always a major concern about the possibility of overdose to the spinal cord. We reduce the possibility of injury by employing junction field wedges. The unwedged 10 MV

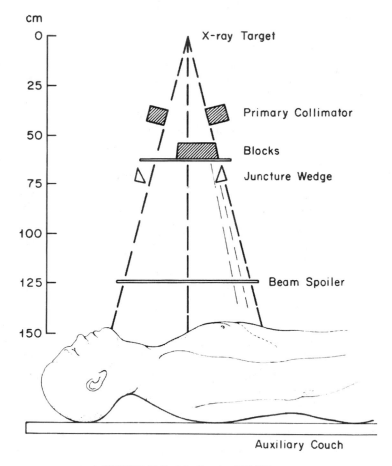

**FIGURE 13-2** Mantle setup 10 MV beam.

## FIELD EDGE MATCHING TECHNIQUE

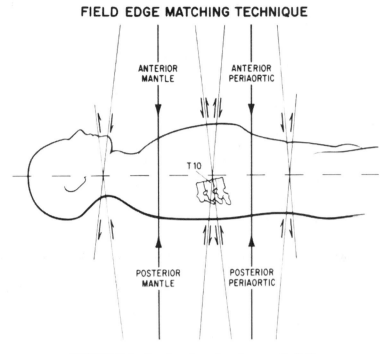

**FIGURE 13-3**    Junction of mantle and para-aortic fields.

photon penumbra at 150 cm is 8 mm; the wedge broadens the penumbra to 5 cm. With broad linearly changing penumbrae, an even dose across the junction will result if the fields are abutted at the 50% width of the relative dose profiles. The wedge is mounted on a sliding carriage with three alternative positions. In position 2, the field light edge generated by the edge of the wedge corresponds to the 50% width in the beam profile. Once the patient has been positioned and the wedge aligned, the carriage is locked and the wedge is moved to position 3, where the collimator jaws define the broad penumbra. By viewing the light field on the patient, one can verify that the collimator jaws have been opened until they are aligned with the edge of the wedge. At that time, the wedge then moves to position 1, the treatment position. Either one or both wedges can be used, and if only one is required the other can be moved outside the field entirely. When one is treating the para-aortic field, wedges are used to broaden both the superior and the inferior field edges.

We have encountered only two difficulties with these wedges: first, mechanical constraints prevent fields less than 15.5 cm in height from using both superior and inferior wedges; second, if the splenic hilum or spleen is included in the para-aortic node field, a modification to the lung blocks must be considered to ensure an appropriate dose distribution to the volume of interest from the mantle field. Details of the wedge system are shown in Figure 13-4. In arranging field matches, we calculate a junction of the fields at the midplane, with the anterior mantle lower border matching the superior border of the posterior para-aortic field edge. Similarly, the inferior margin of the posterior mantle field corresponds to the superior margin of the anterior para-aortic field. A typical mantle field design is shown in Figure 13-5. If a patient is difficult to position, immobilization casts can be made, or small cord blocks can be used (about 2 cm long and wide) on one of the fields. These reduce the risk of

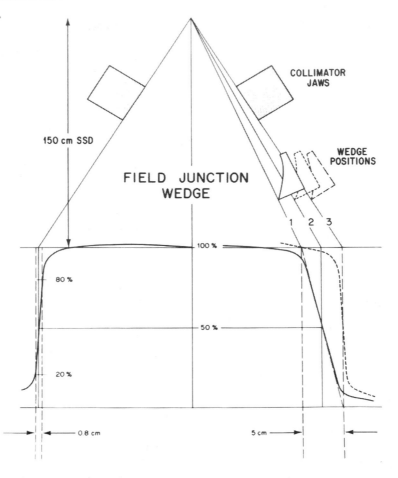

**FIGURE 13-4**   Dose distribution at field junctions.

field overlap over the spinal cord without substantially reducing the mediastinal or para-aortic dose.

### The Para-aortic Field

The superior border of the para-aortic field is defined by the inferior border of the mantle field with a skin gap to avoid overdosing the spinal cord as described above. The inferior border is set up at the L4-5 disc space. The lateral borders are defined by 2 cm margins from the edge of the vertebral bodies to adequately cover the para-aortic nodes, and are typically a minimum of 8 cm and a maximum of 10 cm wide in the adjuvant setting. The portal design for a para-aortic field is shown in Figure 13-6. If the patient had a prior splenectomy, the surgical clips marking the splenic hilar region are included in the field. If the patient has an intact spleen, the entire spleen should be encompassed in the field. When a para-aortic field is required in a patient with an intact spleen, the mantle field inferior margin should be placed above the diaphragm, unless there is a need to cover the lower cardiac boarder in the mantle field. High placement of the junction aids in preventing overlap of the cardiac tissues adjacent to the two fields. The classic subdiaphragmatic radiation field, the "inverted Y," is rarely used for patients presenting with supradiaphragmatic disease. It is used in patients presented with early stage in-

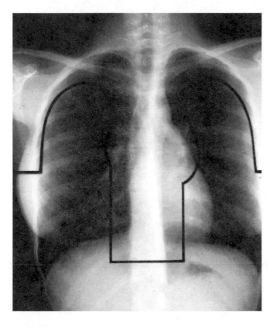

**FIGURE 13-5** Portal design for mantle field.

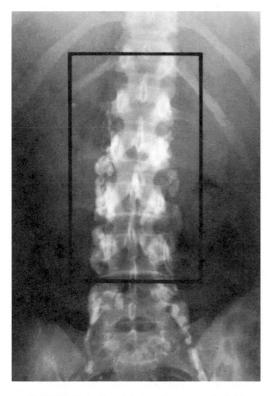

**FIGURE 13-6** Portal design for para-aortic field.

fradiaphragmatic disease, and the field setup may encompass the pelvic lymph nodes with or without the inclusion of the inguinal/femoral nodes. The same technical principles have been applied entirely satisfactorily to the inverted-Y distribution, and safe junctions with para-aortic fields have been achieved.

## NON-HODGKIN LYMPHOMA

Pathologists distinguish more than two dozen malignant proliferations of lymphocytes in which tissue involvement predominates.[31] Each lymphoma subtype represents the clonal expansion of a development compartment of one or another lymphocyte lineage or sublineage, and each is the result of distinct pathogenic mechanisms.[32,33] The complexity of the non-Hodgkin lymphomas accurately reflects the complexity of the lymphoid system. The subtypes of non-Hodgkin lymphoma with widely differing natural histories require diverse therapeutic approaches and present a far more complex problem than Hodgkin disease.[34,35]

Overall 5-year survival for non-Hodgkin lymphoma in the United States is only about 50%,[1,2] and many of the 5-year survivors have indolent lymphoma to which they eventually succumb. In 1994 non-Hodgkin lymphomas were responsible for 94% of the total lymphoma deaths, in contrast to 1950 when Hodgkin disease accounted for 30% of the total.[1] The 3% to 4% annual increase of non-Hodgkin incidence over the time period contributes to its increasing dominance in total lymphoma mortality.

Four considerations dominate our approach to non-Hodgkin lymphoma management[32,34]:

1. Histologic subtype (classification) (Table 13-5), which is the best indication of aggressiveness and dissemination.
2. Primary disease site in lymphomas of extranodal origin.
3. Extent of disease (stage).
4. Age and the presence of complicating disease.

**TABLE 13-5   A Clinician's List of the Non-Hodgkin Lymphomas**

| | Percent of Nodal Lymphoma | Median Survival (years)[a] |
|---|---|---|
| *Nodal B Lineage* | | |
| Low grade malignancy | | |
| Small lymphocytic (includes B-CLL) | 5–8 | 5.5–6 |
| Lymphoplasmacytic/lymphoplasmacytoid | 3–5 | 4 |
| Follicular small cell | 15–20 | 6.5–7 |
| Follicular mixed small and large cell | 10–15 | 4.5–5 |
| Intermediate grade malignancy | | |
| Follicular large cell | 1–5 | 2.5–3 |
| Mantle cell | 4–8 | 3–5 |
| Diffuse large cell | 20–25 | 1–2 |
| Immunoblastic | 5–8 | 0.5–1.5 |
| High grade malignancy | | |
| Burkitt and Burkitt-like | 3–5 | 0.5–1 |
| *T Lineage* | | |
| Lymphoblastic (thymic/prethymic) | 3–5 | 0.5–2 |
| Peripheral T-cell lymphoma: adult T-cell leukemia/lymphoma; angioimmunoblastic lymphoma, nasal/angiocentric lymphoma; lymphomatoid granulomatosis; anaplastic large-cell lymphoma; mycosis fungoides/ Sezary syndrome; intestinal T-cell lymphoma; and other (pleomorphic; small, medium, and large cell) | 5–15 | 1–2 |
| *Extranodal Lymphoma* | | |
| Classified separately by site: many are marginal zone B-cell lineage of MALT (mucosa-associated lymphoid tissue) type | | |

[a]Figures based on 2535 cases from various sources seen between 1952 and 1979.[32,34]

While in Hodgkin disease the extent of disease is the dominant factor, in the non-Hodgkin lymphomas histologic subtype and primary extranodal site are frequently more important considerations. Furthermore, since many patients with non-Hodgkin lymphomas are elderly, age and complicating illness play a more important role in management than they do in Hodgkin disease.

The non-Hodgkin lymphomas are less frequently localized than is Hodgkin disease, and chemotherapy has assumed a more predomi-

nant role in its management over the past decade. Convincing evidence of an acceptable long-term control (cure) rate following radiation therapy *alone* probably exists for less than 10% of non-Hodgkin lymphoma patients.[36] This group includes stage IA and limited stage IIA nodal presentations of lymphomas with follicular small-cell, plasmacytic or small lymphocytic histology; and some stage IA$_E$ lymphomas with low or intermediate grade histology presenting in certain extranodal sites (particularly those of MALT, or mucosa-associated lymphoid tissue, lineage). Radiation also plays an adjuvant role to conventional and high dose chemotherapy in a larger number of patients with both localized and advanced disease.

## Histological Classification

The REAL (Revised European–American Classification of Lymphoid Neoplasms) classification of non-Hodgkin lymphomas is being increasingly accepted by pathologists today.[3] It is the first system to integrate knowledge derived from immunophenotype (which closely reflects the lymphocyte lineage or sublineage), and cytogenetics and molecular genetics (which define causal oncogene derangements) into morphologic diagnosis. The REAL classification much more accurately defines lymphoma subtypes than the Rappaport, Lukes–Collins, Lennert,[31] and Working Formulation[37] classifications it is replacing. The REAL classification has the shortcoming for the clinician (not shared by the Lennert system and the Working Formulation) of deemphasizing the natural history of the various lymphoma subtypes. The listing of Table 13-5 attempts to circumvent this objection by grouping the major entities of the REAL classification into prognosis-based groups.

## Staging Classification and Diagnostic Workup

The Ann Arbor Hodgkin disease staging classification[4] (Table 13-2) is also used for the non-Hodgkin lymphomas, but serves less well for the latter conditions. The staging workup employed for the non-Hodgkin lymphomas is less rigorous. CT scans of the chest, abdomen, and pelvis are obtained. A stained peripheral blood smear is always examined and the bone marrow biopsied. Immunophenotyping blood or tissue by means of flow cytometry is routine in many pathology laboratories. An agarose gel electrophoresis is useful in patients with small lymphocytic and lymphoplasmacytic lymphomas, and the spinal fluid is examined in most pediatric patients, as well as many adults with Burkitt, Burkitt-like, lymphoblastic, and HIV-associated lymphomas. Patients with non-Hodgkin lymphoma are not subjected to staging laparotomy.

## Primary Treatment

***General Observations***   While the multiplicity of treatment modalities and acronym-designated regimens may seem daunting, in reality the therapeutic options available in the non-Hodgkin lymphomas are limited in number: they are listed in Tables 13-6 and 13-7. The first, observation, is frequently suitable for indolent lymphomas in elderly patients; the second, radiation therapy, is employed alone or as part of combined modality therapy for the cure of localized disease, or occasionally for palliation or local control of advanced incurable lymphoma. A single alkylating agent, usually chlorambucil or cyclophosphamide, was the standard conservative approach for disseminated low grade lymphomas. At the present time the purine nucleoside analogs are being introduced in low grade lymphomas, either as single agents or as part of combination therapy. The least aggressive of the drug combinations (Tables 13-6 and 13-7) for advanced low grade, and for both localized and advanced intermediate grade lymphomas, are the regimens C-MOPP [cyclophosphamide, vincristine (Oncovin), prednisone, procarbazine] and CVP (cyclophosphamide, vincristine, prednisone), which contain no doxorubicin (Adriamycin). Their use is now largely restricted to patients in whom doxorubicin is contraindicated for cardiac reasons.

Over the past decade, CHOP (cyclophosphamide, doxorubicin, vincristine, and prednisone) has emerged as the principal chemotherapy program for non-Hodgkin lymphoma. We still employ the more complex ProMACE-CytaBOM regimen in some patents with unfavorable prognostic features (see Table 13-7).

Since salvage drug regimens (ICE, ESHAP) rarely cure individuals who fail doxorubicin-containing programs, the former are most effectively employed for cytoreduction prior to high dose therapy with peripheral stem cell support.

**TABLE 13-6   Therapeutic Options in Non-Hodgkin Lymphoma**[a]

1. Observation
2. Radiation (localized disease)
3. Alkylating agents (chlorambucil or cyclophosphamide)
4. Purine analogs (fludarabine, 2-chlorodeoxyadenosine, 2′-deoxycoformycin), interferon
5. Nondoxorubicin combinations (C-MOPP, CVP)
6. Standard doxorubicin combination (CHOP)
7. Third-generation combination (ProMACE-CytaBOM)
8. Salvage regimens (ICE, ESHAP, etc.)
9. High dose therapy with autologous peripheral stem cell/bone marrow transplantation
10. Special regimens for Burkitt, lymphoblastic, and pediatric lymphomas
11. Monoclonal antibodies (rituximab [Rituxan]) experimental: (radiolabeled, anti-idiotype, toxin-conjugated)

[a]See Table 13-7 for abbreviations.

Special regimens for Burkitt lymphoma, lymphoblastic lymphoma, and lymphomas in the pediatric age group are mentioned in a later section. A monoclonal antibody rituximab (Rituxan) is available for the treatment of low grade lymphomas.[38]

### Low Grade Nodal B-Cell Lymphomas

The first three low grade nodal lymphomas of B lineage in Table 13-5 (small lymphocytic, lymphoplasmacytic, and follicular small cell) share a number of common features. All are indolent, with median survivals in excess of 5 years: indeed in each disorder, a subset with survival in excess of 10 years is identifiable by prognostic variables. All three are almost always disseminated at outset, even when routine procedures suggest the opposite. In the great majority of patients who present with advanced disease, after several to many years during which the disease is little more than an inconvenience, it takes on an aggressive and life-threatening quality: in many instances, rebiopsy at that time will disclose transforma-

tion to a nonfollicular and/or large-cell lymphoma.[34] Finally, many patients with all three conditions are elderly, with limited life expectancy irrespective of the lymphoma. Thus, observation rather than treatment is frequently appropriate. Serial observations over the few months following diagnosis often defines the disease tempo and the need for treatment. [With the addition of extranodal B-cell lymphomas or low grade MALT (mucosa-associated lymphoid tissue) lineage (Tables 13-5 and 13-8), the great preponderance of indolent non-Hodgkin lymphoma is encompassed.]

*Follicular Small-Cell Lymphoma*   Follicular lymphomas of small cells make up 15% to 20% of nodal non-Hodgkin lymphoma. They are characterized by a t(14;18) translocation through which the immunoglobulin heavy chain locus on chromosome 14 deregulates the *bcl-2* gene on chromosome 18, thereby impairing apoptosis.[33] Despite recent advances in understanding the molecular mechanism of the disorder, treatment of this frequently encountered condition is unsatisfactory for patient and physician alike. No form of therapy has been demonstrated to alter the relapse pattern or survival curve of the disorder. Nonetheless, we opt for involved field irradiation for the 10% to 20% of patients in *stage IA or IIA with no more than two areas of contiguous disease* because of the excellent disease-free survival reported following such local treatment (approximately 50% disease-free at 20 years).[36]

The 80% to 90% of patients who present with stage III and IV disease are a more difficult problem. The Stanford group[39] propose observation whenever possible for this and other low grade lymphomas. An expectant approach is certainly appropriate for minimal asymptomatic disease in older individuals with follicular small-cell lymphoma. It is also an option that can be offered to younger patients with nonthreatening disease. However, while a reasonable alternative, expectant treatment has not been proven to be the treatment of choice. We treat many patients under age 55 with exten-

TABLE 13-7   Combination Chemotherapy of Non-Hodgkin Lymphoma

A   Formulation and Cycle Information

| | CVP | C-MOPP | CHOP | ProMACE-CytaBOM |
|---|---|---|---|---|
| Cyclophosphamide | × | × | × | × |
| Oncovin | × | × | × | × |
| Prednisone | × | × | × | × |
| Procarbazine | | × | | |
| Adriamycin | | | × | × |
| Bleomycin | | | | × |
| Methotrexate/leucovorin | | | | × |
| Cytosine arabinoside | | | | × |
| Etoposide (VP-16) | | | | × |
| Bactrim | | | | × |
| Cycle length, weeks | 4 | 4 | 3 | 3 |
| Cycle number | 6 | 6 | 6–8 | Variable |

B   Regimens

| | |
|---|---|
| Chlorambucil | 4–6 (or 0.1–0.15) mg/kg, PO, days 1–14 of 28-day cycle, or 15–20 PO, day 1 ± prednisone, 60 days, days 1–5 of 14-day cycle, or 30–40 day 1, ± prednisone, 60 days, days 1–5 of 21- to 28-day cycle; with subsequent dosage adjusted by WBC and platelet counts repeated every 21–28 days depending on WBC and platelet counts |
| Fludarabine | 15 IV, over 30 min, days 1–5 of 28-day cycle |
| Cladibrine (2-CDA) | 0.09 mg/kg, IV, by continuous infusion (CI), days 1–7, for a single cycle |
| CVP | Cyclophosphamide, 400, PO, days 1–5; vincristine, 1.4, IV, day 1; prednisone, 100, PO days 1–5 |
| C-MOPP | Cyclophosphamide, 650, replaces mustard in MOPP |
| CHOP | Cyclophosphamide, 750; vincristine, 1.4; doxorubicin, 50; all IV, day 1; prednisone, 100, PO, days 1–5 |
| ProMACE-CytaBOM | Cyclophosphamide, 650, doxorubicin, 25, and etoposide (VP-16), 120, IV day 1; prednisone, 60, PO, days 1–14; vincristine, 1.4; cytosine arabinoside, 300; and bleomycin, 5, IV, day 8; methotrexate, 120, IV, day 8, followed in 24 h by leucovorin, 25, PO, q6h × 5 |
| ICE | Ifosfamide, 1500, and etoposide, 100, IV, days 1–3; mesna, 300, 30 min before and 3 and 6 after each ifosfamide dose; carboplatin, AUC, 4–7, IV, day 1 (21-day cycle) |
| ESHAP | Methylpresnisolone, 500, IV, push (15 min); etoposide, 40, IV, over 1–2 h; cisplatin, 25 IV (CI), days 1–4; all days 1–4; cytarabine, 2000, IV (over 2 h); after day 4 cisplatin infusion |

[a]Doses expressed in milligrams per square meter unless noted otherwise, except that the maximum total dose of vincristine should not exceed 2.0 mg. Physicians employing these programs should be familiar with the dose, action, and side effects of each drug.

sive, bulky, symptomatic or progressive stage III or IV follicular small-cell lymphoma with combination chemotherapy, most frequently with CHOP. We also opt for CHOP at the time of diagnosis when the pathologist has difficulty distinguishing between follicular small-cell and follicular mixed histology, particularly in younger individuals.

**TABLE 13-8  Ground Rules for Primary Non-Hodgkin Lymphoma Treatment**[a]

| Lymphoma | Stage I/I$_E$ Localized | Stage II/II$_E$ Regional | Stage III/IV Disseminated |
|---|---|---|---|
| *Primary Nodal* | | | |
| B-lineage | | | |
| Small lymphocytic, lymphoplasmacytic, follicular small cell | RT | RT | O or CT or SA |
| Follicular mixed small and large cell | CT and/or RT | CT and/or RT | CT |
| Diffuse large cell, immunoblastic, follicular large cell, mantle cell | CT + RT | CT + RT | CT |
| Burkitt | Special chemotherapy programs (see text) | | |
| T-lineage | | | |
| Lymphoblastic | Special chemotherapy programs (see text) | | |
| Peripheral T-cell | Special programs (see text) | | |
| *Pediatric Lymphomas* | | | |
| | Special chemotherapy programs (see text) | | |
| *Primary Extranodal* | | | |
| Low grade MALT of skin, lung,[b] orbit, salivary gland, cervix | RT | RT ± CT | CT |
| Intermediate grade of preceding above, and thyroid, testis,[b] bone, breast, tonsil, mediastinum, sinus[c] | CT + RT | CT + RT | CT ± RT |
| Stomach,[d] intestine except IPSID, localized and submucosal or less | XC or RT | | |
| Other | XC + RT or CT | RT and/or CT ± XC | CT ± RT ± XC |
| CNS (brain, spinal cord, retina) | RT + CT[e] | | |

[a]Abbreviations: RT, radiation therapy; CT, CHOP or equivalent combination chemotherapy; SA, single agent (chlorambucil or cyclophosphamide); O, observe; IPSID, immunoproliferative small intestinal disease; XC, excise (resect).
[b]Resect.
[c]CNS prophylaxis.
[d]Trial of antibacterial chemotherapy for *Helicobacter pylori* positive tumors.
[e]Special chemotherapy program.

A single agent, usually chlorambucil or cyclophosphamide, or a nondoxorubicin combination such as CVP, are reasonable alternatives for nonurgent clinical situations in patients with advanced (clinical stage III and IV) and/or recurrent follicular small-cell lymphoma. The therapeutic role of the purine analogs in this subtype is being explored. As mentioned earlier, most nodular lymphomas eventually undergo a transition to aggressive, invasive, and less responsive diffuse and/or large-cell lymphomas.

*Small Lymphocytic and Lymphoplasmacytic Lymphomas*  Lymph nodes involved by small lymphocytic lymphoma and by chronic lymphocytic leukemia (CLL) cannot be distinguished on morphological grounds. The occasional non-leukemic patient presenting with a localized process should receive involved field irradiation as primary treatment. In the remainder of non-leukemic patients, treatment is usually instituted because of one or more of the following: deterioration of the level of one of the formed elements of the blood, systemic complaints, cosmetic considerations, organ involvement, or adenopathy that is progressive and/or threatening in size or location. Fludarabine is replacing chlorambucil with or without prednisone as the initial treatment of choice, or a doxorubicin or nondoxorubicin combination can be employed. Asymptomatic CLL patients without anemia or thrombocytopenia do not require treatment.

The approach to plasmacytic/plasmacytoid lymphomas (rearranged *pax-5*)[33] is similar to that of small lymphocytic lymphomas. The plasmacytoid morphology is likely to contribute the associated syndromes of Waldenström's macroglobulinemia, monoclonal gammopathy, Coomb's positive hemolytic anemia, or cryoglobulinemia, which may require special treatment.

### Follicular Mixed Small- and Large-Cell Lymphoma

Our experience agrees with that of the several investigators who report extended (> 10 years) disease-free survival following combination chemotherapy in approximately half of patients with follicular *mixed* lymphomas.[40,41] The evidence is sufficiently convincing to support the use of CHOP or C-MOPP as primary treatment of follicular mixed lymphoma patients with stage III or IV disease, and to provide an attractive alternative to radiation therapy as primary treatment of those in early stage. Further, because follicular mixed and follicular small-cell lymphomas may be difficult to distinguish, it is reasonable to offer combination chemotherapy to some younger individuals in whom the evidence of small-cell histology is less than conclusive.

### Intermediate Grade Lymphoma Nodal B-Cell Lymphoma

*Diffuse large-cell lymphoma* is an aggressive neoplasm once considered uniformly fatal. On the basis of clinical behavior, morphology, immunophenotype, and cytogenetics and molecular genetics (rearranged *bcl-2,* rearranged *bcl-6,* or neither[33]), we consider diffuse large-cell lymphoma to be a heterogeneous disorder. It is a major subtype of non-Hodgkin lymphoma, constituting approximately one-quarter of the total incidence of nodal B-cell neoplasms. With a short median survival of untreated disease (Table 13-5), and a 30% to 40% cure rate after combination chemotherapy, this subtype provides the major contribution of treatment to increased non-Hodgkin lymphoma survival. Furthermore, diffuse large-cell lymphomas serve as a paradigm for most other intermediate grade lymphomas [*follicular large cell, mantle cell* (rearranged *bcl-1*), and *immunoblastic*], and for low grade follicular mixed small- and large-cell lymphomas as well. It also has been intensely studied with respect to competing drug regimens and prognostic factors.

CHOP [cyclophosphamide, hydroxydoxorubicin (Adriamycin), vincristine (Oncovin), and prednisone] has regained its position as the combination drug program of choice for the treatment of non-Hodgkin lymphoma (Tables 13-6, 13-7). In the 1980s, increasingly complex (including bleomycin, etoposide, cytarabine, and methotrexate, with or without leucovorin rescue) and dose-intensive regimens were introduced. Only in the past few years has CHOP been compared against its competitors in prospective randomized trials. In a recent multi-institutional investigation, CHOP was found to be as effective as m-BACOD (methotrexate/ leucovorin, bleomycin, doxorubicin, cyclophosphamide, vincristine, and dexamethazone), ProMACE-CytaBOM (Table 13-7) and MACOP-B (methotrexate/ leucovorin, doxorubicin, cyclophosphamide, vincristine, and prednisone), and caused less fatal toxicity.[42] Thus CHOP is now our standard program for patients in low and intermediate prognostic groups. We reserve ProMACE-CytaBOM,[42] a well-tolerated and easily administered third-generation regimen, for some young or middle-aged individuals with prognostically unfavorable disease or re-fractory histology.

Factors that influence the prognosis of diffuse large-cell lymphoma continue to interest clinicians. However, the conclusions that emerge from extensive study are intuitively obvious: prognosis depends on the amount of tumor, how widely it has spread, and how well the patient can tolerate the required treatment. Thus, prognosis deteriorates with advanced stage, increased tumor bulk (diameter $> 7$ or 10 cm), and extranodal spread of nodal lymphoma (particularly to more than one extranodal site, or to the central nervous system or gastrointestinal tract). Many features, such as systemic symptoms (fever, sweats, chills, weight loss) and elevated lactic dehydrogenase and $\beta_2$-microglobulin are surrogate markers of tumor bulk. Age is an adverse prognostic factor insofar as older patients poorly tolerate or do not receive aggressive chemotherapy, and are more likely to die of treatment complications: important considerations in a real world. Performance status reflects both host and tumor.

In 1993 a four-part international prognostic index based on age, tumor stage, serum lactic dehydrogenase, performance status, and number of extranodal sites was devised for patients with aggressive non-Hodgkin lymphomas.[43] Five-year survival of patients classified by the index was 73% for the low risk group (0 or 1 risk factors), 51 for the low–intermediate group (2 risk factors), 43% for the high–intermediate group (3 risk factors), and 26% for the high risk group (4 or 5 risk factors). These prognostic criteria may also be applicable to low grade lymphomas.

CHOP or equivalent chemotherapy is appropriate for advanced (stage III and IV) large-cell lymphoma. A 50% to 70% complete remission rate,[32,35] followed by a relapse rate of 7% per year for years 2 through 5,[44] results in the cure of 30% to 40%. The data suggest that the somewhat higher complete remission rate obtained with the newer regimens (m-BACOD, ProMACE-CytaBOM, MACOP-B) is balanced by a higher relapse rate in years 2 to 5 (7%/year vs. 2%),[45] resulting in similar disease-free sur-vivals at 5 years. Most investigators supplement chemotherapy with involved field radiation for early disease, reporting 80% to 85% 5-year disease-free survival (90–95% for stage I and 50–75% for stage II[46]). This approach is also appropriate for *immunoblastic lymphoma* and *follicular large-cell* lymphoma. We have had little success with CHOP in mantle cell lymphoma and are exploring more aggressive approaches.

***Extranodal Lymphoma*** Primary extranodal lymphomas[34,36,47] constitute one-quarter of the non-Hodgkin lymphoma incidence in the United States (up to one-half in parts of Europe and the Far East). Unlike primary nodal lymphoma, where knowledge of histological subtype and stage suffice, each extranodal site exhibits special clinical characteristics and treatment requirements as well. Most extranodal lymphomas are of B lineage, and approximately half arise in the gastrointestinal tract.

Accumulating evidence supports the concept that many extranodal lymphomas arise from marginal zone B cells, a lineage distinct from those that predominate in nodal lymphomas. This lineage serves as an alternative lymphoid system referred to as the *mucosa-associated lymphoid tissue* (*MALT*) system. The characteristic histopathology of MALT lymphomas, centrocyte-like cells and lymphoepithelial lesions, was clarified only in the past decade. These lymphomas have been identified in many extranodal sites: eye (orbit and conjunctiva), stomach, large and small intestine, Waldeyer's ring, thyroid, salivary gland, lung, breast, and skin. In the past, many of these tumors were termed *pseudolymphomas,* but immunophenotype and receptor gene analysis indicates their clonal, hence neoplastic, nature, as does extended follow-up.

Extranodal lymphomas of various sites differ greatly in their natural history. Lymphomas of the skin, orbit, lung, and salivary gland, by definition localized at outset, are among the most indolent human lymphomas in their evolution. *Response to radiation therapy is excellent,* but very late relapse is always a hazard.

Extranodal lymphomas of the thyroid, testis, bone, breast, Waldeyer's ring, and mediastinum (mediastinal large-cell lymphoma is derived from a B lymphocyte of the thymic cortex and is appropriately classified as an extranodal lymphoma) constitute an intermediate group in which prognosis is critically dependent on stage or extent of disease. Superficial or confined lesions are readily cured, but spread beyond the boundaries of the organ frequently results in progressive lymphoma. They usually present as low stage, but at least half recur when primary treatment does not include CHOP or equivalent chemotherapy. When the latter treatment precedes radiation, high cure rates have been reported for early stage primary lymphoma of several extranodal sites (testis, thyroid, bone, Waldeyer's ring, and mediastinum[48]). Because of the excellent local control of Waldeyer's ring lymphoma achieved at the MGH in the past, we continue to initiate combined treatment of early disease of this subset with radiation therapy.[49] Our experience supports the evidence of others that CHOP or similar regimens are much less effective as primary therapy of patients who present with advanced (stage III and IV) extranodal lymphoma than in improving the cure rate of those irradiated for early (stage I and II) disease. In lymphomas of the testis and lung, resection is usually required for diagnosis.

Primary lymphoma of the central nervous system (and retina) and nasal accessory sinus constitute extranodal lymphomas with particularly poor outlook. At the MGH[50] and elsewhere, preirradiation chemotherapy with methotrexate has somewhat improved the dismal survival of CNS lymphoma, but lymphoma of the nasal accessory sinus remains intractable even with CNS prophylaxis.

The frequent gastric lymphomas of MALT lineage that present as low grade lesions localized to the mucosa or submucosa are usually cured by irradiation, combination chemotherapy, or subtotal gastrectomy.[51,52] We are evaluating the role of eradication of *Helicobacter pylori* via antibiotics on the permanent control of these neoplasms.[53]

The prognosis is much less good for more extensive gastric and intestinal lymphomas, which frequently require either irradiation or chemotherapy, or both, and may merit debulking subtotal gastrectomy. Total gastrectomy is never indicated, and the role of less extensive resections is argued. Adverse prognostic factors include high grade MALT or non-MALT histology, involvement of distant abdominal lymph nodes [para-aortic and paracaval (stage $IIE_2$), penetration of serosa to adjacent structures (stage $II_E$), and disseminated disease or supradiaphragmatic node involvement (stage IV)].[54,55]

### Lymphomas of High Grade Malignancy

*Burkitt lymphoma* is a rare condition in the temperate world, where it most frequently presents as an abdominal tumor. It is a formidable neoplasm, with the shortest doubling time of any human malignancy, and is often accompanied by a tumor lysis syndrome (hyperuricemia, hyperkalemia, hyperphosphatemia, hypocalcemia, and acidosis) of catastrophic proportions. Preservation of renal function and initial correction of acidosis are frequently necessary for survival.

Burkitt and Burkitt-like lymphomas differ in morphology (Burkitt-like tumors do not exhibit the monotonous uniformity of nuclear size and contour), clinical characteristics (Burkitt patients are younger and more likely to present with extranodal disease, particularly in the gastrointestinal tract), and molecular genetics (the c-*myc* rearrangements uniformly present in Burkitt are usually absent in Burkitt-like tumors). Most Burkitt lymphoma seen in the United States and Europe is of the sporadic (nonendemic) form characterized by a lower (15–20%) Epstein–Barr virus positivity and molecular genetic abnormalities which differ slightly from those of African (endemic) Burkitt lymphoma.

Most successful adult treatment programs for Burkitt and Burkitt-like lymphomas are modeled after pediatric protocols, and employ brief pulses of high dose alkylating agent therapy coupled with intermediate or high dose methotrexate, vincristine, anthracyclines, epipodophyllins, and cytarabine chemotherapy, and CNS prophylaxis, which may or may not include cranial irradiation.[34,35,56] Patients with limited disease (localized extra-abdominal or completely excised abdominal disease) have an excellent prognosis (close to 100% cure) with 6 months or less of such intensive treatment.[56] Patients with unresectable abdominal disease treated in this manner experience cure rates of 60% to 90%.

In the past, survival was poor (10–40%) in patients with Murphy stage IV (CNS or bone marrow involvement). However recently, excellent outcomes (70–80% event-free survival at 2–7 years) have been reported with several modified intense, short-duration protocols in these patients as well.[56] Results are sufficiently encouraging to raise doubts of the wisdom of high dose/peripheral stem cell consolidation of patients in first remission, even in subgroups with unfavorable prognostic features at diagnosis.

### Lymphomas of T Lineage

*Lymphoblastic Lymphoma*   This thymic/prethymic T-cell lymphoma frequently arises in the mediastinum of older children and young adults. It is closely related to the T-cell variant of acute lymphoblastic leukemia, and its treatment is closely modeled after the treatment of that disease. Emergency problems associated with these aggressive mediastinal masses frequently include airway obstruction, superior vena caval obstruction, and pericardial tamponade. Many regimens effective in Burkitt and Burkitt-like lymphomas are less successful in extensive lymphoblastic lymphomas. Alkylating agents are of less importance here, and longer treatment programs (15–24 months) are needed.[35,56]

Remarkable cure rates have been achieved in the past decade with the protocols of Memorial Sloan-Kettering (LSA$_2$-L$_2$)[57] and of the Berlin–Frankfurt–Munster (BFM) group.[58] Recent modifications of the former (10 different drugs employed in induction, consolidation, and prolonged maintenance phases, with CNS prophylaxis) have produced 60% to 80% long-term actuarial survival in patients with extensive disease (extensive intrathoracic tumor, or widely disseminated disease usually involving the bone marrow) and 90% or more in those with limited disease. The equally complex BFM protocol for acute lymphocytic leukemia/non-Hodgkin lymphoma requires 24 months for completion, and has resulted in 78% predicted disease-free survival at 7 years for a patient population of which more than 90% presented with advanced disease.

*Peripheral T-Cell Lymphoma*   Peripheral T-cell lymphomas deserve special comment.[32,34] Lymphomatoid granulomatosis may respond to CHOP or equivalent chemotherapy, and the subgroup of nasal/angiocentric lymphomas to radiation, as well. Many anaplastic large-cell lymphomas are reported to respond to CHOP or similar programs, but some recognized subtypes of peripheral T-cell lymphoma, including adult T-cell leukemia/lymphoma, are not cured reliably with these or other programs. A minor fraction of those with angioimmunoblastic lymphadenopathy with dysproteinemia will be improved by adrenal corticoids. However, the outlook for most patients with angioimmunoblastic T-cell lymphoma is poor even with conventional aggressive drug treatment. Putative T-cell lymphomas that do not fit into the listed T-cell syndromes are treated with CHOP or similar regimens with results that are variously reported to be equal or inferior to large cell lymphomas of B lineage.[32,35] Our institutional experience with documented (by unequivocal immunophenotype and/or T-cell receptor gene rearrangement) T-cell lymphomas has been discouraging. The International Prognostic Factor Index is reported to be applicable to peripheral T-cell lymphoma.[59]

### Pediatric Non-Hodgkin Lymphomas

Non-Hodgkin lymphomas are infrequently encountered in children (< 100 deaths occurred in the United States in 1993). Although most are high grade and a major fraction are of T lineage, in recent years cure rates have been much higher (approximately 70% cured) than in adults.[2]

Burkitt and Burkitt-like lymphomas (B-cell lineage) constitute approximately one-half (40–50%) of the total pediatric non-Hodgkin lymphoma incidence, and lymphoblastic lymphomas (85% T-cell lineage) another one-third (30–35%)[56,60]: the treatment of these two, which constitute about 80% to 85% of the pediatric total, are briefly discussed above. The remaining 15% to 20% are composed of large-cell lymphomas: diffuse large cell (B lineage), and the recently recognized anaplastic large cell (predominantly T lineage). The diffuse and anaplastic large-cell lymphomas of children are treated successfully, usually with protocols similar to those employed for Burkitt and Burkitt-like neoplasms.

In children with non-Hodgkin lymphoma, special staging classifications devised at the St. Jude Hospital and the National Cancer Institute have replaced the Ann Arbor system, though the same treatment programs produce similar results in pediatric and adult populations with the same histology.

In recent years, chemotherapy has come to occupy an increasingly central place and radiation therapy an increasingly peripheral one in the management of pediatric non-Hodgkin lymphoma. Central nervous system relapse, always an important consideration in non-Hodgkin lymphoma in the pediatric age group, is usually managed by prophylactic intrathecal methotrexate and/or cytarabine and systemic medium or high dose methotrexate, usually without cranial irradiation because of the late toxicity of the latter. Finally, because pediatric non-Hodgkin lymphomas require treatment with the complex and toxic protocols employed in acute childhood leukemia, they are best managed at centers with specialized knowledge and experience.[56]

### Recurrent Disease/Salvage Therapy

Patients with recurrent low grade lymphomas who fail to respond to conventional single-agent and combination chemotherapy frequently respond to the purine nucleoside analogs fludarabine[61,62] or cladibrine (2-chlorodeoxyadenosine, 2-CDA).[63,64] Remission rates of 40% to 50% (most partial) are reported, with median duration of about a year. The relative merits of these drugs have not been established, nor have their therapeutic role in combination with older agents and their spectrum of toxicity been fully evaluated. The interferons in moderate dose achieve modest results in recurrent low grade lymphomas, but at the cost of distressing flu-like side effects.

A number of salvage programs that utilize a variety of active newer agents (cisplatin, mitoxantrone, etoposide, ifosfamide, CCNU, BCNU, and cytarabine) have been developed for non-Hodgkin lymphoma patients who fail conventional regimens (see Table 13-7). Few patients are cured with these programs, and treatment mortality may approach 10%. However, response rates of 40% to 50%, lasting several months to a year or more, are obtained. Salvage programs are also useful in reducing tumor bulk prior to bone marrow transplantation. We find the ICE[65] and ESHAP[66] regimens (Table 13-7) satisfactory.

### High Dose Therapy with Autologous Peripheral Stem Cell Transplantation

PST has opened a multitude of new possibilities in lymphoma management.[67] In contrast to Hodgkin disease, in which some relapsed patients are cured without transplantation, PST offers the only chance of cure for the individual with non-Hodgkin lymphoma who relapses following chemotherapy. The least controversial application is in the patient with intermediate or high grade lymphoma who fails conventional therapy.[68,69] Approximately 40% to 50% of individuals with good performance status in either drug-sensitive relapse or second remission experience 3- to 5-year disease-free survival with a procedure-related mortality of 5% to 10%, survival figures that cannot be approached with other salvage programs. Patients in drug-resistant relapse with disease that exceeds 2 cm in diameter or with poor performance status achieve less than half that survival percentage and may suffer twice that mortality, but may have no other hope of long-term salvage. Radiation therapy is often employed to improve remission status prior to transplantation or to treat residual local disease after the procedure.

The place of PST in the primary therapy of non-Hodgkin lymphoma and for consolidation of first remission remains under investigation and is controversial.[70–72] High dose therapy with PST during remission has been suggested for intermediate grade, and for Burkitt, Burkitt-like, and lymphoblastic lymphomas with unfavorable prognostic features, but the improving outcomes of recent primary treatment programs raise questions about the advisability of up-front transplantation.

High dose therapy with PST has also been employed with curative intent in low grade lymphomas patients in first[73] or later remissions.[74] However, we have not adopted this approach because early publications report a disappointing relapse rate, and a disconcerting incidence of treatment-induced myelodysplasia and acute nonlymphocytic leukemia.[75]

Careful randomized study is sorely needed to evaluate the role of PST as part of the primary therapy of intermediate and high grade non-Hodgkin lymphomas, and in the treatment of low grade tumors.

## Non-Hodgkin Lymphoma Associated with the Acquired Immunodeficiency Syndrome

The epidemic of aggressive and highly lethal non-Hodgkin lymphoma in patients with the acquired immunodeficiency syndrome (AIDS) overshadows the many significant advances in lymphoma management of the past two decades.[32,76,77] A detailed projection placed the number of U.S. cases of AIDS-related non-Hodgkin lymphoma between 3000 and 10,000 in 1992. Furthermore, 2 years into a long-term National Cancer Institute study of antiretroviral therapy with zidovudine, 19% of patients (by actuarial calculation) with severe human im-

munodeficiency virus (HIV) infection had developed non-Hodgkin lymphoma: lymphoma occurrence and CD4 count below 50 mm$^3$ were closely correlated.

HIV-associated lymphomas are almost all of B lineage, the great preponderance being of high grade malignancy.[32,76,77] The predominating morphologies are immunoblastic, Burkitt and Burkitt-like, and diffuse large cell. Three-quarters arise in extranodal sites, and a similar fraction present with advanced disease. Systemic complaints and bone marrow involvement are both frequent. Extranodal lymphomas in AIDS patients differ from those in HIV-negative individuals by their origin in unusual sites. Approximately one-quarter arise in the central nervous system, and an equal number in the gastrointestinal tract, including the mouth and ano/rectal region.

In the past, treatment has been unsatisfactory.[76,77] Median survival for HIV-associated non-CNS lymphomas was 6 to 12 months; those involving the CNS had median survival of about 2 to 3 months. The prognosis is better when non-Hodgkin lymphoma is the presenting AIDS diagnosis than when the neoplasm develops in an individual with clinical AIDS. A markedly depressed CD4 count ($< 100/mm^3$), which limits effective chemotherapy and is a surrogate marker of viral load, is a critical prognostic variable. Age ($\geq$ age 40) and elevated lactic dehydrogenase also predict short survival.

The superiority of special antilymphoma drug regimens in AIDS patients has not been proven. While m-BACOD has received much attention, we feel that the less toxic CHOP program is more suitable for the immunocompromised AIDS patient. Though many individuals required dose attenuation in the past, we are not convinced that half dosage will provide optimal lymphoma control.[78,79] The availability of protease inhibitors and a variety of nucleoside and nonnucleoside reverse transcriptase inhibitors that are less marrow suppressive than zidovudine should improve the outlook of the AIDS patient with non-CNS non-Hodgkin lymphoma. With the improved immunological status possible with the new antiviral agents, the prophylaxis of opportunistic infection, and the availability of G-CSF, GM-CSF, and other cytokines to support granulocytes, platelets, and red cells, it should be possible to *initiate treatment with both optimal antilymphoma treatment (full-dose CHOP) and optimal anti-HIV therapy* (currently two nucleosidase inhibitors and one protease inhibitor[80] in most patients. As with pediatric lymphomas, CNS prophylaxis should always be considered.

Primary AIDS lymphomas of the CNS continue to carry a grim prognosis. We employ whole-brain irradiation.

## OTHER TREATMENT CONSIDERATIONS

Compression of the spinal cord is seen in the non-Hodgkin lymphomas as it is in Hodgkin disease. With the availability of MRI and other new diagnostic techniques, early diagnosis of cord compression, critical for satisfactory functional recovery, has become more feasible. Optimal treatment is usually achieved by irradiation with or without chemotherapy. Laminectomy may still be required for the rare patient who has received extensive prior irradiation and chemotherapy.

Other involvement of the central nervous system by lymphoma at the time of diagnosis or at relapse is of grave prognostic significance. These manifestations usually can be controlled by cranial radiation and intrathecal chemotherapy, but long-term arrest of the disease is rarely achieved.

## CONCLUSION

While the major problem in Hodgkin disease management is reduction in grave treatment complications, the main obstacles to the control of the non-Hodgkin lymphomas is the lack of more effective chemotherapy or biological therapy for systemic disease and the challenge of AIDS-associated lymphomas.

## RADIATION THERAPY CONSIDERATIONS IN NON-HODGKIN LYMPHOMA

The role of radiotherapy as a solitary therapy for non-Hodgkin lymphoma is limited; however, it is critical for optimal combined modality therapy of diffuse large-cell or localized low grade non-Hodgkin lymphomas. It offers cure of disease for truly localized early stage low grade lymphoma, which represents approximately 10% to 15% of all low grade lymphomas. In contrast to Hodgkin disease, the pattern of spread of non-Hodgkin disease does not usually follow the contiguous lymphatic chains. The low grade lymphomas are almost always radioresponsive. Bush et al. report good local control when doses greater than 30 Gy were given.[81] Fuks and Kaplan, in a classic publication, showed a continuous dose response with 50% infield controls at 20 to 30 Gy, and 90% or higher control rates for almost all histology at 40 Gy.[82] While some institutions have advocated extended field or total lymphoid irradiation in patients with early stage disease, it is difficult to be sure that local field is not sufficient. At Stanford University total nodal irradiation resulted in a 10-year freedom from relapse data of 54% of 124 patients, and local field irradiation at the Princess Margaret Hospital resulted in a reported 53% 10-year freedom from relapse data on 190 similar patients. While most of the initial failures at Princess Margaret Hospital were out of field, it is not clear that adjuvant treatment of those fields at Stanford University actually increase survival of this disease, with its very slow natural progression.

We have elected to use limited fields in localized low grade lymphoma: 40 Gy is given to the involved lymph node site and the immediate first-echelon lymphatic. A boost of 5 Gy to a small volume at the site of involved node is sometimes added if the lesion is at a peripheral nodal site. The daily fraction size is 1.8 Gy. There is no clear evidence that chemotherapy is as effective as we would like in low grade lymphomas. Response rates are high, but recurrences are expected with long follow-up. Nevertheless for patients with advanced stage disease (stages III and IV), we have preferred to use a systemic approach in these patients, provided they are well enough to tolerate therapy. Radiation is reserved for localized disease and residual disease in most patients. We have not routinely irradiated sites of bulky disease, although this is a reasonable attitude pursued in some other centers. Likewise, we have not considered low dose whole-body irradiation in these patients, though some others have found this to be effective in previously untreated disease.

As stated in the preceding paragraphs, for intermediate grade lymphoma of early stage (I and II) most investigators supplement chemotherapy with involved field radiation, with a 5-year disease-free survival of 80% to 85%. Randomized studies confirm an improved survival with this combination. We have favored combined modality treatment with CHOP followed by 40 Gy to consolidate control. The results of this approach have been relatively satisfactory; for example, in our first 12 patients with mediastinal disease, 10 individuals first reported in 1982 remain in good control.[83] If a newer but more toxic chemotherapy regimen is to be used instead of CHOP, we are taking the approach that, while radiation can certainly be justified in the care of patients with poor prognostic features, the benefits of adjuvant radiation must be balanced against the risk of short- and long-term toxicity. The need for adjuvant radiation can sometimes be better defined if patients have pre- and then post-chemotherapy gallium scanning.

For patients with head and neck stage I disease, radiation alone historically has been the preferred therapy. Our experience indicates excellent local control (98%) of stage I disease presenting in Waldeyer's ring treated with radiotherapy alone with doses of 45 to 50 Gy to uninvolved cervical nodes and boosts of 5 to 10 Gy to the primary site.[84] Because of higher cure rates reported for early stage primary lymphoma of several extra nodal sites when chemotherapy precedes radiation, we have also initiated chemotherapy prior to radiotherapy for early stage intermediate grade lymphoma in the head and neck region in the recent years.[48]

## REFERENCES

1. Ries LAG, Kosary CL, Hankey BF, Miller BA, Harras A, Edwards BK (eds): *SEER Cancer Statistics Review, 1973–1994,* NIH Publication 97-2789. Bethesda, National Cancer Institute, 1997.

2. Parker SL, Tong T, Bolden S, Wingo PA: Cancer statistics 1997. *CA: Cancer J Clin* 1997;47: 5–25.

3. Harris, NL, Jaffe ES, Stein H, et al: A revised European–American classification of malignant lymphoid neoplasms: A proposal from the International Lymphoma Study Group. *Blood* 1994;84:1361–1392.

4. Carbone PP, Kaplan HS, Musshoff K, et al: Report of the Committee on Hodgkin's Disease Staging Classification. *Cancer Res* 1971;31: 1860–1861.

5. Mauch P, Rosenthal DS, Canellos GP, Come SE, Hellman S: Stage III Hodgkin's disease: Improved survial with combined modality therapy as compared with radiation therapy alone. *J Clin Oncol* 1985;3:1166.

6. Leibenhaut MH, Hoppe RT, Effron B, et al: Prognostic indicators of laparotomy findings in clinical stage I-II supradiaphragmatic Hodgkin's disease. *J Clin Oncol* 1989;7:81–89.

7. Mauch P, Larson D, Osteen R, et al: Prognostic factors for positive surgical staging in patients with Hodgkin's disease. *J Clin Oncol* 1990; 8:257–265.

8. Specht L: Prognostic factors in Hodgkin's disease. *Semin Radiation Oncol* 1996;6:146–161.

9. Tucker MA: Solid second cancers following Hodgkin's disease. *Hematol/Oncol Clin North Am* 1993;7:389–400.

10. Aisenberg AC, Finkelstein DM, Doppke KP, et al: high risk of breast carcinoma after irradiation of young women with Hodgkin's disease. *Cancer* 1997;79:1203–1210.

11. Hancock SL, Tucker MA, Hoppe RT: Factors affecting late mortality from Hodgkin's disease after treatment of Hodgkin's disease. *JAMA* 1993;270:1949–1955.

12. Aisenberg AC: Acute nonlymphocytic leukemia after treatment for Hodgkin's disease. *Am J Med* 1983;75:449–454.

13. Canellos GP, Anderson JR, Propert KJ, et al: Chemotherapy of advanced Hodgkin's disease with MOPP, ABVD, or MOPP alternating with ABVD. *N Engl J Med* 1992;327:1478–1484.

14. Siber GR, Weitzman SA, Aisenberg AC: Antibody response of patients with Hodgkin's disease to protein and polysaccharide antigens. *Rev Infect Dis* 1981;3(suppl):S144–S159.

15. Bonnadonna G: Modern treatment of malignant lymphoma: A multidisciplinary approach. *Ann Oncol* 1994;5(suppl 2):S5–S16.

16. Connors JM: Evaluation and treatment of early-stage Hodgkin's disease, in *American Society of Clinical Oncology Educational Book, 33rd Annual Meeting.* Alexandria, VA: ASCO, 1997, pp 240–243.

17. Cosset J., Henry-Amar M. Meerwaldt J, et al: The EORTC trials for limited stage Hodgkin's disease. *Eur J Cancer* 1992;11:1847–1850.

18. Jones E, Mauch P: Limited radiation therapy for selected patients with pathological stage IA and IIA Hodgkin's disease. *Semin Radiation Oncol* 1996;6:162–171.

19. Lohri A, Barnett M, Fairey RN, et al: Outcome of treatment of first relapse of Hodgkin's disease after primary chemotherapy: Identification of risk factors from the British Columbia experience 1970 to 1988. *Blood* 1991;77:2292–2298.

20. Reece DE, Connors JM, Spinelli JJ, et al: Intensive therapy with cyclophosphamide, carmustine, etoposide ± cisplatin, and autologous bone marrow transplantation for Hodgkin's disease in first relapse after combination chemotherapy. *Blood* 1994;83:1193–1199.

21. Brice P, Bastion Y, Devine M, et al: Analysis of prognostic factors after first relapse of Hodgkin's disease in 187 patients. *Cancer* 1996; 78:1293–1299.

22. Roach M, Kapp DS, Rosenberg SA, et al: Radiotherapy with curative intent: An option in selected patients relapsing after chemotherapy for advanced Hodgkin's disease. *J Clin Oncol* 1987;5:550–555.

23. Mauch P, Tarbell N, Skarin A, et al: Widefield radiation therapy alone or with chemotherapy for Hodgkin's disease in relapse from combination chemotherapy. *J Clin Oncol* 1987;6: 544–549.

24. Yahalom J: Management of relapsed and refractory Hodgkin's disease. *Semin Radiat Oncol* 1996;6:210–214.

25. Nademanee A, O'Donnell MR, Snyder DS, et al: High-dose chemotherapy with or without total body irradiation followed by autologous bone marrow and/or peripheral blood stem cell transplantation for patients with relapsed and refractory Hodgkin's disease: Results in 85 patients with analysis of prognostic factors. *Blood* 1995;85:1381–1390.

26. Horning SJ, Chao NJ, Negrin RS, et al: High-dose therapy and autologous progenitor cell transplantation for recurrent or refractory Hodgkin's disease: Analysis of the Stanford University results and prognostic indices. *Blood* 1997;89:810–813.

27. Mundt AJ, Sibley G, Williams S, et al: Patterns of failure following high-dose chemotherapy and autologous bone marrow transplantation with involved field radiotherapy for relapsed/refractory Hodgkin's disease. *Int J Radiat Oncol Biol Phys* 1995;33:261–270.

28. Willett C, Linggood RM, Meyer J, et al: Results of treatment of stage IA and IIA Hodgkin's disease. *Cancer* 1987;59:1107–1111.

29. Willett C, Linggood RM, Meyer J, et al: Results of treatment of stage IIIA Hodgkin's disease. *Cancer* 1987;59:27–30.

30. Aisenberg AC, Linggood RM, Lew RA: The changing face of Hodgkin's disease. *Am J Med* 1979;67:921–928.

31. Lennert K, Feller AC: *Histopathology of Non-Hodgkin's Lymphomas (based on the updated Kiel classification),* 2nd ed. New York, Springer-Verlag, 1992.

32. Aisenberg AC: Coherent view of non-Hodgkin's lymphoma. *J Clin Oncol* 1995;13: 2656–2675.

33. Gaidano G, Dalla-Favera, R: Lymphomas: Molecular biology, in VT Devita Jr, S Hellman, and SA Rosenberg (eds): *Cancer: Principles and Practice of Oncology,* 5th ed. Philadelphia, Lippincott, 1997, pp 2131–2145.

34. Aisenberg AC: *Malginant Lymphoma: Biology, Natural History and Treatment.* Philadelphia, Lea & Febiger, 1991.

35. Shipp MA, Mauch PM, Harris NL: Non-Hodgkin's lymphomas, in VT Devita Jr, S Hellman, and SA Rosenberg (eds): *Cancer:*

*Principles and Practice of Oncology,* 5th ed. Philadelphia, Lippincott, 1997, pp 2165–2219.

36. Gospodorowicz MK, Sutcliffe SB: The extranodal lymphomas. *Semin Radiat Oncol* 1995; 5:281–300.

37. Non-Hodgkin's Lymphoma Classification Project: National Cancer Institute study of classifications of non-Hodgkin's lymphomas: Summary and description of a working formulation for clinical usage. *Cancer* 1982;49:2112–2135.

38. Maloney DG, Grillo-Lopez AJ, Bodkin DJ, et al: IDEC-C2B8: Results of a phase I multiple-dose trial in patients with relapsed non-Hodgkin's lymphoma. *J Clin Oncol* 1997;15: 3226–3274.

39. Horning SJ, Rosenberg SA: The natural history of initially untreated low-grade non-Hodgkin's lymphoma. *N Engl J Med* 1984;311:1471–1475.

40. Longo DL, Young RC, Hubbard SM, et al: Prolonged initial remission in patients with nodular mixed lymphoma. *Ann Intern Med* 1984;100: 651–656.

41. Peterson BA, Anderson JR, Frizzera G, et al: Combination chemotherapy prolongs survival in follicular mixed lymphoma. *Proc Am Soc Clin Oncol* 1990;9:259 (abstr).

42. Fisher RI, Gaynor ER, Dahlberg S, et al: Comparison of a standard regimen (CHOP) with three intensive chemotherapy regimens for advanced non-Hodgkin's lymphoma. *N Engl J Med* 1993;328:1002–1006.

43. Shipp MA, Harrington DP, Anderson JR, et al: A predictive model for aggressive non-Hodgkin's lymphomas. *N Engl J Med* 1993; 329:987–994.

44. Shipp MA, Yeap BY, Harrington DP, et al: The m-BACOD combination chemotherapy program: Analysis of the completed trial and comparison with the M-BACOD regimen. *J Clin Oncol* 1990;8:84–93.

45. Cabanillas F, Velasquez WS, Hagermeister FB, et al: Clinical, biologic, and histologic features of late relapses in diffuse large cell lymphoma. *Blood* 1992;79:1024–1028.

46. Tondini C, Zanini M, Lombardi F, et al: Combined modality treatment with primary CHOP chemotherapy following locoregional irradiation in stage I and II histologically aggressive non-Hodgkin's lymphomas. *J Clin Oncol* 1993; 11:720–725.

47. Isaacson PG, Norton AJ: *Extranodal Lymphoma.* Edinburgh and New York, Churchill Livingstone, 1994.

48. Jacobson J, Aisenberg AC, Lamarre L, et al: Mediastinal large cell lymphoma: An uncommon subset of adult lymphoma curable with combined modality therapy. *Cancer* 1988; 62: 1893–1898.

49. Wang CC: *Radiation Therapy of Neoplasms of the Head and Neck,* 3rd ed. New York, Wiley, 1997.

50. Glass J, Gruber ML, Cher L, Hochberg FH: Preirradiation methotrexate chemotherapy of primary central nervous system lymphoma: Long-term outcome. *J Neurosurg* 1994;188:81.

51. Cogliatti SB, Schmid U, Schumacher U, et al: Primary B-cell gastric lymphoma: A clinicopathological study of 145 patients. *Gastroenterology* 1991;101:1159–1170.

52. Thirlby RC: Gastrointestinal lymphoma: A surgical perspective. *Oncology* 1993;7:29–38.

53. Roggero E, Zucca E, Pinotti G, et al: Eradication of *Helicobacter pylori* infection in primary low-grade gastric lymphoma of mucosa-associated lymphoid tissue. *Ann Intern Med* 1995; 122:767–769.

54. Azab MB, Henry-Amar M, Rougier P, et al: Prognostic factors in primary gastrointestinal non-Hodgkin's lymphoma: A multivariate analysis, report of 106 cases, and review of the literature. *Cancer* 1989;64:1208–1217.

55. Montalban C, Castrillo JM, Abraira V, et al: Gastric B-cell mucosa-associated lymphoid tissue lymphoma. Clinicopathological study and evaluation of the prognostic factors in 143 patients. *Ann Oncol* 1995;6:355–362.

56. Shad AT, Magrath IT: Diagnosis and treatment of non-Hodgkin's lymphoma in childhood, in PH Wiernik, GP Canellos, JP Dutcher, and RA Kyle (eds): *Neoplastic Diseases of the Blood,* 3rd ed. New York, Churchill Livingstone, 1996, pp 925–961.

57. Patte C, Kalifa C, Flament F: Results of the LMT 81 protocol, a modified LSA$_2$-L$_2$ protocol with high dose methotrexate, on 84 children with non-B-cell (lymphoblastic) lymphoma. *Med Pediatr Oncol* 1992;20:105.

58. Reiter A, Schrappe M, Parwaresch R, et al: Non-Hodgkin's lymphoma of childhood and adolescence: Results of treatment stratified for biologic subtypes and stage—A report of the Berlin–Frankfurt–Munster Group. *J Clin Oncol* 1995;13:359.

59. Ansell SM, Habermann TM, Kurtin PJ, et al: Predictive capacity of the International Prognostic Factor Index in patients with peripheral T-cell lymphomas. *J Clin Oncol* 1997;15: 2296–2301.

60. Kjeldsberg CR, Wilson JF, Berard CW: Non-Hodgkin's lymphoma in children. *Hum Pathol* 1983;14:612–627.

61. Pott-Hoeck C, Hiddemann W: Purine analogs in the treatment of low-grade lymphomas and chronic lymphocytic leukemia. *Ann Oncol* 1995;6:421–433.

62. Tallman MS, Hakimian D: Purine nucloside analogs: Emerging roles in indolent lymphoproliferative disorders. *Blood* 1995;86:2463–2474.

63. Saven A, Piro L: 2-Chlorodeoxyadenosine: A newer purine analog active in the treatment of indolent lymphoid malignancies. *Ann Intern Med* 1994;120:784–791.

64. Saven A, Emanuele S, Kosty M, et al: 2-Chlorodeoxyadenosine activity in patients with untreated indolent non-Hodgkin's lymphoma. *Blood* 1995;86:1710–1716.

65. Fields KK, Zorsky PE, Hiemenz JW, et al: Ifosfamide, carboplatin, and etoposide: A new regimen with a broad spectrum of activity. *J Clin Oncol* 1994;12:544–552.

66. Velasquez WS, McLaughlin P, Tucker S, et al: ESHAP—An effective chemotherapy regimen in refractory and relapsing lymphoma: A 4-year follow-up study. *J Clin Oncol* 1994;12:1169–1176.

67. Yahalom J: High-dose chemotherapy and radiotherapy with bone marrow transplantation in the management of the non-Hodgkin's lymphomas. *Semin Radiat Oncol* 1995;5:316–330.

68. Mills W, Chopra R, McMillan A, et al: BEAM chemotherapy and autologous bone marrow transplantation for patients with relapsed or refractory non-Hodgkin's lymphoma. *J Clin Oncol* 1995;13:588–595.

69. Philip T, Gugielmi C, Hagenbeek A, et al: Autologous bone marrow transplantation as compared with salvage chemotherapy in relapses of chemotherapy-sensitive non-Hodgkin's lymphoma. *N Engl J Med* 1995;333:1540–1545.

70. Haioun C, Lepage E, Gisselbrecht C, et al: Comparison of autologous bone marrow transplantation with sequential chemotherapy for intermediate-grade and high-grade non-Hodgkin's lymphoma in first complete remission: A study of 464 patients. *J Clin Oncol* 1994;12:2543–2551.

71. Pattengell R, Radford JA, Morgenstern GR, et al: Survival benefit from high-dose therapy with autologous progenitor-cell transplantation in poor-prognosis non-Hodgkin's lymphoma. *J Clin Oncol* 1996;14:586–592.

72. Gianni AM, Bregni M, Siena S, et al: High-dose chemotherapy and autologous bone marrow transplantation compared with MACOP-B in aggressive B-cell lymphoma. *N Engl J Med* 1997;336:1290–1297.

73. Freedman AS, Gribben JG, Neuberg D, et al: High-dose therapy and autologous bone marrow transplantation in patients with follicular lymphoma during first remission. *Blood* 1996;88:2780–2786.

74. Bierman PJ, Vose JM, Anderson JR, et al: High-dose therapy with autologous hematopoietic rescue for follicular low-grade non-Hodgkin's lymphoma. *J Clin Oncol* 1997;15:445–450.

75. Stone RM, Neuberg D, Soiffer R, et al: Myelodysplastic syndrome as a late complication following autologous bone marrow transplantation for non-Hodgkin's lymphoma. *J Clin Oncol* 1994;12:2535–2542.

76. Miles SA, Mitsuyasu RI, Aboulafia DM: AIDS-related malignancies, in VT Devita Jr, S Hellman, and SA Rosenberg (eds): *Cancer: Principles and Practice of Oncology,* 5th ed. Philadelphia, Lippincott, 1997, pp 2445–2467.

77. Scadden DT, Groopman JE: AIDS-associated lymphomas, in R Hoffman, EJ Benz Jr, SJ Shattil, B Furie, HJ Cohen, and LE Silberstein (eds): *Hematology: Basic Principles and Practice,* 2nd ed. New York, Churchill Livingstone, 1995, pp 1344–1353.

78. Vaccher E, Tirelli U, Spina M, et al: Age and serum lactate dehydrogenase level are independent prognostic factors in human immunodeficiency virus-related non-Hodgkin's lymphomas:

A single-institute study of 96 patients. *J Clin Oncol* 1996;14:2217–2223.

79. Kaplan LD, Straus DJ, Testa MA, et al: Low-dose compared with standard dose m-BACOD chemotherapy for non-Hodgkin's lymphoma associated with human immunodeficiency virus infection. *N Engl J Med* 1997;336:1641–1648.

80. Hammer SM, Squires KE, Hughes MD, et al: A controlled trial of two nucleoside analogues plus indinavir in persons with human immunodeficiency virus infection and CD4 counts of 200 per cubic milliliter or less. *N Engl J Med* 1997; 337:725–733.

81. Bush RS, Gospodarowicz M, Sturgeon J, et al: Radiation therapy of localized non-Hodgkin's disease lymphoma. *Cancer Treat Rep* 1977; 61:1129–1136.

82. Fuks Z, Kaplan HS: Recurrence rates following radiation therapy of nodular and diffuse malignant lymphomas. *Radiology* 1973;108:615–684.

83. Levitt LJ, Aisenberg ASC, Harris NL, et al: Primary non-Hodgkin's lymphoma of the mediastinum. *Cancer* 1982;50:2486–2492.

84. Shimm DS, Dosoretz DE, Harris NL, et al: Radiation therapy of Waldeyer's ring lymphoma. *Cancer* 1984;54:426–431.

# CHAPTER 14

# PEDIATRIC TUMORS

EDWARD C. HALPERIN and NANCY J. TARBELL

## THE EPIDEMIOLOGY OF CHILDHOOD CANCER

There are 7500 to 8000 new cases of childhood cancer per year in the United States and approximately 1700 cancer deaths. Cancer is the second leading cause of childhood death in the United States among 1- to 14-year-olds—following accidents and preceding congenital anomalies and homicide. The incidence of cancer is 10 to 13 new cases per 100,000 population per year for 5- to 14-year-olds and 19 to 21 new cases per 100,000 per year for zero to 4-year-olds and 15- to 19-year-olds.[1-3]

The frequency of the various types of childhood cancer is influenced by whether the data are based on incidence or mortality. It is, furthermore, affected by whether one stratifies for age, gender, or political subdivision. Among the most reliable data for analysis of frequency of the various types of childhood cancer is that of the Surveillance, Epidemiology, and End Results (SEER) program. SEER is a project of the Biometry branch of the U.S. National Cancer Institute. It draws data from population-based cancer reporting systems covering about 10% of the population of the United States.[4] Table 14-1 shows the relative frequency of the common forms of cancer, based on the SEER data. Leukemias, central nervous system tumors, lymphomas, sympathetic nervous system tumors, kidney tumors, and soft tissue and bone sarcomas are the most frequent childhood cancers. The common epithelial tumors of adults are rare in children.

Over the last 40 years, the survival rate from childhood cancer has improved considerably in the United States (Table 14-2). In 1960–1963 the 5-year cancer survival rate for children was 28%. For the time cohort 1986–1990, it had risen to 71%.

## A CHILDREN'S CANCER CENTER

The management of cancer in children should be conducted by a coordinated group of medical and surgical specialists. The complete pediatric cancer center will be staffed by pediatric medical oncologists, pediatric radiation oncologists; pediatric general surgeons; surgeons with pediatric expertise in neurosurgery, urology, and orthopedic surgery; pathologists with expertise in the pathology of tumors in children and adolescents; and pediatric subspecialists in anesthesiology, diagnostic radiology, intensive care, infectious disease, cardiology, endocrinology, nephrology, and neurology. The allied health staff will include pediatric nurses, social workers, psychologists, pharmacists, and physical and occupational therapists.[5] The institution should be committed to a regularly scheduled multidisciplinary pediatric tumor board and should

*Clinical Radiation Oncology: Indications, Techniques, and Results, 2nd ed.* Edited by C.C. Wang.
ISBN: 0-471-23803-1   Copyright © 2000 Wiley-Liss, Inc.

offer access to ongoing clinical protocols via one of the cancer treatment groups such as the International Society of Pediatric Oncology (SIOP), Children's Cancer Group (CCG), or Pediatric Oncology Group (POG). The practice of pediatric radiation oncology is not for the amateur or dilettante. Radiation oncologists should not hesitate to refer children with cancer to centers with the appropriate infrastructure and expertise.

## ACUTE LEUKEMIA

Leukemia represents about 31% of all pediatric cancers in the United States. It is the most common form of childhood cancer. Approxi-

mately 2500 new cases are diagnosed annually in the United States, representing an incidence of 3.1 cases per 100,000 children under the age of 14 years. Acute lymphoblastic leukemia (ALL) is the most common form of leukemia in children—accounting for 75% to 80% of all childhood leukemia. The remaining 20% to 25% of cases comprise acute nonlymphoblastic leukemia, most often acute myelogenous leukemia (AML).[6-8] Chronic leukemia is rare in children.

The mean age at diagnosis of ALL is 4 years. ALL may be thought of as a clonal expansion of dysregulated, immature lymphoid cells. Blasts cells are characterized by a particular cytochemistry, immunologic surface markers, and chromosome receptor gene re-

TABLE 14-1    Childhood Cancer in the United States: Percent Distribution by Histology, SEER Data, 1973–1987

| Cancer | (%) | (%) |
|---|---|---|
| Leukemias | 31 | |
|    Acute lymphocytic leukemia | | 24 |
|    Acute nonlymphocytic leukemia | | 51 |
|    Chronic myeloid leukemia | | <1 |
| Lymphomas | 12 | |
|    Hodgkin disease | | 5 |
|    Non-Hodgkin lymphoma | | 4 |
|    Burkitt lymphoma | | 2.1 |
| Central nervous system | 18 | |
| Sympathetic nervous system | 8 | |
| Retinoblastoma | 3 | |
| Wilms tumor | 6 | |
| Hepatic tumors | 1 | |
| Bone tumors | 5 | |
|    Osteosarcoma | | 3 |
|    Ewing sarcoma | | 2 |
| Soft tissue sarcoma | 7 | |
| Rhabdomyosarcoma, embryonal sarcoma, and soft tissue Ewing tumor | | 4 |
| Other soft tissue sarcomas | | 4 |
| Germ cell, trophoblastic, and other gonadal neoplasms | 3 | |
| Carcinoma and other malignant epithelial neoplasms | 4 | |

*Source:* Data compiled from Miller RW, Young Jr JL, Navakovic B: Childhood cancer. *Cancer* 1994;75:395.

TABLE 14-2  Trends in 5-Year Cancer Survival Rates for Children Under 15 Years of Age in the United States, 1960–1992

| | Year at Diagnosis | |
|---|---|---|
| Site | 1960–1963 | 1986–1992 |
| All sites[a] | 28% | 71% |
| Acute lymphocytic leukemia | 4% | 79% |
| Acute myeloid leukemia | 3% | 33% |
| Bones and joints | 20%[b] | 65% |
| Brain and other nervous system | 35% | 61% |
| Hodgkin disease | 52%[b] | 92% |
| Neuroblastoma | 25% | 63% |
| Non-Hodgkin lymphoma | 18% | 71% |
| Soft tissue | 38%[b] | 72% |
| Wilms' tumor | 33%[b] | 93% |

[a]Excludes basal and squamous cell skin cancer and in situ carcinomas except bladder.

[b]The standard error of the survival rates is between 5% and 10%.

*Source:* Data was compiled from Wingo PA, Tong T, Bolden S: Cancer statistics 1995. *CA: Cancer J Clinic* 1995;45:8, and Parker SL, Tong T, Bolden S, Wingo PA: Cancer statistics 1997. *CA: Cancer J Clinic* 1997;47:5–27.

arrangement. Approximately 80% to 85% of childhood ALL cases are B-cell lineage. Of these B-cell lineage cases, approximately 2% to 3% are B cell, 20% to 25% have pre-B-cell characteristics, and 55% to 60% of cases appear to be derived from the clonal growth of early pre-B-cell lines.[9]

B-cell precursor ALL may be separated into prognostic groups. Patients 1 to 10 years of age with a white blood cell count below 2,000 are *standard risk.* Patients with a white blood cell count of 25,000 to 50,000 to 75,000 and/or with worrisome cytogenetic findings are *intermediate risk.* Patients 10 years of age and older with a white blood cell count of 50,000 to 75,000 or above are *high risk.* Other important prognostic signs in B-cell ALL are ploidy and the presence or absence of initial involvement of the central nervous system.

T-cell ALL accounts for 15% to 20% of childhood ALL. T-cell ALL is characterized by older age, marked elevation of the white blood cell count, mediastinal mass, and palpable peripheral lymph nodes. The majority of T-cell ALL is considered *high risk* because of the elevated white blood cell count, older age, and/or bulk disease.[7]

The clinical presentation of ALL is explicable on the basis of the proliferation of abnormal lymphoblasts and their tendency to crowd out normal hematopoietic cells. This can result in neutropenia with frequent or recurrent infections, thrombocytopenia with bruising or bleeding, and anemia with generalized malaise. The diagnosis of ALL is based on bone marrow biopsy and aspiration. Central nervous system involvement is assessed by cerebrospinal fluid cytology.

The fundamental elements of ALL therapy include *initial remission and induction, intensification–consolidation* therapy designed to eliminate residual blasts cells, *prevention* of overt nervous system disease, and *continuation therapy.*[7] The total course of chemotherapy usually lasts from 2.5 to 3 years. For high risk ALL, intermittent intensification or reinduction is an important component of therapy. The most commonly used chemotherapeutic agents are prednisone or dexamethasone, vincristine, L-asparaginase, 6-mercaptopurine, methotrexate, and VM 16.

Radiotherapy has several potential roles in the management of ALL. Initial chemotherapeutic trials achieved a striking rate of remission that exceeded 80%. There was, however, only limited long-term survival, largely related to central nervous system relapse.[10] A series of clinical trials established the efficacy of preventive or prophylactic treatment of the central nervous system (CNS), early in the course of therapy, to deal with this sanctuary site.[11] The initial studies utilized craniospinal irradiation (CSI) or cranial irradiation in combination with intrathecal chemotherapy.[12–14]

While CSI, or cranial irradiation with intrathecal chemotherapy, was able to substantially reduce the rate of isolated central nervous system relapse, the use of cranial irradiation and CSI led to the development of late effects on neurocognitive, growth, and neuroendocrine function, which in turn led to numerous trials testing alternative strategies for CNS therapy.[15] The available data indicate that for patients with low risk ALL, treatment programs incorporating intensive systemic chemotherapy with intrathecal chemotherapy achieve high rates of overall hematological remission with adequate CNS control. Some recent studies suggest that the same is true for intermediate risk ALL, although some investigators continue to favor prophylactic cranial irradiation in these patients. For patients with high risk ALL, there is a significantly higher likelihood of controlling occult meningeal leukemia with the addition of prophylactic irradiation in combination with intrathecal chemotherapy. The favorite dose of cranial irradiation to the whole brain and meningeal surfaces down to C2 of the cervical spine is 18 Gy at 1.5 to 2 Gy per fraction, 5 days per week, with parallel opposed lateral fields.[16] The radiotherapist should take care not to use an excessively high photon energy, lest the meninges be underdosed at the entrance of the beam.

The management of overt CNS ALL is less controversial than the choice of preventive therapy. CNS leukemia at diagnosis is present in 3% to 5% of children with ALL. Effective treatment includes chemotherapy and CSI. Following bone marrow and CNS induction with systemic and intrathecal chemotherapy, the dose is 24 to 30 Gy at 1.5 to 2 Gy per fraction. The spinal field is given 15 to 24 Gy.[17]

Historically, there was a debate over whether the testes were a sanctuary site where leukemic cells were protected from chemotherapy. It now appears that testicular involvement with leukemia is a barometer for extramedullary leukemia, foretelling a general recurrence. If there is overt testicular disease at diagnosis, it appears to respond adequately to systemic chemotherapy without requiring subsequent testicular irradiation. Testicular relapse during or after chemotherapy, however, is managed with reinduction systemic therapy plus local irradiation to a dose of 24 to 25 Gy at 1.5 to 2 Gy per fraction.

The cure rate for ALL is 60% to 80%. Unfortunately, the cure rate for AML is 20% to 40%. Current drug regimens for AML incorporate cytosine arabinoside and daunorubicin. The overall incidence of CNS involvement in AML is similar to the high rate seen in ALL without preventive therapy to the CNS at diagnosis. Initial therapy addresses life-threatening presenting symptoms such as infection, hemorrhage, leukostasis, or tumor lysis syndrome. Initial chemotherapy is high dose cytosine arabinoside, daunorubicin, thioguanine, and etoposide. Intrathecal chemotherapy and prophylactic irradiation have reduced the risk of CNS relapse.[8]

Many investigators believe that bone marrow transplantation is indicated for AML in first remission where there it is a suitable donor. In ALL, bone marrow transplantation is utilized for children who relapse or those with particularly unfavorable clinical or cytogenic factors such as Philadelphia chromosome positive ALL in first remission. Most children in the preparative program for bone marrow transplantation for ALL or AML receive total body irradiation (TBI) and high dose chemotherapy. A considerable body of data indicates that programs that utilize TBI plus melphalan are at least equivalent to non-TBI-containing programs such as busulfan and cyclophosphamide and may be superior in certain clinical situations.[18,19]

Many factors can be varied in TBI for bone marrow transplantation. These include dose per fraction, total number of fractions, dose rate, use of partial or full attenuation blocks, use of boost fields to a particular body site, patient position, beam arrangements, and beam energy. Among the more common programs are 1.5 Gy BID in 9 fractions (= 13.5 Gy), 1.25 Gy TID in 12 fractions (= 15 Gy), 2 Gy BID in 6 fractions (= 12 Gy), or 2.25 Gy daily in 5 fractions (= 11.25 Gy). With radiation administered in multiple fractions per day, the normal tissue-sparing effect of low dose rate is less noticeable and 10 to 30 cGy/min is frequently used.[20]

# CENTRAL NERVOUS SYSTEM TUMORS

Radiation therapy is the most common and effective adjuvant modality employed after neurosurgery for the treatment of childhood brain tumors. The indication for radiation therapy in the treatment of pediatric patients demands special attention to both the benefits and the potential long-term toxicities unique to the developing central nervous system. Radiation therapy is used with a curative intent for a majority of different histologies such as craniopharyngioma, optic glioma, medulloblastoma, and ependymoma.

The types and indications for radiation therapy of pediatric brain tumors fall into three categories: (1) those requiring local treatment with focal, noninfiltrating tumors such as craniopharyngiomas, (2) those requiring more extensive irradiation for infiltrating malignant tumors such as malignant gliomas, and (3) tumors such as medulloblastoma, which require CSI for widespread potential spread of disease throughout the craniospinal axis.

For the well-circumscribed tumors such as optic gliomas and craniopharyngiomas, radiation is usually indicated when there is residual disease (craniopharyngioma) or when the tumor is progressive (optic glioma). Here, the recent developments of three-dimensional irradiation techniques and the greater precision in the delivery of conventional radiation therapy, as well as improvements in the precision of immobilization devices, have clearly changed the standard fields used for pediatric patients. CT and MRI scans now provide much improved delineation of CNS neoplasms, and three-dimensional treatment planning systems are available. These technological advances allow for a more focal and precise delivery of radiotherapy.

The adaptation of linear accelerators for accurate small-field precision radiotherapy has been made possible with the modification of stereotactic equipment and sophisticated computer-generated three-dimensional treatment planning systems. Applications of stereotactic technology in radiation therapy include the use of highly collimated, narrow beams of stereotactically directed radiation delivered as a single fraction, and stereotactic radiosurgery (SRS) or multiple fractions, stereotactic radiotherapy (SRT). SRS requires an invasive localization frame and delivers a single fraction of focal radiation with a precise dose distribution and a sharp dose gradient. Over 200 facilities in the United States are treating patients with radiosurgery.

Although the SRS approach is precise in the administration of large single fractions, it is limited by complications associated with larger volumes (> 3 cm) and certain locations (brain stem, visual pathways).

While radiosurgery appears to be therapeutically useful in the treatment of many intracranial lesions, the complication rates that are accepted for SRS are generally larger than those accepted for conventional radiotherapy. In pediatrics, SRS is largely used as a "boost" following conventionally fractionated radiation therapy or for recurrent brain tumors already treated with conventional radiation therapy.[21-24]

To provide highly focal and precise dose delivery to larger lesions or lesions located within certain regions of the CNS without producing significant morbidity, fractionation is required. Stereotactic radiotherapy is defined as the use of stereotactic radiosurgery hardware and software (stereotactic head frame and support system, small field collimators, three-dimensional planning, etc.) employing routine fractionation (180–200 cGy/day) or some form of altered fractionation such as hypofractionation (a few fractions of 400–800 cGy). To perform stereotactic radiotherapy, a repeat head fixation and localization system is necessary.

In many ways, stereotactic radiotherapy is a marriage of conventional radiotherapy and stereotactic radiosurgery. The term *conformal* or *focal radiotherapy* provides a better and more easily understood description of this technique. Dose optimization studies using stereotactic radiotherapy are being performed for lesions that are currently well controlled with conventional radiotherapy.[25–27] These techniques may become standard treatment for many diseases such as craniopharyngioma, pituitary adenoma, and small optic system tumors. The dose to nearby non–target volume structures that are vital for memory (mesial temporal lobe), endocrine function (hypothalamic–pituitary axis), and normal structural development (skull, mandible, and soft tissues of the scalp) is markedly reduced with these techniques. Dose optimization will be particularly important for the pediatric population.

All stereotactic technology produces highly focal dose distributions, making the treatment ideal for treating localized lesions that are not widely infiltrative. Tumors well suited for treatment with stereotactic technology are small, generally 5 cm or less, noninvasive, radiographically distinct, and known to be well controlled with conventional radiation therapy. The goals of stereotactic technology are delivery of a high rate of tumor control and minimization of normal tissue exposure, goals that are ideally suited for treatment of pediatric patients. Conditions are currently eligible for such focal techniques include craniopharyngioma,[26,28] low grade astrocytoma (LGA),[27] and completely resected ependymoma. The usual indications for adjuvant treatment for children with LGA include, recurrent tumors after initial complete resection or symptomatic tumors that have been incompletely excised. In addition, in tumors with demonstrated growth on follow-up imaging, even in the absence of symptoms, treatment is generally recommended. In balancing the optimal treatment, however, the relative efficacies of surgery, chemotherapy, and irradiation must be balanced by a consideration of the potential complications of therapy. The potential risks of delayed intervention include irreversible neurologic impairment. For example, in the close follow-up frequently used in young patients with optic system tumors, there is the risk of permanent visual loss if treatment is delayed.

A small number of institutions are currently using stereotactic techniques to provide treatments with fractionated irradiation. Much of the published experience utilizes unconventional fractionation schemes of 500 to 800 cGy fractions (hypofractionation). The primary reason for hypofractionation was the lack of an available dedicated radiation facility as well as a lack of noninvasive relocatable stereotactic frames. Normal tissue tolerance is unknown when these hypofractionation schemes are used, and such regimen should be considered experimental at this time. The primary indication should be that a patient has failed more conventional therapies.

Between 1992 and 1997, approximately 150 children were treated with SRT at the Brigham and Women's Hospital in Boston.[25,26] Approximately 75 patients were enrolled prospectively on a dose-optimization protocol at the Dana Farber Cancer Institute. The objectives of the protocol were to compare the efficacy of SRT with conventional irradiation and to compare the neurobehavioral outcomes in children treated with three-dimensional irradiation to small target volumes. (Cumulative doses have ranged from 50.4 to 60 Gy.)

For patients with LGA, posttreatment MRI was obtained at 3- to 12-month intervals after the conclusion of therapy. In reporting the first 28 patients treated, Bakardiev et al. noted that approximately 40% of patients had an increase in one or more of following imaging parameters: size, signal intensity, enhancement, cysts or cavitation, and edema or mass effect.[27] These changes were always confined to the treatment volume; they occurred primarily between 9 and 12 months after the beginning of SRT and decreased after this time interval. It is important to differentiate these changes from tumor progression. Most benign tumors respond slowly to radiotherapy and need many years of follow-up to determine control rates and patterns of failure. Clinical end points such as neurobehavioral outcomes are needed to determine whether this new technology results in fewer late effects.

Conventional large-field radiotherapy is integral to the treatment of many infiltrating brain tumors. For example, in malignant gliomas, the irradiated volume includes a significant amount of "normal" tissue, but the radiobiologic advantage of fractionation is incorporated to reduce the potential early and late complications. The radiation field must cover not only the tumor bed (tumor volume) but also tissue felt to be at risk for microscopic disease and a margin for inconsistency in daily treatment setup (target volume). The tolerance of the normal brain parenchyma becomes the limiting parameter of external beam therapy, and risks of late sequelae are dose-limiting factors. Permanent radiation injury can include pituitary–hypothalamic dysfunction, as well as various learning disabilities.[29,30] Late effects appear in a predictable manner in terms of dose, volume, and fractionation. Sheline et al.[30] have shown that frank radiation necrosis is a function of total dose and fraction size, with threshold doses of approximately 45 Gy in 10,

60 Gy in 35, and 70 Gy in 60 fractions, respectively. Thus, small volumes, low daily doses, and multiple fractions decrease the overall incidence of late effects associated with conventional external beam therapy. The total dose required for tumor control is largely dependent on the number of tumor clonagens that are present and the specific tumor in question. Table 14-3 shows some examples of the total dose used for various pediatric brain tumors.

Modification of the total dose may be justified by age-related toxicity. The age at which irradiation should be employed depends on the tumor type, the alternative options available and, probably, on the size and dose of irradiation required for that particular tumor. In general, delay of irradiation or dose reductions in the treatment of brain tumors in very young children (<3 years) have been recommended. This is because myelinization is incomplete, and the functional impairment in this age group is of great concern. In this case, lower control rates may be justified by the decrease in complications. Alternatively, radiation is often delayed in children when there are alternative treatments.[31] For children ages 7 and under with low grade pilocytic tumors, chemotherapy has been used successfully to delay irradiation.[32]

As techniques to improve dose distribution with photons are becoming more commonly available, there are similar efforts in improving the techniques of proton radiotherapy. Interest in proton radiotherapy as a technique to reduce exposure of nontarget tissue results from the

**TABLE 14-3  Total Radiation Dose Used for Various Brain Tumors**

| Tumor | Radiation Dose (Gy)[a] | Field |
|---|---|---|
| Medulloblastoma | | Wide |
|   RT alone | 36 CSI, 54–55 posterior fossa | |
|   Combined modality | 23–25 CSI, 54–55 posterior fossa | |
| Craniopharyngioma | 52–60 Gy | Local |
| Low grade astrocytomas | 50–60 Gy | Local |
| Germinoma | | |
|   RT alone | 50 Gy | Local |
|   Combined modality | 30–45 Gy | ? Local |

[a] CSI, craniospinal irradiation.

physical fact that the proton range in tissue is finite. Accordingly, the dose deep to the target can be zero for each beam. The dose distributions of proton beams are dramatically different from those for conventional therapy beams, and their superiority provides a significant potential to achieve improved clinical outcomes for children with brain tumors. Beam for beam, protons have physical advantages over x-rays. In modern proton therapy facilities that have isocentric gantries and sophisticated beam delivery and control systems, proton therapy techniques are equivalent to that for state-of-the-art, conformal therapy using x-rays with respect to numbers of beams, beam directions, and complex delivery techniques such as intensity modulation. Future protocols will address the role of protons for pediatric brain tumors (see Chapter 15A).

## Controversies Associated with Pediatric CNS Tumors

The management of intracranial germ cell tumors remains one of the most controversial areas. In particular, the germinomas are variably managed and deserve special mention. Most intracranial germ cell tumors (GCT) arise in the pineal or the suprasellar area. The exceptions to this general guideline include patients with an elevated leval of α-fetoprotein (AFP) and possibly the rare multiple midline germinoma. After the diagnosis has been confirmed, the management options include combined modality approaches as well as radiation therapy (RT). The results with chemotherapy alone are clearly inferior to either RT alone or combined therapy with platinum-based chemotherapy and radiation therapy.[33,34]

When RT alone is considered, the volume and dose required are still controversial. CSI offers excellent survival but with significant morbidity in the young. Excellent disease-free and overall survival rates have been obtained at the University of California San Francisco,[35] with whole-brain irradiation and a local boost to approximately 45 Gy in patients with germinoma appropriately staged with negative CSF cytology and a negative MRI of the spine.

A combined chemotherapy plus irradiation is being tested in the Pediatric Oncology Group, but close attention to late effects in such a highly curable disease will be essential if we are to agree on the standard treatment for this relatively rare disease.

## CNS Complications

Complications may be acute, subacute, or long-term. In general, tolerance to the acute and subacute effects of irradiation is improved in pediatric patients, but children are susceptible to a wider range and larger number of late complications.

Acute reactions develop as a consequence of radiation damage to proliferating cell renewal systems and are, therefore, most noticeable in tissues with rapid turnover. The skin and hair follicles are examples of tissues that require continued cellular proliferation for their function and generally show an early acute reaction to irradiation. Subacute toxicities usually occur in more slowly proliferating tissues. An example of a subacute effect is the somnolence syndrome seen following cranial irradiation in patients with acute lymphoblastic leukemia or with brain tumors. Approximately 50% of children will develop some degree of lethargy or irritability typically between 4 and 8 weeks after cranial irradiation.

In contrast to acute reactions, the late effects of radiation are observed from months to years following irradiation. In addition, acute reactions are not a reliable guide to late effects. Although the exact mechanism is unknown, late radiation complications have been thought to be related either to vascular endothelial damage or to damage to parenchymal stem cells of the irradiated organ.[29,30] Each organ appears to have a unique radiation tolerance, and thus vascular injury may not entirely explain the long-term effects of radiation. The late complications of radiation therapy are often the most critical dose considerations in clinical practice.

In the child, irradiation prior to full development of various tissues can result in failure to develop normally. This is most evident in neurocognitive sequelae in brain tumor survivors.[29] In addition, bone growth may be affected. The severity of growth retardation is related primarily to the age at treatment, the dose of radiation used, and the location treated. Doses of over 20 Gy generally have a significant effect on bony growth.[36] However, the younger the patient, the greater the effect, since there is more growth remaining. The entire craniospinal axis is treated in some brain tumors with the potential for affecting the CSF such as medulloblastoma. With such treatment, the growth retardation is manifested primarily as a reduction in sitting height.[36] In addition, irradiation to the brain can result in a decrease in growth hormone, with resulting short stature.[29]

## HODGKIN DISEASE

Hodgkin disease in the pediatric cohort is similar to adult Hodgkin disease with some noteworthy exceptions (see Chapter 13). The greatest difference is in the management, with the majority of children receiving combined modality therapy. This is largely because there are concerns about the effects of higher dose irradiation on bony growth.[37] Among these late effects is profound musculoskeletal retardation, including intraclavicular narrowing, shortened sitting height, decreased mandibular growth, and decreased muscle development in the treated volume. Staging system and workup and histological subtyping are identical, regardless of patient age. Overall survival is slightly better in the pediatric cohort, and thus the emphasis is on decreasing the late effects of therapy.[38,39] Other noteworthy differences include male/female predominance in the cohort under 10 years of age, with an approximately 4:1 ratio of boys to girls. In the United States, the age-specific incidence curves are bimodal.[40]

Current treatment generally includes chemotherapy for children who have not completed their growth, in conjunction with lower doses of radiation and less extensive volumes.[41]

## NON-HODGKIN LYMPHOMA (NHL)

Malignant lymphomas are the third most common malignancy in children under 15 years of age. They are rare under the age of 3 years, peaking in incidence from age 7 to 11 years. There is a male-to-female ratio of approximately 3:1. Lymphomas account for approximately 10% of all childhood cancers; 60% are NHL and 40% are Hodgkin disease. The role of Epstein–Barr Virus in the pathogenesis of Burkitt lymphoma and other malignancies is unknown. NHL occurs in association with genetically determined immunodeficiency syndromes (such as X-linked lymphoproliferative syndrome, ataxia telangiectasia, Wiscott–Aldrich syndrome, common variable immune deficiency disease), presumably as a result of host defects in immunoregulation or gene rearrangement.[42] Immunosuppressive therapy and acquired immunological disorders including acquired immunodeficiency secondary to HIV infection also increase the risk for NHL. These are predominantly large B-cell or Burkitt in subtype.

Symptoms leading to diagnosis are usually of short duration. Approximately 25% of children with NHL present with mediastinal disease (usually lymphoblastic histology with T-cell markers), with malaise and cough progressing to dyspnea. The majority of these patients are adolescents, and their presentation may pose a medical emergency. Involvement of the bone marrow at diagnosis is common, occurring in 20% to 30% of patients with undifferentiated or lymphoblastic histology. Overt CNS involvement at diagnosis is most frequent in children with head and neck sites, advanced disease, or endemic (African) Burkitt lymphoma. African Burkitt lymphoma usually presents in the jaw, in contrast to the abdominal presentation typical of nonendemic Burkitt lymphoma.

### Staging and Classification

The Murphy system recognizes typical patterns of disease presentation and has greater prognostic utility than the Ann Arbor system in pediatric patients. In Burkitt lymphoma the Ziegler staging system is used. It classifies patients according to tumor burden, which correlates with prognosis.[43] Almost all pediatric NHL is diffuse and high grade. The most common subtypes are diffuse lymphoblastic lymphoma (30% of cases), diffuse small noncleaved cell lymphoma (including undifferentiated Burkitt and non-Burkitt types deriving from relatively mature B cells: 35–40% of cases), and large-cell (diffuse histiocytic or immunoblastic) lymphoma (usually B-cell or non-B-, non-T-cell; sometimes T-cell: 25–30% of cases). Lymphoblastic lymphomas share many clinical and biologic features with acute lymphoblastic leukemia (ALL). When the bone marrow is involved with lymphoblasts, the distinction between lymphoma and leukemia is difficult and generally is determined by the percentage of blast cells in the bone marrow, with 25% the most commonly used cutoff.

CNS involvement will develop in 30% to 35% of children with NHL, particularly lymphoblastic subtypes. Therefore, prophylactic CNS treatment is required.[43–45] This is especially true in patients at high risk of CNS disease, such as those with advanced stage lymphoblastic lymphoma. Overt CNS involvement may present with headache, increased intracranial pressure, and focal neurologic deficits.

Because of the high likelihood of disseminated disease, all children, regardless of stage or histology, receive systemic chemotherapy. Childhood NHL responds to a wide range of agents, but different combinations and schedules are optimal for particular histologies, stages, and primary sites. Active drugs include doxorubicin, methotrexate, vincristine, prednisone, mercaptopurine, cyclophosphamide, and cytosine arabinoside.

Approximately 30% of pediatric large-cell lymphomas are classified as anaplastic large-cell lymphomas (ALCL) in the REAL classification. The remainder are diffuse large B-cell, and the rare peripheral T-cell lymphoma. Children with localized large-cell lymphoma have a very favorable prognosis. The COMP and CHOP regimens that are effective in early

stage lymphoblastic and Burkitt lymphoma also result in 85% survival for these children. The results of CHOP with and without involved irradiation were similar.

Most protocols for children with advanced stage large-cell lymphoma do not include involved field radiotherapy, but no controlled trials have addressed this issue. For advanced stage large-cell histology APO, CHOP, and modified ACOP regimens are also effective. Pediatric Oncology Group (POG) study 8615 compared APO [adriamycin, prednisone, vincristine, 6-mercaptopurine, asparaginase, and intrathecal (IT) and intravenous (IV) methotrexate] to ACOP+ (APO with cyclophosphamide but without asparaginase) in large-cell NHL. The 2-year disease-free survival is 79% for APO and 70% for ACOP+.[46]

The role of radiotherapy in the management of all childhood NHL has decreased as chemotherapeutic regimens have become more effective. Recent reports from POG demonstrate successful local and systemic control with chemotherapy alone for children with Murphy/SJCRH stages I and II disease regardless of histology.[47] There also does not appear to be any benefit to the addition of radiation therapy either to the primary site or for CNS prophylaxis for Burkitt NHL.[44,45] The addition of localized radiation therapy to chemotherapy has also shown no benefit for patients with advanced stage disease.

The role of radiation therapy for primary NHL of bone in children has also diminished. These cases were specifically excluded from the POG randomized trials of early stage pediatric NHL, which showed no benefit to local irradiation.[47] In this study, all patients with bone NHL received local radiation therapy. There are data demonstrating good results for pediatric NHL of bone when radiotherapy is omitted.

The current indications for RT outside the CNS in pediatric NHL are as follows: emergency treatment for mediastinal disease or spinal cord compression (a hyperfractionated regimen should be considered), treatment for patients who fail to obtain a complete remission after induction chemotherapy, palliation of pain or mass effect, and for consolidation to regions of local disease prior to or following bone marrow transplantation in patients with recurrent disease.

The CNS requires prophylactic treatment in the majority of children with NHL, thereby reducing the otherwise high risk of CNS relapse.[45] The results of a randomized trial of CNS prophylaxis in stage II–IV pediatric NHL confirm this view. Mandell et al.[44] reported only one isolated CNS relapse in 58 evaluable children treated with an $LSA_2$-$L_2$-based protocol that used IT methotrexate without cranial irradiation regardless of histology or stage. In a Children's Cancer Study Group report of children treated with COMP or a modified $LSA_2$-$L_2$ protocol using IT methotrexate without cranial irradiation, the incidence of isolated CNS relapse was only 6% in patients without CNS disease at diagnosis.[48] Thus, cranial irradiation is not warranted for the majority of patients. Indications for 18 to 24 Gy of cranial irradiation are currently limited to patients with overt CNS lymphoma at diagnosis or relapse and patients with leukemic transformation at diagnosis.[45] These indications are based on a high rate of CNS relapse with chemotherapy alone and the proven efficacy of IT methotrexate plus cranial radiation in these settings. Finally, patients with cranial nerve palsies at diagnosis or subsequently should receive radiation to the skull base or whole cranium. This may improve both survival and functional recovery.[49]

On rare occasions, there is failure to achieve a complete remission on chemotherapy, or relapse with local disease only. Some of these patients will be irradiated to regions of local residual disease.

# RETINOBLASTOMA

Retinoblastoma is the most common malignant intraocular tumor of childhood. There are approximately 200 to 350 new cases per year in the United States and 50 per year in the United Kingdom. The retinoblastoma protein is in-

volved in the control of the cell cycle. This protein, a product of a gene on the long arm of chromosome 13, is a tumor suppressor gene. Retinoblastoma may be inherited from an affected parent or may be the result of sporadic mutations.[50,51] While most cases are sporadic, between 25% and 40% are familial (i.e., inherited from an infected parent who has survived retinoblastoma, a nonaffected gene-carrying parent with no clinical signs of retinoblastoma, or a parent with a new germ line mutation). The disease commonly presents with a white pupillary light reflex, termed leucocoria.

The most widely used grouping system for retinoblastoma is that of Reese and Ellsworth (Table 14-4). This system does not do well at

**TABLE 14-4    The Reese–Ellsworth System of Classifying Retinoblastoma**

GROUP I: VERY FAVORABLE

A. Solitary tumors, less than 4 disc diameters (DD)[a] in size, at or behind the equator.
B. Multiple tumors, none larger than 4 DD in size, all at or behind the equator.

GROUP II: FAVORABLE

A. Solitary tumors, 4–10 DD in size, at or behind the equator.
B. Multiple tumors, 4–10 DD in size, all at or behind the equator.

GROUP III: DOUBTFUL

A. Any lesion anterior to the equator.
B. Solitary tumors, larger than 10 DD in size, behind the equator.

GROUP IV: UNFAVORABLE

A. Multiple tumors, some larger than 10 DD.
B. Any lesion extending anterior to the ora serrata.

GROUP V: VERY UNFAVORABLE

A. Massive tumors involving more than half the retina.
B. Vitreous seeding.

---

[a] The optic nerve's exit (the optic nerve "head" or "disc") is approximately 1.5 mm in diameter. The disc diameter (DD) is often used as a ruler to describe tumor dimensions (i.e., so many DD in size).

discriminating survival probability but does serve as a guide to the chance of vision preservation with conservative therapy.

The primary goal of retinoblastoma therapy is, obviously, cure. Because this disease infrequently metastasizes, the chance of cure is excellent (> 80%). It is appropriate to assert that a secondary treatment goal is the preservation of vision in the affected eye. Forms of therapy available include enucleation, exenteration, cryotherapy, photocoagulation, laser hyperthermia, radioactive plaque application, systemic chemotherapy, and external beam irradiation.[52,53] In recent years there has been a considerable movement away from external beam irradiation and toward focal therapy, often in conjunction with chemotherapy, in an attempt to reduce the substantial risk of treatment-associated second malignant neoplasm in children with a malignant diathesis due to the chromosome abnormality associated with heritable retinoblastoma.[54]

Radioactive plaque applications are appropriate as primary treatment for children with 2 to 16 mm basilar diameter unilateral lesions located within 3 mm of the optic disc or fovea, generally with a thickness under 10 mm, or for two lesions that are small enough and close enough to be covered with one plaque. This therapy can serve as primary treatment, also for the "boost" of disease that is partially responsive to chemotherapy and for local failure following other therapy. Plaques may be constructed of radioactive iodine, iridium, cobalt, or ruthenium. One generally allows 1.5 to 2 mm of margin on either side of basal diameter of the tumor for the plaque, and a dose of approximately 40 Gy to the tumor apex is administered in 4 to 5 days.

External beam irradiation is utilized in treatment programs that do not rely on chemotherapy plus focal treatment, or for failure of chemotherapy when tumor is multifocal and/or close to the macula or optic nerve. The goal of external beam irradiation is to provide a homogeneous and tumorcidal dose to the retinal anlage without exceeding the tolerance of normal tissue structures.[55] There are a variety of photon techniques employed including a single lateral field, a direct anterior field, a half-beam-blocked lateral field, a two-field technique with a lateral and an anterior field, a precision lateral technique with specially devised equipment referred to as the Schipper device, and proton beam treatment.[56,57] The typical dose administered is 40 to 50 Gy at 1.8 to 2 Gy per fraction, 5 days per week, for 4.5 to 5 weeks.[58,59] Anesthesia and a rigid head stabilization device are almost always required in the management of these cases with external beam radiation.[60]

## NEUROBLASTOMA

Neuroblastoma constitutes 10% of all cases of childhood cancer and is the most common malignancy of infants. The tumor arises from primitive adrenergic neuroblasts of the neural crest. This small, blue, round-cell tumor contains a mixture of neuroblasts and mature ganglion cells. The clinical presentation depends on the site along the sympathetic nervous system chain from which the primary tumor develops, as well as the existence of metastatic disease. The abdomen is the most common primary tumor location—tumor may arise from the adrenal or a paraspinal location. Extra-abdominal locations include the sympathetic ganglia of the neck, posterior mediastinum, and pelvis. Neuroblastoma is often associated with an increased or abnormal production of catecholamines and their metabolites (e.g., epinephrine, vanyllmandellic acid, 3 methoxy-4- hydroxylphenol glycol, and/or homovanillic acid), which may be measured in the urine.[61,62]

Several systems have been used for staging of neuroblastoma. The system now generally accepted as proper is the International Neuroblastoma Staging System (Table 14-5). In addition to staging, several clinical and biologic characteristics are associated with prognosis. These include the age at diagnosis (with infants < 12–18 months of age faring better than children older with the same stage), ferritin

**TABLE 14-5    The International Neuroblastoma Staging System**

---

### Stage 1

Localized tumor with complete gross excision, without microscopic residual disease; representative ipsilateral lymph nodes negative for tumor microscopically (nodes attached to and removed with the primary tumor may be positive)

### Stage 2A

Localized tumor with incomplete gross excision; representative ipsilateral nonadherent lymph nodes negative for tumor microscopically

### Stage 2B

Localized tumor with or without complete gross excision, with ipsilateral nonadherent lymph nodes positive for tumor. Enlarged contralateral lymph nodes must be negative microscopically.

### Stage 3

Unresectable unilateral tumor infiltrating across the midline, with or without regional lymph node involvement; or localized unilateral tumor with contralateral regional lymph node involvement; or midline tumor with bilateral extension by infiltration (unresectable) or by lymph node involvement.

### Stage 4

Any primary tumor with dissemination to distant lymph nodes, bone, bone marrow, liver, skin and/or other organs (except as defined for stage 4S).

### Stage 4S

Localized primary tumor (as defined for stage 1, 2A or 2B) with dissemination limited to skin, liver, and/or bone marrow (limited to infants < 1 year of age).

---

*Source:* Brodeur GM et al. *J Clin Oncol* 1988; 6:1874.

level, neuron-specific enolase level, lactate dehydrogenase level, DNA index, n-myc amplification, the presence or absence of growth factor receptor, and chromosome 1 deletion.[63]

Twenty to 40% of children present with localized disease. In these cases an attempt at resection is warranted. Postoperative radiotherapy is unnecessary if the primary tumor is completely excised in low risk, localized, lymph node negative neuroblastoma. Total surgical excision cures the majority of these children regardless of age, catecholamine status, or histologic pattern. For patients with intermediate risk disease (i.e., International System stage II or III disease), chemotherapy is generally administered.[64] The most commonly employed agents are cyclophosphamide, doxorubicin, cisplatin, and teniposide.[65] In these children, the value of postoperative irradiation is undetermined. Staging systems based on biologic markers such as oncogene amplification may determine which patients require adjuvant radiotherapy. While a randomized study of the Pediatric Oncology Group demonstrated benefits to radiation therapy in localized node-positive disease, these results were obtained prior to the use of biologic markers, and the use of radiotherapy for localized disease is now considered an open question.[66] When RT is employed for such purposes, approximately 20 to 30 Gy is given to the tumor bed with a margin.

The majority of children with neuroblastoma present with metastatic disease. In these cases, current management favors induction chemotherapy and myeloablative chemotherapy or total-body irradiation prior to bone marrow transplantation. The majority of available data supports the use of "boost" doses of radiation to sites of bulk disease either prior to the bone marrow transplantation or following the procedure. When radiation is employed in this manner, it is most often given twice a day at 1.5 Gy per fraction or daily at 1.8 to 2 Gy per fraction to a total dose of approximately 21 Gy.[67,68]

Among the peculiarities of neuroblastoma is the occurrence of what was formerly called Evans–D'Angio stage IVS disease (S for special). This occurs in infants with localized primary neuroblastoma and metastasis to liver, bone marrow, and skin. These children have a surprisingly good prognosis and often require minimal therapy. Occasionally massive involvement of the liver can produce upward pressure on the diaphragm and threaten the child's life via respiratory compromise. In these cases, palliation of hepatomegaly may be achieved by 3 to 6 Gy in two to four fractions. It is occasionally necessary to repeat the course of treatment.

## EWING SARCOMA

Ewing sarcoma is a small round-cell tumor of childhood originating in the bone, usually associated with a soft tissue mass. Cytogenetically, Ewing shows a distinctive reciprocal translocation of chromosome 22 at the 12q locus. The t(11;22) translocation is felt to be specific for Ewing sarcoma and primitive neuroectodermal tumors (PNET). Since these tumors share this specific translocation, most centers now use the same approach to treat both entities.

The relative roles of surgery and radiation therapy for the local treatment of Ewing sarcoma are controversial. With advances in surgical technique including allograft procedures and overall improvements in limb-sparing procedures, there has been a renewed interest in surgery for management of the local disease.[69] In addition, there have been reports of Ewing sarcoma—in particular, osteogenic sarcoma—occurring in the irradiated bone.[70] There is little possibility of a randomized trial, since many physicians believe strongly in the superiority of one treatment or the other in the primary management of this relatively rare disease. Thus, general guidelines at the present include surgery as the preferred treatment for easily resectable, small primary sites. In addition, surgery following initial chemotherapy is generally preferred for rib lesions, even when these are initially quite large. This unique site is frequently associated with large soft tissues masses, which make primary irradiation quite difficult, and the soft tissue mass usually responds dramatically to chemotherapy, thus allowing definitive surgery. In this situation, there is usually a need for postoperative irradi-

ation, as well, but lower doses (4500 cGy) for microscopic disease than those used for gross disease (5,500 cGy) can be delivered to smaller volumes that have been surgically defined. The same basic principles that apply to the discussion of rhabdomyosarcomas hold for Ewing: a multidisciplinary approach is critical for optimal patient care.

The local control with irradiation alone has been variable[69,71] and depends on the primary size of the tumor. Tumors exceeding >8 cm in greatest diameter led to approximately a 30% local failure rate, in contrast to a 10% local failure rate in tumors under 8 cm.[72] In addition, magnetic resonance imaging and computed tomography scans together have allowed much better definition of the target volume at risk. Using newer imaging techniques should improve radiation delivery. The use of definitive irradiation as the primary local treatment should be balanced against the functional consequences of surgery. This decision is frequently difficult, because it is not clear why the survival for those with large tumors at presentation is still poor: Would survival be improved by adding more aggressive surgery to full-dose irradiation either preoperatively or postoperatively, or are these patients at such a high risk for metastatic disease that further improvements in local control would have little impact on the overall survival? For the present, selection of the optimal management of Ewing sarcoma usually generates a great deal of discussion. Again, newer radiation techniques will allow for a decrease in the amount of normal tissue irradiated, which could have a significant effect on the deleterious effects of large volumes of irradiation to high total doses.

## OSTEOSARCOMA

Osteosarcoma is the most common primary malignant bone tumor in children. It usually occurs in the metaphyses of the long bones, especially around the knee joint. There is no widely used staging system. The classic definitive operative procedure is either an amputation above the region of the affected bone or a disarticulation at the joint above the lesion. Limb-sparing operations may be selected in certain cases. The long-term survival with radical surgical ablation is approximately 20%. Clinical trials have now demonstrated that the use of adjuvant chemotherapy, frequently including doxorubicin, cyclophosphamide, and methotrexate, can achieve a survival rate of 50% to 70%. Radiation therapy is rarely employed in the management of osteosarcoma save for the patient with inoperable disease requiring palliation, the patient who absolutely refuses appropriate surgery and in whom radiotherapy is employed in the small hope of achieving local control (neutrons have been used in this situation), and in some patients research protocols involving combinations of preoperative or postoperative irradiation and limb sparing surgery.[73-76]

## RHABDOMYOSARCOMA

Rhabdomyosarcoma (RMS) is the most common soft tissue sarcoma in children, and accounts for 4% to 8% of all pediatric malignancies in children less than 15 years of age. Although the peak age range for this disease is 2 to 5 (similar to Wilms tumor and neuroblastoma), approximately 30% of all cases occur in children older than 10. One unusual characteristic of RMS is the great heterogeneity in anatomic location for the tumor, and the apparent differences in long-term disease survival found among similarly treated patients with different primary sites.[77] Thus, patients with RMS of the orbital region (representing approximately 10% of all RMS cases) have a long-term survival expectation of approximately 90%, while patients with RMS primary sites located elsewhere in the head and neck (approximately 25% of cases, including parameningeal sites) have a much lower overall survival rate of approximately 50%. Patients with retroperitoneal RMS primary sites (approximately 10% of all cases) have even longer long-term survivals (on the order of 30% to 40%). While it is assumed that part of this rela-

tionship between primary site and apparent disease aggressiveness represents a difference in tumor bulk and/or resectibility, the true explanation is not clear. Moreover, RMS represents a heterogeneous mixture of histologies, the most common being the generally favorable "embryonal" RMA (approximately 50% to 60% of all RMS cases, when one includes the "botryoid" variant) and the generally unfavorable "alveolar" RMS (20% to 25% of all RMS cases). Since some anatomic sites are more likely to harbor rhabdomyosarcoma tumors of certain histological subtypes (e.g., genitourinary RMS is virtually always embryonic type). The site-specific and histology-specific characteristics of RMS behavior have contributed to the difficulty of defining treatment, particularly the role of surgery and/or radiotherapy for many clinical presentations of this disease.

The role of radiotherapy in the treatment of RMS depends heavily on the details of the individual case under consideration. Doses used for RMS are somewhat higher than those used for other common intra-abdominal pediatric malignancies, approximately 40 Gy for microscopic diseases and approximately 55 Gy for treatment of gross residual tumor. Chemotherapy is an important part of the overall management plan for virtually all cases of RMS, and it usually involves some variation of the "VAC" (vincristine/actinomycin-D or Adriamycin/Cytoxan) regimen. For virtually all nonmetastatic patients, the first major step in therapy involves an attempt at gross total resection of the tumor. Radiotherapy considerations will depend heavily on pathologic staging information obtained at surgery and the degree of resection that has been accomplished. For patients with completely resected disease and no lymphatic involvement [Intergroup Rhabdomyosarcoma Study (IRS) group I patients], the IRS-I randomized trial suggested that radiotherapy offered no benefit in overall survival, at least for the patients having favorable histology.[78] These patients are no longer treated with adjuvant radiotherapy, although care should be taken to be sure that the margins are inked at the time of surgery and that all margins are truly free of tumor.

For resectable tumors with local–regional spread (IRS group II) and for patients with gross residual disease (IRS group III), radiotherapy remains an important part of the treatment approach. In IRS study II, local relapse rates for patients irradiated with 4000 to 5000 cGy were found to be 10% for group II and 30% for group III. Although complete radiologic disappearance of all residual tumor in the primary site was commonly observed after chemotherapy and radiation doses of 45 to 55 Gy, rates of local relapse for patients with locally infiltrative group III tumors were unacceptably high (25–50%). For that reason, the IRS-IV study randomized group III patients between conventionally fractionated radiotherapy (5040 cGy in 180 cGy daily fractions) versus hyperfractionated radiotherapy (5940 cGy in 110 cGy twice-daily fractions).[79] The goals of this approach are twofold—to increase the local control rates for these unresectable tumors, and to decrease the late musculoskeletal toxicity and growth arrest commonly seen in children undergoing high dose radiotherapy prior to adolescence.

Several clinical scenarios require special mention. For patients with orbital RMS, conventional radiotherapy to doses of 40 to 45 Gy appears capable of producing excellent local control with tolerable late effects, even in patients with gross residual disease.[80] It is unclear whether unconventional radiotherapy fractionation schemes are necessary or desirable in this favorable group. For patients with head and neck region tumors that occur in parameningeal sites, the initial IRS-I study suggested that approximately one-third of all group II or III patients would eventually develop meningeal extension, and therefore prophylactic whole-brain or whole-neuraxis irradiation was initially recommended. However, a careful analysis of the radiotherapy field arrangements in patients experiencing a central nervous system relapse showed that target volumes in these patients were often inadequate, and it now appears that patients with no evidence of intracranial extension of cerebrospinal fluid involvement do not require CNS irradiation,[81] but do require extensive local fields to adequately cover the initial extent of disease. Patients with head and neck primary tumors who demonstrate extensive bony erosion on their radiologic studies appear to be at increased risk of local failure (30–50%) and may benefit from more aggressive radiotherapy "boost" techniques or craniofacial surgery.[82]

Finally, patients with RMS of the genitourinary systems present a special therapeutic dilemma: local control rates for patients treated with chemotherapy and radical surgical resections or exenterations are generally excellent (in some cases >90%), but bladder and/or reproductive organ function is lost. Organ-sparing approaches employing minimal surgery followed by chemotherapy and high dose pelvic irradiation initially appeared to result in equivalent survivals and increased rates of bladder function, but, unfortunately, longer follow-up periods revealed that local recurrences and late bladder toxicity continued to occur as these data matured,[83] eventually falling to a level below the radical surgery group. Thus, the optimal treatment approach for the patient with genitourinary RMS remains one of the most vexing problems in clinical pediatric oncology. This group of children is likely to benefit significantly from advances in the delivery of radiation through techniques that incorporate three-dimensional treatment planning, also referred to as "conformal" therapy.

Other experimental radiotherapeutic approaches currently being developed to address these problems include novel brachytherapy (radioactive implantation) techniques, pharmacological and cytotoxic radiosensitizers, planned surgical "nidusectomy" prior to tumor bed radiotherapy, and novel radiation dose fractionation schemes.[83]

## SOFT TISSUE SARCOMAS OTHER THAN RHABDOMYOSARCOMA

Nonrhabdomyosarcoma soft tissue sarcoma constitutes 2% to 4% of childhood cancer. The histologic groups include neurogenic sarcoma, synovial sarcoma, liposarcoma, fibrosarcoma, leiomyosarcoma, epithelioid sarcoma, alveolar soft part sarcoma, extraskeletal Ewing sarcoma, peripheral primitive neuroectodermal tumor, and undifferentiated sarcoma.[84,85]

Most cases of nonrhabdomyosarcoma soft tissue sarcoma present as a painless swelling. The disease may be staged by the rhabdomyosarcoma grouping system. The histologic tumor grade is quite important in the management of soft tissue sarcoma, and it is not considered in the rhabdomyosarcoma system. Therefore, for many clinicians, the system of the American Joint Cancer Committee for Staging is preferable.[86] Stage is determined by histologic grade, tumor size, and the presence or absence of distant metastasis.

Therapy for nonrhabdomyosarcoma soft tissue sarcoma often begins with complete surgical excision. There are many patients, however, for whom limb-sparing treatments may be considered: that is, removal of the tumor while the extremity is preserved with a satisfactory functional and cosmetic result. Most limb-sparing procedures involve the use of pre- or postoperative external beam radiation therapy, brachytherapy, and/or intra-arterial or systemic chemotherapy.

When radiotherapy is employed in the management of nonrhabdomyosarcoma soft tissue sarcoma, the tumor or tumor bed is irradiated with a wide margin with external beam. Local control is strikingly improved in cases of marginal excisions or in attempts for limb sparing with the combination of radiation and more limited surgery. For the management of microscopic nonrhabdomyosarcoma soft tissue sarcoma in children, investigators favor a dose of 50 to 60 Gy, utilizing a progressive shrinking field technique. In some institutions, excision in combination with brachytherapy is the preferred technique. If external beam radiation is combined with brachytherapy, the brachytherapy boost is generally 10 to 20 Gy at 50 cGy/hr. If brachytherapy is the sole form of radiotherapy, then 40 to 50 Gy is given.[87-90]

The role of adjuvant chemotherapy in nonrhabdomyosarcoma soft tissue sarcoma is a matter of considerable controversy. There are a large number of randomized trials and meta-analyses, largely considering the value of doxorubicin in the prevention of metastatic disease. Most randomized trials are negative. Some of the meta-analyses hint at a possible benefit of chemotherapy in certain patient subgroups.

## WILMS TUMOR

Wilms tumor is an embryonic kidney tumor. There are approximately 500 new cases per year in the United States. The tumor is a triphasic embryonal neoplasm that has blastemal, epithelial, and stromal elements. The disease may be grouped into *favorable histology,* defined as having typical histologic features of Wilms tumor without anaplastic or sarcomatous components, and *unfavorable histology* including anaplastic Wilms tumor, clear cell sarcoma, and rhabdoid tumor (some authorities now consider these latter two not to be variants of Wilms tumor but to be better treated as distinct entities).

A variety of staging systems have been used for Wilms tumor including those developed by Cassady et al., the National Wilms Tumor Study Group, and the International Society of Pediatric Oncology.[91] The National Wilms Tumor Study Group staging system is shown in Table 14-6.

A considerable body of information has been compiled concerning the management of Wilms Tumor by cooperative groups. The development of these clinical trials for Wilms tumor and their results have been reviewed.[92-98] In brief, the International Society of Pediatric Oncology Trials (SIOP) began with the presumption that treatment, prior to definitive surgery, would render a Wilms tumor less vulnerable to intraoperative rupture and surgery-related tumor seeding. It was hoped that by downstaging the tumor one could reduce treatment related morbidity and reduce the total amount of treatment. In contrast, the National Wilms Tumor strategy was to forego preoperative therapy in order to obtain

**TABLE 14.6 Staging System Used in National Wilms Tumor Study 3 and 4**

I. Tumor limited to kidney and completely excised. The surface of the renal capsule is intact. Tumor was not ruptured before or during removal. There is no residual tumor apparent beyond the margins of resection.

II. Tumor extends beyond the kidney but is completely removed. There is regional extension of the tumor—that is, penetration through the outer surface of the renal capsule into perirenal soft tissues.

  Vessels outside the kidney substance are infiltrated or contain tumor thrombus. The tumor may have been biopsied, or there has been local spillage of tumor confined to the flank. There is no residual tumor apparent at or beyond the margins of excision.

III. Residual nonhematogenous tumor confined to abdomen. Any one or more of the following occur:

   a. Lymph nodes on biopsy are found to be involved in the hilus, the periaortic chains, or beyond.

   b. There has been diffuse peritoneal contamination by tumor such as by spillage of tumor beyond the flank before or during surgery, or by tumor growth that has penetrated through the peritoneal surface.

   c. Implants are found on the peritoneal surfaces.

   d. The tumor extends beyond the surgical margins either microscopically or grossly.

   e. The tumor is not completely resectable because of local infiltration into vital structures.

IV. Hematogenous metastases: deposits beyond stage III (e.g., lung, liver, bone, and brain).

V. Bilateral renal involvement at diagnosis: an attempt should be made to stage each side according to the criteria above on the basis of extent of disease before biopsy.

Staging, which is on the basis of gross and microscopic tumor distribution, is the same for tumors with favorable and with unfavorable histologic features. The patient should be characterized, however, by a statement of both criteria—for example, stage II (favorable histologic features) or stage III (unfavorable histologic features).

  Tumors of unfavorable type are those with focal or diffuse anaplasia, or those of sarcomatous histology.

the maximum amount of information concerning prognostic factors and tailor therapy accordingly. The current SIOP trial classifies patients into groups based on histologic subtype. Patients with Stage I low grade histology receive four weeks of preoperative chemotherapy and then no further therapy after surgery. Patients with stage I intermediate or high grade tumors are randomized to four weeks of postoperative vincristine plus actinomycin vs. a six week program. All stage II and III patients receive chemotherapy and local irradiation.

  In the current NWTS, patients with Stage I favorable and anaplastic histology and Stage II favorable histology receive actinomycin D and vincristine. Stage I favorable histology in children <24 months of age and a tumor weight <550 grams are treated with surgery alone. Stage III and IV favorable histology and Stage II–IV focal anaplastic tumors are treated with 24 weeks of actinomycin, vincristine, and adriamycin and local abdominal irradiation (generally on the order of 10 Gy) and whole lung irradiation when appropriate. Stage II–IV diffuse anaplastic and Stage I–IV clear cell sarcoma of the kidney are treated with cyclophosphamide, vincristine, adriamycin, and etoposide, along with local and whole lung irradiation as appropriate. Rhabdoid tumor of the kidney, Stages I–IV, is treated with carboplatinum, etoposide, cyclophosphadmide, and irradiation.

## TUMORS OF THE LIVER

Primary malignant liver tumors of childhood constitute between 0.5% and 2% of pediatric cancer. Hepatoblastoma is the most common primary malignant liver tumor occurring in the first twenty years of life and may be subclassified into the more favorable fetal cell pattern and other less favorable histologic subgroups. Hepatocellular carcinoma is the second most primary malignant tumor of children and it accounts for 25-33% of pediatric hepatic malignancies.[99–101]

  Localized hepatoblastoma or hepatocellular carcinomas are curable with complete surgical excision. Tumor resectability is determined by the size of the tumor and the presence or absence of bilobar involvement, vascular invasion, or distant metastases. Most cases are managed with preoperative chemotherapy to reduce the tumor burden prior to an attempt at resection. The commonly employed chemotherapeutic drugs include vincristine, actinomycin D, cyclophosphamide, doxorubicin, 5 flurouracil, and cisplatin.[102–105] Radiotherapy is occasionally employed preoperatively in an attempt to improve the resectibility of the tumor or postoperatively for difficult resections or for palliation. When radiotherapy is employed, 25 to 45 Gy is appropriate to a limited area for microscopic disease and 35 to 45 Gy for bulkier disease. Liver transplantation has also been employed.

Event-free survival for early stage hepatoblastoma is better than 85%. For advanced disease survival is reported to be between 20% and 60%.

## GERM CELL TUMORS

Malignant germ cell tumors occur in fewer than 300 children under 15 years of age each year in the United States. They may arise in the ovaries, testes, sarcococcygeal region, retroperitoneum, and mediastinal areas. The main histologic types are germinoma, embryonal carcinoma, yolk sac tumor (endodermal sinus tumor), malignant mixed germ cell tumors, and malignant teratomas (referred to by some authorities as immature teratomas). The general management principles are as follows:

1. Ovarian nondysgerminoma germ cell tumors are potentially lethal malignancies. Surgery followed by postoperative chemotherapy has considerably improved survival.

2. Ovarian dysgerminoma, in the past, was treated postoperatively with radiation therapy. It is now possible to identify early cases that may be managed by surgery alone. For more advanced cases, where one can manage with either

chemotherapy or irradiation, most authorities now favor chemotherapy.

3. Testicular germ cell tumors are most commonly yolk sac tumors. Most stage I testicular yolk sac tumors may be treated with orchiectomy alone. More extensive disease is managed with postoperative chemotherapy.

4. Sacrococcygeal germ cell tumors include the benign teratomas, which are treated with surgery alone. Malignant disease is managed with surgery and chemotherapy. Radiation therapy is employed in rare cases of patients with persistent disease following chemotherapy. The expectations are limited, but 45 to 50 Gy may be employed in an attempt to salvage the patient.[106–118]

## JUVENILE NASOPHARYNGEAL ANGIOFIBROMA

Juvenile nasopharyngeal angiofibroma is a rare tumor that arises from the nasopharynx and may extend into the nasal cavity, the maxillary and sphenoid sinuses, the orbit, the anterior and middle cranial fossae, the infratemporal region, or the pterygopallatine fossa. It is more common in males than in females. These firm, red masses present with nasal obstruction and/or bleeding. The definitive therapies are surgery and external beam radiotherapy. The treatment of smaller juvenile nasopharyngeal angiofibromas is generally surgical. More extensive disease is treated with external beam radiation. While a considerable range of doses of external beam radiotherapy have been employed, most of the available data support a total dose of 30 to 36 Gy with parallel opposed lateral fields, a three-field technique, or arcs.[119–122]

## LANGERHANS CELL HISTIOCYTOSIS

A confusing nomenclature has been employed for Langerhans cell histiocytosis, including histiocytosis X, eosinophilic granuloma, Hand–

Schuller–Christian disease, and Letterer–Siewie disease. In normal physiology the Langerhans cell is involved in presenting antigens introduced via epithelial surfaces to T cells. The annual incidence of Langerhans cell histiocytosis is 0.5 to 2 cases per 100,000 per year. In children under 2 years of age there may be a widespread seborrheic rash, as well as liver, lung, gastrointestinal, or bone marrow involvement. In children over 2 years of age, the most common presenting symptoms relate to bone involvement with localized pain, with or without an associated soft tissue mass. Diabetes insipidus is the most common CNS problem associated with Langerhans cell histiocytosis. The mechanism of injury is thought to be either infiltration of the meninges adjacent and posterior to the hypothalamic–pituitary axis or direct involvement of the brain itself.

In many cases Langerhan cell histiocytosis takes an indolent course and no therapy is warranted. The pediatric radiation oncologist will most commonly be consulted in cases of bone involvement. These lesions, which may be painful or may interfere with function, may be managed with observation alone, curettage alone, intralesion installation of steroids, local irradiation, or systemic prednisone, etoposide, vinblastine, or cyclosporine (although these drugs are usually used for multifocal disease with organ dysfunction). If radiotherapy is chosen, then a total dose of 6 to 10 Gy in two to five fractions is usually adequate for bone disease. In an attempt to treat diabetes insipidus, emergent radiotherapy may be employed with 5 to 15 Gy. The response rate is poor.[123–125]

## HEMANGIOMAS

Hemangiomas are common developmental vascular abnormalities. These benign blood vessel tumors have a natural history, most commonly, of increasing size during the first few months of life followed by a period of slower growth and involution. No therapy is required.

In rare cases hemangiomas will warrant therapy because of rapid progression, which produces unacceptable symptoms. If a decision is made to treat a hemangioma, radiotherapy is rarely employed because of the long-term risks of inducing a second malignant neoplasm. More commonly used therapeutic options include steroids, interferon, estrogen compounds, therapeutic embolism, vasoligation, cryotherapy, laser therapy, and surgical excision.[126–130]

## REFERENCES

1. Miller RW, Young Jr JL, Navakovic B: Childhood cancer. *Cancer* 1994;75:395.

2. Parkin DM, Stiller CA, Draper GJ, Bieber CA, Terracini B, Young JD, eds: *International Incidence of Childhood Cancer.* Lyon: World Health Organization, International Agency for Research on Cancer, 1988, pp.101–107.

3. Wingo PA, Tang T, Bolden S: Cancer statistics 1995. *CA: Cancer J Clini* 1995;45:8.

4. National Institutes of Health: *SEER Cancer Statistics Review, 1973–1992. Tables and Graphs.* Bethesda, MD: U.S. Department of Health and Human Services (NIH Publication 96-2789), 1995, p 57.

5. Hematology/oncology guidelines for the pediatric cancer center and role of such centers in diagnosis and treatment. *Pediatrics* 1997;99:139–141.

6. Young JL, Percy CL, Asire AJ, eds: Surveillance, Epidemiology, and End Results: Incidence and mortality data, 1973–77. *Natl Cancer Inst Monogr* 1981;57:98–101.

7. Kun LE: Acute lymphoblastic leukemia. *Semin Radiat Oncol* 1997;7:185–194.

8. Ebb DH, Weinstein HJ: Diagnosis and treatment of childhood acute myelogenous leukemia. *Pediatr Clin North Am* 1997;44:847–862.

9. Rubinitz JE, Crist WM: Molecular genetics of childhood cancer: Implications for pathogenesis, diagnosis and treatment. *Pediatrics* 1997;100:101–107.

10. Dahl GV, Simone JV, Hustu HO, Mason C: Preventive central nervous system irradiation in children with acute non-lymphocytic leukemia. *Cancer* 1978;42:2187–2192.

11. Leukemia and the central nervous system (editorial). *Lancet* 1985;i:1196.

12. Nesbit ME Jr, Robinson LL, Littman PS, Sather HN, Ortega J, D'Angio GJ, Hammond GD: Presymptomatic central nervous system therapy in previously untreated childhood acute lymphoblastic leukaemia: comparison of 1800 rad and 2400 rad: A report for Children's Cancer Study Group. *Lancet* 1981;1:461–466.

13. Nesbit ME Jr, Sather HN, Ortega J, D'Angio GJ, Robinson LL, Donaldson M, Hammond GD: Effect of isolated central nervous system leukaemia on bone marrow remission and survival in childhood acute lymphoblastic leukaemia. A report for Children's Cancer Study Group. *Lancet* 1981;2:1386–1389.

14. Nesbit ME, Sather HN, Robinson LL, et al: Sanctuary therapy: A randomized trial of 724 children with previously untreated acute lymphoblastic leukemia. *Cancer Res* 1982;42:674–680.

15. Bleyer WA: Neurologic sequelae of methotrexate and ionizing radiation. A new classification. *Cancer Treat Rep* 1981;65: 89–98.

16. Belasco J, Goldwein J, Lange B, et al: Monthly low-dose cranio-spinal (C-S) radiotherapy (RT) to 18 Gy after CNS relapse in children with acute lymphoblastic leukemia (ALL). *Proc Am Soc Clin Oncol* 1996;15:368.

17. Cherlow JM, et al: Craniospinal irradiation for acute lymphoblastic leukemia with CNS disease at diagnosis—A report from the Children's Cancer Group. *Int J Radiat Oncol Biol Phys* 1996;36:19–27.

18. Blume KG, et al: A prospective randomized comparison of total body irradiation etoposide versus busulfan–cyclophosphamide as preparatory regimens for bone marrow transplantation in patients with leukemia who were not in first remission. *Blood* 1993;81:2187–2193.

19. Chao NJ, Forman SJ: Allogeneic bone marrow transplantation for acute lymphoblastic leukemia, in Forman SJ, Blume KG, and Thomas ED (eds), *Bone Marrow Transplantation*. Boston: Blackwell Scientific Publications, 1994, pp. 618–628.

20. Shank B: Can total body irradiation be supplanted by busulfan in cytoreductive regimens for bone marrow transplantation? *Int J Radiant Oncol Biol Phys* 1995;31:195–196.

21. Goumnerova LC, Loeffler JS, Moriarty T, et al: Radiosurgery in the management of recurrent and residual intracranial ependymomas. *J Neurosurg* 1998;

22. Patrice SJ, Tarbell NJ, Goumnerova LC, et al: Results of radiosurgery in the management of recurrent and residual medulloblastoma. *Pediatr Neurosurg* 1995;22:197–203.

23. Aggarwal R, Kun L: Efficacy or feasibility of SRS in the primary management of unfavorable pediatric ependymoma. *Radiother Oncol* 1997;43:269–273.

24. Stokes MA, Sulpicio GS, Tarbell NJ, et al: Anesthesia for stereotactic radiosurgery in children. *J Neurosurg Anesthiol* 1995;7: 100–108.

25. Shrieve, DC, Tarbell NJ, Alexander E, et al: Stereotactic radiotherapy: A technique for dose optimization and escalation for intracranial tumors. *Acta Neurochir* 1994;62:55–60.

26. Tarbell NJ, Scott RM, Goumnerova LC, et al: Craniopharyngioma: Preliminary results of stereotactic radiation therapy. *Radiosurgery* 1995:75–82.

27. Bakardjiev AI, Barnes PD, Goumnerova LC, et al: Magnetic resonance imaging changes after stereotactic radiation therapy for childhood low grade astrocytoma. *Cancer* 1996;78: 864–873.

28. Hetelekidis M, Barnes Pd, Tao M, et al: Twenty-year experience in childhood craniopharyngioma. *Int J Radiat Oncol Biol Phys* 1993;17:189–195.

29. Glauser TT and Packer RJ: Cognitive deficits in long term survivors of childhood brain tumors. *Child's Nervous System* 1991;7:2–12.

30. Sheline GE, Wara WM, Smith V: Therapeutic irradiation and brain injury. *Int J Radiat Oncol Biol Phys* 1980;6:1215–1228.

31. Duffner PK, Cohen ME, and Sandford RA: Postoperative chemotherapy and delayed radiation in children less than 3 years of age. *New Eng J Med* 1993;328:1725–1731.

32. Garvey M and Packer RJ: An integrated approach to the treatment of chiasmatic-hypothalamic gliomas. *J Neuro-Oncology* 1996;28: 167–183.

33. Harrigan-Hardenbergh PM, Golden JA, Billett A, et al: Intracranial germinoma: The case for

low dose radiation therapy. *Int J Radiat Oncol Biol Phys* 1997;39:419–426.

34. Balmaceda C, Heller G, Rosenblum M, et al: Chemotherapy without irradiation—A novel approach for newly diagnosed CNS germ cell tumors: Results of an international cooperative trial. *J Clin Oncol* 1996;14:2908–2915.

35. Lindstadt D, Wara W, Edwards M, et al: Radiotherapy of primary intracranial germinomas: The case against routine craniospinal irradiation. *Int J Radiat Oncol Biol Phys* 1988; 15:291–297.

36. Silber JH, Littman PS, Meadows AT: Stature loss following skeletal irradiation for childhood cancer. *J Clin Oncol* 1990;8: 304–312.

37. Mauch PM, Weinstein H, Botnick L, et al: An evaluation of long-term survival and treatment complications in children with Hodgkin's disease. *Cancer* 1983;51:925–932.

38. Cleary S, Link M, Donaldson S: Hodgkin's disease in the very young. *Int J Radiat Oncol Biol Phys* 1994;28:77–84.

39. Mauch P, Tarbell NJ, Weinstein H, et al: Stage IA-IIA supradiaphragmatic Hodgkin's disease: Prognostic factors in surgically staged patients. *J Clin Oncol* 1988;6:1576–1583.

40. MacMahon B: Epidemiological evidence on the nature of Hodgkin's disease. *Cancer* 1957; 10:1045–1054.

41. Donaldson SS, Link MP: Combined modality treatment with low-dose radiation and MOPP chemotherapy for children with Hodgkin's disease. *J Clin Oncol* 1987;5:742–749.

42. Filipovich AH, Mathur A, Kamat D, Shapiro RS: Primary immunodeficiencies: Genetic risk factors for lymphoma. *Cancer Res* 1992; 52(Suppl):5465s–5476s.

43. Weinstein HJ, Tarbell NJ: Leukemias and lymphomas of childhood, in: DeVita VT, Hellman S, and Rosenberg SA (eds): *Cancer, Principles and Practice of Oncology,* 5th ed. Philadelphia: Lippincott-Raven, pp 2145–2164.

44. Mandell LR, Wollner N, Fuks Z: Is cranial radiation necessary for CNS prophylaxis in pediatric NHL? *Int J Radiat Oncol Biol Phys* 1987;13(3):359–363.

45. Murphy SB, Bleyer WA: Cranial irradiation is not necessary for central nervous system prophylaxis in pediatric non-Hodgkin's lymphoma. *Int J Radiat Oncol Biol Phys* 1987;13: 467–468.

46. Pick T, Weinstein HJ, Schwenn M, et al: Treatment of advanced stage large cell non-Hodgkin's lymphoma in childhood: A Pediatric Oncology Group study (8615). *Blood* 1993;82:333a.

47. Link M, Donaldson S, Berard C, Shuster JJ, Murphy S. Results of treatment of childhood localized non-Hodgkin's lymphoma with combination chemotherapy with or without radiotherapy. *N Engl J Med* 1990;322:1169–1174.

48. Anderson J, Jenkin D, Wilson D, et al. Long-term follow-up of patients treated with COMP or LSA$^2$L$^2$ therapy for childhood NHL: A report of CCG-551 from the CCG. *J Clin Oncol* 1993;11.

49. Ingram LC, Fairclough DL, Furman WL, et al: Cranial nerve palsy in childhood acute lymphoblastic leukemia and non-Hodgkin's lymphoma. *Cancer* 1991;67:2262–2268.

50. Varmus H, Weinberg RA: *Genes and the Biology of Cancer.* New York: Scientific American Library, 1993.

51. Weinberg RA: The retinoblastoma gene and gene product. *Cancer Surv* 1992;12:43–57.

52. Gallie BL, Budning A, DeBoer G, Thiessen JJ, Koren G, Verjec Z, Ling V, Chan HSL: Chemotherapy with focal therapy can cure intraocular retinoblastoma without radiotherapy. *Arch Ophthalmol* 1996;114:1321–1328.

53. Dunkel IJ, Mendelsohn M, Bayer L, Finlay JL, McCormick B, Abramson DH: A pilot phase 2 trial of carboplatin in children with intraocular retinoblastoma. *Proc Am Soc Oncol* 1996; 15:459.

54. Roarty JD, McLean IW, Zimmerman LE: Incidence of second neoplasms in patients with bilateral retinoblastoma. *Ophthalmology* 1988;95:1583–1587.

55. Foote RL, Garretson BR, Schamberg PJ, et al: External beam irradiation for retinoblastoma: Patterns of failure and dose—response analysis. *Int J Radiat Oncol Biol Phys* 1989;116: 823–830.

56. Schipper J: An accurate and simple method for megavoltage radiation therapy of retinoblastoma. *Radiother Oncol* 1983;1:31–41.

57. Schipper J, Tan KEWP, Van Peperzeel HA: Treatment of retinoblastoma by precision

megavoltage radiation therapy. *Radiother Oncol* 1985;3:117–132.

58. Toma NMG, Hungerford JL, Plowman PN, Kingston JE, Doughty D: External beam radiotherapy for retinoblastoma: II. Lens-sparing technique. *Br J Ophthalmol* 1995;79: 112–117.

59. Weiss DR, Cassady JR, Peterson R: Retinoblastoma: A modification in radiation therapy technique. *Radiology*: 1975;114:705–708.

60. Cassady JR, Sagerman RH, Tretter P, Ellsworth RM: Radiation therapy in retinoblastoma. *Radiology* 1969;93:405–409.

61. Castleberry RP: Neuroblastoma. *Eu J Cancer* 1997;33:1430–1438.

62. Castleberry RP: Biology and treatment of neuroblastoma. *Pediatr Clin North Am* 1997;44: 919–937.

63. Castleberry R: Clinical and biologic features in the prognosis and treatment of neuroblastoma. *Curr Opin Oncol* 1992;4:116–123.

64. Matthay KK: Neuroblastoma: a clinical challenge and biologic puzzle. *CA: Cancer J Clini* 1995;45:179–192.

65. Castleberry R, Kun L, Shuster J, et al: Radiotherapy improves the outlook for patients older than 1 year with Pediatric Oncology Group stage C neuroblastoma. *J Clin Oncol* 1991;9:789–795; and letter to editor, *J Clin Oncol* 1991;9:2076–2077.

66. Castleberry R, Shuster J, Altshuler G: Infants with neuroblastoma and regional lymph node metastases have a favorable outlook after limited postoperative chemotherapy: A Pediatric Oncology Group study. *J Clin Oncol* 1992;10: 1299–1304.

67. Kushner B, O'Reilly R, Mandell L, Gulati S, LaQuaglia M, Cheung N: Myeloablative combination chemotherapy without total body irradiation for neuroblastoma. *J Clin Oncol* 1991;9:274–279.

68. Matthay KK: Impact of myeloablative therapy with bone marrow transplantation in advanced neuroblastoma. *Bone Marrow Transplant* 1996; 18 Suppl.3:S21–S24.

69. Dunst J, Jürgens H, Sauer R, et al: Radiation therapy in Ewing's sarcoma: An update of the CESS 86 trial. *Int J Radiat Oncol* 1995;32: 919–930.

70. Tucker MA, D'Angio GJ, Boice JD, et al: Bone sarcomas linked to radiotherapy and chemotherapy in children. *N Engl J Med* 1987;317:588–693.

71. Hayes FA, Thompson E, Meyer WH, et al: Therapy for localized Ewing's sarcoma of bone. *J Clin Oncol* 1989;7:208–213.

72. Marcus RB Jr, Million RR: The effect of primary tumor size on the prognosis of Ewing's sarcoma. *Int J Radiat Oncol Biol Phys* 1984; 10:88–96.

73. Winkler K, Beran G, Delling G, Heise U, Kabisch H, Purfurts C, Berger J, Ritter J, Jurgens H, Gerein V, et al: Neoadjuvant chemotherapy of osteosarcoma: Results of a randomized cooperative trial (Coss-82) with salvage chemotherapy based on histological tumor response. *J Clin Oncol* 1988;6: 329–337.

74. Winkler K, Bielack SS, Belling G, Jurgens H, Kotz R, Salzer-Kuntschik M: Treatment of osteosarcoma: Experience of the cooperative osteosarcoma study group (COSS), in Humphrey GB, Koops HS, Molenaar WM, and Postma A, (eds): *Osteosarcoma in Adolescents and Young Adults: New Developments and Controversies.* Boston: Kluwer Academic Publishers, 1993;269–272.

75. Taylor WF, Ivins JC, Pritchard DJ, Dahlin DC, Gilchrist GS, Edmonson JH: Trends and variability in survival among patients with osteosarcoma: 7 year update. *Mayo Clin Proc* 1985;60:91–104.

76. Souhami RL, Craft AW, Vander Ei, Ken JW, Nooi M, Spooner D, Bramwell VHC, Wierzbicki R, Malcolm AJ, Kirpatrick A, Uscinska BM, Van Glabbeke M, Machin D: Randomized trial of two regimens of chemotherapy in operable osteosarcoma: A study of the European Osteosarcoma Intergroup. *Lancet* 1997;350:911–917.

77. Newton WA Jr, Soule EH, Hamoudi AB, et al: Histopathology of childhood sarcomas, Intergroup Rhabdomyosarcoma Studies I and II: Clinicopathologic correlation. *J Clin Oncol* 1988;6:67–75.

78. Maurer HM, Beltangady M, Gehan EA, et al: The Intergroup Rhabdomyosarcoma Study—I: A final report. *Cancer* 1988;61:209–220.

79. Maurer HM, Christ W, Wharam M, et al: IRS Study IV (protocol). 893.

80. Mandell L, Ghavini F, Peretz T, et al: Radiocurability of microscopic disease in childhood rhabdomyosarcoma with radiation doses less than 4,000 cGy. *J Clin Oncol* 1990;8: 1536–1542.

81. Tefft M, Fernandez C, Donaldson M, et al: Incidence of meningeal involvement by rhabdomyosarcoma of the head and neck in children: A report of the Intergroup Rhabdomyosarcoma Study (IRS). *Cancer* 1978;42: 253–258.

82. Mandell LR, Ghavimi F, Exelby P, et al: The influence of extensive bone erosion on local control in non-orbital rhabdomyosarcoma of the head and neck. *Int J Radiat Oncol Biol Phys* 1989;17:649–653.

83. Raney RB Jr, Gehan EA, Hays DM, et al: Chemotherapy with or without radiation therapy and/or surgery for children with localized sarcoma of the bladder, prostate, vagina, uterus, and cervix. *Cancer* 1990;66:2072–2081.

84. Dillon P, Maurer J, Jenkins J, Krummel T, Parham D, Webber B, Salzberg A: A prospective study of nonrhabdomyosarcoma soft tissue sarcomas in the pediatric age group. *J Pediatr Surg* 1992;27:241–245.

85. Coffin CM, Dehner LP: Peripheral neurogenic tumors of the soft tissues in children and adolescents: A clinicopathologic study of 108 examples in 103 patients. *Pediatr Pathol* 1989; 11:559–588.

86. Sobin LH, Wittekind C. *TNM Classification of Malignant Tumours, Fifth Edition.* NY: Wiley-Liss, 1997.

87. Sommelet-Olive D. Non-rhabdo malignant mesenchymal tumors in children. *Med Ped Oncol* 1995;25:273.

88. Bramwell V, Rouesse J, Steward W, Santoro A, Schraffordt-Koops H, Buesa J, Ruka R, Priario J, Wagener T, Burgers M, Van Unmik J, Contesso G, Thomas D, van Glabbeke M, Markham D, Pinedo H: Adjuvant CYVADIC Chemotherapy for adult soft tissue sarcomareduced local recurrence but no improvement in survival: A study of the European Organization for Research and Treatment of Cancer Soft Tissue and Bone Sarcoma Group. *J Clin Onc* 12:1137–1149.

89. Alvegard TA, Sigurdsson H, Mourdisen H, Solheim O, Unsgaard Ringbord U, Dahl O, Nordentoft AM, Blomkvist C, Rydholm Stener B, Ranstam J: Adjuvant chemotherapy with doxyrubicin and high grade soft tissue sarcoma: a randomized trial of the Scandanavian Sarcoma Group. *J Clin Oncol* 1989;7: 1504–1513.

90. Shiu MH, Hilaris BS, Harrison LB, Brennan MF. Brachytherapy and function-saving resection of soft tissue sarcoma arising in the limb. *Int J Radiat Oncol Biol Phys* 1991;21: 1485–1492.

91. D'Angio GJ: SIOP and the management of Wilms tumor (editorial). *J Clin Oncol* 1983;1:595–596.

92. D'Angio GJ, Evans AE, Breslow N, et al: The treatment of Wilms tumor: Results of the National Wilms' Tumor Study. *Cancer* 1976;38: 633–646.

93. D'Angio GJ, Tefft M, Breslow N, Meyer JA: Radiation therapy of Wilms tumor: Results according to dose, field, post-operative timing and histology. *Int J Radiat Oncol Biol Phys* 1978;4:769–780.

94. D'Angio GJ, Evans A, Breslow N, et al: The treatment of Wilms tumor: Results of the Second National Wilms' Tumor Study. *Cancer* 1981;47:2302–2311.

95. D'Angio GJ, Breslow N, Beckwith JB, Evans A, Barum E, DeLorimier A, Fernbach D, Hrabovsky E, Jones B, Kelalis P, Othersen HB, Tefft M, Thomas PPM: Treatment of Wilms tumor: Results of the Third National Wilms Tumor Study. *Cancer* 1989;64:349–360.

96. Green DM, Thomas PRM, Shochat S: The treatment of Wilms tumor: results of the national Wilms tumor studies. *Hematol Oncol Clin North Am* 1995;9:1267–1274.

97. Green DM, Finkelstein JZ, Breslow NE, Beckwith JB: Remaining problems in the treatment of patients with Wilms tumor. *Pediatr Clin North Am* 1991;38:475–588.

98. Green DM, Coppes MJ: Future directions in clinical research in Wilms tumor. *Hematol Oncol Clinic North Am* 1996;27:218.

99. Ablin A, Kraila M, Hass J, Rogers P, Campbell J, Tefft M, Land V, Viettis T, Hammond D: Hepatoblastoma and hepatocellular carcinoma in children: A report from the Children's Cancer Study Group (CCG) and the Pediatric Oncology Group (POG). *Med Pediatr Oncol* 1988; 16:417.

100. Bellani FF, Massimino M: Liver tumors in childhood: Epidemiology and clinics. *J Surg Oncol Suppl* 1993;3:119–121.

101. Berry CL, Keeling JW: Hepatoblastoma, in Berry CL (ed): *Pediatric Pathology.* Berlin: Springer-Verlag, 1981, pp 660–662.

102. Black CT, Cangir A, Choroszy M, et al: Marked response to pre-operative high dose *cis*-platinum in children with unresectable hepatoblastoma. *J Pediatr Surg* 1991;26:1070–1073.

103. Bowman LC, Riely CA: Management of pediatric liver tumors. *Surg Oncol Clin North Am* 1996;5(2):451–459.

104. Clatworth HW Jr, Schiller M, Grosfeld JL: Primary liver tumors in infancy and childhood: 41 cases variously treated. *Arch Surg* 1974;109:143–147.

105. Cohen MD, Bugaieski EM, Haliloglu M, Faught P, Siddiqui AR: Visual presentation of the staging of pediatric tumors. *Radiographics* 1996;16(3);523–545.

106. Noseworthy J, Lack EE, Kozakewich HPW, Vawter GF, Welch KJ: Sacrococcygeal germ cell tumors in childhood: an updated experience with 118 patients. *J Pediatr Surg* 1981; 16:358–364.

107. Raney RB, Sinclair L, Uri A, Schnaufer L, Cooper A, Littman P: Malignant ovarian tumors in children and adolescents. *Cancer* 1987;59:1214–1220.

108. Red E. Study: save contralateral ovary in girls with ovarian malignancy. *Oncol Times* 1986;8: 1–16.

109. Slayton RE, Park RC, Silverberg SG, Shingleton H, Creasman WT, Blessing J: Vincristine, dactinomycin, and cyclophosphamide in the treatment of malignant germ cell tumors of the ovary: a gynecologic oncology group study (a final report). *Cancer* 1985;56:243–248.

110. Tewfik HH, Tewfik FA, Lataurette HB: A clinical review of seventeen patients with ovarian dysgerminoma. *Int J Radiat Oncol Biol Phys* 1982;8:1705–1709.

111. Thomas WJ, Kelleher JF, Duval–Arnould B: Successful treatment of metastatic extragonadal endodermal sinus (yolk sac) tumor in childhood. *Cancer* 1981;48:2371–2374.

112. Valdiserri RO, Yunis EJ: Sacrococcygeal teratomas: Review of 68 cases. *Cancer* 1981;48: 217–221.

113. Vassai G, Falmant F, Caillaud JM, Demeoca F, Nihoul-Fekete C, Lemerle J: Juvenile granulosa cell tumor of the ovary in children: A clinical study of 15 cases. *J Clin Oncol* 1988;6: 990–995.

114. Vogelzang NJ, Anderson RW, Kennedy BJ: Successful treatment of mediastinal germ cell/endodermal sinus tumors. *Chest* 1985;88:64–69.

115. Wells RG, Sty JR: Imaging of sacrococcygeal germ cell tumors. *RadioGraphics* 1990;10: 701–713.

116. Wollner N, Exelby PR, Woodruff M, et al: Malignant ovarian tumors in childhood. Prognosis in relation to initial stage. *Cancer* 1976;37: 1953–1964.

117. Hawkins EP, Finegold MJ, Hawkins HK, Krischer JP, Starling KA, Weinberg A: Nongerminomatous malignant germ cell tumors in children: a review of 89 cases from the Pediatric Oncology Group, 1971–1984. *Cancer* 1986;58:2579–2584.

118. Huddart SN, Mann JR, Gornall P, Pearson D, Barrett A, Raafat F, Barnes JM, Wallendus KR. The UK Children's Cancer Study Group: testicular malignant germ cell tumours 1979–1988. *J Pediatr Surg* 1990;25:406–410.

119. Jacobsson M, Petruson B, Svedsen P, Berthelsen B: Juvenile nasopharyngeal angiofibroma: a report of eighteen cases. *Acta Otolaryngol (Stockh)* 1988;105:132–139.

120. Garcia-Cervigan E, Bien S, Rufenacht D, Thurel C, Reizine D, Tran Ba Huy P, Merland JJ: Pre-operative embolization of nasopharyngeal angiofibromas: report of 58 cases. *Neuroradiology* 1988;30:556–560.

121. Fields JN, Halverson KJ, Devinein VR, Simpson JR, Perez CA: Juvenile nasopharyngeal angiofibroma: efficacy of radiation therapy. *Radiology* 1990;176:263–265.

122. Iannetti G, Belli E, DePonte F, Cicconetti A, Delfini R: The surgical approaches to nasopharyngeal angiofibroma. *J Cranio-Maxillo-Facial Surg* 1994;22:311–316.

123. Willis B, Ablin A, Weinberg V, Zager S, Wara WM, Matthay KK: Disease course and late sequelae of Langerhans cell histiocytosis: 25-year experience at the University of Caliornia, San Francisco. *J Clin Oncol* 1996;14:2073–2082.

124. Willman CL, Busque L, Griffith BB, Favara BE, McClain KL, Duncan MH, et al: Langerhans cell histiocytosis (histiocytosis X): A clonal proliferative disease. *N Engl J Med* 1994;331:154–160.

125. Selch MT, Parker RG: Radiation therapy in the management of Langerhans cell histiocytosis. *Med Pediatr Oncol* 1990;18:97–102.

126. Dutton SC, Plowman PN: Paediatric haemangiomas: The role of radiotherapy. *Br J Radiol* 1991;64:261–269.

127. Morelli JG: Hemangiomas and vascular malformations. *Pediatri Ann* 1996;25:91–96.

128. Furst CJ, Lundell M, Holm LE: Radiation therapy of hemangiomas, 1909–1959. A report based on 50 years of clinical practice at Radiumhemmet, Stockholm. *Acta Oncol* 1987;26: 33–36.

129. Furst CJ, Lundell M, Holm L-E, Silfversward C: Cancer incidence after radiotherapy for skin hemangioma: A retrospective cohort study in Sweden. *Natl Cancer Inst* 1988;80: 1387–1392.

130. Lindberg S, Karlsson P, Arvidsson B, Holmberg E, Lundberg LM, Wallgran A: Cancer incidence after radiotherapy for skin haemangioma during infancy. *Acta Oncol* 1995;34: 735–740.

# CHAPTER 15

# NOVEL RADIOTHERAPEUTIC APPROACHES

## A. Use of Particle Radiation Therapy -

JOHN E. MUNZENRIDER

## INTRODUCTION

External beam radiotherapy techniques involve the transfer of energy from the radiation source to the target of interest, generally a neoplasm involving a specific anatomic site. Ideally, all that energy should be deposited in the target, giving little or no dose to adjacent normal tissues. However, normal tissues surrounding the target always receive some radiation dose, and tolerance of adjacent organs may limit the dose that can safely be delivered to the target. This dose limitation potentially decreases the probability of achieving the desired therapeutic goal, be that tumor inactivation, elimination of abnormal blood flow in an arteriovenous malformation (AVM), or some other desired effect. If a smaller volume of normal tissue is irradiated, the likelihood of treatment-related morbidity is diminished, since radiation injury cannot develop in nonirradiated tissues.

The use of charged particles (proton or heavier ion beams) has great potential for reducing dose to normal tissues, while delivering the desired dose to the target. This part of the chapter focuses on the rationale for using light ions (protons or helium ions) in clinical radiotherapy, and the favorable results obtained at selected tumor sites with those particles. In this discussion, protons and helium ions will be considered to be comparable in terms of the dose distributions that can be achieved with either particle.

Charged particles that are heavier than protons and helium ions, such as neon, argon, silicon, carbon, and negative $\pi$ mesons (pions) have also been used in clinical radiotherapy. Such beams produce better dose distributions than those obtained with high energy supervoltage photons, but also have some high linear energy transfer (LET) properties, resulting theoretically in both a physical and a biological advantage over low LET radiations. Neutron beams have also been used clinically. These beams of neutral particles have dose distribution in tissue similar to x-rays, but also have high LET properties, giving these beams a potential biological advantage relative to x-rays. Discussions of the rationale for, and clinical experience with particles heavier than protons and helium ions, and with neutrons, were reviewed in 1998.[1]

## NEED FOR BETTER RADIATION THERAPY

### Local Tumor Control

Local failure rates for intermediate and advanced stages of disease [Stages T2–T4] range

*Clinical Radiation Oncology: Indications, Techniques, and Results, 2nd ed.* Edited by C.C. Wang.
ISBN: 0-471-23803-1   Copyright © 2000 Wiley-Liss, Inc.

from about 10% to 90%, depending on tumor type, tumor volume, and anatomic site.[2–6] In patients with local tumor progression after radiation therapy, cure rates rarely exceed 30% in patients suitable for aggressive salvage surgery.[7] Local failure, often associated with substantial morbidity and ultimately death due to local tumor progression, is also usually accompanied by an increased rate of distant metastasis, which presumably originates in the locally recurring tumor.[8–10] Tumor control probability (TCP) increases with increasing radiation dose: the slope of the dose–response curve defines the gain in TCP for a specified increment in dose, and can be numerically described in terms of a gamma factor $g$, the percent point increase in TCP for a 1% increase in dose.[11] The $g$ factor is greatest at the 37% point on the dose–response curve and decreases toward the end of this curve. The $g_{50}$ is the factor at the midportion of the dose–response curve, and approximates 2 for human tumors, a value derived by reviewing slopes of dose–response curves from published clinical experiences.[12] A positive slope to a tumor dose–response curve indicates that any improvement in technique that permits the administration of a higher tumor dose will yield an incremental increase in TCP.

## Normal Tissue Damage

Clinically significant normal tissue damage is seen relatively infrequently, since treatment techniques and doses employed are usually designed to limit significant morbidity rates to 5% or less, with acceptance of whatever TCP can be achieved with the administered dose. Frequency and severity of treatment-related morbidity are closely related to the volume of critical tissues/organs included in the treatment volume, the dose delivered to those tissues, and their initial functional capacity. Although quantitative knowledge of the relationship between dose and the probability of normal tissue damage is less secure than that of the relationship between dose and tumor control probability, dose reduction to normal tissues will most cer-

tainly result in fewer and less severe treatment-related injuries. Patients cannot help but benefit, in terms of decrease morbidity, from efforts and resources applied to improving technical aspects of treatment planning and delivery. Such efforts may also lead to improved rates of uncomplicated local tumor control if the tumor can safely be given a higher dose.

Margins must always be added to the target volume, as defined by appropriate imaging studies, to ensure that it will be included in three dimensions at each treatment session. This explicitly allows for inaccuracies in treatment planning, target misalignment with respect to treatment beams, and change in patient position, patient contour, or target position during each individual treatment session or over the course of the treatment. Physical characteristics of radiation beams also constrain the ability to conform dose distributions in three dimensions to the defined target. The ongoing challenge to radiation physicists and oncologists is to reduce the volume of normal tissue irradiated, while still delivering the prescribed dose to the target.[13]

Nontarget tissues most frequently develop symptomatic radiation injury.[14] Patients treated for uterine, bladder, rectal, or prostatic carcinoma may incur radiation injury to small and large bowel, pelvic bones, and/or lumbosacral nerves. These structures, not usually directly involved by tumor, are included in the high dose volume because of proximity to the target. Injury to the spinal cord may appear following treatment of head and neck, thoracic, and upper abdominal tumors. Uninvolved kidneys and/or liver may be injured during treatment of abdominal or retroperitoneal tumors. Brain, brain stem, eye, ear, jaw, and salivary glands may manifest injury after treatment of head and neck and skull base tumors.

## Limits to Improvements in Dose Distributions

There are limitations to the degree of improvement that can be expected with the higher doses that technical advances in radiation therapy might allow: increases in radiation dose potentially achievable by reducing dose to normal tissue probably will not exceed 10% to 20% for most tumors. An absolute limit to improvement will be reached when the volume receiving the prescribed dose conforms exactly to the target volume. Approaching this ideal situation for some anatomic sites may be more possible with heavy charged particle radiation therapy than with state-of-the-art x-ray techniques.[15]

The ability to distinguish target from non-target tissues has improved remarkably in the past decade, largely because imaging techniques, specifically CT and MRI scans, have improved. Along with this enhanced ability to define the clinical target volume (CTV) from the images, an awareness has emerged about the need to formally and systematically incorporate all interfraction and intrafraction variations in CTV into the definition of planning target volumes (PTV). This will ensure that adequate margins are included in definition of the PTV, so that the CTV will receive the prescribed dose. Portable software tools have been developed which allow three-dimensional PTVs to be rapidly, consistently, and automatically generated from CTVs.[16] This improved knowledge of target location and configuration, when incorporated into three-dimensional treatment planning systems, has both limited the likelihood of local failure due to inadequate target definition and greatly enhanced the ability of newer techniques, such as heavy charged particle radiation therapy, to improve the probability of achieving uncomplicated local control of human tumors at various sites in the body.

# CHARGED PARTICLE BEAM THERAPY—BETTER DOSE DISTRIBUTIONS

## Charged Particles Versus X-Rays

Charged particle beams are potentially advantageous for clinical radiotherapy because bet-ter dose distributions can be achieved with such particles than with megavoltage x-ray beams. This advantage is almost exclusively due to the qualitatively different depth–dose characteristics of the two types of radiation. The following discussion relates specifically to proton beams but is generally applicable to helium and heavier ion beams as well. A proton has mass roughly 1835 times that of an electron and carries a single positive charge. The precisely predictable range of a proton beam in a specific tissue is determined by both the beam's energy and the density of that tissue. In contrast, a photon (x- or $\gamma$-ray) beam loses energy exponentially and is much less influenced by tissue inhomogeneities. Figure 15-1 shows depth–dose curves for a 10 MeV x-ray beam from a linear accelerator and for both monoenergetic and modulated-energy 160 MeV proton beams. The proton beam shows a typical "Bragg peak" configuration; with a low dose in the entrance region, a maximum dose at depth as energy is lost near the end of the beam's range, and a rapid fall-off to a zero dose: **tissues distal to the beam are not irradiated**. In contrast, tissues distal to an x-ray beam continue to be irradiated as beam intensity decreases exponentially until the beam exits the body. As an added advantage, dose to tissues proximal to the target will never be greater than the dose delivered to the target, while normal tissues in the entrance path of a photon beam usually receive a greater dose than does the target.

## Spread-Out Bragg Peak and Dose Uniformity

A monoenergetic proton beam is of limited clinical value owing to the narrow region of high dose in the Bragg peak. The high dose region can be made broad enough to be clinically useful, or "spread out" (modulated), by appropriate selection of a distribution of proton energies. This produces a spread-out Bragg peak (SOBP), a uniform region of full dose at the depth of interest in the patient. However, the entrance dose rises as additional Bragg peaks

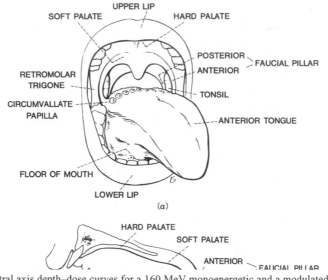

**FIGURE 15-1**   Central axis depth–dose curves for a 160 MeV monoenergetic and a modulated ("spread-out") proton beam, shown with the depth–dose curve for a 10 MV linear accelerator beam; SOBP, spread-out Bragg peak.

are added together, so that an SOBP proton beam may have relatively greater entrance dose, specifically in the buildup region of a megavoltage x-ray beam (Figure 15-1). However, deep to the buildup region, x-ray beams usually deliver to the tissues proximal to the target a greater dose than would be obtained from a corresponding proton beam. X-ray beams also are associated with a dose gradient across the target, and they deliver unnecessary dose to normal tissues distal to the target. Proton beams have neither of these undesirable characteristics.

Elegant dose distributions can be achieved by using multiple x-ray beams and complex field angles, as well as by varying field sizes, beam energies, intensities, and modifiers. Equally elegant or superior dose distributions can readily be achieved with less complexity and perhaps fewer fields by means of proton beams. In no tumor–normal tissue configuration examined to date have dose distributions achieved with relatively simple proton plans been inferior to those achieved with photon plans (see below). The primary virtues of proton beams for clinical radiation therapy are the lower doses to tissues in the entrance region, uniform doses across the target from each portal, and most importantly, the absence of an exit dose.

## Relative Biologic Effectiveness (RBE) and Linear Energy Transfer (LET)

Both protons and photons are low LET radiations; that is, they lose relatively little energy by ionization and excitation of atoms and molecules along the beam's path. The rate of energy loss is less than 1 kV/mm of beam path length for both protons and photons. At the end of a proton beam's range, a rapid loss of energy occurs, associated with production of a limited zone of high LET radiation (dense ionization). This results in the characteristic Bragg peak of the monoenergetic 160 MeV proton beam shown in Figure 15-1. The regions of dense ionization occurring in the Bragg peak may be distributed throughout the spread-out Bragg peak and may account for an increased biological effectiveness (> 1.0 for proton beams), which has been observed in multiple biological systems.[17,18] An RBE of 1.1 has been used clinically for the Harvard Cyclotron Laboratory (HCL) beam and for most other proton clinical treatment programs. Proton doses are defined in terms of cobalt-Gy equivalents, or CGE (CGE = proton Gy $\times$ 1.1). Use of 1.1 as a "universal proton RBE" has been described by Miller as a "practical means of bringing photon beam and proton beam clinical response into rough agreement. Application of a different RBE for each clinical response endpoint is beyond the current state of the art."[19]

## History of Proton Beam Therapy

Over half a century ago R. Wilson suggested that protons offered several advantages for use in clinical radiotherapy because of their physical characteristics.[20] Comparative dose distributions for protons, photons, and electrons were presented in 1972 by Koehler and Preston.[21] Potential advantages of protons for para-aortic irradiation were proposed in 1974 by Archambeau et al.[22] Clinical studies were first reported from the University of California at San Francisco (UCSF) and the Lawrence Berkeley Laboratory (LBL) in 1955,[23,24] from the University of Uppsala, Sweden, in 1957,[25] from the Massachusetts General Hospital and the Harvard Cyclotron Laboratory in 1961,[26-28] and from the Physics Research Institute at Dubna, Russia, in 1964 and the Institute for Experimental and Theoretical Physics (ITEP) in Moscow in 1969.[29] As of July 1998, eighteen centers throughout the world were actively engaged in clinical proton beam therapy. In excess of 22,000 patients have been treated with protons, as shown in Table 15-1.[30]

Particle accelerators (cyclotrons or synchrotrons) designed for basic particle physics research were initially used for clinical proton beam therapy. Beams from those accelerators all had a fixed horizontal or vertical beam, requiring alignment of the patient to the beam, rather than the beam to the patient, the technique

**TABLE 15-1   Patients Treated by Proton Beams**

| Center | Dates | Number of Patients |
| --- | --- | --- |
| UCSF/LBL, U.S. | 1995–1992 | 30 |
| Uppsala, Sweden | 1957 | 220 |
| MGH/MEEI/HCL, U.S. | 1961 | 7,694 |
| Dubna, Russia | 1964 | 124 |
| Moscow, Russia | 1969 | 3,039 |
| St. Petersburg, Russia | 1975 | 1,029 |
| Chiba, Japan | 1979 | 96 |
| Tsukuba, Japan | 1983 | 576 |
| PSI, Switzerland | 1984 | 2,496 |
| Clatterbridge, U.K. | 1989 | 817 |
| Loma Linda, U.S. | 1990 | 3,433 |
| Louvain, Belgium | 1991 | 21 |
| Nice, France | 1991 | 1,010 |
| Orsay, France | 1991 | 956 |
| NAC, South Africa | 1993 | 263 |
| Indiana University, U.S. | 1993 | 1 |
| UC-Davis, U.S. | 1994 | 162 |
| TRIUMF, Vancouver, BC, Canada | 1995 | 37 |
| Berlin, Germany | 1998 | 3 |
| | | 22,107 |

that has been standard practice with clinically configured isocentric megavoltage linear accelerators for the past three to four decades. Relatively low energy beams with sufficient range in tissue to treat only relatively superficial targets are available at six of the facilities listed in Table 15-1. Those centers are limited to treating tumors involving some head and neck sites, and intracranial or ocular lesions. Some of the other beams have higher energies and are able to treat more deeply seated tumors, but their penetration is still insufficient to treat lesions at all sites in the human body. These technical factors and the interests of participating clinicians explain why the majority of patients treated with protons have had intracranial lesions (benign pituitary tumors and arteriovenous malformations) or uveal melanomas. A significant number of patients with skull base tumors and with prostate cancer have also been treated. Because of the distribution of patients treated, a critical appraisal of the efficacy of proton beam radiation therapy can be made for only a few tumor sites.

Loma Linda University Medical Center in California began treating patients with protons accelerated by a 270 MeV synchrotron in 1990. That facility has both fixed and isocentric beam capabilities, and the accelerator has sufficient energy to treat tumors at any site in the body. Techniques used for routine photon therapy are being employed there for treating patients with various tumor categories.[31] A gantry-equipped proton facility became available for patient treatment at Paul Shirer Institute (PSI) in Switzerland in 1997. Similarly configured cyclotrons initiated treatment in Boston and in Kashiwa, Japan, during 1999. A more definitive assessment of the role of proton beam therapy in human clinical oncology must await future efforts at these and other centers that may be activated within the next decade.

## DOSE DISTRIBUTIONS WITH PROTONS

A special issue of the *International Journal of Radiation Oncology Biology and Physics* published selected papers that had been presented at a workshop sponsored by the National Cancer Institute on "Potential Gains by Use of Superior Dose Distribution."[32] Articles addressed the general question of improved dose distributions in relation to gains in therapeutic results,[33] dose escalation,[34] normal tissue complication probabilities,[35] and imaging techniques.[36] Treatment plans comparing dose distributions with protons and with x-rays were presented for patients with glioblastoma multiforme,[37] for pediatric brain tumors,[38,39] for maxillary sinus carcinoma,[40] for tonsillar carcinoma,[41] for cervical cancer,[42–44] for rectal cancer,[45] and for retroperitoneal pediatric tumors.[46] Comparative treatment plans for x-rays and protons have also been published for nasopharyngeal cancer,[47] arteriovenous malformations,[48] medulloblastoma,[49] and esophageal carcinoma.[50] Proton dose distributions were superior to those achieved with x-rays in all cases.

A National Cancer Institute–sponsored multi-institutional working group has also published an NCI monograph summarizing its findings from evaluations of treatment plans with various charged and uncharged (neutrons) particle beams.[51] Intriguing dose distributions that could potentially be useful in treating surface lesions have recently been described with proton arcs.[52]

## CONFORMAL THREE-DIMENSIONAL TREATMENT PLANNING

Dose distribution with both proton beams and x-rays can be precisely predicted in homogeneous material such as tissue or water. However, bone or air cavities, or other tissue inhomogeneities, produce much greater dose distribution perturbations with protons than are recorded with x-ray beams. Therefore, it is more important to know tissue density in the volume to be irradiated if protons are to be used. This is particularly true if marked tissue inhomogeneity is present in the target region, so that accurate compensation may be made for tissue inhomogeneities, both in treatment planning and in proton beam delivery.[53–55] Accurate alignment of the patient with the compensator at the time of treatment is also essential to assure that the dose delivered to the target will be distributed as planned. The paragraphs that follow describe patient immobilization, treatment planning, aperture and compensator specification and fabrication, and treatment techniques used for proton beam therapy at the Harvard Cyclotron Laboratory.

Patients are immobilized in the treatment position[56,57] with various combinations of an individualized bite block, a thermoplastic face mask, and, if indicated, an individualized body mold. The treatment planning CT scan is performed on the immobilized patient in the treatment position, except that scans taken in the supine position have been used for treatment of patients who may receive a portion of their treatment of skull base or intracranial lesions in a seated position. The CT scan data then are transferred to the treatment planning computer, and target and normal tissue contours are manually drawn on serial CT sections throughout the treatment volume. In this work radiologists use information from referring surgeons, operative notes, and pre- and postoperative imaging studies, specifically CT and MRI scans to accurately define the target and nearby dose-limiting normal tissues.

The interactive treatment planning program incorporates a "beams-eye view" feature, which is used to define optimal beam directions for treatment of the defined target volume, while geometrically minimizing dose received by defined normal tissues.[58] Each field is defined with a brass or Cerrobend aperture; a multileaf collimator also could be employed. Dose penetration at depth for each portal is defined with a portal-specific Lucite compensator. Brass apertures and Lucite compensators are individually machined for each field (apertures > 17.5 cm in diameter are cast from Cerrobend). As few as one and as many as 12 aperture–compensator sets are fabricated for each patient. The HCL beam has been available only 4 days per week for the fractionated proton therapy program. To follow a conventional fractionation schedule of 5 days per week, most patients receive some treatment through two or more x-ray portals. Some skin sparing is also achieved with

the x-rays employed. Three-dimensional dose distributions throughout the volume of interest are reviewed prior to plan implementation, so that unexpected dose variations can be corrected prior to actual treatment.

## TREATMENT TECHNIQUES AND DOCUMENTATION

The patient is positioned for treatment with the same immobilization device used for the treatment planning scan. Radiographic verification of patient position is achieved for each treatment by aligning the position of the beam center and the edges of the field aperture seen on a portal radiograph with bony or metallic fiducials previously identified on a digital radiograph, which has been reconstructed from the planning CT scan data. Setup accuracy and reproducibility, which is ± 2 mm with skeletal fiducials,[56] can be as little as ± 1 mm when small metallic screws or BBs surgically placed in the skull serve as fiducials.[57] The importance of precise patient positioning to obtain maximum benefit from the dose-localizing properties of the proton beam, during treatment of targets adjacent to or abutting dose-limiting normal tissues, has been demonstrated.[59]

Full three-dimensional dose distributions are calculated and can be displayed on the computer monitor or printed out as hard copy, showing either conventional isodose lines or color shades with the appropriate scale displayed. As many as four different plans can be viewed simultaneously for plan comparison purposes. **Dose–volume histograms** can be produced for any structure that has been defined on the planning scan. A full data set for each patient is archived at the completion of treatment and can be recalled for clinical or research purposes at any time after treatment has been completed.[60,61]

## CURRENT INDICATIONS FOR PROTON THERAPY AT HARVARD

Patients treated at the Harvard cyclotron have generally had relatively superficial tumors, as

**TABLE 15-2  Population Treated at HCL Through September 1998**

| Category | Number | Percent |
|---|---|---|
| CNS (radiosurgery) | 3347 | 43 |
| Uveal melanoma | 2568 | 33 |
| Macular degeneration | 193 | 2 |
| Other eye | 183 | 2 |
| Prostate | 215 | 3 |
| Chordoma–chondrosarcoma | 622 | 8 |
| Other bone | 125 | 2 |
| CNS | 126 | 2 |
| Head and neck | 126 | 2 |
| Other | 449 | 7 |
| | 7811 | |

dictated by the maximum penetration in tissue of 16 cm for the 160 MeV beam. Ocular targets, such as uveal melanomas, choroidal angiomas, hemangiomas, metastases, retinoblastomas, and subfoveal neovascular membranes in patients with age-related macular degeneration are generally treated with protons only. Intracranial, skull base, vertebral and paravertebral tumors, and paranasal sinus and nasopharyngeal carcinomas have received the majority of their treatment with the proton beam. A proton boost after large-field x-ray therapy is employed for patients with prostatic carcinomas, and some soft tissue and bone sarcomas. Patients with small intracranial lesions continue to be treated with single-fraction stereotactic radiosurgery.[26–28] Table 15-2 describes the patient population treated through September 1998.

## CLINICAL RESULTS FROM PROTON THERAPY

A major portion of the clinical experience with fractionated proton beam therapy at HCL and indeed worldwide has been in patients with uveal melanomas, skull base chordomas and chondrosarcomas, and prostate cancer. The subsections that follow discuss clinical indications, treatment outcome, and current treatment protocols in these patients, and for patients with malignant gliomas, benign, atyp-

ical, and malignant meningiomas, and paranasal sinus carcinomas treated in whole or in part with fractionated proton beam therapy.

## Ocular Neoplasms

Fewer than 1% of all human malignancies arise in the eye. The most common primary ocular tumor, uveal melanoma, afflicts mainly adults. Retinoblastomas occur much less frequently, with almost all cases occurring in infants and young children. Blindness following progressive visual morbidity can result from growth or complications of benign blood vessel tumors, such as angiomas and hemangiomas. Choroidal metastases can lead to severe deterioration in the quality of life for patients, who usually have a relatively limited life span because of progressive cancer.

The potential for the conservative treatment of ocular tumors, specifically uveal melanomas, was first demonstrated with episcleral radionuclide $^{60}$Co plaque brachytherapy by Stallard and associates, who achieved eye preservation in almost two-thirds of surviving patients.[62] In recent years, conservative treatment of uveal melanoma patients has become commonplace, with either radionuclide plaques[62–67] or charged particle beams.[68–75] This part of the chapter discusses the latter technique, concentrating principally on techniques employed and results obtained in patients treated at the Harvard Cyclotron Laboratory.

Since charged particle beams can be made to focus their dose in the target, while largely sparing noninvolved intraocular and orbital structures, such beams are ideal for treating ocular tumors in general, and uveal melanomas in particular. A large number of ocular tumors have been treated in a most fruitful collaborative effort between the Radiation Oncology Department of Massachusetts General Hospital (MGH), the Retina Service of the Massachusetts Eye and Ear Infirmary (MEEI), and the Harvard Cyclotron Laboratory (HCL), as shown in Table 15-2. Uveal melanomas have also been treated in the former Soviet Union,[68] at Clatterbridge, England,[70] at the Paul Shirer

Institute (PSI, formerly the Swiss Institute for Nuclear Research, SIN) in Villingen, Switzerland,[72] at the Gustav Werner Institute in Uppsala, Sweden, in Brussels, Belgium, in both Nice and Orsay, France, in Chiba, Japan,[74] and at Loma Linda University in California. A collaborative effort between the Radiation Oncology Department and the Ocular Oncology Unit of the University of California–San Francisco (UCSF), and the Lawrence Berkeley Laboratory, using helium ions, was unfortunately terminated in 1992 when the accelerator at Berkeley was shut down. Patients from UCSF are currently being treated with protons at the University of California–Davis.[75] Planning and treatment techniques developed at HCL for charged particle therapy of ocular lesions, and results of such treatments largely at HCL, are presented below.

***Preclinical Studies*** Normal eyes and simulated ocular tumors in monkeys were treated with single proton doses of 50 to 100 Gy, using 7 or 10 mm diameter beams. Areas of edematous retina and choroid developed within 20 hours in the treated eyes, while immediately outside the irradiated volume the retina and choroid appeared entirely normal.[76] Fractionation had a marked effect: 125 Gy in 5 fractions produced the same effect at 24 hours and at 1 year as 30 Gy in a single pulse.[77] Chorioretinal changes persisted within the irradiated area at 45 to 51 months; normal retinal architecture was preserved immediately outside the discrete retinal proton scar.[78]

***Planning and Treatment Techniques*** A computerized treatment planning program has been used for all patients.[79] Required input data include axial eye length and tumor height from ultrasound, and tumor configuration drawn manually on the computer screen from tumor sketches and/or fundus photographs (Figures 15-2A, B). Most uveal melanoma patients undergo surgical tumor localization,[79–81] at which time 2 mm diameter tantalum rings are sutured to the sclera around the perimeter of the tumor as defined by transillumination or indirect ophthalmoscopy. Ring position for the planning program is determined from measurements taken during surgery, and from radiographs taken in the treatment position on the second or third day after surgery. A transparency with appropriate magnification is used for treatment setup, and shows the desired clip position (Figure 15-2C) and the light field projected through the proton aperture onto the front of the eye (Figure 15-2D). Dose–volume histograms for the globe, lens, ciliary body, retina, macula, and disc are also available. A computer-controlled milling machine is used to fabricate an individualized brass aperture for each patient, as specified by the treatment planning program. Treatment portals are relatively small, ranging from 10 to 35 mm in diameter. Tissue compensators are not used for the ocular treatments.

Anterior ciliary body and peripheral choroidal lesions are treated with a light field setup only, verifying tumor location for treatment by transillumination after initial computerized planning from fundus photographs, tumor sketches, and ultrasound. A light field setup is also used for treating angiomas and hemangiomas, choroidal metastases, and in patients with subfoveal neovascular membranes, primarily those with age-related macular degeneration. All patients are treated in a seated position, the head immobilized with an individually molded face mask and a bite block. Eyelids are retracted for treatment, to reduce or eliminate eyelid exposure. The eye fixates voluntarily on an external light source during treatment, after initial radiographic or light field setup. Treatment times approximate 1 to 2 minutes, with setup being accomplished in 5 to 10 minutes. During treatment, eye position is monitored by a video camera. Mean movement during treatment was $0.5 \pm 0.3$ mm during 41 treatments in 11 patients, with maximum movement of 1.2 mm.[56]

***Uveal Melanomas*** Melanomas of the uveal tract are relatively rare; approximately 1500 cases are diagnosed annually in the United States. Equally common in males and

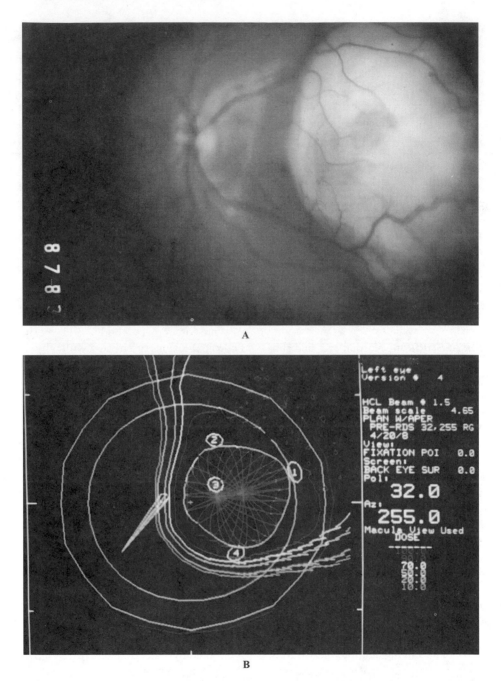

**A**

**B**

**FIGURE 15-2** **(A)** Narrow-angle fundus photograph showing a large choroidal melanoma. The macula is seen as the dark spot immediately to the left of the midportion of the tumor. The optic disc and retinal vessels are also shown. **(B)** Tumor shown in **(A)**, modeled on the eye treatment planning program.[79] Optic disc shown as cone-shaped structure to the right, with the macula being at the end of the blue line just inside the tumor edge. Clips placed surgically to mark the tumor are shown. Clip 3 was not able to be placed at the posterior tumor edge due to the extreme posterior location of the tumor. Iso-dose curves are shown on the unfolded retina of the patient. Dose is prescribed to the 90% isodose line, which is placed 1.5 mm from the edge of the modeled tumor.[79] Macula (small purple cross) and tumor receive full dose, while the 50% isodose line passes through the center of the disk. **(C)** "Beam's eye view" of the proton beam on the anterior eye with patient in treat-

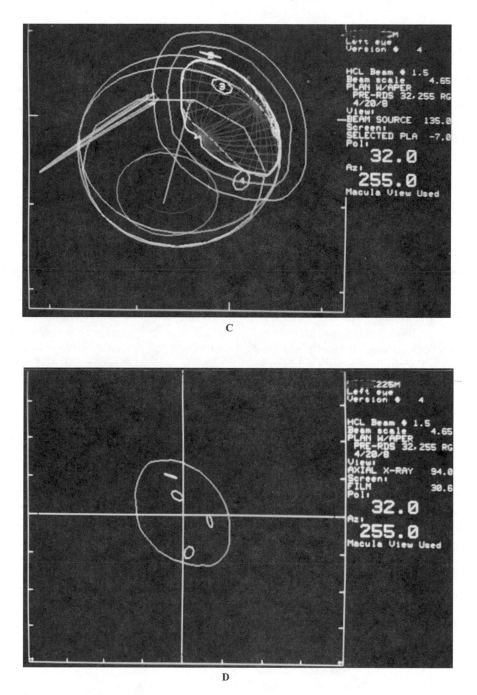

**C**

**D**

ment position. Eye is voluntarily fixated on an inferior and slightly medial point, as indicated by the projection of the optic axis (blue line) connecting the center of the lens with the macula. The 50% and 90% isodose lines are shown in yellow and red, respectively, as outlined by the aperture. A field light projected through the treatment aperture onto the eye would outline the 50% yellow isodose line and allow verification of patient setup after radiographic alignment had been achieved. **(D)** Schematic of the desired position of the tumor-marking clips relative to the central axis of the beam and the aperture edge. A transparency of this schematic with the same magnification as a portal x-ray can be directly superimposed on the portal x-ray, to verify proper position of the eye during treatment setup. Figures also appear in Color Figure section.

females, they are much less common than cutaneous melanoma and infrequently occur in blacks. Historically, eyes thought to contain melanoma were enucleated. Diagnostic accuracy of current noninvasive techniques is so high that treatment decisions can routinely be based on clinical evaluation only. In a multi-institutional study, 413 eyes with a clinical diagnosis of choroidal melanoma, established by indirect ophthalmoscopy, fundus photography, fluorescein angiography, and ultrasonography, were enucleated. The diagnosis was correct on histological examination of 411 patients (99.5%). The other two patients, respectively, had a hemangioma and a magnocellular nevus (melanocytoma).[82]

Through September 1998, 2568 uveal melanoma patients were treated at HCL. The standard dose currently is 70 CGE delivered in five fractions over 7 to 9 days. Approximately half the patients are females. When HCL patients are classified according to the Collaborative Ocular Melanoma Study (COMS) size categories,[82] approximately 20% are found to have small tumors, 50% medium tumors, and 30% large tumors.

*Acute Reaction*   Acute reaction is limited to moist eyelid desquamation, seen in patients whose eyelid cannot be completely retracted from the irradiation field. This typically involves a relatively small lid segment (2–5 mm × 8–15 mm). Although this condition heals in 2 to 4 weeks, there is usually permanent eyelash loss with late atrophy and scarring in the desquamated area.

*Local Control*   Local control of the tumor within the treated eye was 96.3 ±1.5% and 95.4 ± 3.3% at 60 and 84 months, with 236 and 82 patients available for follow-up at those intervals, respectively. Two failures occurred after 48 months. Two tumors recurred in the full dose (70 CGE) region, while 10 were at the margin of the previously irradiated volume.[83] These remarkably high local control rates can be attributed to the large dose per fraction and high total dose delivered, the accuracy of the tumor localization and treatment techniques employed, and the relatively small tumor size, relative to the average size of tumors usually treated in clinical radiation oncology.

*Survival*   At 5 years, survival is approximately 80%.[84,85] Proton-treated patients survive at least as well as patients treated primarily with enucleation. A survival comparison was carried out between 556 proton-treated patients and two groups treated with enucleation: 238 patients enucleated during the same 10-year period in which the irradiations took place (July 1975 to December 1984) and 275 enucleated during the preceding decade (January 1965 to June 1975). With median follow-up for the three patient groups of 5.3, 8.8, and 17.0 years, respectively, estimated Kaplan–Meier survival rates at 5 years were 81 ±2%, 68 ± 3%, and 74 ± 3% and at 10 years 63 ± 5%, 53 ±4%, and 50 ±3%, respectively, for irradiated patients, patients enucleated in the later period, and those enucleated in the earlier period respectively.[86,87]

Patients were classified in each treatment group by means of risk factors known to have prognostic significance in both irradiated[84] and enucleated[88] patients. Lower risk patients were those with relatively small posterior tumors and were younger; higher risk patients were older and had larger tumors involving the ciliary body, while intermediate risk patients had tumors extending anterior to the equator, but not involving the ciliary body, and were intermediate in both tumor size and age. In all three risk categories, estimated survival probabilities were better for proton-treated patients than for either of the enucleated groups. Treatment choice appeared to have little overall influence on survival in these uveal melanoma patients.[86]

Patients requiring enucleation for local tumor recurrence did appear to have decreased survival relative to those whose eyes were removed because of radiation complications. Survival in the latter group did not differ from that of patients treated with radiation alone. One hundred thirty-seven of 1541 patients (median follow-up, 8 years) were enucleated for complications (103) or tumor progression (34). Patients enucleated for tumor growth were almost four times as likely to die of metastasis than those losing the eye because of complications (rate ratios 3.8 vs. 0.9, 95% confidence limits 2.3–6.3 and 06.–1.4, respectively). Probability of eye retention at 10 years was 89 ±2%.[89]

Patients with cutaneous melanoma at high risk for recurrence who were randomized to receive interferon$\alpha$-2b (IFN) had significantly greater median survival and median relapse-free survival than those randomized to observation only.[90] Because of the increased risk of metastatic death in high risk uveal melanoma patients, those with one or more risk factors (tumor $\geq$ 15 mm diameter, ciliary body involvement, and age $>$ 65) are currently offered IFN treatment in a nonrandomized clinical trial. Metastatic and survival rates in the IFN-treated patients will be compared to a historical control group of patients matched for known prognostic factors who were treated with protons only. Through September, 1998, 109 patients had started treatment with IFN following standard dose proton beam radiotherapy.

*Eye Retention Probability*    This depends on tumor size, being 97%, 93%, and 78% for patients with small, intermediate, and large tumors, respectively. Significantly greater enucleation rates were observed in patients with large tumors (tumor height $>$ 8 mm, tumor diameter $>$ 16 mm) and with tumor involvement of the ciliary body ($p = <0.0001$ for all comparisons). Independent risk factors associated with greater likelihood of eye loss were identified by multivariate analysis as involvement of the ciliary body, tumor height exceeding 8 mm, and distance between the posterior tumor edge and the fovea. The high risk group (208 patients) had two or more risk factors, the moderate risk group (569 patients) had only one, while the low risk group (213 patients) had no risk factor. Eye retention rates at 5 years were 99 ±1% and 92 ± 2% for the low and intermediate risk groups, respectively. Even the patients in the highest risk group had

a 76 ±7% probability of retaining the irradiated eye 5 years after treatment.[91] Pathological changes in eyes enucleated after proton beam treatment have been described.[92–95]

*Late Complications*    These may involve anterior or posterior ocular structures, or both. **Radiation injuries to anterior structures** include rubeosis iridis with neovascular glaucoma and cataract formation, both of which have some potential for visual preservation or restoration with successful treatment.[75,96] Lens changes after proton beam therapy have been studied. In 388 patients with clear lenses initially, posterior subcapsular opacities (PSC) developed in 42% of patients within 3 years of treatment. Probability of PSC formation was related to lens dose, tumor height, and older age.[97] Lens opacities were present in 494 of the 1171 patients (42%) treated through December 1987. Eighty-four of the patients with opacities underwent cataract extraction between 2 months and 11 years after treatment. Visual acuity one year after surgery was 20/100 or better in approximately half the patients, and 20/40 or better in approximately one-third of patients. Larger tumor size was highly correlated with poorer visual outcome after cataract extraction. Six of the patients were later enucleated, five because of painful blind eyes, and one because of a "ring melanoma" diagnosed after surgery.[96]

*Late Radiation Injury to Posterior Ocular Structures*    In contrast to injuries to anterior structure, posterior ocular structures are largely untreatable if late radiation injury is sustained. Radiation-induced macular edema, maculopathy, papillopathy, and optic atrophy can be associated with significant loss of visual function. Although visual acuity after treatment is unchanged or better than initial acuity in more than 50% of treated eyes, visual morbidity is greater in eyes with larger and with more posteriorly placed tumors. Posttreatment visual prognosis is significantly associated with tumor height, distance of the posterior tumor margin from the optic dose and/or fovea, pretreatment retinal detachment involving the macula, initial visual acuity, and radiation dose to disc, fovea, and lens.[98] Leading causes of visual loss in patients with useful vision (visual acuity 20/200 or better) before treatment were retinal detachment, cataract, and radiation retinopathy. Useful vision was preserved at 36 months in 67% of 199 patients with tumor edge more than 3 mm from both the optic disc and the fovea, and in 39% of 363 patients with tumor edge 3 mm or less from either structure. The disc and/or fovea received a high dose (> 35 CGE) in only 9% of the former, and in 83% of the latter group.[99]

Because of the visual morbidity associated with treatment of posteriorly located tumors, a **randomized dose de-escalation trial** was conducted between October 1989 and July 1994 in patients with small and medium melanomas involving the posterior pole of the eye. These patients were randomized to receive either the standard dose (70 CGE) or the experimental dose (50 CGE) in five fractions over 7 to 9 days. Study subjects had eyes with tumors 5 mm or less high and 15 mm or less in diameter located within 6 mm of the optic disc and/or fovea, known to be at high risk of developing significant visual morbidity with the standard dose of 70 CGE in five fractions. Because of the relatively small size and posterior location of the tumors, these patients had a relatively low risk of developing metastatic disease or of losing the eye because of radiation complications. These prognostically favorable characteristics would predict that the treated eye in most patients would be available for follow-up. End points for the trial were visual loss, retinopathy, and local control. An interim report on this trial was scheduled for 1999.

Equally encouraging results have been seen in patients treated at Lawrence Berkeley Laboratory with helium ions[69,73,100] and in patients treated with protons at PSI.[72] Patients with melanomas less than 10 mm in height and less than 15 mm in diameter were randomized by the LBL-UCSF group to receive either 70 Gy in five treatments with helium ions, or 70 Gy to the tumor apex with [125]I plaque brachytherapy.

In the initial report of this trial, significantly higher local failure and enucleation rates were observed in plaque-treated patients, but anterior segment complications were more common in particle-treated patients.[101]

***Retinoblastoma*** The dose localization properties of protons are also most attractive for the treatment of retinoblastomas. Patients with the hereditary form of that disease are at high risk of developing a second primary malignancy.[102,103] Proton techniques should lead to a reduced incidence of radiation-induced tumors in these patients because the volume of normal tissue irradiated is significantly reduced. These children are also likely to have abnormal facial bone growth, attributed to the treatment received in their infancy.[104] Reduction of the volume treated to a high dose may be associated with improved cosmesis because facial and orbital development in such children is more nearly normal.

The beam can be targeted to individual tumors, to the retina posterior to the equator, or to the entire retina with a single lateral portal. Regardless of the target size, anterior normal tissues and those across the midline, as well as the brain, hypothalamus, and pituitary gland receive no radiation, whereas some or all of those tissues usually receive some dose with whatever photon technique is employed.

The three-dimensional CT-based treatment planning system described above is used for these patients. They are immobilized, scanned for treatment planning, and treated under general anesthesia. Infants with previously untreated retinoblastoma have shown good acute tolerance and tumor regression following proton beam therapy with doses of 40 to 46 CGE in 20 to 23 fractions at 2 CGE per fraction.[105] Dose distributions for treatment of retinoblastoma with a single lateral proton beam are shown in Figure 15-3. The sheer elegance of the simple proton beam technique, in terms of limiting dose to bone, anterior ocular structures, and the contralateral eye, is readily apparent. Refinements to the beam line have decreased the lateral beam penumbra (80% to

20%) from 6 mm to 3 mm. A scanned proton beam could allow use of variable modulation, which would also reduce unnecessary dose in the entrance region, further improving the conformality of dose to the target.[106] Availability of a gantry in the new facility (New England Particle Tumor Clinic; NEPTC) which initiated treatment in 1999, also allows greater flexibility and treatment approaches to such patients.

***Angiomas, Hemangiomas, and Metastatic Tumors*** Planning and treatment techniques similar to those used for ocular melanomas have been employed for patients with angiomas, hemangiomas, and metastatic intraocular tumors. A light field technique is appropriate for most patients in this category. The treatment plan is prepared from fundus photographs, tumor sketches, and ultrasound, which can be obtained at the first clinic visit. A treatment aperture is fabricated, and the first of the scheduled treatments can be given at the initial visit to the particle facility. Doses have been 25 to 35 CGE in four to five fractions for the blood vessel tumors. This treatment is also effective, appropriate, and efficient for the palliation of ocular symptoms in patients with choroidal metastasis, who receive 28 CGE in two fractions. Conventional palliative treatment might require at least 11 patient visits (one for initial evaluation and for 10 treatments). The importance of such economical use of the time, energy, and resources of patients and their families should not be minimized.

***Age-Related Macular Degeneration*** Age-related macular degeneration is the leading cause of severe visual morbidity in the United States, afflicting over 750,000 older Americans.[107] Although significant loss of central vision can occur in the "dry" variety, more severe visual loss accompanies the "wet" or exudative form, in which a choroidal neovascular membrane develops in the subfoveal area. Such membranes are effectively treated with laser photocoagulation, but such treatment in the macular region causes immediate and permanent central vision loss. The rationale for the use of radiotherapy in treating these choroidal neovascular membranes was reviewed in 1998; both fractionated x-rays and single-fraction x-rays or protons have shown some benefit in treating the exudative variety.[108]

A two-fraction dose-searching protocol was initiated in September 1995 in patients with subfoveal neovascular membranes, most of whom have had age-related exudative macular degeneration (AMD), although patients with the same pathological process due to myopic degeneration, fungus infection, choroiditis, and pseudoxanthoma elasticum have also been included. Patients meeting study criteria are randomized to receive either 16 or 24 CGE in two treatments, usually given on consecutive days. A light field setup is used, similar to that described above for patients with blood vessel tumors and choroidal metastasis. Accrual of the planned 200 patients was to have been achieved in late 1998. Initial results have been encouraging, but full assessment of the treatment's benefit must await longer follow-up of treated patients. The same economical use of both time and resources discussed above for patients with choroidal metastasis applies equally to these patients, who also require only three visits for both initial evaluation and treatment.

## Summary: Indications for Particle Therapy of Ocular Tumors

Uveal melanomas and other ocular neoplasms can be efficiently and successfully treated conservatively with proton beam techniques. Uveal melanoma patients have good expectations for visual preservation and eye retention. Even very large tumors can be treated if vision is poor or absent in the fellow eye. Although the expectation for visual preservation in such cases is low, approximately 80% of such eyes can be salvaged with some degree of visual function. Survival clearly has not been compromised, local control is achieved in almost all treated eyes, and useful vision is preserved in the majority of patients.

Successfully treating uveal melanoma without removal of the involved eye is one of the

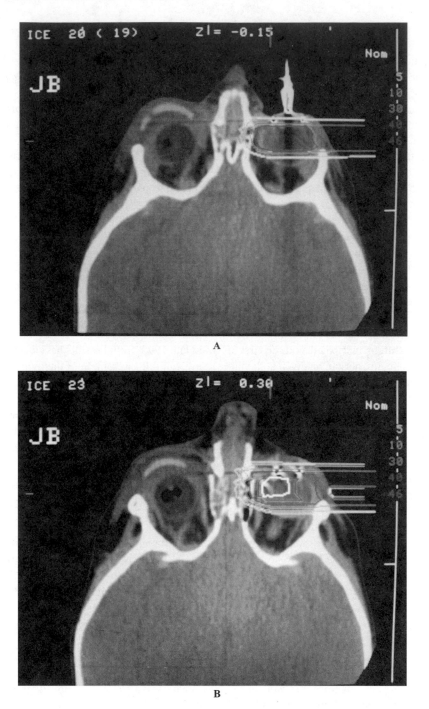

**FIGURE 15-3** **(A)** Dose distribution to a retinoblastoma patient with a single direct lateral proton portal. Scan section is 1.5 mm superior to top of lesion, with dose of 40 CGE delivered at this level. Note stem of suction cup used to fix eye in place for treatment, with artifact in central globe from metallic stem. Radiopaque circles anteriorly are cross sections of a circular wire embedded in the plastic contact lens, which adheres to the cornea by suction during the treatment. The wires in the contact lens define the anterior margin of the eye and are used for radiographic patient setup. Patient has prosthesis with anterior shell in right eye. Prescribed dose (46 CGE, green isodose line) is given to all the tumor defined on this slide. **(B)** Scan 3

major oncologic triumphs of the latter part of the twentieth century. Very high rates of local control can be achieved with either heavy charged particle external beam radiotherapy or radioisotope episcleral plaque brachytherapy, with preservation of a functionally useful eye in many patients. Conservative treatment with charged particle beams achieves local control rates similar or superior to those achieved with radiation therapy alone in other commonly treated solid tumors, including early stage carcinomas of the breast, vocal cord, and prostate. Excellent results in the eye melanoma patients

demonstrates also that almost all the patients can successfully cooperate in their treatment by voluntarily fixating the eye upon a particular point during treatment, so that their tumor is positioned properly in the beam during treatment. Continued careful follow-up of conservatively treated patients will be essential for obtaining better understanding of the effects of proton beam radiation therapy both on uveal melanomas and on normal ocular structures.

It is also impressive that these gains have not been achieved at a cost of increased mortality: survival rates in irradiated patients are at least

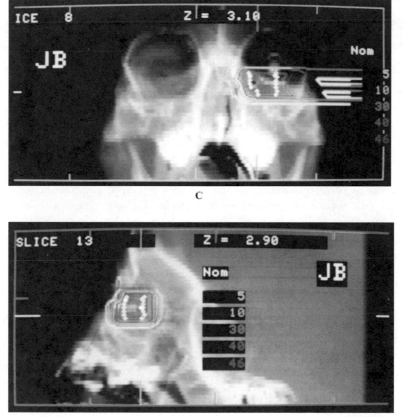

mm inferior to scan in (A), showing small punctate calcification in tumor medially, and outline of tumor in white. The prescribed dose of 46 CGE conforms to virtually all of the defined tumor on this slice. Entrance dose is 40 CGE or less. **(C)** Coronal reconstruction of the planning CT scan. Conformality of prescribed dose (46 CGE) to target is again noted. A small portion of the inferior left lateral orbit is included in the 40 CGE isodose line. **(D)** Sagittal reconstruction of the planning CT scan. Conformality of prescribed dose (46 CGE) to target is again noted, with the dose on this scan appearing to be concentrated solely in the globe. A small portion of the inferior left lateral orbit is included in the 40 CGE isodose line. Figures also appear in Color Figure section.

as good as those reported after enucleation.[86,87] Further observation will reveal whether these initial dramatic and encouraging results will be maintained. Ultimately, the COMS study may provide additional data in this regard, at least regarding survival after brachytherapy relative to enucleation.[82] However, it will not clarify indications for the two types of radiotherapy (brachytherapy and charge particle therapy), nor will it allow direct comparisons of acute and chronic ocular effects of those therapeutic modalities. The UCSF-LBL trial mentioned above, which compared helium ion therapy with [125]I episcleral plaque treatment,[101] has documented the superiority of charged particle therapy to plaque therapy in terms of local tumor control and eye retention.

The distant failures and metastatic deaths in uveal melanoma patients, most common in those with larger and more anteriorly located tumors, are most distressing. A randomized clinical trail of adjuvant systemic therapy is clearly indicated, but has not been mounted because the results obtained with systemic therapy in patients with metastatic melanoma have been relatively poor. The recent report of improved survival in cutaneous melanoma patients at high risk for metastasis who were treated with interferon is encouraging.[90] Our nonrandomized study described above, which administers interferon following proton eye irradiation, may also demonstrate some improvement in this regard.

Additional clinical experience and possibly clinical trials will be required to clarify the role of particle beam therapy relative to other conservative techniques in the treatment of other ocular tumors, such as retinoblastomas, vascular tumors, and metastatic lesions, and in patients with subfoveal neovascular membranes (age-related macular degeneration).

## Skull Base and Cervical Spine Chordomas and Chondrosarcomas

Skull base and cervical spine tumors are estimated to represent between 3% and 11% of primary bone tumors.[109] The skull base and its foramina are in close proximity to numerous vital normal tissues, including the brain stem, the inferior surfaces of the frontal, temporal, parietal, and occipital lobes of the brain and the cerebellum, as well as the cranial nerves and the cerebral blood vessels. Ninety-seven skull base patients (49 chordomas and 48 chondrosarcomas) presented predominantly with initial symptoms of headache and intermittent diplopia (67% and 49%, and 75% and 78%, respectively). Other presenting symptoms in those patients included decreased hearing or visual acuity, tinnitus, dysphagia, and dysarthria.[110]

Histologically, osteosarcoma and chondrosarcoma are the most common primary bone tumors. Osteosarcoma is seen relatively infrequently at the skull base, although it not uncommonly involves the maxilla or the mandible. Chordomas are rare tumors thought to originate in rests of the embryonal notochord and always involve the midline, with 35% to 40% occurring in the skull base.[111] Atypical and malignant meningiomas, and benign tumors such as pituitary adenomas, craniopharyngiomas, acoustic neuromas, and meningiomas, can also be seen in the skull base. Histological diagnosis of most skull base tumors is relatively straightforward, although the cartilaginous tumors can present a special challenge. Histology on 255 patients referred for proton beam therapy was reviewed at the Massachusetts General Hospital (MGH). Forty percent of patients referred with a diagnosis of chordoma were reclassified as having chondrosarcomas, leading to an almost equal proportion of each tumor type being included in the 125 chordomas and 130 chondrosarcomas studied.[112] Special immunohistochemical stains have proven helpful in the classification of these tumors.[113]

Invasive skull base tumors present a formidable management problem, regardless of presenting symptoms or histology. Total resection usually cannot be accomplished because of the involvement of adjacent critical normal structures (optic nerves and chiasm, cranial nerves, major blood vessels, and brain and brain stem).[114,115] The benign tumors listed above are usually treated to relatively lower doses (54–60 Gy), which can be delivered with relative safety using conventional supervoltage techniques. Radiation modalities and techniques that can best localize the dose delivered to the defined target are especially attractive for epithelial and sarcomatous tumors, which require much higher doses (68–76 Gy) to achieve local control.

Fractionated particle beam therapy has been shown to offer a significant advantage for patients with cartilaginous tumors of the skull base.[116,117] The maximum penetration of the Harvard cyclotron's fixed horizontal 160 MeV proton beam of 16.0 cm is particularly well suited for skull base tumors, regardless of histology. Techniques developed for treating patients with chordomas and low grade chondrosarcomas of the skull base and cervical spine, results of that treatment, and current protocols in that patient population are discussed in the subsections that follow.

**Population and Treatment** Four hundred thirty-three patients with chordomas and chondrosarcomas of the skull base, and **95** with cervical spine tumors were treated between 1975 and May 31, 1997. In the **skull base category,** 218 males and 215 females ranged in age from 1.3 to 80 years (mean 39 years). Two hundred fifty-one (58%) had chordoma, and 182 (42%) had chondrosarcoma. All were ambulatory, none had been irradiated or known to have metastasis. Estimated tumor volume at initiation of treatment ranged from 3.3 to 318 mL, with a median volume of 40 mL for skull base and 70 mL for cervical spine tumors.

Diagnosis is confirmed for all patients by a single pathologist. Patients not having primary surgery at MGH are assessed to determine whether additional surgery might facilitate treatment, in terms not only of reducing tumor bulk but also of improving tumor–normal tissue geometry to allow better treatment of residual disease and to limit dose to adjacent normal tissues. Endocrine, auditory, and ophthalmological status are formally assessed prior to initiation of treatment. Children younger than 4 years of age are generally treated under general anesthesia. Almost all patients received some portion of the treatment with high energy (4 or 10 MV) x-rays, to allow patients to be treated five times per week. Prescribed doses have ranged from 56.8 to 80 CGE, delivered in most patients at 1.8 CGE per fraction, with five fractions per week. Figure 15-4 shows radiological images and dose–volume histograms for a young patient with low grade chondrosarcoma of the clivus.

### Local Control and Survival

SKULL BASE  Local control has been defined as neurological improvement or stability, and absence of demonstrable enlargement of treated tumor on follow-up imaging studies; imaging studies performed after treatment are almost always abnormal, reflecting surgical changes or the persistence of an unregressed and/or calcified tumor mass.[118] With median follow-up of approximately 5 years, local control was significantly better for chondrosarcoma patients (165) than for chordoma patients (169): 97% versus 64% at 5 years, respectively, as shown in Figure 15-5 (Liebsch et al., unpublished data).

No gender difference in outcome was seen in chondrosarcoma patients, while males with skull base chordomas were surprisingly found to have significantly better local control and survival than females with that histology. In 132 adult chordoma patients with median follow-up of 46 months (range 2–158 months), local control for males was estimated to be 77 ±11%, versus 40 ±13% for females at 5 years ($p = 0.0003$). In non–chondroid chordoma patients, **survival** was also strongly gender dependent, being 84 ±9% and 75 ±12%, versus 82 ±9% and 17 ±15% for females at 5 and 8 years, respectively ($p = 0.008$).[119] Possible explanations for the influence of gender on treatment outcome have were reviewed in 1995.[120]

CERVICAL SPINE  **Local control** has been less good in patients with cervical spine tumors than in those with skull base tumors (62 ±16%

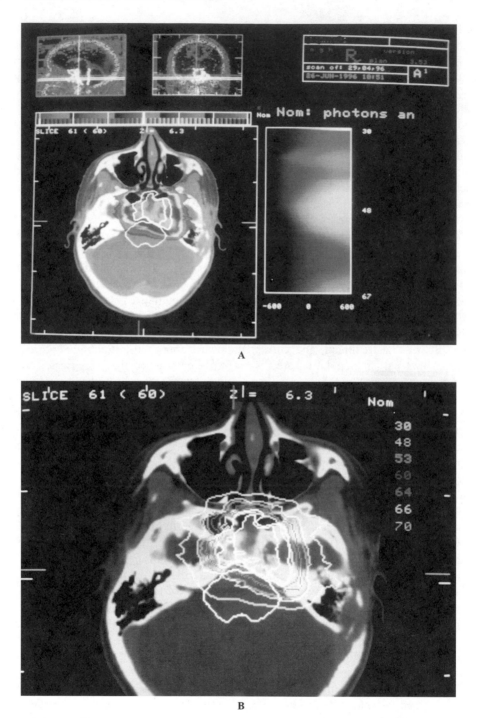

**FIGURE 15-4**   **(A)** Contours shown in white outline the smaller and the larger clinical target volumes (CTVs) defined on this CT image of the planning scan of a 13-year-old girl with a low grade chondrosarcoma of the clivus. The smaller volume is gross residual tumor seen on imaging studies, and the larger contour represents target enlargement to allow for uncertainty in target definition on planning scan, and for microscopic extension. Area shown in magenta received the prescribed dose of 66.6 CGE. Note sparing of the right internal auditory canal, the right cochlea, and the right acoustic

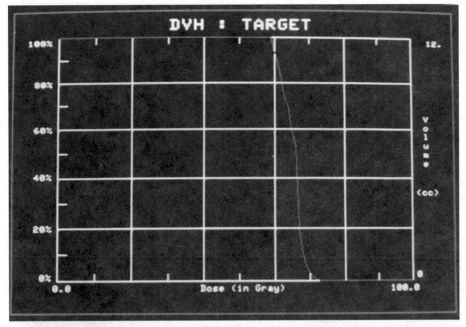

C

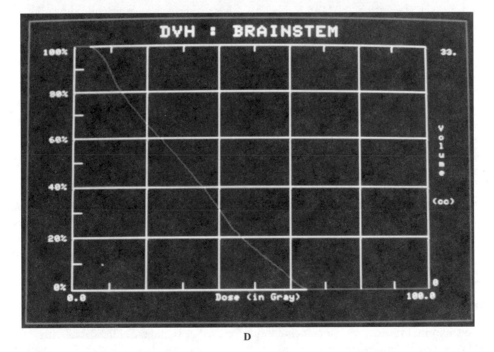

D

nerve, each of which receives less than 30 CGE. **(B)** Same scan as in **(A)**, showing isodose lines instead of color-wash display. **(C)** Dose–volume histogram (DVH) for primary target (gross residual tumor) of patient shown in **(A)** and **(B)**. Volume of outlined structure is given as 12 cc. Minimum dose of approximately 59 CGE reflects constraints applied in treatment planning for tumor abutment to optic nerves and chiasm, and to the brain stem. Approximately 90% of the target receives 60 CGE. **(D)** Dose–volume histogram (DVH) for brain stem shown in Figures 15-2A and 15-2B. Mean dose is less than 30 CGE, while maximum dose is approximately 64 CGE, the constraint dose defined for the brain stem in this patient. Figures also appear in Color Figure section.

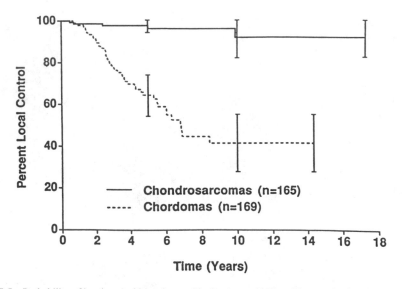

**FIGURE 15-5** Probability of local control in patients with chordomas (169) and low-grade chondrosarcomas (165) of the skull base.

vs. 76 ± 6%) at 5 years, $p = 0.0444$). Neither a gender difference nor one related to tumor histology was found. **Survival** is also better for skull base tumor patients than for those with cervical spine tumors.

*Recurrence Sites, Failure Patterns, and Outcome After Relapse* Imaging studies were available for analysis of **recurrence sites** in 26 patients. More than half the failures (15 of 26) occurred in a dose gradient region, which was the result of the normal tissue constraints imposed in developing the treatment plan because of target proximity to the brain stem and/or optic nerves and chiasm. Approximately one-quarter of the recurrences (6 of 26) were judged to have occurred in regions of the tumor that received the prescribed dose (67–72 CGE, mean 69 CGE). Tumor regrowth adjacent to but outside the initially defined target volume (marginal failure) was documented in three patients, and surgical pathway failure attributable to tumor seeding at surgery, but away from the initial tumor volume, was observed in two patients.[61]

**Failure patterns and outcome after relapse** were studied in 204 patients with skull base and cervical spine chordomas. There were identified 45 relapses in skull base and 18 in cervical spine patients. The predominant failure pattern was local tumor regrowth, seen in 60 (95%) patients. Local failure only occurred in 49 patients (78%). Three patients had "seeding" into the operative bed, and two had nodal relapse. Thirteen patients, 20% of the total, developed metastasis, with lung and bone being the most common distant sites (in 7 and 6 cases, respectively). Postrelapse survival was 43% and 7% at 3 and 5 years, respectively. Salvage treatment, given to 49 patients, included subtotal tumor resection in 44, total resection in 2, and chemotherapy, radiation, and combined chemotherapy and radiation in one patient each. The majority of patients receiving salvage therapy (26 of 49, 53%) had initial improvement but later deteriorated. Progressive neurologic deterioration despite treatment occurred in 16 patients (33%), and only 7 patients (14%) remained stable or improved neurologically during the observation period after salvage therapy. Some patients may have benefited from postrelapse treatment, since their survival at 2 and 5 years was 63% and 6%, respectively, versus 21% at 2 years for patients receiving supportive therapy only, as shown in Figure 15-6.[120]

*Treatment-Related Toxicity*  Relatively few significant complications have been observed, considering the high doses delivered, and the proximity of these tumors to dose-limiting normal structures. Observed morbidity that could be attributed to the treatment included functional and anatomical abnormalities in the brain, brain stem, and cervical spine, as well as deficits of neuropsychiatric, visual, auditory, and endocrine function.

BRAIN STEM TOXICITY  This condition was evaluated in 367 skull base tumor patients treated between 1974 and 1995. Prescribed doses ranged from 63.0 to 79.2 CGE (mean 67.8 CGE), with dose to the surface and the center of the brain stem being constrained to $\leq 64$ and $\leq 53$ CGE, respectively. These constraints resulted in a dose gradient in most tumors at the brain stem–tumor interface, which ranged from the constraint dose (53–64 CGE) to the prescribed dose. Follow-up ranged from 6 months to 21.4 years (mean 42.5 months) in the 195 chordoma

and 172 chondrosarcoma patients studied. In patients without local failure, 6% (17 of 282) developed signs and symptoms of brain stem injury, which led to death in three patients. Probability of surviving free of significant brain stem toxicity was 92% and 87% at 5 and 10 years after treatment, respectively. Three factors were significant predictors of brain stem injury by multivariate analysis: number of prior surgical procedures ($p < 0.001$), volume of brain stem receiving more than 60 CGE ($p < 0.007$), and the presence of diabetes ($p < 0.05$). Brain stem tolerance in these patients was a steep function of the volume of brain stem included in the high dose region, rather than of maximum brain stem dose.[121]

CERVICAL SPINAL CORD TOXICITY  This condition was evaluated in 78 patients with cervical spine chordomas (66) and chondrosarcomas (12) treated through March 1996. Prescribed doses ranged from 64.5 to 79.2 CGE, and treatment plans were developed with dose constraints to the surface and the center of the spinal cord of $\leq 64$ and $\leq 53$ CGE, respectively. These constraints resulted in a dose gradient in most

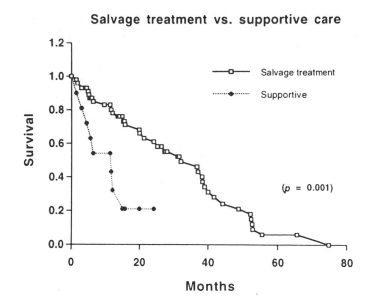

**FIGURE 15-6**  Probability of survival after relapse in skull base and cervical spine chordoma patients who received salvage therapy (49 patients) or supportive case only (14 patients).[120]

tumors at the cord–tumor interface, which ranged from the constraint dose to the pre-scribed dose. Follow-up ranged from 3 to 157 months (mean 46.4 months): more than 80% of patients had follow-up of 12 months or more. Eleven patients developed radiographic signs and/or clinical symptoms that were attributed to radiation effects on the spinal cord: six pa-tients with Lhermitt syndrome, four with imag-ing changes, three with sensory deficits only, and one with motor deficits.

The single patient who developed motor weakness was the only one not treated with the constraints described above. That patient had received 9 Gy in three fractions elsewhere be-cause of an initial diagnosis of lymphoma. Af-ter pathology review returned a diagnosis of chordoma, which was confirmed at MGH, the patient underwent partial tumor resection and spinal cord decompressions, followed by frac-tionated proton–photon therapy in the usual fashion. Total dose was 70.2 CGE, including the initial 9 Gy given prior to referral to MGH. In that patient, spinal cord dose (62 CGE and 69 CGE to the cord surface and center, respec-tively) exceeded the usual cord tolerance levels of 53 and 64 CGE, respectively. Experi-ence in these 78 patients strongly affirms the safety of the techniques and doses employed, since significant myelopathy occurred in only 3.9% of patients receiving very high doses to tumors abutting or compressing the cervical spinal cord.[122]

TEMPORAL LOBE DAMAGE   Normal brain, espe-cially the inferior and medial portions of the temporal lobes, may receive doses approach-ing those prescribed for these skull base tu-mors. **Temporal lobe damage** was identified in 10 of 96 chordoma patients. One had only asymptomatic imaging changes, but the other nine had both clinical symptoms and imaging abnormalities. Eight of the injuries were mod-erate to severe. Temporal lobe dose was not constrained because of tumor proximity to that structure, although the constraints de-scribed above were applied for the brain stem, and if appropriate, the optic nerves and chi-asm. Doses prescribed for the injured patients were 66.6 and 72 CGE in four and six pa-tients, respectively; doses prescribed for the total population ranged from 64.8 to 72 CGE (median 68.4 CGE). Conservative treatment with corticosteroids and/or anticonvulsive medication was employed initially, but three patients with persistent or progressive imag-ing changes and clinical deterioration under-went temporal lobe resection. Radiation necrosis was documented pathologically in all three patients. Seven patients improved neu-rologically following medical or surgical treatment. Two patients had significant and persistent neurological deficit, and one patient whose neurological deficit remained stable later died of locally recurrent tumor. The **probability of temporal lobe injury** was 8% and 13% at 2 and 5 years, respectively. Multi-ple tumor or host-related characteristics were evaluated, but only male gender proved to be a significant predictor of injury by both univari-ate and stepwise Cox regression analysis.[123]

NEUROPSYCHOLOGICAL EFFECTS   A battery of standard psychological tests designed to exam-ine specific cognitive functions was adminis-tered to 38 patients prior to and at specified intervals after treatment. Brain adjacent to the tumor volume received the prescribed dose, which ranged from 66.6 to 72 CGE (median 68.4 CGE). Seventeen patients were restudied 48 or more months after treatment. Cognitive function was not adversely affected. Tests of verbal and nonverbal learning and memory, si-multaneous attention and concentration, and language and visuospatial processing either were stable or showed slight improvement over time, although these results could have been due to repetition of the tests. Statistically sig-nificant psychomotor slowing of reaction time and motor speed was shown for the group as a whole. Self-reported assessments documented progressive improvement in anxiety, depres-sion, and self-perceived cognitive efficiency, while fatigue levels remained stable over the course of observation. Following treatment, pa-tients appeared to either stabilize or improve from an emotional standpoint, and to develop some degree of motor slowing.[124]

Treatment techniques have been modified, to try to decrease the frequency of brain injury. In addition to direct lateral portals, a greater number and variety of beam directions are being employed, including simple and compound angles of posterior, oblique, or superior portals. A minimum of two portals are usually treated each day, to decrease the daily dose increment delivered to nontarget tissues in the entrance region. Additional decreases in dose to nontarget brain in the entrance region would be possible with scanned proton beams.[106]

VISION   It is routine to monitor the vision of patients who have been treated for tumors involving the upper clivus that approach, abut, or displace the optic nerves and/or chiasm.[125] Visual function was studied in 274 patients who received 40 CGE or more to the optic structures. Doses to optic structures were constrained in treatment planning as described above, with prescribed tumor doses ranging from 61 to 76 CGE. With minimum follow-up of 12 months, 12 patients developed optic neuropathy (4.4%). One had unilateral hemianopsia only, while nine and two patients developed unilateral and bilateral blindness, respectively. Median time to injury was 12 months (range 7–40 months). Maximum dose to the optic structures in injured patients ranged from 50.21 to 69.6 CGE (median 59.43 CGE).

Comparisons were made between dose distributions and dose–volume histograms of the 12 patients with neuropathy, and a matched control group of 24 patients without toxicity. Various parameters were examined for prognostic value, including minimum, mean, and maximum dose to optic structures; the volume receiving 50, 55, and 60 CGE; the presence or absence of diabetes and/or hypertension; the number of surgical procedures; and use of a "patching technique" in which a portion of the target volume is treated with one portal, and the rest with another portal, to contour the dose around a critical structure, such as the brain stem. With that technique, a small "hot spot"

occurs, in which one field "ranges out" (stops) in the tissue (target) that is receiving full dose from the other portal. Use of the "patching" technique was the only parameter found to significantly be related to the development of optic neuropathy.[126] Treatment plans incorporating the patch technique are now carefully scrutinized prior to implementation, to assure that "hot spots" will not occur in or near the optic structures.

HEARING   A study of the relationship between audiological outcome and dose to auditory pathways assessed hearing in 33 patients. Patients studied had a normal baseline audiogram, received at least 15 CGE to the auditory structures, were free of recurrent tumor near those structures, and had had follow-up audiogram. Audiographic documentation of significant hearing loss was obtained in 15 patients: at 2 years in three, 3 years in one, at 4 years in ten, and at 5 years in one. Almost two-thirds of patients receiving 60 CGE or more to either cochlea or auditory nerve manifested significant loss, while no loss was observed in patients receiving 59 CGE or less to those structures. Progression to severe hearing loss was usually quite rapid after onset.[127] Doses to the eighth nerve and cochlea are currently constrained to 60 CGE or less on at least one functional side, unless the target–normal tissue configuration is such that tumor coverage would be compromised by adopting that constraint.

CRANIAL NEUROPATHY   This condition was documented in 15 of 27 patients studied following high dose irradiation given for chordomas (14), chondrosarcomas (11), an acoustic neuroma, and a meningioma. The cranial nerve dysfunction that developed following treatment in those 15 patients could not be attributed to tumor progression. Dose delivered to the nerve predicted the likelihood of injury, which rose from an estimated probability of 1% at 60 CGE (0.5–3%, 95% CL) to 5% at 70 CGE (64–81 CGE, 95% CL). The dose–response curve slope at 50% was 3.2 (2.2–5.4, 95% CL). Dose delivered to the nerve or its nucleus had no significant relation to the latency period for appearance of nerve dysfunction.[60] Doses to brain stem, optic nerves and chiasm, and auditory nerves and cochlea are constrained as noted above; dose constraints are not employed for the other cranial nerves.

ENDOCRINOPATHY   Since the pituitary gland receives the same dose as the tumor in centrally placed upper clival lesions, endocrinopathy may follow treatment to skull base tumors.[128] Relatively lower pituitary doses would generally be received by patients with lower clival tumors and chondrosarcoma patients with tumors arising in the temporal bone. Endocrine function before and after treatment has also been evaluated in 79 skull base sarcoma patients who received 40 CGE or more to the pituitary gland. Prescribed doses to those patients ranged from 48.6 to 75.6 CGE (median 68.4 CGE). Thirty-two patients (40%) developed endocrinopathy after treatment. Deficiencies in luteinizing hormone, prolactin, and thyroid-stimulating hormone and cortisone were detected in between 12 and 18 patients (15–23%) (Renard et al., unpublished data).

The latent period for endocrinopathy has been long, with deficiencies developing as late as **8 to 10 years** after treatment. Patients whose hypothalamic–pituitary axis has received 40 CGE or more must undergo lifelong endocrine surveillance, since undiagnosed and untreated hormone deficiencies can be disabling and even fatal. Although injections are necessary for testosterone replacement, most hormonal deficiencies are readily treated with oral replacement therapy. Fertility in males appears to be less severely impaired than in females. Although secondary amenorrhea is not uncommon, at least two such women have delivered healthy full-term infants following pituitary stimulation; three others also spontaneously conceived and had equally happy outcomes, carrying those pregnancies to term.

*Clinical Trial: PROG 85-26*   MGH-HCL and Lawrence Berkeley Laboratory (LBL) collaborated to initiate a randomized prospective clinical trial in 1985, supported by the NCI through the Radiation Therapy Oncology Group (RTOG). End points for the study were local tumor control and normal tissue effects, with patients randomly assigned to receive doses of either 66.6 or 72 CGE, given with protons and x-rays at MGH-HCL and with helium ions at LBL. However, as the study progressed it became apparent there were two separate groups in this population, in terms of the risk of both local failure and survival. **Lower risk** patients (male skull base chordomas and all skull base chondrosarcomas) had a significantly better treatment outcome than did **higher risk** patients (female skull base chordomas and all cervical spine patients), as shown in Figure 15-7.

The initial protocol was modified in May 1993 in recognition of these differences. Lower risk patients continued to be randomized between the original dose levels (66.6 vs. 72 CGE), using the original normal tissue dose constraints, while higher risk patients (female skull base chordomas and cervical spine tumors of either sex or histology) were randomized between 72 and 79 CGE. Normal tissue dose constraints were increased by 5% for patients randomized to the 79.2 CGE arm. Three hundred twenty-eight patients had been randomized through September 1998: 271 at MGH-HCL, 24 at UCSF-LBL (prior to discontinuation of that program in 1992), and 33 at Loma Linda University Medical Center. An interim report on the initial phase of the study, dealing with patients randomized before May 1993, is being prepared, as is a preliminary report on patients randomized since May 1993.

## Discussion and Summary

Most patients treated with conventional radiotherapy after surgery die with locally progressive disease.[129] The **local recurrence-free survival** achieved with the techniques described by Catton et al.[129] are markedly superior to results described in the literature. The improved results described can be attributed to the higher doses delivered, because of the

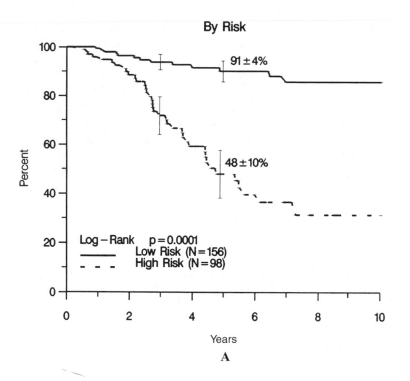

A

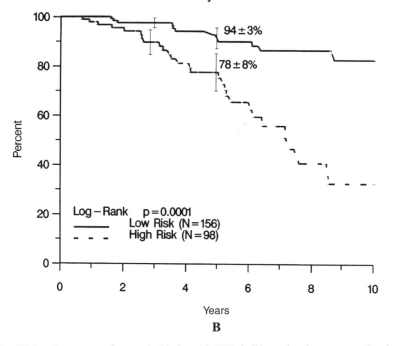

B

**FIGURE 15-7** **(A)** Local recurrence-free survival in low risk (156 skull base chondrosarcoma and male chordoma) and high risk (98 cervical spine and female chordoma) patients. **(B)** Overall survival in same set of low risk and high risk patients.

improved dose-localization characteristics of the proton beam, and the computerized three-dimensional treatment planning employed. Similar encouraging results have been reported from LBL.[117]

**Complications** observed have been acceptable, given the major morbidity and invariably fatal outcome associated with uncontrolled tumor growth in such patients. The neurological, visual, endocrine, and auditory problems detailed above can appear at any time after treatment, mandating the indefinite continuation of initial multidisciplinary surveillance of treated patients by clinicians experienced in those areas, so that tumor recurrence, extension, or metastasis, as well as treatable complications, can be identified promptly and managed by the initiation of appropriate treatment.

In summary, high dose radiation therapy such as can be delivered by means of three-dimensional planned proton–photon techniques following appropriate surgical management appears to represent the best management policy currently available for patients with chordomas and low grade chondrosarcomas of the skull base and cervical spine. Such treatment is potentially hazardous, expensive, time-consuming, and demanding for patients, their families, and those involved in their care. Nonetheless, such therapy does appear to offer significantly improved outcome over that to be expected with conventional supervoltage x-ray techniques. The role of stereotactic radiosurgery or intensity-modulated conformal x-ray therapy remains to be assessed in these patients.

## Other Tumors

*Prostate Cancer*   These patients have received three-dimensional conformal radiation therapy at HCL through a perineal portal, in combination with whole pelvic photon irradiation given at MGH. Initial results of a single-institution phase I/II trial were encouraging. In 66 patients doses ranged up to 75 CGE, 10% to 20% greater than those then being given with conventional supervoltage x-ray techniques. Rectal and bladder morbidity appeared to be similar to that expected after conventional supervoltage x-ray treatment.[130,131]

In 1981 a phase III randomized dose-searching clinical trial based on that experience was initiated. The trial closed in June 1992, having enrolled 203 patients with T3-4 Nx-0 M0 disease. All patients initially received 50.4 Gy in 1.8 Gy fractions with x-rays to the pelvis, and were randomly assigned to receive either a perineal proton boost to a total of 75.6 CGE, or an x-ray boost through opposed lateral portals to a total of 67.4 Gy, a 12.5% dose increase for the proton boost arm. The boost was given at 2.1 CGE or Gy, delivered 4 days per week. A 7- to 14-day break between completion of the photon treatment and initiation of the boost was allowed by the protocol. This break had been found necessary in the pilot study to allow the rectal reaction from the photon treatment to subside so that patients could tolerate the probe used both for alignment and to position in the rectum a balloon which, when inflated, would displace the posterior rectal wall away from the beam.[130]

With median follow-up of 61 months (range 3–139 months), **local control** was significantly better for proton-boosted patients with poorly differentiated tumors (94% and 84% vs. 64% and 19% for x-ray-boosted patients at 5 and 8 years, respectively, $p = 0.0014$). Local control was also higher in patients completing the trial and randomized to the proton boost, but the difference did not achieve statistical significance (92% and 77% for the 93 proton-boosted patients and 80% and 60% for 96 x-ray-boosted patients at 5 and 8 years, respectively, $p = 0.089$).[72]

**Overall survival** was not improved, perhaps reflecting the relatively advanced stage of the patient population. **Complications** were higher in the patients receiving higher dose: grades 1 and 2 rectal bleeding and urethral stricture occurred more commonly in the proton-boosted patients; the difference was significant only for rectal bleeding ($p = 0.002$ and $p = 0.07$, respectively).[132]

Dose–volume histogram analysis in 41 patients has demonstrated that the total volume of anterior rectum receiving more than 75 CGE was significantly related to the probability of remaining free of rectal bleeding. No rectal bleeding was experienced by 80% of 27 patients in whom more than 40% of the anterior rectum received more than 75 CGE, while only 40% of 14 patients in whom more than 40% of the anterior rectum received more than 75 CGE remained free of rectal bleeding.[133] Hartford et al. have reviewed and updated that data set, using logistic regression to seek individual combinations of dose and irradiated volume that would separate patients with a high risk of rectal bleeding from those with a low risk, thereby allowing an accurate prediction of the probability of rectal bleeding from the dose–volume histogram of a specific treatment plan.[134] Of

128 dose–volume combinations examined, 10 were found to be significant predictors of rectal bleeding. Three groups were identified, corresponding to low, intermediate, and high risk of rectal injury. Good correlation was observed between the model-derived normal tissue complication probability (NTCP) and the frequency of rectal bleeding actually observed in that patient population. Calculated NPTC for the low risk category was $0.100 \pm 0.08$; only one of 12 (0.08) patients in that group had bleeding. In the moderate and high risk groups, 5 of 17 (0.29) and 8 of 12 (0.67) patients had bleeding; calculated NTCPs were $0.35 \pm 0.15$ and $0.58 \pm 0.18$, respectively, as shown in Figure 15-8.[134] With appropriate modification, the general technique employed would appear to be applicable to risk assessment in other normal tissues.

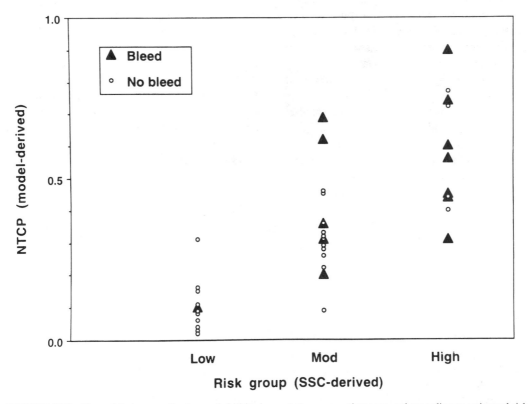

**FIGURE 15-8**   Normal tissue complication probabilities in prostate cancer patients grouped according to estimated risk for rectal bleeding as determined by dose–volume histogram analysis. Most complications (rectal bleeding) are seen in the higher risk groups.[134]

A second randomized phase III dose-searching clinical trial was initiated in prostate cancer patients with less advanced disease (stage T1-2b, PSA ≤ 15) in 1996, also in collaboration with Loma Linda University Medical Center (LLUMC). Patients are randomized to receive either 70.2 or 79.2 CGE. PROG 95-09 differs from the earlier phase III clinical trail in that it not only enrolls patients with earlier stage disease, but also gives both groups the proton prostate boost initially, followed by x-ray treatment to a larger volume including the prostate and seminal vesicles. An additional difference is that the newer protocol does not incorporate a break between the proton and the x-ray treatments. Proton boost levels are either 19.8 or 28.8 CGE; all patients received 50.4 Gy to the larger volume with x-rays. MGH patients use the perineal portal for the boost, while at LLUMC opposed lateral portals are employed.[135] The latter technique allows better shielding of the rectum, but the HCL beam lacks sufficient range to deliver the boost from a lateral approach. The required sample size for PROG 95-09 is 390 patients; through September 1998, 269 had been randomized, 221 from LLUMC and 48 from MGH.

A new collaborative trial is being planned between MGH and LLUMC, for patients with more advanced disease (T3-4). That trial will combine initial androgen suppression with a dose-searching study similar to the other two trials. Dose escalation trials using three-dimensional conformal x-rays with or without intensity modulation are in progress at several U.S. centers. In the future, outcome comparisons between results of state-of-the-art x-ray treatment and proton treatment may become possible. A clinical trial directly comparing the two modalities has not been proposed.

### Central Nervous System (CNS) Targets

Techniques developed for treating patients with skull base chordomas and chondrosarcomas can be used to good effect on CNS targets. Both fractionated and single-fraction (radiosurgery) treatments have been employed for treating patients with discrete CNS lesions, in-

cluding gliomas, benign, atypical, and malignant meningiomas, functioning and nonfunctioning pituitary adenomas, acoustic neuromas, craniopharyngiomas, metastatic lesions, and vascular malformations. The MGH–Harvard experience with high grade and meningiomas and gliomas is reviewed next.

*Benign Meningiomas* A possible trend toward improved local control in patients treated with three-dimensional planning and combined photon–proton techniques was reported in 36 benign meningioma patients treated at MGH between 1968 and 1986. Six of 25 patients (24%) treated with conventional planning and supervoltage techniques experienced recurrence, compared to none of 11 patients treated with combined photon and proton techniques ($p = 0.14$). Four of the six complications in the total population, including one case of bilateral blindness, occurred in the 25 patients treated with photons alone. The other major complication occurred in a patient treated early in the proton project who received 71.6 CGE for a massive recurrent meningioma, compressing the brain stem and extending through the jugular foramen to the parapharyngeal area and ipsilateral neck. Localized brain stem injury developed in the high dose area at 9 months, unilateral cerebellar necrosis at 75 months, and unilateral hearing loss at 78 months.[136] The patient was alive at last follow-up (192 months) with significant but stable neurological deficit.

In a more recent analysis, 46 patients with incompletely excised or recurrent benign intracranial meningiomas were treated at HCL to doses ranging from 53.1 to 73.1 CGE (median 59 CGE) with combined proton and photon treatment. Median age of the patients was 50 years (range 11–74 years), and median follow-up was 53 months (range 12–207 months). Benign histology in all patients was confirmed at MGH. There were five deaths, none from meningioma progression. Four patients died from other causes, and one of brain stem necrosis at 22 months. It was unclear whether basilar artery thrombosis found to be present at autopsy was caused by the radiation the patient had received. Local tumor progression was documented in three patients at 61, 95, and 125 months; the patient who experienced local recurrence at 61 months had had "drop" metastases to the lumbar region at 21 months and to the cervical region at 88 months. **Overall survival** was 93% and 77%, and **local recurrence-free survival** was 100% and 88% at 5 and 10 years, respectively. **Grade 3 or 4 toxicities** occurred in eight patients: four had visual loss, four had brain or brain stem toxicity, and two had hearing loss.[137]

It is difficult to compare toxicity in these proton-treated patients with that seen in photon-treated patients, since the patient populations may be quite different, particularly with respect to tumor site. Patients treated for tumors in the skull base or the orbit would be likely to receive higher doses to radiation-sensitive structures, such as the brain stem, and the optic nerves and chiasm. Forty-four of the 46 HCL patients (91%) had skull base lesions; the other two had orbital tumors. In one large photon-treated series, patients with cortical or parasagittal lesions, who are at lower risk for optic tract or brain stem toxicity, comprised 50% of the total population. In that series, the complication rate was lower, but the progression-free survival rate was also lower.[138]

A dose-searching randomized phase III clinical trial was initiated in 1995 to prospectively evaluate local control and morbidity after three-dimensional conformal proton–photon therapy of incompletely resected or recurrent benign meningiomas. In PROG 95-03, patients are randomized to receive either 55.8 or 63.0 CGE. Doses to the optic structures are constrained to 54 CGE or less, and to the brain stem surface and center to 63 and 53 CGE or less, respectively. Through September 1998, a total of 30 patients were entered into PROG 95-03: 25 from MGH and 5 from LLUMC.

*Atypical and Malignant Meningioma* Patients with incompletely excised or recurrent tumors have also been treated at HCL. Outcome has been assessed in 15 patients treated with photons only, and in 16 patients who received three-dimensional planned proton-photon irradiation, using techniques similar to those employed for skull base tumor patients. Doses ranged up to 72 CGE in the combined modality group. Mean age of the patients was 49 years, ranging from 6 to 79 years. Mean follow-up was 59 months (range 7–155 months). Histology was classified at MGH in all patients according to the WHO criteria.[139] Patients receiving proton–photon treatment had local control rates significantly improved over those treated with photons only (80% vs. 17% at 5 years, $p = 0.003$). Target doses of 60 CGE or more were also predictive of improved local control for patients with both atypical and malignant histology ($p = 0.025$ and $p = 0.0006$, respectively). At time of the analysis, 14 of the 15 atypical meningioma patients (93%) and 6 of the 16 malignant meningioma patients (38%) were alive. **Overall survival** was 89% for atypical and 51% for malignant meningiomas, respectively, at both 5 and 8 years. A significant survival benefit was documented for patients receiving proton–photon treatment and for patients receiving 60 CGE or more ($p = 0.008$ and $p = 0.025$, respectively). All three patients who developed metastasis had malignant histology. Three patients developed symptomatic brain damage after doses of 59.3, 68.4, and 72 CGE.[140]

This retrospective analysis suggested a dose–response relationship for patients with both atypical and malignant meningiomas, and provided support for developing the phase I/II nonrandomized protocol currently employed for patients with these histologies. Under MGH Protocol M7-11, doses to patients with atypical and malignant meningiomas are 68.4 and 72 CGE, respectively. Enrollment is open to patients from both MGH and LLUMC.

*Glioblastomas* In a pilot study, 90 CGE in 50 fractions was given at 1.8 CGE or Gy twice daily over 5 to 5.5 weeks to the CT-enhancing volume of patients with glioblastoma multiforme. This program was well tolerated acutely, with all nine patients entering the protocol completing the treatment. Survival was not improved. Tumor recurrence occurred in the lower dose volume immediately outside the 90 CGE volume. This suggested that the CT-enhanced volume underestimated tumor extent and perhaps contributed to local failure in the patients treated.

A subsequent protocol combined CT, MRI, and PET scanning in the initial definition of the target volume, and used the dose fractionation schedule described above. Twenty-three adult patients were enrolled, all of whom had unilateral supratentorial MGH-verified grade IV/IV astrocytoma (Daumas-Duport classification), 60 mL or less of residual tumor, and Karnofsky performance score of 70 or better. Median survival was 20 months, and estimated survival at 2 and 3 years was 34% and 18%, respectively. Four patients were surviving at the time of analysis. Recurrent tumor was again most commonly seen in the volume receiving 60 to 70 CGE, suggesting that the dose-fractionation pattern employed prevented regrowth in most patients within the 90 CGE volume.[141] Necrosis was seen in several patients, suggesting that brain tolerance to the dose-fractionation pattern employed may well limit further attempts at dose escalation or target enlargement in patients with glioblastomas. New approaches are needed for this deadly tumor. Glioblastomas have also been treated with heavy ions at LBL, with similar relatively disappointing results.[142,143]

PARANASAL SINUS AND NASAL ANTRUM TUMORS These tumors have been treated with a hyperfractionated accelerated protocol, used twice daily. Eligible histologies include squamous cell, undifferentiated, adeno-, adenoid cystic, and mucoepidermoid carcinomas. A dose of 76 CGE is given, with a morning dose of 1.5 CGE or Gy, followed by an afternoon or evening dose of 1.8 CGE given 6 or more hours later. The evening dose treats the gross residual tumor mass, while the morning dose is given to a larger volume, including tissues potentially involved with microscopic disease. Initial results in 30 patients have been encouraging in terms of both acute and chronic tolerance, and tumor regres-

sion. Three patients failed locally, with actuarial local control and disease-specific survival at 3 years being 80% and 62%, respectively.[144] Patients with primitive neuroectodermal tumors (PNET) and esthioneuroblastomas have also been treated with this fractionation pattern with most encouraging results. Lower doses, in the order of 68 CGE, are combined with induction and postradiation chemotherapy.[145]

MALIGNANT ORBITAL TUMORS These tumors can be treated with limited surgery and postoperative irradiation, as an alternative to orbital excenteration. Ten patients with tumors requiring doses of 60 Gy or more have been treated, including six with adenoid cystic carcinoma, and one each with adenocarcinoma, mucoepidermoid carcinoma, malignant schwannoma, and malignant melanoma. No local recurrences have been observed, with a median dose at 70.9 CGE and median follow-up of 2.1 years. All eyes remain in place, and seven have functional vision. MRI temporal lobe changes were seen in two patients, one of whom developed temporal lobe seizures. Although these preliminary results are encouraging, further follow-up will be needed to critically assess the true utility of proton beam therapy for orbital malignancies requiring high doses for local control.[146]

### Connective Tissue Tumors

*Sarcomas of the Axial Skeleton* These sarcomas, primarily osteo- and chondrogenic tumors, present a difficult management challenge similar to problems encountered with skull base and cervical spine sarcomas. Total surgical removal is usually not possible, and the radiosensitivity of adjacent normal tissues can prevent safe delivery of the radiation doses required to achieve local control. Combined proton–photon treatment optimized with three-dimensional planning techniques allows delivery of doses that potentially can achieve improved local control, relative to what can be achieved with x-rays alone. Forty-seven patients with axial skeleton sarcomas (20 with chordomas and chondrosarcomas, 15 with osteogenic sarcomas, and 12 with giant cell tumors and osteo- and chondroblastomas) were treated to doses ranging from 55.3 to 82 CGE with combined proton–photon techniques. Mean doses were 73.9, 69.8, and 61.8 CGE in the three respective patient categories. Local control at 5 years was achieved in 100%, 53%, 59%, and 76% of chondrosarcomas (6 patients), chordomas (14 patients), osteogenic sarcomas (15 patients), and 12 patients with giant cell tumors (8), osteoblastomas (2), and chondroblastomas (2), respectively. Results of this retrospective study affirm that the dose-localizing ability of three-dimensional planned photon–proton therapy can indeed contribute to improved results in the management of these uncommon but challenging tumors.[147]

Treatment of these patients is individualized and involves close cooperation with medical, pediatric, and orthopedic oncologists and neurosurgeons. Generally, spinal and paraspinal tumors have been treated with combined proton–photon radiotherapy, in combination with appropriate surgical treatment. Intraoperative brachytherapy, usually administered prior to combined proton–photon radiotherapy, has also been employed in some patients in this category. The current protocol for patients with tumors in the lower lumbar spine and sacrum, M7-10, prescribes doses of 77.4 and 704 CGE to the gross and the subclinical disease, respectively, delivered at 1.8 CGE on a once-daily basis in 10 weeks or less. The cauda equina receives the prescribed tumor dose in many of these patients, and its radiation tolerance is currently being assessed.[148]

Combining posterior and lateral portals to treat the anterior portion of the body and the posterior elements, respectively, has allowed us to conform the dose quite well to target volumes that involve the vertebral body and also extend posteriorly in the cervical spine. Thoracic and upper lumbar vertebral body and paravertebral tumors are problematic, since cord tolerance, as well as that of the lungs, heart, liver, kidneys, and gut, must be respected. Posterior and lateral spinal elements can be treated with a posterior portal, but the HCL beam lacks sufficient energy to treat the anterior portion of the vertebral body with a lateral portal. The ability to treat such tumors was enhanced in 1999 when the Northeast Proton Therapy Center became operational in Boston.

*Head and Neck Tumors* These are well treated with protons, with techniques employed for treatment of skull base and cervical spine tumors. **Head and neck sarcomas** are particularly challenging, since both total surgical removal and radical radiotherapy are limited by the proximity of adjacent normal tissues. Optimized three-dimensional planning techniques and combined proton–photon treatment have resulted in local control rates that appear to be improved, relative to what would have been expected with x-ray treatment alone. Twenty-seven patients with primary (18) and recurrent (9) sarcomas received doses ranging up to 79.2 CGE. Local control at 5 years was achieved in 62%, with both the extent of residual tumor and tumor volume being significantly related to the probability of achieving local control. Ability to localize the radiation dose to the defined target volume contributed to the relatively favorable local control rates achieved with minimal morbidity in these patients. Overall survival was limited by development of distant metastasis, indicating the need for effective systemic therapy to further enhance treatment results in these patients.[149] Advanced nasopharynx cancers have been successfully treated at HCL. Results in both epithelial and connective tissue head and neck tumors treated with heavy charged particles at LBL have been reported.[150,151]

*Other Sites* Patients with lung, esophageal, cervix, prostate, head and neck, and hepatocellular carcinomas have been treated at The National Laboratory for High Energy Physics in Tskuba, Japan, with some benefit being observed.[152,153]

***Treatment of Tumors at Other Sites*** Impressive clinical successes have been achieved with the HCL proton beam, specifically in patients with uveal melanomas, bony and cartilaginous tumors of the skull base and cervical spine, some CNS tumors, and some bone and soft tissue sarcomas of the axial skeleton and head and neck. Protons have also proven to be simple, safe, and effective treatment modalities for dose escalation in prostate cancer. These tumor sites were chosen because they are all relatively superficial, and thus accessible for treatment with the relatively low energy 160 MeV proton beam available there. They were also able to be treated within the limitations imposed by the fixed horizontal beam orientation available at the HCL.

A systematic effort to study proton treatment of tumors of other types at HCL has not been feasible because of several factors besides the limited range of the HCL beam. Lack of a gantry to orient the beam in other than a fixed horizontal direction has prevented the use of some treatment techniques and angles of approach. Beam time for fractionated treatments has been available only 4 days per week, since stereotactic radiosurgery is carried out on the fifth day. Treatment capacity at HCL is limited to 15 to 25 patients per 12-hour day, 4 days per week. These factors, which have dictated that available beam time be allotted to patients shown early in the clinical experience to benefit from the treatment, have effectively precluded significant efforts to treat tumors of other types.

Tumors at other sites are currently being treated at LLUMC, which has both a higher energy beam (270 MeV) and multiple gantries. Those features will be available at the Northeast Proton Therapy Center (NPTC), which opened on the MGH campus in 1999. The NPTC combines a 230 MeV cyclotron, built to MGH specifications by Ion Beam Applications (IBA) of Belgium, with two isocentric gantries. The treatment capabilities and capacity currently being utilized at the HCL are preserved by moving the eye treatment station and the patient positioner currently in use at the HCL into a fixed beam room in the new facility. That resource, together with the two new gantry-equipped rooms, allow treatment of large numbers of additional patients, increasing treatment capacity from the 15 to 25 patients per 12-hour day to 80 to 120 patients per day, three to five times the previous HCL patient load.

## ASSESSING THE VALUE OF PROTON THERAPY: CLINICAL TRIALS

Dose-searching studies involving only MGH and MEEI patients have been completed, including studies on patients with T3-4 prostate cancer, small and medium uveal melanomas, and age-related macular degeneration. Pilot studies have established the feasibility and efficacy of accelerated hyperfractionated treatment of paranasal sinus carcinomas, and of once-daily, high dose conformal treatment for axial skeleton sarcomas and for atypical and malignant meningiomas. A phase I/II trial established that hyperfractionated accelerated proton–photon therapy for glioblastoma multiforme was well tolerated acutely; patient survival was improved only marginally, if at all, however, despite the high dose delivered. Through the NCI-funded Proton Therapy Oncology Group (PROG), six protocols involving collaboration between HCL-MGH and LLUMC are in place, as discussed above. Since the demise of PROG, a mechanism has been established at the Dana Farber Partners Cancer Center in Boston for protocol data collection from both centers on patients treated on common protocols.

New treatment protocols should be developed in concert with other particle therapy centers, as was done initially by the MGH-HCL group and the UCSF-LBL group and, more recently, with LLUMC. Support from the National Cancer Institute initially through the Radiation Therapy Oncology Group (RTOG) and later from the American College of Radiology (ACR) and PROG, has been most helpful in this regard. If NCI funding is not made available for future protocol development and clinical and research collaborative efforts, alternate support must be aggressively pursued. Development of a national or international proton therapy collaborative clinical research program will not only make proton therapy available to cancer patients within the regions or countries served by the collaborating centers, but will also allow collection of data to aid in the assessment of the true role of proton beam therapy in human clinical oncology. Participation in ongoing clinical trials by all proton therapy centers in the United States and the world will be encouraged.

## PROTON THERAPY CENTERS AS REGIONAL/NATIONAL RESOURCES

A proton therapy center is best conceived as a regional or even national facility that will serve a triple function:

- to make available state-of-the-art clinical treatment to patients in its service area
- to undertake clinical research to define the role of proton beam therapy in twenty-first-century oncology
- to provide training to other physicians and scientists interested in radiation oncology in general, and charge particle radiation therapy in particular

Although a proton center must of necessity be located at a particular place, it is essential that it be organized in such a way that protocol-eligible patients can be accepted from any source. The availability of full supportive services, including state-of-the-art imaging facilities (CT, MRI, PET scans), inpatient support, and anesthesia capabilities, is essential. The proton center should also be located in a facility with an active cancer treatment program, specifically in a large and centrally located academic medical center. Active input from radiation oncologists in the region served by the center will greatly enhance protocol development, as well as generate adequate patient referral and appropriate follow-up and aftercare.

Clinical research protocols should be structured in such a way that the clinical care being provided will be reimbursible as clinical care and that appropriate clinical research questions can be addressed with sufficient scientific merit to ensure the securing of support for the research activities.

## NEW PROTON THERAPY CENTERS

Accrual of patients into cooperative clinical trials may be accelerated by the initiation of proton therapy at several new centers, both in the United States and abroad. A new center virtually identical to the NPTC initiated proton therapy in Kashiwa, Chiba Prefecture, Japan, in 1999. It is likely that at least three other "NPTC clones" will be built at major U.S. academic centers early in the twenty-first century. Each of these "clones" will have a 230 MeV IBA cyclotron, three treatment rooms, including two gantries and a fixed beam room, and supporting clinical and administrative functions. Systematic evaluation of proton therapy for multiple new tumor sites is already under way at the LLUMC 270 MeV clinically configured synchrotron. A clinically configured high energy proton facility equipped with an isocentric gantry is already in operation at Paul Shirer Institute (PSI) in Villingen, Switzerland.[154]

A novel approach to beam delivery is being developed at the National Accelerator Center in Faure, South Africa, which has been doing proton therapy with a fixed horizontal beam since 1993. A second treatment room will be equipped with an overhead beam oriented downward at 30° which, when combined with a multifunctional patient couch, will allow many of the treatment angles used with a gantry to be employed. Funding is being sought to further develop a Proton Center at Indiana University in Bloomington, which currently has a single treatment room with a fixed horizontal beam.

Active proton therapy centers, and those anticipating initiation of proton therapy in the rel-

TABLE 15-3 New Proton Beam Therapy Centers

| Where | When | Comment |
|---|---|---|
| NCI, Kashiwa, Japan | 1998 | 235 MeV, gantries, fixed beam |
| NPTC, MGH, Boston | 1999 | 235 MeV, gantries, fixed beam |
| Catania, Italy | 1999 | 70 MeV, eyes, superficial sites |
| Bratislavia, Slovakia | 2000 | 70 MeV, eyes, superficial sites |
| Northern Taiwan | 2001 | 250 MeV, gantries |
| Hyogo, Japan | 2001 | Protons, heavy ions, gantries, fixed beams |
| Faure, South Africa | 2001 | New treatment room; fixed overhead beam, 30° vertical |
| Tskuba, Japan | 2001 | 270 MeV, gantries, research |
| Wakasa Bay, Japan | ?2001 | Multipurpose accelerator, medical program under discussion |
| PROTOX, England | ?2001 | RAL, 250 MeV, 3 gantries |
| Shizuoka Cancer Center, Japan | ?2002 | ?230 MeV, gantries, fixed beam |
| Milan and Pavia, Italy | ?2002 | Synchrotron, gantry, fixed beams |
| ISS, Rome, Italy | ???? | 200 MeV linear accelerator; funded |
| Austron, Austria | ???? | Protons, heavy ions, "ferris wheel" gantries, fixed beams |
| Clatterbridge, England | ???? | Upgrade facility (booster linear accelerator) |
| Krakow, Poland | ???? | 60 MeV, eyes, superficial sites |
| Groningen, Netherlands | ???? | KVI, 200 MeV, gantry, fixed beam |
| Tenant Health Care, U.S.A. | ???? | NPTC "clones," 235 MeV, gantries, fixed beam, three U.S. cities |

*Source:* Ref. 30.

atively near future are listed in Tables 15-1 and 15-3, respectively.

With the availability of greatly enhanced treatment capabilities and capacity anticipated for the first decade of the new century, the challenge will be to determine which tumor categories would be better treated with protons than with state-of-the-art megavoltage x-rays. Successfully meeting that challenge will require that clinical trials be undertaken to determine the true role of proton beam therapy in the radiotherapeutic armamentarium. Clinical experience at the existing and soon-to-exist centers, and at others that appear in the less immediate future, will allow systematic evaluation of the role of proton therapy for tumors involving abdominal, pelvic, and thoracic sites. Clinical trials in general, and radiation therapy trials in particular, require long observation periods to properly assess the end points of local control, patient survival, and acute and chronic morbidity. Even if cooperative clinical trials at additional clinical sites can be mounted in the relatively near future, it is likely that the true efficacy of proton radiation therapy will not be assessed until well into the first or second decade of the twenty-first century. However, the infrastructure will soon be in place to properly implement such trials.

## RELATIVE COSTS: PROTON THERAPY VERSUS X-RAY THERAPY

Costs for proton therapy relative to those for supervoltage x-ray therapy cannot be totally assessed at this time. Charges at newly designed facilities may reflect developmental costs for the accelerators, hence may not be readily comparable to costs for photon treatment delivered with off-the-shelf, state-of-the-art linear accelerators. Rather, proton charges should be compared with conformal optimized three-dimensional planned supervoltage x-ray therapy, rather than with the cost of routine clinical treatments. Initial cost of a proton accelerator, beam transport system, gantry system, and building to house the larger accelerator will undoubtedly be greater for protons. However, x-ray linear accelerators are generally replaced every 10 to 20 years, while a proton accelerator might operate up to three times that long—the HCL became operational in 1948, over a half-century ago, and could continue to be used indefinitely for clinical treatments.

Personnel costs should be quite comparable for proton and photon facilities with similar patient capacity, although some additional engineering staff will be required for the proton facility because of the greater complexity of the accelerator itself. Treatment planning should be similar for both modalities, since treatment planning programs can operate on the same system. The use of custom apertures and compensators for the proton treatment as is practiced at both HCL and LLUMC is undoubtedly more expensive than the standard blocking systems employed in photon therapy. However, multileaf collimators and beam scanning techniques can eliminate the need for individually fabricated apertures and compensators for either modality.[155] The longer useful life of a particle accelerator over time may offset its higher initial cost by a significant factor. Cost increment of protons over conformal optimized three-dimensional planned supervoltage x-ray therapy has been estimated to be a factor of 1.3 to 1.5.[156,157]

## SUMMARY: CLINICAL BENEFITS PREDICTED WITH PROTON BEAM TREATMENTS

Suit and Krengli have tabulated the following clinical gains anticipated from treating smaller volumes of normal tissue with proton beam techniques:

1. Greater patient tolerance
2. A higher radiation dose
3. An increased tumor control probability
4. A reduced frequency and severity of treatment-related morbidity[157]

Some or all of these gains have indeed been achieved in patients treated at the HCL to date, but the future challenge will be to demonstrate that they can also be regularly achieved during routine treatment of patients with more common malignancies.

## SUMMARY AND CONCLUSIONS

Protons are not "magic bullets." Despite impressive results in some tumor categories, proton therapy does not represent a revolutionary development in the treatment of malignant disease. Rather, when combined with three-dimensional treatment planning, proton beam therapy is best considered as an evolutionary advance in radiotherapy practice, similar to dose distribution improvements with supervoltage x-rays, afterloading brachytherapy capabilities, and the availability of electron beam techniques. The efficacy of intensity-modulated photon therapy relative to proton beam therapy must also be assessed. An additional challenge will be the incorporation of sequential or concomitant systemic chemotherapy into treatment protocols, as has been occurring in general radiation oncology practice.

Active participation by radiation oncologists from the region in all phases of planning and operation of the center is essential for protocol development, adequate patient referral, and appropriate follow-up and aftercare. Ideally, protocols should be structured to incorporate clinical research questions into the clinical care being provided, so that adequate financial support for the facility will be available while relevant research questions are being addressed.

Common treatment protocols should be employed at various proton centers, coordinated if at all possible through a national funding agency, such as the NCI. Development of common treatment protocols would have at least two advantages: making proton therapy available to appropriate cancer patients within the region, and allowing for accumulation of data to aid in the assessment of the true role of proton beam therapy in human oncology. In all our efforts in this regard, it is essential that the development and testing of new technologies be based on clinical research of the highest quality; there also must be an ethical basis for the innovations adopted, and scrupulous adherence to ethical principles in the design and implementation of clinical trials.[158] Much has been accomplished in the first century since Roentgen's discovery of x-rays. Equally exciting challenges may well await those who still actively seek to find better ways to use radiation therapy in the treatment of human disease in the twenty-first century.

## REFERENCES

1. Castro JR, Petti PL, Blakely EA, Linstadt DE: Particle radiation therapy, in SA Leibel and TL Phillips (eds): *Textbook of Radiotherapy.* New York: Saunders, 1998.

2. Cancer Treatment Symposia: *Proceedings of the Workshop on Patterns of Failure After Cancer Treatment.* Vol. 2, 1983.

3. DeVita VT, Hellman S, Rosenberg ST: *Cancer: Principles & Practice of Oncology.* Philadelphia, Lippincott, 1989.

4. Fletcher GH: *Textbook of Radiotherapy,* 3rd ed. Philadelphia: Lea & Febiger, 1980.

5. Perez CA, Brady LW: *Principles and Practice of Radiation Oncology.* Philadelphia, Lippincott, 1992.

6. Wang CC: *Clinical Radiation Oncology: Indications, Techniques and Results.* Littleton, MA: PSG Publishing, 1988.

7. Suit HD: Potential for improving survival rates for the cancer patient by increasing the efficacy of treatment of the primary lesion [American Society of Therapeutic Radiology presidential address, October 1981]. *Cancer* 1982;50:1227–1234.

8. Fuks Z, Leibel SA, Wallner KE, et al: The effect of local control on metastatic dissemination in carcinoma of the prostate: Long-term results in patient treated with [125]I implantation. *Int J Radiat Oncol Biol Phys* 1991;21:537–547.

9. Leibel SA, Scott CB, Mohiuddin M, et al: The effect of local–regional control on distant metastatic dissemination in carcinoma of the head and neck: Results of an analysis from the RTOG head and neck database. *Int J Radiat Oncol Biol Phys* 1991;21:549–555.

10. Suit HD: Local control and patient survival. *Int J Radiat Oncol Biol Phys* 1992;23:653–660.

11. Brahme A: Dosimetric precision requirements in radiation therapy. *Acta Radiol [Oncol]* 1984;23(fasc 5):379–391.

12. Suit HD, Walker AM: Predictors of radiation response in use today: Criteria for new assays and methods of verification, in JD Chapman, LJ Peters, and HR Withers (eds): *Prediction of Tumor Treatment Response.* Oxford: Pergamon Press, 1988, pp 3–19.

13. Suit HD, Verhey LJ: Precision in megavoltage radiotherapy. *Br J Radiol* suppl 1988;22:17–24.

14. Suit HD, duBois W: The importance of optimal treatment planning in radiation therapy. *Int J Radiat Oncol Biol Phys* (F Ellis dedicatory issue) 1991;21:1471–1478.

15. Suit HD, Urie MU, Efird JT: Proton beams in clinical radiation therapy. *Princ Pract Oncol* 1992;6:1–15.

16. Austin-Seymour M, Kalet I, McDonald J, Kromhout-Schiro S, Jacky J, Hummel S, Ungar J: Three-dimensional planning target volumes: A model and software tool. *Int J Radiat Oncol Biol Phys* 1995;33:1073–1080.

17. Urano M, Goitein M, Verhey LJ, Tepper JT, Suit HD, Mendiando O, Gragoudas ES: Relative biological effectiveness of modulated proton beams in various murine tissues. *Int J Radiat Oncol Biol Phys* 1984;10:509–514.

18. Yashkin PN, Silin DI, Zolotov VA, Kostjuchenko VI, Nichiporov DF, Feoktistova KS, Minakova YI, Khoroshkov VS, Polonski PB, Zinovyeva LV: Relative biological effectiveness of proton medical beam at Moscow Syn-

chotron determined by the Chinese hamster cells assay. *Int J Radiat Oncol Biol Phys* 1995;31:535–540.

19. Miller DW: A review of proton beam radiotherapy. *Med Phys* 1995;22:1943–1954.

20. Wilson RR: Radiological uses of fast protons. *Radiology* 1946;47:487–491.

21. Koehler AM, Preston WM: Protons in radiation therapy. Comparative dose distributions for protons, photons, and electrons. *Radiology* 1972;104:191–195.

22. Archambeau JO, Bennett GW, Chen ST: Potential of proton beams for total nodal irradiation. *Acta Radiol Ther Phys Biol* 1974;13: 393–401.

23. Raju MR: *Heavy Particle Radiotherapy.* New York: Academic Press, 1980.

24. Tobias CA, Lawrence JH, Born JL, McCombs RK, Roberts JE, Anger HO, Low-Beer BVA, Huggins CB: Pituitary irradiation with high energy proton beams: A preliminary report. *Cancer Res* 1958;18:121–134.

25. Graffman S, Jung B: Clinical trials in radiotherapy and the merits of high energy protons, photons, and electrons. *Acta Radiol Ther Phys Biol* 1970;9:1–23.

26. Kjellberg RN, Shintani A, Frantz AG, et al: Proton beam therapy in acromegaly. *N Engl J Med* 1968;278:689–695.

27. Kjellberg RN, Kliman B: Bragg peak proton treatment for pituitary-related conditions. *Proc R Soc Med* 1974;67:32–33.

28. Kjellberg RN, Kliman B: Lifetime effectiveness—A system of therapy for pituitary adenomas, emphasizing proton hypophysectomy, in JA Linfoot (ed): *Recent Advances in the Diagnosis and Treatment in Pituitary Tumors.* New York: Raven Press, 1979, pp 269–288.

29. Chuvilo IV, Goldin LL, Khoroshkov VS, et al: ITEP synchrotron proton beam in radiotherapy. *Int J Radiat Oncol Biol Phys* 1984;10: 185–195.

30. Sisterson J (ed): *Parti Newsl* 22:July 1998.

31. Slater JM, Archambeau JO, Miller DW, et al: The proton treatment center at Loma Linda University Medical Center: Rationale for and description of its development. *Int J Radiat Oncol Biol Phys* 1992;22:383–389.

32. National Cancer Institute: Potential Clinical Gains by Use of Superior Radiation Dose Distribution. NCI Proton Workshop. *Int J Radiat Oncol Biol Phys* 1992;22:233–390.

33. Urtasun RC: Does improved depth dose characteristics and treatment planning correlate with a gain in therapeutic results? Evidence from past clinical experience using conventional radiation sources. *Int J Radiat Oncol Biol Phys* 1992;22:235–239.

34. Thames HD, Schultheiss TE, Hendry JH, et al: Can modest escalations of dose be detected as increased tumor control? *Int J Radiat Oncol Biol Phys* 1992;22:241–246.

35. Lyman JT: Normal tissue complication probabilities: Variable dose per fraction. *Int J Radiat Oncol Biol Phys* 1992;22:247–250.

36. Henkleman RM: New imaging techniques: Prospects for target definition. *Int J Radiat Oncol Biol Phys* 1991;22:251–257.

37. Tatsuzaki H, Urie MM, Linggood R: Comparative treatment planning: Proton vs x-ray beams against glioblastoma multiforme. *Int J Radiat Oncol Biol Phys* 1992;22:265–273.

38. Archambeau JO, Slater JD, Slater JM, et al: Role for proton beam irradiation in treatment of pediatric CNS malignancies. *Int J Radiat Oncol Biol Phys* 1992;22:287–294.

39. Wambersie A, Gregroire V, Brucher JM: Potential clinical gain of proton (and heavy ion) beams for brain tumors in children. *Int J Radiat Oncol Biol Phys* 1992;22:275–286.

40. Miralbell R, Crowell C, Suit HD: Potential improvement of three dimension treatment planning and proton therapy in the outcome of maxillary sinus cancer. *Int J Radiat Oncol Biol Phys* 1992;22:305–310.

41. Slater JM, Slater JD, Archambeau JO: Carcinoma of the tonsillar region: Potential for use of proton beam therapy. *Int J Radiat Oncol Biol Phys* 1992;22:311–319.

42. Levin CV: Potential for gain in the use of proton beam boost to the para-aortic lymph nodes in carcinoma of the cervix. *Int J Radiat Oncol Biol Phys* 1992;22:355–359.

43. Slater JD, Slater JM, Wahlen S: The potential for proton beam therapy in locally advanced carcinoma of the cervix. *Int J Radiat Oncol Biol Phys* 1992;22:343–347.

44. Smit BM: Prospects for proton therapy in carcinoma of the cervix. *Int J Radiat Oncol Biol Phys* 1992;22:349–353.

45. Tatsuzaki H, Urie MM, Willett CG: 3-D comparative study of proton vs x-ray radiation therapy for rectal cancer. *Int J Radiat Oncol Biol Phys* 1992;22:369–374.

46. Gademann G, Wannenmacher M: Charged particle therapy to pediatric tumors of the retroperitoneal region: A possible indication. *Int J Radiat Oncol Biol Phys* 1991;22:375–381.

47. Brown AP, Urie MM, Chisin R, Suit HD: Proton therapy for carcinoma of the nasopharynx. *Int J Radiat Oncol Biol Phys* 1989;16:1607–1614.

48. Miralbell R, Urie M: Potential improvement of three dimension treatment planning and proton beams in fractionated radiotherapy of large cerebral arteriovenous malformations. *Int J Radiat Oncol Biol Phys* 1993;25:353–358.

49. Miralbell R, Lomax A, Bortfeld T, Rouzaud M, Carrie C: Potential role of proton therapy in the treatment of pediatric medulloblastoma/primitive neuroectodermal tumors: Reduction of the supratentorial target volume. *Int J Radiat Oncol Biol Phys* 1997;38:477–484.

50. Isacsson U, Lennernas B, Grusell E, Jung B, Montelius A, Glimelius B: Comparative treatment planning between proton and x-ray therapy in esophageal cancer. *Int J Radiat Oncol Biol Phys* 1983;41:441–450.

51. Goitein M, Urie MM, Munzenrider JE, et al: Report of the working groups on the evaluation of treatment planning for particle beam radiotherapy. Washington, DC: Division of Cancer Treatment, National Cancer Institute, 1987.

52. Sandison GA, Papiez, Bloch C, Morphis J: Phantom assessment of lung dose from proton arc therapy. *Int J Radiat Oncol Biol Phys* 1997;38:891–897.

53. Goitein M, Abrams M: Multi-dimensional treatment planning: 1. Delineation of anatomy. *Int J Radiat Oncol Biol Phys* 1983;9:777–787.

54. Goitein M: Compensation for inhomogeneities in charged particle radiotherapy using computed tomography. *Int J Radiat Oncol Biol Phys* 1978;4:499–508.

55. Urie M, Goitein M, Wagner M: Compensating for heterogeneities in proton radiation therapy. *Phys Med Biol* 1983;29:553–566.

56. Verhey LJ, Goitein M, Munzenrider JE, Suit HD, McNulty P: Precise positioning of patients for radiation therapy. *Int J Radiat Oncol Biol Phys* 1982;8:289–294.

57. Gall KP, Verhey LJ, Wagner M: Computer-assisted positioning of radiotherapy patients using implanted radiopaque fiducials. *Med Phys* 1993;20:1153–1159.

58. Goitein M, Abrams M, Rowell D, Pollari H, Wiles J: Multi-dimensional treatment planning: II. Beam's-eye view, back projection and projection through CT sections. *Int J Radiat Oncol Biol Phys* 1983;9:789–797.

59. Tatsuzaki H, Urie MM: Importance of precise positioning for proton beam therapy in the base of skull and cervical spine. *Int J Radiat Oncol Biol Phys* 1991;21:757–765.

60. Urie MU, Fullerton B, Tatsuzaki H, et al: A dose response analysis of injury to cranial nerves and/or nuclei following proton beam radiation therapy. *Int J Radiat Oncol Biol Phys* 1992;23:27–39.

61. Austin JP, Urie MM, Cardenosa G, Munzenrider JE: Probable causes of recurrence in patients with chordoma and chondrosarcoma of the base of skull and cervical spine. *Int J Radiat Oncol Biol Phys* 1993;25:439–444.

62. Stallard HB: Malignant melanoblastoma of the choroid. *Mod Probl Ophthalmol* 1966;7:16–38.

63. Cruess AF, Augsburger JJ, Shields JA, et al: Visual results following cobalt plaque radiotherapy for posterior uveal melanomas. *Ophthalmology* 1984;91:131–136.

64. Garretson BR, Robertson DM, Earle JK: Choroidal melanoma treatment with iodine-125 brachytherapy. *Arch Ophthalmol* 1987;105:1394–1397.

65. Lommatzsch PK: β-Irradiation of choroidal melanoma with $^{106}$Ru/$^{106}$Rh applicators. *Arch Ophthalmol* 1983;102:713–717.

66. Marcoe AM, Brady LW, Shields J, et al: Radioactive eye plaque therapy versus enucleation for the treatment of posterior uveal malignant melanoma. *Radiology* 1985;156:801–803.

67. Rotman M, Long RS, Packer S, et al: Radiation therapy of uveal melanomas. *Trans Ophthalmol Soc UK* 1977;97:431–435.

68. Brovkina AF, Zarubei GD: Ciliochoroidal melanomas treated with a narrow medical proton beam. *Arch Ophthalmol* 1986;104:402–404.

69. Char DH, Castro JR, Kroll SM, et al: Five-year follow-up of helium ion therapy for uveal melanoma. *Ophthalmology* 1990;108:209–214.

70. Bonnet DE, Kacperek A, Sheen MA, Goodall R, Saxton TE: The 62 MeV proton beam for the treatment of ocular melanoma at Clatterbridge. *Br J Radiol* 1993;66:907–914.

71. Gragoudas ES, Seddon JM, Egan K, et al: Long-term results of proton beam irradiated uveal melanomas. *Arch Ophthalmol* 1987;94:349–353.

72. Zografos L, Perret C, Egger E, et al: Proton beam irradiation of uveal melanomas at Paul Scherrer Institute (former SIN). *Strahlenther Onkol* 1990;166:114.

73. Castro JR, Char DH, Petti PL, Daftari IK, Quivey JM, Singh RP, Blakely EA, Phillips TL: 15 years experience with helium ion radiotherapy for uveal melanoma. *Int J Radiat Oncol Biol Phys* 1997;39:989–996.

74. Tsunemoto H, Morita S, Kawachi K, et al: Clinical results of proton radiotherapy in Japan. *Proceedings of the Eighth International Congress of Radiation Research*, Edinburgh, 1987, pp 922–927.

75. Daftari IK, Char DH, Verhey LJ, Castro JR, Petti PL, Meecham WJ, Kroll S, Blakely EA: Anterior segment sparing to reduce charged particle radiotherapy complications in uveal melanoma. *Int J Radiat Oncol Biol Phys* 1997;39:997–1010.

76. Constable IJ, Koehler AM, Schmidt RA: Proton irradiation of simulated ocular tumors. *Invest Ophthalmol* 1975;14:547–555.

77. Constable IJ, Goitein M, Koehler AM, et al: Small field irradiation of monkey eyes with protons and photons. *Radiat Res* 1976;65:304–314.

78. Gragoudas ES, Zakov NZ, Albert DM, et al: Long term observations of proton-irradiated monkey eyes. *Arch Ophthalmol* 1979;97:2184–2191.

79. Goitein M, Miller T: Planning proton therapy of the eye. *Med Phys* 1983;10:275–283.

80. Gragoudas ES, Goitein M, Koehler AM, Verhey LJ, Tepper JT, Suit H, Brockhurst R, Constable IJ: Proton irradiation of small choroidal malignant melanomas. *Am J Ophthalmol* 1977;83:655–673.

81. Gragoudas ES, Goitein M, Verhey LJ, Munzenrider JE, Suit H, Koehler AM: Proton beam irradiation: An alternative to enucleation for intraocular melanoma. *Ophthalmology* 1980;87:571–581.

82. The Collaborative Ocular Melanoma Study Group: Accuracy of diagnosis of choroidal melanomas in the Collaborative Ocular Melanoma Study. COMS Report No. 1. *Ophthalmology* 1990;108:1268–1273.

83. Munzenrider JE, Verhey L, Gragoudas ES, Seddon JM, Urie M, Gentry R, Birnbaum S, Ruotolo D, Crowell C, McManus P, Finn S, Sisterson J, Johnson K, Egan K, Lento D, Bassin P: Conservative treatment of uveal melanoma: Dose distribution to tumors with local recurrence after proton beam therapy. *Int J Radiat Oncol Biol Phys* 1989;17:493–498.

84. Gragoudas ES, Seddon JM, Polivogianis LL, Hsieh CC, Egan DM, Goitein M, Verhey L, Munzenrider JE, Austin-Seymour M, Urie M, Koehler A: Prognostic factors for metastasis following proton beam irradiation of uveal melanomas. *Ophthalmology* 1986;93:675–680.

85. Gragoudas ES, Seddon JM, Egan KM, et al: Metastatis from uveal melanoma after proton beam irradiation. *Ophthalmology* 1988;95:992–999.

86. Seddon JM, Gragoudas ES, Albert DM, et al: Comparison of survival rates for patients with uveal melanoma after treatment with proton beam irradiation or enucleation. *Am J Ophthalmol* 1985;99:282–290.

87. Seddon JM, Gragoudas ES, Egan KM, et al: Relative survival rates after alternative therapies for uveal melanoma. *Ophthalmology* 1990;97:769–777.

88. Seddon JM, Albert DM, Lavin P, et al: A prognostic factor study of disease-free interval and survival following enucleation for uveal melanoma. *Arch Ophthalmol* 1983;101:1894–1899.

89. Egan KM, Ryan LM, Gragoudas ES: Survival implications of enucleation after definitive radiotherapy for choroidal melanoma. An example of regression on time-dependent covariates. *Arch Ophthalmol* 1998;116:366–370.

90. Kirkwood JM, Strawderman MH, Ernstoff MS, Smith TJ, Borden EC, Blum RH: Interferon $\alpha$-2b adjuvant therapy of high risk resected cutaneous melanoma: The Eastern

Cooperative Oncology Group Trial EST 1684. *J Clin Oncol* 1996;14:7–17.

91. Egan K, Gragoudas ES, Seddon JM, Glynn R, Munzenrider J, Goitein M, Verhey L, Urie M, Koehler A: The risk of enucleation after proton beam irradiation of uveal melanoma. *Ophthalmology* 1989;96:1377–1383.

92. Ferry AP, Blair CJ, Gragoudas ES, et al: Pathologic examination of ciliary body melanoma treated with proton beam irradiation. *Arch Ophthalmol* 1985;103:1849–1853.

93. Kincaid MC, Folberg R, Torczynski E, et al: Complications after proton beam therapy for uveal malignant melanoma. *Ophthalmology* 1988;95:982–991.

94. Seddon JM, Gragoudas ES, Albert DM: Ciliary body and choroidal melanomas treated by proton beam irradiation: Histopathologic study of eyes. *Arch Ophthalmol* 1983;101:1402–1408.

95. Zinn KM, Stein/Pokorny K, Jakobiec F, et al: Proton beam irradiated epithelial cell melanoma of the ciliary body. *Ophthalmology* 1981;88:1315–1321.

96. Gragoudas ES, Egan KM, Arrigg PG, Seddon JM, Glynn RJ, Munzenrider JE: Cataract extraction after proton beam irradiation for malignant melanoma of the eye. *Arch Ophthalmol* 1992;110:475–479.

97. Gragoudas ES, Egan KM, Walsh SM, Regan S, Munzenrider JE, Taratuta V: Lens changes after proton beam irradiation for uveal melanoma. *Am J Ophthalmol* 1995;119:157–164.

98. Seddon JM, Gragoudas ES, Polivogianis L, Hsieh, Egan KM, Goitein LJ, Verhey LJ, Munzenrider JE, Austin-Seymour, Urie M, Koehler A: Visual outcome after proton beam irradiation of uveal melanoma. *Ophthalmology* 1986;93:666–674.

99. Seddon JM, Gragoudas ES, Egan KM, Glynn R, Munzenrider JE, Austin-Seymour M, Goitein M, Verhey LJ, Urie M, Koehler A: Uveal melanomas near the optic disc or fovea. Visual results after proton beam irradiation. *Ophthalmology* 1987;94:354–361.

100. Kindy-Dedgan NA, Char DH, Castro JR, et al: Effect of various doses of radiation for uveal melanoma on regression, visual activity, complications and survival. *Am J Ophthalmol* 1989;107:114–120.

101. Char DH, Quivey JM, Castro JR, Kroll S, Phillips TL: Helium ions versus iodine-125 brachytherapy in the management of uveal melanoma, a prospective randomized dynamically balanced trial. *Ophthalmology* 1993;100:1547–1554.

102. Smith LM, Donaldson SS, Egbert PR, et al: Aggressive management of second primary tumors in survivors of hereditary retinoblastoma. *Int J Radiat Oncol Biol Phys* 1989;17:499–505.

103. Wong FL, Boice JD, Abramson DH, Tarone RE, Kleinerman RA, Stovall M, Goldman MB, Seddon JM, Tarbell N, Fraumeni JF Jr, Li FP: Cancer incidence after retinoblastoma. Radiation dose and sarcoma risk. *J Am Med Soc* 1998;278:1262–1267.

104. Kaste SC, Chen G, Fontanesi J, Crom DB, Pratt CB: Orbital development in long-term survivors of retinoblastoma. *J Clin Oncol* 1997;15:1183–1189.

105. Mukai S: Management of retinoblastoma. *Semin Ophthalmol* 1993;8:281–291.

106. Urie M, Goitein M: Variable versus fixed modulation of proton beams for treatment in the cranium. *Med Phys* 1989;16:593.

107. American Academy of Ophthalmology: Age-related macular degeneration and choroidal neovascularization (monograph). American Academy of Ophthalmology, 1994.

108. Archambeau JO, Mao XW, Yonemoto LT, Slater JD, Friedrichsen E, Teichman S, Preston W, Slater JM: What is the role of radiation in the treatment of subfoveal membranes: Review of radiobiologic, pathologic, and other considerations to initiate a multimodality discussion. *Int J Radiat Oncol Biol Phys* 1998;40:1125–1136.

109. (a) Dahlin DC, *Bone Tumors,* 2nd ed. Springfield, IL, Charles C Thomas, 1967. (b) Netherlands Committee on Bone Tumors (ed): *Radiologic Atlas of Bone Tumors*, vol 1. Baltimore, Williams & Wilkins, 1966.

110. Volpe NJ, Liebsch NJ, Munzenrider JE, Lessell S: Neuro-ophthalmic findings in chordoma and chondrosarcoma of the skull base. *Am J Ophthalmol* 1993;115:97–104.

111. Halperin EC: Why is female sex an independent predictor of shortened overall survival after proton/photon radiation therapy for skull

base chordomas? *Int J Radiat Oncol Biol Phys* 1997;38:225.

112. O'Connell JX, Renard LG, Liebsch NJ, Efird J, Munzenrider JE, Rosenberg AE: Base of skull chordoma: A correlative study of histologic and clinical features of 62 cases. *Cancer* 1994;74:2261–2267.

113. Rosenberg AE, Brown GA, Bhan AK, Lee JM: Chondroid chordoma: A variant of chordoma: A morphological and immunohistochemical study. *Am J Clin Pathol* 1994;101:36–41.

114. Al-Mefti O, Borba AB: Skull base chordomas: A management challenge. *J Neurosurg* 1997;86:182–189.

115. Raffel C, Wright DC, Gutin PH, Wilson CB: Cranial chordomas: Clinical presentation and results of operative and radiation therapy in twenty-six patients. *Neurosurgery* 1985;17: 703–710.

116. Austin-Seymour M, Munzenrider J, Goitein M, et al: Fractionated proton radiation therapy of chordoma and low grade chondrosarcoma of the base of skull. *J Neurosug* 1989;70: 13–17, 43.

117. Castro JR, Lindstadt DE, Bahary JP, Petti PL, Daftari I, Collier JM, et al: Experience in charged particle irradiation of tumors of the skullbase: 1977–1992. *Int J Radiat Oncol Biol Phys* 1994;29:647–656.

118. Oot RF, Melville GE, New PF, Austin-Seymour M, Munzenrider JE, Spellman JP, Spagnoli M, Shoukimas GM, Momose KJ, Carroll R, Davis KR: The role of MR and CT in evaluating clival chordomas and chondrosarcomas. *Am J Roentgen* 1988:567–575.

119. Munzenrider JE, Hug EB, McManus P, Adams J, Efird J, Liebsch NJ: Skull base chordomas: Treatment outcome and prognostic factors in adult patients following conformal treatment with 3D planning and high dose fractionated combined proton and photon radiation therapy. *Int J Radiat Oncol Biol Phys* 1995; 32(suppl):209.

120. Fagundes MA, Hug EB, Liebsch NJ, et al: Radiation therapy for chordomas of the base of skull and cervical spine: Patterns of failure and outcome after relapse. *Int J Radiat Oncol Biol Phys* 1995;33:579.

121. Debus J, Hug EB, Munzenrider JE, Liebsch NJ, O'Farrell D, Efird J, Suit HD: Brainstem

tolerance to conformal radiotherapy of skull base tumors. *Int J Radiat Oncol Biol Phys* 1997;39:976.

122. Liu MCC, Munzenrider JE, Finkelstein D, Liebsch NJ, Adams J, Hug EB: Radiation myelopathy: Incidence and dose–volume relationships in high dose irradiation of the cervical spinal cord. *Int J Radiat Oncol Biol Phys* 1997;39(suppl 1):272.

123. Santoni R, Liebsch NJ, Finkelstein D, Hug E, Hanssens P, Goitein M, Smith AR, O'Farrell D, Efird J, Fullerton B, Munzenrider JE: *Int J Radiat Oncol Biol Phys* 1998;41:59–68.

124. Glosser G, McManus P, Munzenrider JE, et al: Neuropsychological function in adults after high dose fractionated radiation therapy of skull base tumors. *Int J Radiat Oncol Biol Phys* 1997;38:231.

125. Habrand JL, Austin-Seymour M, Birnbaum S, et al: Neurovisual outcome following proton radiation therapy. *Int J Radiat Oncol Biol Phys* 1989;16:1601–1606.

126. Kim J, Hug EB, Liebsch NJ, Bussiere M, Finkelstein D, Munzenrider JE: Tolerance of optic nerve to high dose fractionated proton and x-ray therapy. *Int J Radiat Oncol Biol Phys* 1997;39:272.

127. Schoenthaler R, Fullerton B, Maas A, et al: Relationship between dose to auditory pathways and audiological outcomes in skull base tumor patients receiving high dose proton/ photon radiotherapy. *Int J Radiat Oncol Biol Phys* 1996;36:291.

128. Slater JD, Austin-Seymour M, Munzenrider J, et al: Endocrine function following high dose proton therapy for tumors of the upper clivus. *Int J Radiat Oncol Biol Phys* 1988;15:607–611.

129. Catton C, O'Sullivan B, Bell R, et al: Chordoma: Long-term follow-up after radical photon irradiation. *Radiother Oncol* 1996;41:67.

130. Shipley WU, Tepper JE, Prout GW Jr, et al: Proton radiation therapy in patients with localized prostatic carcinoma. *JAMA* 1979;241: 1912–1915.

131. Duttenhaver JR, Shipley WU, Perrone TL, et al: Protons or megavoltage x-rays as boost therapy for patients irradiated for localized prostatic carcinoma: An early phase I–II comparison. *Cancer* 1981;51:1599–1604.

132. Shipley WU, Verhey LJ, Munzenrider JE, Suit HD, Urie MM, McManus PL, Young RH, Shipley JW, Zeitman AL, Biggs PJ, Heney NM, Goitien M: Advanced prostate cancer: The results of a randomized comparative trial of high dose irradiation boosting with conformal protons compared with conventional dose irradiation using photons alone. *Int J Radiat Oncol Biol Phys* 1995;32:3–12.

133. Benk VA, Adams JA, Shipley WU, Urie MM, McManus PL, Efird JT, Willett CG: Late rectal bleeding following combined x-ray and proton high dose irradiation for patients with stages T3-T4 prostate carcinoma. *Int J Radiat Oncol Biol Phys* 1993;26:551–557.

134. Hartford AC, Niemierko A, Adams J, Urie MM, Shipley WU: Conformal irradiation of the prostate: Estimating long-term rectal bleeding risk using dose–volume histograms. *Int J Radiat Oncol Biol Phys* 1996;36: 720–730.

135. Slater JD, Yonemoto LT, Rossi CJ, Reyes-Molyneux NJ, Bush DA, Antoine JE, Loredo LN, Schulte RWM, Teichman SL, Slater JM: Conformal proton therapy for prostate carcinoma. *Int J Radiat Oncol Biol Phys* 1998;42: 299–304.

136. Miralbell R, Linggood RM, de la Monte S, et al: The role of radiotherapy in the treatment of subtotally resected benign menigniomas. *J Neuro-Oncol* 1992;13:157–164.

137. Wenkel E, Thornton AF, Finkelstein D, Adams J, Lyons S, de la Monte S, Munzenrider JE: Benign meningioma: Partially resected and recurrent intracranial tumors treated with combined proton and photon radiotherapy. *Int J Radiat Oncol Biol Phys* 1998;42(suppl 1):271.

138. Glaholm J, Bloom HJ, Crow JH: The role of radiotherapy in the management of intracranial meningiomas: The Royal Marsdan Hospital experience with 186 patients. *Int J Radiat Oncol Biol Phys* 1990;18:755–761.

139. Kleihues P, Burger PC, Scheithauer BW: *Histological Typing of Tumors of the Central Nervous System,* 2nd ed. Geneva, World Health Organization/Springer-Verlag, 1993.

140. Hug EB, DeVries A, Thornton AF, Munzenrider JE, Pardo FS, Hedley-Whyte ET, Bussiere MR, Ojemann RG: Management of atypical and malignant meningiomas: Potential role of high dose 3D conformal radiation therapy. *J Neurosurg* (in press).

141. Fitzek MM, Thornton AF, Rabinov JD, Lev M, Pardo FS, Munzenrider JE, Okunieff P, Bussiere M, Braun I, Hochberg FH, Hedley-Whyte T, Liebsch NJ, Harsch GR IV: Results of a phase II study with proton/photon irradiation to 90-cobalt gray equivalent (CGE) in accelerated fractionation for glioblastoma multiforme. *Int J Radiat Oncol Biol Phys* 1997(suppl 2):39.

142. Castro JR, Saunders WM, Austin-Seymour MM, et al: A phase I-II trial of heavy charged particle irradiation of malignant glioma of the brain: A Northern California Oncology Group study. *Int J Radiat Oncol Biol Phys* 1985; 11:1795–1800.

143. Castro JR, Phillips TL, Prados M, Gutin P, Larson DA, Petti PL, Daftari IK, Collier JM, Lillis-Hearne P: Neon heavy particle radiotherapy of glioblastoma of the brain. *Int J Radiat Oncol Biol Phys* 1997;38:257–261.

144. Thornton AF, Fitzek MM, Vavares M, Adams J, Resenthal S, Pollock C, Jackson M, Pilch B-Z, Joseph MP: Accelerated, hyperfractionated proton/photon irradiation for advanced paranasal sinus cancer: Results of a prospective phase I–II study. *Int J Radiat Oncol Biol Phys* 1998;42(suppl 2):222.

145. Bhattacharyya N, Thornton AF, Joseph MP, Goodman ML, Amrein PC: Successful treatment of esthesioneuroblastoma and neuroendocrine carcinoma with combined chemotherapy and proton radiation. *Arch Otolaryngol Head Neck Surg* 1997;123:34–40.

146. Fitzek MM, Thornton AF, Liebsch NJ, Bussiere M, Hug EB, Rubin P, Munzenrider JE: Eye preservation by combined surgery and conformal proton irradiation for malignant tumors of the orbit. *Int J Radiat Oncol Biol Phys* 1998;42(suppl 1):330.

147. Hug EB, Fitzek MM, Liebsch NJ, Munzenrider JE: Locally challenging osteo- and chondrogenic tumors of the axial skeleton: Results of combined proton and photon radiation therapy using three-dimensional treatment planning. *Int J Radiat Oncol Biol Phys* 1995;31: 467–476.

148. Pieters RS, O'Farrell D, Fullerton B, Efird J, Munzenrider JE: Cauda equina tolerance to ra-

diation therapy. *Int J Radiat Oncol Biol Phys* 1996;36(suppl 1):359.

149. Hug EB, Hanssens PE, Liebsch NJ, Thornton AF, Munzenrider JE: Soft tissue sarcomas of the head and neck: Results of combined proton and photon radiation therapy using 3D treatment planning. *Int J Radiat Oncol Biol Phys* 1994;30(suppl 1):222.

150. Castro J, Reimers M: Charged particle radiotherapy for selected tumors in the head and neck. *Int J Radiat Oncol Biol Phys* 1988;14:711–720.

151. Feehan FE, Castro JR, Phillips TL, et al: Recurrent locally advanced nasopharyngeal carcinoma treated with heavy charged particle irradiation. *Int J Radiat Oncol Biol Phys* 1992;23:881–884.

152. Tsujii H, Inada T, et al: Clinical results of fracitonated proton therapy. *Int J Radiat Oncol Biol Phys* 1992;25:49–60.

153. Tanaka N, Matsuzaki Y, Chuganji Y, et al: Proton irradiation for hepatocellular carcinoma. *Lancet* 1992;340:1358–1359.

154. Pedroni E, Bacher R, Blattman H, Bohringer T, Coray A, Lomax A, Lin S, Munkel G, Scheib S, Schneider U, Tourovsky A: The 200 MeV proton therapy project at the Paul Scherrer Institute: Conceptual design and practical realization. *Med Phys* 1995;22:37–53.

155. Chu WT, Ludewigt BA, Renner TR: Instrumentation for treatment of cancer using proton and light ion beams. *Rev Sci Instrum* 1993;64:2055–2122.

156. Gademann G: Cost–benefit considerations of hadrontherapy, in U Amaldi, B Larsson, and Y Lemoigne (eds): *Advances in Hadrontherapy.* Amsterdam, Elsevier, 1997, pp 55–62.

157. Suit HD, Krengli M: Basis for interest in proton beam radiotherapy, in U Amaldi, B Larsson, and Y Lemoigne (eds): *Advances in Hadrontherapy.* Amsterdam, Elsevier, 1997, pp 29–37.

158. Bernier J, Lacombe D, Meunier F: Clinical trials and ethical issues in cancer research, in U Amaldi, B Larsson, and Y Lemoigne (eds): *Advances in Hadrontherapy.* Amsterdam, Elsevier, 1997, pp 73–75.

# B.  Altered Fractionation Radiation Therapy for Head and Neck Cancers - C.C. WANG

## ALTERED FRACTIONATION SCHEMES

In the United States for the past few decades most of the "conventional" or "traditional" fractionation radiation therapy for carcinomas for head and neck cancers consists of 1.8 to 2.0 Gy per fraction per day (Gy/f/day) 5 days a week, for a total of 65 to 70 Gy continuous irradiation. This fractionation scheme was arrived at because of tolerable acute reactions with acceptable late effects. From the standpoint of modern radiobiology, this conventional fractionation radiation therapy may not be optimal in terms of maximal local control of the tumors with minimal late complications.

One of the attempts to improve the therapeutic results is changing the patterns of fractionation. This may involve changes of fraction size, number of daily fractions, total dose, total treatment time, and other treatment variables.

For the past decade and half, a great deal of clinical research has borne fruit in the management of head and neck cancers. The following discussion therefore is focused on head and neck tumor sites.

At the present time altered fractionation programs can be divided into four categories: hypofractionation, split-course radiation therapy, hyperfractionation, and accelerated fractionation.

### Hypofractionation

Hypofractionation implies a larger dose per fraction per day (e.g., 4 or 5 Gy/f, 3 or 4 days per week), for a total dose equal to, or slightly lower than conventional fractionation. The number of weekly fractions is reduced. The overall treatment time can be shortened. Clinical experience indicates that such an approach results in decreased tumor control[1–3] and is associated with severe late effects on normal tissues. The acute effects may be similar to those with the conventional 5 fractions per week, even with identical time–dose–fractionation (TDF) or nominal standard dose (NSD) values; yet late complication rates were higher, indicating a dissociation of responses between acute and late tissue effects to large dose per fraction.

## Split-Course Radiation Therapy

Split-course radiation therapy involves conventional fraction size (1.8–2.0 Gy/f/day) with a midcourse split, or rest period, of 2 to 3 weeks. The overall treatment time of split-course radiation therapy is lengthened. Another split-course approach includes rapid fractionation of 3 Gy/f/day for 10 days with a 2-week treatment break or split, followed by 3 Gy/f/day for 10 more days. The overall treatment course is approximately the same as for conventional radiation therapy with 2 Gy/f. Clinical experience indicates, however, lower tumor control from the split-course approach than with continuous conventional fractionation radiation therapy.[4,5] The inferior results were probably due to excessive repopulation of the tumors during the rest period as well as prolongation of the entire treatment course. Rapid split-course fractionation may show tumor control similar to that with conventional continuous radiation therapy with 2 Gy/f, but with more severe late sequelae such as bone necrosis and severe fibrosis.

## Hyperfractionation

Hyperfractionation is the use of multiple small fractions, two or three times a day with 4 or more hours between fractions. The fraction size may be 1.15 to 1.2 Gy with two treatments per day. This is equivalent to 2 Gy per fraction per day, 5 days a week, and can be given continuously up to 65 to 77 Gy.[6–8] The overall treatment time remains unchanged (e.g., 6–8 weeks). The acute toxicity of such an approach is generally comparable to or slightly more

than the conventional once-daily radiation therapy with 2 Gy/f. The total dose may be increased, since the fraction size has been decreased. The intent is to reduce late effects with an increased total dose, achieving the same late effects and higher tumor control. Experience, however, has showed only slight or no significant improvement of local control after these treatments.[6–8]

## Accelerated Fractionation

The accelerated program uses the conventional dose per fraction (i.e., 2 Gy/2–3 f/day) for a total dose of 60 Gy. The overall treatment time is markedly shortened. The basic intent is to minimize the potential tumor growth or repopulation without changing the late effects, which is possible because the total dose, number of fractions, and dose per fraction are the same as in the conventional program. The difficulties with accelerated fractionation are severe toxicity of the acutely responding tissues (i.e., the mucous membranes), which may necessitate reduction of the total dose or termination of the program early because of poor tolerance. The most common accelerated fractionation schedule includes boost treatment to the primary lesion through the reduced "field-within-field" technique,[9–11] with two or three daily fractions per week, along with the conventional program (1.8–2 Gy/day, 5 days a week). Thus the dose to the primary lesion may amount to a total of 70 Gy delivered over 5 to 6 weeks with somewhat less mucosal toxicity.

Another accelerated approach is to deliver radiation therapy in three fractions of 1.4 to 1.5 Gy/f/day continuously for 12 days (CHART).[12,13] The total dose is limited to 50 to 54 Gy because the mucosal toxicity is severe and patients often require intensive nutritional support and hospitalization.

Radiation therapy delivered by interstitial implant with radioactive isotopes with a dose rate of 0.4 to 0.5 Gy/h may be considered to be another approach to accelerated fractionation. A total dose of approximately 70 Gy is thought of as a sum of numerous fractions of small fraction size. For a standard implant for squamous cell carcinoma, daily dose of 10 Gy for 6 to 7 days is generally given. In spite of unavoidable inhomogeneity of dose distribution from interstitial implant, the local control rates generally are quite satisfactory, and the cosmetic and functional results are often superior to the conventional external beam radiation therapy. To minimize the extent of inhomogeneous dose distribution, interstitial implants are often done in combination with external beam irradiation.

## Accelerated Hyperfractionation

The altered fractionated radiation therapy at the Massachusetts General Hospital (MGH) is a hybrid between accelerated and hyperfractionated programs.[14,15] The scheme consists of 10% to 15% dose reduction per fraction, twice a day (1.6 Gy/f, BID) for a total dose of 67.2 to 70.4 Gy in 6 weeks. The procedure can shorten the total treatment course for about one week, despite the necessity for a break of 10 to 14 days because of severe mucosal toxicity of acutely responding tissues, compared to the once-daily program, and is generally fairly well tolerated.

The treatments of importance are depicted in Figure 15-9.

## RADIOBIOLOGIC CONCEPTS OF ALTERED FRACTIONATION

The principle of altered fractionation radiation therapy for the treatment of human cancers is one of the strategies stemming from the laboratory radiobiologic research. The studies relevant to the understanding and practice of altered fractionated radiation therapy include the results of dose–survival curves of cells, both normal and malignant, and acute- and late-responding tissues, various radiobiologic characteristics of tumor cells and of critical normal tissues, and repair of sublethal damage of both normal and cancer cells after photon irradiation.[16] The biological basis for various dose modification programs has been extensively discussed by Withers et al. and others.[16,17]

It has been observed that the repair of sublethal damage is almost complete in 4 to 6 hours. The shoulder of the survival curve is

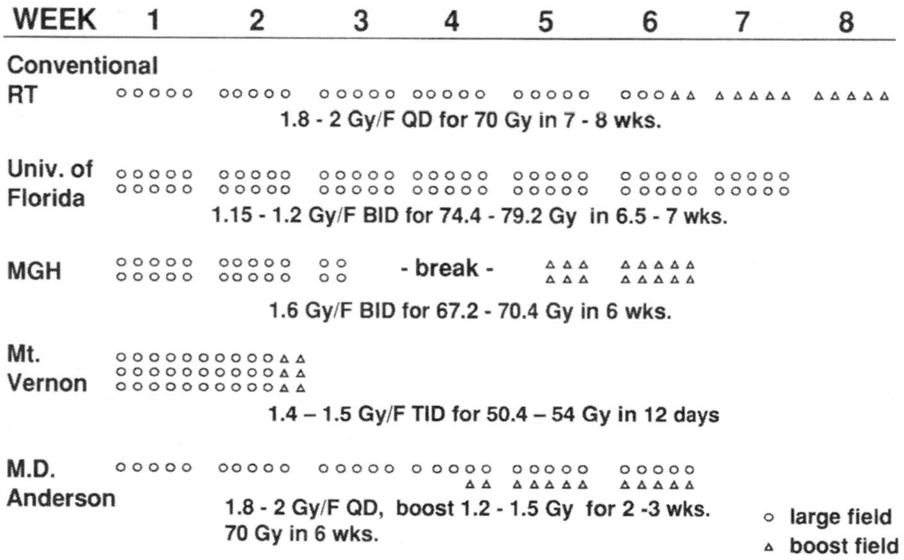

**FIGURE 15-9** Summary of various forms of altered fractionation radiation therapy for head and neck carcinoma.

duplicated, although the degree of repair may be different in various biologic environments and tissues. The acutely responding oxygenated tissues, including skin, mucous membrane of the aerodigestive tract, and testes, have higher capacity of repair of sublethal damage than the chronically hypoxic cancerous cells and late-responding tissues such as vasculoconnective tissues, spinal cord, lung, and kidney. For radiation treatment given in two or three fractions a day, the interval time between fractions should not be less than 4 hours, and preferably 6 hours, if complete repair is achieved. Severe late complications result when interfraction time is shortened to 2 to 3 hours.[18–21]

Various biological tissues respond differently to change of dose per fraction. Withers et al.[22–24] observed that the slopes of the dose–response curve for the late-responding tissues are steeper or curvier than those for the acutely responding tissues (Figure 15-10). The late-responding tissues, therefore, are dependent on the dose per fraction and not on overall treatment time and are much more sensitive to increased fraction size. With identical total dose and treatment time and large fractions, there is marked impairment of repair of sublethal damage, resulting in late complications (Figure 15-11). When smaller sized "common" or conventional radiation therapy dosages ($< 2$ Gy/f) are used, there is preferential sparing of the late-responding tissues relative to the acutely responding tissues. Thus the total dose required to produce a specified level of damage or complications can be increased, perhaps with an increase of local tumor control.

Clinical and experimental studies indicate that both normal and malignant cells are capable of repopulating during and after radiation damage, although to varying degrees. With increased total treatment time, repopulation of tumor cells is increased, followed by decreased tumor control. It is postulated that the best therapeutic strategy is likely to result from delivery of the maximum dose tolerated by late-responding tissues in the minimum time that is consistent with tolerable acute reactions.

## Altered Fractionation

Based on the foregoing knowledge of modern radiobiological observations, altered fractionation is presently centered on two general strategies: use of smaller fraction size ($< 2$ Gy/f, as in conventional radiation therapy) and shortening of overall treatment time. By using a smaller fraction size, especially at doses less than 1.8 to 2 Gy, and shortening the overall treatment course, with total dose maintained at or above conventional fractionation, there is less damage to late-responding tissues (determinants of tolerance for most situations) relative to increased damage to tumor.

It appears that hypofractionation with large daily fractions and split-course radiation therapy programs with prolonged overall treatment time are disadvantageous with regard to severe late normal tissue injuries and inferior tumor control, respectively, and are therefore no

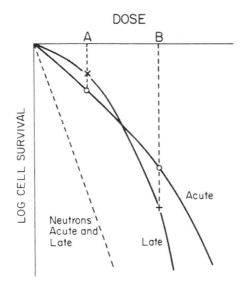

**FIGURE 15-10** Survival curve of late-responding target cells, clearly "curvier" than that of acute-responding cells. With decrease in x-ray dose per fraction, one observes greater sparing of late effects and fewer late complications. (From Withers HR, Thames HD, Peters LJ: *Int J Radiat Oncol Biol Phys* 1982; 8:2071–2076. Used by permission of Withers.)

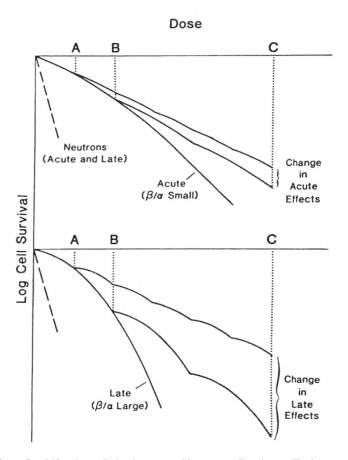

**FIGURE 15-11**    Effects of multifraction radiation in acute and late-responding tissues. The late-responding tissues are more sensitive to change of large fraction size. (From Withers HR, Thames HD, Peters LJ: Differences in fractionation response of acute and late responding tissues. In Karcher KH, Kogeinik HD, Reinartz E (eds): *Progress in Radio-Oncology,* Vol II, New York, Raven Press, 1982, pp 257–296. Used by permission of Withers.)

longer recommended for daily clinical practice. Hyperfractionation with a fraction size of 1.15 to 1.2 Gy may increase the radiation tolerance of late-responding tissues and therefore higher total dose delivered, with perhaps increased local control rates of the tumor, but the overall treatment course is not shortened significantly. Clinical experience with this approach indicated only slight gain in local control in some head and neck tumors.[6] For somewhat higher local control, the total dose is escalated from 75.9 to 82.5 Gy.[7,8]

### The Dilemma of Altered Fractionation Radiation Therapy    Clinically, the extent of

radiation toxicity on acutely responding tissues such as the mucous membranes of the aerodigestive tract is the determinant of the patient's tolerance and is related to fraction size; total daily, weekly, and overall doses; and overall treatment course. If the fraction size is large and the overall treatment course much shortened, there is severe acute toxicity, which may require reduction in total dose, eventually lowering the probability of tumor control.[18,25] Extremely rapid fractionation and high total doses often result in severe radiation complications.[19,20] There is an extremely delicate balance between fraction size, number of fractions per day, and overall total dose and treatment time in selecting the dose fractionation schedule. Figure 15-12 represents an attempt to simplify the interrelationship between changes of acute- and late-responding tissues versus fraction size and overall treatment time relative to toxicity, tolerance, tumor control probability, and complications.

At present, the altered fractionation radiation therapy programs are still undergoing intensive investigation.[21] The programs of considerable promise are summarized as follows.

1. Hyperfractionated program (University of Florida) with 1.15 to 1.2 Gy/f BID, continuously to 74.4 Gy in 6 to 7 weeks.
2. Concomitant boost program (M.D. Anderson Hospital), 1.8/f QD with concomitant boost 1.5 Gy/f for total dose of 69 to 72 Gy in 6 weeks.
3. Accelerated hyperfractionated program (MGH) with 1.6 Gy/f BID for 67.2 to 70.4 Gy in 6 weeks with a midcourse break.
4. CHART program (Mount Vernon Hospital), 1.4 to 1.5 Gy/f continuously for 50.4 to 54 Gy in 12 days.

These treatment schemes were summarized in Figure 15-9.

## Massachusetts General Hospital (BID) Programs

The twice-daily (BID) program for treatment of head and neck carcinomas was initiated at the MGH in 1979 and consists of 1.6 Gy/f, two fractions per day, with a minimum of 4 hours between fractions, for 12 days, 5 days a week. All fields were treated with megavoltage radiation in each session. After 38.4 Gy, patients were given a rest period of approximately 10 days to 2 weeks. After the rest period or "break," the treatment was resumed with a shrinking-field technique. Initially, one fraction of 1.8 Gy/f/day was given, up to 65 to 66 Gy. This is designated as the twice-daily/once-daily (BID-QD) regimen, and did not shorten the overall treatment time compared to the QD program. In August 1982 the twice-daily regimen was resumed after the break, using 1.6 Gy/f for 8 additional days, for a total dose of 67.4 to 70.2 Gy over 6 weeks. In some instances an additional day or two of twice-daily dosing was directed to the primary site through markedly reduced portals as a final boost, for a grand total of 67.2 to 70.4 Gy. This is designated the twice-daily/twice-daily (BID-BID) program, which shortened the overall treatment course of about 7 to 10 days over the QD scheme. The spinal cord dose was excluded after the first 38.4 Gy in 24 fractions of 1.6 Gy each. Figure 15-13 indicates the course of treat-

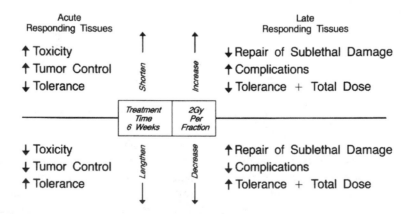

**FIGURE 15-12** Effects of acute and late-responding tissues related to treatment time and dose per fraction.

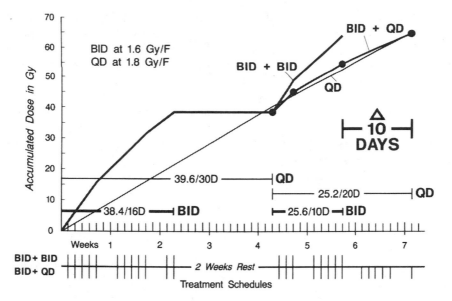

**FIGURE 15-13**    Comparison of accumulated doses before and after midcourse break between BID, BID-QD, and QD radiation therapy programs versus time (days idealized) of the oropharynx and larynx in Tables 15-11 and 15-12.

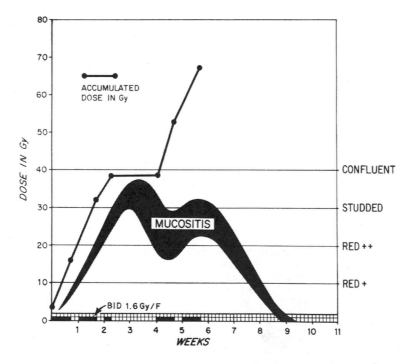

**FIGURE 15-14**    Biphasic mucositis of the oropharynx during twice-daily radiation therapy course versus dose and time. Extent of mucosal reaction shown on right of graph divided into four categories.

ment versus treatment time in the QD, BID-QD, and BID-BID programs at the MGH.

By the end of 1997, a total of 3000 patients had been treated by this BID scheme at the MGH. The results have been periodically published in the literature, and some data analysis is included in this book.

***Acute and Late Effects After Bid Radiation Therapy*** For most patients with head and neck cancers, the acute effects after twice-daily radiation therapy consist mostly of severe sore throat and development of patchy to confluent mucositis. The reactions vary in degree and extent in different anatomic sites, with portal size and irradiated volume, and with the physical condition of the patient. In general, the mucosal reaction follows a rather regular pattern. It occurs rapidly, reaching a peak of studded or confluent mucositis 2.5 to 3 weeks after commencement of therapy. It then decreases rapidly over the 10-day to 2-week therapy break.

TABLE 15-5    5-Year Actuarial Local Control (LC) of Oropharyngeal Carcinoma Related to Treatment Time: 1970–1994

| Lesions | Time (days) | $n$ | LC (%) |
|---|---|---|---|
| T1-2 | <45 | 107 | 88 |
|  | ≥45 | 136 | 75 |
|  |  |  | $p = 0.007$ |
| T3 | <45 | 90 | 67 |
|  | ≥45 | 88 | 44 |
|  |  |  | $p = 0.005$ |

TABLE 15-6    5-Year Actuarial Local Control of Oropharyngeal Carcinoma Related to Total Dose: 1970–1994

| Lesions | Dose (Gy) | $n$ | LC (%) |
|---|---|---|---|
| T1-2 | ≤67 | 149 | 79 |
|  | >67 | 88 | 83 |
|  |  |  | $p = 0.05$ |
| T3 | ≤67 | 113 | 45 |
|  | >67 | 65 | 74 |
|  |  |  | $p = 0.003$ |

TABLE 15-7    5-Year Actuarial Local Control of Supraglottic Carcinoma Related to Treatment Time: 1970–1994

| Lesions | Time (days) | $n$ | LC (%) |
|---|---|---|---|
| T1-2 | ≤45 | 83 | 93 |
|  | >45 | 48 | 84 |
|  |  |  | $p = 0.1381$ |
| T3-4 | ≤45 | 71 | 78 |
|  | >45 | 44 | 56 |
|  |  |  | $p = 0.013$ |

**TABLE 15-8    5-Year Actuarial Local Control of Supraglottic Carcinoma Related to Treatment Dose: 1970–1994**

| Lesions | Dose (Gy) | $n$ | LC (%) |
|---------|-----------|-----|--------|
| T1-2 | >67 | 133 | 78 |
|  | ≤67 | 188 | 73 |
|  |  |  | $p = 0.31$ |
| T3 | >67 | 105 | 73 |
|  | ≤67 | 78 | 57 |
|  |  |  | $p = 0.05$ |
| T4 | >67 | 17 | 65 |
|  | ≤67 | 41 | 37 |
|  |  |  | $p = 0.18$ |

**TABLE 15-9    5-Year Actuarial Local Control of Glottic Carcinoma Related to Treatment Time[28]: 1970–1994**

| Lesions | Time (days) | $n$ | LC (%) |
|---------|-------------|-----|--------|
| T1 | ≤45 | 436 | 92 |
|  | >45 | 220 | 92 |
|  |  |  | $p = 0.67$ |
| T2-2a | ≤45 | 103 | 85 |
|  | >45 | 38 | 78 |
|  |  |  | $p = 0.319$ |
| T2b-3 | ≤45 | 119 | 65 |
|  | >45 | 68 | 47 |
|  |  |  | $p = 0.015$ |

**TABLE 15-10    5-Year Actuarial Local Control of T3 Carcinomas of the Oropharynx and Larynx Related to Treatment Gap**

| Treatment Gap (days) | $n$ (total number of patients/ total at risk) | LC (%) |
|----------------------|-----------------------------------------------|--------|
| ≤ 14 | 80/32 | 80 |
| > 14 | 82/27 | 58 |
|  |  | $p = 0.0073$ |

*Source:* Ref. 27.

Upon resumption of twice-daily radiation therapy, mucositis is reactivated, but to a lesser extent, toward the completion of the course of radiation therapy. With the aid of topical analgesics, the symptoms of mucosal reactions generally are well tolerated. Very few patients require hospitalization or nasogastric intubation or feeding gastrostomy for severe dehydration during the course of irradiation. Figure 15-14 relates the development and subsidence of radiation mucositis of the oropharynx and larynx related to radiation dose and time.

All patients received BID radiation therapy with interfraction time of 4 or more hours, and the late effects were insignificant. The normal tissues were in good condition and showed no undue skin or subcutaneous fibrosis at the irradiated site, nor increased incidence of mucosal ulceration or osteoradionecrosis for observation periods as long as 18 years. No patient has developed radiation myelitis after the twice-daily program as outlined. The few patients who underwent salvage surgery to the primary sites or neck dissection for nodal recurrence or persistent disease did not experience unusually high postoperative complications compared with the patients receiving conventional irradiation.[26]

***Results of Treatment***   To assess the efficacy of the accelerated hyperfractionated radiation therapy program at the MGH, we evaluated the findings of local control and disease-specific survival rates of the patients treated from 1979 to 1996, which were compared in patients with the same diseases and stages arising from various tumor sites treated with conventional once-daily radiation therapy 10 to 15 years prior to the twice-daily schedule. We used the MicroVAX 3600 computer and SAS programs to obtain standard life tables, and we compared the results for statistical difference and extensively published elsewhere as well as in Chapter 5 of this text.

Most importantly the total treatment time and total doses related to the rates of local tumor control of squamous cell carcinoma after accelerated hyperfractionated radiation therapy become apparent.[27,28] The results are also affected by the treatment "gap" during the course of the therapy. Further subdivision of the gaps into periods larger than 11 days ($n = 28$) and 11 to 13 days ($n = 52$) showed local control rates

**TABLE 15-11   5-Year Actuarial Local Control (LC) and Disease-Specific Survival (DSS) Rates for Carcinoma of the Oropharynx After Daily and Twice-Daily Radiation Therapy: 1970–1994**

| Lesion and Treatment Regimen | $n$ | LC (%) | DSS (%) |
|---|---|---|---|
| T1-2 | | | |
| BID | 112 | 87 | 86 |
| QD | 131 | 76 | 65 |
| | $p = 0.006$ | $p = 0.001$ | |
| T3 | | | |
| BID | 98 | 71 | 50 |
| QD | 80 | 38 | 25 |
| | $p = 0.0001$ | $p = 0.0009$ | |
| N0 | | | |
| BID | 101 | 81 | 78 |
| QD | 86 | 69 | 57 |
| | $p = 0.03$ | $p = 0.02$ | |
| N1 | | | |
| BID | 40 | 77 | 66 |
| QD | 52 | 58 | 53 |
| | $p = 0.19$ | $p = 0.14$ | |
| N2-3 | | | |
| BID | 75 | 73 | 43 |
| QD | 88 | 48 | 32 |
| | $p = 0.001$ | $p = 0.009$ | |

**TABLE 15-12   5-Year Actuarial Local Control and Disease-Specific Survival Rates for Carcinoma of the Larynx After Daily and Twice-Daily Radiation Therapy: 1970–1994**

| Lesion and Treatment Regimen | $n$ | LC (%) | DSS (%) |
|---|---|---|---|
| T1 | | | |
| BID | 42 | 84 | 90 |
| QD | 72 | 74 | 76 |
| | | $p = 0.13$ | $p = 0.16$ |
| T2 | | | |
| BID | 126 | 83 | 88 |
| QD | 85 | 61 | 70 |
| | | $p = 0.007$ | $p = 0.002$ |
| T3 | | | |
| BID | 136 | 71 | 70 |
| QD | 47 | 56 | 56 |
| | | $p = 0.07$ | $p = 0.02$ |
| T4 | | | |
| BID | 18 | 84 | 74 |
| QD | 40 | 29 | 21 |
| | | $p = 0.001$ | $p = 0.004$ |
| T1-4 | | | |
| BID | 322 | 78 | 80 |
| QD | 244 | 58 | 60 |
| | | $p = 0.0001$ | $p = 0.0001$ |
| N0 | | | |
| BID | 231 | 82 | 87 |
| QD | 169 | 69 | 76 |
| | | $p = 0.008$ | $p = 0.007$ |
| N1 | | | |
| BID | 32 | 73 | 63 |
| QD | 24 | 43 | 40 |
| | | $p = 0.19$ | $p = 0.28$ |
| N2-3 | | | |
| BID | 58 | 63 | 56 |
| QD | 51 | 27 | 20 |
| | | $p = 0.0001$ | $p = 0.0001$ |

of 87% and 74%, respectively, with $p = 0.0166$ with doses constraint within 65 to 70 Gy.[27]

The data (Tables 15-5 to 15-10) indicate significant improvement in local control by shortening of the total treatment course, treatment gap, and irradiated total doses in patients with advanced (T3-4) carcinoma. With total treatment course completed less than 45 days, the treatment gap less than 14 days or preferably 11 days and total dose of 70 Gy appeared to be optimum

for the local control rates for the advanced carcinoma of the oropharynx and larynx (T3). The deleterious effects of prolonging treatment course and gap are probably due to repopulation of the tumors during irradiation.[26,27]

The results of BID and QD radiation therapy for the major head and neck carcinomas are presented in Chapter 5. Tables 15-11 and 15-12 give details of the results of treating cancers with daily and twice-daily regimens.

## SUMMARY

1. The concept of altered fractionation is one of the major contributions from laboratory basic research that has changed the practice of radiation therapy of the head and neck malignancies.

2. To exploit the radiobiological phenomenon of repair of sublethal damage, a minimal interfraction interval of 4 or more hours is required.

3. The optimum fraction size (1.2 vs. 1.6 Gy), number of daily fractions (two vs. three or more per day), total dose (65–75 Gy or higher), and total treatment time (5 vs. 8 weeks) have not been established scientifically. A randomized clinical trial is required.

4. Because of the high local control thus far achieved without significant late complications, all patients with squamous cell carcinomas of the head and neck, except those with T1 lesions have been currently treated with BID radiation therapy at the Massachusetts General Hospital.

## REFERENCES

1. Greenberg M, Eisert DR, Cox JD: Initial evaluation of reduced fractionation in the irradiation of malignant epithelial tumors. *Am J Roentgen Radium Ther Nucl Med* 1976;126:268–278.

2. Byhardt RW, Greenberg M, Cox JD: Local control of squamous cell carcinoma of the oral cavity and oropharynx with 3 vs. 5 treatment fractions per week. *Int J Radiat Oncol Biol Phys* 1977;2:415–420.

3. Cox JD, Byhardt RW, Komaki R, et al: Reduced fractionation and the potential of hypoxic cell sensitizers in irradiation of malignant epithelial tumors. *Int J Radiat Oncol Biol Phys* 1980;6:37–40.

4. Parsons JT, Bova FJ, Million RR: A re-evaluation of split-course technique for squamous cell carcinoma of the head and neck. *Int J Radiat Oncol Biol Phys* 1980;6:1645–1652.

5. Marcial VA, Hanley JA, Hendrickson F, et al: Split-course radiation therapy of carcinoma of the tongue: Results of a prospective national collaborative clinical trial conducted by the Radiation Therapy Oncology Group. *Int J Radiat Oncol Biol Phys* 1983;9:437–443.

6. Marcial VA, Pajak TF, Chang C, et al: Hyperfractionated photon radiation therapy in the treatment of advanced squamous cell carcinoma of the oral cavity, pharynx, larynx and sinuses using radiotherapy as the only planned modality: Preliminary report by the Radiation Therapy Oncology Group (RTOG). Proceedings of the 27th Annual Meeting of the American Society for Therapeutic Radiology and Oncology, Miami Beach, *Int J Radiat Oncol Biol Phys* 1987;13:41–47.

7. Parsons JT, Cassisi N, Million RR: Preliminary report on results of twice a day irradiation of squamous cell carcinoma of the head and neck at the University of Florida. *Int J Radiat Oncol Biol Phys* 1984;10:2041–2051.

8. Million RR, Parsons JT, Cassisi NJ: Twice-a-day radiation technique for squamous cell carcinoma of the head and neck. *Cancer* 1985;55:2096–2099.

9. Peters LJ, Ang KK, Thames HD: Accelerated fractionation in radiation treatment of head and neck cancer. A critical comparison of different strategies. *Acta Oncol* 1988;27:185–194.

10. Ang KK, Peters LJ: Concomitant boost radiotherapy in the treatment of head and neck cancers. *Semin Radiat Oncol* 1992;2:31–33.

11. Schmidt-Ullrich RK, Johnson CR, Wazer DE, et al: Accelerated superfractionated irradiation for advanced carcinoma of the head and neck: Concomitant boost technique. *Int J Radiat Oncol Biol. Phys* 1991;21:563–569.

12. Dische S, Saunders MI: Continuous hyperfractionated, accelerated radiotherapy (CHART): An interim report upon late morbidity. *Radiother Oncol* 1989;16:65–72.

13. Saunders MI, Dische S, Grosch EJ, et al: Experience with CHART. *Int J Radiat Oncol Biol Phys* 1991;21:871–878.

14. Wang CC, Blitzer PH, Suit HD: Twice-a-day radiation therapy for cancer of the head and neck. *Cancer* 1985;55:2100–2104.

15. Wang CC: Accelerated hyperfractionation, in HR Withers and LJ Peters (eds): *Innovations in*

*Radiation Oncology.* Berlin, Springer-Verlag, 1987, pp 239–243.

16. Withers HR: Biologic basis for altered fractionation schemes. *Cancer* 1985;55:2086–2095.

17. Withers HR, Horiot J: Hyperfractionation, in RH Withers and L Peters (eds): *Innovations in Radiation Oncology.* Berlin, Springer-Verlag, 1985, p 223.

18. Wang CC: The enigma of accelerated hyperfractionated radiation therapy for head and neck cancer. *Int J Radiat Oncol Biol Phys* 1987; 14:209–210.

19. Bourhis J, Fortin A, Dupiis O, Domenge C, Lusinchi A, Marandas P, Schwaab G, Armand JP, Luboinski B, Malaise E, Eschwege F, Wibault P: Very accelerated radiation therapy: Preliminary results in locally unresectable head and neck carcinomas. *Int J Radiat Oncol Biol Phys* 1995;32:747–752.

20. Delaney GP, Fisher RJ, Smee RI, Hook C, Barton MB: Split-course accelerated therapy in head and neck cancer: An analysis of toxicity. *Int J Radiat Oncol Biol Phys* 1995;32: 763–768.

21. Fu KK, Clery M, Ang KK, Byhardt RW, Maor MH, Beitler JJ: Randomized phase 1/11 trial of two variants of accelerated fractionated radiotherapy regimens for advanced head and neck cancer: Results of RTOG 88-09. *Int J Radiat Oncol Biol Phys* 1995;32:589–599.

22. Withers HR, Thames HD, Peters LJ: Differences in fractionation response of acute and late responding tissues, in KH Karcher, HD Kogelnik, and E Reinartz (eds): *Progress in Radio-Oncology,* Vol II. New York, Raven Press, 1982, pp 257–296.

23. Withers HR, Thames HD, Peters LJ: A new iso-effect curve for change in dose per fraction. *Radiother Oncol* 1983;1:187–191.

24. Withers HR, Thames HD, Peters LJ: Biological bases for high RBE volumes for late effects of neutron irradiation. *Int J Radiat Oncol Biol Phys* 1982;8:2071–2076.

25. Nguyen TD, Panis X, Froissart D, et al: Analysis of late complications after rapid hyperfractionated radiotherapy in advanced head and neck cancers. *Int J Radiat Oncol Biol Phys* 1988;14: 23–25.

26. Metson R, Freehling D, Wang CC: Surgical complications following twice-a-day versus once-a-day radiation therapy. *Laryngoscope* 1988;98:30–34.

27. Wang, CC, et al: Local control of T3 carcinomas after accelerated fractionation—A look at the "gap." *Int J Radiat Oncol Biol Phys* 1996; 35:439–441.

28. Wang CC, Efird JT: Does prolonged treatment course adversely affect local control of carcinoma of the larynx? *Int J Radiat Oncol Biol Phys* 1994;29:657–660.

# C. Intraoperative Electron Beam Irradiation -

## CHRISTOPHER G. WILLETT

## INTRODUCTION

In the past 20 years, there has been significant progress in the experimental and clinical application of intraoperative electron beam radiation therapy (IOERT) as a potential treatment modality for selected neoplasms. The National Cancer Institute and Colorado State University have established a framework of knowledge regarding short- and long-term tolerances of normal tissues frequently irradiated with IOERT.[1–12] On the clinical front, American, European, and Japanese investigators have described treatment strategies and experience with IOERT and have explored the potential value and limitations of this modality. More importantly, their efforts have identified disease sites in which IOERT, in combination with surgery and external beam radiation therapy (EBRT), may be of potential value. This part of the chapter describes the radiobiological and laboratory basis of IOERT and summarizes our experience with this modality for patients with locally advanced rectal carcinoma and retroperitoneal sarcoma.

## EXPERIMENTAL IOERT STUDIES

The radiation tolerance of most normal tissues to conventional fractionated EBRT is well understood. Because it is always done during surgery, IOERT is given in a single radiation fraction. IOERT doses usually range from 20 to 40 Gy when given alone and from 10 to 20 Gy when given in combination with EBRT. The biological effectiveness of this single fraction is incompletely understood; however, it is believed to be equivalent to that of a dose at least two times greater given by means of conventional fractionation. Data from canine experiments by Gillette et al. (6–12) indicate that the effectiveness of IOERT may be as high as five times that of an equivalent dose given by means of conventional fractionation in certain normal tissues. Information about normal tissue tolerance after large single doses ($> 10$ Gy) was first provided by canine experiments at the National Cancer Institute.[1-5] A series of experiments was done to evaluate the tolerance of normal retroperitoneal structures including the aorta, vena cava, kidney, ureters, bile duct, and retroperitoneal soft tissues. In addition, attempts were made to define the tolerance of surgically manipulated tissues such as vascular and intestinal anastomoses. Animals were irradiated with doses of 20 to 50 Gy delivered in a single fraction with an 11 MeV electron beam. Dogs were selected as the animal model so that the size of the normal structures would be as close as possible to that in humans. Table 15–13 outlines the results of the experiments.[1-5] The data can be summarized as follows: high doses of radiation are poorly tolerated by functioning organ systems, such as the liver and kidney, and by hollow viscous organs, especially those with small diameter (ureter, bile duct, bowel), while the retroperitoneal soft tissues, vessels, and bones all appear to tolerate even the highest dose without significant complications.

Additional studies were performed to determine the tolerance of surgically manipulated tissues because of the likelihood that manipulated bowel or blood vessels might often be in the radiation field when IORT is combined. These studies (Table 15–14) indicate the feasi-

**TABLE 15-13  Normal Tissue Tolerance to IORT in Dogs**

| Tissue | Maximum Tolerated Dose(Gy) | Tissue Effect |
|--------|---------------------------|---------------|
| Aorta, vena cava | 50 | Wall fibrosis at $> 30$ Gy |
| Kidney | <20 | Atrophy and fibrosis |
| Ureter | 20 | Fibrosis and stenosis |
| Bile duct | <20 | Fibrosis and stenosis |
| Small intestine | <20 | Ulceration, fibrosis, and stenosis at $>20$ Gy |
| Colon | 15 | Ulceration, fibrosis, and stenosis at $>15$ Gy |

*Source:* Refs. 1–5.

**TABLE 15-14  Radiation Tolerance of Surgically Manipulated Tissue of Dogs to IORT**

| Tissue | Maximum Tolerated Dose(Gy) | Tissue Effect |
|--------|---------------------------|---------------|
| Aortic anastomosis | 20 | Fibrosis and stenosis at $> 20$ Gy; no anastomosis or disruption at $> 45$ Gy |
| Biliary anastomosis | <20 | Anatomotic breakdown at $> 20$ Gy |
| Defunctionalized small intestine | 45 | Fibrosis and stenosis at $> 20$ Gy; no suture-line breakdown at $> 45$ Gy |

*Source:* Refs. 1–5.

**TABLE 15-15    Tolerance of Canine Retroperitoneal Tissue to IORT/EBRT from Colorado State University**

| Tissue | End Point | Estimated Maximum Tolerated Dose: IORT + EBRT |
|---|---|---|
| Aorta Wall | Aneurysms | 30 Gy IORT |
| Branch arteries | Thromboses, narrowing | 20 Gy IORT + 50 Gy EBRT |
| Ureter | Radiographic abnormalities | 25 Gy IORT; 17.5 Gy IORT + 50 Gy EBRT |
| Muscle | Muscle fibers decrease, vessel lesions | 20–25 Gy IORT + 50 Gy EBRT |
| Bone | Necrosis | 15–20 Gy IORT + 50 Gy EBRT |

*Source:* Refs. 6–12.

bility of combining IOERT with extensive surgical resections, although there are areas in which significant toxicity can result.[1–5]

Gillete et al. have undertaken prospective long-term studies (2–5 years) of the response of normal tissues in a canine model to IOERT, IOERT with fractionated EBRT, and EBRT alone.[6–12] Beagles were allocated to one of three treatment arms: IOERT only, with single doses of 15 to 50 Gy; IOERT with single doses ranging from 10 to 42.5 Gy; EBRT with 50 Gy given in 2 Gy fractions over 5 weeks; or 60, 70, or 80 Gy given in 30 fractions of 2, 2.33, or 2.67 Gy over 6 weeks. These investigators performed detailed clinical, radiologic, physiologic, and pathologic analysis of irradiated aorta, branch arteries, ureter, bone, and peripheral nerves. The results of these studies (Table 15–15) show that the toxicity of combined IOERT and EBRT is predominantly due to the effect of IOERT, not EBRT, on normal tissues; IOERT doses of 10 to 20 Gy, when combined with EBRT, are the maximum tolerable doses for blood vessels, ureter, bone, and peripheral nerve; and previous experimental and clinical data have probably underestimated the long-term tolerance of normal tissues to IOERT.

## TECHNICAL ASPECTS OF IOERT

At the Massachusetts General Hospital (MGH), there is a dedicated IOERT suite within the operating room (Figure 15–15). This facility simplifies the integration of IOERT with surgery and permits complete operating room capability as well as delivery of IOERT. There is no requirement of a transport process from the operating room to a radiation therapy suite, and operating room personnel (anesthesiogists, OR nursing, and surgeons) remain in a familiar working environment.

The MGH facility employs the Siemens ME accelerator, which provides electron energies ranging from 6 to 18 MeV. This system utilizes a "soft" dock system in which there is no physical contact between the cone and the linear accelerator. In the "soft" dock system, the cone is secured in the patient by a modified Bookwalter retraction system. There is no further movement of the cone in the patient after it has been immobilized. Once the patient is under the radiation therapy machine, geometric alignment of the treatment cone with the gantry head is achieved by a laser alignment system with appropriate couch movement and gantry rotation.

A large variety of applicators of different sizes and geometries are available to tailor the treatment to the individual anatomy and topography of the tumor bed. For treatment of the tumors that are commonly irradiated (rectal cancer with pelvic sidewall or sacral involvement, pancreas, bile duct, gastric bed, and abdominal or pelvic lymph node diseases), round cylinders are available at 6, 7, 8, and 9 cm, both with no bevel on the edge of the cylinder and with a 15° and a 30° bevel for each of the nominal cylinder diameters. Small diameter cylinders of 3 and 4 cm are sometimes useful but have a more limited application. For treatment of some pancreatic tumors and for intra-abdominal tumors such as gastric carcinoma,

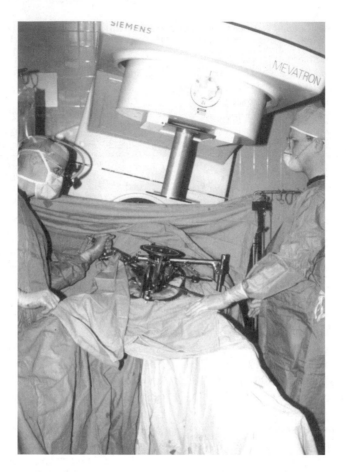

FIGURE 15-15    Intraoperative radiation therapy setup for a patient with rectal cancer in the full-time dedicated IORT suite at the Massachusetts General Hospital.

retroperitoneal sarcomas, and colonic tumors, either rectangular or elliptical applicators should be available. Elliptical applicators of 12 × 9 cm$^2$ and 9 × 7 cm$^2$ have been very helpful and are easier to position than rectangular ones. An applicator called the "squircle," which has one end circular and the other end rectangular simplifies the problem of field abutment in patients who require more than one IOERT field.

At the time of surgery, the tumor volume (tumor bed after resection or unresectable tumor) to be irradiated is defined by the surgeon and the radiation oncologist, and marking sutures are placed around the perimeter of the lesion. An applicator is then selected that encompasses the tumor bed, usually with a 1 cm margin. A margin of at least 1 cm is optimal to allow for both dose and tumor variabilities. When one is visualizing the tumor or tumor bed through the cone, the marking sutures should be readily identified well within the perimeter of the cone, thus ensuring adequate coverage of the the tumor volume.

If a cone with a bevel is used, it is easy to overestimate the beam coverage toward the heel of the bevel (depth of penetration is less at heel versus toe end of beveled cone). Because tissues directly below the heel may be underdosed, the treatment cylinder must be carefully placed. In addition, the bevel decreases the total beam penetration from what would be obtained without a bevel.

Although the IOERT cone can often function adequately as a normal tissue retractor to hold sensitive normal structures out of the IOERT field, patient respiration or spontaneous movement of the bowel can allow normal tissues to move under the cone, insinuating themselves inside the intraoperative field. The cone must be observed to confirm that this is not occurring. If there is evidence that bowel or other normal tissues are slipping into the IOERT field, surgical packing must be used to hold them out of the way. It is important that the packing itself does not itself enter into the field because this would decrease the electron beam penetration, resulting in underdosage of a portion of the tumor volume.

In certain situations, normal tissues cannot be physically moved out of the radiation field. Thus, it is essential that a technique be available for secondary shielding. We have available standard lead sheets, which can be cut to the appropriate shape and an appropriate number used to attenuate 90% of the radiation beam. The lead is covered with saline-soaked gauze and placed over the normal tissues. Lead shielding is often essential if abutting IOERT fields are to be used. Other methods for secondary collimation may be employed, but we have found this method to be effective.

IOERT is currently utilized as a component of a comprehensive treatment program of pre- or postoperative external beam irradiation (45–54 Gy in 25–28 fractions), frequently with concurrent chemotherapy and surgery for a locally advanced malignancy. Because most patients have received a course of full dose external beam irradiation, IOERT doses usually are in the range of 7.5 to 20 Gy. The selection of dose as well as electron energy depends on the amount of residual tumor remaining after maximal resection. Guidelines are as follows: resection margin negative but narrow, 7.5 to 10 Gy; margin microscopically positive or res(m), 10 to 12.5 Gy; gross residual, res(g), 2 cm or less in largest diameter, 15 Gy, unresected or res(g) of 2 cm or greater, 17.5 to 20 Gy. Doses of 20 Gy or higher are not utilized unless there have been limitations of delivery of external beam irradiation.

## RESULTS OF SELECTED CLINICAL STUDIES USING IOERT

### Locally Advanced Rectal Cancer

In an effort to improve local control and survival in patients with locally advanced rectal carcinoma, investigators at MGH, Mayo Clinic, and other centers have used a combination of high dose preoperative radiation therapy, surgical resection, and IOERT in patients with residual disease, positive surgical margins, or persisting tumor adherence.[13–15] Because of the propensity of rectal cancer to remain localized in a substantial number of patients, this seemed to be an excellent site in which to test the utility of this approach.

Patients eligible for this protocol were thought by their respective referring surgeons to have disease that was locally advanced and beyond the realm of surgical resection with curative intent. Generally, the area of adherence and fixation was on the pelvic sidewall or the sacrum, but occasionally it was on the prostate. These patients were treated with preoperative radiation therapy by a four-field technique to the pelvis to a total dose of 45 Gy in 25 fractions over 5 weeks. With reduced fields, additional irradiation to the primary tumor was usually given to a total dose of 50.4 Gy. During the early period of this study (1978–1985), patients did not receive 5-fluorouracil (5-FU) during the course of external beam irradiation. Beginning in 1986, patients received 5-FU (500 mg/m$^2$/d) for 3 consecutive days during the first and last weeks of irradiation, usually the first 3 and last 3 days. More recently, the administration of 5-FU has changed. Since 1994, patients received 5-FU as a protracted venous infusion (225 mg/m$^2$/24h) throughout the 5- to 6-week course of preoperative radiation therapy.

Four to six weeks after completion of radiation therapy, patients underwent laparotomy. At surgery, the abdomen was examined, and diversion or resection was performed if any metastoses were found. These patients were excluded from analysis. Patients without metastases underwent either an abdominoperineal resection, low anterior resection, or exenteration. In most patients, gross removal of tumor was carried out. In the remainder, subtotal resection was carried out, leaving as little residual cancer at the points of adherence as feasible. Close attention was paid to sites of tumor adherence during the resection. For patients undergoing gross total resection of their tumor, the specimen was taken to the frozen section pathology laboratory, where the tumor was grossly and microscopically examined for margin status. Patients who were found to have no tumor adherence and had negative margins did not receive IOERT. Patients with residual tumor or patients with positive or close ($<$ 5 mm) margins were then evaluated for IOERT.

The technique of IOERT at the Massachusetts General Hospital has been described elsewhere.[13,15] The area at highest risk was defined jointly by the surgeon and the radiation oncologist, with the most common site being the pelvic sidewall or the sacrum. From our library of cones with various angles and sizes, an appropriate cone was selected to direct the electron beam to the tumor bed in the pelvis. By 9 to 15 MeV electon beam, a dose of 10 to 20 Gy was delivered to the tumor bed. The lower doses were given for minimum residual disease and the higher doses for gross residual cancer after resection.

The 5-year actuarial local control and disease-specific survival for 45 patients with primary locally advanced rectal cancer undergoing complete resection with IOERT was 89% and 63%, respectively.[13] For patients undergoing partial resection, local control and disease-specific survival correlated with the extent of residual cancer: 68% and 40%, respectively, for microscopic residual disease, and 57% and 14%, respectively, for gross residual disease. The results have been less satisfactory for patients with recurrent rectal cancer, regardless of extent of resection.[15] The 5-year actuarial local control and disease-free survival of 27 patients undergoing complete re-resection (7 patients with microscopic residual) was 47% and 21%, respectively. By contrast, the outcome of 14 patients undergoing partial resection was poor, with 5-year local control and survival of 21% and 7%, respectively.

The combined use of high dose preoperative EBRT, surgical resection, and IOERT has generally been well tolerated. The perineal wounds usually heal without difficulty in patients with primary disease, and there is no detectable increase in the complication rate over that in patients treated with surgery and EBRT alone. In patients with locally advanced recurrent disease, the complication rate is higher. Potential morbidity includes peripheral neuropathy and soft tissue injury.

In summary, data from the MGH and Mayo Clinic give good evidence of the beneficial effect of IOERT when combined with high dose EBRT and surgical resection in patients with locally advanced primary rectal carcinoma and show a meaningful salvage rate in the patients with locally advanced recurrent disease.

## Retroperitoneal Sarcomas

Despite impressive advances in surgery and radiation therapy, the management of patients with retroperitoneal sarcoma remains a therapeutic challenge.[16,17] Published series of surgical resection alone for retroperitoneal sarcoma have shown poor local control rates and survival rates. Because of the infiltrative nature of these tumors and and their anatomic origin, it is frequently difficult to obtain macroscopically and microscopically clear resection margins. The efficacy of EBRT after resection is unclear from published reports. Because of the large size of these tumors, significant volumes of normal tissue (liver, small bowel, stomach, kidney, or spinal cord) may be within the EBRT field, and treatment is frequently limited to 45 to 50 Gy in 1.8 Gy or 2 Gy fractions. It is not surprising that the local failure rate remains unacceptably high after postoperative irradiation because of the dose limitations of normal tissue to EBRT and the likelihood of at least microscopic residual disease after resection. In an effort to improve the local control and survival in patients with retroperitoneal sarcoma, treatment strategies employing IOERT with preoperative or postoperative EBRT and surgery have been explored.

The current treatment approach at the Massachusetts General Hospital for patients with nonmetastatic retroperitoneal sarcoma is to utilize moderate dose preoperative irradiation (40–50 Gy), surgical resection, and IOERT (if technically feasible).[16,17] The preoperative EBRT approach is favored for many reasons. First, a high dose preoperative regimen sterilizes a large percentage of tumor cells and may minimize the risk of tumor implantation in the peritoneal cavity after the marginal resection has been performed. Second, partial regression obtained from EBRT may allow a more complete resection to be performed. Third, these large tumors usually displace abdominal and retroperitoneal viscera to a degree that large volumes of radiosensitive organs such as the stomach and small bowel can be effectively excluded from the preoperative EBRT field. Because of this reduction of normal tissue irradiation by the tumor's displacement of viscera outside the radiation field, it is usually feasible to give daily doses of 1.8 Gy with excellent tolerance, an approach that may not be feasible if contemplated postoperatively.

Anterior–posterior and posterior–anterior fields with 5 cm margins are commonly used, since these tumors frequently extend from the retroperitoneal surface to the anterior abdominal wall. Occasionally, oblique fields are helpful in minimizing the dose to normal structures such as the spinal cord and kidney. Patients with right-sided or left-sided lesions sometimes can receive a portion or all of their treatment in the decubitus position to displace small bowel loops away from the tumor bed. If tumor bed irradiation requires the inclusion of one kidney to doses beyond tolerance, blood urea nitrogen and creatinine levels should be obtained. An intravenous pyelogram (IVP), CT scan with IV contrast, or renal scan is useful to document normal contralateral renal function.

Four to six weeks after completion of EBRT, exploratory laparotomy is performed in the dedicated IOERT suite. At surgery, the abdomen–pelvis is carefully examined for metastases to the liver and/or peritoneal surfaces. If no metastases are found, the patient undergoes resection of the tumor, leaving as little residual sarcoma as possible. If no gross tumor remains, frozen section pathologic analysis is carried out on the specimen from areas at greatest risk for residual disease. Biopsy specimens are obtained to examine for the presence of residual sarcoma in the tumor bed. The areas at highest risk for local tumor recurrence are defined by the surgeon and radiation oncologist.

To direct the IOERT, applicators (circular, elliptical, or rectangular) are used. Applicator geometry and size are carefully selected to fully cover the high risk area. The electron energy is selected according to the desired depth of penetration and ranges typically between 9 and 15 MeV. The dose is dependent on amount of residual disease and volume treated. For patients with completely resected tumors and negative margins, an IOERT dose of 10 Gy is usually selected, whereas a grossly resected tumor bed with positive microscopic margins will receive 12.5 to 15 Gy (depending on volume treated). For gross residual disease, doses will range from 15 to 20 Gy, depending on the extent of residual tumor and volume treated.

The Massachusetts General Hospital experience of IOERT in the management of retroperitoneal sarcoma in a group of 20 patients with either primary ($n = 14$) or recurrent ($n = 6$) disease has been reviewed.[16] In contrast to other institutions, these patients routinely received preoperative EBRT, which was followed by exploratory laparotomy and IOERT. Seventeen of the 20 patients underwent laparotomy and 14 had a complete resection. Three patients had a partial resection, and distant metastasis developed during EBRT in 3 patients. IOERT was given to 12 of the 14 patients. The 4-year actuarial local control and disease-free survival of the 14 patients undergoing complete resection was 81% and 64%, respectively. Doses used were 40 to 50 Gy EBRT at 1.7 to 2.0 Gy per fraction and 10 to 20 Gy IOERT with 9 to 15 MeV electrons. The time interval between EBRT and surgery was 4 to 6 weeks. In this series five patients developed complications: two with hydronephrosis, two (17%) with sensory neuropathy, and one with a small-bowel obstruction. Based on this experience, the current treatment policy is to limit the IOERT dose to 10 to 15 Gy for microscopic residual and 17 to 20 Gy for macroscopic residual disease.

## SUMMARY

In the past 20 years, there has been significant laboratory and clinical experience in the use of IOERT. Because of this experience, single high doses of radiation therapy can be delivered to a tumor volume in appropriate clinical situations without producing significant normal tissue morbidity. Most important, this high dose of additional radiation treatment appears to improve local control of selected tumors. A combination of EBRT, surgical resection, and IOERT for patients with locally advanced rectal carcinoma and retroperitoneal sarcoma has yielded excellent local control and higher survival. The future of IOERT will be in the successful integration of this therapy into multimodality treatment programs of chemotherapy, external beam irradiation, and surgery for locally advanced head and neck, thoracic, abdominal, and pelvic malignancies.

## REFERENCES

1. Tepper JE, Sindelar W, Travis EL, et al: Tolerance of canine anastomoses to intraoperative radiation therapy. *Int J Radiat Oncol Biol Phys* 1983;9:987–992.

2. Sindelar W, Tepper JE, Travis EL: Tolerance of bile duct to intraoperative irradiation. *Surgery* 1980;2:533–542.

3. Sindelar WF, Kinsella T, Tepper JE, et al: Experimental and clinical studies with intraoperative radiotherapy. *Surg Gynecol Obstet* 1983; 157:205–218.

4. Sindelar WF, Tepper JE, Travis EL. Tolerance of retroperitoneal structures to intraoperative radiation. *Ann Surg* 1981;5:601–608.

5. Kinsella TJ, Sindelar WF, Deluca AM, et al: Tolerance of peripheral nerve to IORT: Clinical and experimental studies. *Int J Radiat Biol Oncol Phys* 1985;11:1579–1585.

6. Ahmadu-Suka F, Gillette EL, Withrow SJ, et al: Pathologic response of the pancreas and duodenum to experimental intraoperative irradiation. *Int J Radiat Oncol Biol Phys* 1988;14:1197–1204.

7. Gillette EL, Powers BE, McChesney SL, et al: Aortic wall injury following intraoperative irradiation. *Int J Radiat Oncol Biol Phys* 1988;15:1401–1406.

8. LeCouteur RA, Gillette EL, Powers BE, et al: Peripheral neuropathies following experimental intraoperative radiation therapy (IORT). *Int J Radiat Oncol Biol Phys* 1989;17:583–590.

9. Hoopes PJ, Gillette EL, Withrow SJ, et al: Intraoperative irradiation of the canine abdominal aorta and vena cava. *Int J Radiat Oncol Biol Phys* 1989;17:583–590.

10. McChesney SL, Gillette EL, Powers BE, et al: Ureteral injury following experimental intraoperative radiation therapy. *Int J Radiat Oncol Biol Phys* 1989;17:791–798.

11. Powers BE, Gillette EL, McChesney SL, Gillette EL, et al: Bone necrosis and tumor induction following experimental intraoperative irradiation. *Int J Radiat Oncol Biol Phys* 1989;17: 599–567.

12. Powers BE, Gillette EL, McChesney SL, et al: Muscle injury following experimental intraoperative irradiation. *Int J Radiat Oncol Biol Phys* 1991;20:463–471.

13. Nakfoor BM, Willett CG, Shellito PC, Kaufman DS, et al: The impact of 5-fluorouracil and intraoperative electron beam radiation therapy on the outcome of patients with locally advanced primary rectal and rectosigmoid cancer. *Ann of Surg* (in press).

14. Gunderson LL, Nelson H, Martenson JA, et al: Locally advanced primary colorectal cancer: Intraoperative electron and external beam irradiation + 5-FU. *Int J Radiat Oncol Biol Phys* 1997;37:601–614.

15. Wallace HJ, Willett CG, Shellito PC, Coen JJ, Hoover HC: Intraoperative radiation therapy for locally advanced recurrent rectal or rectosigmoid cancer. *J Surg Oncol* 1995;60: 122–127.

16. Willett CG, Suit HD, Tepper JE, et al: Intra-operative electron beam radiation therapy for retroperitoneal sarcoma. *Cancer* 1991;68: 278–283.

17. Gunderson LL, Nagorney DM, McIlrath DC, et al: External beam and intraoperative electron irradiation for locally advanced soft tissue sarcomas. *Int J Radiat Oncol Biol Phys* 1993;25: 647–656.

# D. 3D Conformed Radiation Therapy -

JULIAN G. ROSENMAN

## INTRODUCTION

The concept of radiation treatment planning, that is, the modeling of a treatment plan before it is implemented, is quite old, perhaps dating to the 1930s.[1] Radiation portals were designed mainly by using external patient anatomic landmarks to determine the location of the tumor. The dose calculations had to be done by hand, and thus were often limited to a single point or, at most, a midplane dose. As a result, the number of alternative treatment plans that could be produced for clinical consideration was necessarily quite limited. By 1970, the advent of computerized dosimetry made it possible to calculate the dose at many points within a plane, and connect points of equal radiation dosage into isodose lines, which greatly aided the understanding of a complex 2-D treatment plan. It was also possible to consider many alternative treatment plans, and thus individualize treatment somewhat.

CT scanning, available after 1975, significantly changed the way radiation treatment planning was performed. At first CT scans were used mainly to assist the radiation oncologist in identifying the volume to be treated. By the 1980s a technique known CT-based treatment planning, which overlayed CT slices with the radiation dose distribution, made it possible to know in detail how much radiation dose would be delivered to any given organ.[2]

Full 3-D treatment planning systems that allowed one to build and manipulate 3-D patient models, and design and display entire 3-D treatment plans first became available in the 1990s.[3] Such systems could calculate a "beam's-eye view"[4] which shows the clinician exactly which organs and tissue volumes are included within the beams, and allows the clinician to be sure that the tumor target drawn on the simulation film is the proper projection of the tumor as seen on the planning CT. State-of-the-art treatment planning systems now allow data from multiple imaging studies to be utilized in the planning process,[5] and permit one to shape or "conform" radiation dose distributions around the desired tumor target, while substantially limiting the dose to nearby dose-sensitive normal tissue.[6] These new capabilities have introduced changes into the practice of radiotherapy that are as profound as those wrought by the advent of the simulator and linear accelerator. However, as many radiation oncologists are not yet familiar with some of the basic concepts involved in 3-D planning, it is the goal of this chapter to explain these ideas and show how they can be used to solve everyday problems that emerge during everyday clinical practice.

## THE PLANNING PROCESS

### Acquiring the CT

3-D planning begins by acquiring a CT scan of the patient in the treatment position.[7] This is important, because tumor and normal anatomy can move substantially, depending on the patient's position. Ideally the patient should be scanned and treated in the same immobilization device. An insert into the CT table should be used to make it flat, much like the treatment table. Marks must be placed onto the cast to indicate the position of the first (or any other selected) scan in anticipation of the eventual need to correlate the CT data with the actual patient. Scanning must be done over a wide area, encompassing the suspected tumor volume with generous superior and inferior margins. Beams placed out of the transverse plane will not exit (or worse, enter) through volumes that have not been scanned. In addition, care must be taken to ensure that organs at risk for radiation damage are scanned in their entirety. For example, in the treatment of lung cancer the entire lung volume must be scanned so that one may determine what percentage of the *whole* lung will be destroyed by the radiation. Some institutions prefer to simulate the patient with approximate fields before the CT scanning, but we have found the use of a scout view on the scanner sufficient to determine upper and lower scanning borders. Typically 80–100 4-mm-thick CT slices will be obtained, but thicker slices away from the tumor can be used to reduce the size of the data set, and ultra-thin slices (2 mm) may sometimes be helpful over the tumor itself. All CT slices should be contiguous. Once this data is obtained the patient can be sent home. All subsequent work will be done on the model generated from this data.

### Image segmentation

To simplify the planning process, the enormous amount of data collected by the CT scanner must be organized and managed. The first step is to *segment* the CT image into tumor and critical normal structures. Formally, image segmentation means assigning regions of the CT image to named objects. For example, in lung cancer, one might draw contours around the lungs, heart, and spinal cord. This data may be used later, for example to calculate what percentage of the lung receives more than 2000 cGy, what percentage of the heart receives more than 4000 cGy, and what is the highest dose any of the spinal cord receives. Unfortunately, much of this segmentation must be done by hand. Implementation of an accurate, automatic method of image segmentation for all but the most highly contrasted organs remains an elusive goal of computer scientists who work on image processing.[8]

Tumor identification remains the quintessential task of the radiation oncologist—it is unlikely that this task can ever be satisfactorily automated. In general at least three distinct volumes must be identified. Following the recommendations of the ICRU 50[9] report, we call the first of these volumes the "gross tumor volume" or GTV. The GTV is defined as the lump, or abnormality seen on the planning CT. Sometimes the GTV will consist only of the primary tumor, other times it may also include the lymph nodes or other sites of tumor spread. In some cases, for example, in post-operative rectal cancer, there may be no GTV at all.

The second volume, the "clinical tumor volume" or CTV is much more difficult to determine than the GTV. The CTV includes all the volume that the clinician thinks might reasonably be involved with tumor, gross or microscopic. Obviously the CTV must take into account the history and physical examination, tumor grade, location, and other clinical data. In some cases, the CTV may be little more than the GTV, expanded slightly to allow for microscopic direct spread. In other cases, it may be much bigger than the GTV.

The third volume is the "planning target volume" or PTV. The PTV includes the CTV plus a margin for both internal organ motion and patient motion. In the past, clinicians used to simply allow 0.5 to 1.0 cms for motion in all directions, but new work has enabled us to draw PTVs in a more sophisticated fashion.[10] For example, it is now known that the prostate can move in anteriorly or posteriorly, but rarely left or right. A PTV can drawn to take advantage of that knowledge. Note that the PTV does not take into account radiation field penumbra. The actual radiation portals (treatment volume or TV) will have to be expanded slightly over the PTV to be sure the tumor dosimetry is acceptable.

### Portal Design

Once the planning CT data is properly segmented, it can then be used as a model for the planning process. We have found three distinct visualizations of this data to be useful in this regard.[11] First, of course, are the CT slices and contours themselves. Ultimately, all proposed radiation beams, and the resultant dose distribution must be overlaid on this data set. (The upper middle panel in Figure 15–16 shows a CT slice with beams overlaid.) However, the CT slices are a poor visualization on which to design the beams. Not only would it be awkward to specify the beams on all 80 slices, but it would actually be impossible to do, unless the CT slices were parallel to the beam at each level, which they cannot be because of beam divergence, let alone if a nontransverse planar beam were used.

A second visualization, that of the beam's-eye view, is much more useful for construction of radiation portals. In its simplest form the beam's-eye view takes the form of a collection of "wireloops" or contours that can be 3-D rotated in real time. The contours represent the tumor or normal tissue that is seen by the radiation beam (in the radiation beam), hence the name "beam's-eye view." In theory, this display should suffice for beam design as the PTV contains all the volume to be treated as determined from the planning CT. In practice the plane radiograph, and its bony landmarks are sometimes indispensable for determining the PTV, especially when the PTV is large compared to the GTV, as, for example, in head and neck cancer. As a result, fields designed strictly around the PTV contours often look odd and incomplete when projected onto the simulation film.

We have found that the beam's-eye view becomes entirely satisfactory only when the PTV contours are displayed on top of a synthetic simulation film. Such a display, known technically as a "digitally reconstructed radiograph" or DRR[12] is formed by mathematically casting rays through the stack of CT slices and adding up the sum of the CT densities each ray passes through. (The direction of the rays is determined by the geometry of the beam's-eye

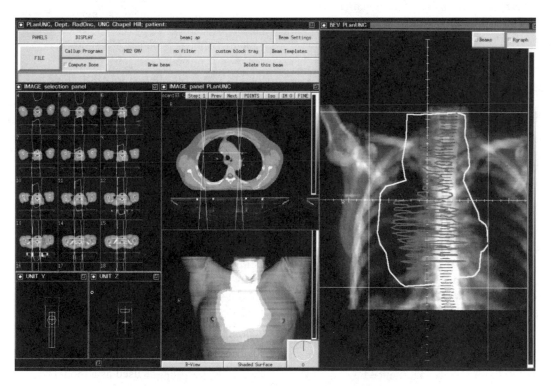

**FIGURE 15–16** Portal design using a 3-D treatment planning system.

view.) After some heuristic adjustment for the fact that CT scanner typically use higher energies than do planar x-rays, the sum of CT densities can be represented as a gray-scale color image. This image looks remarkably like an ordinary x-ray, which is not surprising as its mathematical construction models what actually happens when an x-ray is taken. The resultant "contours + DRR display" seen in the right panel of Figure 15–16 is a natural and easy image on which to draw portal outlines.

With the advent of cheap, fast computer hardware and sophisticated image processing algorithms, it is possible to produce displays such as Figure 15–16 at interactive rates.[13] The clinician can then "rotate the gantry" to any desired angle and see the resultant DRR + contours, almost as on a fluoroscopy unit. The computer, of course, can be programmed to draw a portal outline a specified distance from the PTV, and even to avoid certain specified anatomic structures. The resultant portal outline then twists and reshapes itself as the clinician tries out a number of beam angles to determine what is best for the patient. At any time he can also see how these beams overlay the original CT data.

A third display that is sometimes useful is shown in the center bottom panel of Figure 15–16. A mathematical alteration of the DRR algorithms makes surfaces appear (an x-ray or DRR normally shows no surfaces). The resultant image, known as a "volume rendering" looks remarkably like the patient and can show the beam orientations on the skin.[14] This display is often helpful as a final check of the treatment plan, much as going into the room and seeing the beam on the patient is helpful. Over the years it has alerted us to such undesirable errors as having the external auditory canal in a head and neck portal, not covering the entire breast surface in a treatment for breast cancer, or having the penis in the field during treatment for prostate cancer. In each case this information could have been obtained in other ways (from the DRR, or directly from the CT data) but the volume rendering made it much more explicit, and therefore likely to be noticed.

## Output of a 3-D Planning System

We now skip over the difficult issue of dose calculation, display, and optimization to address the issue of accurately implementing a given radiation treatment plan. Ultimately there must be some way to deliver each radiation beam that has been designed with certainty that it is being done correctly. We accomplish this task by having the planning system print out a stylized set-up instruction set, and the DRR itself. The DRR is printed by the same kind of printer that makes CT scan pictures and can be treated like an ordinary x-ray. The patient then undergoes an ordinary simulation (check-film simulation) using the set-up instructions. The resulting simulation film should match the DRR within a few millimeters as shown in Figure 15–17. In our experience this is usually the case, especially if the patient has been well immobilized. In cases of less than adequate immobilization, some adjustment of the patient position during check-film simulation needs be done to make the real film match the computed one. It has been suggested by some that if adequate immobilization has been used, this step could be skipped altogether with the resultant cost savings. In our institution we usually compare the port film to the DRR, not the simulation film; likewise if shaping blocks are to be used they can be cut from the DRR as well (multileaf collimator settings are sent directly from the planning system to the treatment machines).

## Naming Radiation Fields

Because any beam angle may be chosen in a 3-D planning system, even ones not in the transverse plane, some systematic way to name the fields is needed. Diagnostic radiology uses terms such as "right anterior oblique," which not only is the name for all beams angled from 1–89 degrees, but is reversed from what radiation oncologists usually mean as an RAO. Such nomenclature also does not informatively name a beam that comes in from 20 degrees superiorly, for example.

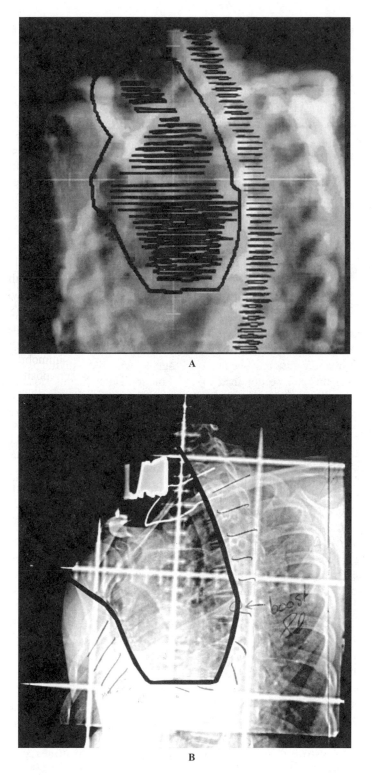

**FIGURE 15.17(A)**    A DRR of a lung simulation film. **(B)** The corresponding conventional simulation film.

At our institution we name each radiation beam by how many degrees away from a primary direction it is angled. The six primary directions are anterior, posterior, right (not right, lateral), left, superior, and inferior. So a beam angled twenty degrees to patients right would be called an "anterior, right 20" or A2OR for short. An A6OR would, rather, be called an R30A. A beam 20 degrees to the right, 15 degrees superior would be called A20R05S. A typical "oblique pair" for treating lung cancer would be A20R, P20L.[15]

## Multimodality Imaging

Suppose the planning CT fails to show the GTV. This can happen for several reasons: because the tumor has been removed surgically or cytoreduced by chemotherapy, or because CT is not the best imaging modality as often is the case for brain tumors, for example. To use such images the digital imaging data must be available. In some cases this can be obtained directly from the imaging machine (CT or MRI), but if the scan has been done at an outside institution, the digital data is probably not obtainable. In that case the films can be scanned, and the digital data reconstituted. Great care must be taken with this data (and all multimodality data) to allow for the many artifacts that are introduced when diagnostic films are obtained.[16] These artifacts include, but are not limited to arbitrary changes in pixel size, z-spacing, image center, and table height. Diagnostic studies are sometimes not obtained contiguously. Sometimes certain slices are missing and must be reconstructed using linear interpolation. A particularly dangerous situation can arise when a CT study is obtained with *gantry tilt.* When the gantry is tilted the z-axis (which lies in the plane of the table) is no longer perpendicular to the scan plane and *shear* is introduced into the image. To use this data it must be de-sheared by resampling the image. A further caution is that MR slices, as opposed to CT, are usually not entirely space-filling in the sense that the slices do not extend upwards and downwards enough to touch their neighbors. The opposite problem is occasionally seen in CT where the slices can be overlapping.

Once the multimodality data is obtained it must be registered with the planning CT. Many commercial systems offer rudimentary ways to do this; most such methods fail outside the brain. This is particularly unfortunate because sophisticated registration methods have been available in the non-medical world for a long time, and much is known about how to achieve good registrations.[17] For the physician who feels that registration of images is not necessary for radiation treatment plan we point out that all of treatment planning require registration of outside images with the planning CT, of the planning CT with the simulation film, and of the simulation film to the patient. The only question is whether this registration is to be done explicitly on the computer, or in the mind of the physician only. In any event, once an image is registered with the planning CT it is possible to display beams, doses, or all other data upon it.

How much value is this use of multimodality imaging? The answer is not completely known[18-19] but difference in tumor placement can reach 5 cm between CT and MR in the brain.[20] In Figure 15–18 the tumors defined by these two modalities is quite different. Which is correct? Our policy is to perform a mathematical *union* between the CT- and MR-defined tumors and use the composite tumor as the correct one. Another way of viewing this is saying that if a given volume is thought to be tumor on any study, it should be considered tumor.

In the future, radiation treatment planning should not be limited to only CT and MR imaging. Nuclear medicine studies,[21-22] [Gritters 1993, Marks 1995], PET,[23] and nuclear resonance spectroscopy imaging all hold out promise for better tumor definition.[24]

## Conformal Dose Distributions

The ultimate goal of any treatment planning system should result in a treatment that gives a high, uniform dose to the tumor while sparing

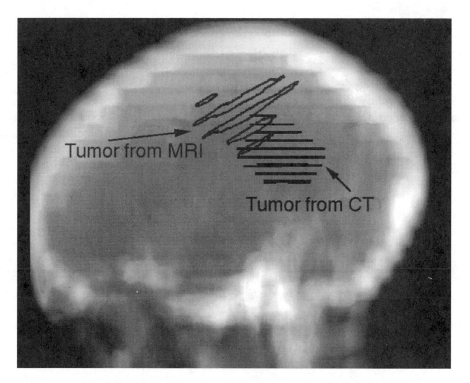

**FIGURE 15–18**    Comparison of tumor projected from MRI and CT.

normal tissue as much as possible. A dose distribution that mimics the shape of the PTV is said to be "conformal" from the mathematical term meaning "shape preserving." It is important to point out that conformal therapy does not necessary imply small, tight radiation fields. The term only implies that the dose is correctly shaped around the planning target volume, which might, in fact, be quite generous compared to the CTV or GTV.

How can a radiation dose distribution that conforms to the PTV be achieved? The answer is that multiple, properly shaped radiation beams are needed. These beams should be preferably well separated, but enter and exit through logical locations.[25] So far, this is not different from the approach with 2-D planning, except in 3-D the beams are not necessarily limited to the axial or transverse plane. 2-D planned beams that are not opposed often have to be wedged to reduce the hot spots that may occur between the beams. The formula relating

the hinge angle to wedge angle is well known, and the wedges are oriented with their thick edge toward each other. In addition, wedges are sometimes used to make up for "missing tissue." In 3-D the situation is much more complex. The reader might try to image how he would orient wedges for three perpendicular beams, for example. In 3-D "the missing tissue" problem also becomes more complex, and it seems doubtful that anything as simple as a wedge could adequately compensate for this. An obvious solution is to generalize the concept of a wedge by building a free-form shape that would compensate for both missing tissue and non-opposed beams to ensure a uniform tumor dose.

It is not enough just to have the radiation dose conform to the PTV. Sometimes there are nearby critical normal structures that must receive very little radiation dose. Consider the situation wherein there is painful metastatic disease throughout a vertebral body, but spinal cord, which is completely surrounded by bone, has already received its maximum tolerable dose. Is there a way to treat the vertebral body, but not the cord? At first, this might seem impossible, but consider a plan wherein seven planar beams are used with a cord block on each one. The cord now receives only the scatter dose (probably less than 20%), but the vertebral body receives a "patchy" dose, hot where all seven beams contribute, cold where fewer than 7 contribute (because of the cord blocks). Can modulating the intensity of one or more of the seven radiation beams smooth out the dose on the vertebral body, just as it did for missing tissue, or non-orthogonal beams? The experimental answer seems to be "yes," the vertebral body dose can be made quite uniform. Figure

15–19 shows a curve known as a cumulative dose-volume histogram (DVH) taken from the seven field vertebral body example. It shows that about 60% of the vertebral body is receiving 100% of the dose *or more*. None of the body is receiving more than 110%, and about 90% of the vertebral body receives at least 80% of the dose. DVHs are often much easier to understand than isodose curves in a full 3-D plan, because for a typical 3-D plan, 80–100 CT slices might be used. The DVH reduces all this data into a single diagram. Of course, like any statistic, there is a price to be paid for this data reduction. The DVH also shows that about 2% of the vertebral body receives only 40% of the dose. This is acceptable, if it is bone just adjacent to the cord—it is due to the penumbra

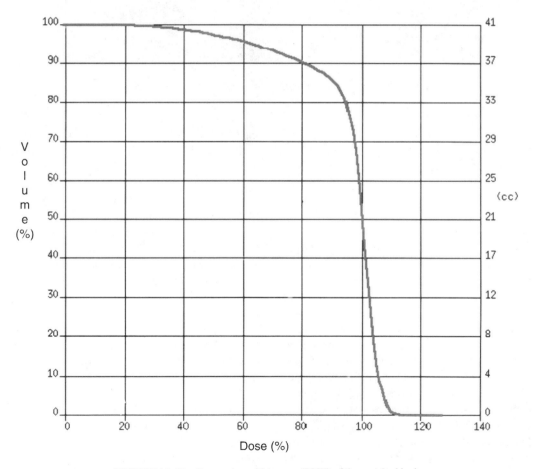

**FIGURE 15–19**    Dose-volume histogram (DVH) of the vertebral body.

effect of the blocks (this, in fact, *is* what is happening here, and the situation can be improved by making the cord block thinner). But the cold spot could be somewhere in the bone, perhaps in tumor. There is no way to tell from the DVH. The lesson here is that the DVH and isodose curves supplement each other; neither is satisfactory alone.

## Intensity Modulation and Dose Optimization

The previous example suggests a useful way to even further generalize the concept of a wedge. In addition to asking for a uniform tumor dose, could one also specify a desired dose distribution over the entire PTV and modulate the radiation beams to achieve it? This is known as the inverse problem,[26] and formal solutions to it are known. Unfortunately, in general, such solutions require that some of the radiation beams have negative weights. Put another way, many dose distributions cannot be obtained by any means. Using pure inverse methods, the clinician would have to sequentially ask for less and less until a solution could be reached with only positive beam weights. Such an approach to optimization can be slow and clumsy.

Forward planning presupposes that the clinician or the computer knows how to set up the ideal beam arrangement in advance.[27] The radiation beams are then modulated to make the dose uniform over the tumor. Certain dose restrictions could be placed on the doses received by other organs. However, to satisfy these secondary constraints, some dose homogeneity over the tumor has to be sacrificed. If the hot and cold spots over the tumor are deemed unacceptable then the restrictions on normal tissue need to be relaxed, or, perhaps, another beam arrangement picked. This, too, can be clumsy and time consuming, although with experience, certain beam arrangements for a given tumor site can be proven to be optimal, and then stored in the computer for routine use.

Elements of both the inverse and forward method of treatment planning can be combined into a single approach. One way to do this is to forward plan by picking a limited range of possible beam arrangements and then specifying limits on normal tissues, again sacrificing tumor homogeneity for normal tissue sparing. Then beam weights will always be positive, but those with a very small contribution to the treatment can be eliminated. If the beam range includes all, or most reasonable beam arrangements, there is no need to search further using other beam arrangements. Again, a trade-off between normal tissue sparing and tumor homogeneity must be made. One popular commercial system, the Peacock$^{TM28}$ has adopted this approach.

Earlier we said that radiation beams could be modulated by building generalized devices that act as wedges. This approach is certainly reasonable, but requires custom construction of a modulator for each patient, and, as for the case with custom blocks, it requires the therapist to physically change the modulator for each radiation beam. Another approach is to use the multileaf collimator as the beam intensity modulator.[29] Through the use of field shaping leaves, each radiation port can be replaced by a series of ports within a port that have the effect of treating the entire radiation beam unequally. Figure 15–20 illustrates how a modulator shape can be calculated, digitized, and converted into field shapes that can be rapidly delivered in an automatic fashion.

## Evaluation of Treatment Plans

The power of a 3-D treatment planning system to target a tumor in a number of ways raises the obvious question of which way is best. Put another way, how does one evaluate the merit of a given treatment plan?[30] Generally speaking, most treatment plans will either use just a few beams, and expose a moderate amount of normal tissue to very high radiation doses, or use many beams, and expose a lot of normal tissue to a rather low dose. Superimposed cumulative dose volume histograms for two such competing plans will always cross, as shown in Figure 15–21. Which curve will lead to the lowest normal tissue complication probability (NTCP)?

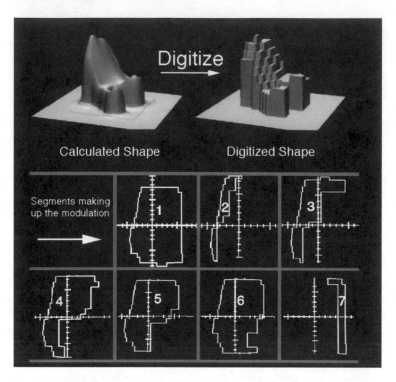

**FIGURE 15–20**    Changing physical to virtual modulators.

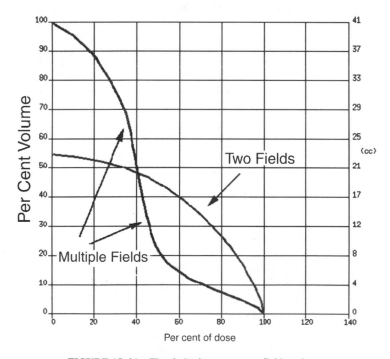

**FIGURE 15–21**    The choice between many fields and two.

There is a great deal of literature on NTCP[31–33] which attempts to model the probability of organ damage based on clinical information, and a detailed physiologic knowledge of the organ. However, all NTCP models to date must be regarded with caution by clinicians, as the work is still in the experimental phase.

Finally, it is not enough just to evaluate the NTCP for one tissue or organ. Rather, one must calculate NTCPs for all the organs at risk, and somehow combine these into a figure of merit (FOM) for the entire treatment. Evaluating the FOM for a treatment plan today remains very much a clinical judgment.

## CLINICAL USE OF 3-D TREATMENT PLANNING

Hard clinical data has not yet been accumulated to prove either that 3-D planning leads to higher tumor control or reduced treatment-related complications. However, some data is available that suggests that both these advantages of 3-D treatment planning may result in better patient outcome. Below is a brief summary of some of the better established clinical results.

### Brain

There is probably more experience treating brain tumors with 3-D treatment planning than for any other site. This is probably because it has been long recognized that locating brain tumors requires CT or MR, non-axial beams are easy to implement in the brain, and gliomas, at least, require doses for sterilization far beyond what can be safely achieved with normal planning techniques. There is now published data to suggest that conformal treatment to some parts of the brain might allow doses as high as 8000 cGy without undue complications. However, no improvement in survival in glioblastoma has yet been demonstrated at this dose level,[34–37] or in lower grade gliomas.[38] Doses in excess of 800 cGy are probably possible in some cases, so sterilization of glioblastoma

with external beam radiation may yet prove to be possible.

The brain is an important area of multi-modality targeting as the T1 weighted MRI often shows disease unsuspected on CT, and the T2 weighted MRI is the best way to image edema, thought by some to also harbor tumor cells.

### Head and Neck

Tumors of the base of floor of mouth or larynx probably do not need 3-D planning for tumor targeting. However, 3-D planning has revealed subtle effects of the junctioned fields, and has proved novel approaches to treating patients in whom a midline cord block is inappropriate.[38] 3-D treatment planning is also helpful (or even essential) to boost tumors of the base of tongue if a submental approach is used to spare the mandible. 3-D planning tumors of the sinuses can also be quite useful in targeting the tumors and potential pathways of spread, and in defining such structures as the floor of orbit. In addition, for some patients, novel beam arrangements made possible by 3-D planning can offer substantial benefits over conventional plans.[39–40]

Perhaps the most exciting use of 3-D planning for patients with head and neck cancer is parotid sparing through the use of novel beam arrangements and intensity modulation. Ongoing studies suggest that this is possible for many patients without a decrease in local tumor control. Furthermore, the technique results in substantial reduction in xerostomia, and a measurable increase in quality of life.[41–43]

### Lung

It is now known that conventional doses in the treatment of non-small cell lung cancer (NSCLC) of 6000 cGy are completely inadequate for local control.[44] Doses as high as 9000 cGy or more can be safely given to small, peripheral lesions.[45] At our institution we now routinely deliver 7400 to large central lesions with neoadjuvant and concomitant drug.[46] Of course great care must be taken not to overdose the esophagus and heart; dose-volume histograms of these organs must be obtained and found acceptable for such treatment to be safe. The relationship between the probability of developing severe radiation pneumonitis and dose-volume data is still poorly understood.[47] However, higher doses are still probably possible, although intensity modulation will probably be required. The survival advantage of these very high doses has not yet been demonstrated, although several trials are ongoing and should provide information on this question.[48–50]

## Breast

One would think that 3-D planning would not be needed for as obvious a target as breast cancer. It is our observation, however, that many patients suffer from sore spots in the breast or chest wall following radiation treatment. Some of this discomfort may be due to hot spots in the 3-D dose distribution.

It has been known for some time that the use of a wedge with the medial lateral tangent will often increase scatter to the contralateral breast.[51] While it is not known if this contalateral breast dose is harmful, the increased use of radiation for the treatment of DCIS must reduce our tolerance for inducing a cancer in the uninvolved breast. To reduce the dose to the contralateral breast some workers have suggested using only a single lateral wedge, but in many cases this worsens the dose inhomogeneity across the treated breast. Intensity modulation, even if used just with the lateral field, can produce a more homogeneous dose than can be obtained from two wedges.[52–53] This is because the wedges correct only for missing tissue in the anterior/posterior direction but not in the superior/inferior direction. Figure 15–22 is in a *differential* dose-volume histogram which compares the dose distribu-

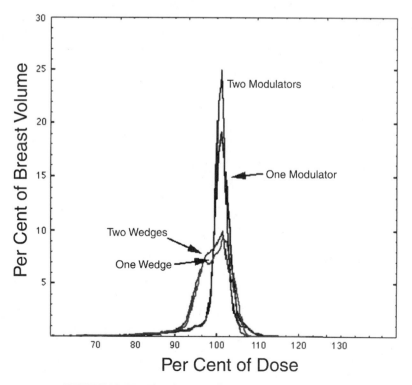

**FIGURE 15–22**    The advantage of modulation of a breast treatment.

tion across a breast for a one wedge, two wedge and one modulator and two modulators, showing the substantial improvement possible with intensity modulation.

## Prostate

After brain tumors, 3-D treatment planning probably has been most heavily used in the treatment of prostate cancer because it has been realized for a long time that traditional radiation doses were not sufficient for advanced disease.[54] In addition, the treatment of prostate cancer requires that a number of generic 3-D treatment planning problems be solved.

Perhaps the most fundamental problem to be solved in radiation treatment planning is tumor definition. Although the prostate seems to be seen well on CT, Wilder et al. have demonstrated that the prostate apex, determined by urethrogram, was often different than that determined by CT. There now are some data supporting the use of MRI as a better imaging modality for localizing prostate.[56-58] In addition to difficulties in localizing the prostate, motion of that organ is now well recognized,[59] requiring one to design an adequate PTV from the CTV. External patient motion is also a problem if one is to use highly conformal radiation fields (which are needed if the dose is to be escalated).[60-62]

The treatment of prostate cancer offers a good test for dose optimization techniques and the prostate is surrounded by several dose critical structures including rectum, femoral heads, and bladder.[63-67] No one method of treatment has yet emerged as a clear standard.

Although not conclusive, it now seems likely that 3-D planning does allow for the safe use of prostate doses of 7500 cGy or more.[68-71] Whether or not such elevated doses improve local control or survival is still investigational. Two centers, the University of Michigan[72] and Memorial Sloan-Kettering,[73-74] have now had considerable experience in phase I/II trials, as have had a national cooperative group of institutions.[75] A phase III trial comparing high versus conventional dose external beam irradi-

ation as mono-therapy for patients with Stage T3–T4 prostate cancer has been carried out by Shipley et al.[76] The results of using 67.2 of x-ray alone was compared to 75.6 cobalt Gray equivalent using a conformal perineal proton boost for the last 25.2 Gy. Significantly improved local control was seen for the higher dose patients with poorly differentiated tumors. However, there was no increase in overall survival, disease-specific survival, or total recurrence-free survival in any subgroup. It now seems likely that higher radiation doses will benefit only certain subsets of prostate cancer patients, perhaps those with advanced disease, but low PSAs. There is some evidence that treating these patient subsets will even be cost effective.[77-78]

## Miscellaneous

3-D treatment planning is of value wherever the target is difficult to define, dose sensitive normal tissue is nearby, or there is a need to escalate the dose past usual levels. In soft tissue sarcomas, magnetic resonance scanning is known to be superior to CT in defining the gross tumor volume.[79] 3-D planning systems are necessary to take full advantage of these images. Pancreatic cancer is surrounded by dose sensitive structures such as the liver, stomach, and kidneys. Sometimes clever beam arrangements to limit dose to these organs can be worked out using 3-D planning.[80] Malignancies of the external auditory canal are difficult to control without high radiation doses, but exquisite care must be taken to avoid overdosing temporal bone and deeper structures.

Although clinical trials for these clinical situations will probably never be done, the value of sophisticated treatment planning is self-evident.

## CONCLUSION

3-D treatment planning offers better targeting, better radiation beam design and intensity modulation. If it is accepted that better radiation will lead to better outcomes, then the use of 3-D treatment planning should become universal.

## REFERENCES

1. Tod MC, Meredith WJ: A dosage system for use in the treatment of cancer of the uterine cervix. *Bri J Radiol* 1938;11:809–824.

2. Tepper JE, Padikal TN: The role of computed tomography in treatment planning. In: Radiation Therapy Planning, edited by NM Bleehen, E Glatstein, and JL Haybittle, New York, Marcel Dekker Inc., 1983, pp 139–158.

3. Rosenman JG, Chaney EL, Sailer S, Sherouse GW, Tepper JE: Recent advances in radiotherapy treatment planning. *Cancer Investigation* 1991;9:465–481.

4. Goitein M, Abrams M, Rowell D, et al: Multidimensional treatment planning: II. Beam's-eye view, back projection, and projection through CT sections. *Int J Radiat Oncol Biol Phys* 1983;9:789–797.

5. Rosenman J, Miller E, Cullip T, Tracton G: Image registration: An essential part of radiation therapy treatment planning. *Int J Radiat Oncol Biol Phys* 1998;40(1):197–205.

6. Liebel SA, Kutcher GJ, Mohan R, Harrison LB, Armstrong JG, Zelefsky MJ, LoSasso TJ, Burman CM, Mageras GS, Chui CS, Brewster LJ, Masterson ME, Lo YC, Ling C, Fuks Z: Three-dimensional conformal radiation therapy at the Memorial Sloan-Kettering Cancer Center. *Sem Radiat Oncol* 1992;2:274–289.

7. Rosenman J, Sherouse, GW, Chaney EL, Tepper, JE: Virtual Simulation: Initial Clinical Results. *Int J Radiat Oncol Biol Phys* 1991;20: 843–851.

8. Chaney EL, Pizer SM: Defining anatomical structures from medical images. *Sem Radiat Oncol* 1992;2: 215–225.

9. ICRU Report 50: Prescribing, Recording, and Reporting Photon Beam Therapy, International Commission on Radiation Measurements and Units, Washington, DC, 1994.

10. Austin-Seymour M, Chen GTY, Rosenman J, Michalski J, Lindsley K, Goitein M: Tumor and target delineation: Current research and future challenges. *Int J Radiat Oncol Biol Phys* 1995;33(5):1041–1052.

11. Cullip TJ, Symon JR, Rosenman JG, Chaney EL: Digitally reconstructed fluoroscopy and other interactive volume visualizations in 3-D treatment planning. *Int J Radiat Oncol Biol Phys* 1993;27:145–151.

12. Sherouse GW, Novins K, Chaney EL: Computation of digitally reconstructed radiographs for use in radiotherapy treatment design. *Int J Radiat Oncol Biol Phys* 1990;18:651–658.

13. Cullip TJ, Symon JR, Rosenman JG, Chaney EL: Digitally reconstructed fluoroscopy and other interactive volume visualizations in 3-D treatment planning. *Int J Radiat Oncol Biol Phys* 1993;27:145–151.

14. Levoy M: Display of surfaces from volume data. In: IEEE Computer Graphics and Applications 1998;8:29–37.

15. Sailer S, Bourland D, Rosenman J, Sherouse G, Chaney E, Tepper J: 3D beams need 3D names. *Int J Radiat Oncol Biol Phys* 1990;19:797–798.

16. Tracton GS, Miller EP, Rosenman J, Chang SX, Sailer S, Boxwala A, Chaney E: Preparing diagnostic 3D images for image registration with planning CT images. *Int J Radiat Oncol Biol Phys* 1997;39(2):340.

17. Brown LG: A survey of image registration techniques. *ACM Computing Surveys* 1992;24: 325–376.

18. Heesters, MA, Wijrdeman HK, Struikmans H, Witkamp T, Moerland MA: Brain tumor delineation based on CT and MR imaging. Implications for radiotherapy treatment planning. *Strahlenther-Onkol* 1993;169(12):729–733.

19. Suit H, Regaud Lecture, Granada 1994. Tumors of the connective and supporting tissues. *Radiother Oncol* 1995;34(2):93–104.

20. Rosenman J, Miller E, Cullip T, Tracton G. Image registration: An essential part of radiation therapy treatment planning. *Int J Radiat Oncol Biol Phys* 1998;40(1):197–205.

21. Gritters LS, Wahl RL: Single photon emission computed tomography in cancer imaging. *Oncol* 1993;7(7):59–63.

22. Marks LB, Spencer DP, Sherouse GW, Bentel G, Clough R, Vann K, Jaszczak R, Coleman RE, Prosnitz LR: The role of three-dimensional functional lung imaging in radiation treatment planning: the functional dose-volume histogram. *Int J Radiat Oncol Biol Phys* 1995; 33(1):65–75.

23. Pietrzyk U, Herholz K, Fink G, Jacobs A, Mielke R, Slansky I, Wurker M, Heiss WD: An interactive technique for three-dimensional image registration: validation for PET, SPECT, MRI and CT brain studies. *J Nucl Med* 1994; 35(12):2011–2018.

24. Houkin K, Kamada, K, Sawamura Y, Iwasaki Y, Abe H, Kashiwaba T: Proton magnetic resonance spectroscopy (1H-MRS) for the evaluation of treatment of brain tumours. *Neuroradiol* 1995;37(2):99–103.

25. Sailer SL, Rosenman JG, Symon JR, Cullip TJ, Chaney EL: The tetrad and hexad: Maximum beam separation as a starting point for noncoplanar 3-D treatment planning: Prostate cancer as a test case. *Int J Radiat Oncol Biol Phys* 1994;30(2):439–446.

26. Goitien M: The inverse problem. *Int J Radiat Oncol Biol Phys* 1990;18:489–491.

27. Niemierko A, Urie M, Goitein M: Optimization of 3D radiation therapy with both physical and biological end points and constraints. *Int J Radiat Oncol Biol Phys* 1992;23:99–108.

28. Meeks SL, Buatti JM, Bova FJ, Friedman WA, Mendenhall WM, Zlotecki RA: Potential clinical efficacy of intensity-modulated conformal therapy. *Int J Radiat Oncol Biol Phys* 1998; 40(2):483–495.

29. Mohan R, Wu Q, Wang X, Stein J: Intensity modulation optimization, lateral transport of radiation, and margins. *Med Phys* 1996;23(12): 2011–2021.

30. Goitein M: The comparison of treatment plans. *Sem Radiat Oncol* 1992;2:246–256.

31. Lyman JT: Complication probability as assessed from dose-volume histograms. *Rad Res* 1985;104:S13–S19.

32. Burman C, Kutcher GJ, Emami B, Goitein M: Fitting of normal tissue tolerance data to an analytic function. *Int J Radiat Oncol Biol Phys* 1991;21:123–135.

33. Niemierko A, Goitein M: Modeling of normal tissue response to radiation: the critical volume model. *Int J Radiat Oncol Biol Phys* 1993; 25(1):135–145.

34. Sandler HM: 3-D conformal radiotherapy for brain tumors. The University of Michigan experience. *Frontiers of Radiat Ther Oncol* 1996;29:250–254.

35. Nakagawa K, Aoki Y, Fujimaki T, Tago M, Terahara A, Karasawa K, Sakata K, Sasaki Y, Matsutani M, Akanuma A: High-dose conformal radiotherapy influenced the pattern of failure but did not improve survival in glioblastoma multiforme. *Int J Radiat Oncol Biol Phys* 1998; 40(5):1141–1149.

36. Fitzek M, Thornton A, Rabenow J, Lev M, Pardo F, Bussiere M, Braun L, Finklestein D, Hochberg F, Cosgrove GR, Okunieff P, Munzenrider J, Liebsch N, Harsh G: Results of 90 Gy proton/photon radiation therapy for glioblastoma multiforme. *Int J Radiat Oncol Biol Phys* 1997;39(2):139.

37. Radany EH, Sandler HM, Ten Haken RK, Marsh LH, Parker P, Greenberg HS, Junck L, Page M, Lichter AS: 3D conformal radiotherapy for malignant astrocytomas. Dose escalation to 90 Gy. *Int J Radiat Oncol Biol Phys* 1997;39(2):140.

38. Morris D, Miller EP, Rosenman J, Sailer S, Tepper J: A comparison of radiation treatment techniques for carcinomas of the larynx and hypopharynx using 3-D dose distributions and intensity modulation. *Int J Radiat Oncol Biol Phys* 1997;39(2):236.

38. Pu AT, Sandler HM, Radany EH, Blaivas M, Page MA, Greenberg HS, Junck L, Ross DA: Low grade gliomas: preliminary analysis of failure patterns among patients treated using 3D conformal external beam irradiation. *Int J Radiat Oncol Biol Phys* 1995;31(3):461–466.

39. Sheldon JM, Forster LB, Harrson RR, Woode HJ, Lee CM, Burman CS, Chui WR, Lutz WR, Spirou SV, Kutcher GJ, Fuks ZY, Leibel SA, Ling CC: Dose escalation for maxillary sinus cancer using intensity-modulatied radiation therapy (IMRT). *Int J Radiat Oncol Biol Phys* 1997;39(2):237.

40. Verhey U, Xia P, Akazawa P: Clinically practical intensity modulation for complex head and neck lesions using multiple, static, MLC fields. *Int J Radiat Oncol Biol Phys* 1997;39(2) 237.

41. Eisbruch A, Ship JA, Martel MK, Ten Haken RK, Marsh LH, Wolf GT, Esclamado RM, Bradford CR, Terrell JE, Gebarski SS, Lichter AS: Parotid gland sparing in patients undergoing bilateral head and neck irradiation: techniques and early results. *Int J Radiat Oncol Biol Phys* 1996;36(2):469–480.

42. Emami B, Purdy JA, Simpson JR, Harms W, Gerber R, Wippold JF: 3-D conformal radiotherapy in head and neck cancer. The Washington University experience. *Frontiers of Radiation Therapy & Oncology* 1996;29:207–220.

43. Yaparpalvi R, Fontenla DP, Tyerech SK, Boselli LR, Beitler JJ: Parotid gland tumors: a comparison of postoperative radiotherapy techniques using three-dimensional (3D) dose distributions and dose-volume histograms (DVHS). *Int J Radiat Oncol Biol Phys* 1998;40(1):43–49.

44. Le Chevalier T, Arriagada R, Quoix E, Ruffie P, Martin M, Tarayre M, Lancombe-Terriere MJ, Douillard JY, Laplanche A: Radiotherapy alone versus combined chemotherapy and radiotherapy in non-resectable non-small cell lung cancer: first analysis of a randomized trial in 353 patients. *J Natl Cancer Inst* 83:417–423;1991.

45. Robertson JM, Ten Haken RK, Hazuka MB, Turrisi AT, Martel MK, Pu AT, Littles JF, Martinez FJ, Francis IR, Quint LE, Lichter AS: Dose escalation for non-small cell lung cancer using conformal radiation therapy. *Int J Radiat Oncol Biol Phys* 1997;37(5):1079–1085.

46. Socinski MA, Clark JA, Halle J, Steagall A, Kaluzny B, Rosenman JG: Induction therapy with carboplatin/paclitaxel followed by concurrent carboplatin/paclitaxel and dose-escalating conformal radiotherapy in the treatment of locally advanced, unresectable non-small cell lung cancer: preliminary report of a phase I trial. *Sem Oncol* 1997;24(4 Suppl 12).

47. Martel MK, Ten Haken RK, Hazuka MB, Turrisi AT, Fraass BA, Lichter AS: Dose-volume histogram and 3-D treatment planning evaluation of patients with pneumonitis. *Int J Radiat Oncol Biol Phys* 1994;28(3):575–581.

48. King SC, Acker JC, Kussin PS, Marks LB, Weeks KJ, Leopold KA: High-dose, hyperfractionated, accelerated radiotherapy using a concurrent boost for the treatment of nonsmall cell lung cancer: unusual toxicity and promising early results. *Int J Radiat Oncol Biol Phys* 1996;36(3):593–599.

49. Graham MV, Purdy JA, Emami B, Harms W, Matthews J: 3-D conformal radiotherapy for lung cancer. The Washington University experience. *Frontiers of Radiat Ther Oncol* 1996;29:188–198.

50. Armstrong J, Raben A, Zelefsky M, Burt M, Leibel S, Burman C, Kutcher G, Harrison L, Hahn C, Ginsberg R, Rusch V, Kris M, Fuks Z: Promising survival with three-dimensional conformal radiation therapy for non-small cell lung cancer. *Radiother Oncol* 1997;44(1):17–22.

51. Kelly CA, Wang XY, Chu JC, Hartsell WF: Dose to contralateral breast: a comparison of four primary breast irradiation techniques. *Int J Radiat Oncol Biol Phys* 1996;34(3):727–732.

52. Hansen VN, Evans PM, Shentall GS, Helyer SJ, Yarnold JR, Swindell W: Dosimetric evaluation of compensation in radiotherapy of the breast: MLC intensity modulation and physical compensators. *Radiother Oncol* 1997;l 42(3):249–256.

53. Dubal N, Chang S, Cullip T, Tracton G, Rosenman J: Intensity modulation for tangential breast treatment. *Int J Radiat Oncol Biol Phys.* (To appear, 1998.)

54. Hanks GE, Martz KL, Diamond JJ: The effect of dose on local control of prostate cancer. *Int J Radiat Oncol Biol Phys* 1988;15(6):1299–1305.

55. Wilder RB, Fone PD, Rademacher DE, Jones CD, Roach M 3rd, Earle JD, White RD: Localization of the prostatic apex for radiotherapy treatment planning using urethroscopy. *Int J Radiat Oncol Biol Phys* 1997;38(4):737–741.

56. Roach M 3rd, Faillace-Akazawa P, Malfatti C, Holland J, Hricak H: Prostate volumes defined by magnetic resonance imaging and computerized tomographic scans for three-dimensional conformal radiotherapy. *Int J Radiat Oncol Biol Phys* 1996;35(5):1011–1018.

57. Lau HY, Kagawa K, Lee WR, Hunt MA, Shaer AH, Hanks GE: Short communication: CT-MRI image fusion for 3D conformal prostate radiotherapy: use in patients with altered pelvic anatomy. *Bri J Radiol* 1996;69(828):1165–1170.

58. Kagawa K, Lee WR, Schultheiss TE, Hunt MA, Shaer AH, Hanks GE: Initial clinical assessment of CT-MRI image fusion software in localization of the prostate for 3D conformal radiation therapy. *Int J Radiat Oncol Biol Phys* 1997;38(2):319–325.

59. Roach M 3rd, Faillace-Akazawa P, Malfatti C: Prostate volumes and organ movement defined by serial computerized tomographic scans during three-dimensional conformal radiotherapy. *Radiat Oncol Invest* 1997;5(4):187–194.

60. Bieri S, Miralbell R, Nouet P, Delorme H, Rouzaud M: Reproducibility of conformal radiation therapy in localized carcinoma of the

prostate without rigid immobilization. *Radiother Oncol* 1996;38(3):223–230.

61. Ragazzi G, Mangili P, Fiorino C, Cattaneo GM, Bolognesi A, Reni M, Calandrino R: Variations of tumor control and rectum complication probabilities due to random set-up errors during conformal radiation therapy of prostate cancer. *Radiother Oncol* 1997;44(3):259–263.

62. Hanley J, Lumley MA, Mageras GS, Sun J, Zelefsky MJ, Leibel SA, Fuks Z, Kutcher GJ: Measurement of patient positioning errors in three-dimensional conformal radiotherapy of the prostate. *Int J Radiat Oncol Biol Phys* 1997;37(2):435–444.

63. Oldham M, Neal A, Webb S: A comparison of conventional "forward planning" with inverse planning for 3D conformal radiotherapy of the prostate. *Radiother Oncol* 1995;35(3):248–262.

64. Akazawa PF, Roach M 3rd, Pickett B, Purser P, Parkinson D, Rathbun C, Margolis L: Three-dimensional comparison of blocked arcs vs. four and six field conformal treatment of the prostate. *Radiother Oncol* 1996;41(1):83–88.

65. Burman C, Chui CS, Kutcher G, Leibel S, Zelefsky M, LoSasso T, Spirou S, Wu Q, Yang J, Stein J, Mohan R, Fuks Z, Ling CC: Planning, delivery, and quality assurance of intensity-modulated radiotherapy using dynamic multileaf collimator: a strategy for large-scale implementation for the treatment of carcinoma of the prostate. *Int J Radiat Oncol Biol Phys* 1997;39(4):863–873.

66. Hanks GE, Schultheiss TE, Hanlon AL, Hunt M, Lee WR, Epstein BE, Coia LR: Optimization of conformal radiation treatment of prostate cancer: report of a dose escalation study. *Int J Radiat Oncol Biol Phys* 1997;37(3):543–550.

67. Reinstein LE, Wang XH, Burman CM, Chen Z, Mohan R, Kutcher G, Leibel SA, Fuks Z: A feasibility study of automated inverse treatment planning for cancer of the prostate. *Int J Radiat Oncol Biol Phys* 1998;40(1):207–214.

68. Teshima T, Hanks GE, Hanlon AL, Peter RS, Schultheiss TE: Rectal bleeding after conformal 3D treatment of prostate cancer: time to occurrence, response to treatment and duration of morbidity. *Int J Radiat Oncol Biol Phys* 1997;39(1):77–83.

69. Mantz CA, Song P, Farhangi E, Nautiyal J, Awan A, Ignacio L, Weichselbaum R, Vijayaku-

mar S: Potency probability following conformal megavoltage radiotherapy using conventional doses for localized prostate cancer. *Int J Radiat Oncol Biol Phys* 1997;37(3):551–557.

70. Schultheiss TE, Lee WR, Hunt MA, Hanlon AL, Peter RS, Hanks GE: Late GI and GU complications in the treatment of prostate cancer. *Int J Radiat Oncol Biol Phys* 1997;37(1):3–11.

71. Widmark A, Fransson P, Franzen U, Littbrand B, Henriksson R: Daily-diary evaluated side-effects of conformal versus conventional prostatic cancer radiotherapy technique. *Acta Oncologica* 1997;36(5):499–507.

72. Fukunaga-Johnson N, Sandler HM, McLaughlin PW, Strawderman MS, Grijalva KH, Kish KE, Lichter AS: Results of 3D conformal radiotherapy in the treatment of localized prostate cancer. *Int J Radiat Oncol Biol Phys* 1997;38(2):311–317.

73. Leibel SA, Kutcher GJ, Zelefsky MJ, Burman CM, Mohan R, Ling CC, Fuks Z: 3-D conformal radiotherapy for carcinoma of the prostate. Clinical experience at the Memorial Sloan-Kettering Cancer Center. *Frontiers of Radiat Ther Oncol* 1996;29:229–237.

74. Zelefsky MJ, Leibel SA, Kutcher GJ, Fuks Z: Three-dimensional conformal radiotherapy and dose escalation: where do we stand? *Sem Radiat Oncol* 1998;8(2):107–114.

75. Purdy JA, Harms WB, Michalski J, Cox JD: Multi-institutional clinical trials: 3-D conformal radiotherapy quality assurance. Guidelines in an NCI/RTOG study evaluating dose escalation in prostate cancer radiotherapy. *Frontiers of Radiat Ther Oncol* 1996;29:255–263.

76. Shipley WU, Verhey LJ, Munzenrider JE, Suit HD, Urie MM, McManus PL, Young RH, Shipley JW, Zietman AL, Biggs PJ, et al: Advanced prostate cancer: the results of a randomized comparative trial of high dose irradiation boosting with conformal protons compared with conventional dose irradiation using photons alone *Int J Radiat Oncol Biol Phys* 1995;32(1):3–12.

77. Perez CA, Michalski J, Ballard S, Drzymala R, Kobeissi BJ, Lockett MA, Wasserman TH: Cost benefit of emerging technology in localized carcinoma of the prostate. *Int J Radiat Oncol Biol Phys* 1997;39(4):875–883.

78. Kobeissi BJ, Gupta M, Perez CA, Dopuch N, Michalski JM, Van Antwerp G, Gerber R, Wasserman TH: Physician resource utilizatior

in radiation oncology: a model based on management of carcinoma of the prostate. *Int J Radiat Oncol Biol Phys* 1998;40(3):593–603.

79. Suit H, Regaud Lecture, Granada 1994. Tumors of the connective and supporting tissues. *Radiother Oncol* 1995;34(2):93–104.

80. Higgins PD, Sohn JW, Fine RM, Schell MC: Three-dimensional conformal pancreas treatment: comparison of four- to six-field techniques. *Int J R Oncol Biol Phys* 1995;31(3): 605–609.

# INDEX

# CLINICAL RADIATION ONCOLOGY

Second Edition